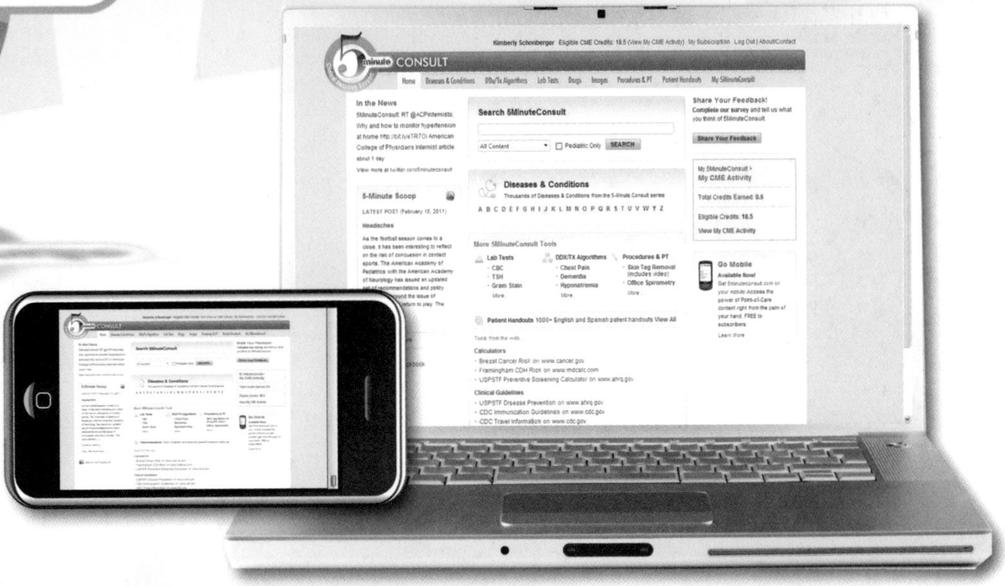

Wills Eye Institute

5-Minute Ophthalmology Consult

Wills Eye Institute
5-Minute Ophthalmology Consult

Senior Editors:

Joseph I. Maguire, MD
Attending Surgeon
Retina Service
The Wills Eye Institute
Associate Professor of Ophthalmology
Thomas Jefferson University
Philadelphia, Pennsylvania

Ann P. Murchison, MD, MPH
Attending Surgeon
Oculoplastic and Orbital Surgery Service
Co-Director Wills Eye Emergency Room
The Wills Eye Institute
Assistant Professor of Ophthalmology
Thomas Jefferson University
Philadelphia, Pennsylvania

Edward A. Jaeger, MD
Professor of Ophthalmology
Jefferson Medical College
Thomas Jefferson University
Attending Surgeon
The Wills Eye Hospital
Philadelphia, Pennsylvania

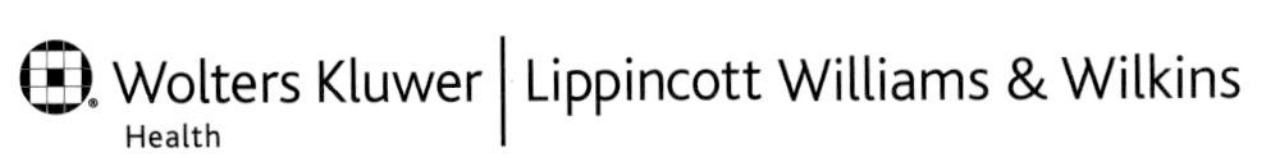

Philadelphia • Baltimore • New York • London
Buenos Aires • Hong Kong • Sydney • Tokyo

Senior Executive Editor: Jonathan W. Pine, Jr.
Senior Product Manager: Emilie Moyer
Vendor Manager: Alicia Jackson
Senior Manufacturing Manager: Benjamin Rivera
Marketing Manager: Lisa Lawrence
Designer: Theresa Mallon
Production Service: Aptara, Inc.

Two Commerce Square
2001 Market Street
Philadelphia, PA 19103 USA
LWW.com

Printed in China

Library of Congress Cataloging-in-Publication Data

Maguire, Joseph I.
Wills Eye Institute 5-minute ophthalmology consult / senior editors,
Joseph I. Maguire, Ann P. Murchison, Edward A. Jaeger.
p. ; cm. – (5-minute consult series)
Wills Eye Institute five-minute ophthalmology consult
5-minute ophthalmology consult
Includes bibliographical references and index.
ISBN 13: 978-1-60831-665-6 (alk. paper)
ISBN 10: 1-60831-665-3 (alk. paper)
I. Murchison, Ann P. II. Jaeger, Edward A. III. Title. IV. Title:
Wills Eye Institute five-minute ophthalmology consult. V. Title:
5-minute ophthalmology consult. VI. Series: 5-minute consult.
[DNLM: 1. Eye Diseases–Handbooks. 2. Eye Abnormalities–Handbooks.
WW 39] 617.7–dc23 2011036417

Care has been taken to confirm the accuracy of the information presented and to describe generally accepted practices. However, the authors, editors, and publisher are not responsible for errors or omissions or for any consequences from application of the information in this book and make no warranty, expressed or implied, with respect to the currency, completeness, or accuracy of the contents of the publication. Application of the information in a particular situation remains the professional responsibility of the practitioner.

The authors, editors, and publisher have exerted every effort to ensure that drug selection and dosage set forth in this text are in accordance with current recommendations and practice at the time of publication. However, in view of ongoing research, changes in government regulations, and the constant flow of information relating to drug therapy and drug reactions, the reader is urged to check the package insert for each drug for any change in indications and dosage and for added warnings and precautions. This is particularly important when the recommended agent is a new or infrequently employed drug.

Some drugs and medical devices presented in the publication have Food and Drug Administration (FDA) clearance for limited use in restricted research settings. It is the responsibility of the health care providers to ascertain the FDA status of each drug or device planned for use in their clinical practice.

To purchase additional copies of this book, call our customer service department at (800) 638-3030 or fax orders to (301) 223-2320. International customers should call (301) 223-2300.

Visit Lippincott Williams & Wilkins on the Internet: at LWW.com. Lippincott Williams & Wilkins customer service representatives are available from 8:30 am to 6 pm, EST.

10 9 8 7 6 5 4 3 2 1

CCS1011

To the Wills Eye family, whose physicians, graduates, and staff define excellence in patient care

CONTRIBUTORS

Fatima K. Ahmad, MD
Resident Physician, 2009–2012
Wills Eye Institute
Department of Ophthalmology
Thomas Jefferson University Hospital
Philadelphia, Pennsylvania

Anthony J. Aldave, MD
Resident Physician, 1997–2000
Wills Eye Institute
Philadelphia, Pennsylvania
Associate Professor of Ophthalmology
Director, Cornea Service, Cornea and Refractive Surgery Fellowship
The Jules Stein Eye Institute
Los Angeles, California

Amro Ali, MD
Instructor
Ophthalmology
Casey Eye Institute–Oregon Health & Science University
Portland, Oregon

David R. P. Almeida
Department of Ophthalmology Queen's University
Hotel Dieu Hospital
Kingston, Ontario, Canada

Rizwan Alvi, MBBS, MD
Research Assistant
Pediatric Ophthalmology and Ocular Genetics
Wills Eye Institute
Philadelphia, Pennsylvania

Nicholas G. Anderson, MD
Fellow, Retina and Vitreous Surgery, 2003–2005
Wills Eye Institute
Philadelphia, Pennsylvania
Associate Clinical Professor
Department of Surgery
University of Tennessee Medical Center
Southeastern Retina Associates
Knoxville, Tennessee

David B. Auerbach, DO
Volunteer
Faculty of the University of Central Florida, College of Medicine
Medical Education
University of Central Florida College of Medicine
Active Staff
Ophthalmology
Orlando Regional Medical Center
Orlando, Florida

Brandon D. Ayres, MD
Instructor
Ophthalmology
Jefferson Medical College
Assistant Surgeon
Cornea Service
Wills Eye Institute
Associate
Ophthalmology
Thomas Jefferson University Hospital
Philadelphia, Pennsylvania

Avni Badami, BS
Medical Student
Jefferson Medical College
Philadelphia, Pennsylvania

Robert S. Bailey, Jr., MD
Clinical Associate Professor
Ophthalmology
Jefferson Medical College
Director
Cataract and Primary Eye Care Services
Wills Eye Institute
Chief, Division of Ophthalmology
Surgery, Division of Ophthalmology
Chestnut Hill Hospital
Philadelphia, Pennsylvania

Steven T. Bailey, MD
Assistant Professor and Attending Physician
Department of Ophthalmology
Casey Eye Institute–Oregon Health and Science University
Portland, Oregon

Paul S. Baker, MD
Retina Service
Wills Eye Institute
Jefferson Medical College
Philadelphia, Pennsylvania

Brad Ballard, MD
Resident in Ophthalmology
Madigan Army Medical Center
Tacoma, Washington

Alok S. Bansal, MD
Fellow, Vitreoretinal Surgery, 2010–2012
Retina Service
Wills Eye Institute
Philadelphia, Pennsylvania

Behin I. Barahimi, MD
Resident, 2008–2011
Ophthalmology
Wills Eye Institute
Philadelphia, Pennsylvania
Oculoplastics Fellow
Ophthalmology
University of Minnesota
Minneapolis, Minnesota

Michael J. Bartiss, OD, MD, FAAO, FAAP, FACS
Fellow
Pediatric Ophthalmology and Strabismus, 1991–1992
Wills Eye Institute
Philadelphia, Pennsylvania
Medical Director
Pediatric Ophthalmology Services
Departments of Surgery and Pediatrics
First Health of the Carolinas
Pinehurst, North Carolina

Darrell E. Baskin, MD
Vitreoretinal Fellow
Retina Service
Wills Eye Institute
Philadelphia, Pennsylvania

Caroline R. Baumal, MD
Former Fellow
Vitreoretinal Dieseases and Surgery and Intraocular Tumors Wills Eye Institute
Philadelphia, Pennsylvania
Assistant Professor of Ophthalmology
Tufts University School of Medicine
Boston, Massachusetts

Gitanjali B. Baveja, MD
Comprehensive Ophthalmology
Ashburn, Virginia

Stephanie A. Baxter, MD
Fellow, 2003–2004
Cornea/External Disease
Wills Eye Institute
Philadelphia, Pennsylvania
Assistant Clinical Professor
Queens University Hospital
Kingston, Ontario, Canada

Edward H. Bedrossian, Jr., MD, FACS
Attending Surgeon,
Ophthalmic Plastic and Reconstructive Surgery Department
Wills Eye Institute
Assistant Clinical Professor of Ophthalmology
Jefferson Medical School
Director, Ophthalmic Plastic and Reconstructive Surgery
Associate Clinical Professor of Ophthalmology
Temple University School of Medicine
Philadelphia, Pennsylvania
Chief of Ophthalmology
Delaware County Memorial Hospital
Drexel Hill, Pennsylvania

Robert D. Behar, MD
Attending Surgeon
Cataract and Primary Eye Care Service
Wills Eye Institute
Jefferson Medical College
Philadephia, Pennsylvania

Raed Behbehani, MD, FRCSC
Consultant Ophthalmologist
Neuro-Ophthalmology/Orbit Service
Al-Bahar Ophthalmology Center
Kuwait City, Kuwait

Irina Belinsky, MD
Resident in Ophthalmology
New York University
New York, New York

Michael J. Belliveau, MD
Resident
Queen's University Department of Ophthalmology
London, Ontario, Canada

Robert L. Bergren, MD
Resident, 1988–1991 and Retina Fellow, 1991–1993
Wills Eye Institute
Philadelphia, Pennsylvania
Clinical Instructor
Department of Ophthalmology
University of Pittsburgh Medical Center
Pittsburgh, Pennsylvania

Chris S. Bergstrom, MD, OD
Assistant Professor
Ophthalmology
Emory University
Atlanta, Georgia

Stephen Best, MD
Fellow, 1991–1992
Neuro-ophthalmology
Wills Eye Institute
Philadelphia, Pennsylvania
Clinical Senior Lecturer
Eye Department
University of Auckland
Ophthalmologist
Eye Department
Greenlane Clinical Centre
Auckland, New Zealand

Carlos Bianciotto, MD
Fellow
Ophthalmology
Jefferson Medical College
Ocular Oncology
Wills Eye Institute
Philadelphia, Pennsylvania

Jurij R. Bilyk, MD
Associate Professor
Ophthalmology
Wills Eye Institute and Jefferson University Hospital
Attending Surgeon
Oculoplastic and Orbital Surgery Service
Wills Eye Institute
Philadelphia, Pennsylvania

Gil Binenbaum, MD
Division of Ophthalmology
Children's Hospital of Philadelphia
Philadelphia, Pennsylvania

Mark H. Blecher, MD
Assistant Clinical Professor
Ophthalmology
Jefferson Medical College
Attending Surgeon
Co-Director, Cataract and Primary Eye Care
Wills Eye Institute
Philadelphia, Pennsylvania

Jeffrey P. Blice, MD
Retina Fellow, 1995–1997
Wills Eye Institute
Philadelphia, Pennsylvania
Assistant Professor
Surgery
Uniformed Services Health Sciences University
Staff Ophthalmologist
Ophthalmology
Walter Reed National Military Medical Center Bethesda
Bethesda, Maryland

Benjamin H. Bloom, MD
Cataract and Primary Eye Care Service
Wills Eye Institute
Philadelphia, Pennsylvania

Louis C. Blumenfeld, MD
Fellow, 1995
Neuro-ophthalmology
Wills Eye Institute
Philadelphia, Pennsylvania
Volunteer Faculty
College of Medicine
University of Central Florida
Department of Ophthalmology
Arnold Palmer Hospital of Children
Orlando, Florida

J. Luigi Borrillo, MD
Ophthalmologist
San Mateo, California

Christopher J. Brady, MD
Resident
Department of Ophthalmology
Wills Eye Institute
Philadelphia, Pennsylvania

Gary Brown, MD, MBA
Ophthalmologist
Glenside, Pennsylvania

Vatinee Y. Bunya, MD
Assistant Professor, Cornea & External Disease
Ophthalmology
Scheie Eye Institute, University of Pennsylvania
Philadelphia, Pennsylvania

William A. Cantore, MD
Associate Professor
Ophthalmology and Neurology
Penn State College of Medicine
Hershey, Pennsylvania

Jacqueline R. Carrasco, MD
Assistant Professor, Oculoplastic Surgery
Wills Eye Institute
Philadelphia, Pennsylvania

Christopher B. Chambers, MD
Assistant Professor of Ophthalmology
Northwestern University
Northwestern Memorial Hospital/
Children's Memorial Hospital
Chicago, Illinois

Eric Chen, MD
Retina Consultants of Houston
The Methodist Hospital
Houston, Texas

Hall F. Chew, MD, FRCSC
Clinical Fellow, 2007–2008
Cornea, External Disease, & Refractive Surgery
Wills Eye Institute
Philadelphia, Pennsylvania
Assistant Professor
Department of Ophthalmology & Vision Sciences
University of Toronto
Staff Physician
Department of Ophthalmology
Sunnybrook Health Sciences Centre
Toronto, Ontario, Canada

Lan Chen, MD, PhD
Clinical Associate Professor
Medicine
University of Pennsylvania
Attending Physician
Medicine
Penn Presbyterian Medical Center
Philadelphia, Pennsylvania

Allen Chiang, MD
Vitreoretinal Fellow, 2009–2011
Retina Service
Wills Eye Institute
Philadelphia, Pennsylvania

Hyung Cho, MD
Retina Fellow
Ophthalmology
Tufts/New England Eye Center
Boston, Massachusetts

Colleen Christian, MD
Ocular Oncology Service
Wills Eye Institute
Thomas Jefferson University
Philadelphia, Pennsylvania

Christine W. Chung, MD
Resident, 1996—1999
Fellow, Corneal & External Disease, 1999–2000
Wills Eye Institute
Philadelphia, Pennsylvania

Jennifer E. Cohn, MD, MPH
Assistant Professor
Infectious Diseases
University of Pennsylvania School of Medicine
Philadelphia, Pennsylvania

Brian P. Connolly, MD
Retina Service
Wills Eye Institute
Philadelphia, Pennsylvania

Mary Ellen P. Cullom, MD
Department of Surgery
Riverside Regional Medical Center
Newport News, Virginia

Melissa B. Daluvoy, MD
Cornea External Disease Fellow, 2009–2010
Wills Eye Institute
Philadelphia, Pennsylvania
Ophthalmologist
Veterans Affairs Hospital
Washington, DC

Helen V. Danesh-Meyer, FRANZCO
Associate Clinical Professor
Sir William and Lady Stevenson Associate Professor of Ophthalmology
Department of Ophthalmology
University of Auckland
Auckland, New Zealand

John B. Davies, MD
Ophthalmologist
St. Paul, Minnesota

Matthew R. Debiec, MD
Resident in Ophthalmology
Madigan Army Medical Center
Tacoma, Washington

Emily A. DeCarlo, MD
Tri-County Eye Physicians
Southampton, Pennsylvania

Char DeCroos
Associate Faculty Member
Wills Eye Institute
Philadelphia, Pennsylvania

Michael A. DellaVecchia, MD, PhD, FACS
Cataract and Primary Eye Care Service
Wills Eye Institute
Co-Director, Wills Eye Emergency Department at Jefferson Hospital
Assistant Professor of Ophthalmology
Jefferson Medical College of Thomas Jefferson University
Philadelphia, Pennsylvania

Kristin DiDomenico, MD
Resident
Wills Eye Institute
Philadelphia, Pennsylvania

Harminder S. Dua, MD, FRCOphth, PhD
Henry and Corrine Bower Research Scholar, 1990–1991
Fellow, Cornea 1992–1993
Wills Eye Institute
Philadelphia, Pennsylvania
Chair and Professor of Ophthalmology
Ophthalmology and Visual Sciences
University of Nottingham
Consultant Ophthalmologist
Queens Medical Centre, University Hospital
Nottingham, England

Ryan P. Edmonds, OD
Low Vision/Contact Lens Service
Wills Eye Institute
Philadelphia, Pennsylvania

Scott A. Edmonds, OD
Adjunct Instructor
Public Health
Salus University
Elkins Park, Pennsylvania
Co-Director
Low Vision/Contact Lens Service
Wills Eye Institute
Philadelphia, Pennsylvania
Specified Health Professional
Lankenau Hospital
Wynnewood, Pennsylvania

Susan E. Edmonds, OD
Low Vision/Contact Lens Service
Wills Eye Institute
Philadelphia, Pennsylvania
Specified Health Professional, Ophthalmology
Lankenau Hospital
Wynnewood, Pennsylvania

Justis P. Ehlers, MD
Chief Resident, 2007–2008 and Resident, 2005–2008
Wills Eye Institute
Philadelphia, Pennsylvania
Staff Physician, Vitreoretinal Service
Cole Eye Institute
Cleveland Clinic Foundation
Cleveland, Ohio

J. Mark Engel, MD
Assistant Clinical Professor
Pediatric Ophthalmology
University of Medicine and Dentistry of New Jersey
Newark, New Jersey

Anthony W. Farah, MD
Resident
Wills Eye Institute
Philadelphia, Pennsylvania

Christopher M. Fecarotta, MD
Resident
Wills Eye Institute
Philadelphia, Pennsylvania

Brad H. Feldman, MD
Attending Surgeon
Cornea and Cataract & Primary Eye Care
Wills Eye Institute
Instructor
Department of Ophthalmology
Jefferson Medical College
Philadelphia, Pennsylvania

Mark M. Fernandez, MD
Duke Eye Center
North Carolina

Mitchell S. Fineman, MD
Retina Service
Wills Eye Institute
Assistant Professor of Ophthalmology
Jefferson Medical College
Philadelphia, Pennsylvania

Thomas A. Finley, MD
Fellow, Retinal Consultants of Alabama
Retina/Vitreous Surgery
Homewood, Alabama

David Fintak, MD
Division of Emergency Medicine
Washington University in St. Louis
School of Medicine
St. Louis, Missouri

Robert Fintelmann, MD
Former Resident in Ophthalmology
Wills Eye Institute
Philadelphia, Pennsylvania
Cornea Fellow
Proctor Institute
University of California–San Francisco
San Francisco, California

Brian J. R. Forbes, MD, PhD
Assistant Professor of Ophthalmology
The University of Pennsylvania
Assistant Professor of Ophthalmology
Pediatric Ophthalmology
The Children's Hospital of Philadelphia
Philadelphia, Pennsylvania

Alan R. Forman, MD
Wills Eye Institute
Faculty Member
Assistant Professor of Ophthalmology
Jefferson Medical College
Philadelphia, Pennsylvania

Rod Foroozan, MD
Resident, 1998–2001
Fellow, 2001–2002
Neuro-Ophthalmology
Wills Eye Institute
Philadelphia, Pennsylvania
Assistant Professor of Ophthalmology
Baylor College of Medicine
Houston, Texas

Nicole R. Fram, MD
Co-Chief Resident, 2007
Ophthalmology
Thomas Jefferson University
Philadelphia, Pennsylvania
Clinical Instructor
Department of Ophthalmology
University of California Los Angeles
Associate Staff
Ophthalmology
Cedars Sinai Medical Center
Los Angeles, California

Kathryn Burleigh Freidl, MD
Fellow, Glaucoma Service, Wills Eye Institute, 2010–2011
Philadelphia, Pennsylvania
Fellowship-trained Glaucoma Specialist
Florida Eye Specialists
Jacksonville, Florida

Scott J. Fudemberg, MD
Glaucoma Service
Wills Eye Institute
Philadelphia, Pennsylvania

Sunir J. Garg, MD, FACS
Associate Professor of Ophthalmology
The Retina Service of Wills Eye Institute
Thomas Jefferson University
Fellow, 2004
The Retina Service
Wills Eye Institute
Philadelphia, Pennsylvania

Adam T. Gerstenblith, MD
Resident, 2008–2011
Vitreoretinal Surgery Fellow
Wills Eye Institute
Thomas Jefferson University Hospital
Philadelphia, Pennsylvania

Neelofar Ghaznawi, MD
Fellow, 2009–2010
Cornea and External Disease
Wills Eye Institute
Philadelphia, Pennsylvania
Clinical Instructor
Department of Ophthalmology
New York University
Attending
Department of Ophthalmology
New York University Medical Center
New York, New York

Ahmara V. Gibbons, BA
Thomas Jefferson University
Philadelphia, Pennsylvania

Katherine G. Gold, MD
Resident Class of 2010
Ophthalmology
Wills Eye Institute, Thomas Jefferson University
Philadelphia, Pennsylvania
Fellow—Ophthalmic Plastic Surgery
Ophthalmology
New York University School of Medicine
Assistant Clinical Professor
Ophthalmology
New York University Medical Center
New York, New York

Scott M. Goldstein, MD
Adjunct Clinical Assistant Professor
Department of Ophthalmology
Jefferson Medical College
Oculoplastic Attending
Assistant Professor, Oculoplastic Surgery
Wills Eye Institute
Philadelphia, Pennsylvania

Matthew Gorski, MD
Resident
Ophthalmology
SUNY Downstate Medical Center
Brooklyn, New York

Robert J. Goulet, III, MD
Glaucoma Fellow, 2010–2011
Wills Eye Institute
Philadelphia, Pennsylvania

Robert J. Granadier, MD
Fellow, Neuro-Ophthalmology, 1988–1989
Wills Eye Institute
Philadelphia, Pennsylvania
William Beaumont Eye Institute
Royal Oak, Michigan

Florin Grigorian, MD
Pediatric Ophthalmology
Children's Mercy Hospital
Kansas City, Missouri

Paula Grigorian, MD
Pediatric Ophthalmology
Children's Mercy Hospital
Kansas City, Missouri

Deepak P. Grover, DO
Fellow, 2009–2010
Neuro-Ophthalmology
Wills Eye Institute
Philadelphia, Pennsylvania
Ophthalmologist on Staff
Lehigh Valley Hospital
Allentown, Pennsylvania
Ophthalmologist on Staff
St. Luke's Hospital
Bethlehem, Pennsylvania

Lili Grunwald, MD
Medical Retina
Private Practice
Philadelphia, Pennsylvania

Kammi Gunton, MD
Assistant Professor
Pediatric Ophthalmology
Wills Eye Institute
Philadelphia, Pennsylvania

Shelly R. Gupta, MD
Fellow, 2010–2011
Glaucoma
Wills Eye Institute
Philadelphia, Pennsylvania
Assistant Professor
Ophthalmology
The Ohio State University
Columbus, Ohio

Carlos Gustavo, MD
Oncology Service
Wills Eye Institute
Philadelphia, Pennsylvania

Colleen Halfpenny, MD
Resident, 2002–2005
Fellow, Corneal & External Disease, 2005–2006
Member, Cornea Service
Clinical Instructor, Cornea
Wills Eye Institute
Assistant Professor, Ophthalmology
Jefferson Medical College
Philadelphia, Pennsylvania

Kristin M. Hammersmith, MD
Wilmer Eye Institute
Johns Hopkins Hospital
Baltimore, Maryland

Sadeer B. Hannush, MD
Assistant Professor
Ophthalmology
Jefferson Medical College
Attending Surgeon
Cornea Service
Wills Eye Institute
Philadelphia, Pennsylvania

Dorothy H. Hendricks, MD
Clinical Instructor
Ophthalmology
Jefferson University Hospital
Philadelphia, Pennsylvania
Clinical Instructor
Pediatric Ophthalmology
Al DuPont Hospital for Children
Wilmington, Delaware

Lawrence Y. Ho, MD
Staff Physician
Ophthalmology
Holy Spirit Hospital/Pinnacle Hospital
Mechanicsburg/Harrisburg, Pennsylvania

Susan Hoch, MD
Clinical Associate Professor of Medicine
Department of Rheumatology
University of Pennsylvania
Philadelphia, Pennsylvania

Elizabeth M. Hofmeister, MD
Assistant Professor
Department of Surgery
Uniformed Services University of the Health Sciences
Bethesda, Maryland
Refractive Surgery Advisor for Navy Ophthalmology
Head, Navy Refractive Surgery Center San Diego
Naval Medical Center San Diego
San Diego, California

Douglas S. Holsclaw, MD
Assistant Clinical Professor
Department of Ophthalmology
Francis I. Proctor Foundation
University of California, San Francisco
San Francisco, California

Eliza Hoskins, MD
Resident, 2005–2008
Wills Eye Institute
Philadelphia, Pennsylvania
Cornea Fellow
University of California, San Francisco
San Francisco, California

Jason Hsu, MD
Clinical Instructor
Ophthalmology
Thomas Jefferson University
Assistant Surgeon
Retina Service
Wills Eye Institute
Philadelphia, Pennsylvania

Denise Hug, MD
Assistant Professor
Ophthalmology
University of Missouri-Kansas City School of Medicine
Pediatric Ophthalmologist
Surgery, Section of Ophthalmology
Children's Mercy Hospital and Clinic
Kansas City, Missouri

Saunders L. Hupp, MD
Fellow, 1984–1985
Neuro-Ophthalmology
Wills Eye Institute
Philadelphia, Pennsylvania
Clinical Professor
Neurology
University of South Alabama
Attending
Surgery
Providence Hospital
Mobile, Alabama

Parul Ichhpujani, MD
Former Clinical Research Fellow in Glaucoma
Wills Eye Institute
Philadelphia, Pennsylvania
Assistant Professor
Government Medical College and Hospital
Chandigarh, India

Edsel Ing, MO, FRCS
Associate Professor
Ophthalmology and Vision Sciences
University of Toronto
Attending Staff
Ophthalmology
Toronto East General Hospital
Toronto, Ontario, Canada

Suzanne K. Jadico, MD
Chief Resident, 2009–2010 and Resident, 2007–2010
Ophthalmology
Wills Eye Institute
Philadelphia, Pennsylvania
Associate Ophthalmologist
Department of Surgery
University Medical Center of Princeton
Princeton, New Jersey

Edward A. Jaeger, MD
Professor of Ophthalmology
Jefferson Medical College
Attending Surgeon
Comprehensive Ophthalmology Service/Medical Education
Wills Eye Institute
Active Staff Member
Ophthalmology
Thomas Jefferson University Hospital
Philadelphia, Pennsylvania

Annie Jensen
Department of Environmental Health Institute of Public Health
University of Copenhagen
Copenhagen, Denmark

Jing Jin, MD, PhD
Clinical Assistant Professor
Ophthalmology and Pediatrics
Thomas Jefferson University
Pediatric Ophthalmology
Wills Eye Hospital
Philadelphia, Pennsylvania
Pediatric Ophthalmologist
Surgery
Nemours/Alfred I. duPont Hospital for Children
Wilmington, Delaware

Brandon B. Johnson, MD
Resident
Ophthalmology
Wills Eye Institute
Thomas Jefferson University Hospital
Philadelphia, Pennsylvania

Paul B. Johnson, MD
Attending Ophthalmologist
Emergency Department
Wills Eye Institute
Associate Oculoplastic Surgeon
Ophthalmology
Soll Eye Associates
Philadelphia, Pennsylvania

Rick S. Kaiser, MD
Associate Professor
Ophthalmology
Jefferson Medical College
Associate Surgeon
Retina Service
Wills Eye Institute
Philadelphia, Pennsylvania

Steven J. Kanoff, MD
Clinical Instructor
Wills Eye Institute
Philadelphia, Pennsylvania

Tulay Kansu, MD
Professor
Neurology
Hacettepe University School of Medicine
Professor
Neurology, Neuro-ophthalmology Unit
Hacettepe University Hospitals
Ankara, Turkey

L. Jay Katz, MD
Glaucoma Service
Wills Eye Institute
Philadelphia, Pennsylvania

Matthew D. Kay, MD
Fellow, 1991–1992
Neuro-Ophthalmology
Wills Eye Institute
Philadelphia, Pennsylvania
Assistant Clinical Professor
Ophthalmology
Florida International University College of Medicine
Miami, Florida

Bhairavi V. Kharod, MD
Clinical Associate
Cornea and Refractive Surgery Service
Duke University Eye Center
Durham, North Carolina

Monica R. Khitri, MD
Department of Ophthalmology
Scheie Eye Institute, University of Pennsylvania
Attending Physician
Department of Surgery
Philadelphia VA Medical Center
Philadelphia, Pennsylvania

Hyunjin J. Kim, MD
Clinical Fellow, 2010–2011
Ocular Oncology
Wills Eye Institute
Clinical Instructor
Ophthalmology
Thomas Jefferson University Hospital
Philadelphia, Pennsylvania

Terry Kim, MD
Department of Ophthalmology
New York University Medical Center
New York, New York

Robert A. King, MD
Fellow, 1985–1986
Pediatric Ophthalmology
Wills Eye Institute
Philadelphia, Pennsylvania
Children's Eye Physicians
Wheat Ridge, Colorado

Harold P. Koller, MD, FAAP, FACS
Professor of Ophthalmology
Jefferson Medical College
Attending Surgeon
Pediatric Ophthalmology
Attending Surgeon
Ophthalmology
Wills Eye Institute
Philadelphia, Pennsylvania

Susan M. Ksiazek, MD
Neuro-Ophthalmology Fellow, 1987–1988
Department of Ophthalmology, Section of Neuro-Ophthalmology
Wills Eye Hospital
Philadelphia, Pennsylvania
Associate Professor
Department of Surgery, Section of Ophthalmology and Visual Science
University of Chicago
Residency Program Director
Department of Surgery, Section of Ophthalmology and Visual Science
University of Chicago Hospitals
Chicago, Illinois

Kenneth C. Kubis, MD
Captain Medical Corps, United States Navy
Fellow, 1998–1999
Neuro-Ophthalmology
Wills Eye Institute
Philadelphia, Pennsylvania
Assistant Professor, Uniformed Services University
Department of Ophthalmology
Naval Medical Center
Chairman
Department of Ophthalmology
Naval Medical Center San Diego
Director, Neuro-Ophthalmology
San Diego, California

Peter R. Laibson, MD
Director Emeritus
Cornea Service
Wills Eye Institute
Professor of Ophthalmology
Thomas Jefferson University
Philadelphia, Pennsylvania

David R. Lally, MD
Resident Physician
Ophthalmology
Wills Eye Institute
Philadelphia, Pennsylvania

Sara Lally, MD
Oncology Service
Wills Eye Institute
Philadelphia, Pennsylvania

Andrew Lam, MD
Resident, 2003–2006, and Retina Fellow, 2006–2008
Wills Eye Institute
Philadelphia, Pennsylvania
New England Retina Consultants
Attending Surgeon
Department of Surgery
Baystate Medical Center
Springfield, Massachusetts

Katherine A. Lane, MD
Resident, 2004–2007
Wills Eye Institute
Philadelphia, Pennsylvania
Attending Surgeon
Fletcher Allen Hospital Center
Burlington, Vermont

Judith B. Lavrich, MD
Department of Pediatric Ophthalmology
Wills Eye Institute
Jefferson Medical College
Philadelphia, Pennsylvania

Esther Lee, MD
Preliminary Residency in Internal Medicine
Drexel/Hahnemann University
Philadelphia, Pennsylvania

Sharon S. Lehman, MD
Clinical Professor
Ophthalmology and Pediatrics
Jefferson Medical College
Assistant Surgeon
Pediatric Ophthalmology
Jefferson Medical College/Wills Eye Institute
Philadelphia, Pennsylvania
Chief
Pediatric Ophthalmology
Nemours Children's Clinic/Al Dupont Hospital for Children
Wilmington, Delaware

Alex V. Levin, MD, MHSc, FRCSC
Professor
Ophthalmology and Pediatrics
Jefferson Medical College
Chief, 2008-Current
Pediatric Ophthalmology and Ocular Genetics
Wills Eye Institute
Professor
Ophthalmology and Pediatrics
Thomas Jefferson University Hospital
Philadelphia, Pennsylvania

Brett Levinson, MD
Corneal, External Disease, and Refractive Surgery Fellow, 2006–2007
Wills Eye Institute
Philadelphia, Pennsylvania
Director of Anterior Segment Surgery and Contact Lenses
Select Eye Care
Active Staff
Department of Ophthalmology
Sinai Hospital of Baltimore
Baltimore, Maryland

Mimi Liu, MD
Resident, Graduated 2003
Retina Fellow, Graduated 2005
Wills Eye Institute
Philadelphia, Pennsylvania
Attending Surgeon
Ophthalmology
Porter Adventist Hospital
Denver, Colorado

Wayne R. Lo, MD
Staff Physician
Department of Ophthalmology
Northwest Permanente
Portland, Oregon

Nikolas London, MD
California Pacific Medical Center
San Francisco, California

Caesar Luo, MD
Ophthalmologist
Royal Oak, Michigan

Margaret MacClary, DO

Assumpta Madu, MD
Department of Ophthalmology
Glaucoma Service Montefiore Medical Center
Albert Einstein College of Medicine
Bronx, New York

Joseph I. Maguire, MD
Attending Surgeon
Retina Service
The Wills Eye Institute
Associate Professor of Ophthalmology
Thomas Jefferson University
Philadelphia, Pennsylvania

Naresh Mandava, MD
Professor and Chair
Department of Ophthalmology
University of Colorado–Denver
Anschutz Medical Campus
Aurora, Colorado

Donelson Manley, MD
Pediatric Ophthalmology
Wills Eye Institute
Philadelphia, Pennsylvania

Anand V. Mantravadi, MD
Glaucoma Service
Wills Eye Institute
Instructor in Ophthalmology
Jefferson Medical College
Philadelphia, Pennsylvania

Stephanie J. Marioneaux, MD
Former Wills Eye Resident and Cornea Fellow
Hospital Authority of Chesapeake Regional Medical Center
Chesapeake Regional Medical Center
Chesapeake, Virginia
Assistant Professor
Department of Ophthalmology
Eastern Virginia Medical School
Norfolk, Virginia

Bruce J. Markovitz, MD
Clinical Instructor
Cataract and Primary Eye Care Service
Wills Eye Institute
Philadelphia, Pennsylvania
Ophthalmology Program Director
Surgery
Cooper University Hospital
Camden, New Jersey

Arman Mashayekhi, MD
Assistant Professor
Ophthalmology
Thomas Jefferson University
Staff Physician
Oncology Service
Wills Eye Institute
Philadelphia, Pennsylvania

John O. Mason III, MD
Retina Consultants
Birmingham, Alabama

Amanda Matthews, MD
Resident Physician
Ophthalmology
Wills Eye Institute
Philadelphia, Pennsylvania

Marlon Maus, MD, MPH
Former Residency Director
Oculoplastics
Thomas Jefferson University/Wills Eye Institute
Philadelphia, Pennsylvania
DrPH Candidate
School of Public Health
University of California, Berkeley
Berkeley, California

J. Arch McNamara, MD*
Assistant Professor
Department of Ophthalmology
Jefferson Medical College
Attending Surgeon
Retina Service
Wills Eye Institute
Philadelphia, Pennsylvania

Eugene Milder
Fellow, Retina Service, 2009–2011
Wills Eye Institute
Philadelphia, Pennsylvania
Vitreoretinal Surgeon
Ophthalmology
Dewitt Army Community Hospital
Fort Belvoir, Virginia

Ammar Miri
School of Clinical Sciences
Division of Ophthalmology and Visual Sciences
University of Nottingham, United Kingdom
Department of Surgery
College of Medicine
The University of Basrah
Basrah, Republic of Iraq

Dan P. Montzka, MD
Retina Fellow, 1994–1995
Wills Eye Institute
Philadelphia, Pennsylvania
Gulf Coast Retina
Port Richey, Florida

Edward Moss, MD
Resident in Ophthalmology
Queen's University Hospital
Kingston, Ontario, Canada

Mark L. Moster, MD
Fellow, 1983–1984
Attending Surgeon
Neuro-Ophthalmology
Wills Eye Institute
Professor
Neurology and Ophthalmology
Jefferson Medical College
Philadelphia, Pennsylvania

Marlene R. Moster, MD
Professor of Ophthalmology
Jefferson Medical College
Attending Surgeon
Ophthalmology
Wills Eye Institute
Philadelphia, Pennsylvania

Ann P. Murchison, MD, MPH
Attending Surgeon
Oculoplastic and Orbital Surgery Service
Co-Director Wills Eye Emergency Room
The Wills Eye Institute
Assistant Professor of Ophthalmology
Thomas Jefferson University
Philadelphia, Pennsylvania

Jonathan S. Myers, MD
Glaucoma Service
Wills Eye Institute
Philadelphia, Pennsylvania

Parveen K. Nagra, MD
Assistant Professor
Department of Ophthalmology
Jefferson Medical College
Cornea Service
Wills Eye Institute
Philadelphia, Pennsylvania

Sarkis M. Nazarian, MD, FAAN, FNANOS
Associate Professor
Departments of Neurology & Ophthalmology
University of Arkansas for Medical Sciences
Chief
Neurology Service
Central Arkansas Veterans Hospital
Little Rock, Arkansas

Leonard B. Nelson, MD, MBA
Pediatric Ophthalmology
Wills Eye Institute
Philadelphia, Pennsylvania

Mark L. Nelson, MD
Retina Fellow, 2001–2003
Wills Eye Institute
Philadelphia, Pennsylvania
Assistant Professor of Surgery
Uniformed Services University of the Health Sciences
Bethesda, Maryland
Attending Surgeon
Allenmore Hospital
Tacoma, Washington

Melissa D. Neuwelt, MD
Resident, 2007–2010
Wills Eye Institute
Philadelphia, Pennsylvania
Retinal Fellow
Williams Beaumont Hospital
Royal Oak, Michigan

Erin M. Ney, MD, FACP
Clinical Assistant Professor
Jefferson Medical College
Assistant Program Director
Internal Medicine Residency
Thomas Jefferson University Hospital
Philadelphia, Pennsylvania

Joshua J. Ney, MD
Resident
Ophthalmology
Scheie Eye Institute
Philadelphia, Pennsylvania

**Deceased*

Rachel M. Niknam, MD
Glaucoma Service
Wills Eye Institute
Philadelphia, Pennsylvania

Thaddeus S. Nowinski, MD
Clinical Associate Professor
Ophthalmology
Jefferson Medical College
Attending Surgeon
Oculoplastic Service
Wills Eye Institute
Philadelphia, Pennsylvania

Mary O'Hara, MD
Professor
Ophthalmology, Pediatrics
University of California, Davis
Chief, Pediatric Ophthalmology & Strabismus
UC Davis Health System Eye Center
Sacramento, California

Linda H. Ohsie, MD
Resident, 2007–2010
Fellow (Neuro-ophthalmology), 2010–2011
Wills Eye Institute
Philadelphia, Pennsylvania
Wisda Eye Center
Vineland, New Jersey
Comprehensive Ophthalmology
Staff Physician
Surgery
South Jersey Healthcare Elmer Hospital
Elmer, New Jersey

Scott E. Olitsky, MD
Professor of Ophthalmology
University of Missouri-Kansas City School of Medicine
Chief of Ophthalmology
Children's Mercy Hospitals and Clinics
Kansas City, Missouri

Scott C. N. Oliver, MD
Assistant Professor
Ophthalmology
University of Colorado School of Medicine
Faculty Physician
Ophthalmology
Children's Hospital Colorado
Partner
Ophthalmology
University of Colorado Hospital
Aurora, Colorado

Jeffrey L. Olson, MD
Retina/Vitreous Surgery
University of Colorado Hospital
Aurora, Colorado

Sriranjani P. Padmanabhan, MD
Resident in Ophthalmology
Scheie Eye Institute
University of Pennsylvania
Philadelphia, Pennsylvania

Vasudha A. Panday, MD
Associate Professor
Department of Ophthalmology
San Antonio Uniformed Services Health Education Consortium
San Antonio, Texas
Former Resident
Department of Ophthalmology
Thomas Jefferson Medical College
Philadelphia, Pennsylvania
Chief, Cornea/External Disease and Refractive Surgery
Department of Ophthalmology
Wilford Hall Medical Center
Lackland Air Force Base, Texas

Kristina Yi-Hwa Pao, MD
Resident, July 2009-present
Ophthalmology
Wills Eye Institute
Philadelphia, Pennsylvania

Britt J. Parvus, DO
Clinical Fellow, 2008–2010
Ocular Oncology
Wills Eye Institute
Philadelphia, Pennsylvania
Affiliate Faculty
Ophthalmology
Philadelphia College of Osteopathic Medicine
Affiliate Staff
Ophthalmology
Riddle Memorial Hospital
Media, Pennsylvania

Apurva K. Patel, MD
Retina Fellow
New York Eye and Ear Infirmary
New York, New York

Chirag P. Patel, MD, MPH
Resident, 2005–2008
Retinal Fellow, 2008–2010
Wills Eye Institute
Philadelphia, Pennsylvania

Jayrag A. Patel, MD
Wills Eye Institute
Philadelphia, Pennsylvania

Robert B. Penne, MD
Assistant Clinical Professor
Ophthalmology
Jefferson Medical College
Philadelphia, Pennsylvania

Jared D. Peterson, MD
Resident
Ophthalmology
Wills Eye Institute
Thomas Jefferson University Hospital
Philadelphia, Pennsylvania

Arun Prasad, MD
Former Clinical Fellow, 2007–2008
Glaucoma Department
Wills Eye Institute
Philadelphia, Pennsylvania
Glaucoma Specialist
Eye Care Center of Napa Valley
Napa, California

Michael J. Pro, MD
Glaucoma Service
Wills Eye Institute
Philadelphia, Pennsylvania

Anam Quershi, MD
Resident
Crozer-Chester Hospital
Chester, Pennsylvania

Irving M. Raber, MD
Clinical Assistant Professor
Ophthalmology
Jefferson Medical College
Attending Surgeon
Cornea Service
Wills Eye Institute
Associate Staff
Ophthalmology
Thomas Jefferson University Hospital
Philadelphia, Pennsylvania

Michael P. Rabinowitz, MD
Resident Physician, 2008–2011
The Wills Eye Institute
Clinical Instructor
Department of Ophthalmology
Thomas Jefferson University Hospital
Philadelphia, Pennsylvania

Rajesh K. Rajpal, MD
Fellow, 1991–1992
Corneal Service
Wills Eye Institute
Philadelphia, Pennsylvania
Associate Clinical Professor
Georgetown University Hospital
Washington, DC
Cornea/External Disease/Refractive Surgery
McLean, Virginia

Kamalesh Janaksinh Ramaiya, MD
Vitreoretinal Surgeon
Eye Associates of New Mexico
Albuquerque, New Mexico

Aparna Ramasubramanian, MD
Former Fellow, Oncology Service, 2008–2009
Wills Eye Institute
Philadelphia, Pennsylvania
Resident in Ophthalmology
Indiana University
Indianapolis, Indiana

P. Kumar Rao, MD
Associate Professor
Ophthalmology and Visual Sciences
Washington University
St. Louis, Missouri

Christopher J. Rapuano, MD
Professor
Ophthalmology
Jefferson Medical College
Director, Cornea Service
Ophthalmology
Wills Eye Institute
Philadelphia, Pennsylvania

Mahta Rasouli, MD
Retinal Fellow
University of Alberta
Edmonton, Alberta, Canada

M. Reza Razeghinejad, MD
Research Glaucoma Fellow, 2009–2010
Glaucoma
Wills Eye Institute
Philadelphia, Pennsylvania
Associate Professor
Ophthalmology
Shiraz University of Medical Sciences
Director of Glaucoma Service
Ophthalmology
Khalili Hospital
Shiraz, Iran

Swathi C. Reddy, MD, MPH
Resident
Ophthalmology
Montefiore Medical Center
Bronx, New York

Carl D. Regillo, MD, FACS
Professor of Ophthalmology
Ophthalmology
Jefferson Medical College
Attending Surgeon
Retina Service
Wills Eye Institute
Philadelphia, Pennsylvania

David S. Rhee, MD
Retinal Fellow, 2007–2009
Wills Eye Institute
Philadelphia, Pennsylvania

Melvin Roat, MD, FACS
Clinical Associate Professor
Ophthalmology
Jefferson Medical College
Assistant Surgeon
Cornea
Wills Eye Institute
Philadelphia, Pennsylvania

Kathleen Romero, BS, MS, MD
Resident in Ophthalmology
University of California San Diego
San Diego, California

Brett J. Rosenblatt, MD
Kellogg Eye Center
Department of Ophthalmology and Visual Science
University of Michigan
Ann Arbor, Michigan

Julie M. Rosenthal, MD
Resident, 2007–2010
Ophthalmology
Wills Eye Institute
Philadelphia, Pennsylvania
Fellow, Vitreoretinal Surgery
Casey Eye Institute
Oregon Health and Science University
Portland, Oregon

Christine G. Saad, MD
Cornea Fellow, 2006–2007
Cornea and External Disease/Cornea Service
Wills Eye Institute
Philadelphia, Pennsylvania
Ophthalmologist
Department of Surgery
Lehigh Valley Hospital
Allentown, Pennsylvania

Dalia G. Said
Division of Ophthalmology and Visual Sciences
University of Nottingham
Nottingham, United Kingdom

Arvind Saini, MD, MBA
Cornea Fellow, 2004–2010
Wills Eye Hospital
Philadelphia, Pennsylvania
Milwaukee Eye Care Associate
Milwaukee, Wisconsin

Jonathan H. Salvin, MD
Clinical Assistant Professor
Departments of Ophthalmology & Pediatrics
Jefferson Medical College of Thomas Jefferson University
Philadelphia, Pennsylvania
Division of Ophthalmology
Nemours/Al duPont Hospital for Children
Wilmington, Delaware

Rob Sambursky, MD
Former Resident, 2001–2004
Cornea Fellow, 2004–2005
The Wills Eye Institute
Philadelphia, Pennsylvania

Lov Sarin, MD
Wills Eye Institute
Philadelphia, Pennsylvania

Andrea K. Sawchyn, MD
Clinical Glaucoma Fellow, 2009–2010
Wills Eye Institute
Philadelphia, Pennsylvania
Assistant Professor
Ophthalmology
The Ohio State University
Columbus, Ohio

Emil Anthony T. Say, MD
Research Fellow, 2009–2010
Ocular Oncology
Wills Eye Institute
Philadelphia, Pennsylvania
Retina Fellow, 2010–2012
Department of Ophthalmology
University of North Carolina
Chapel Hill, North Carolina

Anita P. Schadlu, MD
Wills Eye Hospital
Philadelphia, Pennsylvania

Ramin Schadlu, MD
Scheie Eye Institute
University of Pennsylvania
Abington, Pennsylvania

Joseph W. Schmitz, MD
Resident
Ophthalmology
Naval Medical Center San Diego
San Diego, California

Bruce Schnall, MD
Pediatric Ophthalmology
Wills Eye Institute
Philadelphia, Pennsylvania

Herman D. Schubert, MD
Professor of Clinical Ophthalmology and Pathology
Columbia University
Attending
Ophthalmology
New York Presbyterian Hospital
New York, New York

Geoffrey P. Schwartz, MD
Glaucoma Service
Wills Eye Institute
Jefferson Medical College
Philadelphia, Pennsylvania

Kelly D. Schweitzer, MD
Department of Ophthalmology
Queen's University Hospital
Kingston, Ontario, Canada

Margaret E. M. Scott, DO
General Medical Officer
Ophthalmology
Naval Medical Center San Diego
San Diego, California

Vikram J. Setlur, MD
Resident
Ophthalmology
Wills Eye Institute
Philadelphia, Pennsylvania

Chirag P. Shah, MD, MPH
Vitreoretinal Surgery Fellow, 2008–2010, Co-Chief Resident, 2007–2008, and Resident, 2005–2008
Wills Eye Institute
Philadelphia, Pennsylvania
Vitreoretinal Surgeon
Ophthalmic Consultants of Boston
Associate Professor
Harvard Medical School and Tufts New England Medical Center
Boston, Massachusetts

Gaurav K. Shah, MD
Retinal Consultants of Arizona
Phoenix, Arizona

Rajiv Shah, MD
Department of Ophthalmology
St Vincent's Hospital
Sydney, Australia

Raza M. Shah, MD
Resident
Ophthalmology
Drexel Eye Physicians
Philadelphia, Pennsylvania

Sumit P. Shah, MD
Tufts Medical Center
Department of Ophthalmology
Boston, Massachusetts

Tiffany Shiau, MHS
Medical Student
Jefferson Medical College
Philadelphia, Pennsylvania

Carol L. Shields, MD
Co-Director
Oncology Service
Wills Eye Institute
Philadelphia, Pennsylvania

Jerry A. Shields, MD
Co-Director
Oncology Service
Wills Eye Institute
Professor of Ophthalmology
Jefferson Medical College
Philadelphia, Pennsylvania

Gary Shienbaum, MD
Resident, 2008
Ophthalmology
Wills Eye Institute
Philadelphia, Pennsylvania
Vitreoretinal Fellow
Ophthalmology
Bascom Palmer Eye Institute
Miami, Florida

Olga A. Shif, MD
Resident, Internal Medicine
Pennsylvania Hospital
Philadelphia, Pennsylvania

Magdalena F. Shuler, MD, PhD
Retina Fellow, 2000–2002
Retina Service
Wills Eye Hospital
Philadelphia, Pennsylvania
Vitreoretinal Surgeon
Department of Surgery
Gulf Coast Medical Center
Panama City, Florida

Arunan Sivalingam, MD
Wills Eye Institute
Philadelphia, Pennsylvania

Bradley T. Smith, MD
Ophthalmology Resident, 2003–2006
Wills Eye Institute
Philadelphia, Pennsylvania
Clinical Instructor
Department of Ophthalmology & Visual Sciences
Washington University School of Medicine
Vitreoretinal Specialist
The Retina Institute
St. Louis, Missouri

Rachel K. Sobel, MD
Former Resident, 2007–2010
Ophthalmology
Wills Eye Institute
Philadelphia, Pennsylvania
Fellow
Department of Oculoplastics
University of Iowa
Iowa City, Iowa

Riz Somani
Department of Ophthalmology
Royal Alexandra Hospital
University of Alberta
Alberta, Edmonton, Canada

George L. Spaeth, MD
Professor
Ophthalmology
Jefferson Medical College
Resident, 1963
Attending Surgeon
Glaucoma
Director, Research Center
Glaucoma Service
Wills Eye Institute
Philadelphia, Pennsylvania

Justin M. Spaulding, OMS III
Medical Student
Rocky Vista University College of Osteopathic Medicine
Parker, Colorado

Benjamin D. Spirn, MD
Attending
Ophthalmology
Riverview Medical Center
Red Bank, New Jersey

Marc J. Spirn, MD
Retina Service
Wills Eye Institute
Philadelphia, Pennsylvania

Erin D. Stahl, MD
Assistant Professor of Ophthalmology
University of Missouri School of Medicine
Kansas City, Missouri

Eliza S. Stroh, MS
Ocular Genetics Counselor
Pediatric Ophthalmology and Ocular Genetics
Wills Eye Institute
Philadelphia, Pennsylvania

Tak Yee Tania Tai, MD
Fellow, 2010–2011
Glaucoma
Wills Eye Institute
Philadelphia, Pennsylvania
Department of Ophthalmology
New York Eye and Ear Infirmary
New York, New York

Matthew S. Tennant, BA, MD, FRCSC
Retina Fellow, 2003
Wills Eye Hospital
Philadelphia, Pennsylvania
Associate Clinical Professor
Ophthalmology
University of Alberta
Associate Clinical Professor
Ophthalmology
Royal Alexandra Hospital
Edmonton, Alberta, Canada

Alex B. Theventhiran, BSE, MS, MD
Resident
Department of Ophthalmology
Temple University
Temple University Hospital
Philadelphia, Pennsylvania

Michael D. Tibbetts, MD
Harvard Medical School
Boston, Massachusetts

Patrick Tiedeken, MD
Glaucoma Service
Wills Eye Institute
Philadelphia, Pennsylvania

Richard Tipperman, MD
Attending Surgeon
Cataract and Primary Eye Care
Wills Eye Institute
Philadelphia, Pennsylvania

Ethan H. Tittler, MD
Intern
Medicine
University of Utah
Salt Lake City, Utah
Subintern
Glaucoma
Wills Eye Institute
Philadelphia, Pennsylvania

Elyse Trastman-Caruso, MD
Glaucoma Fellow, 2008–2009
Glaucoma Service
Wills Eye Institute
Attending/Clinical Instructor
Glaucoma/Ophthalmology
Wills Eye Institute
Philadelphia, Pennsylvania

Tara A. Uhler, MD
Assistant Professor
Director of Resident Education
Ophthalmology
Jefferson Medical College
Medical Staff
Ophthalmology
Thomas Jefferson University Hospital
Philadelphia, Pennsylvania

Scott Uretsky, MD
Neuro-Ophthalmology Section
Neurological Surgery PC
Lake Success, New York

James F. Vander, MD
Wills Eye Institute
Philadelphia, Pennsylvania

G. Atma Vemulakonda, MD
Assistant Professor
Vitreoretinal Disease and Surgery
Department of Ophthalmology
University of Washington
Attending Physician
Vitreoretinal Disease and Surgery
Department of Ophthalmology
University of Washington Medical Center and Harborview Medical Center
Seattle, Washington

Frederick B. Vivino, MD, FACR
Associate Professor of Clinical Medicine
University of Pennsylvania School of Medicine
Chief of Rheumatology
Penn Presbyterian Medical Center
Director, Penn Sjögren's Syndrome Center
Philadelphia, Pennsylvania

Avni Vyas, MD
Resident, 2006–2009
Co-Chief Resident, 2008–2009
Wills Eye Institute
Philadelphia, Pennsylvania
Clinical Instructor
Ophthalmology
University of Pittsburgh
Pittsburgh, Pennsylvania

Rudolph S. Wagner, MD
Fellow, 1982–1983
Pediatric Ophthalmology and Adult Motility
Wills Eye Hospital
Philadelphia, Pennsylvania
Clinical Professor
Department of Ophthalmology
UMDNJ—New Jersey Medical School
Director of Pediatric Ophthalmology
Institute of Ophthalmology & Visual Science
University Hospital
Newark, New Jersey

Daniel Warder, MD
Resident in Ophthalmology
Queen's University Hospital
Kingston, Ontario, Canada

Barry Wasserman, MD
Clinical Instructor
Pediatric Ophthalmology
Wills Eye Institute
Philadelphia, Pennsylvania

Daniel T. Weaver, MD
Fellow, 1991–1992
Wills Eye Institute
Philadelphia, Pennsylvania
Pediatric Ophthalmology
Billings, Montana

Hong Wei, MD
Research Fellow, 2009–2010
Glaucoma Research Center
Wills Eye Institute
Philadelphia, Pennsylvania
Lecturer
Ophthalmology Department
Sichuan University
Physician
Ophthalmology Department
West China Hospital
Chengdu, Sichuan, P.R. China

Christian Wertenbaker, MD
Associate Clinical Professor
Ophthalmology and Neurology
Albert Einstein College of Medicine
Director, Neuro-Ophthalmology Service
Montefiore Medical Center
Bronx, New York

James H. Whelan, MD, FRCSC
Fellow, 1998–2000
Retina/Vitreous Surgery
Wills Eye Institute
Philadelphia, Pennsylvania
Comprehensive Ophthalmology
St. John's, Newfoundland, Canada

Susan Whitmer, MD
Resident, Ophthalmology
Naval Medical Center San Diego
San Diego, California

Douglas M. Wisner, MD
Co-Chief Resident
Ophthalmology
Wills Eye Institute
Co-Chief Resident
Ophthalmology
Thomas Jefferson University Hospital
Philadelphia, Pennsylvania

Andre J. Witkin, MD
Vitreoretinal Surgery Fellow
Wills Eye Hospital
Thomas Jefferson University
Philadelphia, Pennsylvania

Jeremy D. Wolfe, MD, MS
Vitreoretinal Surgery Fellow, 2008–2010
Wills Eye Institute
Philadelphia, Pennsylvania
Assistant Professor
Oakland University William Beaumont School of Medicine
Attending Surgeon
Associated Retinal Consultants
Royal Oak, Michigan

Vladimir Yakopson, MD, MAJ, Medical Corps, US Army
Fellow, Oculoplastic and Orbital Surgery, 2009–2011
Oculoplastic and Orbital Surgery Service
Wills Eye Institute
Philadelphia, Pennsylvania
Chief, Ophthalmology Service
Department of Surgery
Carl R. Darnall Army Medical Center
Fort Hood, Texas

Jacky Y. T. Yeung
Practicing Ophthalmologist Peterborough, Ontario, Canada

William O. Young, MD
Adjunct Assistant Professor
Family Medicine
University of North Carolina School of Medicine
Chapel Hill, North Carolina
Surgery
Greensboro, North Carolina

Omaya H. Youssef
Wills Eye Institute
Thomas Jefferson University
Philadelphia, Pennsylvania

FOREWORD

Five minutes worth of advice from a colleague who knows as much about the topic as anyone in the world? What could be better?

The *Wills Eye Institute 5-Minute Consult in Ophthalmology* provides just that type of targeted, focused advice; a quick curbside consult with an expert from Wills regarding a patient there in your office.

Wills Eye has been in the business of providing exactly this sort of help to physicians worldwide since we opened the doors of our first hospital through a gift to the City of Philadelphia from James Wills, a Quaker merchant and grocer, who died in 1825 leaving his money to build a hospital to care for the "indigent blind." As a result, in 1839, the first ophthalmology residency was inaugurated at Wills, the beginning of a long and storied history of training physicians in our field.

Our Wills history and experience with patient care and education translates into "right to the bottom line" clinical decision-making and advice. Drs. Maguire, Murchison, and Jaeger have organized this superb volume to provide just this type of very practical support: the maximum help within a minimum of time.

This volume will be a well-thumbed, front-of-the-bookshelf addition for the busy practitioner who is absorbed with following Osler's great dictum for prioritizing the crush of clinical care, "The best preparation for tomorrow is to do today's work superbly well." This superb tome will help in that time-honored and noble task!

Julia A. Haller, MD
Ophthalmologist-in-Chief
Wills Eye Institute
Professor and Chair of Ophthalmology
Jefferson Medical College of
Thomas Jefferson University
Philadelphia, Pennsylvania

PREFACE

To see a World in a Grain of Sand
And a Heaven in a Wild Flower
Hold Infinity in the palm of your hand
And Eternity in an hour
William Blake

We have a privileged position, as ophthalmologists, of specializing in an anatomic structure so constructed that even Darwin considered it an exemption from evolution.

Its visceral importance is measured by a position in romantic poetry equal only to the human heart.

As both the portal to our souls and our window onto the world, it holds a unique spot not only in the practice of medicine but in our psyches; there is no greater primal fear than loss of vision.

We tell our residents and fellows that if it happens in the body, it can happen in the eye and its adnexae. That is a developmental fact. What other organ has features of neuroectoderm, mesoderm, and epidermis?

This is vast territory, and to orient ourselves we must necessarily start with large concepts and move to the small.

In an increasingly real-time world, with its explosion of medical and scientific information related to patient care and research, it is a constant struggle to keep abreast of new data and innovations in one's own specialty yet alone compensate for the breakneck pace of change in others. One can become easily adrift and lost in this data equivalent of the metaphorical "forest for the trees."

It is therefore helpful to have a starting point, a chassis to which additional facts and information can be melded over time and as needed. We feel that the *Wills Eye Institute 5-Minute Ophthalmology Consult* format, with more than 300 topics and 45 algorithms, fills this void admirably. The eye's optical construct is ideally suited for photography and the multitude of accompanying photographs will be an additional rapid and invaluable resource.

We hope that this inaugural edition will serve as a primer and valuable resource that informs, validates, and even comforts the ophthalmologist, internist, general practitioner, resident, intern, and emergency room physician in the hustling pace of daily practice and the isolation of the nights loneliest hours.

Joseph I. Maguire, MD
Ann P. Murchison, MD, MPH
Edward A. Jaeger, MD

ACKNOWLEDGMENTS

We extend our thanks to the associate editors and contributing authors who made this first edition of the Wills Eye Institute 5-Minute Ophthalmology Consult possible.

CONTENTS

CONTENTS–BY SUBSPECIALTY

Neuro-Ophthalmology

Oculoplastics

Retina/Vitreous

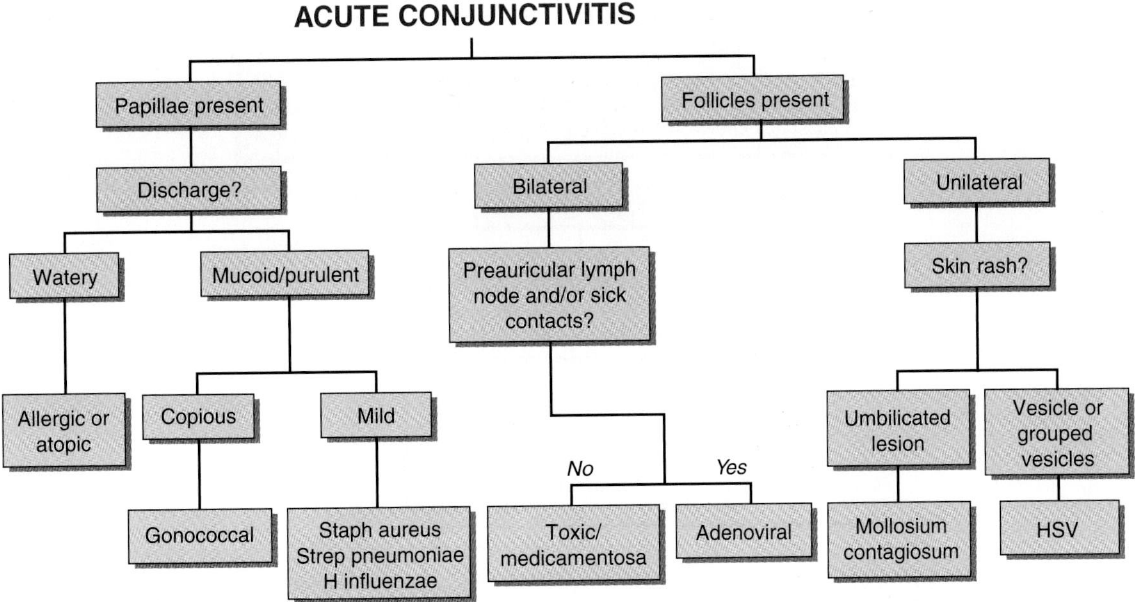

Colleen Halfpenny

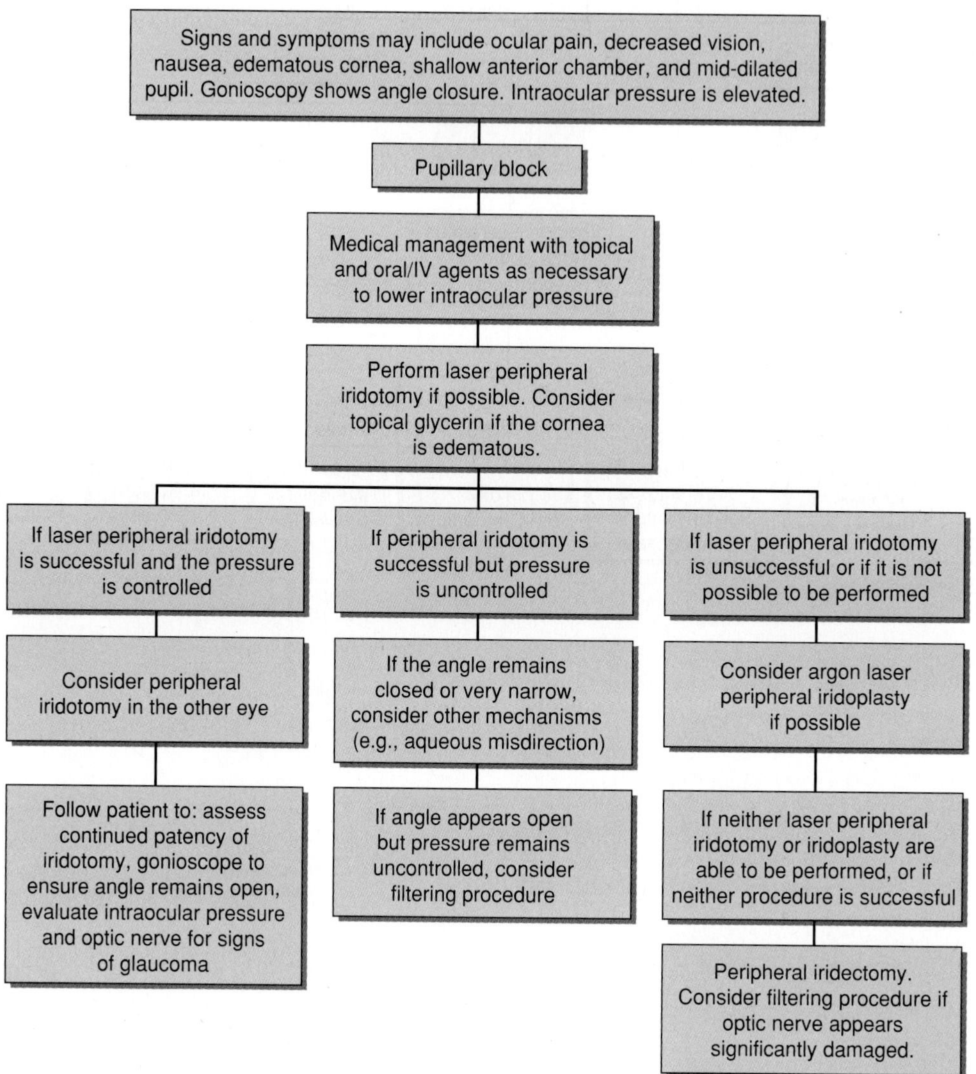
ACUTE PRIMARY ANGLE CLOSURE GLAUCOMA
Signs and symptoms may include ocular pain, decreased vision, nausea, edematous cornea, shallow anterior chamber, and mid-dilated pupil. Gonioscopy shows angle closure. Intraocular pressure is elevated.
Pupillary block
Medical management with topical and oral/IV agents as necessary to lower intraocular pressure
Perform laser peripheral iridotomy if possible. Consider topical glycerin if the cornea is edematous.
If laser peripheral iridotomy is successful and the pressure is controlled
Consider peripheral iridotomy in the other eye
Follow patient to: assess continued patency of iridotomy, gonioscope to ensure angle remains open, evaluate intraocular pressure and optic nerve for signs of glaucoma
If peripheral iridotomy is successful but pressure is uncontrolled
If the angle remains closed or very narrow, consider other mechanisms (e.g., aqueous misdirection)
If angle appears open but pressure remains uncontrolled, consider filtering procedure
If laser peripheral iridotomy is unsuccessful or if it is not possible to be performed
Consider argon laser peripheral iridoplasty if possible
If neither laser peripheral iridotomy or iridoplasty are able to be performed, or if neither procedure is successful
Peripheral iridectomy. Consider filtering procedure if optic nerve appears significantly damaged.

Tak Yee Tania Tai

BLEPHARITIS

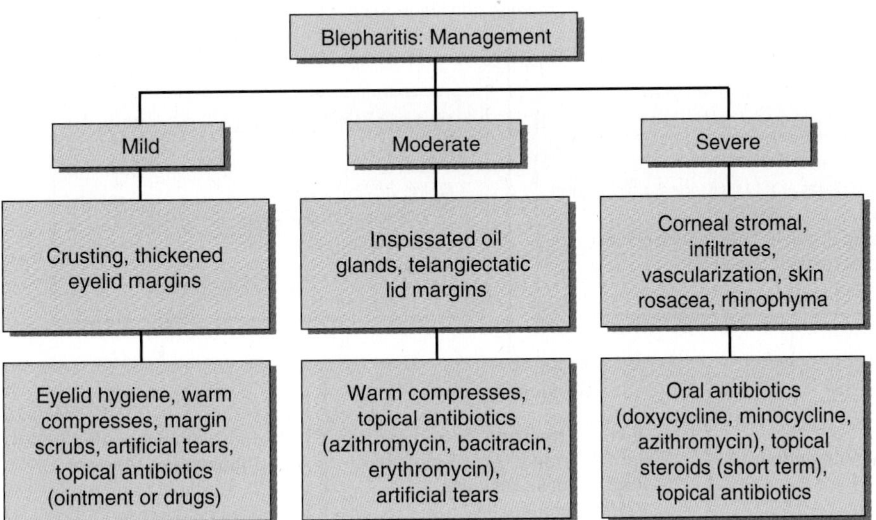
Blepharitis: Management
Mild
Moderate
Severe
Crusting, thickened eyelid margins
Inspissated oil glands, telangiectatic lid margins
Corneal stromal, infiltrates, vascularization, skin rosacea, rhinophyma
Eyelid hygiene, warm compresses, margin scrubs, artificial tears, topical antibiotics (ointment or drugs)
Warm compresses, topical antibiotics (azithromycin, bacitracin, erythromycin), artificial tears
Oral antibiotics (doxycycline, minocycline, azithromycin), topical steroids (short term), topical antibiotics

Colleen Halfpenny

BULL'S EYE MACULOPATHY

Description: Central foveal hyperpigmentation surrounded by a ring area of hypopigmentation

Key History:
- Age
- Symptoms (central visual acuity (VA) loss, color vision, photophobia)
- PMH (rheumatologic diseases, neurologic disease)
- Systemic and herbal meds (plaquenil)
- Family history of vision loss

Key Ophthalmic Exam & Ancillary Tests:
- Visual acuity
- Color vision
- Fluorescein angiogram
- Electroretinogram
- Visual field

Ocular Diseases:
1. **Cone dystrophy**
2. **Stargardt's (findus flavimaculatus)**
3. **Age-related macular degeneration (ARMD)**
4. Central areolar choroidal dystrophy
5. Benign concentric annular macular dystrophy
6. Fenestrated sheen macular dystophy
7. Leber's congenital amaurosis

Systemic Diseases:
1. **Juvenile neuronal ceroid lipofuscinosis (aka; Spielmeyer-Vogt-Sjögren disease, Batten disease, JNCL)**
2. Bardet-Biedl syndrome
3. Hallervorden-Spatz syndrome
4. Fucosidosis
5. Leigh disease

Medication Toxicity:
1. **Hydroxychloroquine (Plaquenil)**
2. **Chloroquine (Aralen)**
3. Clofazimine (Lamprene)
4. Uva ursi (tea extract)

Cone Dystrophy
- Age < 30
- Central VA loss
- Abnormal color VA
- Photophobia
- Dilated fundus examination (DFE): normal early in disease; later "Bull's Eye" changes
- Electroretinogram (ERG): Subnormal cone function

Stargardt's
- Age < 50
- Central VA loss
- Aut Rec > Aut Dom.
- Accum. of liposfucin
- DFE: yellow flecks or "Bull's Eye" later in disease
- Fluorescein angiogram (FA): "Silent choroid"
- ERG: normal in early stages of disease

ARMD
- Age > 50
- Dry or Wet
- DFE: Drusen, retinal pigment epithelium (RPE) changes, geographic atrophy, subretinal fluid, subretinal hemorrhage
- FA: choiroidal neovascular membrane (CNVM)

JNCL
- Ages 4-8
- Neurodegenerative lysosomal storage disease
- Rapidly progressive VA loss
- Seizures, ataxia
- DFE: "Bull's Eye"
- ERG: Electronegative early in the disease

Hydroxychloroquine or Chloroquine
- Dose-dependent effect
  - Plaquenil: >6.5mg/kg/day
  - Chloroquine: >3mg/kg/day
  - Based on ideal body weight
- Central VA loss
- DFE: Early RPE changes, later "Bull's Eye" changes
- Humphrey visual field (HVF): 10-2 red stimulus; paracentral scotoma
- Retinopathy may progress despite cessation of medication

Alok S. Bansal, Joseph I. Maguire

CATARACT

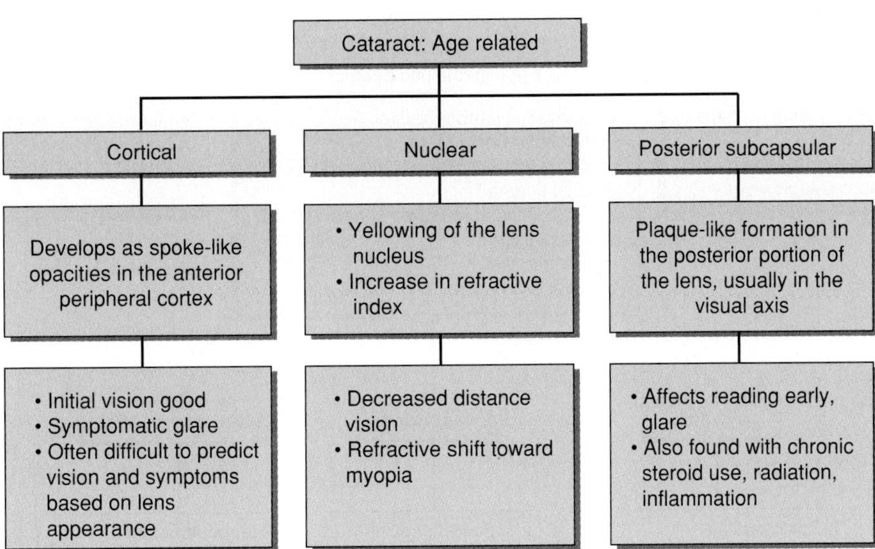
Cataract: Age related
Cortical
Nuclear
Posterior subcapsular
Develops as spoke-like opacities in the anterior peripheral cortex
• Yellowing of the lens nucleus
• Increase in refractive index
Plaque-like formation in the posterior portion of the lens, usually in the visual axis
• Initial vision good
• Symptomatic glare
• Often difficult to predict vision and symptoms based on lens appearance
• Decreased distance vision
• Refractive shift toward myopia
• Affects reading early, glare
• Also found with chronic steroid use, radiation, inflammation

Edward A. Jaeger

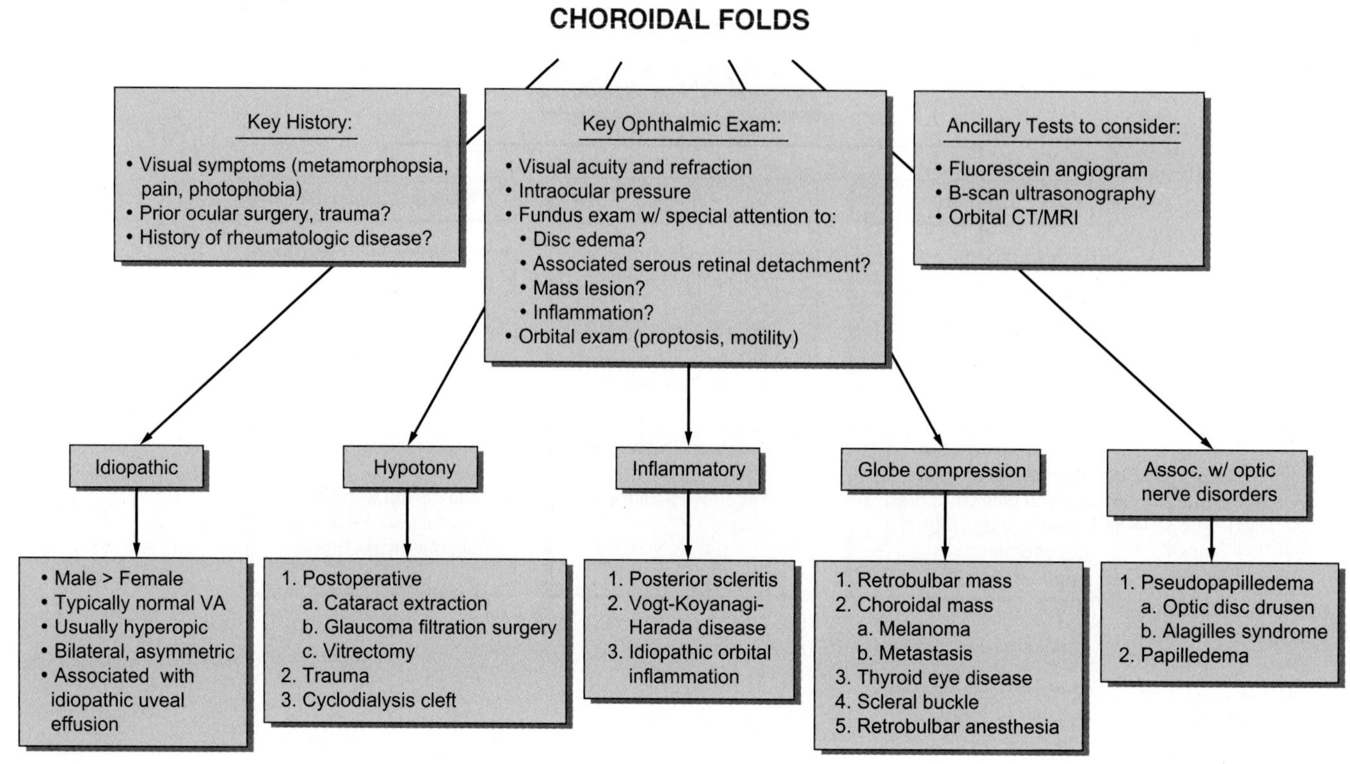

CHOROIDAL FOLDS
Key History:
• Visual symptoms (metamorphopsia, pain, photophobia)
• Prior ocular surgery, trauma?
• History of rheumatologic disease?
Key Ophthalmic Exam:
• Visual acuity and refraction
• Intraocular pressure
• Fundus exam w/ special attention to:
• Disc edema?
• Associated serous retinal detachment?
• Mass lesion?
• Inflammation?
• Orbital exam (proptosis, motility)
Ancillary Tests to consider:
• Fluorescein angiogram
• B-scan ultrasonography
• Orbital CT/MRI
Idiopathic
• Male > Female
• Typically normal VA
• Usually hyperopic
• Bilateral, asymmetric
• Associated with idiopathic uveal effusion
Hypotony
1. Postoperative
a. Cataract extraction
b. Glaucoma filtration surgery
c. Vitrectomy
2. Trauma
3. Cyclodialysis cleft
Inflammatory
1. Posterior scleritis
2. Vogt-Koyanagi-Harada disease
3. Idiopathic orbital inflammation
Globe compression
1. Retrobulbar mass
2. Choroidal mass
a. Melanoma
b. Metastasis
3. Thyroid eye disease
4. Scleral buckle
5. Retrobulbar anesthesia
Assoc. w/ optic nerve disorders
1. Pseudopapilledema
a. Optic disc drusen
b. Alagilles syndrome
2. Papilledema

Alok S. Bansal, Joseph I. Maguire

CHOROIDAL TUMORS

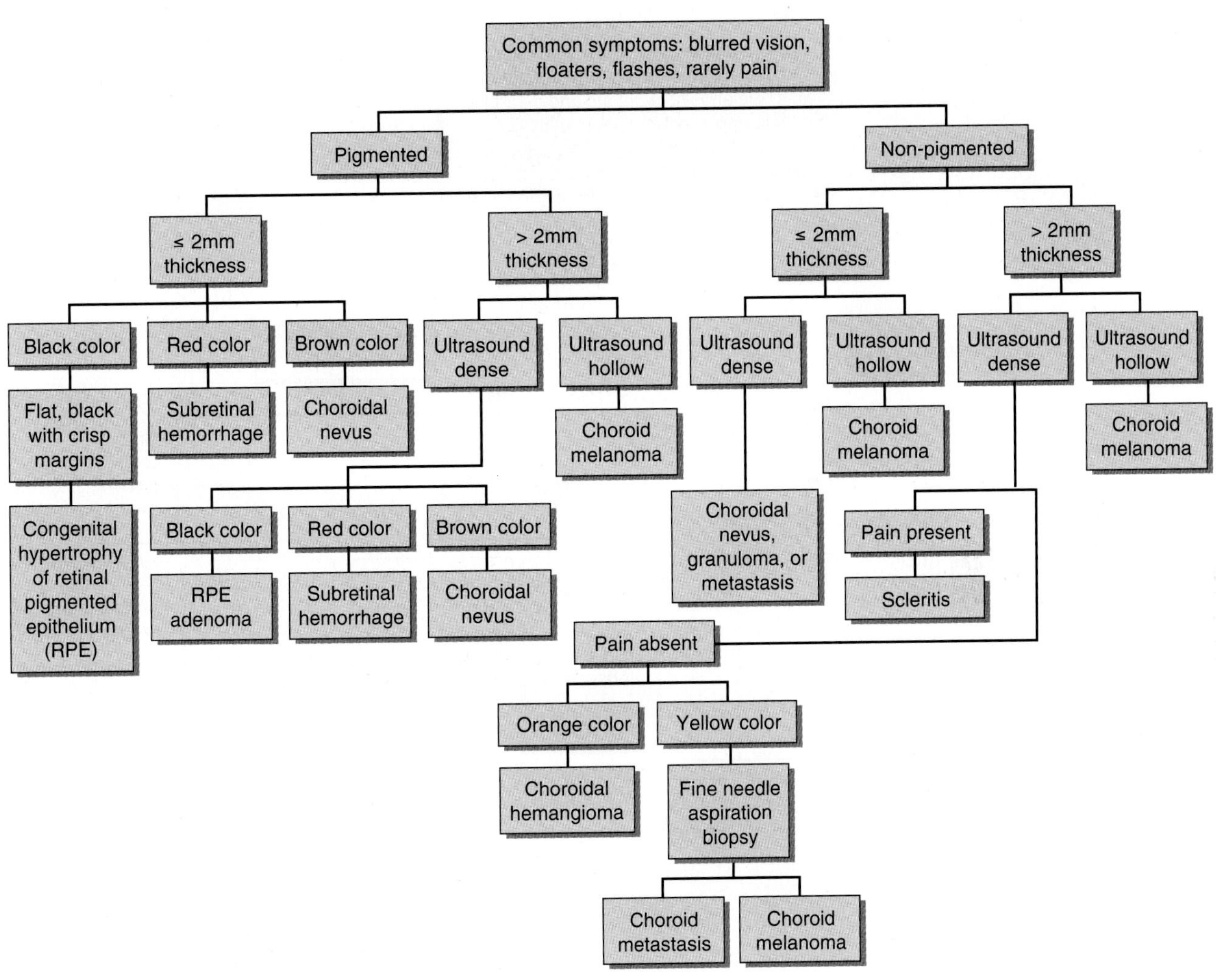

Carol Shields

CONJUNCTIVAL LESIONS

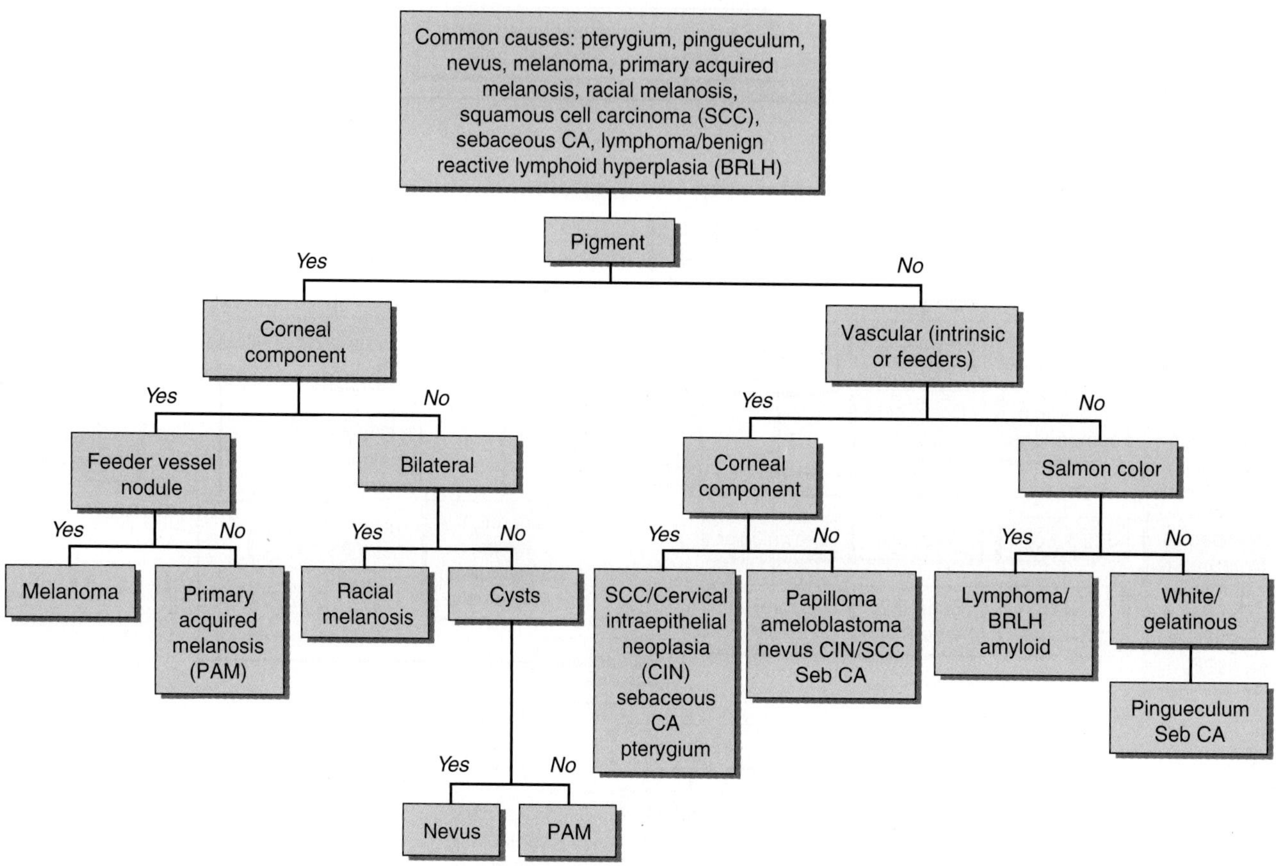
Common causes: pterygium, pingueculum, nevus, melanoma, primary acquired melanosis, racial melanosis, squamous cell carcinoma (SCC), sebaceous CA, lymphoma/benign reactive lymphoid hyperplasia (BRLH)
Pigment
Yes
No
Corneal component
Vascular (intrinsic or feeders)
Yes
No
Feeder vessel nodule
Bilateral
Yes
No
Corneal component
Salmon color
Yes
No
Melanoma
Primary acquired melanosis (PAM)
Yes
No
Racial melanosis
Cysts
Yes
No
Nevus
PAM
Yes
No
SCC/Cervical intraepithelial neoplasia (CIN) sebaceous CA pterygium
Papilloma ameloblastoma nevus CIN/SCC Seb CA
Yes
No
Lymphoma/ BRLH amyloid
White/ gelatinous
Pingueculum Seb CA

Sara Lally

CONJUNCTIVAL TUMORS

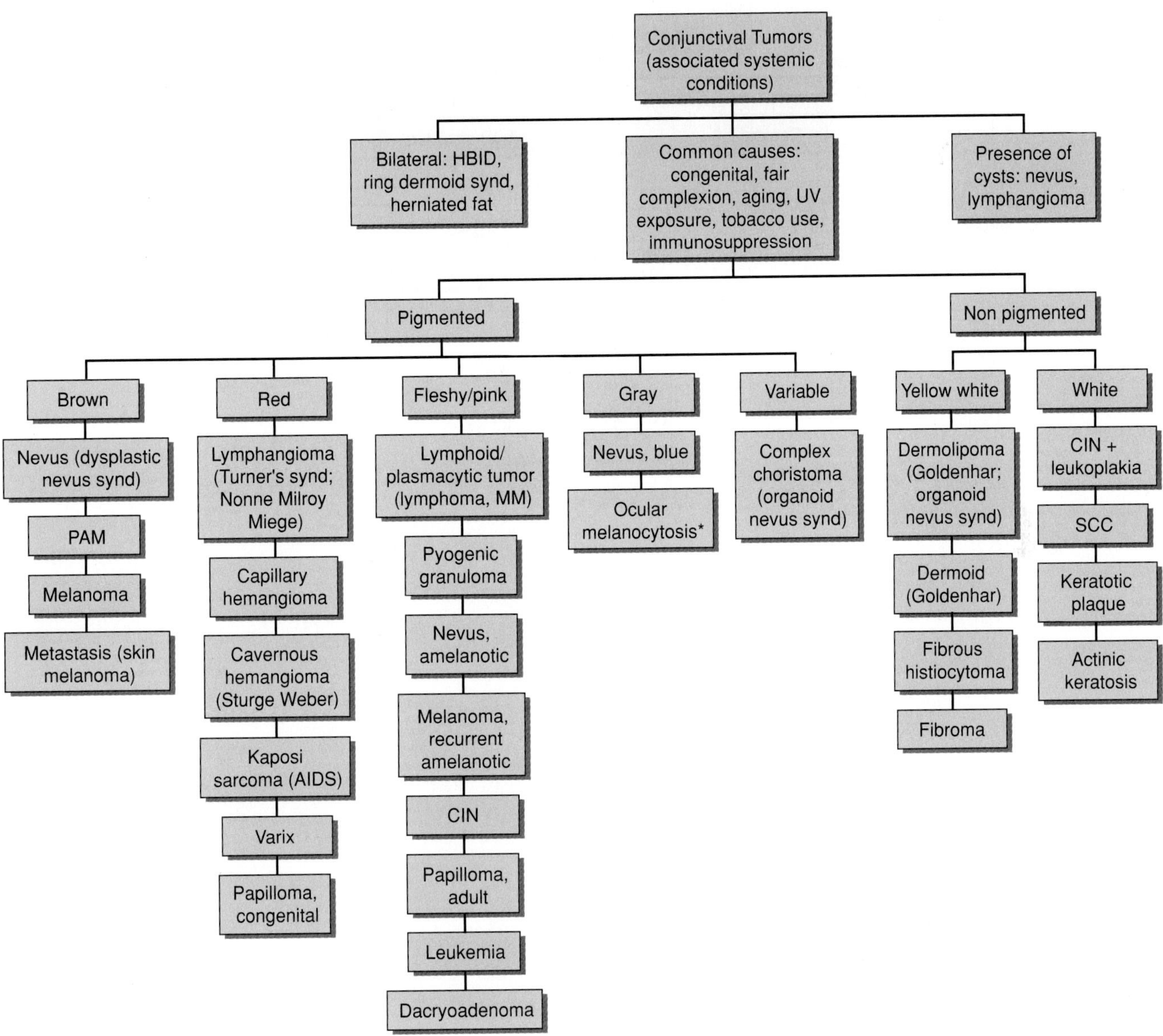

CIN = conjunctival intraepithelial neoplasia
HBID = hereditary benign intraepithelial dyskeratosis in Haliwa Indians
MM = multiple myeloma
PAM = primary acquired melanosis
SCC = squamos cell carcinoma
Synd = syndrome

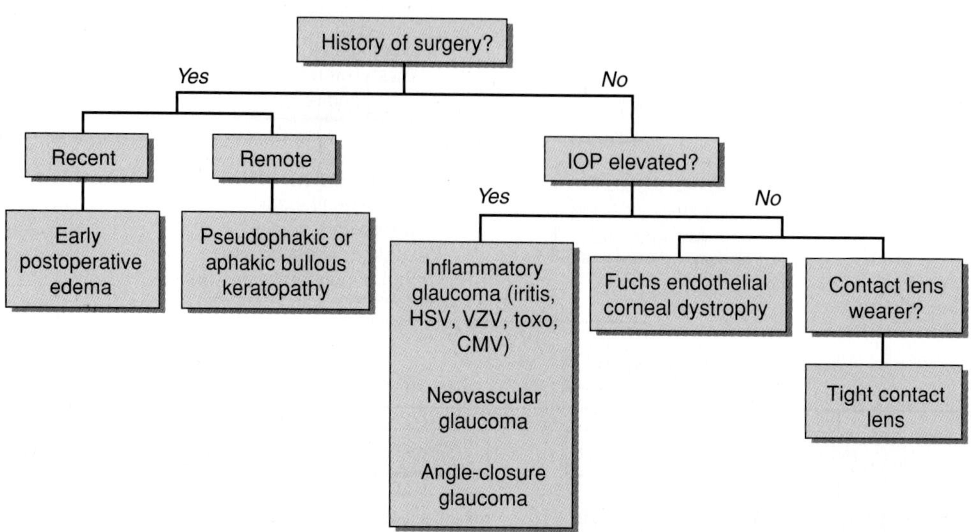

Michael J. Pro

COTTON WOOL SPOTS

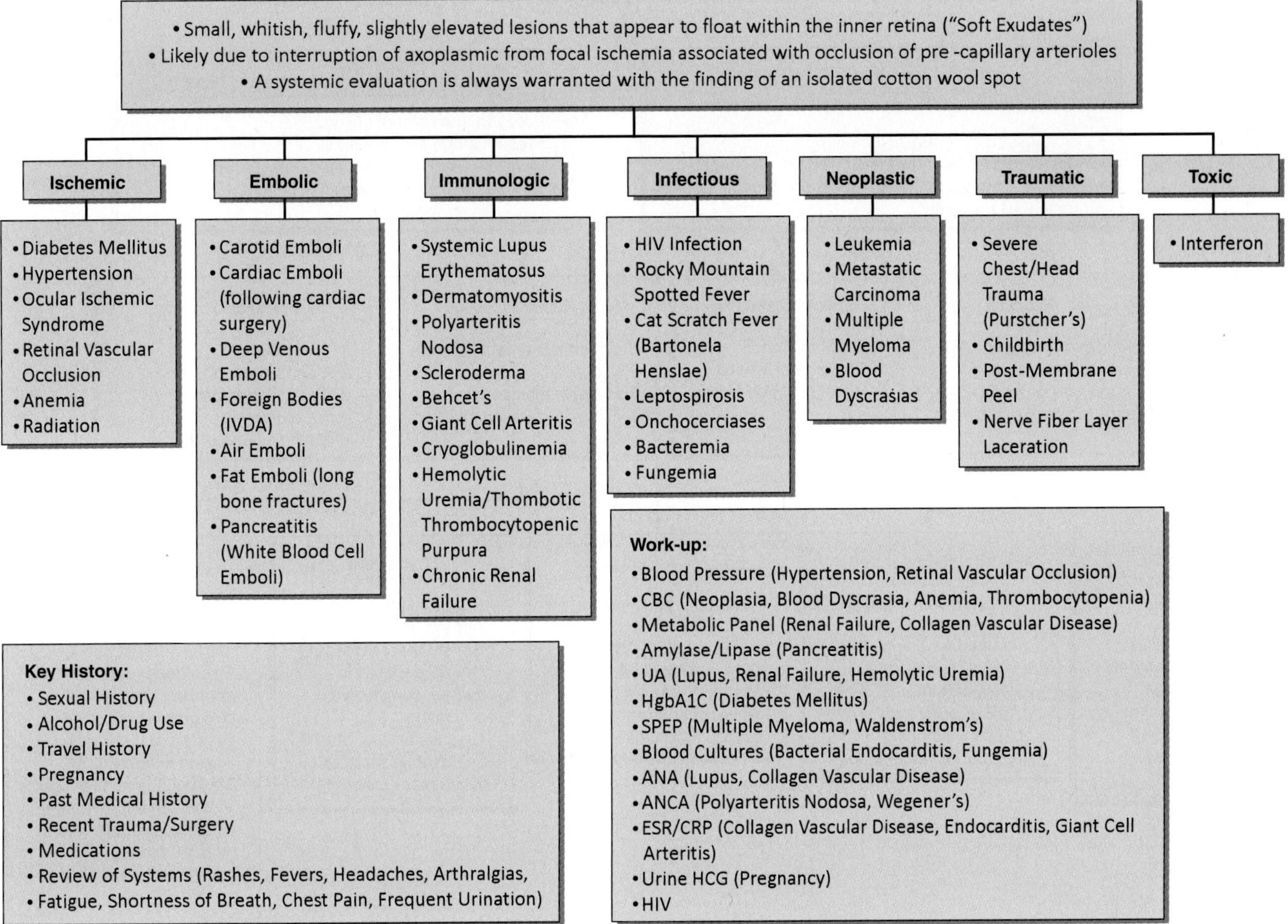

• Small, whitish, fluffy, slightly elevated lesions that appear to float within the inner retina ("Soft Exudates")
• Likely due to interruption of axoplasmic from focal ischemia associated with occlusion of pre -capillary arterioles
• A systemic evaluation is always warranted with the finding of an isolated cotton wool spot
Ischemic
• Diabetes Mellitus
• Hypertension
• Ocular Ischemic Syndrome
• Retinal Vascular Occlusion
• Anemia
• Radiation
Embolic
• Carotid Emboli
• Cardiac Emboli (following cardiac surgery)
• Deep Venous Emboli
• Foreign Bodies (IVDA)
• Air Emboli
• Fat Emboli (long bone fractures)
• Pancreatitis (White Blood Cell Emboli)
Immunologic
• Systemic Lupus Erythematosus
• Dermatomyositis
• Polyarteritis Nodosa
• Scleroderma
• Behcet's
• Giant Cell Arteritis
• Cryoglobulinemia
• Hemolytic Uremia/Thombotic Thrombocytopenic Purpura
• Chronic Renal Failure
Infectious
• HIV Infection
• Rocky Mountain Spotted Fever
• Cat Scratch Fever (Bartonela Henslae)
• Leptospirosis
• Onchocerciases
• Bacteremia
• Fungemia
Neoplastic
• Leukemia
• Metastatic Carcinoma
• Multiple Myeloma
• Blood Dyscrasias
Traumatic
• Severe Chest/Head Trauma (Purstcher's)
• Childbirth
• Post-Membrane Peel
• Nerve Fiber Layer Laceration
Toxic
• Interferon

Key History:

- Sexual History
- Alcohol/Drug Use
- Travel History
- Pregnancy
- Past Medical History
- Recent Trauma/Surgery
- Medications
- Review of Systems (Rashes, Fevers, Headaches, Arthralgias,
- Fatigue, Shortness of Breath, Chest Pain, Frequent Urination)

Work-up:

- Blood Pressure (Hypertension, Retinal Vascular Occlusion)
- CBC (Neoplasia, Blood Dyscrasia, Anemia, Thrombocytopenia)
- Metabolic Panel (Renal Failure, Collagen Vascular Disease)
- Amylase/Lipase (Pancreatitis)
- UA (Lupus, Renal Failure, Hemolytic Uremia)
- HgbA1C (Diabetes Mellitus)
- SPEP (Multiple Myeloma, Waldenstrom's)
- Blood Cultures (Bacterial Endocarditis, Fungemia)
- ANA (Lupus, Collagen Vascular Disease)
- ANCA (Polyarteritis Nodosa, Wegener's)
- ESR/CRP (Collagen Vascular Disease, Endocarditis, Giant Cell Arteritis)
- Urine HCG (Pregnancy)
- HIV

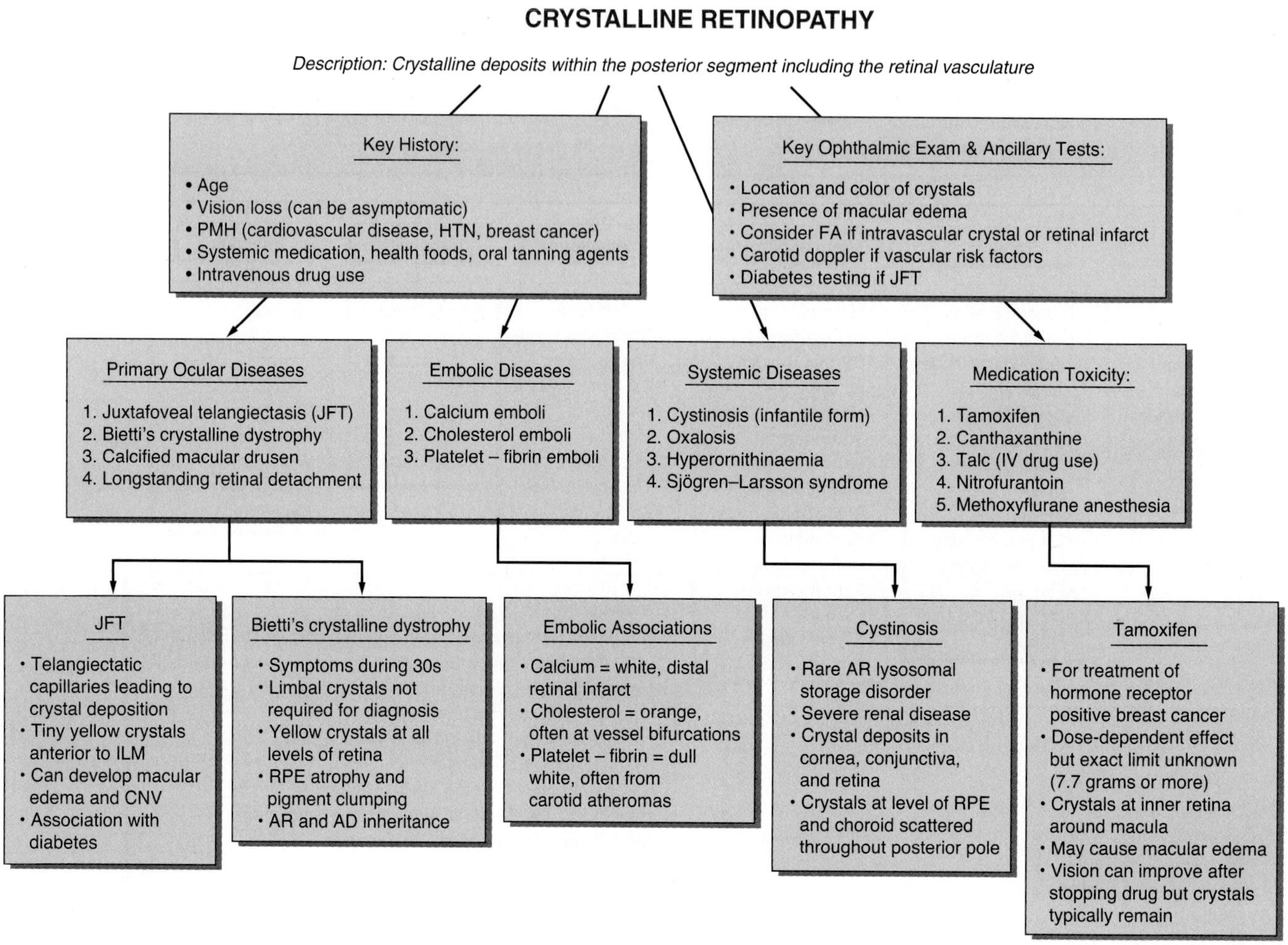

CRYSTALLINE RETINOPATHY

Description: Crystalline deposits within the posterior segment including the retinal vasculature

Key History:

- Age
- Vision loss (can be asymptomatic)
- PMH (cardiovascular disease, HTN, breast cancer)
- Systemic medication, health foods, oral tanning agents
- Intravenous drug use

Key Ophthalmic Exam & Ancillary Tests:

- Location and color of crystals
- Presence of macular edema
- Consider FA if intravascular crystal or retinal infarct
- Carotid doppler if vascular risk factors
- Diabetes testing if JFT

Primary Ocular Diseases

1. Juxtafoveal telangiectasis (JFT)
2. Bietti's crystalline dystrophy
3. Calcified macular drusen
4. Longstanding retinal detachment

Embolic Diseases

1. Calcium emboli
2. Cholesterol emboli
3. Platelet – fibrin emboli

Systemic Diseases

1. Cystinosis (infantile form)
2. Oxalosis
3. Hyperornithinaemia
4. Sjögren–Larsson syndrome

Medication Toxicity:

1. Tamoxifen
2. Canthaxanthine
3. Talc (IV drug use)
4. Nitrofurantoin
5. Methoxyflurane anesthesia

JFT

- Telangiectatic capillaries leading to crystal deposition
- Tiny yellow crystals anterior to ILM
- Can develop macular edema and CNV
- Association with diabetes

Bietti's crystalline dystrophy

- Symptoms during 30s
- Limbal crystals not required for diagnosis
- Yellow crystals at all levels of retina
- RPE atrophy and pigment clumping
- AR and AD inheritance

Embolic Associations

- Calcium = white, distal retinal infarct
- Cholesterol = orange, often at vessel bifurcations
- Platelet – fibrin = dull white, often from carotid atheromas

Cystinosis

- Rare AR lysosomal storage disorder
- Severe renal disease
- Crystal deposits in cornea, conjunctiva, and retina
- Crystals at level of RPE and choroid scattered throughout posterior pole

Tamoxifen

- For treatment of hormone receptor positive breast cancer
- Dose-dependent effect but exact limit unknown (7.7 grams or more)
- Crystals at inner retina around macula
- May cause macular edema
- Vision can improve after stopping drug but crystals typically remain

Char DeCroos

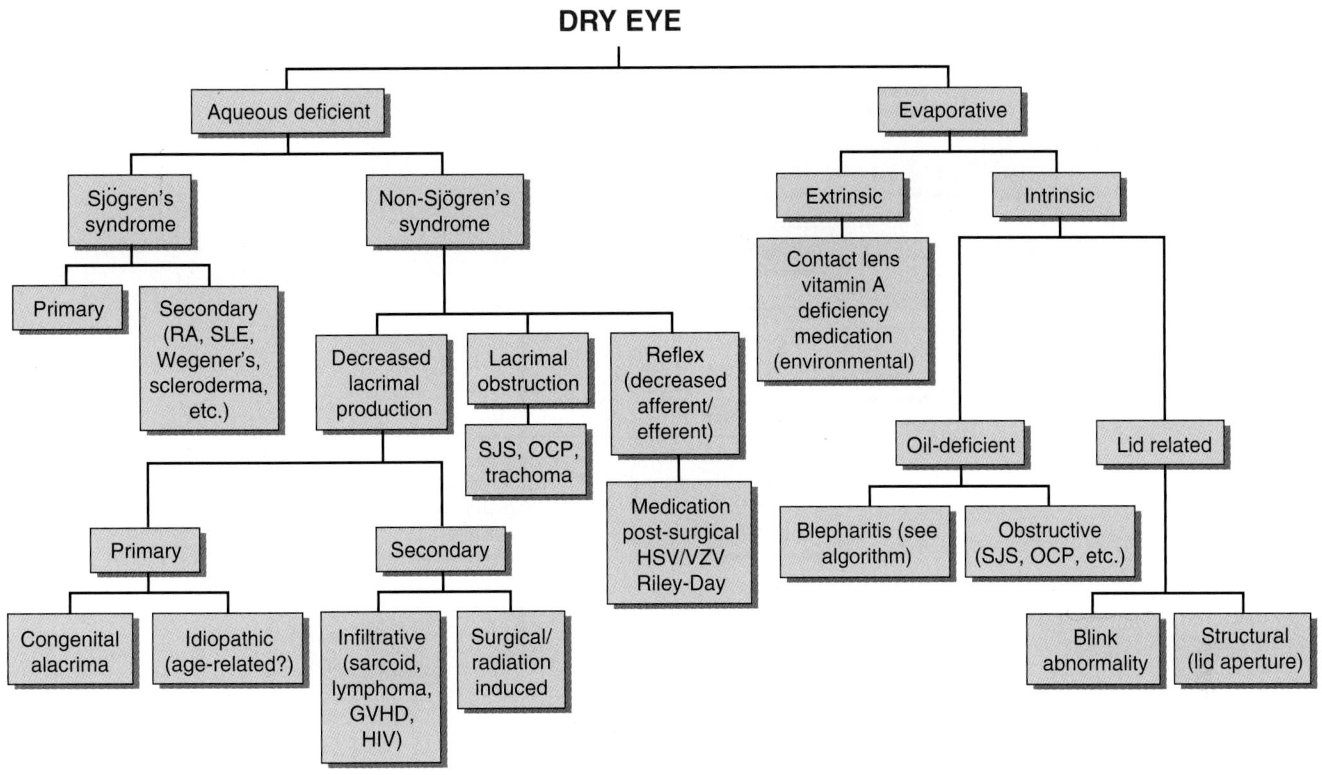

Colleen Halfpenny

ENOPHTHALMOS

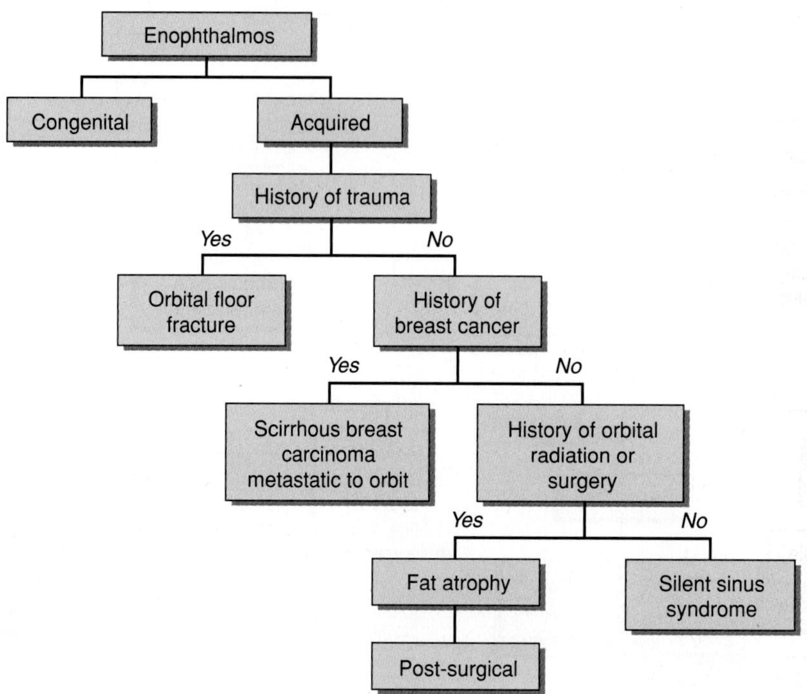

Katharine G. Gold

ESOTROPIA

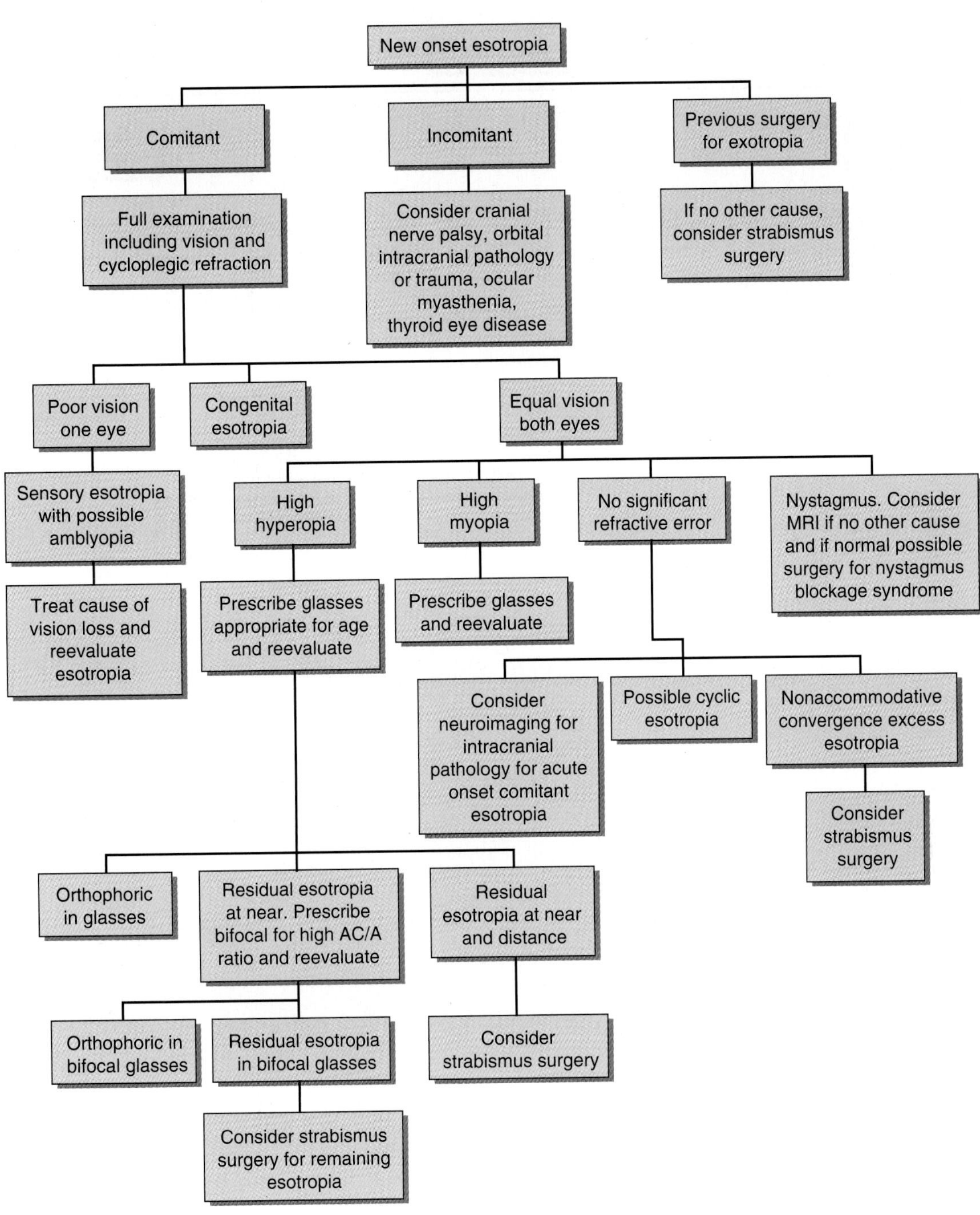

Barry Wasserman, David Lally

EYELASH LOSS

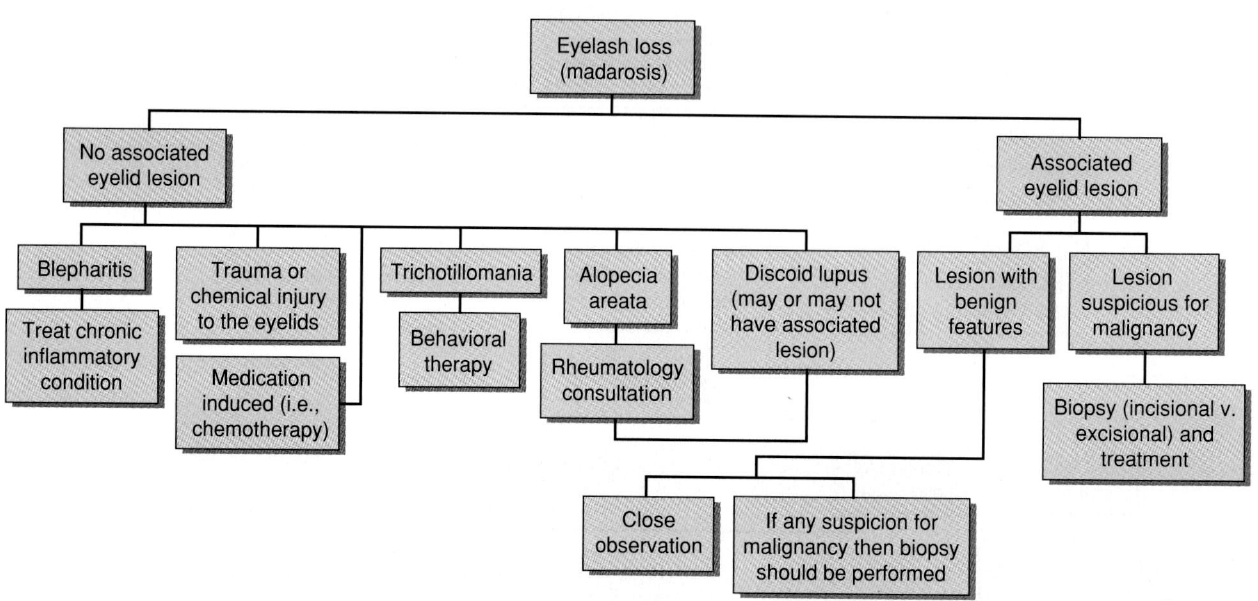

Amanda Matthews

EYELID SWELLING

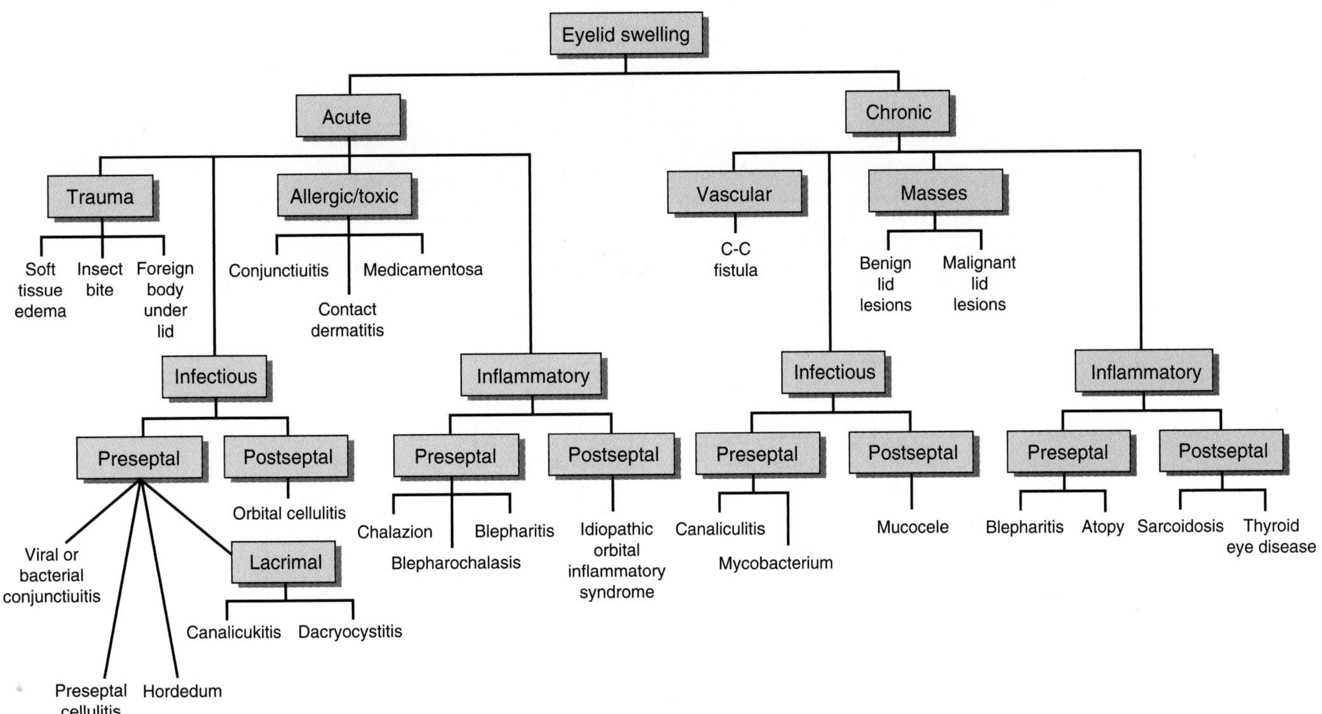

Michael Rabinowitz

HIGH IOP IN CHILDREN

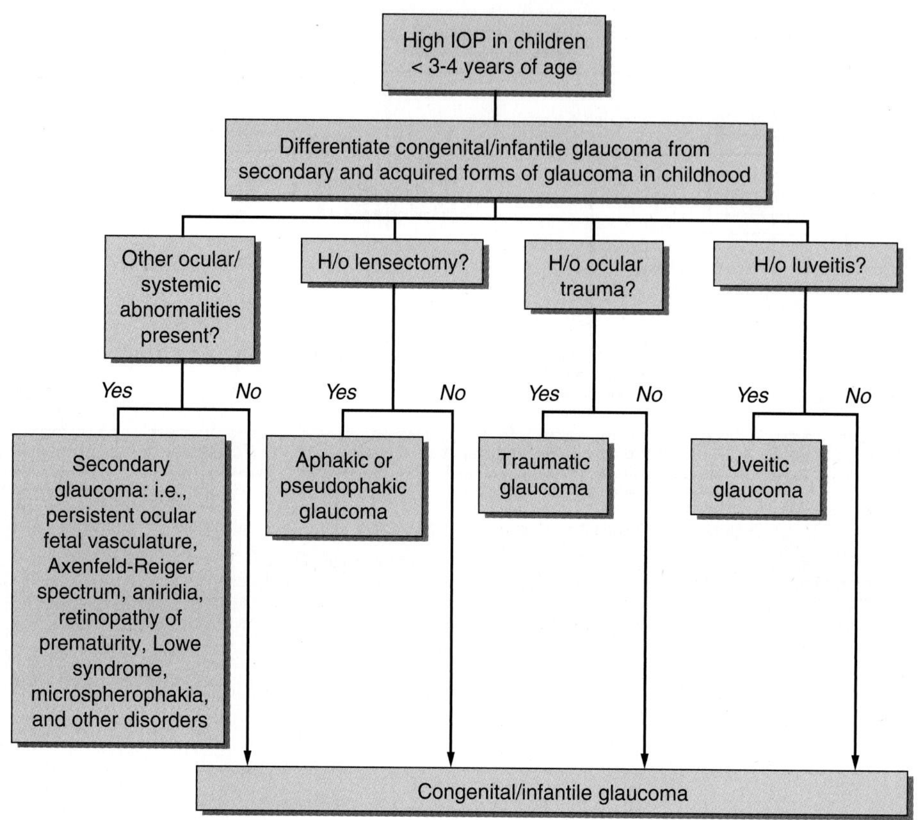

Andrea Knellinger Sawchyn

IRIDOCORNEAL ENDOTHELIAL SYNDROME

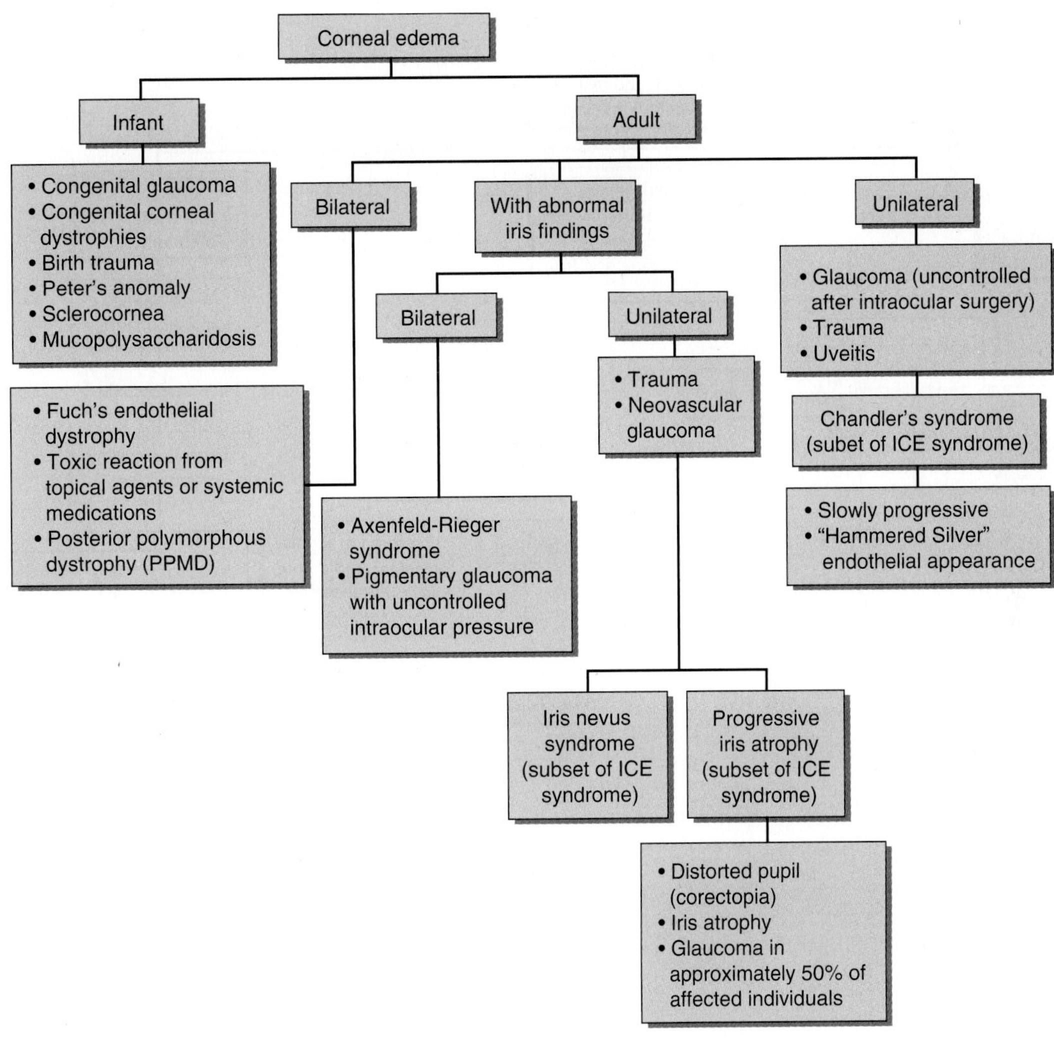

Michael J. Pro

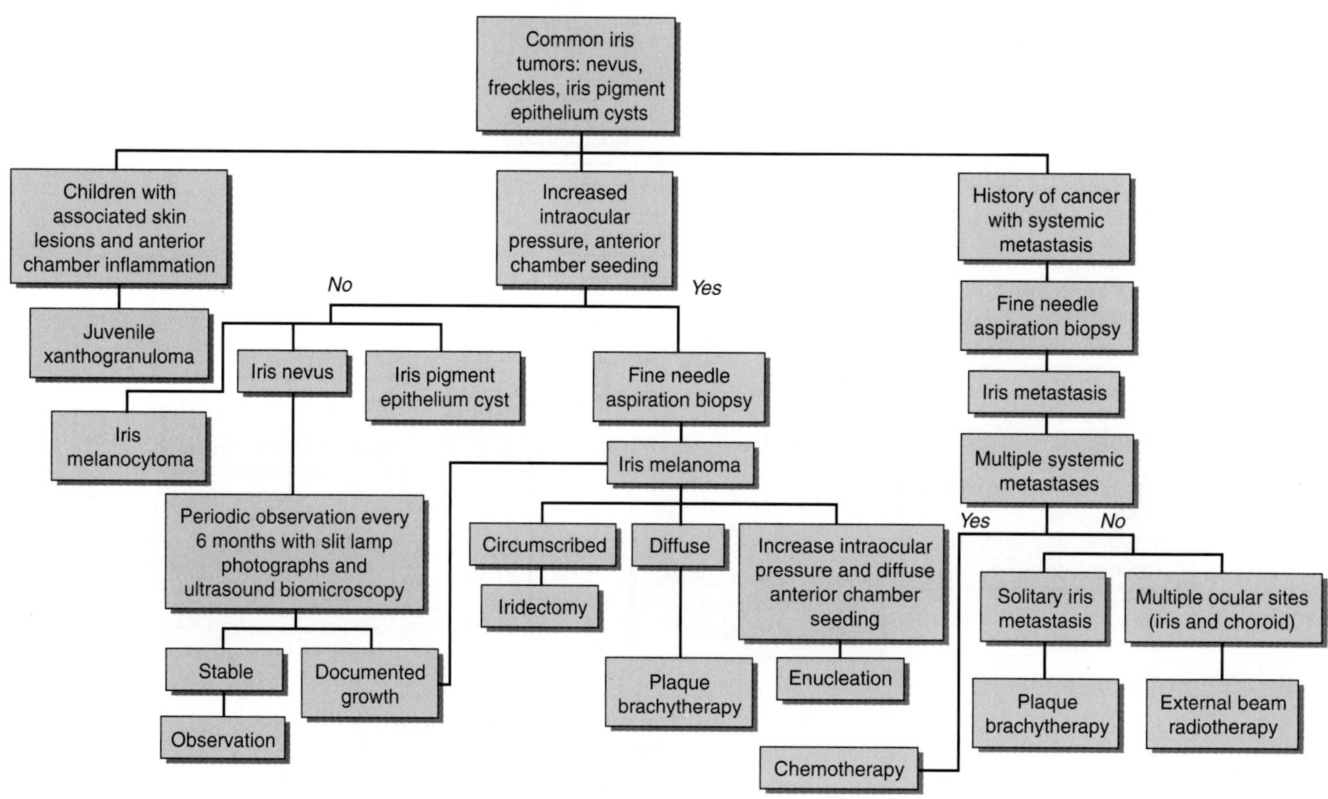

Carlos Gustavo

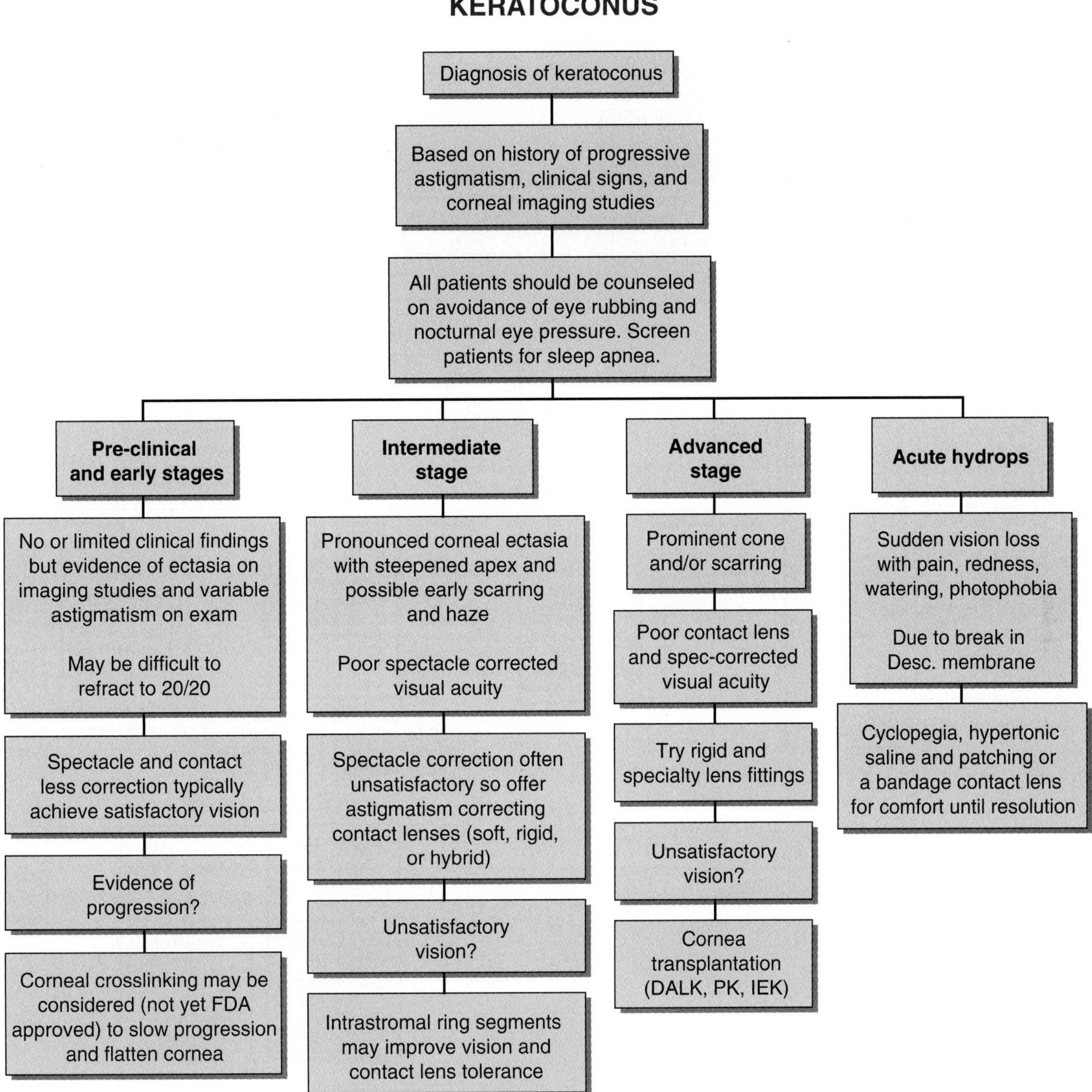
KERATOCONUS
Diagnosis of keratoconus
Based on history of progressive astigmatism, clinical signs, and corneal imaging studies
All patients should be counseled on avoidance of eye rubbing and nocturnal eye pressure. Screen patients for sleep apnea.
Pre-clinical and early stages
No or limited clinical findings but evidence of ectasia on imaging studies and variable astigmatism on exam
May be difficult to refract to 20/20
Spectacle and contact less correction typically achieve satisfactory vision
Evidence of progression?
Corneal crosslinking may be considered (not yet FDA approved) to slow progression and flatten cornea
Intermediate stage
Pronounced corneal ectasia with steepened apex and possible early scarring and haze
Poor spectacle corrected visual acuity
Spectacle correction often unsatisfactory so offer astigmatism correcting contact lenses (soft, rigid, or hybrid)
Unsatisfactory vision?
Intrastromal ring segments may improve vision and contact lens tolerance
Advanced stage
Prominent cone and/or scarring
Poor contact lens and spec-corrected visual acuity
Try rigid and specialty lens fittings
Unsatisfactory vision?
Cornea transplantation (DALK, PK, IEK)
Acute hydrops
Sudden vision loss with pain, redness, watering, photophobia
Due to break in Desc. membrane
Cyclopegia, hypertonic saline and patching or a bandage contact lens for comfort until resolution

Brad Feldman

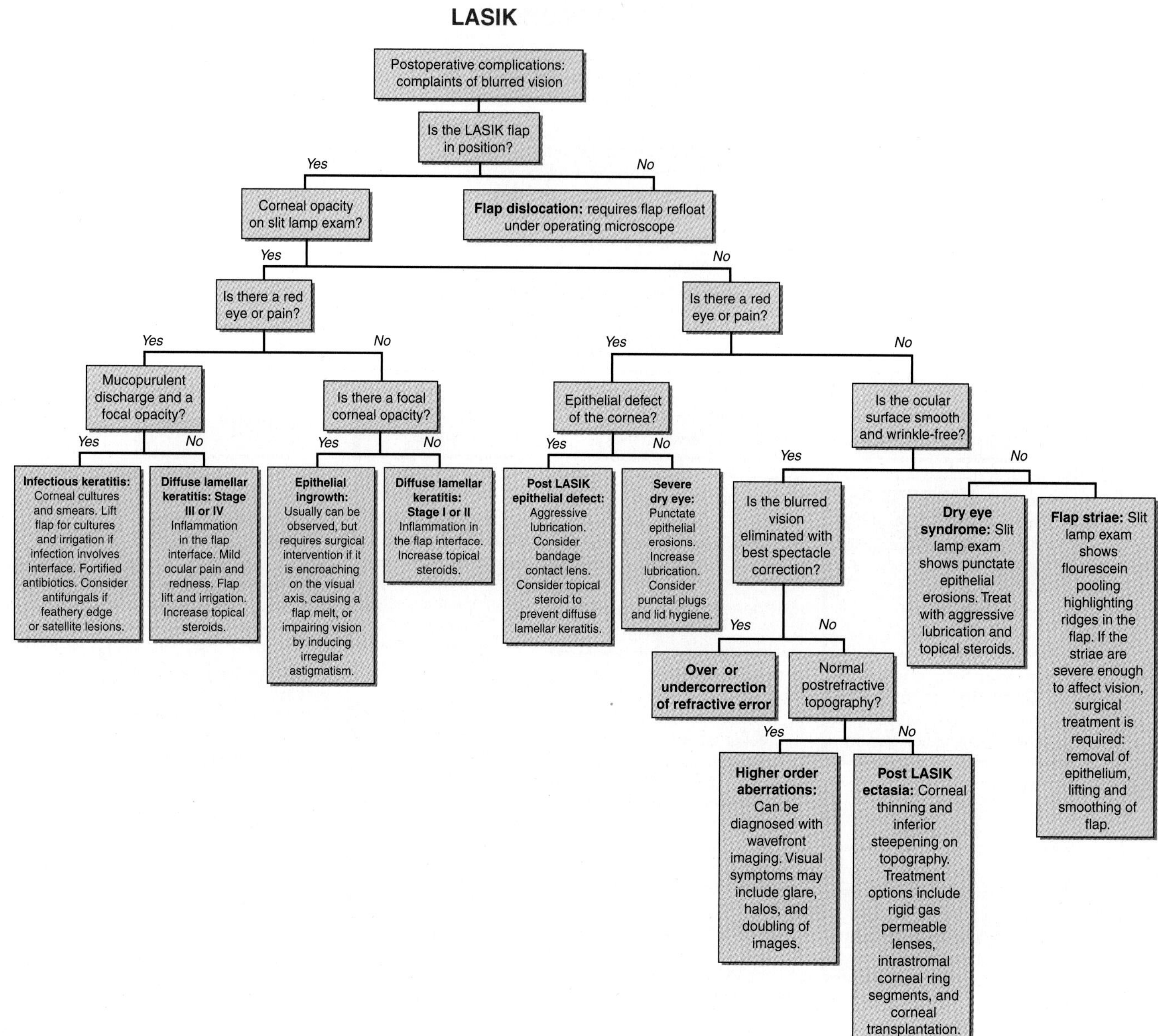

Elizabeth Hofmeister

LENS RELATED GLAUCOMA

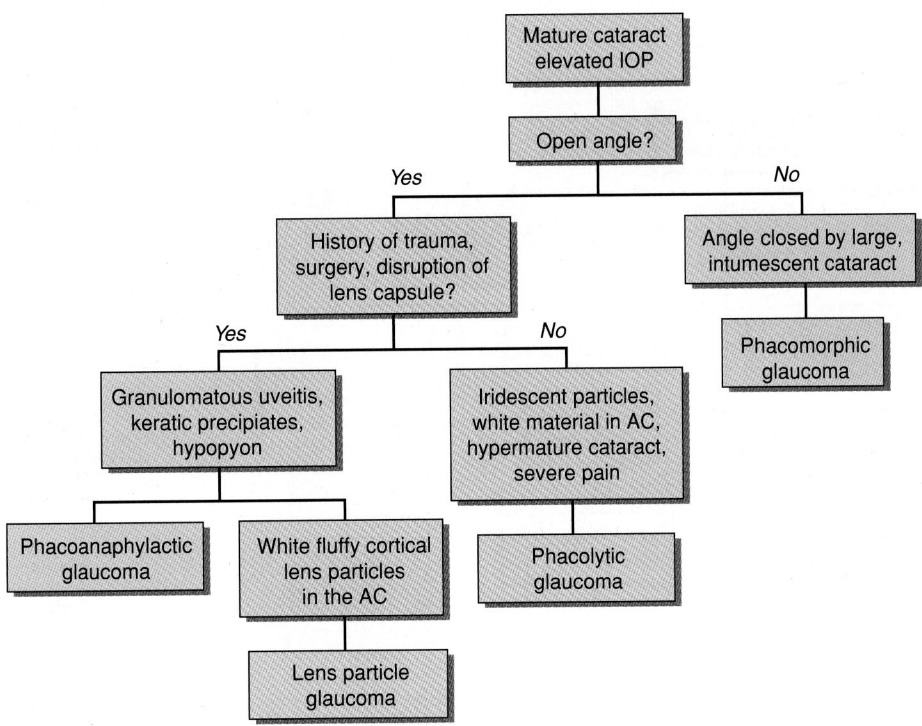

Rachel M. Niknam

LEUKOCORIA

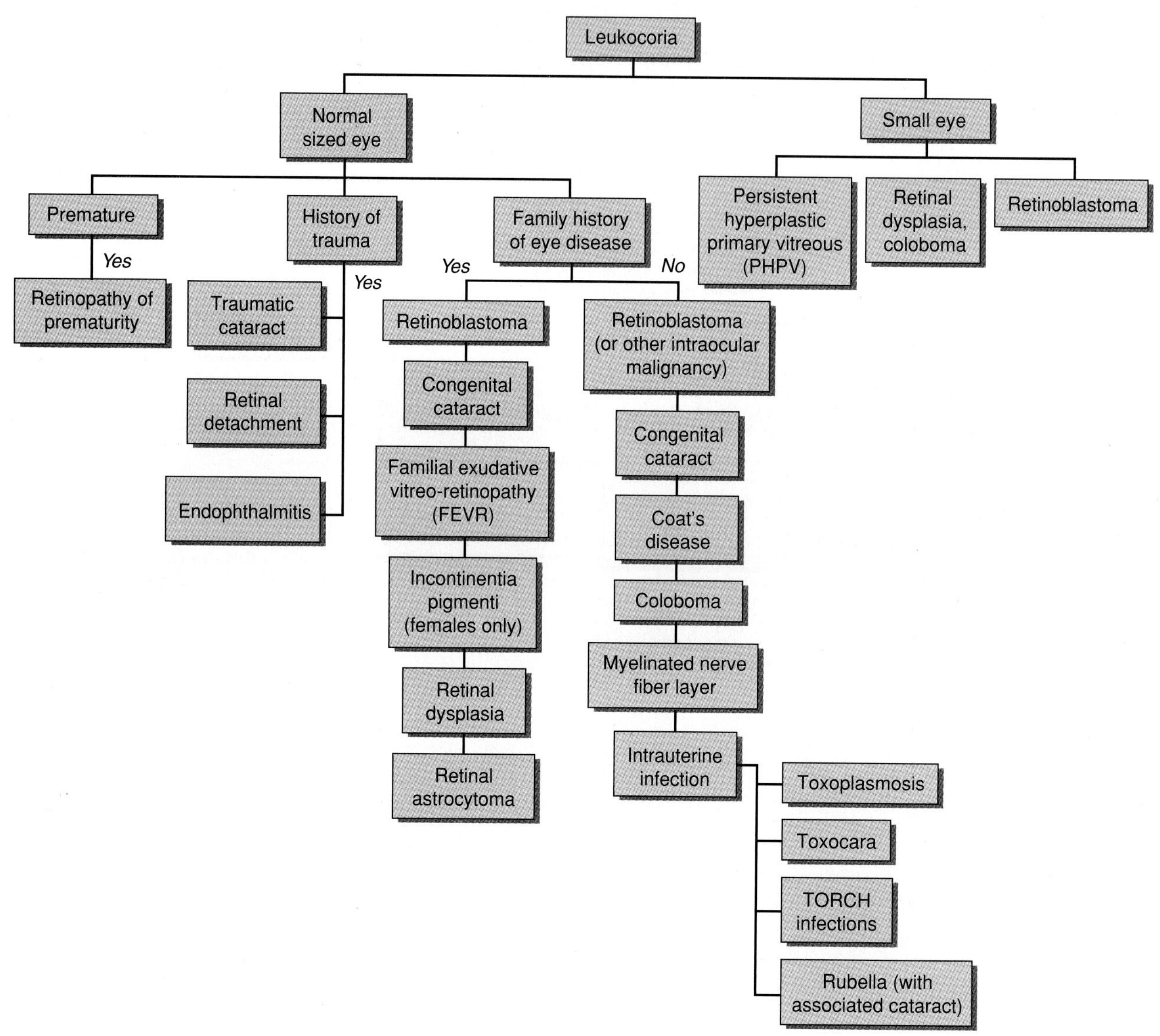

Jonathan Salvin

LOW VISION MANAGEMENT

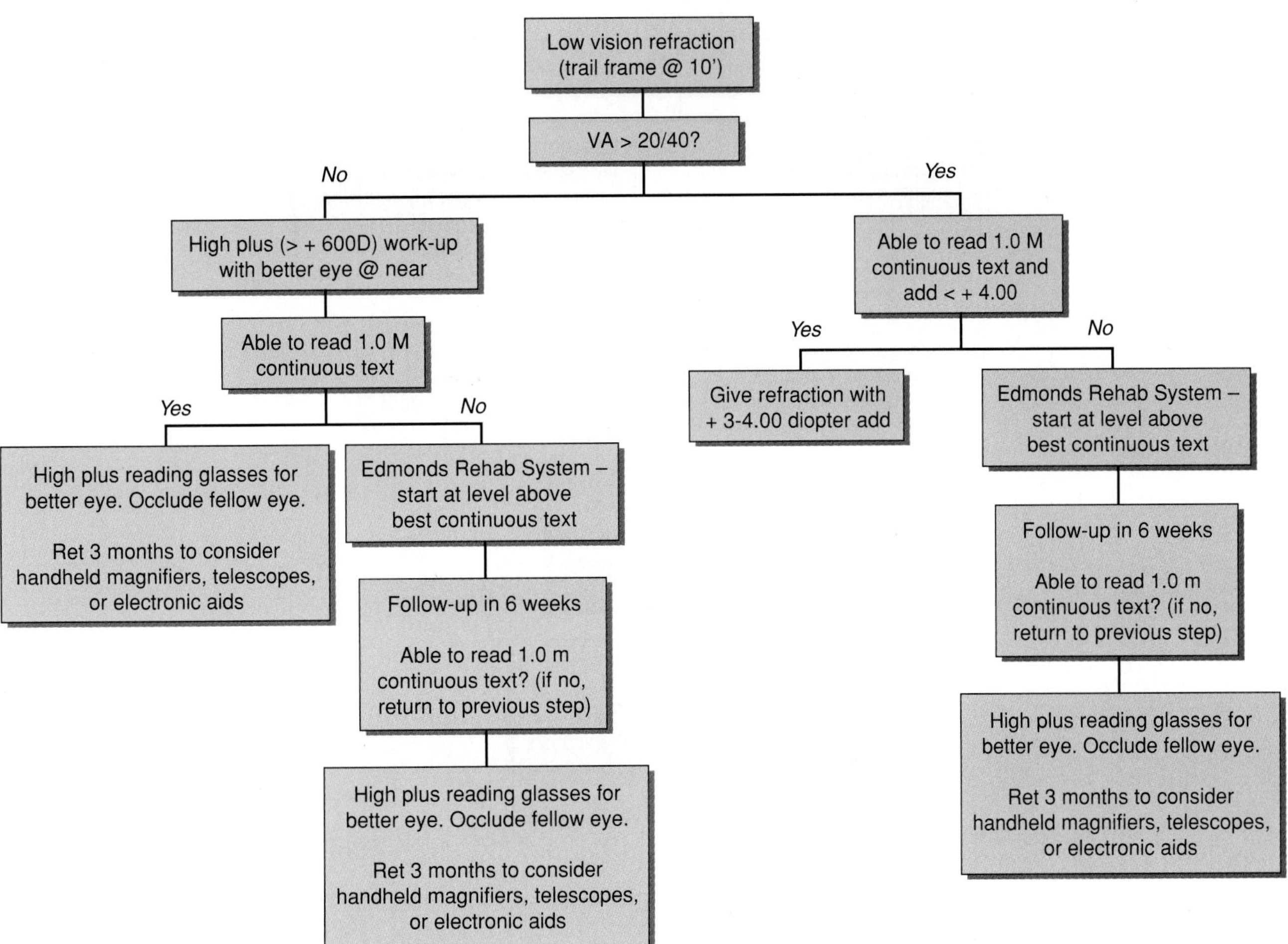

Scott Edmonds

MALIGNANT GLAUCOMA

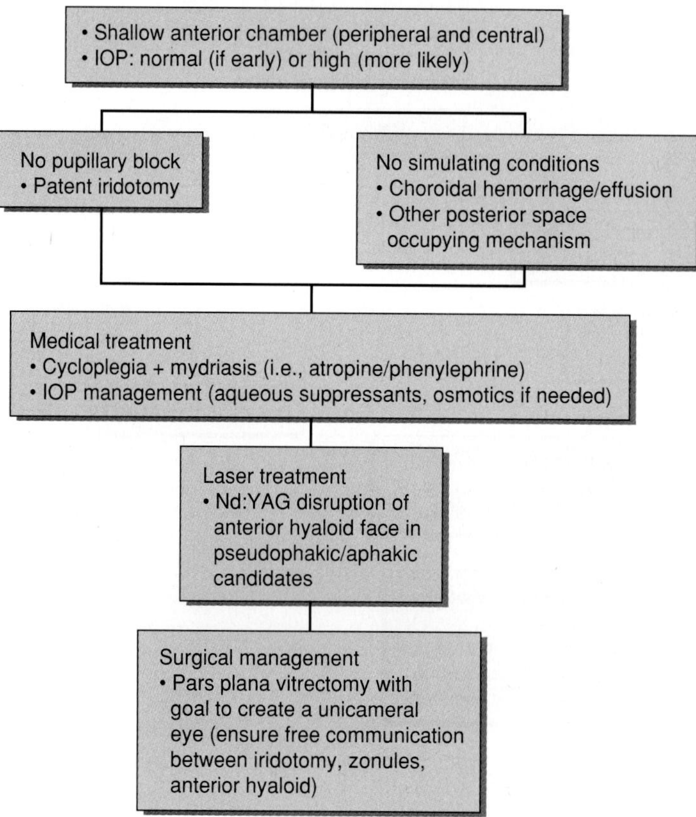
• Shallow anterior chamber (peripheral and central)
• IOP: normal (if early) or high (more likely)
No pupillary block
• Patent iridotomy
No simulating conditions
• Choroidal hemorrhage/effusion
• Other posterior space occupying mechanism
Medical treatment
• Cycloplegia + mydriasis (i.e., atropine/phenylephrine)
• IOP management (aqueous suppressants, osmotics if needed)
Laser treatment
• Nd:YAG disruption of anterior hyaloid face in pseudophakic/aphakic candidates
Surgical management
• Pars plana vitrectomy with goal to create a unicameral eye (ensure free communication between iridotomy, zonules, anterior hyaloid)

Anand Mantravadi

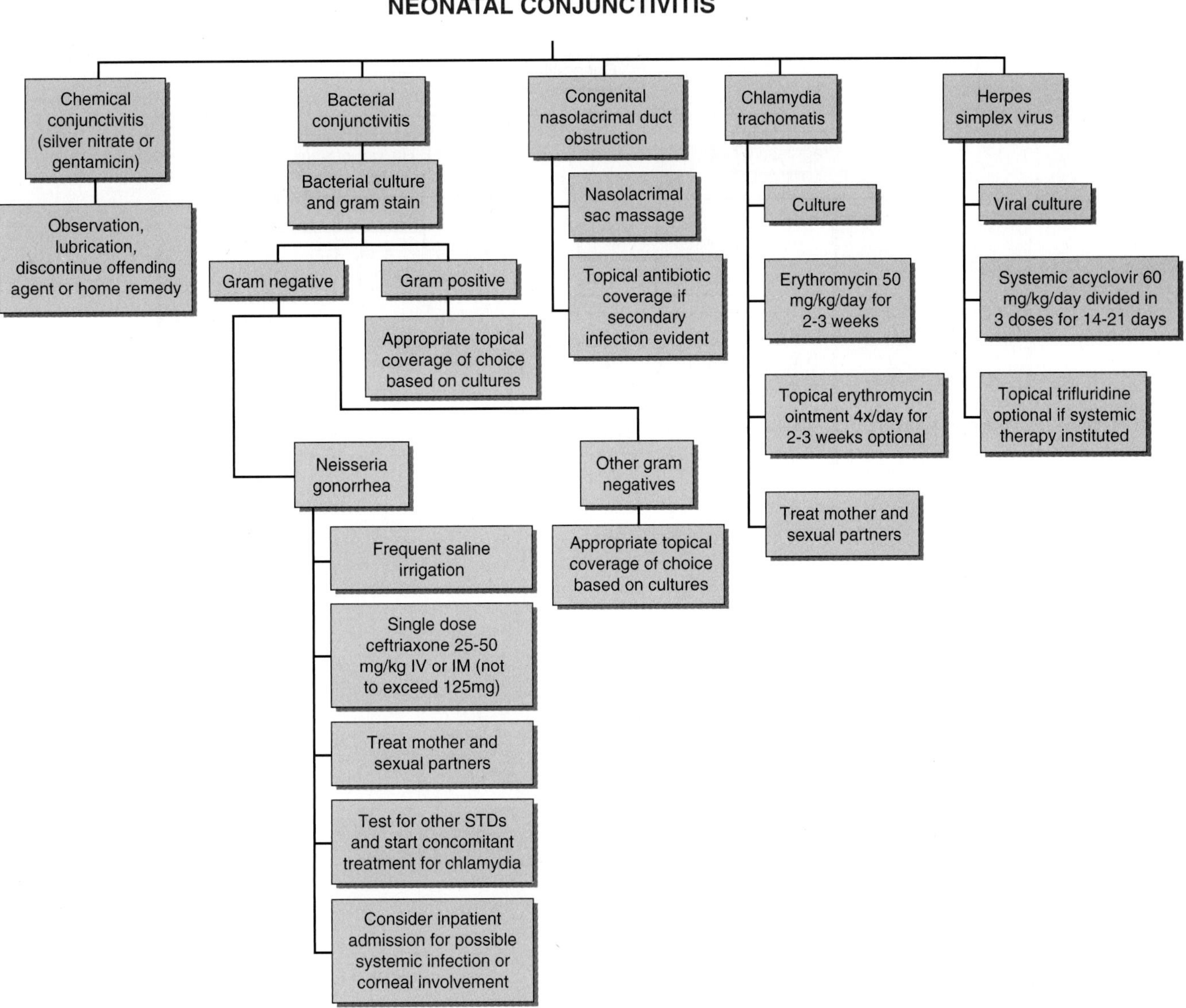
NEONATAL CONJUNCTIVITIS
Chemical conjunctivitis (silver nitrate or gentamicin)
Observation, lubrication, discontinue offending agent or home remedy
Bacterial conjunctivitis
Bacterial culture and gram stain
Gram negative
Gram positive
Appropriate topical coverage of choice based on cultures
Neisseria gonorrhea
Frequent saline irrigation
Single dose ceftriaxone 25-50 mg/kg IV or IM (not to exceed 125mg)
Treat mother and sexual partners
Test for other STDs and start concomitant treatment for chlamydia
Consider inpatient admission for possible systemic infection or corneal involvement
Other gram negatives
Appropriate topical coverage of choice based on cultures
Congenital nasolacrimal duct obstruction
Nasolacrimal sac massage
Topical antibiotic coverage if secondary infection evident
Chlamydia trachomatis
Culture
Erythromycin 50 mg/kg/day for 2-3 weeks
Topical erythromycin ointment 4x/day for 2-3 weeks optional
Treat mother and sexual partners
Herpes simplex virus
Viral culture
Systemic acyclovir 60 mg/kg/day divided in 3 doses for 14-21 days
Topical trifluridine optional if systemic therapy instituted

Jonathan Salvin and Sharon Lehman

NIGHT BLINDNESS (NYCTALOPIA)

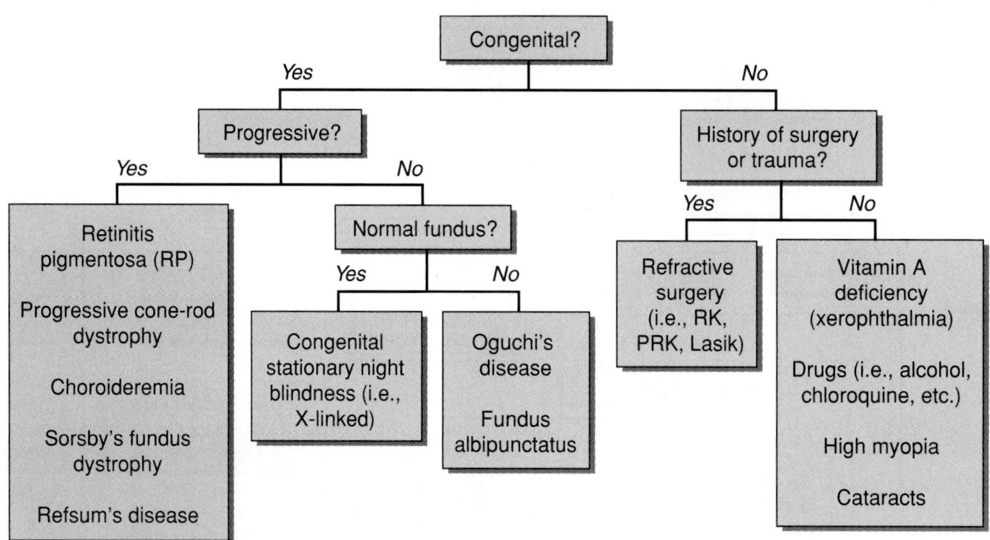

OCULAR HYPERTENSION

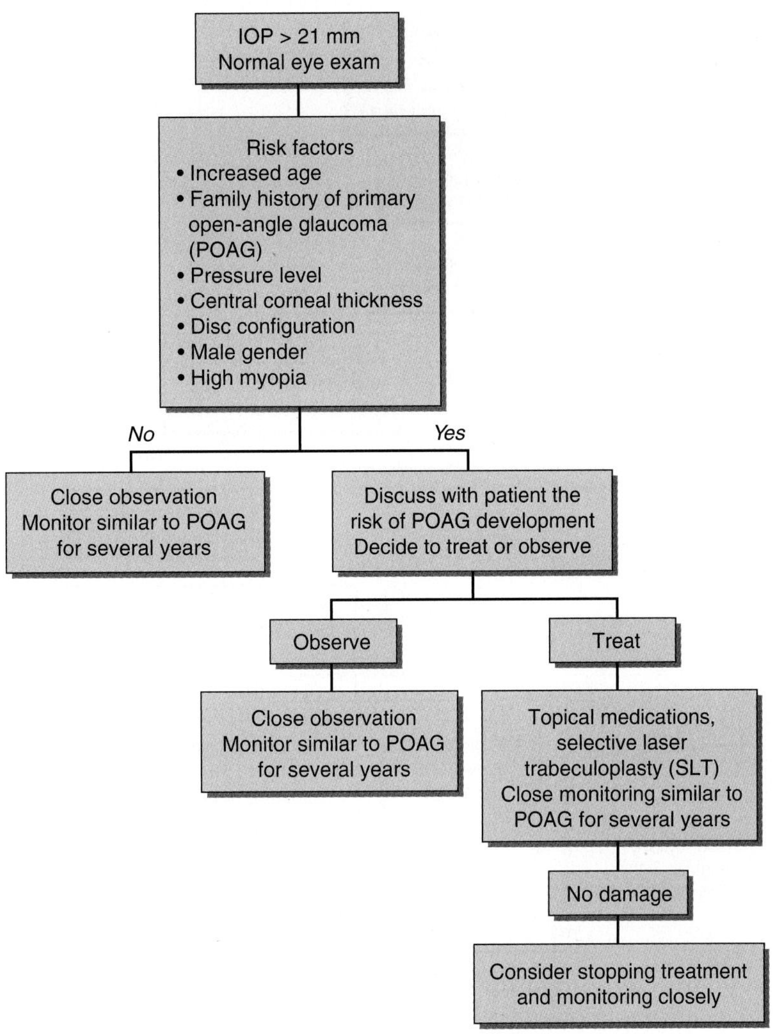

Tara A. Uhler

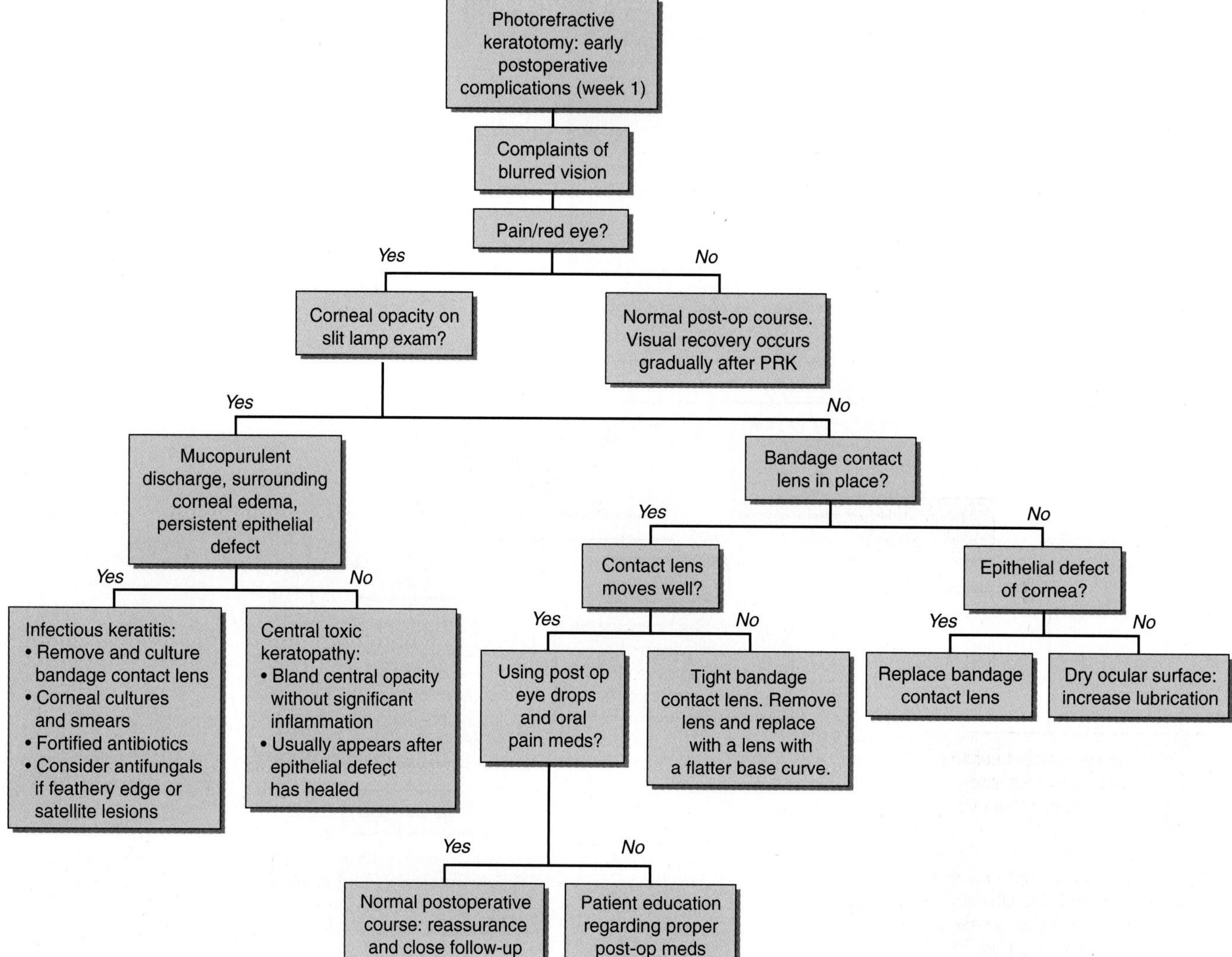

Elizabeth Hofmeister

Photorefractive Surgery Complications (Late)

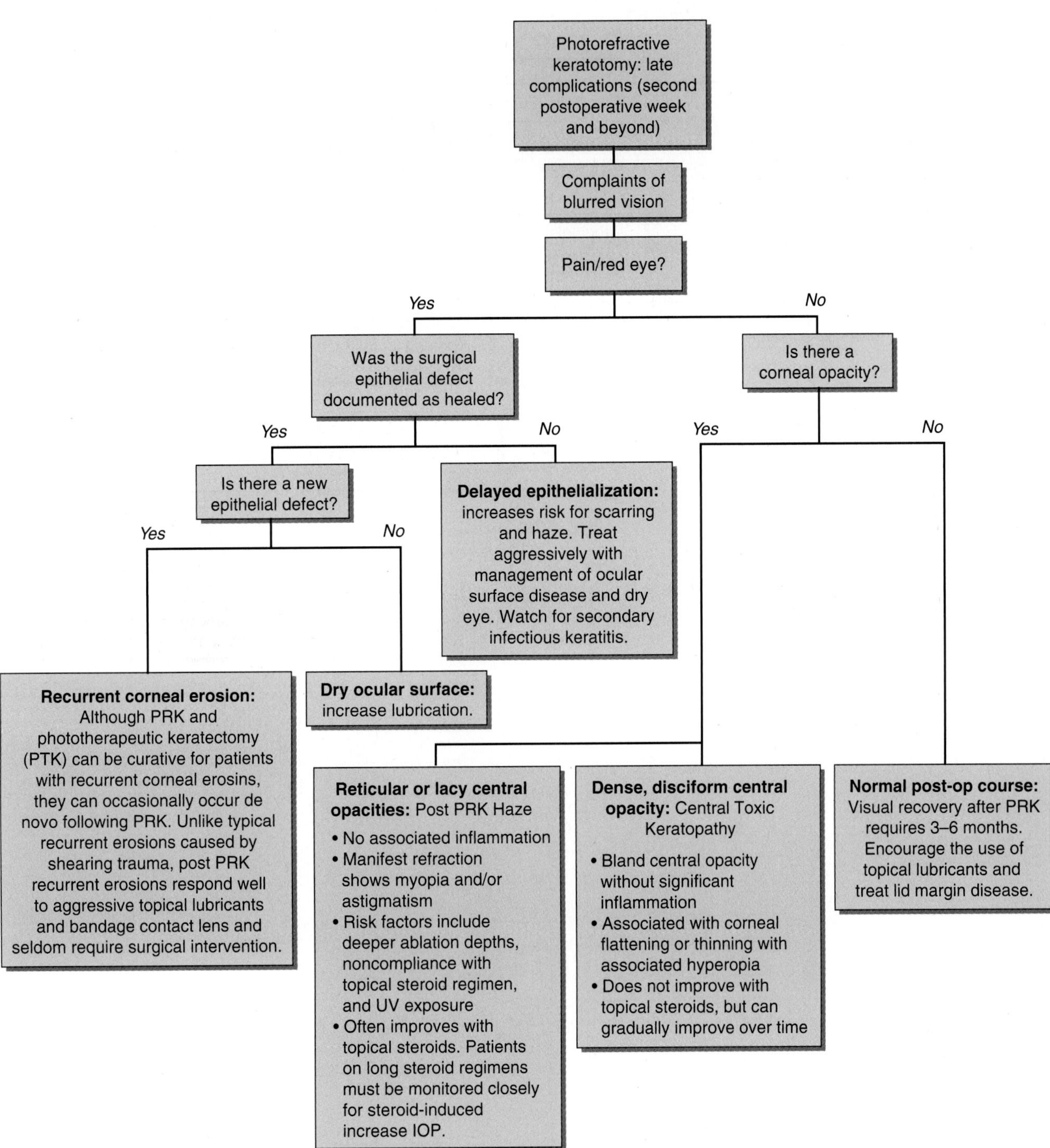

Photorefractive keratotomy: late complications (second postoperative week and beyond)
Complaints of blurred vision
Pain/red eye?
Yes
No
Was the surgical epithelial defect documented as healed?
Is there a corneal opacity?
Yes
No
Yes
No
Is there a new epithelial defect?
Delayed epithelialization: increases risk for scarring and haze. Treat aggressively with management of ocular surface disease and dry eye. Watch for secondary infectious keratitis.
Yes
No
Recurrent corneal erosion: Although PRK and phototherapeutic keratectomy (PTK) can be curative for patients with recurrent corneal erosins, they can occasionally occur de novo following PRK. Unlike typical recurrent erosions caused by shearing trauma, post PRK recurrent erosions respond well to aggressive topical lubricants and bandage contact lens and seldom require surgical intervention.
Dry ocular surface: increase lubrication.
Reticular or lacy central opacities: Post PRK Haze
• No associated inflammation
• Manifest refraction shows myopia and/or astigmatism
• Risk factors include deeper ablation depths, noncompliance with topical steroid regimen, and UV exposure
• Often improves with topical steroids. Patients on long steroid regimens must be monitored closely for steroid-induced increase IOP.
Dense, disciform central opacity: Central Toxic Keratopathy
• Bland central opacity without significant inflammation
• Associated with corneal flattening or thinning with associated hyperopia
• Does not improve with topical steroids, but can gradually improve over time
Normal post-op course: Visual recovery after PRK requires 3–6 months. Encourage the use of topical lubricants and treat lid margin disease.

Elizabeth Hofmeister

PIGMENTED CONJUNCTIVAL LESION(S)

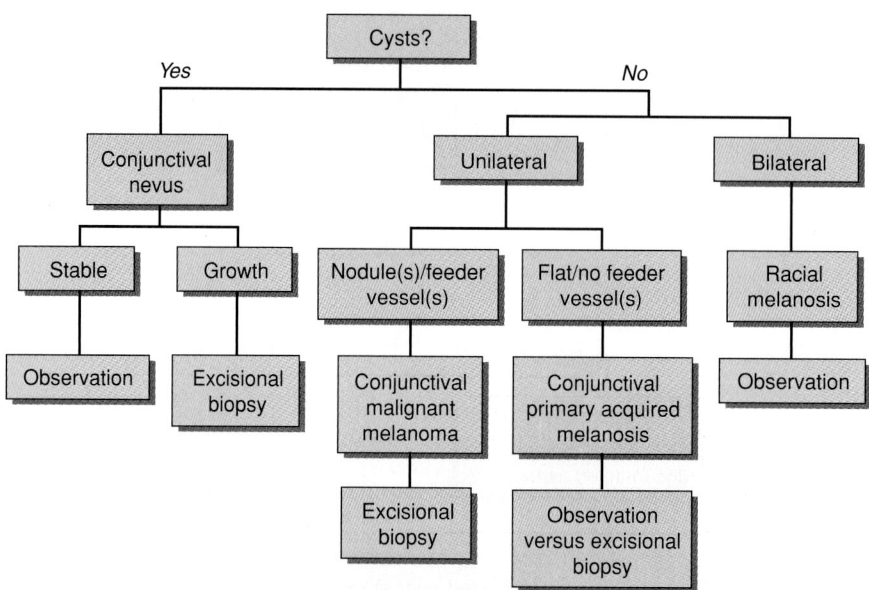

Britt Parvus

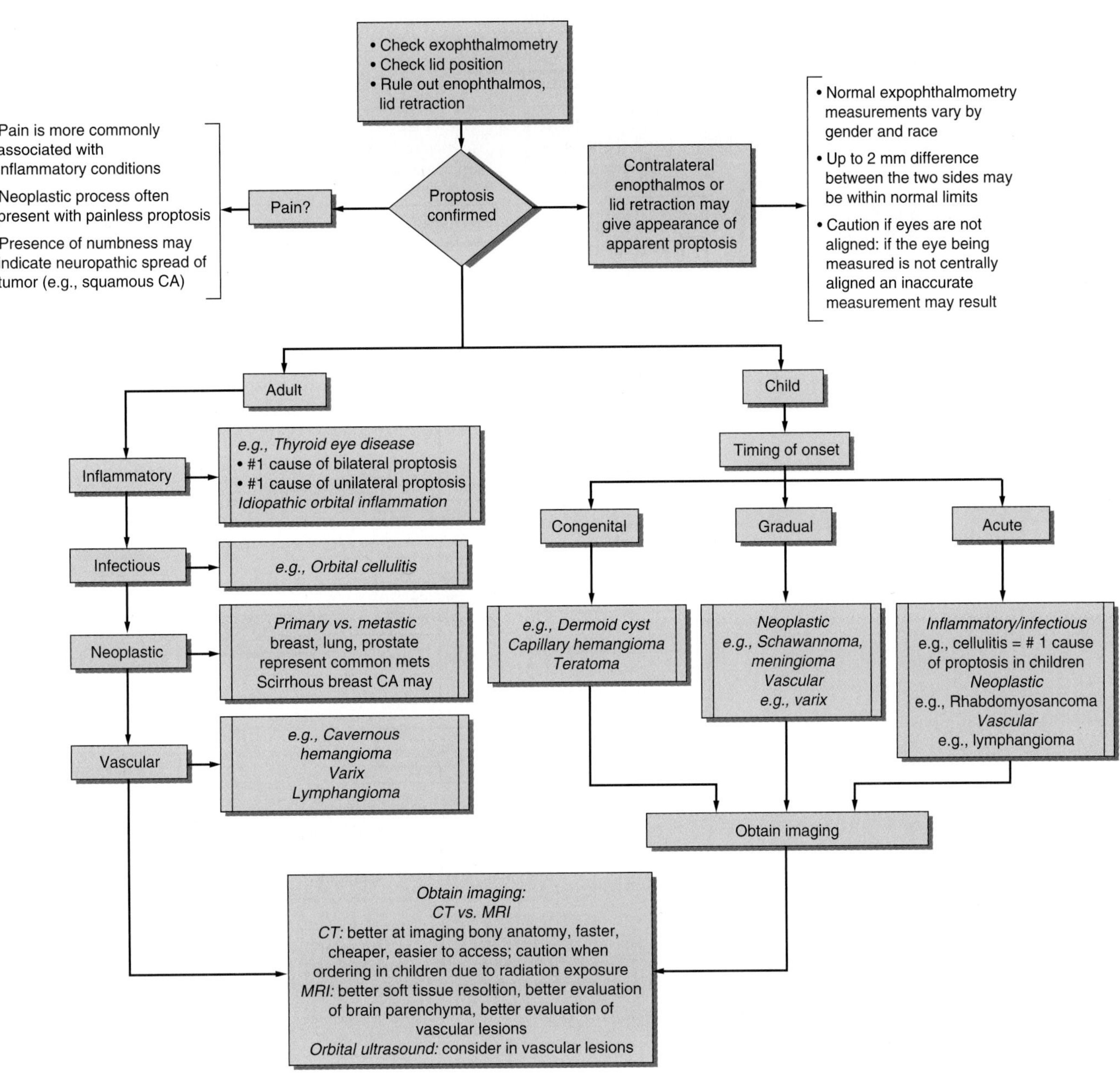
PROPTOSIS
• Check exophthalmometry
• Check lid position
• Rule out enophthalmos, lid retraction
Proptosis confirmed
Pain?
• Pain is more commonly associated with inflammatory conditions
• Neoplastic process often present with painless proptosis
• Presence of numbness may indicate neuropathic spread of tumor (e.g., squamous CA)
Contralateral enopthalmos or lid retraction may give appearance of apparent proptosis
• Normal expophthalmometry measurements vary by gender and race
• Up to 2 mm difference between the two sides may be within normal limits
• Caution if eyes are not aligned: if the eye being measured is not centrally aligned an inaccurate measurement may result
Adult
Child
Inflammatory
e.g., Thyroid eye disease
• #1 cause of bilateral proptosis
• #1 cause of unilateral proptosis
Idiopathic orbital inflammation
Infectious
e.g., Orbital cellulitis
Neoplastic
Primary vs. metastic
breast, lung, prostate represent common mets
Scirrhous breast CA may
Vascular
e.g., Cavernous hemangioma
Varix
Lymphangioma
Timing of onset
Congenital
Gradual
Acute
e.g., Dermoid cyst
Capillary hemangioma
Teratoma
Neoplastic
e.g., Schawannoma, meningioma
Vascular
e.g., varix
Inflammatory/infectious
e.g., cellulitis = # 1 cause of proptosis in children
Neoplastic
e.g., Rhabdomyosancoma
Vascular
e.g., lymphangioma
Obtain imaging
Obtain imaging:
CT vs. MRI
CT: better at imaging bony anatomy, faster, cheaper, easier to access; caution when ordering in children due to radiation exposure
MRI: better soft tissue resoltion, better evaluation of brain parenchyma, better evaluation of vascular lesions
Orbital ultrasound: consider in vascular lesions

Vladimir Yakopson

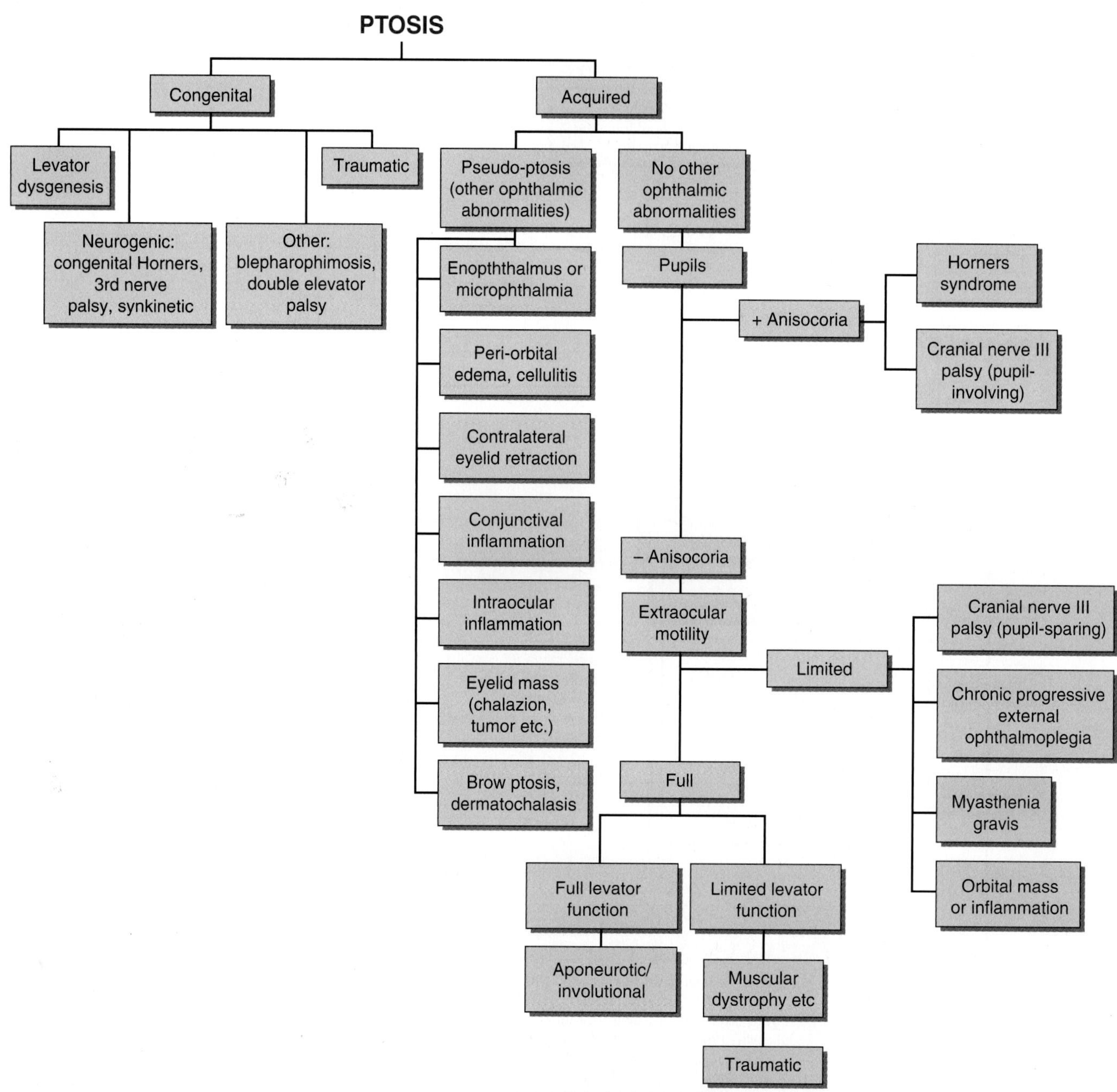

Katherine A. Lane

RECURRENT CORNEAL EROSION SYNDROME

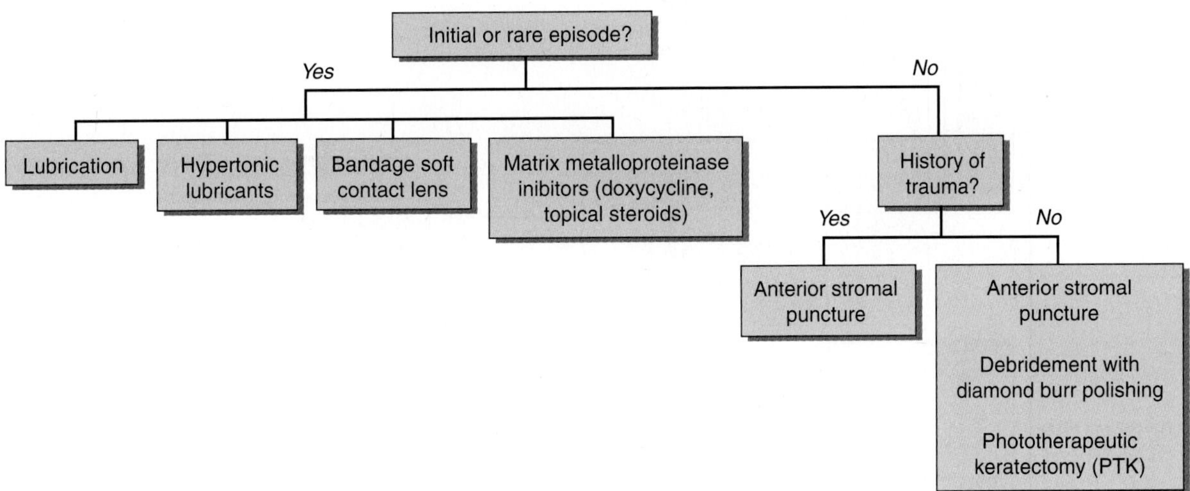

Colleen Halfpenny

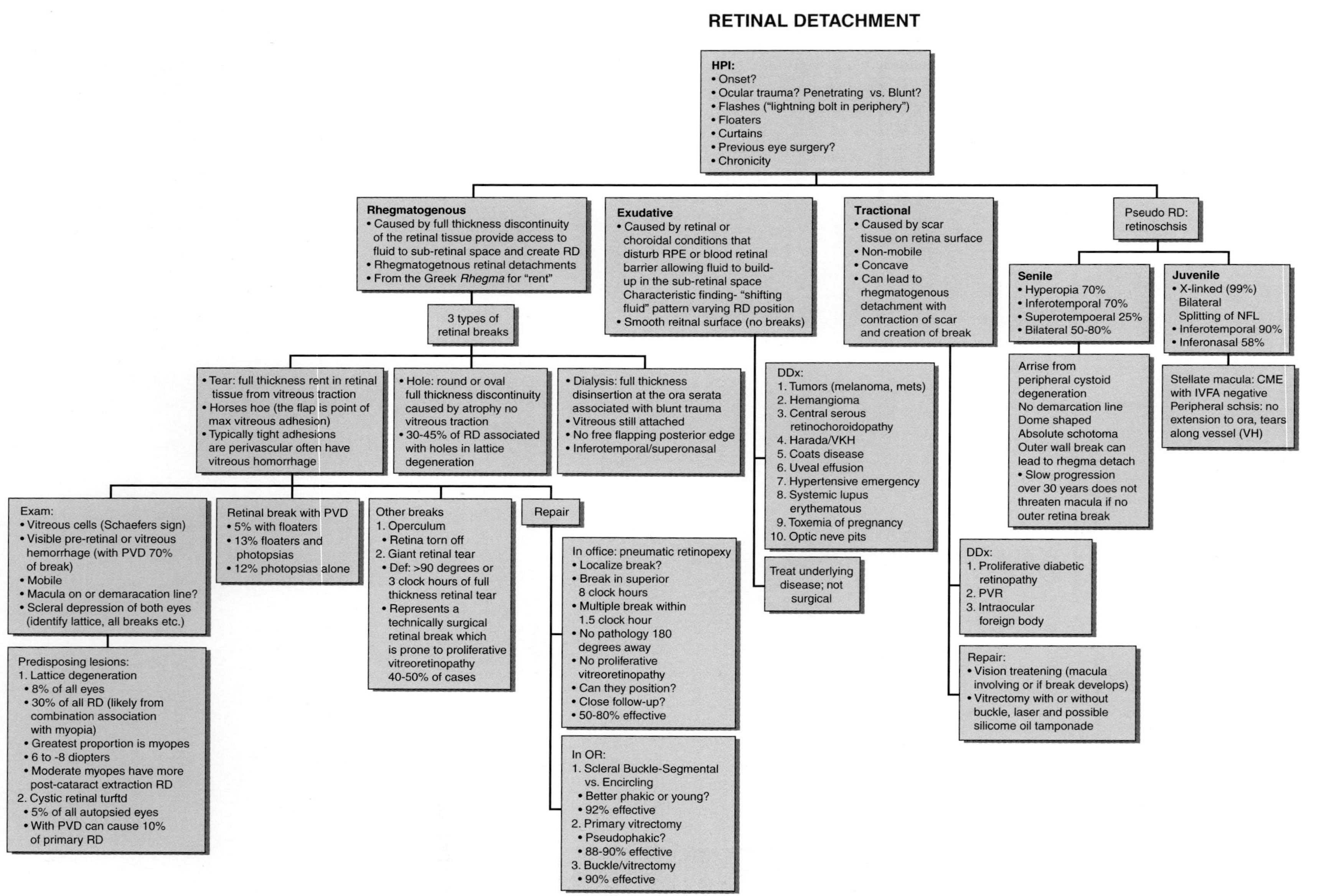
RETINAL DETACHMENT
HPI:
• Onset?
• Ocular trauma? Penetrating vs. Blunt?
• Flashes ("lightning bolt in periphery")
• Floaters
• Curtains
• Previous eye surgery?
• Chronicity
Rhegmatogenous
• Caused by full thickness discontinuity of the retinal tissue provide access to fluid to sub-retinal space and create RD
• Rhegmatogetnous retinal detachments
• From the Greek Rhegma for "rent"
Exudative
• Caused by retinal or choroidal conditions that disturb RPE or blood retinal barrier allowing fluid to build-up in the sub-retinal space Characteristic finding- "shifting fluid" pattern varying RD position
• Smooth reitnal surface (no breaks)
Tractional
• Caused by scar tissue on retina surface
• Non-mobile
• Concave
• Can lead to rhegmatogenous detachment with contraction of scar and creation of break
Pseudo RD: retinoschsis
Senile
• Hyperopia 70%
• Inferotemporal 70%
• Superotempoeral 25%
• Bilateral 50-80%
Juvenile
• X-linked (99%) Bilateral Splitting of NFL
• Inferotemporal 90%
• Inferonasal 58%
Arrise from peripheral cystoid degeneration No demarcation line Dome shaped Absolute schotoma Outer wall break can lead to rhegma detach
• Slow progression over 30 years does not threaten macula if no outer retina break
Stellate macula: CME with IVFA negative Peripheral schsis: no extension to ora, tears along vessel (VH)
3 types of retinal breaks
• Tear: full thickness rent in retinal tissue from vitreous traction
• Horses hoe (the flap is point of max vitreous adhesion)
• Typically tight adhesions are perivascular often have vitreous homorrhage
• Hole: round or oval full thickness discontinuity caused by atrophy no vitreous traction
• 30-45% of RD associated with holes in lattice degeneration
• Dialysis: full thickness disinsertion at the ora serata associated with blunt trauma
• Vitreous still attached
• No free flapping posterior edge
• Inferotemporal/superonasal
DDx:
1. Tumors (melanoma, mets)
2. Hemangioma
3. Central serous retinochoroidopathy
4. Harada/VKH
5. Coats disease
6. Uveal effusion
7. Hypertensive emergency
8. Systemic lupus erythematous
9. Toxemia of pregnancy
10. Optic neve pits
Treat underlying disease; not surgical
DDx:
1. Proliferative diabetic retinopathy
2. PVR
3. Intraocular foreign body
Repair:
• Vision treatening (macula involving or if break develops)
• Vitrectomy with or without buckle, laser and possible silicome oil tamponade
Exam:
• Vitreous cells (Schaefers sign)
• Visible pre-retinal or vitreous hemorrhage (with PVD 70% of break)
• Mobile
• Macula on or demaracation line?
• Scleral depression of both eyes (identify lattice, all breaks etc.)
Predisposing lesions:
1. Lattice degeneration
• 8% of all eyes
• 30% of all RD (likely from combination association with myopia)
• Greatest proportion is myopes
• 6 to -8 diopters
• Moderate myopes have more post-cataract extraction RD
2. Cystic retinal turftd
• 5% of all autopsied eyes
• With PVD can cause 10% of primary RD
Retinal break with PVD
• 5% with floaters
• 13% floaters and photopsias
• 12% photopsias alone
Other breaks
1. Operculum
• Retina torn off
2. Giant retinal tear
• Def: >90 degrees or 3 clock hours of full thickness retinal tear
• Represents a technically surgical retinal break which is prone to proliferative vitreoretinopathy 40-50% of cases
Repair
In office: pneumatic retinopexy
• Localize break?
• Break in superior 8 clock hours
• Multiple break within 1.5 clock hour
• No pathology 180 degrees away
• No proliferative vitreoretinopathy
• Can they position?
• Close follow-up?
• 50-80% effective
In OR:
1. Scleral Buckle-Segmental vs. Encircling
• Better phakic or young?
• 92% effective
2. Primary vitrectomy
• Pseudophakic?
• 88-90% effective
3. Buckle/vitrectomy
• 90% effective

Rajiv Shah

RETINAL HEMORRHAGE

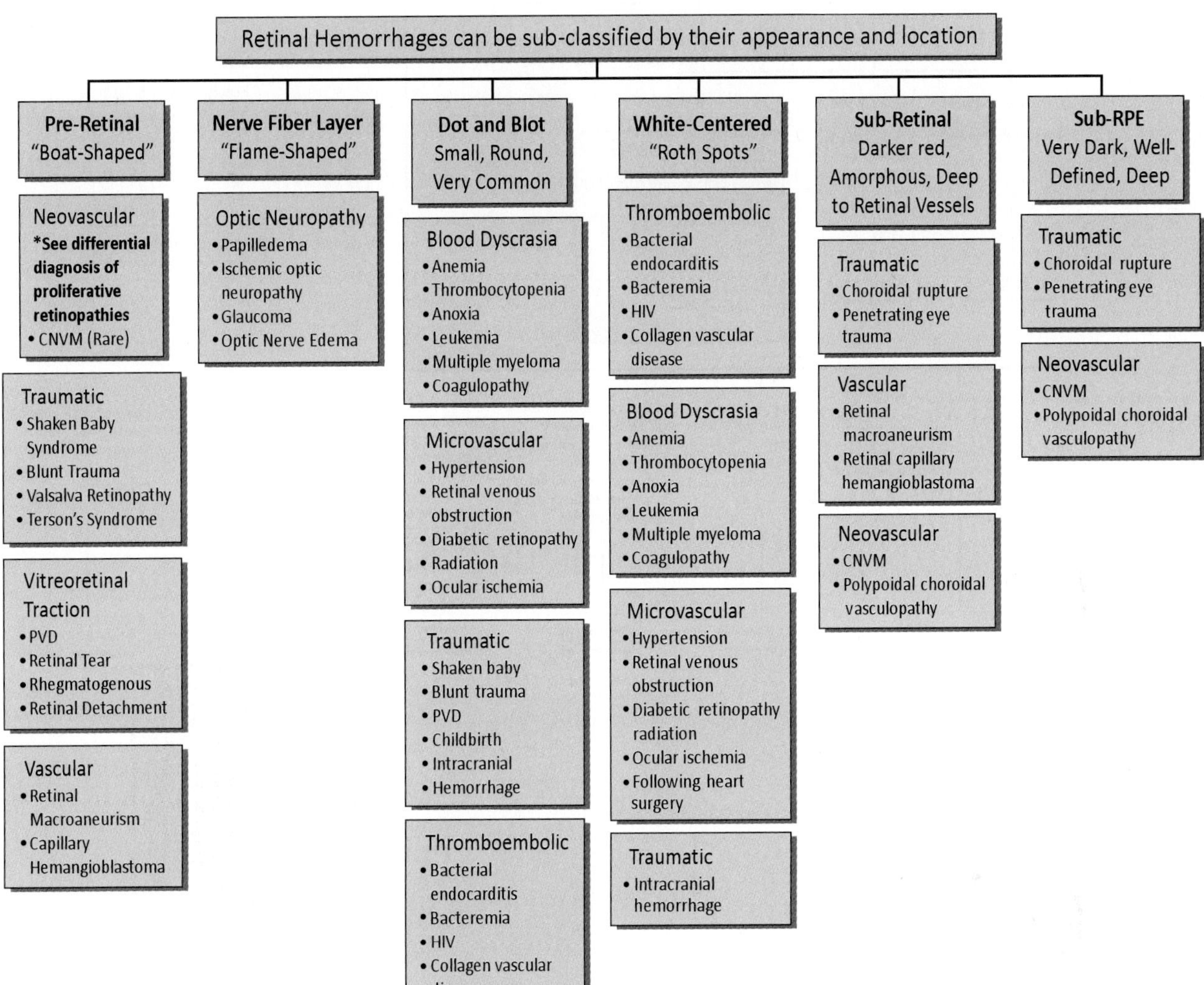

Retinal Hemorrhages can be sub-classified by their appearance and location
Pre-Retinal "Boat-Shaped"
Neovascular *See differential diagnosis of proliferative retinopathies • CNVM (Rare)
Traumatic • Shaken Baby Syndrome • Blunt Trauma • Valsalva Retinopathy • Terson's Syndrome
Vitreoretinal Traction • PVD • Retinal Tear • Rhegmatogenous • Retinal Detachment
Vascular • Retinal Macroaneurism • Capillary Hemangioblastoma
Nerve Fiber Layer "Flame-Shaped"
Optic Neuropathy • Papilledema • Ischemic optic neuropathy • Glaucoma • Optic Nerve Edema
Dot and Blot Small, Round, Very Common
Blood Dyscrasia • Anemia • Thrombocytopenia • Anoxia • Leukemia • Multiple myeloma • Coagulopathy
Microvascular • Hypertension • Retinal venous obstruction • Diabetic retinopathy • Radiation • Ocular ischemia
Traumatic • Shaken baby • Blunt trauma • PVD • Childbirth • Intracranial • Hemorrhage
Thromboembolic • Bacterial endocarditis • Bacteremia • HIV • Collagen vascular disease
White-Centered "Roth Spots"
Thromboembolic • Bacterial endocarditis • Bacteremia • HIV • Collagen vascular disease
Blood Dyscrasia • Anemia • Thrombocytopenia • Anoxia • Leukemia • Multiple myeloma • Coagulopathy
Microvascular • Hypertension • Retinal venous obstruction • Diabetic retinopathy radiation • Ocular ischemia • Following heart surgery
Traumatic • Intracranial hemorrhage
Sub-Retinal Darker red, Amorphous, Deep to Retinal Vessels
Traumatic • Choroidal rupture • Penetrating eye trauma
Vascular • Retinal macroaneurism • Retinal capillary hemangioblastoma
Neovascular • CNVM • Polypoidal choroidal vasculopathy
Sub-RPE Very Dark, Well-Defined, Deep
Traumatic • Choroidal rupture • Penetrating eye trauma
Neovascular • CNVM • Polypoidal choroidal vasculopathy

*All causes of Dot-Blot hemorrhage can also cause nerve fiber layer hemorrhages

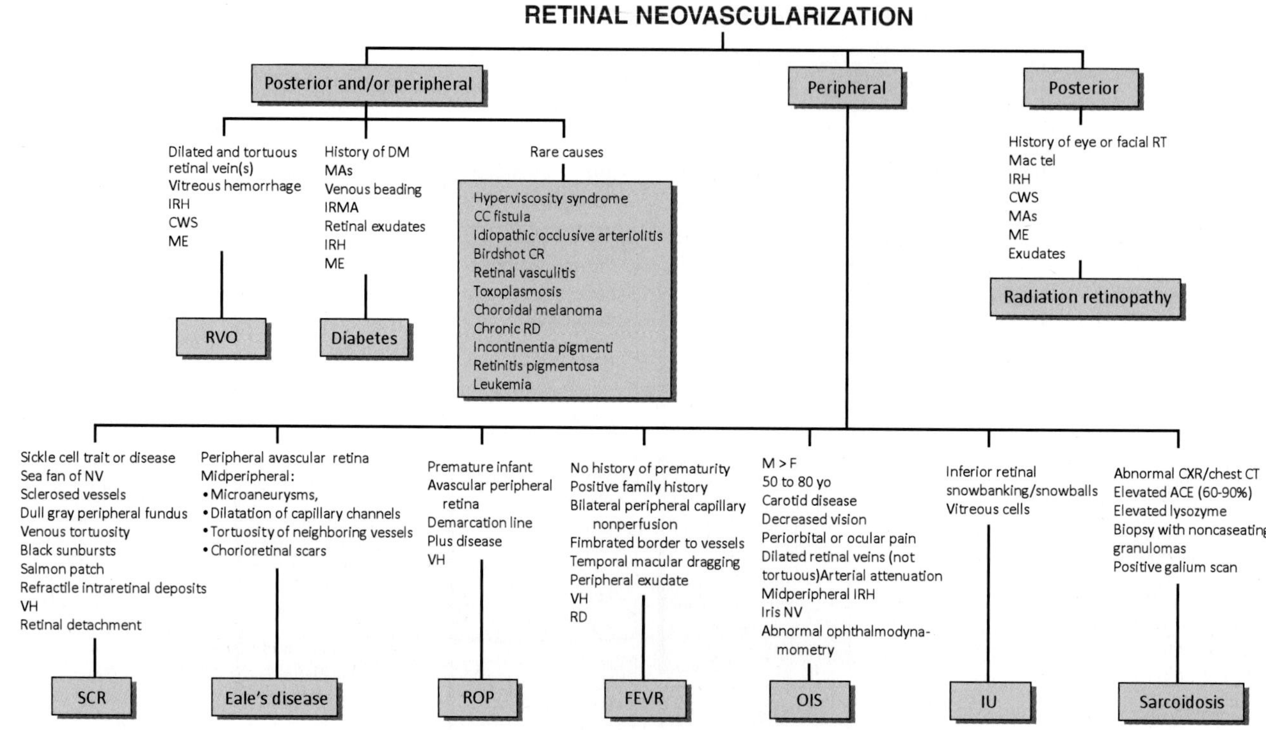
RETINAL NEOVASCULARIZATION
Posterior and/or peripheral
Peripheral
Posterior
Dilated and tortuous retinal vein(s)
Vitreous hemorrhage
IRH
CWS
ME
RVO
History of DM
MAs
Venous beading
IRMA
Retinal exudates
IRH
ME
Diabetes
Rare causes
Hyperviscosity syndrome
CC fistula
Idiopathic occlusive arteriolitis
Birdshot CR
Retinal vasculitis
Toxoplasmosis
Choroidal melanoma
Chronic RD
Incontinentia pigmenti
Retinitis pigmentosa
Leukemia
History of eye or facial RT
Mac tel
IRH
CWS
MAs
ME
Exudates
Radiation retinopathy
Sickle cell trait or disease
Sea fan of NV
Sclerosed vessels
Dull gray peripheral fundus
Venous tortuosity
Black sunbursts
Salmon patch
Refractile intraretinal deposits
VH
Retinal detachment
SCR
Peripheral avascular retina
Midperipheral:
• Microaneurysms,
• Dilatation of capillary channels
• Tortuosity of neighboring vessels
• Chorioretinal scars
Eale's disease
Premature infant
Avascular peripheral retina
Demarcation line
Plus disease
VH
ROP
No history of prematurity
Positive family history
Bilateral peripheral capillary nonperfusion
Fimbrated border to vessels
Temporal macular dragging
Peripheral exudate
VH
RD
FEVR
M > F
50 to 80 yo
Carotid disease
Decreased vision
Periorbital or ocular pain
Dilated retinal veins (not tortuous)Arterial attenuation
Midperipheral IRH
Iris NV
Abnormal ophthalmodynamometry
OIS
Inferior retinal snowbanking/snowballs
Vitreous cells
IU
Abnormal CXR/chest CT
Elevated ACE (60-90%)
Elevated lysozyme
Biopsy with noncaseating granulomas
Positive galium scan
Sarcoidosis

Nikolas London

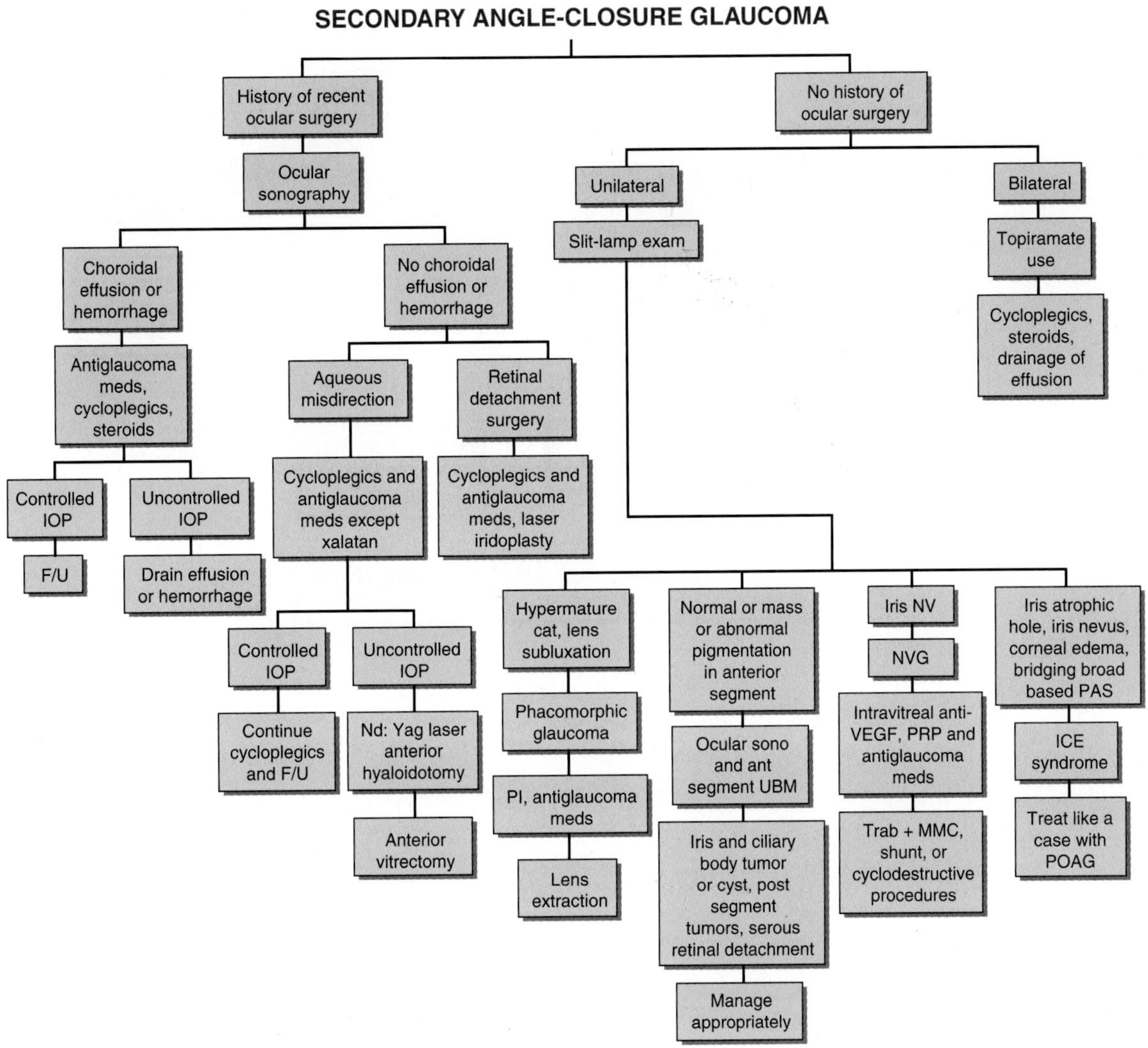

M. Reza Razeghinejad

STROMAL CORNEAL DYSTROPHIES

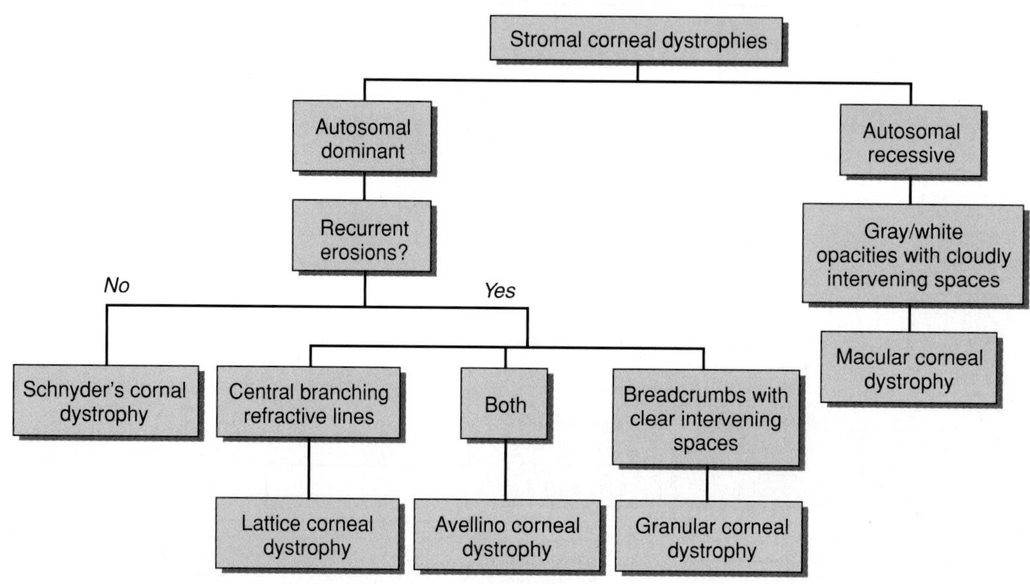

Colleen Halfpenny

SUBLUXATED or DISLOCATED Lens

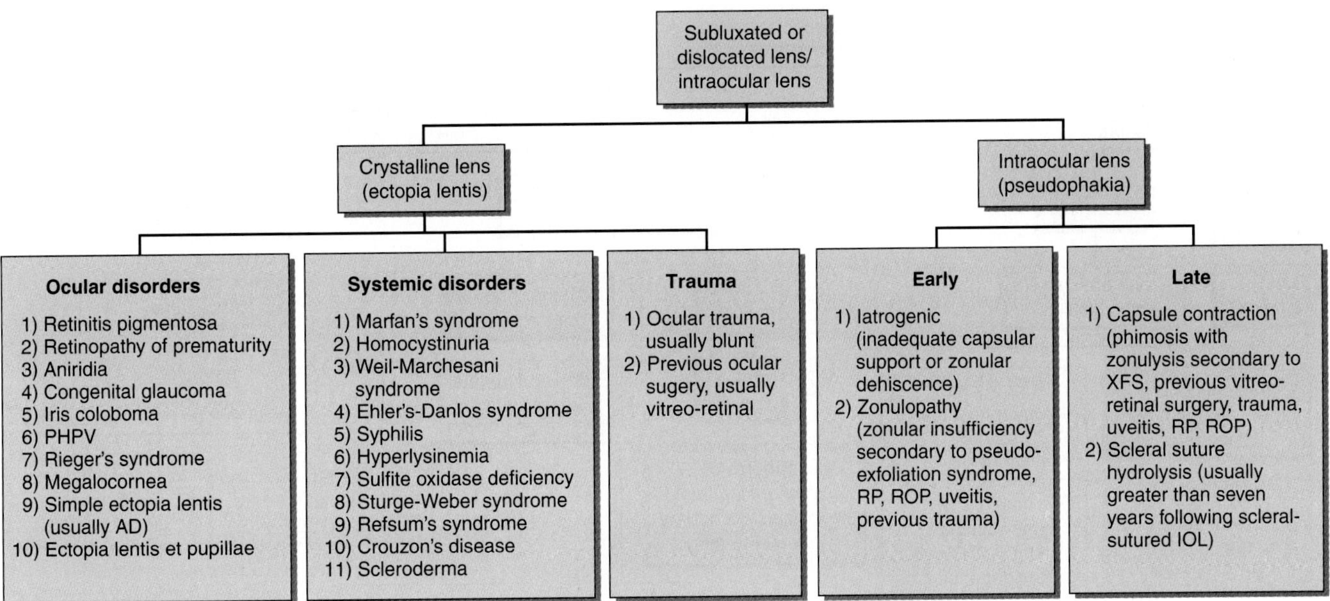

Subluxated or dislocated lens/ intraocular lens
Crystalline lens (ectopia lentis)
Intraocular lens (pseudophakia)
Ocular disorders
1) Retinitis pigmentosa
2) Retinopathy of prematurity
3) Aniridia
4) Congenital glaucoma
5) Iris coloboma
6) PHPV
7) Rieger's syndrome
8) Megalocornea
9) Simple ectopia lentis (usually AD)
10) Ectopia lentis et pupillae
Systemic disorders
1) Marfan's syndrome
2) Homocystinuria
3) Weil-Marchesani syndrome
4) Ehler's-Danlos syndrome
5) Syphilis
6) Hyperlysinemia
7) Sulfite oxidase deficiency
8) Sturge-Weber syndrome
9) Refsum's syndrome
10) Crouzon's disease
11) Scleroderma
Trauma
1) Ocular trauma, usually blunt
2) Previous ocular sugery, usually vitreo-retinal
Early
1) Iatrogenic (inadequate capsular support or zonular dehiscence)
2) Zonulopathy (zonular insufficiency secondary to pseudo-exfoliation syndrome, RP, ROP, uveitis, previous trauma)
Late
1) Capsule contraction (phimosis with zonulysis secondary to XFS, previous vitreo-retinal surgery, trauma, uveitis, RP, ROP)
2) Scleral suture hydrolysis (usually greater than seven years following scleral-sutured IOL)

Robert Behar

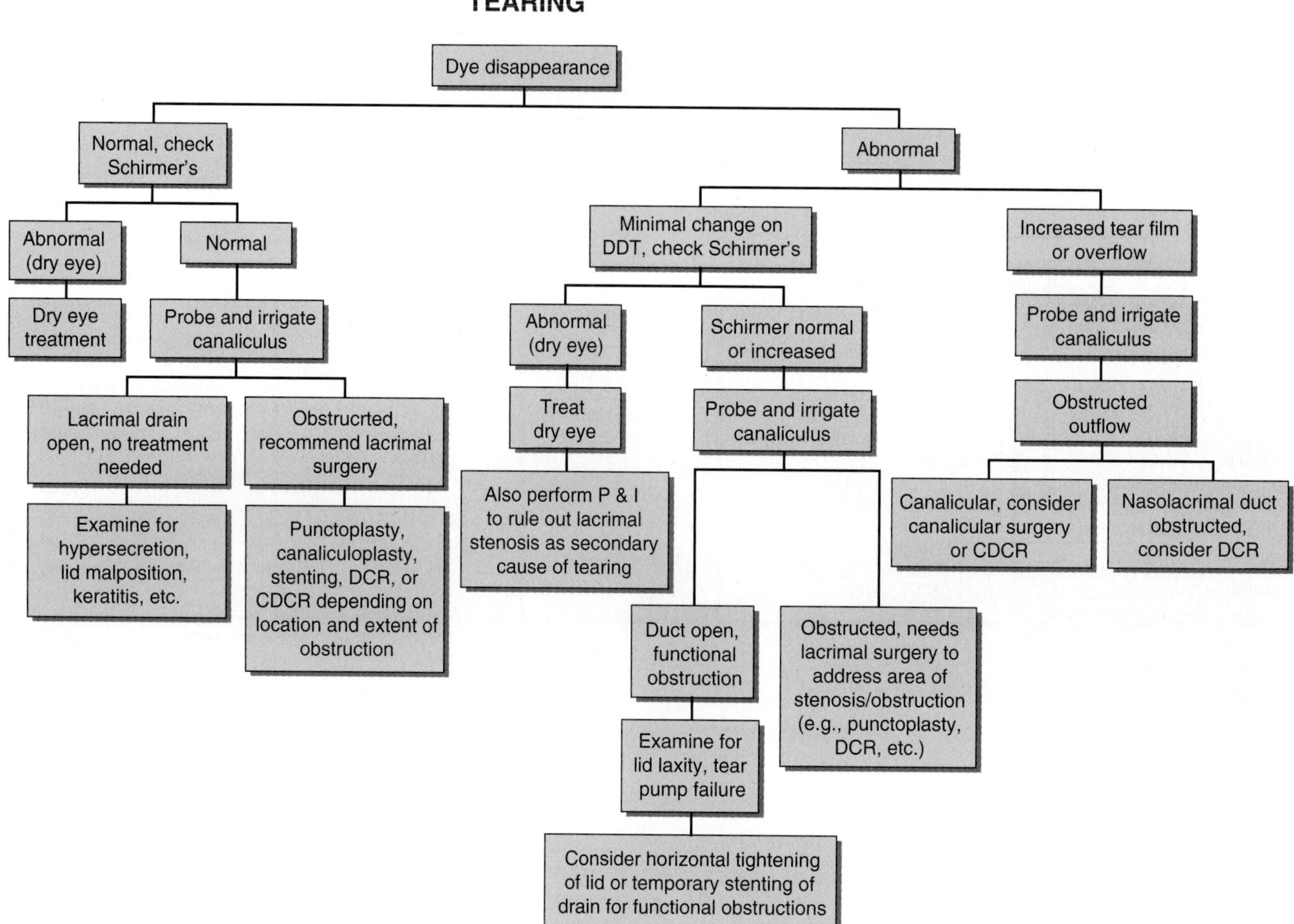

Scott Goldstein

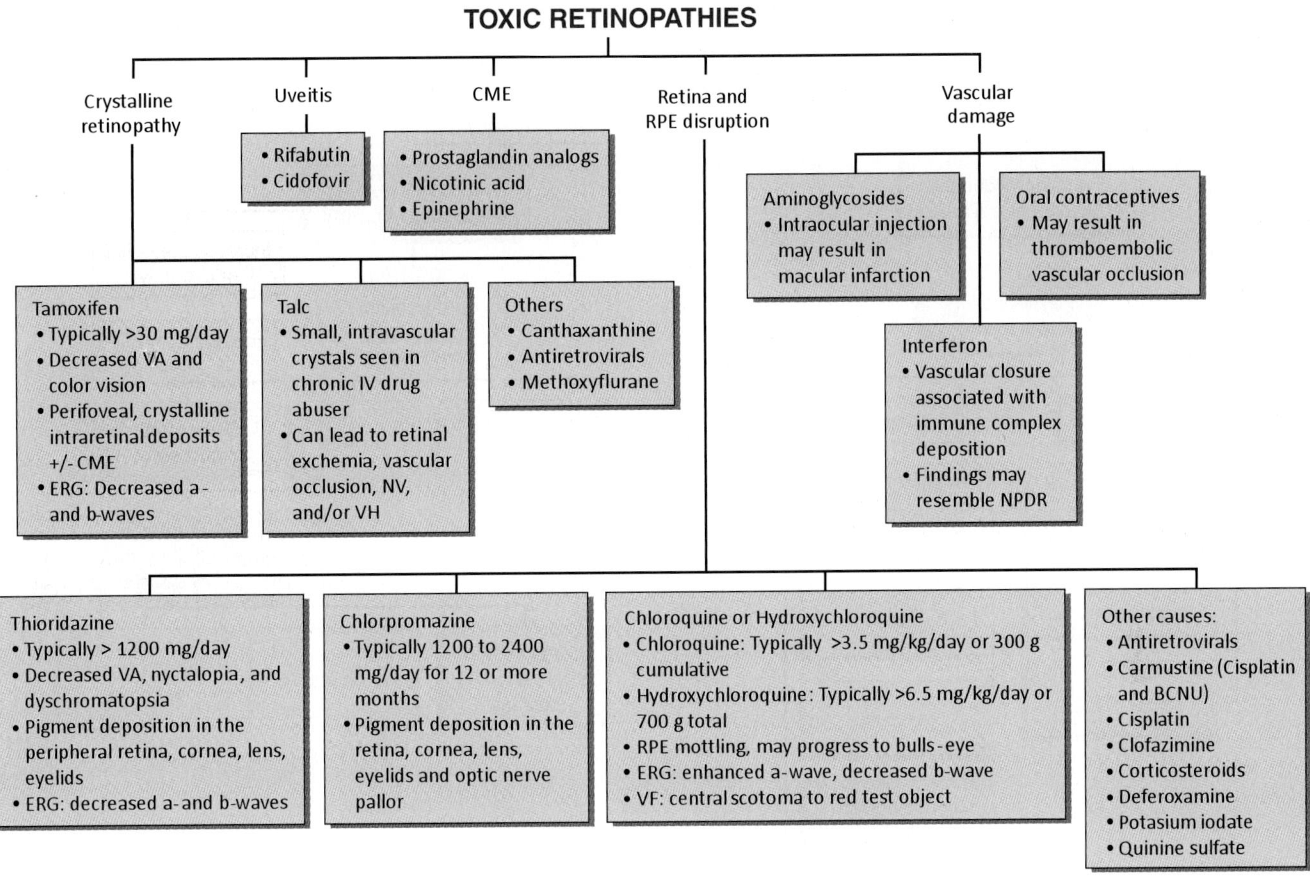
TOXIC RETINOPATHIES
Crystalline retinopathy
Uveitis
CME
Retina and RPE disruption
Vascular damage
• Rifabutin
• Cidofovir
• Prostaglandin analogs
• Nicotinic acid
• Epinephrine
Aminoglycosides
• Intraocular injection may result in macular infarction
Oral contraceptives
• May result in thromboembolic vascular occlusion
Tamoxifen
• Typically >30 mg/day
• Decreased VA and color vision
• Perifoveal, crystalline intraretinal deposits +/- CME
• ERG: Decreased a- and b-waves
Talc
• Small, intravascular crystals seen in chronic IV drug abuser
• Can lead to retinal exchemia, vascular occlusion, NV, and/or VH
Others
• Canthaxanthine
• Antiretrovirals
• Methoxyflurane
Interferon
• Vascular closure associated with immune complex deposition
• Findings may resemble NPDR
Thioridazine
• Typically > 1200 mg/day
• Decreased VA, nyctalopia, and dyschromatopsia
• Pigment deposition in the peripheral retina, cornea, lens, eyelids
• ERG: decreased a-and b-waves
Chlorpromazine
• Typically 1200 to 2400 mg/day for 12 or more months
• Pigment deposition in the retina, cornea, lens, eyelids and optic nerve pallor
Chloroquine or Hydroxychloroquine
• Chloroquine: Typically >3.5 mg/kg/day or 300 g cumulative
• Hydroxychloroquine: Typically >6.5 mg/kg/day or 700 g total
• RPE mottling, may progress to bulls-eye
• ERG: enhanced a-wave, decreased b-wave
• VF: central scotoma to red test object
Other causes:
• Antiretrovirals
• Carmustine (Cisplatin and BCNU)
• Cisplatin
• Clofazimine
• Corticosteroids
• Deferoxamine
• Potasium iodate
• Quinine sulfate

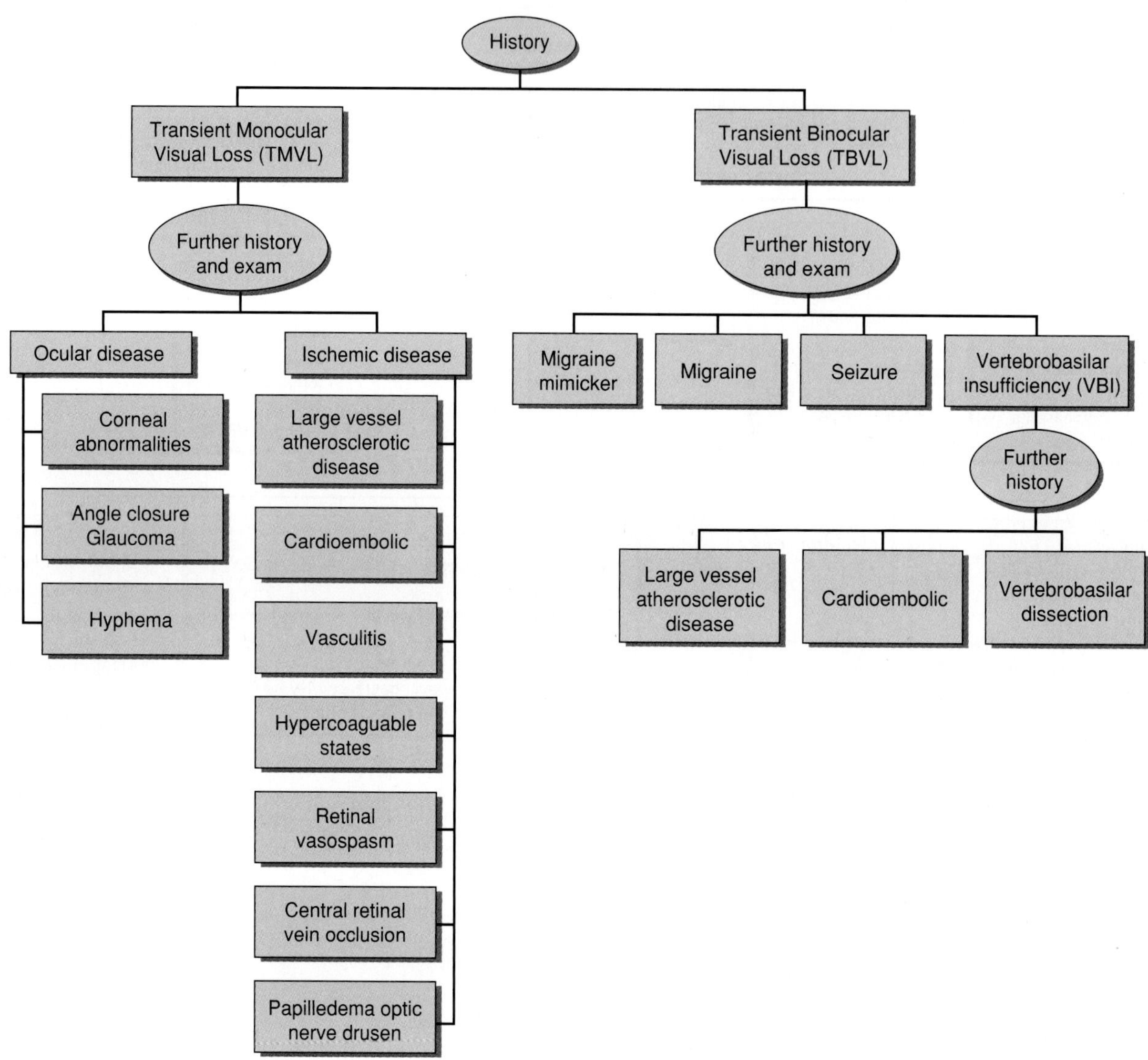

Mary Ellen P. Collum

VASCULITIS

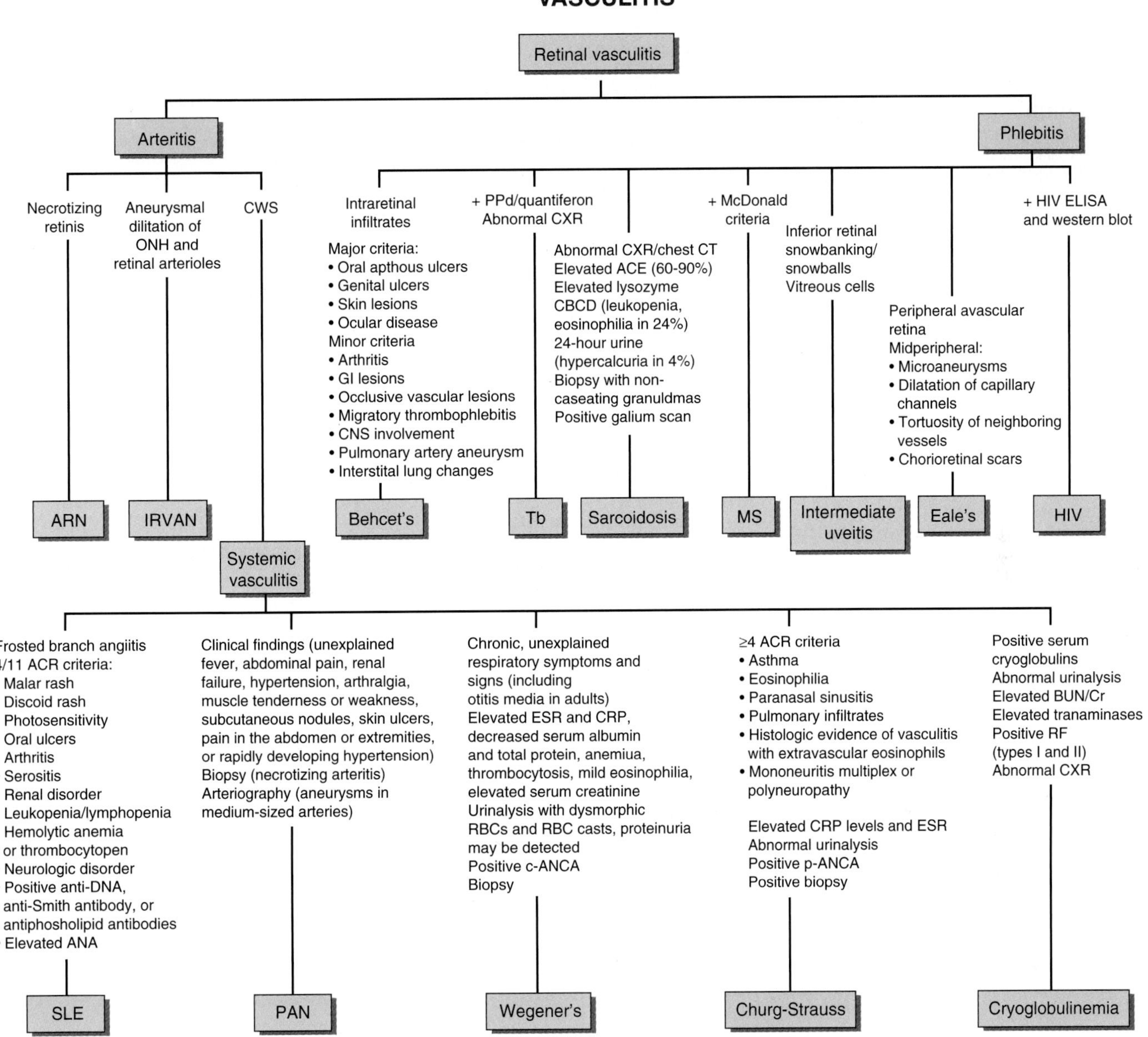

Nikolas London

ABDUCENS/CRANIAL NERVE VI PALSY SIXTH (VI) NERVE PALSY

William A. Cantore

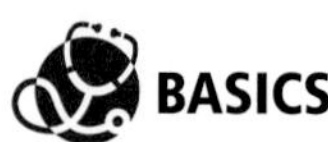

BASICS

DESCRIPTION

- The abducens (VI) nerve (CN VI) innervates the ipsilateral lateral rectus (LR) muscle, abducting the eye. CN VI palsy is the most common isolated cranial nerve palsy. Patients present with binocular horizontal diplopia and esotropia. Children may not complain of diplopia.
- In adults aged over 50 years, CN VI palsies are most often due to microvascular ischemic peripheral nerve injury. In children, CN VI palsies are particularly alarming because of the frequent association with brain tumors.
- The CN VI nucleus is located in the dorsal lower pons. The nuclear complex contains motor neurons to the ipsilateral lateral rectus (LR) muscle and interneurons that project, by the medial longitudinal fasciculus (MLF), to the medial rectus (MR) subnucleus of the contralateral CN III nuclear complex. Therefore, a nuclear lesion will produce an ipsilateral gaze palsy and not a CN VI palsy. The fascicles exit at the pontomedullary junction and the nerve runs along the clivus and travels over the petrous apex of the temporal bone, where it is tethered at the petroclinoid ligament in Dorello's canal. The nerve courses within the cavernous sinus lateral to the internal carotid artery and enters the orbit through the superior orbital fissure.

EPIDEMIOLOGY

- CN VI palsy can occur in all ages; etiology varies depending on age group
- No racial or sex predilection

Incidence

- 11 per 100,000
- Peak incidence in seventh decade

RISK FACTORS

- Diabetes
  - Only independent risk factor linked to ischemic palsies
- Hypertension
- Hyperlipidemia
- Obesity
- Trauma
- Alcohol abuse
  - Wernicke-Korsakoff syndrome is the best known neurologic complication of thiamine (vitamin B1) deficiency.

PATHOPHYSIOLOGY

- Nucleus:
  - A CN VI palsy does not occur with nuclear lesions.
- Fascicle in pons:
  - Demyelinating
  - Infarction
  - Neoplasm
- Nerve root in cerebellopontine angle:
  - Neoplasm (acoustic neuroma)
- Subarachnoid space:
  - Aneurysm
  - Meningitis
  - Inflammation
  - Infection
  - Neoplasm
- Petrous ridge:
  - Recurrent otitis media
  - Nasopharyngeal carcinoma
  - Chondrosarcoma
- Cavernous sinus:
  - Cavernous sinus fistula, thrombosis
  - Neoplasm
  - Internal carotid artery aneurysm, dissection
- Orbital apex:
  - Optic neuropathy
- Orbit:
  - Neoplasm
  - Inflammation
  - Infection

ETIOLOGY

- Ischemic
  - Diabetes
  - Hypertension
    - questionable independent risk factor
- Compressive
- Inflammatory
- Traumatic
  - Unilateral or bilateral
- Intracranial hypertension
  - Unilateral or bilateral
- Intracranial hypotension
  - Post dural puncture, CSF leak
- Multiple sclerosis

Pediatric Considerations

- Congenital
  - Isolated congenital absence of abduction extremely rare
    - Transient CN VI palsy may occur due to birth trauma.
  - **Möbius** syndrome
    - Facial diplegia associated with horizontal gaze abnormalities
    - Etiologies include maldevelopment and intrauterine insults.
  - Duane's retraction syndrome
    - Unilateral or bilateral abduction deficits, variable adduction abnormalities, palpebral fissure narrowing and globe retraction on attempted adduction
    - Congenital absence of 6N neurons with aberrant innervation of LR by branches of CN III
- Most common causes of CN VI palsies in children are tumors (45%), trauma, increased intracranial pressure (ICP).
  - May be post-viral when isolated

COMMONLY ASSOCIATED CONDITIONS

- Nucleus:
  - Conjugate horizontal gaze palsy
- Fascicle in pons:
  - Ipsilateral CN V palsy
  - Ipsilateral CN VII palsy
  - Ipsilateral Horner's syndrome
  - Contralateral hemiparesis (Raymond's syndrome)
- Nerve root in cerebellopontine angle:
  - Ipsilateral deafness or tinnitus
- Petrous ridge:
  - Severe facial and eye pain (Gradenigo's syndrome)
  - Occasionally facial paralysis
- Cavernous sinus:
  - CN III, IV, or V palsy
  - Ipsilateral Horner's syndrome
- Orbital apex:
  - Optic neuropathy
- Orbit:
  - Proptosis
  - Chemosis
  - Lid swelling

DIAGNOSIS

HISTORY

- Abrupt onset when microvascular ischemic
- Purely horizontal diplopia
  - Binocular
  - Worse at distance
  - Worse in direction of action of the paretic LR
- Inquire about headache, pain, hearing loss, trauma, symptoms of giant cell arteritis (GCA)

PHYSICAL EXAM

- Patients may present with a head turn.
- Ipsilateral abduction deficit
- Incomitant esotropia, worse in direction of weak LR
- Exophthalmometry and orbit examination
- Forced duction test
- Assess orbicularis oculi strength to look for myasthenia gravis (MG)

ALERT
- Critical to evaluate function of other cranial nerves
- Look for papilledema

DIAGNOSTIC TESTS & INTERPRETATION

Lab

Initial lab tests

- HbA1c
- ESR, CRP (for GCA)
- Anti-AChR antibodies (for MG)

Imaging

Initial approach

- Insufficient CN VI palsy evidence to support MRI of all patients with 6NP
- Nonisolated
  - Brainstem signs
    - MRI
  - Meningeal signs
    - MRI, LP
  - Orbital signs
    - CT or MRI
  - Elevated ICP signs
    - MRI, MRV, LP
- Isolated
  - Age <15 years
    - Observation, if occurs after viral illness or vaccination
    - Otherwise, MRI
  - Age <50 years
    - MRI
    - LP
  - Age >50 years

MRI if no improvement in 3 months or no identifiable risk factors for microvascular disease (1)

- Bilateral
  - MRI
  - LP

Diagnostic Procedures/Other

- LP
  - Meningeal signs present
  - Elevated ICP signs present

DIFFERENTIAL DIAGNOSIS

- MG
- Thyroid ophthalmopathy
- Medial orbital wall or floor fracture
- Duane's retraction syndrome
  - Patients not diplopic
- Spasm of near reflex

TREATMENT

Most importantly, identify and treat underlying condition if present

MEDICATION

First Line

- Aspirin
  - No scientific data demonstrates reduction in risk of ischemic CN VI palsy

ADDITIONAL TREATMENT

General Measures

- Monocular occlusion
  - Sector occlusion of eyeglass lens with translucent tape may be preferred
  - Alternate patch in children, not necessary in adults
- Fresnel prisms

Issues for Referral

Muscle surgery considered after 6–12 months of stability

Additional Therapies

- Botulinum toxin
  - Inject ipsilateral MR muscle
  - Transient improvement of diplopia
  - No established improvement in recovery rate

SURGERY/OTHER PROCEDURES

- Resection of LR muscle and recession of MR muscle
  - Transposition of vertical rectus muscles may be necessary if no LR function at all
  - 6–12 months of stable measurements

ONGOING CARE

FOLLOW-UP RECOMMENDATIONS

- Patients aged >50 years with microvascular risk factors managed by close observation should have MRI if no improvement in 3 months.
- CN VI palsy that worsens after 2 weeks or becomes associated with a new neurologic finding should have MRI.

Patient Monitoring

In a patient aged >50 years with vasculopathic risk factors in whom microvascular ischemic CN VI palsy is diagnosed, reevaluation in 2 weeks

PROGNOSIS

- Ischemic CN6 lesions usually resolve within 3–4 months.
  - Angle of ocular deviation on presentation may predict recovery (2).
  - In vasculopathic CNVI palsies, 86% completely resolve (3)
- Children with isolated CN VI palsies usually recover within 4 months
- Spontaneous improvement of traumatic CN VI palsies in 30–50%
  - Complete recovery <25%

REFERENCES

1. Chi SL, Bhatti MT. The diagnostic dilemma of neuro-imaging in acute isolated sixth nerve palsy. *Curr Opin Ophthalmol* 2009;20(6):423–429.
2. Park UC, Kim SJ, Hwang JM, et al. Clinical features and natural history of acquired third, fourth, and sixth cranial nerve palsy. *Eye (Lond)* 2008;22(5): 691–696.
3. Sanders SK, Kawasaki A, Purvin VA. Long-term prognosis in patients with vasculopathic sixth nerve palsy. *Am J Ophthalmol* 2002;134(1):81–84.

ADDITIONAL READING

- Brazis PW. Isolated palsies of cranial nerves III, IV, and VI. *Semin Neurol*. Feb 2009;29(1):14–28.

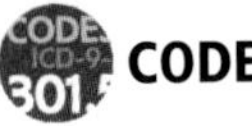

CODES

ICD9

378.54 Sixth or abducens nerve palsy

CLINICAL PEARLS

- Not all abduction deficits are CN VI palsies.
- Because of its location within the substance of cavernous sinus (free from the dural lateral wall), typically first cranial nerve involved by a process there
- When associated with an ipsilateral Horner's syndrome and no other neurological finding, careful investigation of the cavernous sinus is mandatory.
- Bilateral CN VI palsies is not due to ischemia.
- GCA may present as a CN VI palsy.
- Look for papilledema in every CN VI palsy.

ACHROMATOPSIA

Eliza S. Stroh
Alex V. Levin

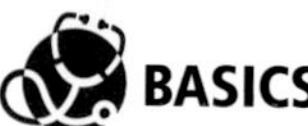

BASICS

DESCRIPTION

- Reduced or absent color discrimination with photophobia, reduced visual acuity, nystagmus, eccentric fixation, and small central scotoma all due to defective cone development
- May be divided into partial (incomplete) versus complete phenotypes

EPIDEMIOLOGY

Incidence

1 per 30,000 individuals (1)[C]

RISK FACTORS

- Consanguineous parents
- Family history

Genetics

- Autosomal recessive inheritance
- ACHM1, gene unknown, chromosome, 14
- ACHM2, alpha subunit cone cGMP gated cation channel (CNGA3), 2q11
- ACHM3 (Pingelap variant), beta subunit cone cGMP gated cation channel (CNGB3), 8q21–22
- ACHM4 cone alpha subunit transducin (GNAT2),1p13

GENERAL PREVENTION

Genetic counseling

PATHOPHYSIOLOGY

Reduced or absent protein expression in cone photoreceptors leads to inhibition of the normal phototransduction cascade and dysfunctional cone development (2)[B]

ETIOLOGY

Mutated gene inherited from each parent

COMMONLY ASSOCIATED CONDITIONS

- None
- Phenotypic heterogeneity includes cone dystrophy and cone-rod dystrophy

DIAGNOSIS

HISTORY

- Family history
  - Typically presents in infancy as fine nystagmus with photophobia
  - Stationary low visual acuity with poor color discrimination
  - Children often referred to as "night owls" due to preference for night time activity and dim illumination

PHYSICAL EXAM

- Full ocular examination
  - Nystagmus is fine, high frequency, often milder with age
  - Assess visual function; best-corrected is typically 20/200 range
  - Hyperopia may be present
  - Photophobia on examination
  - Minimal if any foveal hypoplasia or subtle pigmentary changes, most often normal appearance
  - Fail color vision testing

DIAGNOSTIC TESTS & INTERPRETATION

Lab

Molecular genetic testing available

Imaging

If nystagmus or presentation atypical, consider neuroimaging to rule out intracranial process

Diagnostic Procedures/Other

- Color vision tests show impaired color discrimination along protan, deutan, and tritan axes.
- Full-field ERG shows absent or severely diminished photopic response and typically normal scotopic response.
- Visual field testing may reveal small central scotoma.
- If able, OCT usually normal or shows macular thinning
- If able, multifocal ERG usually isoelectric
- Intravenous fluorescein angiography and fundus autofluorescence normal

Pathological Findings

- Reduced cone number
- Residual cones often abnormal in structure

DIFFERENTIAL DIAGNOSIS

- Incomplete achromatopsia is associated with partial cone function, resulting in some color discrimination, better visual acuity than in complete achromatopsia, and absence of photophobia.
  - Blue-cone monochromatism (X-linked achromatopsia) has similar findings to achromatopsia and can be differentiated by Berson plates or by S-cone function on ERG (4)[C].
  - Cone monochromatism, in which the L- or M-cones are functional.
  - Cone dystrophy is typically associated with normal cone function at birth, with gradual deterioration and progression.
  - Cone-rod dystrophy includes progressive rod dysfunction.
  - Other causes of photophobia and nystagmus
  - Foveal/macular hypoplasia (see chapter)
  - Cerebral achromatopsia is associated with febrile illness or trauma.

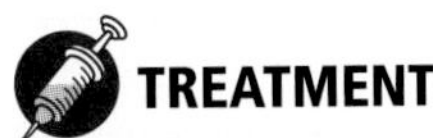

TREATMENT

MEDICATION
None

ADDITIONAL TREATMENT
General Measures
- Dark or Corning filter sunglasses or red-tinted contact lenses (often not tolerated for abnormal appearance) reduce photophobia.
  - Low vision aids
  - Children may benefit from an Individualized Education Plan.

Issues for Referral
- Genetic counseling
  - Low vision evaluation and support as indicated

Additional Therapies
Correction of refractive error

COMPLEMENTARY & ALTERNATIVE THERAPIES
None proven or indicated

SURGERY/OTHER PROCEDURES
None

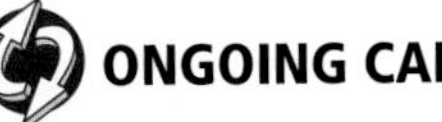

ONGOING CARE

FOLLOW-UP RECOMMENDATIONS
Children should have an ophthalmic evaluation every 6–12 months to monitor refraction and function

PATIENT EDUCATION
- Genetic counseling
- http://www.dailystrength.org/c/Achromatopsia/support-group
- http://www.lowvision.org/achromatopsia_and_color_blindnes.htm
- http://www.achromat.org/

PROGNOSIS
- Visual acuity is usually stable over time on later decades when slow degeneration may occur with natural age related loss of photoreceptors.
  - Nystagmus and photophobia may improve slightly with age.

COMPLICATIONS
- Low vision
  - Photophobia

REFERENCES

1. Rojas CV, Maria LS, Santos JL, et al. A frameshift insertion in the cone cyclic nucleotide gated cation channel causes complete achromatopsia in a consanguineous family from a rural isolate. *Eur J Hum Genet* 2002;10:638–42.
2. Wissinger B, Gamer D, Jagle H, et al. CNGA3 mutations in hereditary cone photoreceptor disorders. *Am J Hum Genet* 2001;69:722–37.
3. Varsanyi B, Wissinger B, Kohl S, et al. Clinical and genetic features of Hungarian achromatopsia patients. *Mol Vis* 2005;11:996–1001.
4. Moskowitz A, Hansen RM, Akula JD, et al. Rod and rod-driven function in achromatopsia and blue cone monochromatism. *Invest Ophthalmol Vis Sci* 2009;50(2):950–8.

ADDITIONAL READING

- http://www.ncbi.nlm.nih.gov/bookshelf/br.fcgi?book=gene&part=achm.

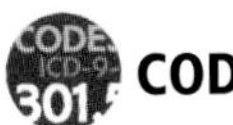

CODES

ICD9
368.54 Achromatopsia

CLINICAL PEARLS

- Consider achromatopsia diagnosis in children with photophobia and nystagmus.
- Color vision may appear remarkably good if patients learn object associations or shades; formal testing is indicated.
- Consider genetic testing and counseling.

ACNE ROSACEA

Swathi Reddy

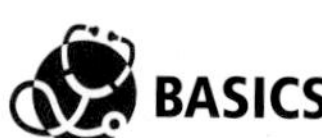

BASICS

DESCRIPTION
Acne rosacea is a chronic acneiform disorder affecting the nose, chin, forehead, or eyelids.

EPIDEMIOLOGY
Prevalence
Affects approximately 1 in 20 Americans.

RISK FACTORS
- Age (usually occurs between the ages of 30–60 years)
- Equal sex distribution
- Suggestion that there is increased prevalence in fair-skinned persons of European or Celtic descent, although not well-substantiated
- Dark pigmentation in black populations may mask presentation.

Genetics
No gene identified as causing rosacea, but tends to run in families.

GENERAL PREVENTION
Rosacea cannot be prevented, although several factors may trigger flare-ups including sun, wind, hot, cold, exercise, stress, and certain foods.

PATHOPHYSIOLOGY
Anomalous vascular response.

ETIOLOGY
- Poorly understood, although infectious, climactic, neurologic, and immunologic factors have been implicated.
- Vasodilation may cause extravasation of plasma, which can induce an inflammatory response.
- *Demodex folliculorum* has also been implicated, but this is largely circumstantial.

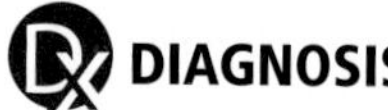

DIAGNOSIS

HISTORY
- Family history
- Symptoms including flushing, persistent erythema, papules, pustules, burning or stinging of the skin, and dryness

PHYSICAL EXAM
- Skin involvement (nose, cheeks, chin, central forehead, neck, and chest)
  - Diffuse erythema
  - Telangiectasias
  - Papules
  - Pustules
  - Hypertrophy of sebaceous glands
  - Rhinophyma (thickening and purplish discoloration of nose skin)
- Ophthalmologic
  - Blepharoconjunctivitis
    - Inspissation of meibomian glands
    - Telangiectasias of lid margin
    - Recurrent hordeolum and chalazion
    - Conjunctival hyperemia and congestion
    - Follicular reaction
    - Papillary hypertrophy
- Corneal (usually involves inferior cornea)
  - Punctuate epithelial keratitis
  - Corneal vascularization
  - Corneal infiltration
  - Corneal ulceration
  - Corneal perforation
- Reports of involvement of episclera, sclera, and iritis, although not widely reported

DIAGNOSTIC TESTS & INTERPRETATION
Lab
No lab testing required

Diagnostic Procedures/Other
Diagnosis is clinical

Pathological Findings
- Vascular dilatation of small vessels
- Perivascular infiltration of histiocytes, plasma cells, and lymphocytes
- Infiltration of conjunctiva and cornea by lymphocytes, epithelioid cells, giant, and plasma cells
- Loss of superficial dermal connective tissues
  - Edema
  - Collagen disruption
  - Elastosis
- Rhinophyma shows increase in sebaceous glands and connective tissue
- Skin biopsies show deposition of complement and immunoglobulin at dermal–epidermal junction

DIFFERENTIAL DIAGNOSIS
- Acne vulgaris
- Lupus erythematosus
- Dermatitis
- Erysipelas
- Seborrheic dermatitis
- Carcinoid syndrome
- Tuberculosis
- Syphilis

TREATMENT

MEDICATION

First Line

- Oral tetracycline (250 mg every 6 hours for 3–4 weeks, with tapering)
- Doxycycline or minocycline (50–100 mg every 12 hours)

Second Line

- Oral erythromycin
- Oral isotretinoin
- Ampicillin
- Metronidazole
- Topical metronidazole (0.75% gel twice daily)
- Azelaic Acid
- Sodium sulfacetamide lotion
- Intensive lid hygiene
- Bacteriostatic ointment at bedtime
- Topical corticosteroids (short-term)
- Electrocautery for telangiectasias

Pediatric Considerations

- Tetracycline not for use in children <8 years old

Pregnancy Considerations

- Tetracycline should not be used during pregnancy
- Isotretinoin is teratogenic and contraindicated during pregnancy – women of childbearing age should be placed on oral contraceptives when warranted

ADDITIONAL TREATMENT

General Measures

- Avoidance of sun exposure
- Daily sunscreen use
- Use of mild soaps
- Avoidance of oil-based cosmetics

Issues for Referral

- Severe ocular involvement (corneal infiltration/ulceration, recurrent chalazia)
- Rhinophyma refractory to standard treatments

COMPLEMENTARY & ALTERNATIVE THERAPIES

- Topical niacinamide
- B vitamins
- Elimination and challenge diet

SURGERY/OTHER PROCEDURES

- Conjunctival flaps, tectonic lamellar keratoplasty, penetrating keratoplasty
- Laser, intense pulse light, photodynamic therapy
- Electrosurgery, surgical steel resculpturing, dermabrasion, or carbon dioxide laser treatment for rhinophyma

ONGOING CARE

FOLLOW-UP RECOMMENDATIONS

- Ophthalmology
- Dermatology

Patient Monitoring

Close ophthalmologic monitoring for corneal thinning, ulceration, infiltration, or perforation

DIET

Limit spicy foods, alcohol, and hot beverages.

PATIENT EDUCATION

The National Rosacea Society (http://www.rosacea.org)

PROGNOSIS

Good prognosis for controlling symptoms, although rosacea is a chronic condition.

ADDITIONAL READING

- van Zuuren EJ, Gupta AK, Gover MD, et al. Systematic review of rosacea treatments. *J Am Acad Dermatol* 2007;56:107.
- Crawford GH, Pelle MT, James WD. Rosacea: I. Etiology, pathogenesis, and subtype classification. *J Am Acad Dermatol* 2004;51:327.
- Webster GF. Rosacea. *Med Clin N Am* 2009;93:1183–1194.

CODES

ICD9

- 372.20 Blepharoconjunctivitis, unspecified
- 374.89 Other disorders of eyelid
- 695.3 Rosacea

CLINICAL PEARLS

- Rosacea may cause chronic ocular symptoms
- History of recurrent hordeolum or chalazion may represent ocular rosacea
- Mainstay of treatment remains topical and oral antibiotics

ACUTE ANTERIOR UVEITIS

Vikram J. Setlur

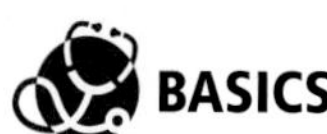

BASICS

DESCRIPTION

Acute anterior uveitis (AAU) involves inflammation of the iris alone (iritis) or iris and ciliary body together (iridocyclitis) of abrupt onset (lasting days to weeks) and limited duration (<3 months).

EPIDEMIOLOGY

Incidence

- 17 cases per 100,000 people in developed countries
- Varying incidence in the general populations depending on the population and country of residence

Prevalence

38 cases per 100,000 people in developed countries

RISK FACTORS

Genetics

HLA-B27 phenotype is a risk factor, seen in 50% of acute anterior uveitis patients in a Caucasian population.

PATHOPHYSIOLOGY

Intraocular inflammation of the iris or iris and ciliary body usually causes pain, redness, blurred vision, and photophobia.

ETIOLOGY

Numerous etiologies can trigger acute anterior uveitis, including: Infections, autoimmune diseases, trauma, surgery, medications, and lens-related disorders. Approximately one-third to half of the cases are idiopathic.

COMMONLY ASSOCIATED CONDITIONS

A number of systemic diseases can be associated with acute anterior uveitis, including HLA-27 associated diseases (Ankylosing spondylitis, inflammatory bowel disease, reactive arthritis, psoriatic arthritis), sarcoidosis, syphilis, Lyme disease, HIV, tuberculosis, collagen vascular diseases, and juvenile idiopathic arthritis.

DIAGNOSIS

HISTORY

- Classic symptoms are pain, redness, photophobia, and blurred vision.
- Detailed review of symptoms and past medical history should be taken with special attention to rheumatologic, dermatologic, gastrointestinal, and autoimmune diseases. Infectious exposures, sexual history, medication usage, and family history (with attention to rheumatologic and inflammatory diseases) should also be included. Ocular history is critical to assess onset and progression of symptoms, history of prior episodes, and success of prior treatments.

PHYSICAL EXAM

- Ciliary flush (perilimbal dilated episcleral vessels are caused by increased blood flow to the ciliary body) is often present.
- Pupillary miosis may be seen.
- Keratic precipitates (KPs) on the corneal endothelium may be fine (non-granulomatous KP) or large and have a "mutton fat" appearance (granulomatous KP).
- Anterior chamber exam may show cell, flare, and rarely, hypopyon (HLA-B27-related and Behçet disease in particular). Iris nodules may be present at the pupillary margin or iris stroma.
- Iris ischemia can cause iris stromal atrophy and may indicate previous episodes.
- Posterior synechiae, which are adhesions between the posterior iris and anterior lens capsule, may be seen. Gonioscopy can reveal peripheral anterior synechiae.
- The intraocular pressure may be high or low.
  - Dilated fundus examination should be performed to look for vitreitis, snowballs, snow banks, optic disc edema and hyperemia, vessel sheathing, perivascular exudates, retinitis, and choroidal infiltrates. Though cystoid macular edema and optic disc edema may be seen in acute anterior uveitis, other posterior segment involvement constitutes panuveitis and changes the differential diagnosis.

DIAGNOSTIC TESTS & INTERPRETATION

Lab

- To evaluate patients for an underlying systemic disease, lab testing is performed for acute anterior uveitis that is one of the following: Severe, recurrent, granulomatous, or bilateral
  - History and examination should guide the selection of lab tests, which may initially include CBC, ESR, PPD, FTA-ABS and VDRL, Lyme antibodies, HLA-B27, ANA, ACE, and HIV testing. Numerous other tests can be helpful as the clinical picture dictates.

Imaging

- Chest x-ray is done to look for pulmonary signs of tuberculosis or sarcoidosis.
  - In cases of suspected sarcoidosis, chest computed tomography (CT) scan has higher sensitivity and specificity than chest x-ray.

DIFFERENTIAL DIAGNOSIS

- The causes of AAU is broad, but the most common causes are:
- Idiopathic (approximately half of all cases of AAU)
- HLA-B27 associated uveitis (ocular disease alone or associated with a systemic syndrome such as reactive arthritis, psoriatic arthritis, ankylosing spondylitis, or inflammatory bowel disease)
- Infectious causes (viral [HSV, VZV, CMV, HIV], bacterial [syphilis, TB, Lyme], fungal, and parasitic)
- Sarcoidosis
- Behçet's disease
- Systemic lupus erythematosus
- Juvenile idiopathic arthritis-related uveitis
- Trauma-related iritis
- Lens-induced uveitis
- Fuchs heterochromic iridocyclitis
- Posner-Schlossman syndrome
- Leukemia, lymphoma (masquerade syndromes)
- Idiopathic

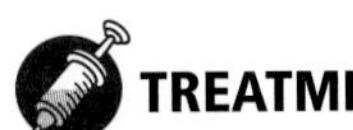

TREATMENT

MEDICATION

First Line

- Corticosteroids are the drug of choice and are dosed based on disease severity
- Topical corticosteroids are easily administered with the least side effects (e.g., prednisolone 1% or Durezol (difluprednate), 1 gtt q1–6 h
- Periocular and/or systemic corticosteroids are indicated for disease unresponsive to topical medication
- Mydriatics/cycloplegics are added to relieve ciliary muscle spasm, prevent posterior synechiae, and help stabilize the blood-aqueous barrier (e.g., cyclopentolate 0.5–2% 1 gtt t.i.d, or atropine 1% or homatropine b.i.d.)

Second Line

- Immunosuppressive agents (e.g., methotrexate, azathioprine, mycophenolate mofetil, cyclosporine, tacrolimus) and biologics (infliximab, adalimumab) are used in corticosteroid-resistant cases or as steroid-sparing agents.
  - The fluocinolone implant (Retisert) or dexamethasone implant (Ozurdex) may be very helpful, but may be associated with an increased rate of cataract or ocular hypertension.

ADDITIONAL TREATMENT

Issues for Referral

Immunosuppressive agents are started in conjunction with an internist/rheumatologist, or uveitis specialist.

Additional Therapies

Elevated intraocular pressure can be treated with topical beta blockers, carbonic anhydrase inhibitors, alpha agonists, or hyperosmolar agents. Prostaglandins should be avoided as they may be proinflammatory. Topical NSAIDs can be used to treat cystoids macular edema.

SURGERY/OTHER PROCEDURES

- Cataract extraction may be done in an eye that is quiet for at least 3 months prior to surgery.
- Glaucoma surgery may be needed for intraocular pressures not responsive to topical therapy.
- Pre- and postoperative systemic and topical steroids are given in the perioperative period to prevent recurrence of inflammation.

IN-PATIENT CONSIDERATIONS

Admission Criteria

Patients with severe vision or life-threatening disease may need to be admitted to provide aggressive immunosuppressive therapy.

ONGOING CARE

FOLLOW-UP RECOMMENDATIONS

Patients require close monitoring until the inflammation is controlled. Then, frequency of medication and follow-up visits may slowly be reduced.

Patient Monitoring

- Patients require measurement of visual acuity and intraocular inflammation at each visit.
- Careful grading of cell and flare at initial and follow-up visits can be used to assess response to treatment.

COMPLICATIONS

Cataract formation may be caused by inflammation and corticosteroids. Glaucoma may be caused by trabeculitis, peripheral anterior synechiae, and iris neovascularization. Hypotony can result from ciliary body shutdown or cyclitic membranes. Cystoid macular edema may also occur.

ADDITIONAL READING

- Agrawal RV, Murthy S, Sangwan V, et al. *Indian J Ophthalmol* 2010;58(1):11–19.
- Weinberg RS. Anterior Uveitis. *Ophthalol Clin N Amer* 1993;6(1):23–28.
- Rothova A, van Veenendaal WG, Linssen A, et al. Clinical feature of acute anterior uveitis. *Amer J Ophthalmol* 1987;103:137–145.
- Pavesio CE, Nozik RA. Anterior and intermediate uveitis. *Int Ophthalmol Clin* 1990;30(4):244–251.

CODES

ICD9

- 364.00 Acute and subacute iridocyclitis, unspecified
- 364.3 Unspecified iridocyclitis

CLINICAL PEARLS

- Classic findings are abrupt onset of pain, redness, blurred vision, and photophobia accompanied by cell and flare in the anterior chamber.
- Targeted work-up can reveal an underlying systemic condition.
- Topical, periocular, and systemic corticosteroids, as well as steroid-sparing agents, are used as needed to control all intraocular inflammation whenever possible.

ACUTE PRIMARY ANGLE-CLOSURE GLAUCOMA

Shelly R. Gupta
Robert J. Goulet III
Kathryn B. Freidl
L. Jay Katz

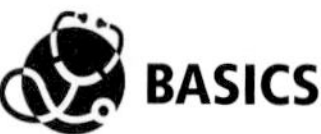

BASICS

DESCRIPTION
- Angle closure is defined by apposition of the iris against the trabecular meshwork. In acute primary angle closure, the intraocular pressure (IOP) rises rapidly due to a sudden increase in trabecular meshwork obstruction by the iris. Glaucomatous optic neuropathy can result from this event (acute primary angle-closure glaucoma).
- The most common cause is pupillary block.

EPIDEMIOLOGY
Incidence
- Primary angle closure incidence ranges from 4.7–15.5/100,000 people/year.
- Inuit > Asians > India/Thai/Malay > Europeans > African/Hispanic
- The fellow eye of a patient suffering an acute attack has a 40–80% chance of developing an acute attack within 5–10 years.

Prevalence
- Prevalence of angle-closure glaucoma in the US is 0.2%.
- Acute angle closure is rare, relative to chronic angle closure.

RISK FACTORS
- Older age
- Female gender
- Race (see above)
- Hyperopia/shorter axial length/shallow
- anterior chamber
- Thick crystalline lens
- Family history

GENERAL PREVENTION
- Screening gonioscopy is necessary to identify patients at risk of having occludable angles.
- Provocative tests (stimulation of mydriasis), have not been shown to be accurately predictive of eyes at risk for acute angle closure.
- Peripheral iridotomy in eyes determined to have anatomically narrow angles can prevent acute attacks and resultant vision loss.

PATHOPHYSIOLOGY
- Physical obstruction of the trabecular meshwork by the iris leads to decreased aqueous drainage and acute elevation of intraocular pressure. The following mechanisms can occur independently or in various combinations.
  - Pupillary block: Iridolenticular touch causes resistance of aqueous flow from the posterior chamber to the anterior chamber. Elevated posterior chamber pressure causes the iris to bow forward and occlude the trabecular meshwork.
  - Phacomorphic: Age-associated lens enlargement or lens dislocation can lead to pupillary block or anterior displacement of the iris. This is traditionally thought of as a secondary angle-closure mechanism but can contribute to primary angle closure.
  - Plateau Iris: Anteriorly displaced ciliary processes push the peripheral iris forward resulting in narrowing of the anterior chamber angle.

ETIOLOGY
- Not all eyes with narrow angles develop angle closure.
  - In normal eyes, there appears to be a decrease in iris volume with mydriasis; it has been proposed that eyes prone to acute angle closure may experience an increase in iris volume with mydriasis.
  - Additionally, eyes prone to angle closure may inadequately regulate choroidal thickness.
    - Clinically imperceptible changes in choroidal thickness may increase intraocular pressure, rotate the ciliary body–iris complex forward, and increase resistance at the iris–lens interface.

COMMONLY ASSOCIATED CONDITIONS
- Small anterior segment (Hyperopia, Nanophthalmos, Microphthalmos)
- Retinal vascular occlusion (as a result of elevated IOP)
- Ischemic optic neuropathy (as a result of elevated IOP)

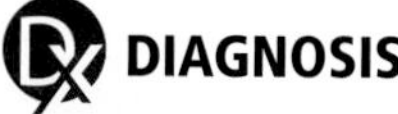

DIAGNOSIS

HISTORY
- Presenting complaints include ocular pain, headache, blurred vision, halos around lights, nausea, and vomiting.
- Prior episodes of headache with blurred vision may signify previous angle-closure events.
- Ophthalmic and medical history should focus on contributory factors:
  - Recent pharmacologic dilation
  - Use of medicines with anticholinergic effects
    - antihistamines, tricyclic antidepressants, MAO inhibitors
  - Causes of ciliary body edema
    - Panretinal photocoagulation
    - Scleral buckle
    - Medications such as sulfonamides and topiramate

PHYSICAL EXAM
- Decreased visual acuity
- Mid-dilated pupil
- Relative afferent pupillary defect (RAPD)
- Elevated intraocular pressure
- Conjunctival injection
- Microcystic corneal edema
- Shallow anterior chamber with mild cell and flare
- Optic nerve swelling and hyperemia
- Retinal arterial pulsations
- Gonioscopy: Closed angle (perform indentation gonioscopy to differentiate between appositional and synechial angle closure)
- Signs of previous acute attack:
  - Lower corneal endothelial cell count compared to the unaffected fellow eye
  - Peripheral anterior synechiae (PAS)
  - Anterior subcapsular lens opacities (glaukomflecken) secondary to ischemia
  - Segmental iris atrophy with pigment release from focal iris stromal necrosis
  - Dilated, irregular pupil from iris ischemia

DIAGNOSTIC TESTS & INTERPRETATION
Imaging
Initial approach
- The diagnosis is made on clinical examination.
- Imaging of the anterior segment is useful in the setting of a patent peripheral iridotomy to delineate causes of non-pupillary block angle closure. One may use:
  - Ultrasound biomicroscopy
  - Optical coherence tomography

Follow-up & special considerations
- It is essential to evaluate the angle of the fellow eye. Iridotomy should be done in the fellow eye as soon as possible due to high risk of subsequent angle closure.
- Need to perform repeat gonioscopy following peripheral iridotomy to confirm narrow angle has resolved.
  - If narrow angle is not resolved with peripheral iridotomy, anterior segment imaging is warranted.

Diagnostic Procedures/Other
Thymoxamine test: Thymoxamine is a selective alpha 1 adrenergic antagonist that blocks the iris dilator muscle, producing miosis. In normal eyes, IOP will not decrease with thymoxamine administration. In angle closure, thymoxamine causes the IOP to decrease as miosis removes iris from the outflow channel. Thymoxamine is not available in the US.

DIFFERENTIAL DIAGNOSIS
- Malignant glaucoma
- Secondary angle closure
- Glaucomatocyclitic crisis (Posner–Schlossman syndrome)
- Herpetic uveitis
- Pigmentary glaucoma
- Pseudoexfoliative glaucoma
- Neovascular glaucoma

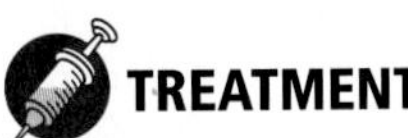

TREATMENT

MEDICATION
First Line
- **Topical ocular hypotensives**
  - Pilocarpine should not be used as a first line agent for angle closure. Despite its miotic effect, pilocarpine may worsen angle closure due to anterior displacement of the lens-iris diaphragm. Additionally, the miotic response may be limited by iris ischemia.
  - Aqueous suppressants
    - β-blockers, alpha 2 agonists, carbonic anhydrase inhibitors
  - Outflow facilitators
    - Prostaglandins
  - Steroids may be helpful in reducing any coincident or contributory inflammatory swelling.
    - Prednisolone, Durezol
- **Systemic carbonic anhydrase inhibitors**
  - Acetazolamide
    - Diamox 125–250 mg PO q.i.d
    - Diamox Sequels 500 mg PO b.i.d
    - Diamox 500 mg IV b.i.d
    - Do not exceed 1g in a 24-hour period.
    - Contraindicated in severe renal disease, hepatic disease, severe pulmonary obstruction, and adrenocortical insufficiency.
  - Methazolamide 50–100 mg PO b.i.d
    - Contraindicated in renal insufficiency.
- **Systemic hyperosmotic**
  - Mannitol 1.5–2 g/kg IV over 30 min period
    - 20% solution (7.5–10 mL/kg)
    - 15% solution (10–13 mL/kg)
    - Do not exceed 500mL in a 24-hour period.
    - Contraindicated in anuria, progressive renal failure, CHF, severe dehydration, or intracranial bleeding.

Second Line
- Analgesic and antiemetic medications can be used to control symptoms of acute IOP rise.
- Topical osmotic medications can temporarily dehydrate a swollen cornea to facilitate laser treatment.
  - Glycerin (apply topical anesthetic first)
- Muro-128

ADDITIONAL TREATMENT
General Measures
Compression gonioscopy may open the angle allowing trabecular flow.

Issues for Referral
Surgical intervention as listed below

Additional Therapies
Pilocarpine is not an alternative to iridotomy.

SURGERY/OTHER PROCEDURES
Intervention is dependent upon the underlying cause of angle closure. Medical management does not correct the pathology in this condition or decrease the risk of recurrent episodes. Laser or surgical intervention is required.

- ***Pupillary Block:***
  - Peripheral laser iridotomy (with Argon or Yag laser) should be done as soon as possible.
    - If attack is broken medically, one may consider waiting for corneal edema to clear to complete iridotomy.
  - Surgical iridectomy should be considered when laser treatment cannot be accomplished.
  - Argon laser peripheral iridoplasty may be used when angle closure is unresponsive to medical therapy, as an alternative to laser iridotomy, or if laser iridotomy fails.
  - Goniosynechialysis
- ***Plateau iris***
  - Argon laser peripheral iridoplasty
  - Peripheral laser iridotomy should be performed in an attempt to eliminate any pupillary block component.
  - Pilocarpine can place the iris on stretch and open the angle.
  - Some cases may be responsive to surgical lens extraction.
- ***Phacomorphic***
  - There is often an element of super-imposed pupillary block, so if possible, peripheral laser iridotomy should be preformed.
  - Surgical lens extraction
- Trabeculectomy or glaucoma drainage device (i.e., tube shunt) placement may be necessary for inadequately controlled IOP after the above measures.

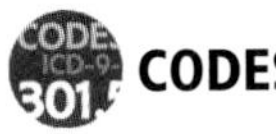

ONGOING CARE

FOLLOW-UP RECOMMENDATIONS
Laser peripheral iridotomy in fellow eye should be done as soon as possible.

Patient Monitoring
- The ischemia caused by acute angle closure may result in decreased aqueous production by the ciliary body. Rebound hypertension or recurrent angle closure may develop if the anatomical problem is not resolved. The patient should be monitored very closely to ensure stability of IOP and unimpeded flow of aqueous from the anterior chamber (open angle, filter, tube shunt, etc.).
- The patient will require life-time monitoring for the development or progression of glaucoma.
- A full examination, including visual fields and optic nerve head/nerve fiber layer imaging, should be completed to assess for glaucomatous changes. A dilated examination should be completed when deemed safe for the patient.

DIET
No dietary modifications are indicated.

PATIENT EDUCATION
The patient should be educated about the nature of his/her disease and concerning symptoms to monitor. Medications that may result in narrowing of the anterior chamber angle (see above) should be discussed with the patient.

PROGNOSIS
- Prompt treatment with adequate IOP reduction minimizes resultant optic neuropathy.
- Continued elevation of intraocular pressure following laser PI may be due to peripheral anterior synechia, incomplete iridotomy, underlying open angle glaucoma, or secondary angle closure. Treat these appropriately.
- Primary angle-closure glaucoma is the leading cause of glaucomatous blindness worldwide.

COMPLICATIONS
- Ischemic optic neuropathy
- Retinal vascular occlusion
- Chronic angle closure (PAS)
- Trabecular meshwork injury
- Accelerated cataract progression
- Corneal decompensation

ADDITIONAL READING

- Aptel F, Philippe D. Optical coherence tomography qualitative analysis of iris volume changes after pharmacologic mydriasis. *Ophthalmology*, 2010;117(1):3–10.
- Foster P, Low S. Primary angle closure glaucoma. In: Shaarawy TM, Shurwood MB, Hitchings RA, et al. Eds. *Glaucoma*, Vol I, Philadelphia: Elsevier; 2009: 327–337.
- Tarongoy P, Ho CL, Walton DS. Angle-closure glaucoma: The role of the lens in the pathogenesis, prevention, and treatment. *Surv Ophthalmol* 2009;54(2):211–225.
- Quigley HA. Editorial: The iris is a sponge: A cause of angle closure. *Ophthalmology*, 2010;116(1):1–2.
- Quigley HA. Angle-closure glaucoma-simpler answers to complex mechanisms: LXVI Edward Jackson Memorial Lecture. *Am J Ophthalmol* 2009;148(5):657–669. e1.

CODES

ICD9
- 365.20 Primary angle-closure glaucoma, unspecified
- 365.22 Acute angle-closure glaucoma
- 365.61 Glaucoma associated with pupillary block

ACUTE RETINAL NECROSIS/NECROTIZING HERPETIC RETINITIS

Matthew Debiec
Mark L. Nelson

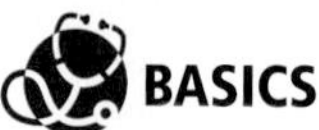

BASICS

DESCRIPTION

- Infectious retinitis caused by members of the herpes virus family, predominantly Varicella Zoster Virus and Herpes Simplex Virus
- Syndrome characterized by anterior uveitis, vitritis, peripheral foci of retinal necrosis that extend posteriorly and circumferentially, retinal vasculopathy, and retinal detachment

EPIDEMIOLOGY

Incidence

- Approximately 1 case in 1.6/2.0 million, although there are few significant epidemiologic studies.
- Generally affects healthy, immunocompetent hosts
- Bimodal distribution with peaks at 20 and 50 years of age

RISK FACTORS

- Previous ocular herpetic infections including HSV keratitis, Herpes Zoster Ophthalmicus; as well as systemic herpetic infections such as cold sores, chickenpox, encephalitis, and shingles
- Immunodeficiency may play a role, although the majority of cases occur in immunocompetent patients.

Genetics

- Vary within different ethnicities: In the US, Caucasian patients often manifest HLA-DQw7 antigen; Japanese patients tend to manifest HLA-Aw33, B44, and DRw6.
- Cases with more fulminant presentation are sometimes associated with HLA-DR9.

PATHOPHYSIOLOGY

- Remains to be fully described; latent viral reactivation and primary infection with Herpes virus have been reported to migrate by axonal transport to the retina and surrounding tissues.
- On histopathology, there is intranuclear accumulation of viral particles at multiple foci, with subsequent granulomatous and non-granulomatous inflammation and necrosis.

ETIOLOGY

Several members of the Herpes virus family cause the inciting infection; VZV accounts for the majority of cases (reported at approximately 50%), but HSV-1, HSV-2, CMV, and EBV have also been reported.

DIAGNOSIS

HISTORY

- Presenting symptoms may be minimal and include irritation, redness, photophobia, periorbital pain, and floaters.
- One epidemiologic study noted sudden visual loss as the main presenting complaint in 85% of cases; photophobia is reported in over half of patients, whereas ocular pain and flu-like symptoms are present in one-quarter of cases; a minority of patients (16%) presented with a red eye.
- It is a clinical diagnosis:
  - The American Uveitis Society criteria include:
    - One or more discrete foci of peripheral retinal necrosis
    - Circumferential spread
    - Occlusive arteriolar retinopathy
    - Prominent vitreous or anterior chamber inflammatory reaction
    - Rapid disease progression in the absence of therapy

PHYSICAL EXAM

- Inspect for anterior uveitis including episcleritis, scleritis, and/or keratic precipitates. At presentation, over 80% of patients have anterior chamber activity, vitreous activity, or peripheral retinal involvement.
- Posterior segment manifestations typically develop within 2 days of initial symptoms and appear as well-defined, multifocal patches of yellowish–white or cream colored retinal infiltrates.
- Vascular sheathing and perivascular intraretinal hemorrhages may develop.
- Retinal necrosis progresses rapidly and spreads circumferentially and posteriorly; the macula is often spared.
- 6–12 weeks after infection, proliferative vitreoretinopathy may lead to retinal holes at the border of normal and affected retina. Rhegmatogenous retinal detachment may occur in over 50% of affected eyes, usually within 1–2 months, although it can occur anytime from 1 week to around 6 months.
- 20% of patients have bilateral infection at presentation. Spread to the contralateral eye typically occurs within 3 months of symptom onset. Systemic antiviral therapy reduces the risk of infection in the second eye from roughly 65–17%.

DIAGNOSTIC TESTS & INTERPRETATION

Lab

Initial lab tests

- Diagnostic confirmation can be made by polymerase chain reaction (PCR) analysis of aqueous sample or vitreous biopsy. PCR has the highest specificity and sensitivity ofavailable laboratory studies.
  - Other laboratory methods that have been used and may suggest an etiologic agent or diagnosis include local and/or systemic antibody titers, Goldmann-Witmer coefficient, fluorescent antibody techniques, or tissue culture. These tests are indicative but not usually considered diagnostic.

Follow-up & special considerations

Detailed examination of the both eyes at each visit is critical as the infectious process can spread bilaterally.

Imaging

Initial approach

Color photographs are useful to follow disease progression.

Pathological Findings

Full-thickness retinal necrosis with eosinophilic intranuclear inclusions. Choroidal inflammation can be granulomatous and usually underlies areas of retinitis. The optic nerve, iris, and ciliary body may be also infiltrated with plasma cells, eosinophils, or macrophages.

DIFFERENTIAL DIAGNOSIS

- Progressive outer retinal necrosis
- Cytomegalovirus retinitis
- Behcet's disease
- Toxoplasmosis retinochoroiditis
- Sarcoidosis
- Large cell lymphoma
- Syphillic neuroretinitis
- *Candida albicans* endophthalmitis

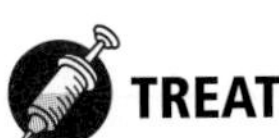

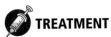

TREATMENT

MEDICATION

First Line

- Historically, ARN was first managed with intravenous acyclovir at 500 mg/m^2 3 times daily for 7–10 days followed by oral acyclovir at 800 mg 5 times daily for up to 14 weeks.
- Newer antivirals have been used in different combinations such as:
  - Valacyclovir 1–2 g 3 times daily
  - Famciclovir 250–500 mg twice daily
  - Valganciclovir 450–900 mg twice daily
  - IV acyclovir with intravitreal injection of foscarnet or ganciclovir
  - Oral valacyclovir or famciclovir followed by IV acyclovir

Second Line

- Intravitreal injections of foscarnet (1.2–2.4 mg per 0.1 mL) and ganciclovir (200–2000 μg per 0.1 mL) have been used as adjunctive therapy.
- Systemic corticosteroids (often prednisone 30–80 mg daily) are used in more than half of patients.
- Most patients receive topical corticosteroids in the initial treatment period anywhere from every 1–6 hours.

ADDITIONAL TREATMENT

Issues for Referral

Patients with suspected ARN require prompt referral to a uveitis/retinal specialist because of the rapid, severe sequelae of untreated infection and due to the possible need for vitrectomy and/or laser retinopexy.

SURGERY/OTHER PROCEDURES

- Prophylactic argon laser retinopexy has been found in some studies to reduce the incidence of secondary RD by approximately half, whereas others find no significant difference.
- Vitrectomy is usually performed for dense vitreous opacities, vitreous hemorrhage, or after secondary retinal detachment.

IN-PATIENT CONSIDERATIONS

Admission Criteria

No clear admission criteria have been elucidated. Such decisions are typically made based on the clinical situation.

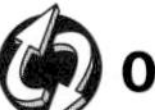

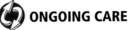

ONGOING CARE

PROGNOSIS

- Risk factors for poor outcomes and worse final visual acuity include initial visual acuity and subsequent retinal detachment.
- Retinal detachment occurs with similar frequency in the newer antiviral era when compared with the acyclovir-only era.
- Final visual acuity of patients with ARN is significantly worsened despite the advent of new antiviral medications and surgical interventions with some studies showing half of patients having acuity worse than 20/200 by 3 months and 75% having acuity worse than 20/200 by 5 years.

COMPLICATIONS

Retinal detachment, optic nerve involvement, vitreous hemorrhage, retinal neovascularization, and blindness.

ADDITIONAL READING

- Tibbetts MD, Shah CP, Young LH, et al. Treatment of acute retinal necrosis. *Ophthalmology* 2010;117(4): 818–824.
- Muthiah MN, Michaelides M, Child CS, et al. Acute retinal necrosis: A national population-based study to assess the incidence, methods of diagnosis, treatment strategies and outcomes in the UK. *Br J Ophthalmol* 2007;91(11):1452–1455.
- Lau CH, Missotten T, Salzmann J, et al. Acute retinal necrosis features, management, and outcomes. *Ophthalmology* 2007;114(4):756–762.
- Hillenkamp J, Nolle B, Bruns C, et al. Acute retinal necrosis: clinical features, early vitrectomy, and outcomes. *Ophthalmology* 2009;116(10): 1971–1975.
- Chang S, Young LH. Acute retinal necrosis: An overview. *Int Ophthalmol Clin* 2007;47(2):145–152.
- Aizman A, Johnson MW, Elner SG. Treatment of acute retinal necrosis syndrome with oral antiviral medications. *Ophthalmology* 2007;114(2): 307–312.

CODES

ICD9

- 053.29 Herpes zoster with other ophthalmic complications
- 364.3 Unspecified iridocyclitis
- 379.29 Other disorders of vitreous

CLINICAL PEARLS

- Acute retinal necrosis can present in an insidious manner and easily be misdiagnosed as an anterior uveitis if a dilated fundus examination is not performed.
- The other eye can frequently become involved, so systemic antiviral therapy and close monitoring of the other eye is very important.
- Diagnosis is made by clinical findings alone, but testing such as PCR can help if there is a diagnostic dilemma.

ADIE TONIC PUPIL

Kenneth C. Kubis
Joseph W. Schmitz

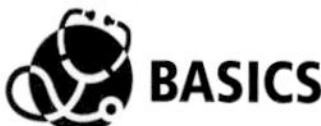

BASICS

DESCRIPTION

- Idiopathic, postganglionic parasympathetic denervation of the iris sphincter, followed by aberrant reinnervation, which results in segmental and sluggish pupillary reaction to light, pupillary light-near dissociation, and slow redilation after accommodation effort
- On initial presentation, 80% of cases are unilateral.
- 4% of unilateral cases per year become bilateral.
- Affected pupil is initially larger but then tends to undergo a gradual miosis becoming smaller than unaffected pupil over years.

EPIDEMIOLOGY

Incidence

Estimated at 4.7 per 100,000 per year

Prevalence

Estimated at 2.0 per 1,000

RISK FACTORS

- Approximately 70% female
- Mean age 32 years

PATHOPHYSIOLOGY

- Postganglionic parasympathetic denervation of iris sphincter
- Aberrant reinnervation of the iris sphincter by ciliary ganglion axons originally destined for ciliary body

ETIOLOGY

Idiopathic

COMMONLY ASSOCIATED CONDITIONS

- Holmes Adie syndrome-
  - Tendon Areflexia
- Ross Syndrome-
  - Holmes Adie syndrome
  - Segmental hypohidrosis

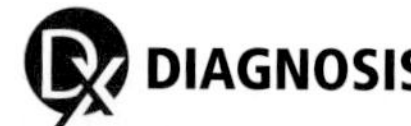

DIAGNOSIS

HISTORY

- Incidental anisocoria
- Blurred near vision
- Photophobia

PHYSICAL EXAM

- Affected pupil constricts more with accommodation than with light and redilates slowly
- If unilateral, anisocoria that is greater in light than dark
- Segmental contraction of pupil sphincter that is best seen at slit-lamp
- Approximately 10% of patients may have no light reaction.
- Deep tendon reflexes to assess for Holmes Adie syndrome
- Relative accommodative weakness compared to contralateral eye

ALERT

Full ophthalmic exam with particular attention to eye motility and ptosis to rule out third nerve palsy and Horner syndrome.

DIAGNOSTIC TESTS & INTERPRETATION

Lab

Usually not indicated unless atypical history or physical examination to rule out other etiology for tonic pupil.

Diagnostic Procedures/Other

- Dilute Pilocarpine drops (0.125%) administered to both eyes will show constriction of effected pupil, and not the normal pupil, due to denervation supersensitivity.
- Positive in 80% of patients

Pathological Findings

Ciliary body has reduced number of ganglion cells.

DIFFERENTIAL DIAGNOSIS

ALERT

Tonic pupil (especially when bilateral) may be secondary to many etiologies and a thorough history and physical should be undertaken to identify potential UNDERLYING disease

- Secondary tonic pupil due to:
  - Inflammation
  - Infection
  - Ischemia
  - Trauma
  - Generalized neuropathy
- Physiologic anisocoria
- Third nerve palsy
- Pharmacologic mydriasis
- Iris damage (traumatic mydriasis, siderosis)

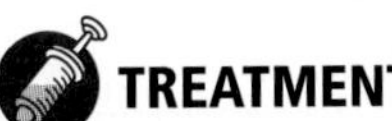

TREATMENT

MEDICATION

Dilute pilocarpine (0.1%) as needed for photophobia due to large pupil.

ADDITIONAL TREATMENT

Issues for Referral

Neurology or neuro-ophthalmology referral if the diagnosis is in doubt.

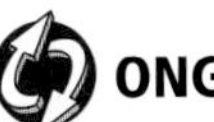

ONGOING CARE

FOLLOW-UP RECOMMENDATIONS

- Acute tonic pupil should be followed periodically for development of light near dissociation.
- Periodic evaluation for identification of underlying etiology

PROGNOSIS

Excellent.

ADDITIONAL READING

- Thompson HS. Adie's syndrome: Some new observations. *Trans Am Ophthalmol Soc* 1977; 75:587–626.
- Weller M, Wilhelm H, Sommer N, et al. Tonic Pupil, areflexia, and segmental anhidrosis: Two additional cases of Ross syndrome and a review of the literature. *J Neurol* 1992; 239:231–234.
- Kardon RH, Corbett JJ, Thompson HA. Segmental denervation and reinnervation of the iris sphincter as shown by infrared videographic transillumination. *Ophthalmology* 1998; 105:313–321.

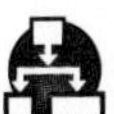

See Also (Topic, Algorithm, Electronic Media Element)

- Anisocoria algorithm

CODES

ICD9

379.46 Tonic pupillary reaction

CLINICAL PEARLS

- Pupil with light-near dissociation
- Slow redilation (tonic) after accommodation
- Approximately 90% show sector palsy of iris sphincter with remainder showing no light reactivity and mimicking pharmacologic dilation.

AGE-RELATED MACULAR DEGENERATION AND POLYPOIDAL CHOROIDAL VASCULOPATHY

G. Atma Vemulakonda

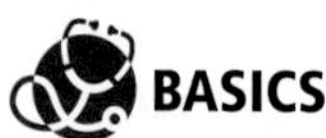

BASICS

DESCRIPTION

- Age-related macular degeneration (AMD) is a leading cause of irreversible blindness among older patients in the developed world (1)
  - AMD is the leading cause of legal blindness in patients ≥65 years in the US
  - 90% of AMD patients have the non-exudative or "dry" form
  - 10% have the exudative or "wet" form
- Polypoidal choroidal vasculopathy (PCV) is a separate disease from AMD, characterized by abnormalities in the inner choroid, external to the choriocapillaris, including a branching network of dilated vessels that leads to serous leakage and hemorrhage.
  - PCV predominately affects patients of African and African American descent and Asian patients, with a lower incidence in Caucasians

EPIDEMIOLOGY

Incidence

- Overall 5-year incidence of late AMD was 0.9% (2)
- Incidence of Early AMD increased from 3.9% in patients aged between 43–54 years to 22.8% in patients >75 years (2)
- No clear incidence data available for PCV

Prevalence

- Total prevalence of any AMD in the 1991 civilian population ≥ 40 years was 9.2% (2)
- In the US, neovascular AMD and/or geographic atrophy in Americans 40 years and older is estimated to be 1.47% (2004 data) (1)
- PCV: Prevalence varies from 4–14%
  - In Asians, men are more affected, usually unilaterally in the macula (3).
  - Rates may be as high as 23–54% in Japanese patients diagnosed with AMD (3)
  - In Caucasians, women are more affected bilaterally in the peripapillary region (3)

RISK FACTORS

- AMD
  - Age
  - Family history
  - Race (Caucasians 5–6 times more frequently affected than African Americans)
  - Cardiovascular risk factors including elevated cholesterol and hypertension
  - Cigarette smoking
  - Gender (women slightly more than men)
  - Obesity
- PCV: Ethnicity and age

Genetics

- Genes associated with increased risk of AMD
  - Complement Factor H (CFH) on 1q32
    - Homozygosity for risk allele increases risk by factor of 7.4 (4)
  - LOC 387715 on 10q26
  - HTRA1 on 10q26
- Genes associated with increased risk of PCV
  - LOC 387715 on 10q26
  - HTRA1 on 10q26

GENERAL PREVENTION

- AMD
  - Smoking cessation
  - Age-related eye disease study (AREDS) vitamins for appropriate patients
    - 25% decrease in progression to advanced AMD in high risk individuals (patients with intermediate or advanced AMD)
    - Vitamins include: Vitamins C&E, zinc, beta carotene, and copper

PATHOPHYSIOLOGY/ETIOLOGY

- AMD most likely a combination of:
  - Senescent retinal pigment epithelium (RPE) accumulates remnants of rod and cone membranes that leads to diminished RPE function and drusen formation
  - Vascular theory proposes that choroidal circulation is diminished leading to retinal ischemia
  - Genetic theory based on findings of AMD specific gene mutations
- PCV results from (5)
  - Inner choroidal vasculature abnormalities (most common type)
  - Polypoidal CNV, expanding rapidly under the RPE, ultimately with polypoidal lesions developing at vessel termini.
  - Radiation associated choroidal neovasculopathy

COMMONLY ASSOCIATED CONDITIONS

- AMD
  - HTN
  - Elevated cholesterol

DIAGNOSIS

HISTORY

- AMD
  - Central blurring, distortion, blind spot, or no symptoms (non-exudative)
- PCV: Central blurring, distortion, blind spot, or no symptoms

PHYSICAL EXAM

- AMD
  - Findings in non-exudative AMD include drusen, retinal pigment epithelial changes, and retinal thinning/atrophy
  - Findings in exudative AMD include vitreous hemorrhage, pigment epithelial detachment (PED), retinal and subretinal hemorrhage, lipid, fluid, and RPE tear
- Suspect PCV in an elderly patient with an exudative maculopathy and:
  - Nonwhite patient
  - Peripapillary CNV
  - Few or no drusen in the fellow eye of a patient with unilateral involvement

DIAGNOSTIC TESTS & INTERPRETATION

Imaging

Initial approach

- AMD: Fluorescein angiography (FA) and optical coherence tomography (OCT)
- PCV: Indocyanine green angiography (ICG), FA, and OCT

Follow-up & special considerations

- AMD
  - OCT to follow disease course and response to treatment
  - FA as needed to help determine end points for treatment
- PCV
  - OCT to follow disease course and response to treatment
  - ICG and FA as needed to help determine end points for treatment

Diagnostic Procedures/Other

- AMD
  - ICG

Pathological Findings

- AMD
  - Non-exudative: Accumulation of rod and cone membranes leading to drusen, RPE pigment changes, and eventual retinal atrophy
  - Exudative: Subretinal and Sub RPE choroidal neovascular membranes
- PCV pathology reveals (6):
  - Large choroidal arterioles with an inner elastic layer
  - Disruption of the inner elastic layer and arteriosclerotic changes of the vessels were identified by light microscopy.
  - Transmission electron microscopy demonstrated increased deposition of basement membrane-like material, together with collagen fibers, in the arteriolar walls

DIFFERENTIAL DIAGNOSIS

- AMD and PCV:
  - Degenerative myopia, angioid streaks, pattern dystrophies, presumed ocular histoplasmosis syndrome, multifocal choroiditis, serpiginous choroiditis, Best's disease, Stargardt's disease, gyrate atrophy, retinitis pigmentosa, choroidal rupture/trauma, idiopathic

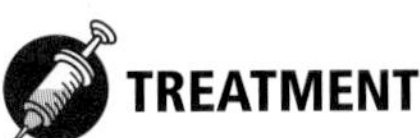

TREATMENT

MEDICATION

First Line

- AMD
  - Intravitreal anti-VEGF injections
    - Bevacizumab
    - Ranibizumab
- PCV:
  - Conventional thermal laser for non subfoveal lesions
  - Photodynamic therapy (PDT) for subfoveal lesions, based on the greatest linear dimension of the choroidal lesion seen on ICG
    - Reduced fluence PDT may be useful in certain cases
  - Intravitreal anti-VEGF injections, appear to be less effective than with AMD based on studies to date
  - Combination therapy of anti-VEGF and PDT appears promising

Second Line

- AMD
  - Intravitreal anti-VEGF injections: Macugen
  - PDT based on the greatest linear dimension of the choroidal lesion seen on FA
  - Conventional thermal laser for non-subfoveal lesions
  - Intravitreal steroid injection
  - Combination treatment
    - Combination of anti-VEGF +/– PDT +/– Intravitreal steroid
    - May be more useful in patients with poor response to treatment

ADDITIONAL TREATMENT

General Measures

- AMD
- AREDS vitamins
- Modifiable risk reduction: Control of HTN, high cholesterol, obesity (high Body mass index), and smoking cessation

Issues for Referral

Refer to retina specialist for evaluation and treatment of both AMD and PCV

SURGERY/OTHER PROCEDURES

- AMD
  - Submacular surgery found to be less helpful in treating exudative AMD

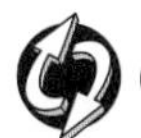

ONGOING CARE

FOLLOW-UP RECOMMENDATIONS

- Retinal specialist
- Low vision evaluation for patients with vision loss

Patient Monitoring

- See follow-up
- Home Amsler Grid

DIET

- AMD
  - AREDS nutrient supplementation for patients with intermediate or advanced AMD
  - Balanced diet
  - Omega-3 fatty acids, lutein, and zeaxanthin currently under investigation in AREDS II trial

PATIENT EDUCATION

AMD: http://www.aao.org/eyesmart/diseases/amd.cfm

PROGNOSIS

Normal lifespan, development, intelligence, and fertility

Pregnancy Considerations

- **PCV:** Concern for toxicity of PDT and anti-VEGF treatments in pregnancy
- **AMD:** Not applicable

COMPLICATIONS

AMD and PCV: Vision loss

REFERENCES

1. Friedman DS, O'Colmain BJ, Munoz B, et al. Prevalence of age-related macular degeneration in the United States. *Arch Ophthalmol* 2004;122(4):564–72.
2. Klein R, Klein BEK, Jensen SC, et al. The five year incidence and progression of age-related maculopathy. *Ophthalmology* 1997;104:7–21.
3. Klein RJ, Zeiss C, Chew EY, et al. Complement factor H polymorphism in agerelated Macular Degeneration. *Science* 2005;308(5720):385–389.
4. Gomi F, Tano Y. Polypoidal choroidal vasculopathy and treatments. *Curr Opin Ophthalmol* 2008;19(3):208–12.
5. Yuzawa M, Mori R, Kawamura A. The origins of polypoidal choroidal vasculopathy. *Br J Ophthalmol* 2005;89(5):602–607.
6. Kuroiwa S, Tateiwa H, Hisatomi T, et al. Pathological features of surgically excised polypoidal choroidal vasculopathy membranes. *Clin Experiment Ophthalmol* 2004;32(3):297–302.

CODES

ICD9

- 362.50 Macular degeneration (senile) of retina, unspecified
- 362.51 Nonexudative senile macular degeneration of retina
- 362.52 Exudative senile macular degeneration of retina

AGE-RELATED (SENILE) RETINOSCHISIS

Adam T. Gerstenblith
Sunir Garg

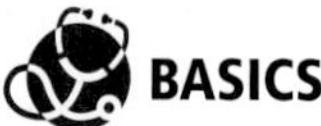

BASICS

DESCRIPTION
Age-related (senile) retinoschisis (SR) is an acquired condition characterized by splitting of the retina into 2 separate layers.

EPIDEMIOLOGY

Incidence
Not clearly defined.

Prevalence
- Ranges from 1.65–7% among persons older than 40 years (1)[C]
- Generally equal in male and females

RISK FACTORS
- Preexisting peripheral retinal cystoid degeneration
- Hyperopia

Genetics
Unknown.

GENERAL PREVENTION
None.

PATHOPHYSIOLOGY
- Vision is not significantly affected when the schisis cavity remains in the periphery
- Visual loss occurs predominantly in 2 circumstances:
  - The area of retinoschisis extends posteriorly toward, or into, the macula (occurs in 3% of cases).
  - An associated rhegmatogenous retinal detachment (RRD) develops.

ETIOLOGY
- Generally develops as a consolidation of intraretinal cysts in an area of peripheral cystoid degeneration
  - Begins anterior at the ora serrata and extends posteriorly
  - The splitting most often occurs in the outer plexiform layer

COMMONLY ASSOCIATED CONDITIONS
- Hyperopia
- An RRD may develop secondarily.

DIAGNOSIS

HISTORY
- Age-related retinoschisis is usually asymptomatic and is detected on routine examination.
- Some patients may have peripheral visual field loss, flashes and floaters, and central vision loss.

PHYSICAL EXAM
- Dilated funduscopic examination shows:
  - A smooth dome-like elevation of the retina that remains fixed in position and does not undulate.
  - Often bilateral (one-fifth to half of the cases) but can be asymmetric.
  - Most commonly located inferotemporally
  - Peripheral cystoid degeneration is seen anterior to the schisis cavity.
  - Inner and/or outer retinal holes may be present.
  - Fine, irregular white dots may be seen on the retinal surface.
  - Sclerotic retinal vessels in the area of schisis
  - The inner layer does not collapse on scleral depression.

DIAGNOSTIC TESTS & INTERPRETATION

Imaging

Initial approach

Photographs to document posterior extent of the area of retinoschisis may be useful for comparison on follow up.

Follow-up & special considerations

Asymptomatic and peripheral age-related retinoschisis can be followed every 2–3 years.

Diagnostic Procedures/Other
Visual field testing reveals an absolute scotoma in the areas of schisis.

Pathological Findings
- There are 2 main types of acquired retinoschisis:
  - Typical degenerative retinoschisis
    - The more common subtype in which the splitting occurs in the outer plexiform layer
  - Reticular degenerative retinoschisis is characterized by cystoid spaces and splitting within the nerve fiber layer
    - Breaks in the outer retina occur in 11–24% of cases, and may lead to rhegmatogenous retinal detachment.

DIFFERENTIAL DIAGNOSIS

- Rhegmatogenous retinal detachment. This is the most important condition to differentiate from age-related retinoschisis. Chronic rhegmatogenous retinal detachments also may appear smooth and domed. The presence of pigment in the vitreous, or a pigmented demarcation line suggests rhegmatogenous detachment.
  - In some cases, differentiating these 2 conditions can be difficult. Two other ways to diagnose them are: 1) Laser retinopexy to the cavity will cause a burn in retinoschisis, but not in a retinal detachment, and 2) Optical coherence tomography (OCT) at the edge of the schisis cavity will show a complete neurosensory retinal detachment in a rhegmatogenous detachment, and a splitting of the neurosensory retina with apposition of the photoreceptors and retinal pigment epithelium in cases of retinoschisis.

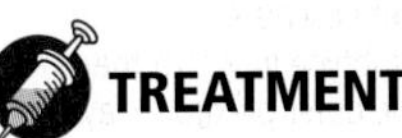

TREATMENT

SURGERY/OTHER PROCEDURES

- The majority of cases only need observation as they progress slowly, if at all (1).
- For SR that extends into the posterior pole, demarcation with cryotherapy or laser retinopexy can be considered (2). However, most of these may be observed as rarely does age-related retinoschisis reach the macula, and cryotherapy may increase formation of retinal detachment.
- If a frank RRD develops, surgical repair with scleral buckle or pars plana vitrectomy is usually necessary (1,2).

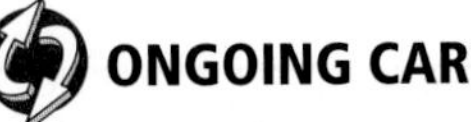

ONGOING CARE

FOLLOW-UP RECOMMENDATIONS

- Dilated fundus examination every 1–3 years for uncomplicated SR without holes
- Patients with multiple retinal breaks or significant posterior extension should be followed more closely.
  - Should a retinal detachment develop or should there be a question of an associated retinal detachment, prompt referral to a retinal specialist is advised.

Patient Monitoring

Patients should be counseled to return to the ophthalmologist if any changes in vision occur.

PROGNOSIS

- Vision is typically unaffected or only minimally affected if the area of retinoschisis remains peripheral.
- The prognosis is significantly worse should a retinal detachment develop.

COMPLICATIONS

- RRD
- Posterior extension of the retinoschisis

REFERENCES

1. Buch H, Vinding T, Nielsen NV. Prevalence and long-term natural course of retinoschisis among elderly individuals: The Copenhagen City Eye Study. *Ophthalmology* 2007;114(4):751–5.
2. Byer NE. Perspectives on the management of the complications of senile retinoschisis. *Eye(London)* 2002;16(4):359–64.

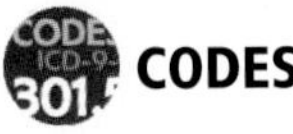

CODES

ICD9

- 361.13 Primary retinal cysts
- 361.19 Other retinoschisis and retinal cysts

CLINICAL PEARLS

- This is an idiopathic acquired condition in older patients characterized by bullous retinal elevation, most often located inferotemporally.
- Usually bilateral but may be asymmetric
- Visual prognosis is often excellent and most cases can be observed.
- The most important consideration is differentiating age-related retinoschisis from an RRD and monitoring for its development.

AICARDI SYNDROME

Scott E. Olitsky
A Paula Grigorian

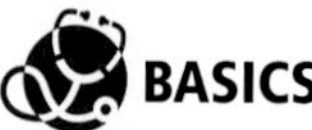

BASICS

DESCRIPTION
- Genetic neurodevelopmental disorder characterized by the triad of:
  - Infantile spasm type seizure disorder
  - Agenesis of corpus callosum
  - Chorioretinal lacunae

EPIDEMIOLOGY
Incidence
Unknown but very rare

Prevalence
Kroner (1) estimated there to be greater than 853 cases in the US and several thousand cases worldwide.

RISK FACTORS
None known, genetic disorder

Genetics
- Presumed X-linked dominant disorder
- Lethal in males, affected surviving males rare and usually have chromosomal aberration of sex chromosomes (e.g., translocation, XXY)
- No gene definitively identified
- Phenocopy del1p36

(NOTE: Not to be confused with Aicardi-Goutières syndrome)

GENERAL PREVENTION
- Unknown, prenatal genetic testing not available
- Prenatal ultrasound can detect corpus callosum abnormalities

PATHOPHYSIOLOGY
Developmental defect presumably of neuroectoderm

ETIOLOGY
Presumed gene mutation

COMMONLY ASSOCIATED CONDITIONS
- Ocular associations
  - Cardinal feature: Chorioretinal lacunae (see below)
  - Congenital optic disc anomalies: Coloboma, hypoplasia, congenital pigmentation
  - Microphthalmia, retinal detachment, nystagmus
- Systemic associations
  - Vertebral malformations: Fused vertebrae, scoliosis, spina bifida, costal malformations (absent ribs, fused or bifurcated ribs)
  - Muscular hypotonia, microcephaly, dysmorphic facies, auricular anomalies
  - Brain anomalies: Dysgenesis of the corpus callosum (complete or partial), cerebral asymmetry with polymicrogyria or pachygyria, periventricular and intracortical gray matter heterotopias, midline arachnoid cysts, choroid plexus papillomas, and ventriculomegaly and intracerebral cysts, often at the third ventricle and in the choroid plexus. Severe mental retardation
  - Gastrointestinal: Constipation, diarrhea, gastroesophageal reflux, difficulty feeding
  - Integument: Vascular and pigmented lesions

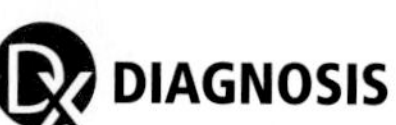

DIAGNOSIS

HISTORY
Infants 3–5 months of age may present with: Decreased visual acuity, amblyopia, or strabismus, but more often present with neurological manifestations of developmental delay, hypotony, and intractable seizures

PHYSICAL EXAM
- Classic triad
  - infantile spasms
  - agenesis of corpus callosum
  - chorioretinal lacunae
- Major features
  - Cortical malformations (mostly polymicrogyria)
  - Periventricular and subcortical heterotopias
  - Cysts around third cerebral ventricle and/or choroid plexus
  - Optic disc/nerve coloboma or hypoplasia
- Supporting features
  - Vertebral and rib abnormalities
  - Microphthalmia
  - "Split-brain" EEG, infantile spasm hypsarrhythmia
  - Cerebral hemispheric asymmetry
  - Vascular malformations or vascular malignancy

ALERT
- All 3 classic features present are diagnostic for Aicardi syndrome.
- 2 classic features plus 2 other major or supporting features are suggestive

DIAGNOSTIC TESTS & INTERPRETATION
Lab
- Routine lab tests–normal
- Karyotype and if normal, microarray, recommended

Imaging
Initial approach

MRI with and without contrast to look for brain malformations

Follow-up & special considerations
- Neurology managements of seizures
- Support for multiple care needs: Usually severe developmental delay and totally care-dependent
- If requires vigabatrin for seizure control, follow protocols for monitoring retinal and optic nerve effects with periodic eye examination, electroretinography, and possibly optical coherence tomography

Diagnostic Procedures/Other

EEG

Pathological Findings

Chorioretinal lacunae represent focal thinning and atrophy of retinal pigment epithelium and choroid. The overlying retinal architecture is severely disrupted and there may also be hyperplastic and ectopic retinal pigment epithelium

DIFFERENTIAL DIAGNOSIS

- Agenesis of the corpus callosum – isolated or in conjunction with other brain malformations and syndromes
- Neuronal migration disorders: Polymicrogyria, pachygyria, heterotopias – isolated or as part of the phenotype associated with other syndromes or chromosome abnormalities
- Oculocerebrocutaneous syndrome: Orbital cysts and anophthalmia or microphthalmia, focal skin defects, brain malformations that include polymicrogyria, periventricular nodular heterotopias, enlarged lateral ventricles, and agenesis of the corpus callosum – predominant in males with pathognomonic mid-hindbrain malformation
- Infantile spasms – isolated or as part of other syndromes, inborn errors of metabolism, or chromosome disorders
- Chorioretinal lacunae are virtually pathognomonic for Aicardi syndrome, but they have also been reported in orofaciodigital syndrome type IX
- Microphthalmia and other developmental eye defects in X-linked dominant disorders, such as Goltz syndrome and microphthalmia with linear skin (MLS) defects
- Chorioretinal lacunae: Congenital toxoplasmosis, coloboma, "macular coloboma" of Leber congenital amaurosis, congenital torpedo maculopathy, prenatal varicella retinitis, prenatal cytomegalovirus, laser scars, trauma (including chorioretinal scars reported with abusive head injury)

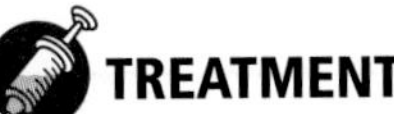

TREATMENT

MEDICATION

- Symptomatic
  - Seizure control: Anti-epileptic drugs (vigabatrin) and vagus nerve stimulators. Physical therapy, occupational therapy, and speech therapy.

ADDITIONAL TREATMENT

General Measures

- Developmental delay usually too severe to justify low vision intervention
- Low vision community support

Issues for Referral

Neurology, gastroenterology, and dermatology, as needed

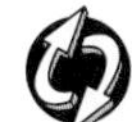

ONGOING CARE

FOLLOW-UP RECOMMENDATIONS

- According to the eye findings
- If patient on vigabatrin follow-up (see above)
- Long-term management by a pediatric neurologist with expertise in management of infantile spasms and medically refractory epilepsy

PATIENT EDUCATION

- Genetic counseling – usually siblings not affected, recurrence risk low if chromosomes normal and mother unaffected
- Support groups: www.aicardisyndrome.org, www.afb.org/CVI
- www.rarediseases.org/search/rdbdetail_abstract.html?disname = Aicardi+Syndrome

PROGNOSIS

- Ocular lesions usually have little effect on vision unless macula is involved
- Usually severe cortical visual impairment
- Survival is highly variable, with the mean age of death about 8.3 years and the median age of death about 18.5 years

COMPLICATIONS

Cause of death is usually intractable seizures, aspiration or morbidity related to severe neurologic delay

REFERENCE

1. Kroner BL, Preiss LR, Ardini MA, et al. New incidence, prevalence, and survival of Aicardi syndrome from 408 cases. *J Child Neurol* 2008;23(5):531–5.

ADDITIONAL READING

- Aicardi J, Lefebvre J, Lerique-Koechlin A. A new syndrome: Spasm in flexion, callosal agenesis, ocular abnormalities. *Electroencephalogr Clin Neurophysiol* 1965;19:609–10.
- Galdos M, Martinez R, Prats JM. Clinical outcome of distinct aicardy syndrome phenotypes. *Arch Soc Esp Oftalmol* 2008;83:29–36.
- McMahon RG, Bell RA, Moore GR, et al. Aicardi's syndrome. A clinicopathologic study. *Arch Ophthalmol* 1984;102(2):250–3.

CODES

ICD9

- 742.2 Congenital reduction deformities of brain
- 743.10 Microphthalmos, unspecified
- 743.57 Specified congenital anomalies of optic disc

CLINICAL PEARLS

- Chorioretinal lacunae
- Infantile spasms
- Agenesis of corpus callosum

ALBINISM

Chirag P. Shah
Alex V. Levin

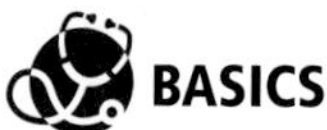

BASICS

DESCRIPTION

- **Oculocutaneous albinism (OCA)** is a group of hereditary diseases marked by absent or decreased melanin biosynthesis within melanocytes, or abnormalities of melanosome formation or function.
  - Hypopigmentation of the hair, skin, and eyes
  - Four types of OCA
    - OCA1: Usually white hair, pale skin, and light irides
    - OCA2: Usually less severe than type 1, more frequent in African Americans, Africans and some Native Americans
    - OCA3: Brown (BOCA) or rufous (ROCA), more frequent in Africa
    - OCA4: Similar to type 2, more frequent in Japan and Turkey
  - Because of phenotypic overlap, the types of OCA are most accurately distinguished by their genetic defects
- **Ocular albinism** (OA) is a disorder marked by abnormal melanosomes (macromelanosomes), though each is fully pigmented.
  - Signs and symptoms are mostly limited to the eye.

EPIDEMIOLOGY

Incidence

- Varies by region, about 1 in 20,000 births worldwide
- The highest incidence in the world is found in the Kuna Indians of the San Blas Islands of Panama
- OCA1 and OA1 are the most common forms

Prevalence

- 1 in 17,000 people have one of the forms of albinism
- 1 in 70 people are carriers for one of the implicated genes
- 1 in 60,000 males is affected by ocular albinism type 1, also known as the Nettleship-Falls type, the most common type of ocular albinism

RISK FACTORS

Genetics

- Oculocutaneous albinism is usually autosomal recessive. Autosomal dominant is rare.
- Patients typically harbor 2 different mutations in 1 gene for oculocutaneous albinism (i.e., compound heterozygotes).
  - Tyrosinase (TYR) – OCA1
  - P-gene – OCA2
  - Tyrosinase-related protein 1 (TRP1) – OCA3
  - Membrane-associated transporter protein (MATP, also called SLC45A2) – OCA4
- Ocular albinism is usually X-linked recessive, female carriers may manifest signs by lyonization
  - G protein-coupled receptor 143 (GPR143, albinism type 1). The gene protein controls the growth and maturation of melanosomes.
  - Autosomal recessive ocular albinism has also been described.
  - Digenic inheritance has also been reported.

GENERAL PREVENTION

- Genetic counseling
- Prenatal molecular diagnosis available when cultural attitudes may result in psychosocial disability

PATHOPHYSIOLOGY

Hypopigmentation in RPE during early gestation leads to macular hypoplasia, which in turn leads to delayed ganglion cell differentiation and abnormal chiasmal decussation.

ETIOLOGY

The different types of oculocutaneous albinism are due to genes involved in the biosynthesis of melanin and melanosomes in melanocytes (see "Genetics").

COMMONLY ASSOCIATED CONDITIONS

- Hermansky-Pudlak syndrome
  - Platelet aggregation deficiency. More prevalent in Puerto Ricans and Swiss. May have accumulation of ceroid throughout the body, leading to pulmonary fibrosis, granulomatous enteropathic disease, and renal failure
- Chediak–Higashi syndrome
  - Impaired bactericidal activity and thus an increased susceptibility to infection
- Griscelli syndrome
  - Large clumps of pigment in hair shafts. Immunodeficiency in one variant; neurologic deficits in another
- Prader-Willi
  - Neonatal hypotonia, hyperphagia, and obesity, small hands and feet, hypogonadism, mental retardation
- Angelman syndrome
  - Neonatal hypotonia, developmental delay, microcephaly, severe mental retardation, ataxic movements, inappropriate laughter

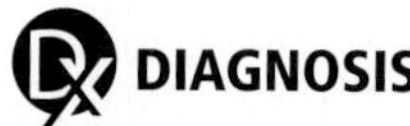

DIAGNOSIS

- Ophthalmic features of oculocutaneous and ocular albinism include various degrees of:
  - Congenital nystagmus
  - Strabismus
  - Iris transillumination
  - Photophobia
  - Hypopigmentation of the fundus
  - Macular hypoplasia
  - Reduced visual acuity (20/40–20/400)
  - Refractive errors
  - Amblyopia due to strabismus or anisometropia
  - Grey optic nerves with or without optic nerve hypoplasia
- Cutaneous features of oculocutaneous albinism include various degrees of:
  - Skin hypopigmentation
  - Hair hypopigmentation
  - May have nevi (ephelides)

HISTORY
- Family history
- Decreased vision
- Photosensitivity
- Review of systems should assess easy bruising and bleeding (Hermansky–Pudlak) and propensity for infection (Chediak–Higashi)

PHYSICAL EXAM
- External examination including hair and skin
- Complete ophthalmic examination including refraction, motility, slit lamp examination (iris transillumination defects), and dilated fundus examination (hypoplastic fovea, hypopigmented retina with highly visible choroidal vasculature)

DIAGNOSTIC TESTS & INTERPRETATION
Diagnostic Procedures/Other
- Prenatal diagnosis possible if gene mutation known
- Albinism is a clinical diagnosis which can be confirmed in some cases with DNA testing
- Optical coherence testing (OCT) demonstrates macular hypoplasia
- Multichannel visual evoked potentials demonstrate excessive decussation of retinal ganglion cell axons at the chiasm in most cases
- Molecular genetic testing may determine the specific mutations and thus helps identify the subtype of oculocutaneous albinism
- Tests for OCA1, OCA2, and OA1 are available clinically
- Tests for other genes only for research purposes

Pathological Findings
- Macromelanosomes may be seen on skin biopsy in OA1, Hermansky–Pudlak syndrome, and Chediak–Higashi syndrome.

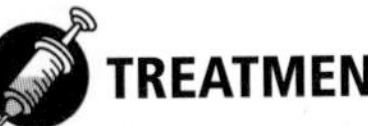

TREATMENT

ADDITIONAL TREATMENT
General Measures
- Address refractive error with glasses or contact lens
- Tinted or polychromic lens for photophobia
- Treat amblyopia, which can result from strabismus or anisometropia
- High contrast reading material and large type fonts
- Distance low vision aids (usually after first grade)
- Suntan lotion (minimum 15 SPF) and other protective measures against UV sunlight exposure

SURGERY/OTHER PROCEDURES
Eye muscle surgery for strabismus or nystagmus

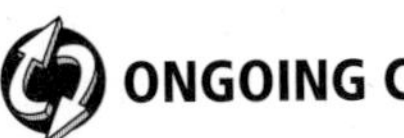

ONGOING CARE

FOLLOW-UP RECOMMENDATIONS
- Ophthalmologist
- Low vision
- Primary care doctor or dermatologist for periodic skin examinations
- Hematology evaluation if Hermansky–Pudlak or Chediak–Higashi syndrome a concern

PATIENT EDUCATION
The National Organization for Albinism and Hypopigmentation (http://www.albinism.org)

PROGNOSIS
- Normal lifespan, development, intelligence, fertility
- Increased risk of skin cancer

COMPLICATIONS
- Visual loss
- Actinic keratosis, squamous cell carcinoma, and basal cell carcinoma in sun-exposed areas

ADDITIONAL READING

- Grønskov K, Ek J, Brondum-Nielsen K. Oculocutaneous albinism. *Orphanet Journal of Rare Diseases* 2007;2:43.
- Okulicz JF, Shah RS, Schwartz RA, et al. Oculocutaneous albinism. *J Eur Acad Dermatol Venereol*. 2003;17(3):251–256.

CODES

ICD9
270.2 Other disturbances of aromatic amino-acid metabolism

CLINICAL PEARLS

- Oculocutaneous albinism (OCA) is a group of hereditary diseases marked by absent or decreased melanin or melanosome synthesis within melanocytes.
- OCA is usually autosomal recessive and affects the eyes, skin, and hair.
- Ocular albinism is an X-linked recessive disorder generally limited to the eye, due to a genetic defect leading to macromelanosomes.
- Visual acuity is usually reduced.

ALLERGIC CONJUNCTIVITIS

Christine G. Saad

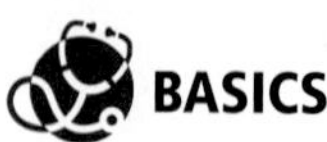

BASICS

DESCRIPTION
- Allergic conjunctivitis is an allergic inflammation of the ocular surface that can be divided into the following categories: seasonal and perennial allergic conjunctivitis (SAC and PAC), vernal keratoconjunctivitis (VKC), atopic keratoconjunctivitis (AKC), and giant papillary conjunctivitis (GPC).
  - SAC: Conjunctival inflammation occurring at a specific time of year
  - PAC: A variant of SAC that occurs throughout the year
  - VKC: Bilateral, chronic inflammatory condition of the conjunctiva with possible corneal involvement
  - AKC: Bilateral, chronic inflammatory condition associated with atopic dermatitis
  - GPC: Inflammatory condition affecting superior tarsal conjunctiva

EPIDEMIOLOGY
- Allergic conjunctivitis affects up to 40% of the population.
- Atopic dermatitis affects up to 3% of the population and ocular involvement occurs in 25–40% of these individuals.

RISK FACTORS
- Personal or family history of atopic conditions including eczema, asthma, hay fever, and allergic rhinitis:
  - Exposure to aeroallergens to which an individual has a known allergy
  - GPC: Use of soft or rigid gas permeable lenses, ocular prosthesis or foreign body

Genetics
Hereditary background of atopic conditions is common.

GENERAL PREVENTION
Avoidance of known allergens

PATHOPHYSIOLOGY
- Activation of mast cells by antigens results in release of chemical mediators (i.e., histamine).
  - SAC/PAC: Type I hypersensitivity reaction
  - AKC/VKC: Type I and IV hypersensitivity reaction
  - GPC: Trauma to upper lid

ETIOLOGY
- SAC: Grass and pollen allergens
- PAC: Indoor allergens such as dust mites and animal dander
- VKC/AKC: Multiple environmental allergens
- GPC: Foreign body causing irritation to upper lid

COMMONLY ASSOCIATED CONDITIONS
Atopic disease

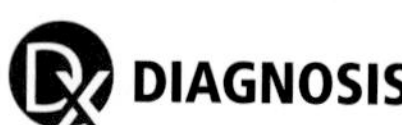

DIAGNOSIS

HISTORY
- Itching, burning, irritation, photophobia, tearing, watery discharge:
  - SAC: Occurs at a specific time to known allergens.
  - PAC: Occurs throughout the year but may be worse at specific times.
  - VKC: Severe itching. Bilateral. Predilection for young males from hot, dry climates (Mediterranean, Africa). Seasonal exacerbation. Affects most prior to puberty and resolves by late teens/early twenties.
  - AKC: Older population. Symptoms may occur year round and is not associated with hot weather.
  - GPC: Contact lens use, suture, foreign body.

PHYSICAL EXAM
- SAC/PAC: Mild conjunctival injection and edema. Papillary reaction, but no giant papillae.
- VKC: Conjunctival injection, giant papillae, involvement of upper palpebral conjunctiva. Limbal thickening, limbal nodules, Trantas' dots. Corneal involvement: punctuate keratopathy, erosions, shield ulcer, plaque, pannus.
- AKC: Conjunctival injection, atopic dermatitis of lids, papillary hypertrophy. Corneal involvement: pannus, ulcer, scarring. Cataract.
- GPC: Giant papillae, upper palpebral conjunctiva.

DIAGNOSTIC TESTS & INTERPRETATION

Lab
- Not typically necessary
  - Conjunctival scraping

Diagnostic Procedures/Other
Conjunctival provocation test

Pathological Findings
Eosinophils on conjunctival scraping

DIFFERENTIAL DIAGNOSIS
Viral conjunctivitis, dry eye, blepharitis, contact dermatitis, toxic/chemical conjunctivitis, floppy eyelid syndrome/eyelid imbrication

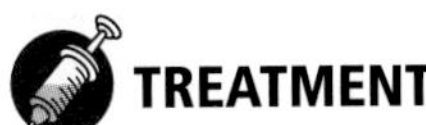

TREATMENT

MEDICATION

First Line

- SAC/PAC: Topical antihistamine-vasoconstrictor eye drops (antazoline/naphazoline 0.5/0.05%: 1 drop q.i.d. PRN)
- SAC/PAC: Topical antihistamine (levocabastine 0.05%, emedastine 0.05% q.i.d. OU), mast cell stabilizer (lodoxamide 0.1% or pemirolast 0.1% q.i.d.), or antihistamine with mast cell stabilizing properties (olopatadine 0.1% b.i.d. or 0.2% per day, azelastineepinastine 0.05%, ketotifen 0.025%, or bepotastine 1.5% b.i.d.)
- VKC/AKC: Topical steroid (prednisolone acetate up to 8 times per day) in addition to mast cell stabilizer or antihistamine with mast cell stabilizing properties. Topical steroids should be tapered to least possible dosing.
- GPC: in mild cases, modification of lens hygiene and use may be sufficient. Contact lens holiday or limitation of use. Antihistamine or mast cell stabilizer may help with symptoms. Use of enzymatic lens cleaners to remove surface debris from contact lenses

Second Line

- SAC/PAC: Topical steroid may be used in severe cases. Oral antihistamines used in systemic disease may help with ocular symptoms.
- VKC/AKC: Oral steroid or antihistamine in addition to the above measures. Topical cyclosporine A (i.e., restasis or up to 2% compound)

ADDITIONAL TREATMENT

General Measures

Avoid allergens. Seek cool climate, air-conditioned environment.

Issues for Referral

Corneal involvement. Vision threatening disease.

Additional Therapies

- Artificial tears to soothe the ocular surface. In VKC or AKC, artificial tears may prevent epithelial breakdown.
  - Preservative-free artificial tears may be used frequently (i.e., every 1–2 h).

SURGERY/OTHER PROCEDURES

VKC/AKC: Superficial keratectomy may be indicated if corneal plaque develops. Occlusive therapy (i.e., tarsorrhaphy) may be helpful in persistent epithelial defect/ulcer refractory to other measures.

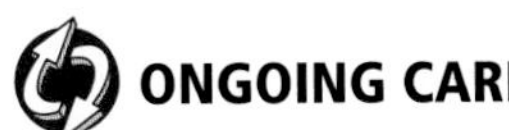

ONGOING CARE

FOLLOW-UP RECOMMENDATIONS

VKC and AKC should be followed closely for corneal involvement and risk to vision.

Patient Monitoring

Monitor vision. With topical steroid use, monitor intraocular pressure and lens changes.

PATIENT EDUCATION

Risks of topical steroid use include glaucoma, cataract formation, and predisposition to infection.

PROGNOSIS

- SAC/PAC/GPC: good prognosis
- VKC/AKC: prognosis can be guarded with corneal involvement.

COMPLICATIONS

- Corneal complications (scarring, pannus). Loss of vision.
  - Most likely to occur with VKC or AKC

REFERENCES

1. Allansmith M, Ross R. Ocular allergy and mast cell stabilizers. *Surv Ophthalmol* 1986;30(4):229–244.
2. Bielory L, Friedlaender M. Allergic conjunctivitis. *Immunol Allergy Clin N Am* 2008;28(1):43–58.
3. Bleik J, Tabbara K. Topical cyclosporine in vernal keratoconjunctivitis. *Ophthalmology* 1991;98(11): 1679–1684.
4. Foster C, Calonge M. Atopic keratoconjunctivitis. *Ophthalmology* 1990;97(8):992–1000.

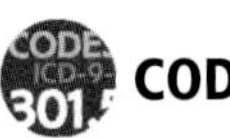

CODES

ICD9

- 372.05 Acute atopic conjunctivitis
- 372.13 Vernal conjunctivitis
- 372.14 Other chronic allergic conjunctivitis

ALPORT SYNDROME

Christopher M. Fecarotta

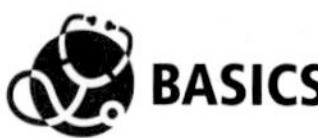

BASICS

DESCRIPTION

- Alport syndrome is a genetic disease characterized by glomerulonephritis, sensorineural hearing loss, and ocular changes.
- Patients often progress to end-stage renal failure and high-tone deafness by age 40.
- Common ocular associations include a dot-and-fleck retinopathy, anterior lenticonus, and posterior polymorphous corneal dystrophy.
- Less common ocular associations include other corneal dystrophies, ulceration, microcornea, arcus, iris atrophy, cataracts, spontaneous lens rupture, spherophakia, a poor macular reflex, fluorescein angiogram hyperfluorescence, electrooculogram and electroretinogram abnormalities, and retinal pigmentation.

EPIDEMIOLOGY

Prevalence

- 1 in 5000 people has one of the forms of Alport syndrome.
- Alport syndrome accounts for approximately 2.1% of pediatric patients with end-stage renal failure.
- Over 85% of Alport syndrome patients are male.

RISK FACTORS

Genetics

- Alport syndrome is usually X-linked recessive.
- Less common autosomal recessive and autosomal dominant forms exist.
- Patients typically harbor a mutation in one of the genes for type IV collagen.
  - COL4A5 (most common)
  - COL4A4
  - COL4A3

GENERAL PREVENTION

Genetic counseling

PATHOPHYSIOLOGY

Type IV collagen is the major structural component of basement membranes found in the glomerulus, cochlea, cornea, and retina.

ETIOLOGY

Many different mutations involving disruption of tertiary and quaternary structure of type IV collagen cause Alport syndrome. The most common mutation involves a substitution for glycine in the a5(IV) chain of type IV collagen that results in a misshapen protein.

COMMONLY ASSOCIATED CONDITIONS

- Hematuria:
  - Most common presenting symptom
- Proteinuria
- Nephrotic syndrome
- End-stage renal failure:
  - Due to chronic glomerulonephritis
  - Associated anemia and osteodystrophy
- Hypertension:
  - Due to chronic renal failure
- High-frequency sensorineural hearing loss:
  - Begins by late childhood or early adolescence
  - Extends to low frequency as the disease progresses
- Myopia
- Posterior polymorphous corneal dystrophy
- Dot-and-fleck retinal dystrophy:
  - Usually asymptomatic
- Anterior lenticonus:
  - Highly suggestive of Alport syndrome once trauma has been excluded
- Other ocular conditions as mentioned above
- Diffuse leiomyomatosis of the esophagus and trachea
- Vulvar and clitoral leiomyomatosis in females

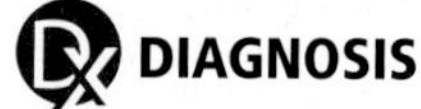

DIAGNOSIS

HISTORY

- Hematuria is the most common presenting symptom.
  - Childhood microscopic hematuria
  - Episodes of gross hematuria associated with upper respiratory infections
- Hearing loss
- Poor vision
- Family history of juvenile renal failure, hearing loss, or vision loss

PHYSICAL EXAM

- Hypertension
- Edema from nephrotic syndrome
- Evidence of known ophthalmic manifestations

DIAGNOSTIC TESTS & INTERPRETATION

Diagnostic Procedures/Other

- Urine analysis:
  - Microscopic or gross hematuria
  - Dysmorphic RBCs with casts
  - Proteinuria
- Electrolytes, BUN, creatinine:
  - Reflect level of renal insufficiency
- Renal ultrasound:
  - Rule out other conditions
  - Normal early in disease course, may show progressive atrophy
- High-frequency audiometry
- Ophthalmologic examination
- Renal biopsy
- Genetic analysis:
  - Can diagnose the carrier state as well

Pathological Findings

Nonspecific renal histology. Electron microscopy, however, reveals a characteristic thickening of the glomerular basement membrane that is directly proportional to the patient's age and severity of proteinuria.

DIFFERENTIAL DIAGNOSIS

- Dot-and-fleck retinopathy must be differentiated from other inherited retinopathies, hypertensive changes, choroidal infarcts, and vasculitic changes.
- Anterior lenticonus must be differentiated from age-related nuclear sclerosis.
- Differential diagnosis of posterior polymorphous corneal dystrophy includes Fuchs corneal dystrophy, congenital hereditary corneal dystrophy, Axenfeld-Rieger syndrome, and congenital glaucoma.

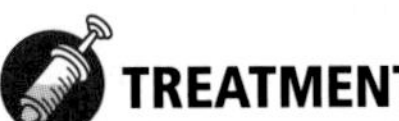

TREATMENT

ADDITIONAL TREATMENT

General Measures

- Address refractive error with glasses or contact lenses
- Cataract surgery for visually significant lenticular changes
- Complications from posterior polymorphous corneal dystrophy should be managed on an individual basis. Some patients are asymptomatic while others require corneal transplantation for severe visual impairment.
- Dot-and-fleck retinal changes are asymptomatic and do not require treatment.
- Kidney transplant or dialysis for renal failure
- Hearing aids for sensorineural hearing loss

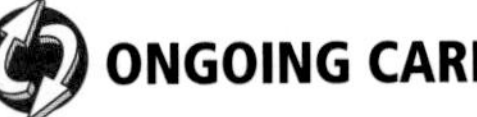

ONGOING CARE

FOLLOW-UP RECOMMENDATIONS

- Ophthalmologist
- Nephrologist
- Audiologist
- Screen family members for microscopic hematuria

PATIENT EDUCATION

- The Alport Syndrome Foundation (http://www.alportsyndrome.org)

PROGNOSIS

- 90% of male patients with X-linked Alport syndrome develop renal failure and are deaf by age 40.
- Progression to renal failure and deafness in females is less likely.
- Visual impairment is variable.

COMPLICATIONS

- Visual loss
- Renal failure
- Sensorineural hearing loss

ADDITIONAL READING

- Govan JA. Ocular manifestations of Alport syndrome: A hereditary disorder of basement membranes. *Br J Ophthalmol* 1983;67:493–503.
- Colville DJ, Savige J. Alport syndrome: A review of the ocular manifestations. *Ophthalmic Genet* 1997;18(4):161–173.
- Flinter F. Alport syndrome. *J Med Genet* 1997;34(4): 326–330.
- Kashtan CE. Alport syndrome and thin glomerular basement membrane disease. *J Am Soc Nephrol* 1998;9(9):1736–1750.

CODES

ICD9

- 362.10 Background retinopathy, unspecified
- 743.36 Congenital anomalies of lens shape
- 759.89 Other specified congenital anomalies

CLINICAL PEARLS

- Anterior lenticonus and posterior polymorphic corneal dystrophy are highly suggestive of Alport syndrome.
- Patients with an established diagnosis of Alport syndrome should have regular ophthalmologic exams.
- Renal failure and sensorineural hearing loss are the most common associations.
- Hematuria is the most common presenting symptom.

AMAURORSIS FUGAX

Brandon B. Johnson
Lov Sarin

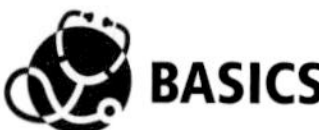

BASICS

DESCRIPTION

Amaurosis fugax is defined as transient monocular visual loss secondary to ischemia or vascular insufficiency.

EPIDEMIOLOGY

Incidence

50,000 new cases a year in the United States (2)[C]

RISK FACTORS

- Hypertension
- Hypercholesterolemia
- Smoking
- Diabetes

GENERAL PREVENTION

Lifestyle choices such as diet, exercise, and smoking cessation can help mitigate risk factors.

PATHOPHYSIOLOGY

- Transient ischemia to the retina or optic nerve results in visual field loss for seconds to minutes.
  - Field loss generally begins in upper field and sometimes in the lower field and periphery.
  - Patchy or sectorial field loss may occur.
  - Recurrent events tend to follow the same pattern.
  - Full visual recovery often occurs.

ETIOLOGY

- Thromboembolic:
  - Transient disruption in the ophthalmic circulation due to atherosclerotic emboli from ipsilateral common carotid artery and its branches.
  - Cardiac embolism may result from valvular disease secondary to rheumatic heart disease, mitral valve prolapse, marantic or infectious endocarditis, and calcific valve disease.
- Hemodynamic:
  - Change in posture, exercise, exposure to bright light in the setting of extensive atherosclerotic arterial occlusive disease especially involving aortic arch branches
  - Hypoperfusion secondary to low cardiac output or acute hypovolemia
  - Alteration of blood flow from systemic disturbance of blood viscosity, cellularity, or coagulability
  - Vasospasm or retinal arterial system leading to retinal migraine
- Ocular vascular disease:
  - Anterior ischemic optic neuropathy due to giant cell arteritis, atherosclerosis, or thrombosis secondary to acute occlusion or severe narrowing of the posterior ciliary arteries leading to acute optic nerve head ischemia
  - Central retinal vein occlusion can begin with amaurotic episodes due to slowing of retinal arterial circulation as the central retinal vein is occluded.
  - Malignant arterial hypertension can cause optic nerve head ischemia.

COMMONLY ASSOCIATED CONDITIONS

- Carotid occlusive disease
- Valvular heart disease

DIAGNOSIS

HISTORY

- Determine if the visual symptoms are consistent with amaurosis.
- Patients describe decreased vision progressing over seconds and lasting for seconds to minutes.
  - Monocular vision loss generally occurs for seconds to minutes and recovers completely.
  - Visual loss may occur like a "curtain."
  - Upper field affected>lower field>periphery.
- Ask for symptoms concerning giant cell arteritis (in patients over 55).
  - Scalp tenderness
  - Fever
  - Weight loss
  - Jaw claudication
  - Proximal muscle weakness

PHYSICAL EXAM

- Measure blood pressure, heart rate, and rhythm
- Auscultation of heart and carotid arteries
- Palpation of temporal arteries
- Complete ophthalmic exam with dilated fundus exam by an ophthalmologist or neuro-ophthalmologist
  - Assess pupillary reactions, and look for afferent pupillary defect
  - Ocular signs of ischemia:
    - Retinal pallor
    - Hemorrhages
    - Distended veins
    - Microaneurysms
    - Cotton wool spots
    - Hollenhorst plaques

DIAGNOSTIC TESTS & INTERPRETATION

Lab

Initial lab tests

- Workup for amaurosis should commence without delay and rule out giant cell arteritis and to evaluate for occult cardiac disease
  - Complete blood count
  - Erythrocyte sedimentation rate
  - C-reactive protein
  - Lipid panel
  - Diabetes workup
  - Consider workup for hypercoagulable state: Factor V Leiden, lupus anticoagulant, deficiency of protein C/protein S/antithrombin III.

Imaging

Initial approach

- Duplex ultrasound of carotid arteries:
  - Identify occlusion, stenosis, and ulceration at carotid bifurcation.
  - Consider cerebral CT or MR angiography to evaluate for embolic disease.
  - Fluorescein angiography can document retinal ischemia if results of initial imaging are negative.
  - Carotid angiography is indicated when duplex reveals stenosis but not when the study is normal (4)[A].
  - Echocardiogram is indicated to identify cardiac embolic sources.

Follow-up & special considerations

Patient should follow up with their primary care physician for a thorough systemic evaluation.

Diagnostic Procedures/Other

Further cardiac workup should include EKG and possible Holter monitor.

Pathological Findings

Atheromatous carotid plaques are generally composed of platelet-fibrin thrombi, cholesterol crystals, calcification, and lipid deposition.

DIFFERENTIAL DIAGNOSIS

- Embolic:
  - Carotid bifurcation thromboembolism
  - Great vessel or distal internal carotid artery atheroembolism
  - Cardiac emboli (valve, mural thrombi, intracardiac tumor)
  - Drug abuse-related intravascular emboli
- Hemodynamic:
  - Extensive atheromatous occlusive disease
  - Inflammatory arteritis (Takayasu's disease)
  - Hypoperfusion (cardiac failure, acute hypovolemia, disturbance of blood viscosity, coagulability, or content)
- Ocular:
  - Anterior ischemic optic neuropathy
  - Central or branch retinal artery occlusion
  - Central retinal vein occlusion
  - Nonvascular (vitreous floaters, hemorrhage, angle closure glaucoma, tumor, congenital anomalies of optic disc such as drusen and staphyloma)
- Neurologic:
  - Brainstem, vestibular, oculomotor lesions
  - Optic neuritis, optic nerve, or chiasm compression
  - Papilledema
  - Multiple sclerosis
  - Migraine
  - Psychogenic
- Idiopathic

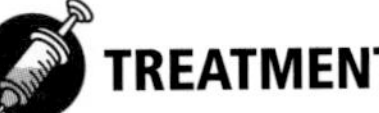

TREATMENT

MEDICATION

- Aspirin 300–325 mg/day reduces stroke prevalence and further transient ischemic attack (TIA) in patients with TIA (4)[A].
  - Address modifiable risk factors such as hypertension, hypercholesterolemia, and smoking
  - Carotid stenosis <50%
  - Aspirin and risk factor treatment (4)[A]
  - Cardio embolism requires appropriate management such as anticoagulation for mural thrombus, aspirin for mitral valve prolapse, etc.
  - Patients with clinical and laboratory evidence of giant cell arteritis (elevated ESR/CRP/platelets) should be placed on high-dose corticosteroids and referred to vascular surgery or oculoplastics for temporal artery biopsy.

ADDITIONAL TREATMENT

General Measures

- It is of upmost importance to recognize ocular vascular diseases that can present with amaurosis.
  - Arteritic anterior ischemic optic neuropathy (giant cell arteritis)
  - Glaucoma (especially angle closure)

SURGERY/OTHER PROCEDURES

- Carotid stenosis 50–70%:
  - Treatment is controversial. Aspirin and risk factor treatment. Carotid endarterectomy is indicated in patients with associated TIA or minor stroke, cerebral infarction on MR or CT, retinal emboli, carotid bulb ulceration, and failure of aspirin therapy (4)[A].
- Carotid stenosis >70%:
  - Carotid endarterectomy is indicated (3)[A].

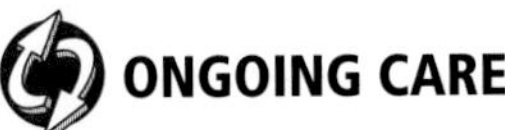

ONGOING CARE

PROGNOSIS

- Annual incidence of stroke in patients with amaurosis is 2% (3).
- 95% of endarterectomy patients are free of ipsilateral stroke for 8 years (1).

COMPLICATIONS

The rate of stroke and death associated with carotid endarterectomy is 6.5% (4).

REFERENCES

1. Berstein EF, Dilley RB. Late results following carotid endarterectomy for amaurosis fugax. *J Vasc Surg* 1987;6:333–340.
2. Brown RD, Petty GW, O'Fallon WM, et al. Incidence of transient ischemic attack in Rochester, Minnesota, 1985–1989. *Stroke* 1998;29:2109–2113.
3. Ferguson GG. The North American Symptomatic Carotid Endarterectomy Trial: Surgical results in 1415 patients. *Stroke* 1999;30:1751–1758.
4. Poole CJM, Ross Russell RW. Mortality and stoke after amaurosis fugax. *J Neurol Neurosurg Psychiatry* 1985;48:902–905.

ADDITIONAL READING

- Benavente O, Eliasziw M, Streifler JY, et al. Prognosis after transient monocular blindness associated with carotid-artery stenosis. *N Engl J Med* 2001;345:1084–1090.
- The Amaurosis Fugax Study Group. Current management of amaurosis fugax. *Stroke* 1990; 23(2):201–208.

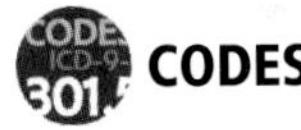

CODES

ICD9

362.34 Transient retinal arterial occlusion

AMBLYOPIA

Kammi B. Gunton

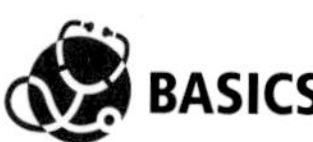

BASICS

DESCRIPTION

- Decreased best-corrected visual acuity not solely attributable to organic pathology affecting one or both eyes:
  - Reduction in vision occurs during the first decade of life and is reversible with treatment during this critical window of visual development.

EPIDEMIOLOGY

Incidence

It is the leading cause of monocular visual loss in young and middle-aged Americans.

Prevalence

- Affects 2–4% of North American population
- Projected lifetime risk of visual loss in patients with amblyopia is 1.2%

RISK FACTORS

- Anisometropia, odds ratio of 29 (1) – if
  - >1.50 diopter (D) hyperopic spherical equivalent
  - >+1.00 D cylinder
  - >–6.00 D myopia
- Strabismus
- High refractive error in both eyes:
  - >+5.00
  - >–10.00 D
  - >3.5 D cylinder
- Organic pathology uncorrected in critical window in the first decade

Genetics

- Follows the pattern of inheritance for the risk factors
- May be familial predisposition for amblyopia but no specific inheritance pattern

GENERAL PREVENTION

- Visual screening of all children during the vulnerable age period allows for detection and treatment.
  - Pediatrician or family physician well child visits
  - School nurses

PATHOPHYSIOLOGY

- Unequal visual competition between eyes leads to the following:
  - Within the lateral geniculate nucleus, cells from the amblyopic eye atrophy
  - Within the primary visual cortex, cells lose ability to respond to stimuli of one or both eyes.

ETIOLOGY

- Strabismus, 38% (2)
- Anisometropia, 37% (2)
- Combined strabismus and anisometropia, 24% (2)
- Organic pathology uncorrected in critical window of visual development
- Congenital media opacities create most dense form of amblyopia.

COMMONLY ASSOCIATED CONDITIONS

- Anisometropia
- Strabismus
- High refractive error
- Asymmetric or unilateral media opacities or other forms of visual pathway interruption

DIAGNOSIS

HISTORY

- Presence of anisometropia, strabismus, combined anisometropia and strabismus, or organic pathology that reduces vision in one eye:
  - Above condition must be present during window of visual development.
  - Subnormal vision unexplained on the basis of physical abnormalities in the eye and in the setting of the condition known to result in amblyopia.

PHYSICAL EXAM

- At least 2 line difference in visual acuity between eyes
- Crowding phenomenon results in reduction in vision when tested by multiple optotypes or crowding bars around isolated line of optotypes.
  - Grating acuity better than expected in strabismic amblyopia
  - Low contrast visual acuity better than expected in strabismic amblyopia
- Testing with single optotypes may show better vision than testing with lines of ootypes.
- Strong fixation preference in preverbal children
- Evaluation for strabismus
- Cycloplegic refraction
- Complete dilated ocular exam to rule out the presence of organic causes of visual loss

DIAGNOSTIC TESTS & INTERPRETATION

Lab

None

Imaging

- Usually none indicated unless ruling out the presence of organic central nervous system cause for subnormal vision.
- OCT may be useful in detecting subtle organic retinal or optic nerve causes of subnormal vision.

Diagnostic Procedures/Other

- Contrast sensitivity testing may be useful.
- Electrodiagnostic testing, especially multifocal electroretinography, may be useful to detect underlying organic retinal disease.
- Visual evoked potentials may be useful in detecting asymmetry or organic deficits.
- In severe amblyopia, asymmetry in the 30-lead visual evoked potential may be seen (test rarely needed).

Pathological Findings

Decrease in the cell size of the parvocellular layer of lateral geniculate nucleus laminae from amblyopic eye

DIFFERENTIAL DIAGNOSIS

- Incorrect refractive correction
- Organic pathology responsible for visual loss
- Failure to comply with patching/penalization results in uncorrected visual deficit.

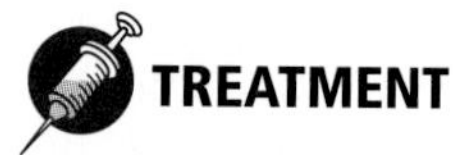

TREATMENT

MEDICATION

First Line

None indicated

Second Line

L-Dopa supplementation during amblyopia treatment under investigation. Improvement of additional 2 lines with L-Dopa supplementation following standard treatment (6). Improvement in the spatial extent of visual cortex activation with stimulation of amblyopic eye with L-Dopa demonstrated on MRI (7). Proper dosage is critical due to frequent side effects of nausea and emesis.

ADDITIONAL TREATMENT

General Measures

- Treatment of etiology of amblyopia
- Refractive correction
- Correction of strabismus
- Correction of organic pathology if possible, e.g. cataract extraction, ptosis repair, corneal transplant
- Amblyopia treatment may still be needed after organic deficit corrected.
- Occlusion of nonamblyopic eye
- Comparing all-day patching to fewer hours of patching revealed faster improvement in visual acuity with greater number of hours of daily patching, but by 6 months, the differences in improvement were not statistically significant (5).
- Atropine penalization to nonamblyopic eye with spectacle correction as applicable: Requires ability to blur better eye to a visual acuity less than the amblyopic eye. Works best for hyperopic eye.
- Improvement in visual acuity 3.6 lines with atropine compared to 3.7 lines with patching at 6 months in children younger than 7 with moderate amblyopia (8)

Issues for Referral

- Refer for surgical correction of organic causes (e.g., cataract)
- May require collaboration with primary care physician regarding behavioral issues secondary to patching and patching compliance issues

Additional Therapies

- There is no additional benefit of adding near activities during amblyopia treatment (9).
- Alternatives to adhesive patch include spectacle-mounted occluder, opaque contact lens, or Bangerter foils.
- Compliance with patching may require adhesion supplements (e.g., benzoin, Tegaderm, tape) or arm immobilization.

COMPLEMENTARY & ALTERNATIVE THERAPIES

- None
- No studies prove efficacy of vision therapy.

SURGERY/OTHER PROCEDURES

Laser refractive correction under investigation in severe anisometropia in noncompliant children.

IN-PATIENT CONSIDERATIONS

Admission Criteria

In-patient admission has rarely been used to facilitate occlusion therapy in recalcitrant children.

ONGOING CARE

FOLLOW-UP RECOMMENDATIONS

Patient Monitoring

- Follow up to ensure compliance and prevent occlusion amblyopia.
- Check vision of both eyes during each visit:
  - With full-time patching, follow-up interval is 1 week for every year of age to a maximum of 4 weeks.
  - With part-time patching, wider intervals are acceptable but not >2–3 months. Younger children require shorter intervals.
  - Consider treatment end point of full correction achieved with the normalization of vision or lack of improvement following 3 successive intervals of compliant treatment.
- Recommend taper of occlusion following maximal improvement in visual acuity (treatment end point).

PATIENT EDUCATION

- Importance of compliance with treatment
- Anticipatory guidance regarding anticipated behavioral resistance to patching and strategies for successful patching (e.g., positive reinforcement, behavioral modification)
- www.pgcfa.org

PROGNOSIS

- 82% of patients maintain increased acuity of within 10 letters after cessation of treatment (10).
- Patching 2 h daily with spectacle correction improves visual acuity 2.2 lines compared to 1.3 lines with spectacle correction alone in children 3–7 years of age (4).
- Improvement in vision of >2 lines is shown with spectacle correction alone with follow-up in 77% patients (3).
- Improvement in vision continues on average 30 weeks before stabilization (3).
- Improvement correlates with less anisometropia and better baseline visual acuity (3).
- 46% of patients achieve 20/25 or better with patching or atropine (11).
- Either 20/30 in amblyopic eye or 3 log-Mar lines of improvement in visual acuity is shown by 6 months with patching or atropine in >74%.
- Moderate amblyopia (vision better than 20/100) has better prognosis.
- Treatment prior to 7 years of age has better prognosis.

COMPLICATIONS

- Occlusion or penalization therapy can uncommonly cause visual loss (usually reversible) in the initially normal eye. Treat by decreasing or discontinuing treatment. May require switching treatment to other eye.
- Patches can cause periocular allergic skin rashes. Consider switching brands.
- Patches can cause periocular skin abrasions. Treat with micropore tape under patch or temporary discontinuation.
- Atropine may cause systemic side effects.
- Psychosocial repercussions of patching or anisometropia from atropine

REFERENCES

1. Huynh SC, Wang XY, Ip J, et al. Prevalence and associations of anisometropic and aniso-astigmatism in a population based sample of 6 year old children. *Br J Ophthalmol* 2006;90: 597–601.
2. Pediatric Eye Disease Investigator Group. The clinical profile of moderate amblyopia in children younger than 7 years. *Arch Ophthalmol* 2002; 120:281–287.
3. Pediatric Eye Disease Investigator Group. Treatment of anisometropic amblyopia in children with refractive correction. *Ophthalmology* 2006; 113:895–903.
4. Pediatric Eye Disease Investigator Group. A randomized trial to evaluate two hours of daily patching for amblyopia in children. *Ophthalmology* 2006;113:904–912.
5. Pediatric Eye Disease Investigator Group. A comparison of atropine and patching treatments for moderate amblyopia by patient age, cause of amblyopia, depth of amblyopia and other factors. *Ophthalmology* 2003;110:1632–1637.
6. Dadeya S, Vats P, Malik KPS. Levodopa/carbidopa in the treatment of amblyopia. *J Pediatr Ophthalmol Strabismus* 2009;46:87–90.
7. Yang C, Yang M, Huang J, et al. Functional MRI of amblyopia before and after levodopa. *Neurosci Lett* 2003;339:49–52.
8. Pediatric Eye Disease Investigator Group. Two-year follow-up of a 6-month randomized trial of atropine vs patching for treatment of moderate amblyopia in children. *Arch Ophthalmol* 2005; 123:149–157.
9. Pediatric Eye Disease Investigator Group. A randomized trial of near versus distance activities while patching for amblyopia in children aged 3 to 7 years. *Ophthalmology* 2008;115:2071–2078.
10. Pediatric Eye Disease Investigator Group. Stability of visual acuity improvement following discontinuation of amblyopia treatment in children 7 to 12 years old. *Arch Ophthalmol* 2007;125:655–659.
11. Pediatric Eye Disease Investigator Group. A randomized trial of atropine versus patching for treatment of moderate amblyopia: Follow-up at 10 years of age. *Arch Ophthalmol* 2008;126: 1039–1044.

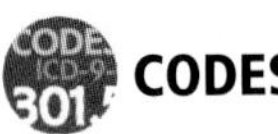

CODES

ICD9

- 368.00 Amblyopia, unspecified
- 368.01 Strabismic amblyopia
- 368.03 Refractive amblyopia

CLINICAL PEARLS

- Screening to detect amblyopia early is of paramount importance.
- Compliance with occlusive treatment is more important than the type of occlusion utilized.
- Appropriate refractive correction is vital to all treatments.
- Treatment of underlying organic etiologies is essential.

AMD-DRY

Brad Ballard
Mark L. Nelson

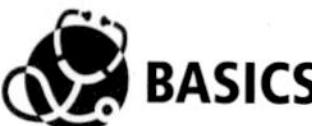

BASICS

DESCRIPTION

- Dry age-related macular degeneration (AMD) is a leading cause of severe vision loss in elderly populations of European descent. Dry AMD causes approximately half of permanent vision loss in older Caucasian patients in the US.
- Retinal findings include drusen, pigmentary changes, and geographic atrophy.
- AMD is a degenerative condition which affects the outer retina, as well as the retinal pigment epithelium (RPE), Bruch's membrane, and the choriocapillaris.

Geriatric Considerations

This is a disease that predominantly affects patients over the age of 65 years. While non-neovascular AMD is less likely to cause severe vision loss than neovascular macular degeneration, it is still a significant cause of legal blindness in patients over 65 years old.

EPIDEMIOLOGY

Incidence

- The 5-year incidence of large drusen or pigmentary changes average 8.7% (ranging from 3.2% in people less than 60 years, and 18.3% in people in their 70s).
- Population studies showed the 5-year incidence of advanced AMD to be 1.1% with 0% in ages less than 60 years, and 5.4% in those older than 80 years.
- Progression of disease from drusen and pigmentary changes to advanced AMD including neovascular AMD increases with age.

Prevalence

Over 8 million people in the US have early AMD of whom 1 million will develop advanced AMD in the next 5 years.

RISK FACTORS

- Age is the most important risk factor
- Family history
- Caucasian ancestry
- Smoking is an important modifiable risk factor
- Studies have been inconsistent about the role of body-mass-index, cardiovascular disease, hypertension, HDL, and total cholesterol.
- Very light pigmentation and blue irides may increase risk.

Genetics

- Population studies with twins and family members have shown a familial component
- Complement Factor H (CFH), complement factor B, HTRA1 on chr. 10q26 all predispose to AMD with CFH being most important.

GENERAL PREVENTION

- AREDS (Age-Related Eye Disease Study) showed antioxidant vitamin supplementation can decrease progression of moderate to severe AMD.
  - Patients with a higher intake of dark, green leafy vegetables and omega-3 fatty acids have a lower risk of developing AMD.
  - Smoking cessation is critical.

PATHOPHYSIOLOGY

- Degenerative changes involving outer portions of the retina, RPE, and Bruch's membrane, and less severely, the choriocapillaris
- The earliest signs may be basal deposits in the RPE and between the RPE and Bruch's membrane.
- Drusen develop because of these deposits and changes in the RPE.
- Hard drusen are PAS-positive nodules between the RPE and Bruch's membrane.
- Soft drusen are eosinophilic deposits adjacent to Bruch's membrane.
- Whether photoreceptor atrophy occurs primarily or secondarily to changes in Bruch's membrane and the RPE, is not known.
- Recent evidence cites A2E, a component of lipofuscin, as a possible pathologic link leading to RPE apoptosis

ETIOLOGY

The nexus of a high photic and oxygen environment in highly metabolic tissue, creates a milieu rife for free radical formation and oxidative damage. Pathologic changes and deposits in Bruch's membrane and the RPE lead to structural changes that lead to AMD. Despite the prevalence of AMD, the etiology is not well understood.

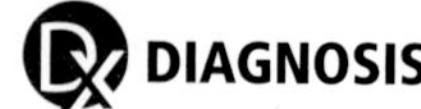

DIAGNOSIS

HISTORY

- Many times patients are asymptomatic and are diagnosed on a routine eye examination.
- Symptoms suggest more advanced disease and include metamorphopsia and gradual impairment of vision over months to years.
- AMD is bilateral but may be asymmetric.
- Sudden visual changes or metamorphopsia in patients with dry AMD may signify progression to exudative AMD.

PHYSICAL EXAM

- Signs of AMD include drusen, RPE changes, incipient and geographic atrophy, and, in cases of exudative AMD, fluid, hard exudates, hemorrhage, and choroidal neovascular membrane (CNV).
- Drusen are classified as small ($<64\ \mu m$), medium ($64–124\ \mu m$), and large ($>124\ \mu m$) or as hard (discrete well demarcated), soft (poorly demarcated), and confluent (contiguous boundaries).
- The RPE shows geographic or non-geographic atrophy and focal hyperpigmentation.
- Geographic atrophy is described as well demarcated areas of RPE loss. Non-geographic atrophy is less well defined and has a more mottled appearance. Focal hyperpigmentation occurs at the outer retina.
- Early AMD is defined as multiple small or intermediate drusen with no evidence of advanced AMD.
- Intermediate AMD is defined as extensive intermediate drusen or 1 large drusen.
- Advanced AMD is defined as presence of geographic atrophy or signs of wet AMD.

DIAGNOSTIC TESTS & INTERPRETATION

Imaging

Initial approach

- Optical coherence tomography (OCT), color photographs, and fluorescein angiography (FA) can be used to document and follow progression of AMD.
- FA can show both hyper- and hypofluorescent areas. Hyperfluorescent lesions include RPE atrophy, RPE tears, CNV, pigment epithelial detachments (PED), and subretinal fibrosis. Hypofluorescent lesions are seen with hemorrhage, lipid deposits, and focal hyperpigmentation. Hemorrhage, fluid, and CNV are hallmarks of exudative (wet) AMD.

- FA can be used when acute visual changes occur to assess for possible progression to exudative AMD.
- OCT can show CNV, edema, subretinal fluid, PED, and drusen as well as delineate areas of RPE atrophy.
- Fundus autofluorescence photography shows areas of RPE loss and surrounding damaged RPE. It is an evolving method of imaging patients with dry AMD.

Follow-up & special considerations

- Risk of progression to wet AMD can be calculated using the AREDS simplified severity score. The score is calculated for each eye
  - Large Drusen – 1 point
  - Pigment abnormalities – 1 point
  - Bilateral intermediate drusen – 1 point
  - Advanced AMD in one eye – 2 points
- 0 factors – 1.5%, 1 factor – 3%, 2 factors – 12%, 3 factors – 25%, 4 factors – 50%

DIFFERENTIAL DIAGNOSIS

Central serous chorioretinopathy, pattern dystrophy of the RPE, Best's disease, idiopathic juxtafoveal telangiectasia, and central areolar dystrophy

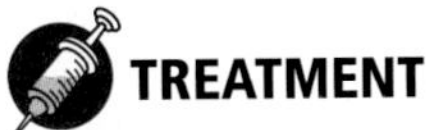

TREATMENT

MEDICATION

First Line

The AREDS study showed vitamins can slow progression of disease. The AREDS formulation is daily administration of 500 mg Vitamin C, 400 IU Vitamin E, 15 mg beta carotene, 80 mg zinc oxide, and 2 mg cupric oxide (to prevent zinc induced anemia).

ALERT

- Use of beta carotene is not recommended in smokers or lung cancer survivors as it may increase risk of lung cancer.
- AREDS showed that patients with intermediate or advanced AMD benefited from vitamin supplementation. There is no data to support a beneficial effect of vitamins in those with no or early AMD.
- Reductions in modifiable risk factors are encouraged, especially smoking cessation. Reducing BMI and controlling cholesterol and cardiovascular risk factors may help reduce the progression of AMD.

Second Line

Lutein, zeaxanthin, and long chain unsaturated fatty acids are currently being investigated in the AREDS 2 study.

ADDITIONAL TREATMENT

General Measures

- Laser photocoagulation
  - Laser photocoagulation has no role in nonexudative AMD. A controlled trial showed that it reduces drusen, but there was no reduction in risk for development of advanced AMD. Laser photocoagulation appears to increase risk of CNV.
- Amsler grid
  - Patients should be given a copy of an Amsler grid and should check the vision in one eye at a time on a regular basis to detect any subtle distortions or blurriness. They should seek ophthalmologic care if changes develop.

Issues for Referral

Patients with drusen, RPE changes, and/or geographic atrophy should have routine dilated examinations.

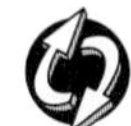

ONGOING CARE

FOLLOW-UP RECOMMENDATIONS

Patients should use their Amsler grid frequently and return for routine care based on AREDS risk. Development of distortion or central blur should lead to prompt evaluation.

DIET

- Patients are encouraged to eat a healthy diet low in saturated fats, as reducing cardiovascular risk factors may help reduce progression of AMD.
  - Foods high in omega 3 fatty acids, as well as dark, green leafy vegetables may reduce the risk of AMD.

PROGNOSIS

- Many patients with early AMD will maintain visual acuity for many years.
- Some patients will progress as they get older to more advanced forms of AMD as part of the natural history of the disease.
- The AREDS simplified severity score can be used to calculate risk of progression to advanced AMD.

ADDITIONAL READING

- Coleman HR, Chan CC, Ferris FL 3rd, et al. Age-related macular degeneration. *Lancet* 2008;372(9652):1835–1845.
- Mitchell P, Wang JJ, Foran S, Smith W. Five-year incidence of age-related maculopathy lesions: The Blue Mountains Eye Study. *Ophthalmology* 2002;109:1092–1097.
- Donaldson MJ, et. al. Treatment of nonexudative (dry) age-related macular degeneration. *Curr Opin Ophthalmol* 2006;17(3): 267–274.
- Age-Related Eye Disease Study Research Group. AREDS report 8. *Arch Ophthalmol* 2001;119:1417–1436.
- Ferris FL, Davis MD, Clemons TE, et al. Age-Related Eye Disease Study (AREDS) Research Group. A simplified severity scale for age-related macular degeneration: AREDS Report No. 18. *Arch Ophthalmol* 2005;123(11):1570–1574.

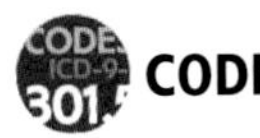

CODES

ICD9

- 362.51 Nonexudative senile macular degeneration of retina
- 362.57 Drusen (degenerative) of retina
- 362.89 Other retinal disorders

CLINICAL PEARLS

- AMD is the most common cause of legal blindness in elderly Caucasian individuals. It affects nearly 8 million people in the US.
- It is a degenerative condition involving the RPE, Bruch's membrane, and the outer retina.
- It is diagnosed by clinical examination showing drusen, pigmentary changes, and exudative markers in the retina-Bruch's membrane-choriocapillaris complex.
- Amsler grid testing, vitamin supplementation, modification of diet, and reduction in smoking are the only therapies to date to show consistent benefit.
- There is much research in the area of laser, micronutrients, neurotophic factors, stem cells, modifiable environmental factors, genetics, and other modalities to help prevent progression of AMD.

AMPPE (ACUTE MULTIFOCAL PLACOID PIGMENT EPITHELIOPATHY)

Marc J. Spirn

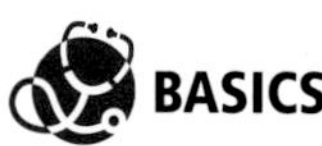

BASICS

DESCRIPTION

- Acquired multifocal inflammatory disorder affecting the retinal pigment epithelium (RPE) and choroid
- Frequently bilateral yellowish–white plaques, often in various stages of resolution

EPIDEMIOLOGY

Incidence

Unknown but rare

RISK FACTORS

Genetics

HLA-B7 and HLA-DR2 have been reported with increased frequency

PATHOPHYSIOLOGY

Believed to result from choroidal vascular obstruction

ETIOLOGY

Etiology is unknown but a viral prodrome occurs in one-third of patients

COMMONLY ASSOCIATED CONDITIONS

- Uveitis
- Retinal vasculitis
- Episcleritis
- Erythema nodosum
- Cerebral vasculitis

DIAGNOSIS

HISTORY

- Painless vision loss
- Viral prodrome occurs in one-third of patients

PHYSICAL EXAM

- Funduscopic examination reveals yellowish–white placoid lesions in the macula
  - Lesions are typically multiple, bilateral, and in various stages of resolution (resolution is denoted by RPE hyperplasia)
  - Lesions reside at the level of the RPE and choroid

DIAGNOSTIC TESTS & INTERPRETATION

Imaging

Fluorescein angiogram shows early hypofluorescence with late hyperfluorescence.

DIFFERENTIAL DIAGNOSIS

- Serpiginous choroiditis
- Relentless/Ampiginous chorioretinitis
- Ocular toxoplasmosis
- Sarcoidosis
- Ocular lymphoma
- Harada disease

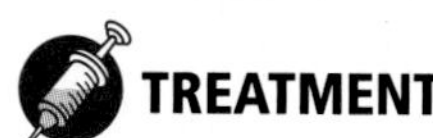

TREATMENT

MEDICATION

- Lesions typically resolve without medical treatment
- If lesions affect the fovea and vision is poor, it is reasonable (but unproven) to consider a short course of oral steroids

ADDITIONAL TREATMENT

Issues for Referral

- Suspected AMPPE should be referred to a retinal specialist to aid in diagnosis and care
- Mental status changes should prompt an immediate referral to a neurologist to rule out cerebral vasculitis

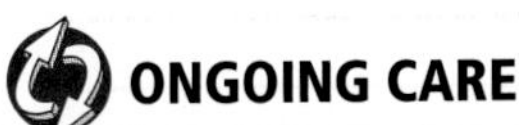

ONGOING CARE

FOLLOW-UP RECOMMENDATIONS

- Spontaneous resolution is the rule.
- Recurrence is possible but is rare. When multiple recurrences occur, a different diagnosis should be considered.

Patient Monitoring

Cerebral vasculitis is a rare associated finding. Mental status changes should prompt an immediate referral to a neurologist.

PROGNOSIS

Spontaneous recovery within 3–4 weeks is the norm. In rare instances, RPE changes in the macula can cause chronic vision loss.

ADDITIONAL READING

- Gass JDM. Acute posterior multifocal placoid pigment epitheliopathy. *Arch Ophthalmol* 1968;80:177–185.
- Heath JD. Acute posterior multifocal placoid pigment epitheliopathy. *Int Ophthalmol Clin* 1995;35(2):93–105.
- O'Halloran HS, Berger JR, Lee WB, et al. Acute multifocal placoid pigment epitheliopathy and central nervous system involvement: Nine new cases and a review of the literature. *Ophthalmology* 2001;108(5):861–8.

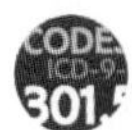

CODES

ICD9

363.15 Disseminated retinitis and retinochoroiditis, pigment epitheliopathy

CLINICAL PEARLS

- AMPPE is a self-limited inflammatory disease of the RPE and choroid
- Rarely AMPPE may be associated with life-threatening complications such as cerebral vasculitis
- Patients often recover significant visual acuity unless there are significant RPE changes in the fovea

ANGIOID STREAKS

Mark L. Nelson
Matthew R. Debiec

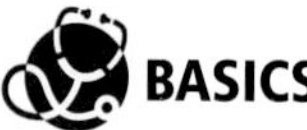

BASICS

DESCRIPTION

Irregular crack-like dehiscences in Bruch's membrane that can be associated with multiple systemic conditions. Significant sequelae include subretinal hemorrhage, choroidal rupture, and possible choroidal neovascularization (CNV).

EPIDEMIOLOGY

Incidence

- Incidence of angioid streaks is based on the underlying condition. Pseudoxanthoma elasticum (PXE), the most common underlying condition, has an incidence of 1 in 160,000.
  – Typically develops between the second and fifth decade of life.

Prevalence

Variable based on the underlying condition. Approximately one-third to half of cases have been reported to occur in patients with PXE. Of patients with PXE, more than 80% tend to have angioid streaks. Approximately 15% of patients with Paget's disease of bone and anywhere from 1–20% of patients with sickle-cell disease develop angioid streaks.

RISK FACTORS

- The most common diseases related to angioid streaks are pseudoxanthoma elasticum, Paget's disease of bone, sickle-cell anemia, and Ehlers-Danlos.
- Other diseases include:
  – Acquired hemochromatosis
  – Acromegaly
  – Diabetes mellitus
  – Acquired hemolytic anemia
  – Hereditary spherocytosis
  – Myopia
  – Neurofibromatosis
  – Sturge-Weber syndrome
  – Hyperphosphatemia
  – Senile elastosis
  – Tuberous sclerosis
  – Some patients have no identifiable systemic disease that can be attributed to angioid streaks and are considered to develop them idiopathically.

Genetics

- Varies based on the underlying condition causing angioid streaks.
  – Pseudoxanthoma elasticum, the most common associated condition, is due to an autosomal recessive or dominant mutation in the ABCC6 transporter gene.

GENERAL PREVENTION

- There are no treatments known to prevent angioid streaks in patients who may be at risk; some reports indicated increased complications following prophylactic laser therapy.
- Patients are susceptible to choroidal rupture following mild trauma and should be educated to wear protective eyewear.

PATHOPHYSIOLOGY

- The crack-like dehiscences are produced by alterations in Bruch's membrane, making it more prone to cracks. Full thickness breaks may allow CNV membranes to form.
- Subretinal hemorrhages can develop regardless of the presence of a CNV. Subretinal hemorrhage can follow traumatic breaks in Bruch's membrane and can disseminate toward the macula.

ETIOLOGY

Underlying genetic predisposition of the aforementioned conditions combined with possible unknown environmental or acquired risk factors lead to angioid streaks.

COMMONLY ASSOCIATED CONDITIONS

See risk factors above.

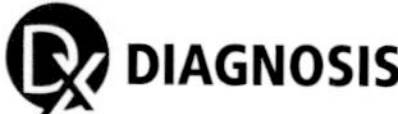

DIAGNOSIS

HISTORY

Angioid streaks are typically asymptomatic although they can present with metamorphopsia and decreased vision.

PHYSICAL EXAM

- Diagnosis is typically based on the characteristic funduscopic appearance, although imaging such as FA or ICG aid in diagnosis.
- Angioid streaks appear on exam as narrow jagged lines, deep to the retina, that radiate out from areas of peripapillary pigment alterations.
- The streaks are almost always bilateral and usually occur in the posterior pole. Width ranges from 50–500 μm. The color of the streaks varies and may range from dark red to brown.
- Eyes of patients with PXE may demonstrate peau d'orange, which is diffused mottling of the retinal pigmented epithelium (RPE) typically found temporal to the macula. These patients may also develop yellowish spots described as salmon spots at the level of the RPE.
- A choroidal neovascular membrane may develop at sites of angioid streaks and full thickness breaks in Bruch's membrane.
- Over two-thirds of patients with angioid streaks develop CNV at some point; however, this rate varies greatly depending on the clinical condition. While patients with PXE have the relative highest probability of macular CNV, patients with sickle-cell anemia tend to have a substantially lower rate of CNV.

DIAGNOSTIC TESTS & INTERPRETATION

Lab

- Laboratory work-up tends to center around evaluating for systemic conditions in those patients that do not have a predisposing diagnosis.
- A focused medical work up may include: Skin biopsy, x-ray imaging, hemoglobin electrophoresis, genetic testing, or blood work.

Imaging

Initial approach

- Fluorescein angiography (FA) is not necessary for diagnosis, but is extremely helpful in establishing the diagnosis in early streaks adjacent to the optic disc and in evaluating the development of CNV.
  – Angioid streaks will appear hyperfluorescent (window defect) in the early phase of FA.
  – CNV shows early hyperfluorescence and late staining.
- Indocyanine Green (ICG) angiography may be employed when both funduscopy and FA are equivocal, for example, in cases of extensive hemorrhages or severe RPE lesions. ICG angiography may show hyperfluorescent lines with pinpoints over their length.

Follow-up & special considerations

Patients with angioid streaks may require on-going follow up with FA to assess for development of CNV.

Pathological Findings

- Characteristic findings include irregular crack-like dehiscences in Bruch's membrane with atrophic degeneration of the overlying RPE.

- Eyes with angioid streaks have shown extensive calcification and thickening of Bruch's membrane with PXE and Paget's disease of bone, although this is not always found in other associated conditions. Bruch's membrane in Sickle hemoglobinopathies has demonstrated iron deposition in addition to calcification.
- The elastic lamina in the middle of Bruch's membrane is often affected with disintegration and fraying of the elastic fibers.

DIFFERENTIAL DIAGNOSIS

- Age-related macular degeneration
- Pathologic myopia
- Histoplasmosis
- Toxoplasmosis
- Retinal vasculitis
- Choroidal rupture

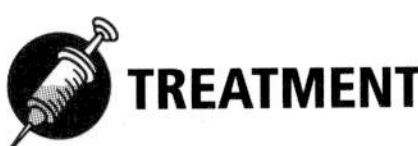

TREATMENT

MEDICATION

First Line

- More recently, off-label use of anti-vascular endothelial growth factor therapy such as pegaptanib, ranibizumab, and bevacizumab has been used to treat CNV.
  - Short-term studies have shown favorable results.
  - One study examining results of bevacizumab up to 24 months after initiation of therapy found recurrence of CNV in up to one-third of patients and new CNV lesions in 20% of patients.
- Risk of intravitreal injections in these eyes is not fully known.

ADDITIONAL TREATMENT

General Measures

- Laser photocoagulation to CNV lesions in patients with angioid streaks has modest results. Argon or Krypton laser photocoagulation is typically considered in eyes with extrafoveal or juxtafoveal CNV. Findings typically show moderate visual loss in eyes treated with laser photocoagulation and greater than 50% rate of persistence and/or recurrence. However, eyes with angioid streaks that are untreated and allowed to naturally progress have a very high rate of poor visual outcome, often with visual acuities of 20/200 or worse.
  - Prophylactic therapy of angioid streaks may actually induce more rapid progression to development of CNV.
- Photodynamic therapy (PDT) with verteporfin may be considered for eyes with subfoveal CNV. This therapy has been attempted in some small retrospective and prospective studies although benefit is limited to a short period and it is often associated with recurrence or subsequent chorioretinal atrophy. Several studies show contradictory results and many consider it as a method to slow, but not prevent the natural course of CNV in angioid streaks.

SURGERY/OTHER PROCEDURES

Macular translocation and submacular surgery has been previously attempted in rare cases of angioid streaks with variable success.

ONGOING CARE

FOLLOW-UP RECOMMENDATIONS

- Patients with angioid streaks should have examinations at least every 6 months to assess for the development of CNV given its relatively high incidence. This follow-up may include FA to assess for CNV.
- Development of symptoms should prompt increased frequency of evaluation to at least every 3 months.
  - Patients that have recently been treated with laser and/or anti-VEGF therapy should be evaluated regularly.
- Patients can be instructed in the use of Amsler grid testing for home monitoring.

PATIENT EDUCATION

Patients should be educated about the importance of protective eyewear as the chance of choroidal rupture or subretinal hemorrhage is high with even minor trauma.

PROGNOSIS

Visual prognosis of eyes with angioid streaks is poor, although this varies based on the underlying diagnosis, time of onset of symptoms, and response to various types of therapy. It appears that in the natural history of untreated eyes, most end up with visual acuity of 20/200 or worse. At present, therapy is directed toward slowing the rate of visual loss and CNV progression.

COMPLICATIONS

Patients with angioid streaks and Pseudoxanthoma Elasticum are at increased risk for cardiovascular disease and spontaneous gastrointestinal bleeding.

ADDITIONAL READING

- Clarkson J, Altman R. Angioid streaks. *Surv Ophthalmol* 1982; 26(5): 235–246.
- Sawa M, Gomi F, Tsujikawa M, et al. Long-term results of intravitreal bevacizumab injection for choroidal neovascularization secondary to angioid streaks. *Am J Ophthalmol* 2009; 148(4): 584–590.
- Lim J, Bressler N, Marsh M, et al. Laser treatment of choroidal neovascularization in patients with angioid streaks. *Am J Ophthalmol* 1993; 116: 414–423.
- Georgalas I, Papaconstantinou D, Koutsandrea C, et al. Angioid streaks, clinical course, complications, and current therapeutic management. *Ther Clin Risk Manag* 2009; 5(1): 81–89.
- Gurwood A, Mastrangelo D. Understanding angioid streaks. *J Am Optometric Assoc* 1997; 68(5): 309–324.

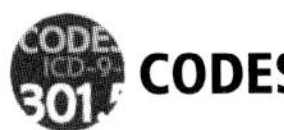

CODES

ICD9

363.43 Angioid streaks of choroid

CLINICAL PEARLS

- Angioid streaks may be a sign of an underlying disease such as pseudoxanthoma elasticum, Ehlers-Danlos syndrome, sickle-cell hemoglobinopathy, or Paget's disease of bone. It may also be idiopathic.
- Angioid streaks make the eye susceptible to severe subretinal hemorrhages from even minor blunt trauma, so patients should wear eye protection at all time.
- Choroidal neovascularization may develop in the areas of angioid streaks; patients need to self-monitor their vision and have regular fundus exams.

ANISOCORIA IN CHILDREN

William O. Young

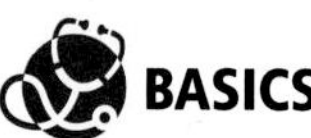

BASICS

DESCRIPTION
Round pupils that differ in size by 0.5 mm or more

EPIDEMIOLOGY
Prevalence
- 15–30% (physiologic)
- Other causes rare

RISK FACTORS
- Physiologic: None
- Trauma (including intraocular or brain surgery)
- Iritis
- Meningitis
- Topical contact with mydriatic or miotic (drop, ointment or plant)
- Paraspinal neuroblastoma
- Birth trauma
- Family history of anterior segment dysgenesis

Genetics
- Physiologic not genetic:
  - Anterior segment dysgenesis may be due to a genetic disorder.

GENERAL PREVENTION
- Physiologic: None
- Genetic counseling for anterior segment dysgeneses
- Avoidance of contact with mydriatics and miotics
- Careful follow-up screening for patients at risk for iritis (e.g., juvenile idiopathic arthritis) to detect inflammation early

PATHOPHYSIOLOGY
- Maldevelopment or dysfunction of the pupillary dilator or sphincter muscle or
- Mechanical impairment of the pupil (e.g., posterior synechia) or
- Idiopathic (physiologic)

ETIOLOGY
- Physiologic/idiopathic (most common)
- Congenital Horner syndrome:
  - Birth trauma including brachial plexus injury
  - Neoplasm rare
- Acquired Horner syndrome

ALERT

Can represent metastatic neuroblastoma:
- Congenital third cranial nerve palsy
- Acquired third cranial nerve palsy:
  - Trauma (most common) – surgical or nonsurgical
  - Meningitis
  - Tumor
  - Aneurysm:
    - Unlikely under age 14
- Traumatic mydriasis (sphincter tears)
- Posterior synechiae due to iritis
- Adie's tonic pupil:
  - Much less common in children than in young women
  - Usually idiopathic
- Pharmacologic mydriasis:
  - Usually cycloplegic (pharmaceutical or environmental)
- Congenital miosis
- Aniridia and other anterior segment dysgenesis

COMMONLY ASSOCIATED CONDITIONS
- None in physiologic anisocoria
- Neoplasm in 23% of pediatric Horner syndrome (1)

ALERT

Note especially neuroblastoma metastatic to cervical sympathetic chain, which can be life threatening and requires urgent workup.

- Other neoplasms causing Horner syndrome in children include benign paraspinal neuroblastoma, rhabdomyosarcoma (2), Ewing sarcoma, and juvenile xanthogranuloma (1).
- Abnormalities of extraocular muscle function and strabismus in third cranial palsy

DIAGNOSIS

HISTORY
- Trauma:
  - Nonocular:
    - Birth trauma
    - Surgical (neck or chest) or other postnatal trauma
  - Ocular blunt trauma
  - Intraocular surgery
- Age of onset:
  - Review old photos
- Duration
- Ptosis:
  - Horner syndrome (1–2 mm or less)
  - Third cranial nerve palsy
- Anhidrosis/hypohidrosis:
  - Seen in some but not all cases of Horner syndrome
- Contralateral facial flushing and ipsilateral hypohidrosis (Harlequin sign):
  - Seen in some but not all cases of Horner syndrome in infants
- Longstanding iris heterochromia in congenital Horner and some anterior segment dysgenesis

PHYSICAL EXAM
- Acuity
- Normal in physiologic anisocoria
- May be decreased due to amblyopia in third nerve palsy and Adie's
- Accommodative amplitudes/dynamic retinoscopy:
  - May be decreased in third cranial nerve palsy and Adie's tonic pupil)
- Pupils:
  - Anisocoria greater in darkness (smaller pupil is abnormal):
    - Physiologic anisocoria
    - Horner syndrome
    - Mechanical restriction
  - Anisocoria greater in light (larger pupil is abnormal):
    - Third cranial nerve palsy
    - Adie's pupil
    - Traumatic mydriasis
    - Pharmacologic mydriasis
  - Dilation lag of smaller pupil:
    - Horner syndrome
  - Light-near dissociation:
    - Adie's tonic pupil
  - Segmental constriction:
    - Adie's tonic pupil
  - Relative difference in pupil size preserved in dim and bright illumination: Physiologic anisocoria
  - Iris heterochromia (lighter iris ipsilateral to smaller pupil):
    - Congenital Horner syndrome

- Eyelids:
  - 1–2 mm (but not more) of upper eyelid ptosis in Horner syndrome, ipsilateral to the smaller pupil
  - More profound ptosis in third nerve palsy, ipsilateral to the larger pupil
  - "Inverse ptosis" (slight elevation of the lower lid of the eye with the small pupil) with Horner syndrome)
- Motility:
  - Normal with all causes of anisocoria except third nerve palsy
  - Limitation of elevation, depression, and adduction in third nerve palsy:
    - The palsied eye is typically "down and out" (exotropic and hypotropic)
- Palpate abdomen and supraclavicular region looking for neuroblastoma or other neoplasm

DIAGNOSTIC TESTS & INTERPRETATION

Lab

- If suspect Horner, with no clear evidence of birth injury: Spot urine for vanillylmandelic acid (VMA) and homovanillic acid (HVA)
- Note: Urine testing may not be as sensitive as imaging (1)[C] in diagnosing neuroblastoma

Imaging

- MRI (with and without gadolinium) of the brain, neck, chest, and upper abdomen if suspect Horner syndrome unless clear evidence of birth trauma (1)[C]:
  - Some recent evidence (3)[C] questions the need for extensive evaluation of patients with Horner syndrome.
- MRI of brain with MRA if suspect third cranial palsy and no clear etiology

Diagnostic Procedures/Other

- Review old photographs to help determine whether anisocoria is congenital or acquired
- Pharmacologic testing for Horner syndrome:
  - Cocaine 5% drops dilate the normal pupil but not the Horner pupil.
  - Apraclonidine 0.5% produces reversal of anisocoria in 30–60 min in Horner syndrome.
    - Effect easier to see in bright than in dim light (4)[C]
  - Hydroxyamphetamine 1% dilates preganglionic but not postganglionic Horner pupil.
- Pharmacologic testing for Adie's tonic pupil: Pilocarpine 0.125% constricts Adie's pupil but not a normal pupil or a pharmacologically dilated pupil.

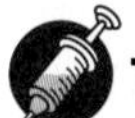

TREATMENT

MEDICATION

- For Adie's tonic pupil: Pilocarpine 0.125% b.i.d.–q.i.d. can be used for cosmesis and to aid accommodation.
- For posterior synechiae due to iritis: Pharmacologic mydriasis (such as atropine 1% drops) to break the synechiae, in addition to topical steroid treatment (with systemic medication as indicated) for the iritis.
- Anisocoria due to other causes is not treated; instead, an underlying cause is identified and treatable.

ADDITIONAL TREATMENT

General Measures

- Amblyopia (most likely with third nerve palsy and Adie's) is treated with refractive correction if needed, and patching or atropine penalization.
- Cosmetic contact lens is used if concerns about appearance in older children.

Issues for Referral

- Patients discovered to have evidence of a neoplasm should be referred without delay to appropriate specialists (oncology, neurosurgery).
- Patients below 12 months of age with Adie's tonic pupil should be referred to pediatric neurology to rule out familial dysautonomia.

ONGOING CARE

FOLLOW-UP RECOMMENDATIONS

- Physiologic: None needed
- Third nerve palsy and Adie's: Follow-up to rule out amblyopia
- Possible Horner syndrome with equivocal clinical and/or pharmacologic findings: Re-examine in 3–6 months, consider repeat urine testing
- Follow-up for glaucoma in anterior segment dysgeneses
- Follow-up for other causes of anisocoria is determined by the underlying cause.

PATIENT EDUCATION

- Reassure parent that anisocoria itself does not affect acuity or visual development (except if accommodation impaired in Aides or third cranial palsy).
- If Horner syndrome is suspected but not proven, instruct the parent to watch for development of ptosis and anhidrosis.

PROGNOSIS

- Physiologic anisocoria: Excellent. No deficit is expected.
- Other causes: Prognosis depends on underlying cause.

REFERENCES

1. Mahoney NR, Liu GT, Menacker SJ, et al. Pediatric Horner syndrome: Etiologies and roles of imaging and urine studies to detect neuroblastoma and other responsible mass lesions. *Am J Ophthalmol* 2006;142(4):651–659.
2. Jeffery AR, Ellis FJ, Repka MX, et al. Pediatric Horner syndrome. *J AAPOS* 1998; 2(3):159–167.
3. Smith SJ, Diehl N, Leavitt JA, et al. Incidence of pediatric Horner syndrome and neuroblastoma threat. *Arch Ophthalmol* 2010;128(3):324–329.
4. Chen PL, Hsiao CH, Chen JT, et al. Efficacy of apraclonidine 0.5% in the diagnosis of Horner syndrome in pediatric patients under low or high illumination. *Am J Ophthalmol* 2006;142(3): 469–474.

ADDITIONAL READING

- Kardon RH, Thompson HS. Congenital and acquired anisocoria in children. In: Cibis GW, Tongue AC, Stass-Isern ML, eds. *Decision Making in Pediatric Ophthalmology*. St. Louis, MO: Mosby-Year Book, 1993:26–27.
- Wright TM, Freedman SF. Exposure to topical apraclonidine in children with glaucoma. *J Glaucoma* 2009;18(5):395–398.

CODES

ICD9

- 364.71 Posterior synechiae of iris
- 379.41 Anisocoria
- 743.46 Other specified congenital anomalies of iris and ciliary body

CLINICAL PEARLS

- Determining whether the anisocoria is greater in darkness or in light is the key first step in determining the cause of anisocoria.
- "Inverse ptosis" (slight elevation of the lower eyelid) and dilation lag are subtle but specific clinical signs of Horner syndrome.
- Iris heterochromia suggests that Horner syndrome is longstanding and usually congenital.
- Old photos can help establish that anisocoria is congenital, and thus less worrisome.

ALERT

- Acquired Horner syndrome is the cause of anisocoria that must not be missed, because of its association with metastatic neuroblastoma.
- Workup for neuroblastoma should be considered for all cases of acquired Horner syndrome, as well as for congenital cases without a clear underlying cause such as birth trauma.

ANISOMETROPIA

Kammi B. Gunton

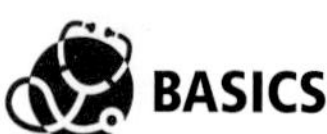

BASICS

DESCRIPTION

- Difference in refractive correction between the two eyes. More amblyogenic if difference is
  - >1.50 diopters (D) hyperopic spherical equivalent
  - +1.00 D cylinder
  - >–6.00 D myopia
- Most common cause of amblyopia
- Two types: Spherical equivalent anisometropia and astigmatic anisometropia

EPIDEMIOLOGY

Incidence

- 25–60% of patients with anisometropia develop amblyopia (1).
- Change in anisometropia with age occurs in >15% children, yet >3D anisometropia more likely to persist (1).

Prevalence

1–11% of population (1)

RISK FACTORS

- Prematurity:
  - retinopathy of prematurity
- Congenital ptosis
- Coloboma
- Lenticular opacities
- Congenital glaucoma
- Asymmetric axial growth or corneal endothelial damage
- Family history
- Any organic cause of monocular poor vision in infancy

Genetics

- No clear inheritance pattern but risk increases by proximity of other affected family members in pedigree.
- Inheritance pattern of underlying disorder prevails.

GENERAL PREVENTION

- Detection at earlier age and treatment of anisometropia can prevent amblyopia.
- Screening
- Photoscreening:
  - Noncycloplegic autorefraction
  - Visual acuity testing by primary care physicians and school nurses
  - 14% one year olds with anisometropia had amblyopia, 40% at 2 years old, 65% at 3 years old, 76% at 5 years old (1).

PATHOPHYSIOLOGY

Amblyopia results from unequal competitive input to visual cortex resulting in a failure of development of the neuronal connections and occipital receptor cells for vision in the non-preferred eye.

ETIOLOGY

Unknown

COMMONLY ASSOCIATED CONDITIONS

- Prematurity:
  - retinopathy of prematurity
- Congenital ptosis
- Coloboma
- Cataract
- Strabismus
- Microphthalmia
- Glaucoma

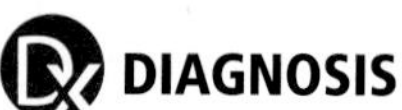

DIAGNOSIS

HISTORY

- Unequal glasses or contact lens prescription between eyes
- Unilateral vision deficit or ocular disorder
- Unequal eye size

PHYSICAL EXAM

- Visual acuity
- Full dilated eye examination to rule out other organic causes of unequal or subnormal vision
- Cycloplegic refraction of each eye to detect interocular difference:
  - Decreased contrast sensitivity in anisometropic amblyopia

DIAGNOSTIC TESTS & INTERPRETATION

Lab

None

Imaging

Usually none required unless ruling out other organic causes of subnormal vision. May be indicated if depth of amblyopia is not proportionate to degree of anisometropia.

Diagnostic Procedures/Other

Function MRI demonstrates suppressed calcarine cortex activation at high spatial frequency and decreased activation of lateral geniculate nucleus, visual cortex from anisometropic amblyopic eye (2).

Pathological Findings

Ocular dominance width size in visual cortex is normal in anisometropia, but binocular driven cells may be reduced (1).

DIFFERENTIAL DIAGNOSIS

- Ocular or cortical pathology is responsible for reduced vision.
- Anisometropia may be caused by asymmetric axial length, lenticular refractive power, corneal refractive power, and retinal elevation.

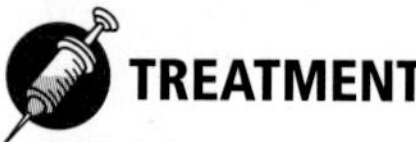

TREATMENT

MEDICATION

No pharmacologic treatment indicated

ADDITIONAL TREATMENT

General Measures

- Refractive correction with spectacles of anisometropia
- In the presence of amblyopia, monitor vision with spectacle correction:
  - Follow-up until resolution of amblyopia, or if no further improvement, begin amblyopia treatment (3).
  - Improvement in vision continues on average 30 weeks before stabilization (3).
- For unresolved amblyopia, occlusion of nonamblyopic eye:
  - Patching from 2 to 6 h daily or atropine penalization of nonamblyopic eye (4)
  - Faster improvement with greater number of hours of patching, but at 6 months equal efficacy (4)

Issues for Referral
If underlying organic cause (e.g., cataract, corneal disease, ptosis) consider referral for surgical intervention.

Additional Therapies
For high degrees of anisometropia, contact lens correction may be preferred both to reduce aniseikonia and for cosmesis.

COMPLEMENTARY & ALTERNATIVE THERAPIES
- None
- No proven efficacy of vision therapy for anisometropia
- Orthokeratology not recommended

SURGERY/OTHER PROCEDURES
Laser refractive surgery in children who fail other means of refractive correction is currently under investigation.

IN-PATIENT CONSIDERATIONS
Admission Criteria
For children extremely recalcitrant to amblyopia therapy, in-patient admission has been rarely used in some centers to facilitate initiation of treatment.

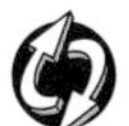

ONGOING CARE

FOLLOW-UP RECOMMENDATIONS
Patient Monitoring
- Follow-up at intervals with refractive correction to monitor improvement of vision in suspected amblyopia until no further improvement. Intervals for follow-up shorter for younger children:
  - When treating amblyopia, treat with patching or atropine for intervals of 1 week for every week of age, and then check vision of each eye (including normal eye for iatrogenic amblyopia).

PATIENT EDUCATION
Focus on prevention of amblyopia

PROGNOSIS
- 2 line or greater improvement in visual acuity by spectacles alone in 77% (3)
- Resolution to 20/20 with spectacles alone in 27% (3)
- Improvement of 1.1 lines with spectacles and patching compared to 0.5 lines with spectacles alone at 5 weeks (5)
- Visual acuity improvement to 20/30 in amblyopic eye occurred with treatment in >74% (6)

COMPLICATIONS
- Occlusion amblyopia can occur in the treated eye.
- High degrees of refractive error, especially if anisometropic; if corrected by spectacles may have adverse psychosocial consequences that make wearing glasses a challenge.

REFERENCES

1. Donahue S. The relationship between anisometropia, patient age, and the development of amblyopia. *Trans Am Ophthalmol Soc* 2005; 103:313–336.
2. Choi MY, Lee KM, Hwang JM, et al. Comparison between anisometropic and strabismic amblyopia using functional magnetic resonance imaging. *Br J Ophthalmol* 2001;85:1052–1056.
3. Pediatric Eye Disease Investigator Group. Treatment of anisometropic amblyopia in children with refractive correction. *Ophthalmol* 2006;113: 895–903.
4. Pediatric Eye Disease Investigator Group. A comparison of atropine and patching treatments for moderate amblyopia by patient age, cause of amblyopia, depth of amblyopia and other factors. *Ophthalmol* 2003;110:1632–1637.
5. Pediatric Eye Disease Investigator Group. A randomized trial to evaluate two hours of daily patching for amblyopia in children. *Ophthalmol* 2006;113:904–914.
6. Pediatric Eye Disease Investigator Group. A randomized trial of atropine versus patching for treatment of moderate amblyopia: Follow-up at 10 years of age. *Arch Ophthalmol* 2008;126: 1039–1044.

CODES

ICD9
- 367.1 Myopia
- 367.31 Anisometropia
- 368.00 Amblyopia, unspecified

CLINICAL PEARLS

- Detection of significant anisometropia at earlier age can prevent amblyopia.
- Spectacle correction alone has significant impact on visual recovery.
- Amblyopia treatment is effective.
- Ongoing follow-up to measure vision and changes in refractive error is essential.

ANOPHTHALMIA

Jing Jin

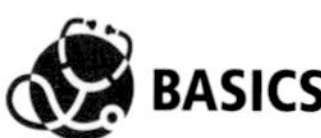

BASICS

DESCRIPTION

- Absence of globe. Must be distinguished from severe microphthalmia in which globe remnants may only be detectable by ultrasound, neuroimaging, or tissue biopsy (e.g., exenteration or autopsy).
- With or without systemic disease

EPIDEMIOLOGY

10–19 per 100,000 newborns (1) (2)[C]

RISK FACTORS

- Chromosomal aberrations, syndromes, and congenital disorders
- Intrauterine factors:
  - Prenatal exposure to teratogenic factors including radiation, alcohol, thalidomide, retinoic acid (3)[C], hydantoin, and lysergic acid diethylamide (LSD)

Genetics

There is no known gene defect specific for true anophthalmia.

GENERAL PREVENTION

- Prenatal ultrasound (4)[C]
- Avoidance of in utero exposures to infection or teratogen

PATHOPHYSIOLOGY

Complete failure in the development of the primary optic vesicle during embryogenesis

ETIOLOGY

- Genetic
- Prenatal exposure to infection or teratogen
- Idiopathic

COMMONLY ASSOCIATED CONDITIONS

- No consistent systemic associations
- Midline craniofacial anomalies
- Developmental delay (often severe) with chromosomal aberration or other systemic syndromic findings
- Craniofacial disproportion with enophthalmic appearance and small palpebral fissures and lids

DIAGNOSIS

HISTORY

- Family history of congenital ocular disease
- Known exposure to infection or teratogen in utero
- Other known associated anomalies or developmental delay

PHYSICAL EXAM

- The condition may affect one or both eyes.
  - Reduced orbital volume with enophthalmic appearance
  - Eyelids may appear normal, small, or partially fused. Lashes, tarsal glands and lacrimal gland and drainage system are usually present.
- Systemic examination for other anomalies, especially brain anomalies
- Complete eye examination of both parents looking for coloboma – if present suggests that the child has severe microphthalmia rather than true anophthalmia

DIAGNOSTIC TESTS & INTERPRETATION

Lab

Initial lab tests

- None if no extraocular findings
- Karyotype/microarray if other congenital anomalies are present
- Molecular genetic testing for mutations in syndromes reportedly associated with anophthalmia

Follow-up & special considerations

- Must follow orbital and periorbital growth
- Follow for developmental delay

Imaging

Initial approach

MRI and CT show the absence of ocular tissue, optic nerve, and extraocular muscles.

Follow-up & special considerations

Serial CT scan may assist in evaluating bony growth.

Pathological Findings

Absence of ocular tissue in orbit

DIFFERENTIAL DIAGNOSIS

- Severe microphthalmia
- Cystic eye
- Acquired anophthalmia following trauma or surgery
- Phthisis (e.g., following infection or trauma)
- Cyclopia/synophthalmia

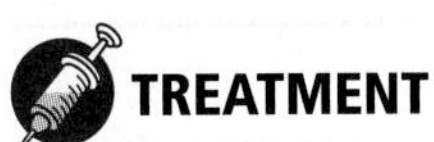

TREATMENT

MEDICATION

None

ADDITIONAL TREATMENT

General Measures

- Safety glasses to protect the good eye in unilateral cases
- Scleral shell to encourage periorbital tissue growth

Issues for Referral

- Genetic consultation
- Special education and referral to services for the blind

SURGERY/OTHER PROCEDURES

Placement of serial enlarging orbital expanders, dermal fat grafting, or intraorbital balloons in severe cases (5)[C]

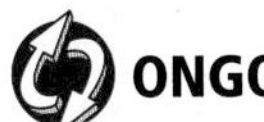

ONGOING CARE

FOLLOW-UP RECOMMENDATIONS

Regular evaluation by an ocularist. Follow orbital and periocular tissue growth especially in first 5 years of life,

Patient Monitoring

- School performance and development
- Patient concerns about appearance

PATIENT EDUCATION

- Genetic counseling
- Blindness interventions
- International Children's Anophthalmia and Microphthalmia Network (http://www.anophthalmia.org)

PROGNOSIS

Depends on associated systemic anomalies

REFERENCES

1. Dolk H, Busby A, Armstrong BG, et al. Geographical variation in anophthalmia and microphthalmia in England, 1988–1994. *Br Med J* 1998;317:905–909.
2. Yoon PW, Rasmussen SA, Lynberg MC, et al. The National Birth Defects Prevention Study. *Public Health Rep* 2001;116(Suppl 1):32–40.
3. Lamer EJ, Chen DT, Hoar RM, et al. Retinoic acid embryopathy. *N Engl J Med* 1985;313:837–841.
4. Wong HS, Parker S, Tait J, Pringle KC. Antenatal diagnosis of anophthalmia by three-dimensional ultrasound: A novel application of the reverse face view. *Ultrasound Obstet Gynecol* 2008;32: 103–105.
5. Schittkowski MP, Guthoff RF. Injectable self inflating hydrogel pellet expanders for the treatment of orbital volume deficiency in congenital microphthalmos: Preliminary results with a new therapeutic approach. *Br J Ophthalmol* 2006; 90(9):1173–1177.

ADDITIONAL READING

- http://www.ncbi.nlm.nih.gov.proxy1.lib.tju.edu:2048/bookshelf/br.fcgi?book=gene&part=anophthalmia-ov
- Stoll C, Alembik Y, Dott B, Roth MP. Congenital eye malformations in 212,479 consecutive births. *Ann Genet* 1997;40(2):122–128.
- Fryns JP, Legius E, Moerman P, et al. Apparently new "anophthalmia-plus" syndrome in sibs. *Am J Med Genet* 1995;58:113–114.
- West B, Bove KE, Slavotinek AM. Two novel STRA6 mutations in a patient with anophthalmia and diaphragmatic eventration. *Am J Med Genet A* 2009;149A(3):539–542.

CODES

ICD9

743.00 Clinical anophthalmos, unspecified

CLINICAL PEARLS

- Check the patient for possible associated systemic findings.
- Examine parents for coloboma.
- Consider genetic consult.
- Prosthesis fitting to ensure orbital and periocular tissue growth

ANTERIOR BASEMENT MEMBRANE DYSTROPHY

Sadeer B. Hannush

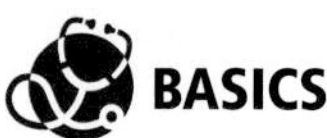

BASICS

DESCRIPTION

Corneal anterior basement membrane dystrophy (ABMD) is the most common corneal dystrophy. It is also known as map-dot-fingerprint, mare's tail, and Cogan's microcystic dystrophy

ALERT

Corneal ABMD is most commonly associated with two clinical presentations: Painful corneal erosions and visual compromise. The treatment of one may differ from that of the other.

EPIDEMIOLOGY

Prevalence

10% of the adult population in the United States has some manifestation of ABMD with a strong predilection for women.

RISK FACTORS

Genetics

The inheritance pattern is autosomal dominant.

PATHOPHYSIOLOGY

Histopathologically, a thickened layer of corneal epithelium is recognized together with reduplication of the epithelial basement membrane and entrapment of debris in cyst-like structures.

ETIOLOGY

As with all corneal dystrophies ABMD is genetically coded for, usually appears in the fourth or fifth decades of life and may worsen over time.

COMMONLY ASSOCIATED CONDITIONS

ABMD may be present with other corneal dystrophies such as Fuchs' endothelial dystrophy and may be exacerbated by chronic blepharitis.

DIAGNOSIS

HISTORY

ABMD is associated with two common presentations:

- Awakening with pain, foreign body sensation, photophobia, and tearing (scenario 1)
- Gradual visual compromise sometimes associated with foreign body sensation (scenario 2)

PHYSICAL EXAM

- Scenario 1: If the patient is symptomatic on presentation, they will likely have a well-demarcated area of loose epithelium in one part of the cornea with the rest of the cornea showing the classical manifestations of ABMD described above.
- Scenario 2: Thickened epithelium and redundant basement membrane over the pupillary aperture in the form of map-dot-fingerprint, mare's tail, microcystic changes, or a combination of the above. This results in an irregular corneal surface over the visual axis.

DIAGNOSTIC TESTS & INTERPRETATION

Visual acuity and slit-lamp biomicroscopy as noted in physical exam

Imaging

- Computerized corneal topography may be an invaluable tool in evaluating the contribution of corneal ABMD to the patient's blurred vision. Irregular mires and an increased surface regularity index (SRI) usually imply that the surface is a significant contributor to the visual compromise.
- More recently, anterior segment ocular coherence tomography (OCT) has been employed to further delineate the epithelial and basement membrane changes.

Diagnostic Procedures/Other

The contribution of the corneal surface to the patient's visual compromise may be further confirmed with a rigid gas-permeable (RGP) contact lens diagnostic evaluation. If the patient's vision improves significantly with an RGP lens, then ABMD may be a significant contributor to the patient's visual compromise.

Pathological Findings

A keratectomy specimen submitted for pathologic examination will usually show thickened epithelium with a redundant basement membrane (it is not uncommon to see basement membrane structures undulating obliquely through multilayered epithelium) with cystic collections of epithelial debris.

DIFFERENTIAL DIAGNOSIS

- Scenario 1 (painful presentation): The differential diagnosis includes keratoconjunctivitis sicca, blepharokeratitis, rosacea keratitis, infectious keratitis, chemical keratitis (and other external factors), trauma, embedded foreign body in the cornea or under the lid, and corneal epithelial edema.
- Scenario 2 (visual compromise): The differential diagnosis includes any condition causing a surface keratopathy including chemical and infectious keratitis, keratoconjunctivitis sicca, other causes of epitheliopathy (edema, Meesmann's dystrophy, and stem cell deficiency), as well as other causes of visual compromise, including other corneal clouding/opacification, cataract, vitreous opacity, maculopathy, and optic neuropathy.

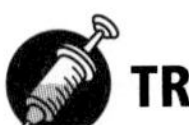

TREATMENT

MEDICATION

First Line

Scenario 1 (Pain)

- Lubrication, lubrication, lubrication! This may include drops, gel, or ointment.
  - Encourage patient to open lids slowly upon awakening followed by instillation of lubricant in the eye

Second Line

- Hypertonic saline especially in ointment form at bedtime:
  - Punctal occlusion to create a wetter surface
  - Therapeutic bandage contact lens to protect the corneal surface, especially the areas(s) of loose epithelium, from the movement of the lid. A prophylactic antibiotic may be considered in this scenario.

COMPLEMENTARY & ALTERNATIVE THERAPIES

Topical nonsteroidal anti-inflammatory medication to control pain and cyclosporine both as an anti-inflammatory and to increase tear production may be added to the first or second line treatments.

SURGERY/OTHER PROCEDURES

- Scenario 1 (pain): Consideration may be given to mechanical keratectomy with a diamond-dusted burr or phototherapeutic keratectomy with the excimer laser. Both techniques have been shown to be equally effective in decreasing the incidence of recurrent erosions.
- Ethanol epitheliectomy has been shown to be equally effective.
- Scenario 2 (visual compromise): When ABMD is visually significant treatment usually consists of a superficial keratectomy. We favor a dull rounded or crescent knife to remove the central 5–6 mm of corneal epithelium overlying the pupillary aperture. The epithelial layer usually cleaves easily off the basement membrane. It is very important to then deliberately remove the irregular, and frequently redundant, basement membrane until Bowman's layer is recognized with its characteristic sheen. Importantly, a diamond-dusted burr is not required in this setting. Since eliminating recurrent erosions is not the focus of treatment, roughening up Bowman's layer to improve adherence is not required (unnecessary diamond-dusted burr polishing of Bowman's layer may result in some fibrosis and visually significant haze). In the same vein, antifibrosis treatment with mitomycin is not necessary. Moreover, there is no real role for excimer laser phototherapeutic keratectomy in the treatment of ABMD in the absence of recurrent erosions.
- In both scenarios a therapeutic bandage contact lens is placed (e.g. Acuvue Oasys). The patient is started on a topical steroid, nonsteroidal anti-inflammatory agent, and fluoroquinolone antibiotic, as is the custom with most surface procedures. Re-epithelialization usually takes place over the next 3–7 days. The bandage contact lens is then removed, the topical nonsteroidal anti-inflammatory agent and antibiotic discontinued, and the steroid tapered rapidly. A couple of weeks later the patient is reevaluated, her visual acuity remeasured, and computerized corneal topography repeated.

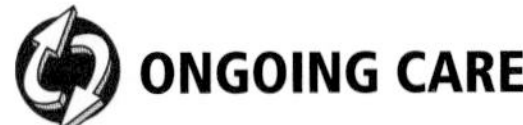

ONGOING CARE

FOLLOW-UP RECOMMENDATIONS

The treatment may be repeated as need.

PROGNOSIS

Excellent in both scenarios

COMPLICATIONS

Secondary infection and subepithelial fibrosis/scar formation

ADDITIONAL READING

- Buxton JN, Fox ML. Superficial epithelial keratectomy in the treatment of epithelial basement membrane dystrophy. A preliminary report. *Arch Ophthalmol* 1983;101(3):392–395.
- Buxton JN, Constad WH. Superficial epithelial keratectomy in the treatment of epithelial basement membrane dystrophy. *Cornea* 1987;6(4):292–297.
- Sridhar MS, Rapuano CJ, Cosar CB, et al. Phototherapeutic keratectomy versus diamond burr polishing of Bowman's membrane in the treatment of recurrent corneal erosions associated with anterior basement membrane dystrophy. *Ophthalmology* 2003;110(9):1855; author reply 1855.
- Wong VW, Chi SC, Lam DS. Diamond burr polishing for recurrent corneal erosions: results from a prospective randomized controlled trial. *Cornea* 2009;28(2):152–156.

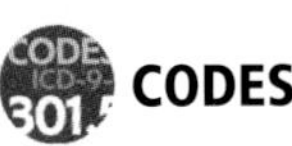

CODES

ICD9

371.52 Other anterior corneal dystrophies

CLINICAL PEARLS

- Corneal ABMD may present as painful corneal erosions or visual compromise.
- The treatment of painful erosions may involve a stepwise approach from lubrication to keratectomy, while visually significant ABMD can usually only be addressed by removal of the abnormal epithelium and basement membrane.

ARCUS SENILIS

Kristin DiDomenico
Alan R. Forman

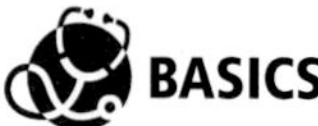

BASICS

DESCRIPTION

- Arcus senilis is a yellowish-white ring of extracellular lipid deposition in the peripheral cornea separated from the limbus by a narrow (<1 mm) clear zone. It is seen most frequently in the elderly, but can present in children and rarely at birth. In younger patients, there is an association with hyperlipidemia and cardiovascular disease risk factors. It does not interfere with vision and requires no treatment.
- Synonyms: Corneal arcus, gerontoxon
  - In children: Arcus juvenilis, anterior embryotoxon

EPIDEMIOLOGY

Prevalence

- Increases with age (1–3)
- Higher in black population (1,3)
- Higher in men (3)
- Estimates of prevalence vary
- Approximately 65% of those 50 years or older (4)

RISK FACTORS

- Older age
- Hypercholesterolemia

Genetics

- Early onset arcus (by age 45) is common in familial hyperlipoproteinemias.
  - Familial hypercholesterolemia is an autosomal dominant inherited defect in lipoprotein metabolism.
    - Homozygotes often present with arcus earlier than heterozygotes (5).

PATHOPHYSIOLOGY

Cholesterol, cholesterol esters, triglycerides, and phospholipids deposit within the cornea causing no functional limitations

ETIOLOGY

- Product of aging and unlikely to represent disturbed metabolism in elderly patients
- In familial hyperlipoproteinemias, development of premature arcus relates to age of patient.
  - In these cases, it is the duration of the dyslipidemic disease, not its severity, that is associated with formation of arcus (6).

COMMONLY ASSOCIATED CONDITIONS

- Most closely associated with aging
- Associated with hyperlipidemia and cardiovascular disease:
  - Early onset arcus (childhood and early adulthood) is seen with familial hypercholesterolemia, and with type III, IV, and V hyperlipoproteinemia.
    - Corneal arcus before the age of 45 is included in the criteria for diagnosing familial hypercholesterolemia (5).
  - Reported as a prognostic factor for cardiovascular disease mortality in hyperlipidemic men aged 30–49 years (1)
  - Also reported as a prognostic factor for coronary artery disease in men aged 30–49 years independent of its association with hyperlipidemia (1)
- When present in children it is called arcus juvenilis:
  - Associated with certain congenital ocular anomalies, such as blue sclera, megalocornea, and aniridia
  - Also associated with familial hyperlipoproteinemias, as stated above

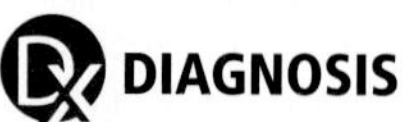

DIAGNOSIS

HISTORY

- Gradual formation of a bilateral white corneal ring. Some patients complain of "changing eye color."
  - For example, a patient with a dark brown iris may state that his or her peripheral iris is becoming lighter.
- Arcus does not cause any visual disturbances.

PHYSICAL EXAM

- A yellowish-white ring is visible in the peripheral cornea with a narrow clear zone separating it from the limbus.
  - While examination is aided by the use of a slit lamp, arcus can be detected by examination with the naked eye and the use of a light source.
- On slit lamp examination, the distribution of lipid deposit is better appreciated.
  - Deposits are most concentrated in the area of Descemet's membrane (a deep corneal layer) and Bowman's membrane (a superficial corneal layer).
  - Appears as two wedge-shaped opacities:
    - One wedge with the base on the superficial membrane and the apex pointing posteriorly into the corneal stroma
    - The other wedge with the base on the deep membrane and the apex pointing anteriorly into the corneal stroma
- Peripheral margin of the arcus forms a sharply defined edge, whereas the central margin is less distinct.

DIAGNOSTIC TESTS & INTERPRETATION

Lab

Patients younger than 50 years require serum lipid measurements (1)[A].

Imaging

In patients less than 50 years of age, consider echocardiogram/stress echocardiogram in the context of other findings.

Diagnostic Procedures/Other

- Any patient younger than 50 years requires detailed work-up for cardiovascular risk factors (1)[A].
  - Assess for history of hypertension, diabetes, family history, symptoms of angina, exercise, and smoking
  - EKG, stress test
- Children must be investigated for dysfunction of lipoprotein metabolism.

Pathological Findings

- Grossly, a white ring of lipid deposit limited to the peripheral cornea with a 0.3–1 mm clear zone separating it from the limbus:
  - Ring begins as two arcs, one near the superior corneal margin and one near the inferior margin. Arcs grow until they meet circumferentially completing a 360° ring.

- Histologically, two concentric rings form within the cornea and extend toward one another in the anterior–posterior plane.
  - Extracellular lipid deposits initially appear in Descemet's membrane forming a triangular shape with the base along Descemet's membrane and the apex extending into the corneal stroma.
  - Lipid deposits also form an anterior triangular shape with the base along Bowman's membrane and the apex extending into the stroma.
  - As more lipid is deposited, the apices of the triangles extend toward one another and eventually fuse forming one ring.
- Deposits consist of cholesterol, cholesterol esters, phospholipids, and triglycerides (2,3).
- Similar lipid deposits also form within the sclera, but cannot be seen clinically because of the normal white scleral color.

DIFFERENTIAL DIAGNOSIS

- Kayser–Fleischer ring: Red, brown, or green ring of abnormal corneal copper deposition forming on Descemet's membrane (deep corneal layer) in Wilson's disease
- Chalcosis: Copper deposition in the cornea from an intra-ocular foreign body
- Band keratopathy: Calcium deposition in the superficial corneal layer; may cause decreased vision and foreign body sensation
- Limbal girdle of Vogt: White semicircular arc causing peripheral opacity in the nasal region of the cornea bilaterally
- Terrien's marginal degeneration: Bilateral thinning of the peripheral corneal stroma forming a 1–2 mm gutter
- Idiopathic furrow degeneration: Thinning of the peripheral cornea; usually requires no treatment
- Staphylococcal marginal keratitis: Infectious corneal infiltrate, often with overlying epithelial defect
- Lecithin-cholesterol acetyltransferase (LCAT) deficiency: Corneal opacity resembling arcus senilis in patients with LCAT gene mutation, associated with anemia, proteinuria, and premature atherosclerosis

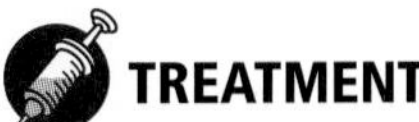

TREATMENT

ADDITIONAL TREATMENT

General Measures

No treatment required

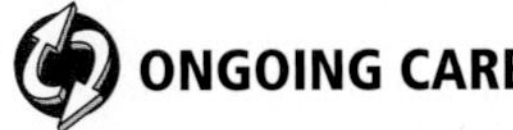

ONGOING CARE

FOLLOW-UP RECOMMENDATIONS

- No follow-up is required for patients older than 50 years.
- Patients younger than 50 years must follow up with a cardiovascular risk factor evaluation with a primary care provider.

PATIENT EDUCATION

- Older patients should be reassured that corneal arcus is a common finding with aging. There are no complications, no treatment is required and it will not interfere with vision.
- Younger patients with arcus should be educated that it may indicate hyperlipidemia and an evaluation is recommended.

REFERENCES

1. Chambless LE, Fuchs FD, Linn S, et al. The association of corneal arcus with coronary heart disease and cardiovascular disease mortality in the Lipid Research Clinics Mortality Follow-up Study. *Am J Public Health* 1990;80:1200–1204.
2. Cogan D, Kuwabawa T. Arcus senilis: It's pathology and histochemistry. *Arch Ophth* 1959;61:353.
3. Barchiesi B, Eckel R, Ellis P. The cornea and disorders of lipid metabolism. *Surv Ophthal* 1991;36(1):1–22.
4. Chua BE, Mitchell P, Wang JJ, et al. Corneal arcus and hyperlipidemia: Findings from an older population. *Am J Ophthalmol* 2004;137:363–365.
5. Civeira F. Guidelines for the diagnosis and management of heterozygous familial hypercholesterolemia. *Atherosclerosis* 2004;173:55–68.
6. Winder AF. Relationship between corneal arcus and hyperlipidaemia is clarified by studies in familial hypercholesterolaemia. *Br J Ophthalmol* 1983; 67:789–794.

ADDITIONAL READING

- Perry H, Cameron J. Arcus senilis. In: Tasman W, Jaeger EA, eds. *Duane's ophthalmology*. Lippincott Williams & Wilkins, 2009:3:9.
- Ehlers JP, Shah CP. *The Wills eye manual: Office and emergency room diagnosis and treatment of eye disease*. Lippincott Williams & Wilkins, 2008.

CODES

ICD9

- 371.41 Senile corneal changes
- 743.43 Other congenital corneal opacities

CLINICAL PEARLS

- Yellowish-white ring in the peripheral cornea separated from the limbus by a narrow clear zone
- Common finding in the elderly
- Does not interfere with vision, has no complications, and requires no treatment
- In patients younger than 50 years may indicate hyperlipidemia and may predict cardiovascular disease:
  - Check serum lipids
  - Evaluate for cardiovascular risk factors

ATAXIA-TELANGIECTASIA (LOUIS-BAR SYNDROME, AT SYNDROME, BODER-SEDGWICK SYNDROME)

David Rhee

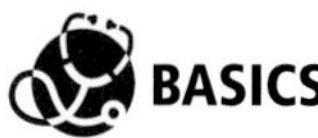

BASICS

DESCRIPTION

- Ataxia-telangiectasia (AT) is a multisystem neurodegenerative and immunodeficiency disorder characterized by cerebellar dysfunction, telangiectasias, immune dysfunction of both B- and T-lymphocytes, radiosensitivity, and lymphoproliferative cancer.
  - Neurodegeneration/cerebellar atrophy results in profound loss of cerebellar function, oculomotor apraxia, progressive dysarthria, and choreoathetoid movements.
  - Immune dysfunction results in recurrent sinopulmonary infections.

EPIDEMIOLOGY

Incidence

Varies by region, in the United States, the highest annual incidence was found to be 11.3 per million in Michigan. In England, the birth frequency has been estimated to be 1 in 300,000 live births.

Prevalence

- Varies by region, in the United States, the estimated prevalence of AT is from 1 in 40,000 to 100,000. In France, the prevalence of AT has been estimated to be 1 in 450,000.
- AT is the most common autosomal recessive ataxic disorder in children <5 years (1)[C].

RISK FACTORS

Genetics

- Autosomal recessive
- The ATM (ataxia-telangiectasia, mutated) gene is localized to 11q22–q23.
- Males and females are equally affected.

GENERAL PREVENTION

- Genetic counseling
- Early diagnosis and referral to appropriate specialists, including neurologists, ophthalmologists, infectious disease specialists, and physical therapists

PATHOPHYSIOLOGY

AT primarily involves severe degeneration of Purkinje fibers in the cerebellar and extrapyramidal areas of the central nervous system; however, the basket and granular cells of the cerebellar cortex may also be involved. Other pathophysiologic changes include diffuse fibrillary gliosis and the degeneration of the anterior horns of the spinal cord.

ETIOLOGY

- Over 400 mutations have been identified in the ATM gene in patients with AT.
  - ATM encodes a protein kinase involved in the biochemical cascade that responds to DNA damage and is required for immune maturation and telomere maintenance.

COMMONLY ASSOCIATED CONDITIONS

- Recurrent sinopulmonary infections
- Lymphomas, leukemias
- Thymic dysplasia

DIAGNOSIS

HISTORY

- Abnormal eye movements (nearly 100%)
- Any episodes of recurrent sinopulmonary infections (48–81%)
- Growth retardation
- Difficulty walking, problems with balance (ataxia) (nearly 100%)
- Abnormal speech
- Choreoathetoid movements (30–90%)
- Abnormal blood vessels on the eyes or skin noticed by the parents

PHYSICAL EXAM

- Clinical diagnosis becomes most apparent after the age of 10 years when most children require a wheelchair, but can be detected in patients <5 years and as early as 3 months.
- Telangiectasias – the interpalpebral bulbar conjunctiva away from the limbus is the most common initial location of telangiectases, appearing at the age of 3–7. Eventually, the telangiectases can involve the entire conjunctiva, resembling conjunctivitis, and can spread to involve malar and orbital, auricular, antecubital and popliteal skin. Classically, these do not hemorrhage (2)[C].
- Positive oculomotor apraxia – slow, hypometric saccades with head-thrusting (1)[C]
- Often abnormalities exist with the optokinetic nystagmus drum.
- Visual acuity (unless there is severe nystagmus), pupillary reflexes, and fundus appearance are usually normal.
- Ataxia can be observed in infancy, as soon as the child is able to walk.
- Stooped position
- Intention tremors that increase with age
- Romberg sign is classically negative because truncal movement is equally pronounced with eyes open or closed.
- Sensation is intact. This finding coupled with the negative Romberg differentiates it from Friedrich's ataxia, which usually presents later in childhood.
- Other signs include premature gray hairs, mask-like faces, inelastic ears, a single café-au-lait spot, large freckles, vitiligo, seborrheic dermatitis, and common warts.

DIAGNOSTIC TESTS & INTERPRETATION

Lab

- More than 95% of AT children have an elevated blood alpha-fetoprotein (AFP) level. Although false positives are rare, in patients <2 years, AFP may be elevated because of the neonatal period (AFP is normally elevated in the pregnant mother) (1)[C].
- Karyotyping – translocations of chromosomes 7 and 14 are common (4)[C].
- Serum immunoglobulin testing reveals deficiencies of IgG2, IgE, and/or IgA.
- Less common – increased sensitivity of colony survival assays to ionizing radiation (5)[C], Western blots to confirm the presence of intracellular ATM protein, protein truncation testing of DNA complementary to the ATM gene is gaining popularity as a fast screening tool (1)[C].

Imaging

- MRI often shows cerebellar atrophy and enlargement of the fourth ventricle, which typically increases with age (3,4)[C].
- Chest radiographs will demonstrate minimal or absent thymic shadow, and changes that may be consistent with cystic fibrosis (1).
- In addition, absent or reduced adenoidal tissue in any area is so common on radiography that the presence of clinical lymphadenopathy is considered suggestive of lymphoma.

Pathological Findings

AT primarily involves severe degeneration of Purkinje fibers in the cerebellar and extrapyramidal areas of the central nervous system; however, the basket and granular cells of the cerebellar cortex may also be involved. Other pathophysiologic changes include diffuse fibrillary gliosis and the degeneration of the anterior horns of the spinal cord.

DIFFERENTIAL DIAGNOSIS

- Friedrich's ataxia
- Cerebral palsy (cerebellar type)
- Familial spinocerebellar atrophies
- GM1 and GM2 gangliosidoses
- Metachromatic leukodystrophy
- Krabbe disease
- Maple syrup urine disease
- Progressive rubella panencephalitis
- Subacute sclerosing panencephalitis
- Postinfectious encephalomyelitis
- Encephalitis
- Other polyneuropathies
- Cerebellar tumor

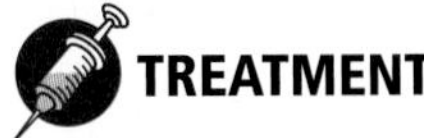

TREATMENT

MEDICATION

- Appropriate antibiotic treatment for recurrent sinopulmonary infections; this treatment should be directed by the infectious disease specialist.
- Periodic administration of immunoglobulin replacement has been reported beneficial for patients with difficulty with vaccine responses. Refer to immunologist, infectious disease.
- No adequate treatment for the neurologic or ophthalmic manifestations has been found.
- Regular surveillance for leukemic or lymphoid malignancies must be observed.

ADDITIONAL TREATMENT

General Measures

- Children will eventually need full-time classroom aides for help with reading.
- Physical therapists and aides are also important for preventing muscle stiffness and position-related issues.
- Parents and guardians should be coached to recognize early signs of pulmonary or respiratory infection.

SURGERY/OTHER PROCEDURES

Muscle surgery if there is a strabismus or nystagmus causing problems with primary gaze or head tilt in primary gaze

ONGOING CARE

FOLLOW-UP RECOMMENDATIONS

- Neurologist to assess progression of ataxia, dysarthria, choreoathetoid movements
- Immunologist to monitor immune dysfunction
- Pulmonologist to monitor for infection
- Ophthalmologist to assess nystagmus and oculomotor apraxia, as well as to follow the conjunctival and palpebral telangiectasias
- Hematologist/oncologist for malignancy

DIET

No nutritional supplement has been shown to have a benefit.

PATIENT EDUCATION

- See "General Measures" and "Follow-up Recommendations"
- http://www.nlm.nih.gov/medlineplus/ency/article/001394.htm
- http://www.nlm.nih.gov/medlineplus/ataxiatelangiectasia.html

PROGNOSIS

- Death is most commonly caused by a recurrent sinopulmonary infection, and most commonly occurs in adolescents, although the life expectancy is quite variable and some have survived to middle age.
- Other common causes of death include malignancy, or a combination of malignancy and infection.

REFERENCES

1. Perlman S, Becker-Catania S, Gatti R. Ataxia-telangiectasia: Diagnosis and treatment. *Semin Pediatr Neurol* 2003;10:173–182.
2. Morrell D, Cromartie E, Swift M. Mortality and cancer incidence in 263 patients with ataxia-telangiectasia. *J Natl Cancer Inst* 1986;77(1):89–92.
3. Tavani F, Zimmerman RA, Berry GT, et al. Ataxia-telangiectasia: The pattern of cerebellar atrophy on MRI. *Neuroradiology* 2003;45(5):315–319.
4. Lavin MF, Gueven N, Bottle S, et al. Current and potential therapeutic strategies for the treatment of ataxia-telangiectasia. *Br Med Bull* 2007;81–82:129–147.
5. Beamish H, Lavin MF. Radiosensitivity in ataxia-telangiectasia: Anomalies in radiation-induced cell cycle delay. *Int J Radiat Biol* 1994;65(2):175–184.

CODES

ICD9

- 334.8 Other spinocerebellar diseases
- 379.51 Congenital nystagmus

CLINICAL PEARLS

- AT is a multisystem neurodegenerative and immunodeficiency disorder.
- It comprises oculomotor apraxia, progressive dysarthria and choreoathetoid movements, telangiectases, lymphoproliferative cancer, and immune dysfunction resulting in recurrent sinopulmonary infections.
- Initial diagnostics features include characteristic findings and elevated blood AFP.
- Treatment involves a multidisciplinary team with neurology, hematology/oncology, pulmonology, immunology, infectious diseases, and ophthalmology.

AXENFELD–RIEGER SYNDROME

Andrea Knellinger Sawchyn
L. Jay Katz

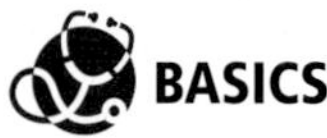

BASICS

DESCRIPTION

- A spectrum of developmental disorders resulting in bilateral iris and angle abnormalities frequently associated with secondary glaucoma and systemic anomalies including dental and facial bone abnormalities
- Nomenclature has changed through the years. Axenfeld anomaly, Rieger anomaly, and Axenfeld–Rieger syndrome have previously been classified separately but now are all considered to be a single entity representing a spectrum of related anterior segment developmental disorders collectively referred to as Axenfeld–Rieger syndrome.

EPIDEMIOLOGY

Incidence

Rare

Prevalence

Unknown

RISK FACTORS

Family history

Genetics

- Autosomal dominant with high penetrance
- Mutations at the following loci have been linked to Axenfeld–Rieger syndrome (1)[B].
  - Paired-like homeodomain transcription factor 2 (PITX2, 4p25): A transcription factor that regulates the expression of other genes in anterior segment structures, dental lamina, and the umbilical cord during embryonic development
  - Forkhead box C1 (FOXC1) – formerly called Forkhead Drosophila homologue-like transcription factor gene – (FKHL7, 6p25): Another transcription factor
  - Gap junction protein, alpha 1 (GJA1, 6q21q23.2): Encodes connexin 43 protein which forms gap junctions
  - Paired box gene 6 (PAX6, 11p13)
  - V-MAF avian musculoaponeurotic fibrosarcoma oncogene (MAF, 16q24)
  - 13q14 (gene unknown)

GENERAL PREVENTION

No known modes of prevention, other than genetic counseling.

PATHOPHYSIOLOGY

- A neural crestopathy resulting from a genetically triggered arrest in anterior segment development during late gestation (2)[C]
- Consequently, the aqueous outflow structures are incomplete and retained primordial endothelium covers the angle and iris (2)[C].

ETIOLOGY

- A genetic developmental disorder
- See "Pathophysiology"

COMMONLY ASSOCIATED CONDITIONS

- The most common systemic anomalies associated with Axenfeld–Rieger syndrome are dental and facial bone abnormalities:
  - Microdontia
  - Hypodontia
  - Oligodontia
  - Anodontia
  - Maxillary hypoplasia
  - Hypertelorism
  - Telecanthus
  - Broad, flat nose
- Other less common systemic associations include:
  - Pituitary anomalies including empty sella syndrome and growth hormone deficiency
  - Redundant periumbilical skin
  - Hypospadias
  - Heart defects
  - Middle ear deafness
  - Mental retardation
- Ocular abnormalities that are not identified as part of the Axenfeld–Rieger spectrum but have been infrequently associated with Axenfeld–Rieger syndrome include:
  - Strabismus
  - Limbal dermoids
  - Cataracts
  - Iris transillumination defects
  - Retinal detachment
  - Macular degeneration
  - Chorioretinal colobomas
  - Choroidal hypoplasia
  - Optic nerve hypoplasia

DIAGNOSIS

HISTORY

- Most cases are identified in infancy or childhood during a routine exam, often prompted by a positive family history.
- Often asymptomatic, but may present with the symptoms of infantile glaucoma such as blepharospasm, epiphora, and/or photophobia
- Glaucoma develops in 50%.

PHYSICAL EXAM

- Typically bilateral
- Ocular findings include a range of the following corneal, angle, and iris anomalies (3)[C]:
  - A prominent, anteriorly displaced Schwalbe's line (posterior embryotoxon) noted 360° or limited to the temporal quadrant with adherent peripheral iris strands.
  - The cornea is usually otherwise normal, although megalocornea, microcornea, and central opacities have rarely been described.
  - On gonioscopy, the iris inserts into the posterior meshwork, obscuring the scleral spur.
  - The iris may be normal or stromal thinning, pseudopolycoria, corectopia, and/or ectropion uvea may be present.
  - Peripheral iris changes usually do not progress after birth, but central iris anomalies have progressed during childhood in a small number of individuals.
  - Elevated intraocular pressure may be present.
  - Optic nerve cupping may develop. When the onset is in childhood, cupping is usually concentric with healthy surrounding disk tissue until late stages.

Pediatric Considerations

- In children, exams under anesthesia are often required. However, all children should also be examined without sedation to screen for amblyopia and monitor ocular motility.
- In children <3 years of age, monitor for the following signs as they may be indicative of the onset of glaucoma:
  - Progressive corneal enlargement
  - Increasing axial length
  - Progressive myopia or rapid loss of hyperopia

DIAGNOSTIC TESTS & INTERPRETATION

Imaging

- Optic disc photos
- Consider optic nerve head imaging (optical coherence tomography, confocal scanning laser ophthalmoscopy, scanning laser polarimetry); hand-held optical coherence tomography (if available) may be used during exams under anesthesia.

Diagnostic Procedures/Other

Visual field (once the child is old enough to complete this test reliably, the age will vary depending on the child)

Pathological Findings

- Peripheral iris strands attached to (or sometimes anterior or posterior to) an anteriorly displaced, prominent Schwalbe's line.
- A monolayer of spindle-shaped cells extends from the cornea to cover the angle and anterior surface of the iris.
- This layer of spindle-shaped cells is frequently seen covering the iris in areas toward which the pupil is displaced.
- The iris stroma may be thin or absent in areas away from the corectopia.
- Iris not adherent to the cornea typically inserts into the posterior aspect of the meshwork.
- The trabecular meshwork is composed of a reduced number of attenuated lamellae.
- Schlemm's canal may be rudimentary or absent.

DIFFERENTIAL DIAGNOSIS

- Iridocorneal endothelial syndrome
- Posterior polymorphous dystrophy (PPMD)
- Posterior embryotoxon
- Peters anomaly

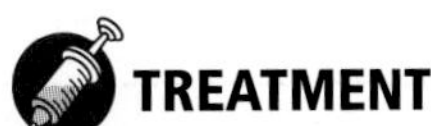

TREATMENT

MEDICATION

First Line

- Observation may be appropriate if no signs of ocular hypertension or glaucoma are present.
- Once elevated intraocular pressure develops, medical therapy should be initiated:
  - Topical beta-blockers (in children, timolol 0.25%, levobunolol 0.25%, or betaxolol are reasonable options)
  - Topical carbonic anhydrase inhibitors (e.g., dorzolamide, brinzolamide)
  - Prostaglandin analogs (e.g., latanoprost, travoprost, bimatoprost)
  - Topical alpha$_2$-agonists (e.g., brimonidine)

ALERT

- Use of alpha$_2$-agonists (e.g., iopidine, brimonidine) in children $<$1 year of age is not recommended due to potential central nervous system depression.

Second Line

Oral carbonic anhydrase inhibitors (in children, acetazolamide 15–30 mg/kg per day, divided into 3 to 4 doses)

ADDITIONAL TREATMENT

General Measures

Treat coexisting amblyopia if present.

Issues for Referral

- All children with Axenfeld–Rieger syndrome should be referred to a pediatrician for a complete physical exam. Subsequent referrals to endocrinology or dentistry are sometimes needed.
- Genetics consultation for counseling and molecular testing
- Referral to a glaucoma specialist or pediatric ophthalmologist experienced with glaucoma may be necessary if/when elevated intraocular pressure develops.

Additional Therapies

Laser trabeculoplasty is usually ineffective and is not recommended.

SURGERY/OTHER PROCEDURES

- When glaucoma progresses inspire of medical management, surgery is indicated.
- With infantile-onset glaucoma, goniotomy or trabeculotomy may be attempted, but results may be suboptimal due to underlying abnormalities of Schlemm's canal (3)[C].
- For all other cases, trabeculectomy (3)[C] or a glaucoma drainage device are the surgical procedures of choice.
- Diode cyclophotocoagulation can be utilized when all other medical and surgical therapies fail.

ONGOING CARE

FOLLOW-UP RECOMMENDATIONS

- All patients require life-long follow-up as glaucoma suspects.
- Once glaucoma develops, patients should be seen every 3–6 months depending on disease severity and age at diagnosis.
- In young children, remember to repeat axial length and corneal diameter measurements as well as streak retinoscopy frequently to monitor for glaucoma progression.
- Optic nerve photos or imaging should be repeated periodically as well.
- Visual fields should be repeated annually in all patients and at least annually in patients with glaucoma (once reliable tests are obtainable).

DIET

No special diets are required.

PATIENT EDUCATION

- The Pediatric Glaucoma and Cataract Family Association www.pgcfa.org
- American Association for Pediatric Ophthalmology and Strabismus www.aapos.org

PROGNOSIS

Development of glaucoma often results in a poor prognosis as this form of secondary glaucoma is typically difficult to control and frequently requires surgical intervention.

COMPLICATIONS

- Glaucomatous visual field loss $\pm$ decreased visual acuity
- Anisometropia
- Myopia
- Amblyopia

REFERENCES

1. Cella W, Cabral de Vasconcellos JP, de Melo MB, et al. Structural assessment of PITX2, FOXC1, CYP1B1, and GJA1 genes in patients with Axenfeld–Rieger syndrome with developmental glaucoma. *Invest Ophthalmol Vis Sci* 2006;47: 1803–1809.
2. Shields MB. Axenfeld–Rieger and iridocorneal endothelial syndromes: Two spectra of disease with striking similarities and differences. *J Glaucoma* 2001;10(Suppl 1):S36–S38.
3. Shields MB, Buckley E, Klintworth GK, Thresher R. Axenfeld–Rieger syndrome. A spectrum of developmental disorders. *Surv Ophthalmol* 1985;29: 387–409.

ADDITIONAL READING

- Alward WL. Axenfeld–Rieger syndrome in the age of molecular genetics. *Am J Ophthalmol* 2000;130: 107–115.
- Shields MB. Axenfeld–Rieger syndrome: A theory of mechanism and distinctions from the iridocorneal endothelial syndrome. *Trans Am Ophthalmol Soc* 1983;81:736–784.

CODES

ICD9

- 365.41 Glaucoma associated with chamber angle anomalies
- 743.44 Specified congenital anomalies of anterior chamber, chamber angle, and related structures

CLINICAL PEARLS

- A bilateral, genetic, developmental disorder of the anterior segment resulting in characteristic corneal, angle, and iris abnormalities
- It may be associated with nonocular anomalies, most commonly dental and facial abnormalities.
- Detection and control of secondary glaucoma, which occurs in 50% of patients, is key to management.
- Glaucoma management can be challenging and often requires surgery.

BAND KERATOPATHY

Christine W. Chung

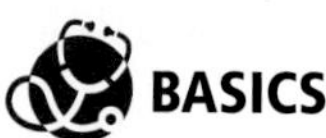

BASICS

DESCRIPTION

A degenerative corneal disorder characterized by a gray or white band of opacity in the interpalpebral fissure, most commonly caused by the gradual precipitation of calcium in the anterior layers of the cornea (Bowman's membrane, epithelial basement membrane, and anterior stroma).

EPIDEMIOLOGY

Incidence

Unknown

Prevalence

Unknown

RISK FACTORS

- Chronic eye disease
- Abnormal calcium and phosphate metabolism
- Mercury exposure
- Ocular surgery using silicone oil
- Gout (causes a pigmented noncalcific band keratopathy)

Genetics

Rare cases of a familial calcific band-shaped keratopathy, probably autosomal recessive, have been reported (1).

GENERAL PREVENTION

Management of chronic eye inflammation or other disease; management of systemic calcium and phosphate abnormalities

PATHOPHYSIOLOGY

Precipitation of calcium below the corneal epithelium, thought to be caused by tear film hypertonicity, pH elevation, or changes in calcium or phosphate concentration. In mercury exposure and silicone keratopathy, calcium deposition occurs because of degenerative corneal changes.

ETIOLOGY

- Chronic eye disease: Chronic uveitis, end-stage glaucoma, phthisis bulbi. Severe dry eye disease may increase risk of band keratopathy because of tear hypertonicity.
- Abnormal calcium and phosphate metabolism or levels: Hyperparathyroidism, malignancy, sarcoidosis, Paget's disease, vitamin D overdose, renal failure, milk-alkali syndrome
- Chemical or drug exposure: Mercury vapor, topical medications containing phosphates or mercurial preservatives, silicone oil
- Gout (causes deposition of urate crystals in the anterior cornea)

COMMONLY ASSOCIATED CONDITIONS

See the Etiology section.

DIAGNOSIS

HISTORY

- Decreased vision (if opacity is in visual axis)
- Foreign body sensation (if epithelium is compromised)
- Ocular and systemic risk factors (see the Risk Factors section)
- Toxic exposures

PHYSICAL EXAM

- Grayish plaque in superficial cornea in the interpalpebral zone, often with clear lacunae, creating a "Swiss-cheese" appearance. Opacity starts at 3 and 9 o'clock positions, separated from the limbus by clear cornea, and slowly progresses centrally. If calcium deposits break through epithelium, fluorescein staining will detect an epithelial defect.
- In gout, the deposits are yellow and crystalline.

DIAGNOSTIC TESTS & INTERPRETATION

Lab

Initial lab tests

- Complete slit lamp examination (see the Physical Exam section for typical features). Look for evidence of underlying ocular disease, including corneal edema, cell and flare in anterior chamber, synechiae, elevated intraocular pressure or hypotony, glaucomatous optic neuropathy, silicone oil, phthisis.
- In the absence of ocular conditions accounting for the band keratopathy, check for elevated serum calcium, phosphate, BUN, creatinine.
- Check for elevated serum uric acid, if gout is suspected.

Follow-up & special considerations

If systemic abnormalities detected, further lab tests may be indicated (e.g., parathyroid hormone level to investigate hypercalcemia).

Pathological Findings

- Basophilic stippling of Bowman's layer, progressing to linear deposits of calcium in the superficial cornea. Calcium deposits are intracellular in hypercalcemia and extracellular in ocular disease.
- In gout, urate crystals are seen in epithelial cell nuclei.

DIFFERENTIAL DIAGNOSIS

- Corneal scar
- Interstitial keratitis
- Calcareous corneal degeneration (posterior stromal or full thickness calcium deposition which may occur in eyes with chronic ocular disease or inflammation)

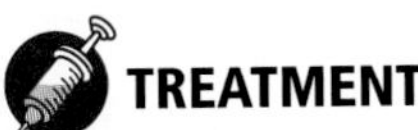

TREATMENT

MEDICATION

- For mild foreign body sensation, topical lubrication with artificial tears or ophthalmic ointments may be helpful. (For decreased vision or more severe foreign body sensation or pain, surgical debridement is indicated. See the Surgery/Other Procedures section below.)
- Medical therapy for underlying ocular or systemic causes as indicated.

ADDITIONAL TREATMENT

Issues for Referral

Follow-up as needed based on symptoms and underlying ocular or systemic disease

SURGERY/OTHER PROCEDURES

- Surgical debridement is indicated if pain or decreased vision becomes significant.
  - Ethylenediamine tetraacetic acid (EDTA) chelation of calcium deposits: Debridement or removal of corneal epithelium, followed by application of EDTA to the exposed corneal surface in order to remove the calcium deposits by chelation (2)[C]
  - Excimer laser phototherapeutic keratectomy (PTK). May be used primarily (3)[C] or in combination with EDTA chelation (4)[C]
  - Mechanical debridement of deposits, e.g., by scraping with a surgical blade (5)[C]

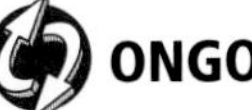

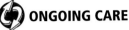

ONGOING CARE

FOLLOW-UP RECOMMENDATIONS

Patient Monitoring

- As needed for symptoms (decreased vision, foreign body sensation)
- As needed for management of underlying ocular or systemic causes
- After EDTA chelation, close follow-up until epithelium is healed, and then as needed.

DIET

As indicated by any systemic etiologies (renal failure, vitamin D overdose, milk-alkali syndrome)

PROGNOSIS

Likely to recur or progress, but because progression is usually very gradual, symptoms of decreased vision and foreign body sensation may not reappear for months to years.

COMPLICATIONS

- Corneal infection due to epithelial breakdown
- Following EDTA chelation, PTK, or other surgical debridement, corneal haze or scarring may develop.
- PTK may cause myopic shift.

REFERENCES

1. Arora R, Shroff D, Kapoor S, et al. Familial calcific band-shaped keratopathy: Report of two new cases with early recurrence. *Indian J Ophthalmol* 2007; 55(1):55–57.
2. Najjar DM, Cohen EJ, Rapuano CJ, et al. EDTA chelation for calcific band keratopathy: Results and long-term follow-up. *Am J Ophthalmol* 2004; 137(6):1056–1064.
3. O'Brart DPS, Gartry DS, Lohmann CP, et al. Treatment of band keratopathy by excimer laser phototherapeutic keratectomy: Surgical techniques and long term follow up. *Br J Ophthalmol* 1993; 77:702–708.
4. Im SK, Lee KH, Yoon KC. Combined ethylenediaminetetraacetic acid chelation, phototherapeutic keratectomy, and amniotic membrane transplantation for treatment of band keratopathy. *Korean J Ophthalmol* 2010;24(2): 73–77.
5. Wood TO, Walker GG. Treatment of band keratopathy. *Am J Ophthalmol* 1975;80:550.

ADDITIONAL READING

- Keratopathy, Band: eMedicine Ophthalmology. http://emedicine.medscape.com/article/1194813-overview
- Stewart OG, Morrell AJ. Management of band keratopathy with excimer phototherapeutic keratectomy: visual, refractive, and symptomatic outcome. *Eye (Lond)* 2003;17(2):233–237.

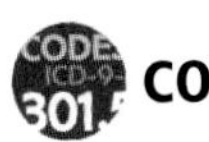

CODES

ICD9

371.43 Band-shaped keratopathy

CLINICAL PEARLS

- Band keratopathy is usually seen in eyes with chronic ocular disease or inflammation.
- When no underlying ocular condition is obvious, check for hypercalcemia or renal abnormalities.

BARTONELLA NEUROREТINITIS

Andrew Lam

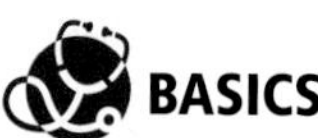

BASICS

DESCRIPTION

- Neuroretinitis is a condition characterized by optic disk swelling and hard exudates distributed in a star pattern centered around the fovea:
  - *Bartonella henselae*, a gram negative bacillus associated with cat-scratch disease, is the most common infectious etiology of neuroretinitis.

EPIDEMIOLOGY

- All ages can be affected
- Most common in third or fourth decade
- No gender predilection

RISK FACTORS

History of contact with cat or kitten

ETIOLOGY

- Infectious causes: *Bartonella henselae*, syphilis, viral, toxoplasmosis, toxocariasis, histoplasmosis, Lyme disease
- Systemic inflammatory conditions such as sarcoidosis

COMMONLY ASSOCIATED CONDITIONS

- Cat-scratch disease
- Syphilis
- Sarcoidosis

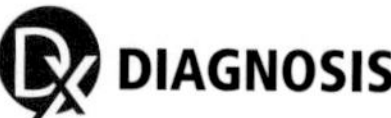

DIAGNOSIS

HISTORY

- Eye complaints: Eye ache, worse with eye movement, blurry vision
- Systemic complaints: Symptoms of cat-scratch disease may include malaise, fever, muscle aches, headache
- Travel history
- Animal contacts
- Sexual history
- Note any ingestion of uncooked food

PHYSICAL EXAM

- Visual acuity varies from normal to light perception
- Abnormal color vision
- Afferent papillary defect
- Optic nerve edema
- Macular hard exudates in star configuration
- Splinter hemorrhages, retinal vessel occlusion may be seen
- Discrete, small yellow-white retinal or choroidal infiltrates
- Vitreous cells/posterior inflammation
- Patients with cat-scratch disease may exhibit lymphadenopathy, arthritis, meningitis, encephalitis, or may be asymptomatic

DIAGNOSTIC TESTS & INTERPRETATION

Lab

- Serologic testing for *Bartonella henselae* and other infectious etiologies
- ELISA for *Bartonella henselae* is available

Imaging

Fluorescein angiogram: Disk swelling/leakage, peripapillary vessel staining may be seen

Diagnostic Procedures/Other

Visual field test – cecocentral scotoma most common defect

DIFFERENTIAL DIAGNOSIS

- Optic neuritis
- Optic neuropathy

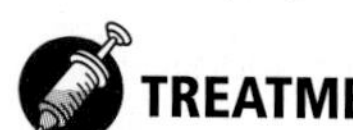

TREATMENT

MEDICATION

First Line

- For cat-scratch disease:
- Ciprofloxacin 750 mg PO b.i.d. for 3 weeks
- Consider erythromycin, azithromycin, doxycycline, rifampin

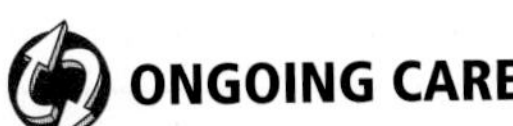

ONGOING CARE

FOLLOW-UP RECOMMENDATIONS

- Primary care doctor or infectious disease specialist
- Ophthalmologist

PROGNOSIS

- Usually a self-limited course with good visual prognosis.
- Optic nerve swelling usually improves over 6–8 weeks. Residual disk pallor may remain.
- Macular exudates resolve over 6–12 months.
- Symptoms of metamorphopsia or blurred vision may persist.
- Most patients do not experience recurrence in the same or fellow eye.

COMPLICATIONS

- Visual loss
- Systemic sequelae of a causative infectious or inflammatory agent

ADDITIONAL READING

- Reed JB, Scales DK, Wong MT, et al. *Bartonella henselae* neuroretinitis in cat scratch disease. Diagnosis, management, and sequelae. *Ophthalmology* 1998;105(3):459–466.
- Ormerod LD, Skolnick KA, Menosky MM, et al. Retinal and choroidal manifestations of cat-scratch disease. *Ophthalmology* 1998;105(6):1024–1031.
- Solley WA, Martin DF, Newman NJ, et al. Cat scratch disease: Posterior segment manifestations. *Ophthalmology* 1999;106(8):1546–1553.
- Ray S, Gragoudas E. Neuroretinitis. *Int Ophthalmol Clin* 2001;41(1):83–102.

CODES

ICD9

363.05 Focal retinitis and retinochoroiditis, juxtapapillary

CLINICAL PEARLS

- Neuroretinitis is characterized by optic nerve swelling and exudative macular star.
- *Bartonella henselae* is the most common infectious cause of neuroretinitis.
- Visual prognosis is often good and disease is self-limited.

BEHÇET'S DISEASE

Alex B. Theventhiran
Sunir J. Garg

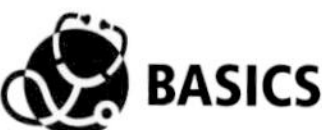

BASICS

DESCRIPTION

- Systemic vasculitis characterized by triad of recurrent oral aphthous ulcers, genital ulcers, and uveitis. Skin lesions are common.
- Uveitis ranges from nongranulomatous anterior uveitis (classically with hypopyon) to chronic retinal vasculitis.

Pediatric Considerations

In Japan, 1.5% of cases of Behçet's disease occur in children. Various forms, including a transient neonatal case, have been documented. In children, there is a greater frequency of uveitis and arthritis, but genital and oral ulcers are less common.

Pregnancy Considerations

Most studies show a good outcome in pregnancy, with the majority of patients showing no change during labor and after delivery, and no worsening of disease symptoms and no significant difference in frequency of congenital malformations, spontaneous abortions, and perinatal death.

EPIDEMIOLOGY

Incidence

- Greatest incidence is in Turkey and Japan, and along the ancient silk route connecting the two.
- More common in young patients (25–35 years), but occurs in all ages.
- Prior studies suggested a higher incidence in men; however, recent reports suggest a more even distribution between men and women.

Prevalence

- Prevalence in Japan is 8–10/100,000 and it comprises 20% of all uveitis cases in Japan. In Turkey, the incidence is 80–300/100,000.
- It is rare in the United States, with prevalence of 4/1,000,000 and comprises 0.2–0.4% of all uveitis cases.

RISK FACTORS

- Occurs most commonly in patients from Turkey, Japan, the Middle East, Pakistan, northern China, and Korea. Rare in North America.
- Poorly defined environmental and infections exposures due to *streptococcus*, HSV type 1, Hepatitis C Virus, and *E. coli* have been suggested.

Genetics

- HLA-B51 phenotype and its subtypes HLA-Bw51 and B*501 have been identified as risk factors.
- HLA-DR1 and HLA-DQw1 have been identified as significantly decreased in Behçet's patients – possibly providing resistance to disease development.

PATHOPHYSIOLOGY

A nonspecific obliterative vasculitis of small blood vessels due to abnormal cellular immune responses including lymphocyte dysfunction

ETIOLOGY

- Unknown. It is postulated that a genetic predisposition combined with an environmental trigger produces the disease.
- *Streptococcus* and viruses (HSV-1, Hepatitis C) have been studied as possible triggers.

DIAGNOSIS

HISTORY

- Behçet's disease is a clinical diagnosis.
- There is no specific laboratory test to confirm the diagnosis.
- There are various systems for diagnosis.
- The International Beḩcet Study Group criteria are:
  - Recurrent oral aphthous ulcers occurring 3 times in 12 months.
  - In addition to oral ulcers, 2 of the following must be present: Recurrent genital ulcers, uveitis, skin lesions, and/or positive pathergy test.
- The Behçet's Disease Research Committee Criteria are:
- 1. Major criteria: Recurrent oral aphthous ulcers, recurrent genital ulcers, skin lesions, and uveitis
- 2. Minor criteria: Arthritis, intestinal ulcers, epididymitis, vascular disease, and neuropsychiatric symptoms
- Complete Behçet's disease requires a history of all 4 major symptoms.
- Incomplete diagnosis requires 3 major symptoms or uveitis with 1 minor symptom.
- Suspect diagnosis requires 2 major symptoms, excluding uveitis.
- Possible diagnosis requires any major symptom.
- The most common symptom is oral aphthous ulcers which occur in 98% of patients. They are discrete white ulcerations with a red border that are 3–15 mm in size.
- Skin lesions are predominately erythema nodosum, superficial thrombophlebitis, and eruptions resembling acne vulgaris or folliculitis.
- Genital ulcers are recurrent and occur in the vagina or vulva in females, the penis or scrotum in males, and in the perianal area in both sexes. They can be painful or painless.
- Uveitis is present in ~79% of patients and manifests as nongranulomatous inflammation with necrotizing obliterative vasculitis.
- Patients often complain of pain, redness, photophobia, and blurred vision.
- The anterior segment often has iridocyclitis without hypopyon. Hypopyon occurs in the "classical presentation"; however, it occurs in less than a third of ocular cases, likely due to more aggressive early treatment.
- Posterior segment involvement leads to greater morbidity. Retinal vasculitis affects both arteries and veins. Vitreitis can occur.
- CNS symptoms (due to vasculitis) may be motor, sensory, or psychiatric. Meningoencephalitis may be the most common manifestation (uncommon overall).
- Neuro-ophthalmic findings include 6th and 7th nerve palsies, central scotomas, and optic disc edema.

PHYSICAL EXAM

- Inspect for oral and genital ulceration, skin lesions, and other criteria listed above.
- Anterior uveitis and presence of a hypopyon. The hypopyon may change position with head movement.
- Posterior segment ocular involvement includes retinal vasculitis affecting both arteries and veins, profound nonperfusion, venous and capillary dilatation with engorgement, patchy perivascular sheathing with inflammatory exudates, yellow-white exudates deep in the retina, neovascularization, and vitreitis.

DIAGNOSTIC TESTS & INTERPRETATION

Lab

Initial lab tests

- None generally necessary.
- Pathergy skin reaction/Behcetine skin test (sterile pustules that develop at the site of spontaneous or induced trauma) is present in 40% of Behçet's patients.
- HLA-B51 typing (present in >50% of Behçet's patients of Mediterranean and Japanese origin) may be used to aid with diagnosis.

- Nonspecific factors of immune system activation: Elevated levels of serum proteins, circulating immune complexes, acute phase reactants, and other complement reactive proteins may be present during the acute phase.

Follow-up & special considerations
Lumbar puncture (not routinely needed) shows pleocytosis of CSF. In addition, MRI and CT imaging may be used to identify possible CNS lesions.

Imaging
Fluorescein angiography (FA) is helpful to analyze the extent of retina vascular damage, to evaluate neovascularization, and to assess response to therapy.

DIFFERENTIAL DIAGNOSIS
- Viral retinitis
- HLA-B27 associated anterior uveitis (hypopyon), especially reactive arthritis
- Sarcoidosis
- Tuberculosis
- Systemic lupus erythematosus (SLE)
- Polyarteritis nodosa (PAN)
- Wegener's granulomatosis (WG)
- Oral ulcers: Stevens–Johnson syndrome, Reiter's syndrome, trauma
- Genital ulcers: Herpetic ulcers, reactive arthritis (Reiter's syndrome)

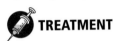

TREATMENT

MEDICATION
First Line
- Medication is based on disease severity. If complete Behçet's disease, severe ocular/retinal involvement, CNS involvement, or other significant vasculitis, aggressive treatment is required. (Men, and people of Turkish/Japanese descent also usually require more aggressive treatment.)
- Oral (1–2 mg/kg per day) or pulse dose corticosteroids have a rapid onset of action. However, Behçet's patients in need of high dose steroids require steroid sparing agents as high dose steroids cannot be used for long periods of time without severe side effects.
- Biologics such as the TNF inhibitors infliximab (Remicade) and adalimumab (Humira) should be considered. Cytotoxic agents (chlorambucil, cyclophosphamide), the antimetabolites azathioprine and mycophenolate mofetil, and the calcineurin inhibitors cyclosporine-A and tacrolimus are used in combination with corticosteroids.

Second Line
- Cyclophosphamide and chlorambucil are useful, especially in cases of severe CNS and gastrointestinal involvement.
- Colchicine and thalidomide can be useful in systemic disease, but do not control uveitis well.
- Neutrophilic apheresis has been shown to be helpful in some patients.

ADDITIONAL TREATMENT
Issues for Referral
- Patients with ocular involvement require prompt referral to a uveitis/retinal specialist as there can be up to a 90% rate of blindness with delayed/inadequate treatment.
- A multidisciplinary team is required to manage the various systemic effects of the disease.

SURGERY/OTHER PROCEDURES
- Surgery for cataracts can occur when visual improvement can be expected and the eye has been inflammation free for 3 months.
- As surgical trauma may induce recurrence of the inflammation, consider prophylaxis with systemic and topical steroids 1 week preoperatively with continuation postoperatively with a slow taper over several weeks. Any systemic immunosuppressive drugs should be continued.
- Laser photocoagulation can be used for retinal neovascularization and does not produce postoperative inflammation.

IN-PATIENT CONSIDERATIONS
Initial Stabilization
High dose oral or pulse dose corticosteroids for rapid anti-inflammatory effect

Admission Criteria
Any severe vision or life-threatening manifestation of Behçet's disease should prompt consideration of hospitalization.

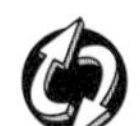

ONGOING CARE

FOLLOW-UP RECOMMENDATIONS
Patients will need very close monitoring until the disease is brought under control. They will also need continuous follow-up with other specialists as needed.

PROGNOSIS
- Prognosis is improved with prompt aggressive treatment, but visual outcomes can be guarded. Even with therapy, legal blindness has been noted to occur in >50% of cases within 4 years (but this was with earlier immunosuppressive agents).
- Systemic prognosis is good in the absence of CNS involvement, vascular involvement, or GI perforation. Remissions increase in duration with time and disease stabilization occurs after ~10 years.
- Prognosis is better in the USA than in Mediterranean or East Asia, possibly due to a less severe form of the disease or more effective treatment.

COMPLICATIONS
- Bilateral vision loss due to ocular inflammation.
- Anterior uveitis can cause cataract formation or glaucoma. Posterior segment inflammation can result in macular and peripheral retinal ischemia, and optic nerve damage.
- Retinal neovascularization, retinal detachment, vitreous hemorrhage, and vitreous traction can also occur.

ADDITIONAL READING

- Kaçmaz RO, Kempen JH, Newcomb C, et al. Ocular inflammation in Behçet disease: Incidence of ocular complications and of loss of visual acuity. *Am J Ophthalmol* 2008;146(6):828–836.
- Marsal S, Falgá C, Simeon CP, et al. Behçet's disease and pregnancy relationship study. *Br J Rheumatol* 1997;36(2):234–238.
- Sakane T, Takeno M, Suzuki N, et al. Behçet's disease. *N Engl J Med* 1999;341:1284–1291.
- Tabbara KF, Al-Hemidan AI. Infliximab effects compared to conventional therapy in the management of retinal vasculitis in Behçet disease. *Am J Ophthalmol* 2008;146(6):845–850.

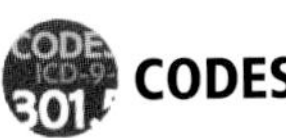

CODES

ICD9
- 136.1 Behçet's syndrome
- 360.12 Panuveitis
- 364.3 Unspecified iridocyclitis

CLINICAL PEARLS

- The characteristic findings are uveitis, oral aphthous ulcers, genital ulcers, and skin lesions.
- As this is a generalized vasculitis, patients have numerous organ and life-threatening complications as a result.
- Prompt and aggressive immunosuppressive control is critical.

BENIGN CONJUNCTIVAL LESIONS

Matthew Gorski
Colleen Halfpenny

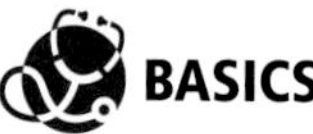

BASICS

DESCRIPTION

Benign conjunctival lesions are a group of tumors, including papilloma (Pap), Kaposi's sarcoma (KS), limbal dermoid (LD), sarcoidosis (Sarc), and pyogenic granuloma (PG) with a low potential for malignant growth and a wide variety of etiologies and management considerations.

EPIDEMIOLOGY

Incidence

- Systemic KS: 4–14% in ocular adnexa (1)[C]
- Ocular KS: 7–18%
- Ocular Sarc: 7–19%

RISK FACTORS

- Pap: Mother with positive human papillomavirus (HPV) history, UV radiation
- KS: Immunocompromised states, including HIV/AIDS, chemotherapy, organ transplantation, elderly males
- LD: <18 years of age
- Sarc: African American race
- PG: transconjunctival surgical incisions (strabismus, retinal surgery), trauma (2)[B]

Genetics

Sarc: HLA-Bw15, HLA-B8, HLA-B13

PATHOPHYSIOLOGY

- Pap: HPV, a double-stranded DNA virus transmitted via direct contact, often through passage of infected birth canal leading to proliferation of fibrovascular connective tissue, acanthosis, and hyperkeratosis
- KS: Dysregulated inflammatory cytokine response due to human herpesvirus-8
- LD: Congenital choristomatous changes due to an unknown process; classified based upon the extent of anterior segment involvement
- Sarc: Inflammatory hyperactivity due to dysregulated cytokine responses following an antigenic stimulus
- PG: Proliferative fibrovascular and inflammatory response usually secondary to aberrant wound healing

ETIOLOGY

- Pap: HPV, most commonly benign types 6 and 11, rarely type 16 or 45
- KS: Human herpesvirus-8 (HHV-8) DNA or Kaposi's sarcoma-associated herpesvirus (KSHV), implicated with patients who are HIV-negative and HIV-positive
- Sarc: Unknown etiology. Suggested causes: Environmental toxins, infectious agents, genetic transmission
- LD: Unknown
- PG: Usually due to prior inflammatory condition or status post trauma or surgery

COMMONLY ASSOCIATED CONDITIONS

- LD: Goldenhar's syndrome
- Sarc: Mikulicz's syndrome: Salivary and lacrimal gland enlargement with keratoconjunctivitis sicca

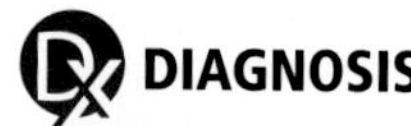

DIAGNOSIS

HISTORY

- Pap, KS, LD, Sarc, PG:
  - often asymptomatic
  - mass effect symptoms
  - foreign body sensation
  - itching
  - tearing
  - mucous
  - ptosis
  - photophobia
  - blurry vision
  - swelling
  - trichiasis
  - poor lid apposition
  - cosmetic effects
- KS: Immune status
- Sarc: Lung and skin nodules, dyspnea, cough malaise, fatigue, lymphadenopathy
- LD: <18 years of age, enlarging since birth, especially after puberty
- PG: History of surgery, inflammatory condition

PHYSICAL EXAM

- Pap: Pedunculated or sessile, pink-red, fleshy, smooth often verrucous appearing on bulbar or palpebral conjunctiva. Viral usually multiple lesions in inferior fornix; single lesions may suggest nonviral etiology and may extend toward the limbus.
- KS: Flat or raised, reddish-purple, oval, nontender mass, or nodular, well-circumscribed lesion
- Sarc: Single or multiple, yellow or salmon colored nodules. Most commonly on palpebral conjunctiva of lower cul-de-sac or plica semilunaris
- LD: Yellowish-white oval-shaped, solid mass involving bulbar conjunctiva, typically near the inferotemporal corneoscleral limbus; may have fine hairs
- PG: well-vascularized, elevated, red-fleshy mass with fibrous stalk
- Secondary findings for all of the above include chemosis, mechanical ectropion, superficial punctuate keratopathy, and corneal dellen.

DIAGNOSTIC TESTS & INTERPRETATION

Lab

- KS: HIV ELISA, HIV Western Blot, CD4
- Sarc: Angiotensin-converting enzyme, calcium, magnesium, phosphorous

Imaging

Sarc: Chest X-ray

Diagnostic Procedures/Other

- Slit lamp, dilated fundus examination, tonometry
- Pap, KS, Sarc, PG: incisional or excisional biopsy, if suspicious for malignancy
- LD: Depth of corneal involvement can be evaluated with ultrasound biomicroscopy (UBM). Examine patient for signs and symptoms of Goldenhar's syndrome, including preauricular skin appendages, hearing loss, lid coloboma, and naso-oro-vertebral anomalies (4)[C].

Pathological Findings
- Pap: Multiple branching fronds with a fibrovascular core lined by thickened, acanthotic, squamous epithelium with or without koilocytosis
- KS: Thin, dilated, endothelial-lined vascular channels surrounded by spindle cells and inflammatory reaction
- LD: Conjunctival epithelium with epidermal appendages surrounding simple choristomatous tissue including hair follicles, sebaceous glands, muscle, adipose, teeth, bone, and cartilage
- Sarc: Noncaseating granulomas
- PG: Granulation tissue, chronic inflammation, small blood vessels

DIFFERENTIAL DIAGNOSIS
- Pap: Conjunctival intraepithelial neoplasia, squamous cell carcinoma, amelanotic melanoma, lymphoma
- KS: Subconjunctival hemorrhage, hemangiopericytoma, pyogenic granuloma, capillary and cavernous hemangioma, lymphoma, malignant melanoma, pingueculitis, bacillary angiomatosis
- Sarc: Chalazia, pyogenic granuloma, conjunctival intraepithelial neoplasia, mycobacterial infections, fungal infection, foreign body granuloma, papilloma
- DL: Pterygium, pinguecula, juvenile xanthogranuloma, staphyloma, foreign body reaction, sclerocornea
- PG: Foreign body granuloma, chalazion, sarcoidosis, papilloma, lymphoma

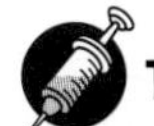

TREATMENT

MEDICATION
First Line
- Pap: Observation for spontaneous resolution
- LD: Topical lubrication, removal of irritating hairs
- KS: Highly active antiretroviral therapy (HAART) (1)[B]
- Sarc: Topical steroid
- PG: Observation for spontaneous resolution

Second Line
- Pap: Topical interferon-alpha-2b, mitomycin C, oral cimetidine (3)[C]
- KS: Local chemotherapy (vinblastine and vincristine), low dose radiotherapy, topical interferon-alpha, human choriogonadotropin
- PG: Low-dose plaque radiotherapy for recurrent PG (4)[C]

ADDITIONAL TREATMENT
Issues for Referral
LD: If clinically suspicious for Goldenhar's syndrome, consult pediatrician with genetics specialty

SURGERY/OTHER PROCEDURES
- Pap: Excisional biopsy with or without cryotherapy if symptomatic, or if concern for malignancy
- KS: Surgical excision, if refractory to HAART, with 1–2 mm margins
- LD: Superficial sclerokeratectomy with or without lamellar graft
- Sarc: Surgical excision, if symptomatic
- PG: Surgical excision, if symptomatic

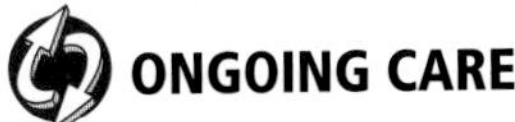

ONGOING CARE

FOLLOW-UP RECOMMENDATIONS
- Outpatient care for periodic observation of lesions and surgical excision of benign conjunctival masses
- Inpatient care for systemic management of complicating illness

PROGNOSIS
Highly favorable prognosis

COMPLICATIONS
- Lesions may reoccur after excision
- Secondary to surgical excision, including scaring, infection, bleeding, blindness
- LD: Refractive error; cornea may remain opacified from scar after surgery
- Systemic complications of underlying conditions

REFERENCES

1. Curtis TH, Durairaj VD. Conjunctival Kaposi sarcoma as the initial presentation of human immunodeficiency virus infection. *Ophthal Plast Reconstr Surg* 2005;21:314–315.
2. Ferry AP. Pyogenic granulomas of the eye and ocular adnexa: A study of 100 cases. *Trans Am Ophthalmol Soc* 1989;87:327–347.
3. Tseng SH. Conjunctival papilloma. *Ophthalmology* 2009;116:1013.
4. Shields CL, Shields JA. Tumors of the conjunctiva and cornea. *Surv Ophthalmol* 2004;49:3–24.

ADDITIONAL READING

- Mannis MJ, Macsai MS, Huntley AC. *Eye and Skin Disease*. Philadelphia: Lippincott-Raven Publishers, 1996.

CODES

ICD9
224.3 Benign neoplasm of conjunctiva

CLINICAL PEARLS

- Excisional biopsy should be considered for papillomatous changes to rule out squamous cell carcinoma and for sarcoidosis to rule out lymphoproliferative disease.
- Clinical evidence of Kaposi sarcoma mandates initiation/optimization of HAART.
- Excision of limbal dermoid with lamellar graft can give excellent cosmetic results, but may not lessen induced astigmatism.

BEST'S VITELLIFORM MACULAR DYSTROPHY

Alok S. Bansal
Marc Spirn

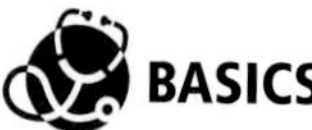

BASICS

DESCRIPTION

- Best's disease (vitelliform macular dystrophy) is a rare, autosomal dominant, bilateral, central retinal dystrophy.
- It is caused by mutations in the BEST1 (formerly VMD2) gene on chromosome 11q13 that encodes the bestrophin-1 protein.
- Age of onset is variable, although most commonly presents in early teenage years.
- It is clinically characterized by a classic yellow, "egg-yolk" (i.e., vitelliform), appearance in the central macula between the neurosensory retina and the retinal pigment epithelium (RPE).
- Visual function tests demonstrate a normal full-field electroretinogram (ERG) coupled with an abnormal electrooculogram (EOG).

EPIDEMIOLOGY

Due to the rarity and variable expressivity of the disease, the true incidence or prevalence is unknown.

RISK FACTORS

Family history of Best's disease

Genetics

- Autosomal dominant
- BEST1 gene on chromosome 11q13 encodes the bestrophin-1 protein
- Multiple different mutations (>100) responsible for variable expressivity and genotype–phenotype correlations (1)[A]

PATHOPHYSIOLOGY

- Bestrophin-1 is a transmembrane protein located on the basolateral membrane of the RPE cell that functions as a Ca^{2+}-activated Cl^{-} channel.
- The abnormal bestrophin-1 protein causes impaired ion transport across the RPE leading to accumulation of lipofuscin between the neurosensory retina and the RPE (1)[C].

ETIOLOGY

Mutations in BEST1 gene

COMMONLY ASSOCIATED CONDITIONS

Best's disease is not associated with any systemic conditions.

DIAGNOSIS

HISTORY

- Family history of retinal dystrophy
- Blurry vision
- Metamorphopsia

PHYSICAL EXAM

- Normal ocular anterior segment
- Classic fundus findings include bilateral "egg-yolk" (i.e., vitelliform) lesions in central macula.
- Previously characterized by the following stages (2)[C]:
  - Stage 0: Normal fundus or subtle RPE changes
  - Stage 1: Definite RPE changes
  - Stage 2 (vitelliform stage): Classic yellow "egg-yolk" lesion
  - Stage 2a (scrambled-egg or vitelliruptive stage): Multiple irregular yellow subretinal deposits
  - Stage 3 (pseudohypopyon stage): Layering of yellowish material in vitelliform cyst
  - Stage 4a (atrophic stage): Absence of yellow deposits leaving atrophic RPE
  - Stage 4b (Cicatricial stage): White fibrous subretinal scar
  - Stage 4c (Choroidal neovascularization stage): Subretinal hemorrhage, serous retinal detachment
- NOTE: There may be great variation in lesion appearance between patients, between the two eyes of the same patient, and even within the same eye of a patient over time.
- Patients may not progress through all stages of disease.

DIAGNOSTIC TESTS & INTERPRETATION

Lab

Genetic testing for BEST1 gene mutations

Imaging

- Fundus photography to document progression of vitelliform lesions
- Fundus fluorescein angiography (FFA):
  - Hypofluorescence due to blockage from vitelliform lesions
  - Hyperfluorescence due to either window defects from RPE atrophy or leakage from choroidal neovascularization (if present)
- Fourier-domain optical coherence tomography (FD-OCT):
  - Thickened hyper-reflective band between photoreceptor outer segments and RPE/Bruch's complex (3)[C]
- Fundus autofluorescence (FAF):
  - Hyper-autofluorescence of vitelliform lesions (3)[C]

Diagnostic Procedures/Other
- Full-field electroretinogram (ERG): Measures total photoreceptor (rod and cone) function:
  - Characteristically *normal* in Best's disease
- Electrooculogram (EOG): Measures standing potential of RPE:
  - Characteristically *abnormal* in Best's disease even in the absence of fundus findings
- Arden ratio (light peak/dark trough ratio):
  - Normal = 1.8; Best's disease <1.5

Pathological Findings
Accumulation of lipofuscin in RPE cells

DIFFERENTIAL DIAGNOSIS
- Adult-onset vitelliform dystrophy
- Pattern dystrophy
- Age-related macular degeneration
- Choroidal neovascularization

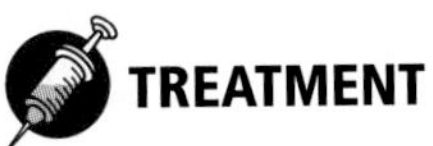

TREATMENT

MEDICATION
No medical treatment is indicated for patients with Best's disease.

SURGERY/OTHER PROCEDURES
- For cases complicated by choroidal neovascularization, consider:
  - Photodynamic therapy (4)[C]
  - Intravitreal anti-VEGF agents (i.e., bevacizumab) (5)[C]

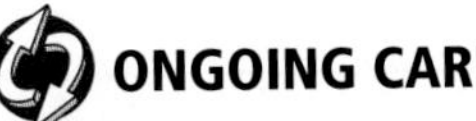

ONGOING CARE

FOLLOW-UP RECOMMENDATIONS
- Serial fundus ophthalmoscopy with retina specialist
- Low vision aids for decreased vision

PATIENT EDUCATION
Genetic counseling for family members of affected patients

PROGNOSIS
Most patients retain 20/40 or better vision (2)[C].

COMPLICATIONS
Choroidal neovascularization

REFERENCES

1. Boon C, Klevering BJ, Leroy BP, et al. The spectrum of ocular phenotypes caused by mutations in the BEST1 gene. *Prog Retin Eye Res* 2009;28:187–205.
2. Mohler CV, Fine SL. Long-term evaluation of patients with Best's vitelliform dystrophy. *Ophthalmol* 1981;88:688–692.
3. Ferrara DC, Costa RA, Tsang S, et al. Multimodal fundus imaging in Best vitelliform macular dystrophy. *Graefes Arch Clin Exp Ophthal* 2010
4. Andrade RE, Farah ME, Costa RA. Photodynamic therapy with verteporfin for subfoveal choroidal neovascularization in Best's disease. *Am J Ophthalmol* 2003;136:1179–1181.
5. Rishi E, Rishi P, Mahajan S. Intravitreal bevacizumab for choroidal neovascular membrane associated with Best's vitelliform dystrophy. *Indian J Ophthalmol* 2010;58:160–162.

ADDITIONAL READING

- Gass JD. Heredodystrophic disorders affecting the pigment epithelium and retina. In Gass JD (ed.), *Stereoscopic atlas of macular diseases: Diagnosis and treatment*. St. Louis: CV Mosby, 1997:304–325.

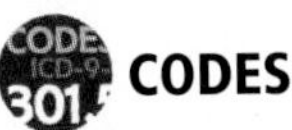

CODES

ICD9
- 362.70 Hereditary retinal dystrophy, unspecified
- 362.76 Dystrophies primarily involving the retinal pigment epithelium

CLINICAL PEARLS
- Best's disease is a rare, autosomal dominant, bilateral, central retinal dystrophy that presents in the early teenage years.
- Classic ophthalmoscopic findings include a yellow "egg-yolk" appearance in the central macula.
- Normal ERG with an abnormal EOG
- Highly variable expressivity
- Most patients retain good vision.

BIRDSHOT CHORIORETINOPATHY

Andre J. Witkin
Sunir J. Garg

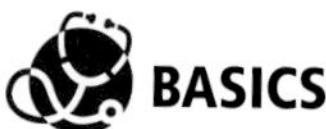

BASICS

DESCRIPTION
- Chronic, bilateral, posterior uveitis
- The characteristic lesions are yellow-white spots at the level of the choroid that "radiate" from the optic nerve.
- Over 90% of patients are HLA-A29 positive.

EPIDEMIOLOGY
Incidence
Very rare eye disease

Prevalence
- In the population, it affects <1/200,000
- It affects 1% of patients in uveitis clinics and 5–7% of all patients with posterior uveitis.

RISK FACTORS
- Most common in Caucasian patients
- Equal male/female distribution
- Mean age of onset ~50 years old

Genetics
- No strong familial association (although disease has been reported in monozygotic twins)
- Very strong association with HLA-A29 allele (birdshot has the highest association between HLA class I alleles and any disease)
- 90% of patients with disease have HLA-A29 compared with 7% of general population.

GENERAL PREVENTION
None

PATHOPHYSIOLOGY
- Likely autoimmune process
- Some similarities between birdshot and murine models of retinal S-antigen-induced uveitis

ETIOLOGY
Autoimmunity, likely involving type IV hypersensitivity

COMMONLY ASSOCIATED CONDITIONS
None known

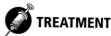

DIAGNOSIS

HISTORY
- Gradual, painless vision loss
- Floaters are common.
- Symptoms are usually bilateral.
- Nyctalopia, peripheral visual field constriction, abnormal color vision, photopsias, and photophobia may also occur.

PHYSICAL EXAM
- The eyes are usually painless and appear white and noninflamed.
- The anterior segment has no to mild inflammation.
- A mild to moderate diffuse vitreitis is common.
- The characteristic lesions are cream colored hypopigmented spots in the choroid with relatively indistinct borders.
- These lesions are suggestive of scattering of "birdshot" from a shotgun.
- The choroidal spots may not appear until later in the disease course, delaying diagnosis.
- Cystoid macular edema (CME) is a common cause of decreased visual acuity.
- Retinal vasculitis involving veins and arteries is sometimes seen, as is optic disc edema.

DIAGNOSTIC TESTS & INTERPRETATION
Lab
- None are absolutely required for diagnosis; however, HLA-A29 is a reliable marker of disease (~95% specificity and sensitivity).
- Must rule out other treatable causes of posterior uveitis, including syphilis, tuberculosis, lyme disease, ocular lymphoma, and sarcoidosis.

Imaging
Initial approach
- Fluorescein angiography (FA) shows early hypofluorescence and late hyperfluorescence of choroidal lesions, as well as hyperfluorescence of the disk, vascular leakage, and CME (when present).
- Indocyanine green angiography (ICGA) often demonstrates more lesions than seen on either clinical exam or FA. ICG shows early hypofluorescence of choroidal lesions.
- Optical coherence tomography (OCT) can be useful to detect macular edema.
- Electroretinograms (ERG) are often abnormal, typically showing a decrease in both photopic and scotopic amplitudes; Initially, B-wave may be affected more than the A-wave.
- Peripheral visual field testing may show constriction.

Follow-up & special considerations
- FA useful to monitor amount of inflammation and to follow response to therapy
- OCT useful to evaluate patients for macular edema, and for evaluating response to treatment

Pathological Findings
There are limited reports in the literature; however, lymphocytic aggregates in the choroid and retinal vasculature have been noted.

DIFFERENTIAL DIAGNOSIS
- White dot syndromes (acute posterior multifocal placoid pigment epitheliopathy, multifocal choroiditis and panuveitis, multiple evanescent white dot syndrome, AZOOR)
- Infectious posterior uveitis (tuberculosis, syphilis, and presumed ocular histoplasmosis syndrome)
- Masquerade syndromes (leukemia and ocular lymphoma)
- Sarcoidosis

TREATMENT

MEDICATION
First Line
- Ocular and systemic steroids have been the mainstay of therapy; however, the typical chronicity of this disease warrants consideration of nonsteroidal immunomodulatory therapy early in the disease course.
- Dramatic improvement of ocular inflammation can often be seen with systemic steroids (prednisone 1 mg/kg per day); however, long-term toxicity of steroids limits this approach.
- Cyclosporine, mycophenolate mofetil, azathioprine, cyclophosphamide, and methotrexate have all been used as nonsteroidal immunomodulatory therapies.

Second Line
- Periocular and intravitreal triamcinolone acetate has been used to treat severe inflammation and/or macular edema.
- More recently, use of antitumor necrosis factor alpha drugs and intravenous immunoglobulin has been reported.

ADDITIONAL TREATMENT

Issues for Referral

- Management of birdshot retinochoroidopathy often requires referral to a uveitis and/or retina specialist.
- Consultation with a rheumatologist or hematologist may be required when immunomodulatory agents are used.

SURGERY/OTHER PROCEDURES

- As with other types of ocular inflammation, cataract formation may be accelerated in patients with birdshot; cataract surgery is best delayed until the patient is free of inflammation for at least 3 months.
- Glaucoma filtration or shunting surgery may be required in some patients with uncontrolled glaucoma.
- In the near future, implantable drug delivery devices may play a major role in the treatment of this disease.

IN-PATIENT CONSIDERATIONS

Initial Stabilization

Pulse intravenous steroids may be considered in severe cases with profound bilateral vision loss.

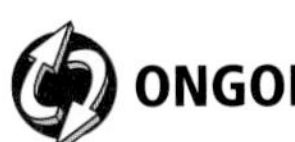

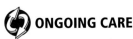

ONGOING CARE

FOLLOW-UP RECOMMENDATIONS

The course of birdshot is often progressive over a number of years, with intermittent exacerbations of disease activity; therefore, patients should be monitored closely by a specialist familiar with the treatment of the disease.

Patient Monitoring

- Visual acuity may be normal until late in the disease course.
- Careful biomicroscopic examination should be undertaken at regular intervals.
- Ancillary testing such as FA, ICGA, OCT, peripheral visual field testing and ERG testing should also be taken at regular intervals to monitor disease activity.

PATIENT EDUCATION

- Patients should be aware of the chronic progressive nature of birdshot chorioretinopathy, and the associated need for close monitoring and long-term treatment of the disease.
- Patients should also be aware that a variety of immunomodulatory treatments are available, and not be discouraged if one treatment modality is insufficient to treat their disease.

PROGNOSIS

- Because of the chronic progressive nature of the disease, visual prognosis is guarded over time.
- Patients often need to be treated with immunomodulatory agents that have side effects.
- Visual function can often be impaired to a greater extent than the visual acuity indicates.

COMPLICATIONS

- CME is the most common cause of decreased visual acuity.
- Epiretinal membranes (ERM) are also common.
- Glaucoma may be seen in up to 20% of patients and is likely a secondary effect from systemic and ocular steroid treatments.
- Choroidal neovascular membranes (CNVM) can occur in areas of chronic choroidal inflammation.
- Retinal neovascularization is uncommon, but can result from retinal vascular inflammation and secondary retinal ischemia.
- Optic nerve atrophy is rare, but has been reported.

ADDITIONAL READING

- Ryan SJ, Maumenee AE. Birdshot retinochoroidopathy. *Am J Ophthalmol* 1980;89(1):31–45.
- Jap A, Chee SP. Immunosuppressive therapy for ocular diseases. *Curr Opin Ophthalmol* 2008;19(6):535–540.
- Monnet D, Brézin AP. Birdshot chorioretinopathy. *Curr Opin Ophthalmol* 2006;17(6):545–550.
- Kiss S, Anzaar F, Foster SC. Birdshot retinochoroidopathy. *Int Ophthalmol Clin* 2006;46(2):39–55.
- Shah KH, Levinson RD, Yu F, et al. Birdshot chorioretinopathy. *Surv Ophthalmol* 2005;50(6):519–541.

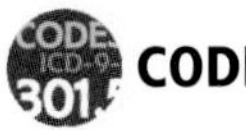

CODES

ICD9

363.20 Chorioretinitis, unspecified

CLINICAL PEARLS

- Chronic, progressive, bilateral posterior uveitis
- Characteristic peripapillary choroidal lesions and associated vitreitis are usually present. Choroidal lesions are often delayed in onset.
- Very strong association with HLA-A29
- Common cause of decreased visual acuity is cystoid macular edema.
- Electroretinograms are usually abnormal.
- Patients are often initially responsive to steroids but often require maintenance with nonsteroidal immunomodulatory agents.

BIRTH TRAUMA TO THE EYE

Sumit P. Shah

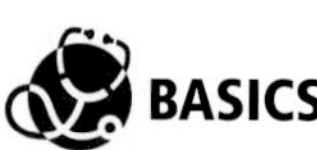

BASICS

DESCRIPTION

Birth trauma to the eye is a result of ocular, adnexal, or facial injuries due to mechanical forces during childbirth.

EPIDEMIOLOGY

Incidence

- 6–8 injuries (ophthalmic and nonophthalmic) per 1000 live births
- 2% of neonatal deaths and still births are due to traumatic injury at the time of birth

RISK FACTORS

- Large baby size:
  - Especially >4500 g
  - May be seen in a mother with gestational diabetes
- Instrument assisted deliveries:
  - Forceps and vacuum assisted
  - Abnormal or excessive traction during delivery
- Prolonged labor:
  - Use of induction medications to promote stronger contractions
  - Vaginal breech delivery
  - Cephalopelvic disproportion (when a baby's head or body is too big to fit through the mother's pelvis), maternal pelvic abnormalities
  - Oligohydramnios (deficiency of amniotic fluid)

GENERAL PREVENTION

- One can consider caesarean section as an alternative to vaginal deliveries when there is a high risk for the need for obstetric instrumentation.
  - Does not guarantee an injury free birth and can pose different or additional risks to the newborn and mother.

PATHOPHYSIOLOGY

Visual deprivation in affected eye due to amblyogenic insult such as irregular astigmatism or ptosis

ETIOLOGY

- Primary trauma to the eye or ocular adnexa
- Secondary ocular injury due to central nervous system, cranial nerve, vascular, or facial bone injuries

COMMONLY ASSOCIATED CONDITIONS

- Midcavity forceps
- Vacuum extraction
- Fetal macrosomia
- Abnormal presentation
- Prolonged labor

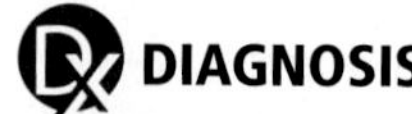

DIAGNOSIS

PHYSICAL EXAM

- Pertinent features of birth trauma relating to ophthalmic involvement include:
  - Vertical or oblique breaks in Descemet's membrane of the cornea due to forceps injury at birth
  - Asymmetric red reflex
  - Eyelid soft tissue ecchymosis, abrasions, or lacerations
  - Conjunctival chemosis
  - Subconjunctival hemorrhage
  - Retinal hemorrhage can be seen in the setting of head injury during delivery such as intracranial hemorrhage or skull fracture. This may result from instrument assisted deliveries.
  - Cranial nerve exam: Facial nerve palsy suggested by inability to close the eyelid on the affected side or facial asymmetry during crying.
  - Ptosis may result due to multiple underlying causes including: (1) mechanical, i.e., soft tissue ecchymosis; (2) neurologic, i.e., injury to sympathetic chain or cranial nerve III; (3) aponeurotic ptosis, i.e., traumatic levator dehiscence.

DIAGNOSTIC TESTS & INTERPRETATION

Imaging

Initial approach

Consider neuroimaging if neurologic symptoms are present

Follow-up & special considerations

Consultation with a pediatric ophthalmologist

Pathological Findings

Histologic examination of corneal birth trauma typically reveals vertical or oblique breaks in Descemet's membrane.

DIFFERENTIAL DIAGNOSIS

- Corneal trauma with or without Descemet's membrane tear
- Corneal abrasion
- Conjunctival chemosis or laceration
- Subconjunctival hemorrhage
- Eyelid laceration
- Cranial nerve injury affecting eyelid function

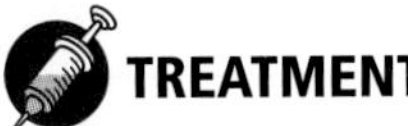

TREATMENT

ADDITIONAL TREATMENT

General Measures

- Directed to the underlying diagnosis:
  - Descemet's tear: Can result in corneal hydrops (edema and clouding). Generally resolves within weeks with observation alone. Monitor for corneal scarring and visual deprivation.
  - Abrasions and lacerations: Careful cleaning, application of antibiotic ointment, and observation. Steri-strips may be used or lacerations may require suturing. Lacerations involving the canalicular system (for tear drainage) warrant consultation with an oculoplastics specialist for surgical reconstruction and repair
  - Facial nerve palsy: Management consists of preventing exposure keratitis by protecting the open eye with frequent lubrication with ointment and artificial tears, and if necessary, limited patching.
  - Ptosis: Directed to the underlying cause initially. Various surgical techniques can be utilized in order to prevent deprivation or refractive amblyopia.

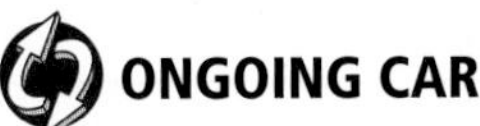

ONGOING CARE

FOLLOW-UP RECOMMENDATIONS

- Early pediatric ophthalmology referral for evaluation and treatment of amblyogenic conditions
- Frequency dictated by underlying condition

PROGNOSIS

Excellent if amblyogenic causes are detected and treated early

COMPLICATIONS

- Amblyopia due to visual deprivation
- Ptosis
- Exposure keratopathy

ADDITIONAL READING

- Moczygemba CK, Paramsothy P, Meikle S, et al. Route of delivery and neonatal birth trauma. *Am J Obstet Gynecol* 2010.
- Schullinger JN. Birth trauma. *Pediatr Clin North Am* 1993;40(6):1351–1358.

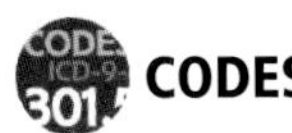

CODES

ICD9

- 371.33 Rupture in descemet's membrane
- 772.8 Other specified hemorrhage of fetus or newborn
- 767.8 Other specified birth trauma

CLINICAL PEARLS

- Breaks in Descemet's membrane may result from forceps injury.
- Frequent ocular lubrication to prevent exposure keratitis is a must in cases of facial nerve injury.
- Monitor babies for amblyopia; visual prognosis is generally excellent.

BLEBITIS

Justin M. Spaulding
Scott J. Fudemberg

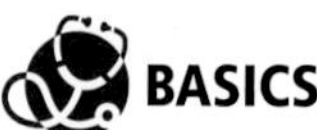

BASICS

DESCRIPTION

- Presumed infection in or around filtering bleb.
- Filtering bleb is a subconjunctival pocket of fluid created intentionally in glaucoma surgery to drain aqueous humor or inadvertently after other types of eye surgery:
  - Classification: Blebitis (no vitreous involvement) and bleb-associated endophthalmitis (BAE) (vitreous involvement)
  - BAE: Early-onset (within 1 month of surgery) and late-onset (occurs more than 1 month after surgery)

EPIDEMIOLOGY

Incidence

- After superiorly located trabeculectomy with mitomycin c
- Blebitis: 5.7% (1)
- Early-onset BAE: 0.124%
- Late-onset BAE: 0.8–4%

RISK FACTORS

- Inferior bleb
- Thin bleb
- Bleb leak
- Antifibrotic agents (mitomycin c, 5-fluorouracil)
- Major complications in early postoperative period following trabeculectomy (flat anterior chamber, early wound leak, suprachoroidal hemorrhage)
- Prior conjunctivitis/upper respiratory infection
- Blepharitis
- History of prior bleb infection
- Chronic use of antibiotics
- Bleb manipulation
- Multiple filtration surgeries

Genetics

Many forms of glaucoma are hereditary, but predisposition to bleb-related infection is not known to be genetic.

GENERAL PREVENTION

- Surgical techniques that promote low diffuse blebs and minimize highly elevated, avascular, thin blebs
- Rapid diagnosis and management of bleb leaks
- Avoidance of eye rubbing in eyes with bleb
- Treatment of blepharitis in eyes with bleb
- Avoid chronic use of topical antibiotic drops

PATHOPHYSIOLOGY

- Early-onset BAE: Likely introduction of normal flora during surgery
- Late-onset BAE: Likely penetration of bleb by transiently present organisms through area of unhealthy tissue or bleb leak

ETIOLOGY

- Blebitis: Most studies report *Staphylococcus epidermidis* and *S. aureus*.
- Early-onset BAE: Most studies report *S. epidermidis* and *S. aureus*.
- Late-onset BAE: Strep species most commonly reported, followed by *Haemophilus influenzae* and gram negatives.
- Organisms that cause late-onset BAE are more virulent, produce exotoxins, may penetrate intact conjunctiva, may rapidly spread into anterior chamber and vitreous.

COMMONLY ASSOCIATED CONDITIONS

Conjunctivitis, uveitis, bleb leak, glaucoma

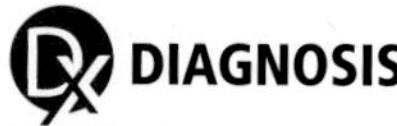

DIAGNOSIS

HISTORY

- Typically, late-onset BAE causes sudden onset red eye followed by photophobia, eye pain, discharge, and decreased vision:
  - Prodrome in blebitis may be of several days or longer while in BAE may progress very rapidly over course of hours to devastating infection.

PHYSICAL EXAM

- Conjunctival injection localized to area of bleb (though may progress to diffuse injection)
- Milky, turbid appearance of bleb
- Frank purulent material in or leaking from bleb
- Bleb leak (may resolve during the course of infection as a result of scarring and/or blocking of leak with debris)
- Inflammatory cells in the anterior chamber (blebitis)
- Inflammatory cells in the vitreous (key differentiating feature between blebitis and BAE)
- Hypopyon in the presence of signs of external bleb infection is endophthalmitis until proven otherwise.

DIAGNOSTIC TESTS & INTERPRETATION

Lab

Initial lab tests

- Gonioscopy may be needed to identify microhypopyon.
- B-scan ultrasound of vitreous is needed if view is obscured by anterior segment inflammation.
- Utility of conjunctival cultures may be limited: If frank purulent material consider swab for gram stain, culture/sensitivities.
- Anterior chamber tap may be used to collect sample for gram stain and culture/sensitivity, but we generally favor low threshold for vitreous tap/inject.

Follow-up & special considerations

- Early diagnosis, prompt treatment, and very close follow-up are critical because progression of blebitis to BAE and BAE to devastating outcomes may be rapid.
- Follow-up of blebitis may be daily with low threshold for multiple exams per day.
- Follow-up of BAE may be multiple times per day with low threshold for hospital admission.
- There is no formally established protocol for follow-up of these conditions.

Pathological Findings

- Thin (1–2 layer) conjunctival epithelium (4)[B]
- Goblet cell depletion resulting in decreased production of mucin, which is a crucial biological/physical barrier of the cornea and conjunctiva (4)[B]
- Presence of hyalin in bleb (4)[B]

DIFFERENTIAL DIAGNOSIS

- Endophthalmitis (not bleb-associated)
- Uveitis
- Scleritis
- Episcleritis
- Sterile inflammatory response (intraocular foreign body, surgical manipulation, intraocular injection)

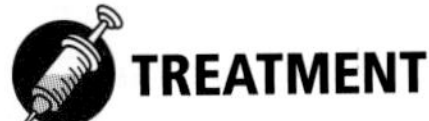

TREATMENT

MEDICATION

First Line

- Blebitis: Fortified vancomycin (25–50 mg/mL) and tobramycin (14 mg/mL) or cefazolin (50 mg/mL); apply alternating topical drops every half hour post loading dose (1 drop every 5 min for a total of 4 drops) (2)[A] (5)[A].
- BAE: Intravitreal administration of vancomycin (1 mg/0.1 mL) and ceftazidime (2.25 mg/0.1 mL) (2)[A] (5)[A].
- BAE (if intolerant to ceftazidime): Intravitreal administration of vancomycin (1 mg/0.1 mL) and amikacin (0.4 mg/0.1 mL) (keep in mind the use of an aminoglycoside such as amikacin that can cause macular infarction and should be used cautiously) (2)[A] (5)[A].
- Intravitreal antibiotics may be repeated every 48–72 h.
- Use of steroids may be needed to control inflammation, but should be used with great caution (1)[C] (2)[A].

Second Line

For mild blebitis only: Fourth-generation fluoroquinolones (gatifloxacin 0.3% or moxifloxacin 0.5%) apply topical drops every hour post loading dose (2)[A] (5)[A]

ADDITIONAL TREATMENT

General Measures

- Oral concentrations of fluoroquinolones (moxifloxacin 400 mg per day) reach significantly higher intravitreal concentrations than the topical counterpart; therefore, these drugs can be used as an adjunct to current therapy and as a prophylaxis for vitreous involvement (3)[B].
- With bleb leak or low intraocular pressure: No eye rubbing, shield when sleeping (or at all times except when taking eyedrops in those that cannot avoid physical contact with the eye), no bending, no straining.
- Worsening signs/symptoms should prompt immediate re-evaluation (redness, blurred vision, discomfort, tearing).

Issues for Referral

If blebitis is suspected immediately refer patient to an ophthalmologist.

SURGERY/OTHER PROCEDURES

- Vitreous tap/inject and vitrectomy should be strongly considered in all patients with BAE.
- Results of the Endophthalmitis Vitrectomy Study may not be extrapolated to included patients with BAE, which may progress more rapidly than late-onset postcataract endophthalmitis.
- Additional glaucoma surgery to control intraocular pressure may be needed following blebitis/BAE because subsequent filtration failure is common.

IN-PATIENT CONSIDERATIONS

Admission Criteria

Low threshold for admission in patients who progress rapidly and in those patients who are noncompliant or likely unable to follow intense regimen of medication administration

ONGOING CARE

FOLLOW-UP RECOMMENDATIONS

- No firmly established and generalizable guidelines
- Close follow-up guided by circumstances of infection and recovery

PATIENT EDUCATION

- Signs and symptoms of infection including redness, discomfort, and blurred vision should be detailed with patient.
- Patient should be instructed to return immediately for development or worsening of these symptoms.

PROGNOSIS

- Blebitis due to Staphylococcus species has a good prognosis with full resolution and decreasing chances of evolution into endophthalmitis.
- BAE has poor prognosis despite aggressive medical intervention and final visual acuity is often 20/200 or less.

COMPLICATIONS

- Bleb failure
- Pain
- Vision loss
- Blurred vision
- Loss of eye
- Elevated intraocular pressure
- Growth of more virulent/resistant infecting organisms
- Conjunctival scarring
- Intraocular scarring (such as posterior synechiae, peripheral anterior synechiae)
- Cataract
- Retinal detachment

REFERENCES

1. Ah-Chan JJ, Molteno ACB, Bevin TH. Anti-inflammatory fibrosis suppression in threatened trabeculectomy bleb failure. *Arch Ophthalmol* 2006;124:603.
2. Kernt M, Kampik M. Endopthalmitis: Pathogenesis, clinical presentation, management, and perspectives. *Clinical Ophthalmology* 2010;121–135.
3. Hariprasad SM, Shah GK, Mieler WF, et al. Vitreous and aqueous penetration of orally administered moxifloxacin in humans. *Arch Ophthalmol* 2006; 124:178–182.
4. Matsuo H, Tomita G, Araie M, et al. Histopathological findings in filtering blebs with recurrent blebitis. *Br J Ophthalmol* 2002;86:827.
5. Prasad N, Latina MA. Blebitis and endophthalmitis after glaucoma filtering surgery. *International Ophthalmol Clinics* 2007;47(2):85–97.

ADDITIONAL READING

- Ba'arah BT, Smiddy WE. Bleb-related endophthalmitis: Clinical presentation, isolates, treatment and visual outcome of culture-proven cases. *Middle East Afr J Ophthalmol* 2009;1:20–24.
- Sharan S, Trope GE, Chipman M, et al. Late-onset bleb infections: Prevalence and risk factors. *Canadian J Ophthalmol* 2009;44:279–283.

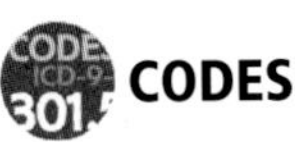

CODES

ICD9

- 379.63 Inflammation (infection) of postprocedural bleb, stage 3
- 379.99 Other ill-defined disorders of eye

BLEPHARITIS

Melvin I. Roat

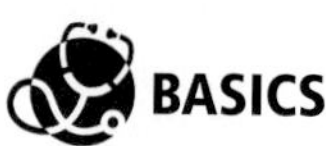

BASICS

DESCRIPTION
- Chronic, recurrent inflammation of the eyelid margin
- Synonyms:
  - Seborrheic blepharitis: Anterior blepharitis, granulated eyelids
  - Meibomian gland dysfunction: Posterior blepharitis, ocular rosacea, meibomianitis

EPIDEMIOLOGY
Prevalence
Common, 37–47% of patients in an ophthalmology or optometry practice

RISK FACTORS
More common in Caucasian from Northern Europe, but found in all races

Genetics
More common if parents had blepharitis

PATHOPHYSIOLOGY
- Seborrheic blepharitis: Large scales of skin form at the surface of the anterior eyelid margin. Secondary bacteria colonization of the area leads to inflammation.
- Meibomian gland dysfunction: An abnormal composition of the meibomian gland lipid secretion leads to inflammation.

ETIOLOGY
- Seborrheic blepharitis: Tends to be inherited and may be due to colonization of the eyelid margin skin with yeast of the *Malassezia* genus
- Meibomian gland dysfunction: Tends to be inherited

COMMONLY ASSOCIATED CONDITIONS
- Evaporative dry eye and staphylococcal hypersensitivity marginal keratitis/ulcers, phlyctenulosis
- Seborrheic blepharitis tends to be associated with seborrheic dermatitis.
- Meibomian gland dysfunction tends to be associated with acne rosacea and chalazia.

DIAGNOSIS

HISTORY
- Itching and burning of the eyelid margins. Redness of the eyelid margin and conjunctiva. Symptoms fluctuate through the day and through the weeks. Many patients are symptomatic of an evaporative dry eye (see topic Dry Eye Syndrome).
- Patients with seborrheic blepharitis also complain of large flakes of skin at the base of the eyelashes.
- Patients with meibomian gland dysfunction also complain of rounded, protruding, creamy-hard white–yellow deposits at the eyelid margin just posterior to the eye lashes.

PHYSICAL EXAM
- Seborrheic blepharitis: Large scales of skin form at the anterior eyelid margin, hyperemia of the anterior eyelid margin, debris in the tear film, inferior punctate keratitis.
- Meibomian gland dysfunction: White–yellow viscous-waxy plugs in meibomian gland orifices, hyperemia of the entire eyelid margin, eyelid margin vessels crossing the gray line, appearance of a thin lipid layer of the tear film, inferior punctate keratitis. There may also be associated chalazia and skin findings of acne rosacea.

DIAGNOSTIC TESTS & INTERPRETATION
Lab
Seborrheic blepharitis: Bacteria can be cultured from the eyelid margin. Small quantities and usually nonvirulent strains may be significant.

Pathological Findings
- Seborrheic blepharitis: The anterior eyelid epidermis shows acanthosis, hyperkeratosis, and/or parakeratosis; lymphocyte and plasma cell infiltrate.
- Meibomian gland dysfunction: Obstruction, dilatation with squamous metaplasia and abnormal keratinization of ducts, enlargement of acini with cystic degeneration and an inflammatory cell infiltrate.

DIFFERENTIAL DIAGNOSIS
Acute bacterial ulcerative blepharitis (usually *Staphylococcus aureus*), acute viral blepharitis (herpes simplex or herpes zoster)

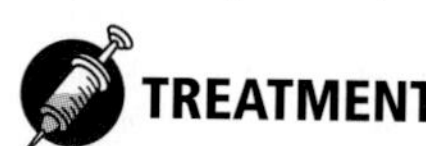

TREATMENT

MEDICATION
First Line
- Seborrheic blepharitis: If the primary treatment of eyelash scrubs, i.e., gently cleaning the base of the eyelashes with a cotton swab dipped in a dilute solution of baby shampoo (e.g., 2–3 drops in $\frac{1}{2}$ cup of hot water) b.i.d., is insufficient, an antibiotic ointment q.h.s. can be used. The antibiotic should be chosen based on eyelid culture results. Treatment with topical antibiotics may need to be used continuously for up to 3 months and may be needed recurrently.
- Meibomian gland dysfunction: If the primary treatment of ocular hot compresses, i.e., gel or bead filled microwaveable hot compresses (not wash cloth hot compresses) 3–4 times per day for 10–15 min, is insufficient, an antibiotic topical azithromycin or oral doxycycline 100 mg b.i.d. may need to be used recurrently for 3–4 months.

Pediatric Considerations
Doxycycline, tetracycline, and derivatives should not be used in children <8 years of age.

Pregnancy Considerations
Doxycycline, tetracycline, and derivatives should not be used in pregnant or nursing mothers.

Second Line

- The secondary evaporative dry eye usually causes more symptoms than the primary seborrheic blepharitis or meibomian gland dysfunction. Therefore, treating the secondary evaporative dry eye results in more symptomatic improvement than treating the blepharitis and is often instituted first. Only if there are unacceptable residual symptoms after treating the secondary evaporative dry eye, would the seborrheic blepharitis or meibomian gland dysfunction be treated. Treatment for the secondary evaporative dry eye can include moderately viscous and viscous artificial tears, punctal plugs, and topical cyclosporin A drops.
- Oral Omega-3 fatty acid dietary supplements, oral fluconazole, topical azithromycin, rarely topical steroid drops, and/or ointment should be used very rarely, because only short-term improvement results, continuous monitoring is required, and severe vision threatening problems such as glaucoma or steroid enhanced herpes simplex keratitis may result.

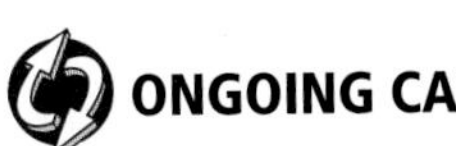

ONGOING CARE

FOLLOW-UP RECOMMENDATIONS

Patient Monitoring

- In seborrheic blepharitis, it can take 2 weeks to know if the eyelash scrubs are helping and 4 weeks to know if the q.h.s. antibiotic ointments are helping.
- In meibomian gland dysfunction, it can take 2 weeks to know if the ocular hot compresses are helping and 4 weeks to know if the doxycycline is helping.

DIET

A diet high in Omega-3 fatty acids will probably improve the symptoms of meibomian gland dysfunction.

PROGNOSIS

Seborrheic blepharitis and meibomian gland dysfunction are lifelong, chronic, recurrent conditions that will respond well to treatment and then will reoccur. Uncomplicated seborrheic blepharitis and meibomian gland dysfunction have an excellent visual prognosis with no visual loss expected.

COMPLICATIONS

Evaporative dry eye and staphylococcal hypersensitivity marginal keratitis/ulcers, phlyctenulosis are complications of seborrheic blepharitis and meibomian gland dysfunction. Meibomian gland dysfunction can be complicated by chalazia.

ADDITIONAL READING

- Shine WE, McCulley JP, Pandya AG. Minocycline effect on meibomian gland lipids in meibomianitis patients. *Exp Eye Res* 2003;76:417–420.
- Souchier M, Joffre C, Grégoire S, et al. Changes in meibomian fatty acids and clinical signs in patients with meibomian gland dysfunction after minocycline treatment. *Br J Ophthalmol* 2008;92:819–822.
- Jackson WB. Blepharitis: Current strategies for diagnosis and management. *Can J Ophthalmol* 2008;43:170–179.
- Macsai MS. The role of Omega-3 dietary supplementation in blepharitis and meibomian gland dysfunction. *Trans Am Ophthalmol Soc* 2008;106:336–356.

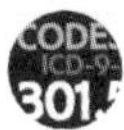

CODES

ICD9

- 370.49 Other keratoconjunctivitis, unspecified
- 373.00 Blepharitis, unspecified
- 373.12 Hordeolum internum

CLINICAL PEARLS

- Treating the secondary evaporative dry eye may lead to more symptomatic improvement than treating the seborrheic blepharitis and meibomian gland dysfunction.
- Use a very dilute solution of baby shampoo for the eyelash scrubs.
- Do not use eyelash scrubs in meibomian gland dysfunction.
- Use gel or bead filled microwaveable hot compresses, wash cloth hot compresses do not stay hot enough for long enough and don't work

BLEPHAROSPASM AND HEMIFACIAL SPASM

Susan M. Ksiazek

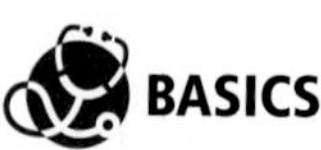

BASICS

DESCRIPTION

- Involuntary closure of both eyelids (blepharospasm) or muscles innervated by facial nerve unilaterally (hemifacial spasm):
  - Blepharospasm:
    - Essential (without associated disease)
    - Blepharospasm-oromandibular dystonia or Meige syndrome (dystonia of face, jaw, and neck)
    - Secondary – due to ocular irritation
  - Hemifacial spasm
- System(s) affected: Nervous; musculoskeletal

EPIDEMIOLOGY

- Predominant age: Middle age (40–60 years)
- Predominant sex: Female > Male (2–4:1)

Incidence

2000 cases of blepharospasm diagnosed annually in the USA (1)

Prevalence

- 1.6–13.3/100,000 for blepharospasm
- 7.4–14.5/100,000 for hemifacial spasm

RISK FACTORS

- Blepharospasm:
  - Head or facial trauma
  - Specific eye disease, e.g., blepharitis and keratoconjunctivitis
  - Family history of dystonia or tremor (2)
  - Cigarette smoking was considered a negative risk factor earlier, but not in recent studies (3,4).
- Hemifacial spasm has no known risk factors.

Genetics

- Most sporadic, yet familial variety with autosomal dominance and incomplete penetrance in blepharospasm
- No genetic relationships known with hemifacial spasm

PATHOPHYSIOLOGY

- Blepharospasm:
  - Two opposing muscle groups, protractors (orbicularis, corrugator, and procerus) and retractors (levator palpebra superioris and frontalis), fire at the same time.
  - Sensitization of the trigeminal system via photophobia (2)
  - Theory of ion channelopathy (5)
- Hemifacial spasm:
  - Ephaptic transmission

ETIOLOGY

- Hemifacial spasm:
  - Vascular compression of the facial nerve by an abnormal artery
  - Rarely tumors of the posterior fossa compressing the facial nerve (6)

COMMONLY ASSOCIATED CONDITIONS

- Blepharospasm:
  - Dry eyes
  - Movement disorders, strokes

DIAGNOSIS

HISTORY

- Blepharospasm (1)[C]
  - Increase blinking progresses to involuntary spasms of eyelids, initially unilateral:
    - Increases in severity and frequency
    - Often has ocular irritation
- History of drug use with tardive dyskinesia
- Hemifacial spasm:
  - Involuntary eye closure that progresses over months to years to other facial muscles on the same side

PHYSICAL EXAM

- Blepharospasm:
  - Nonvolitional contraction of multiple muscles (both protractors and retractors), not just orbicularis
  - Careful exclusion of ocular causes
  - Observation for other tics which are more brief, may involve winking
- Hemifacial spasm:
  - Synchronous spasm of multiple facial muscle ipsilaterally

DIAGNOSTIC TESTS & INTERPRETATION

Lab

- MRI brain
- MRI/MRA brain with attention to the posterior fossa

Pathological Findings

Abnormal blood vessels: aneurysms, dolichoectasia, etc.

DIFFERENTIAL DIAGNOSIS

- Blepharospasm:
  - Ocular myokymia
  - Associated with lesions of brainstem and basal ganglia (Parkinson disease, Huntington disease, Wilson disease, Creutzfeldt–Jakob disease, progressive external ophthalmoplegia)
  - Reflex (due to temporoparietal strokes)
  - Ocular (irritative ocular disease, e.g., entropion)
  - Tardive dyskinesia
  - Facial tics (Tourette syndrome)
  - Functional
  - Focal seizures
- Hemifacial spasm:
  - Tardive dyskinesia
  - Myokymia
  - Tics
  - Dystonia
  - Functional

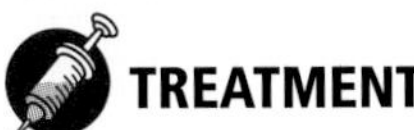

TREATMENT

MEDICATION

First Line

- Treat underlying etiology in secondary etiologies.
- Botulinum toxin injection (7)[B], (8)[A]:
  - Every 3–4 months

Second Line

- Oral medications (carbamazepine, anticholinergics, baclofen, clonazepam, haloperidol):
  - Often sedating and not helpful

ADDITIONAL TREATMENT

Issues for Referral

Socially upsetting to sight impairment

SURGERY/OTHER PROCEDURES

- Blepharospasm:
  - Orbicularis myectomy
  - Differential section of the facial nerve
  - Superior cervical ganglion block
- Hemifacial spasm:
  - Microvascular decompression

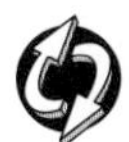

ONGOING CARE

FOLLOW-UP RECOMMENDATIONS

- 1 month after botulinum injections
- If well reinjection every 3 months or longer

PATIENT EDUCATION

- Benign Essential Blepharospasm Research Foundation found to be helpful and other therapies
- Patient and family fact sheet (9)
- Reduce coffee intake

PROGNOSIS

90% improve with botulinum injections

COMPLICATIONS

With microvascular surgery can have facial weakness and hearing loss.

REFERENCES

1. Ben Simon GJ, McCann JD. Benign essential blepharospasm. *Int Ophthalmol Clin* 2005;45: 45–79.
2. Hallett M, Evionger C, Jankovic J, Stacy M. Update on blepharospasm. Report from the BEBRF International Workshop. *Neurology* 2008;71: 1275–1282.
3. Defazio G, Martino D, Abbruzzese G, et al. Influence of coffee drinking and cigarette smoking on the risk of primary late onset blepharospasom: evidence from a multicentre case control study. *J Neurol Neurosurg Psychiatry*. 2007;78:877–879.
4. Hall TA, McGwin G, Searcey K, et al. Benign essential blepharospasm: risk factors with reference to hemifacial spasm. *J Neuroophthalmol* 2005;25:280–285.
5. Leon-Sarmiento FE, Bayona-Prieto J, Gomez J. Neurophysiology of blepharospasm and multiple system atrophy: clues to its pathophysiology. *Parkinsonism and Related Disorders* 2005;11: 199–201.
6. Han I-B, Chang JH, Chang JW, et al. Unusual causes and presentations of hemifacial spasm. *Neurosurgery* 2009;65:130–137.
7. Quagliato EMAB, Carelli EF, Viana MA. Prospective, randomized, double-blind study, comparing botulinum toxins type A Botox and Prosigne for blepharospasm and hemifacial spasm treatment. *Clin Neuropharmacol* 2010;33:27–31.
8. Costa J, Espirito-Santo C, Borges A, et al. Botulinum toxin type A therapy for blepharospasm (Review). *Cochrane Database Syst Rev* 2005;1: 1–11.
9. Whitney CM. Benign essential blepharospasm *The Neurologist* 2005;11:193–194.

ADDITIONAL READING

- Tan N-C, Chan L-L, Tan E-K. Hemifacial spasm and involuntary facial movements. *Q Med J* 2002:95: 493–500.
- Jordan DR, Patrinely JR, Anderson RL, Thiese SM. Essential blepharospasm and related dystonias. *Surv Ophthalmol* 1989;34:123–132.
- Defazio G, Livrea P. Epicemiology of primary blepharospasm. *Mov Disord* 2002;17:7–12.

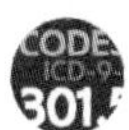

CODES

ICD9

- 333.81 Blepharospasm
- 351.8 Other facial nerve disorders
- 728.85 Spasm of muscle

CLINICAL PEARLS

- Blepharospasm is a diagnosis of exclusion.
- Botulinum toxin is a excellent therapy for both.
- Serious neurologic diseases may cause hemifacial spasm.

BLIND BABY

Jing Jin

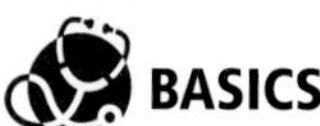

BASICS

DESCRIPTION

The World Health Organization's classification defines blindness as corrected visual acuity of <20/200 in the better eye or visual field ≤10 degrees around the central fixation.

EPIDEMIOLOGY

Incidence

- 0.3/1000 under 5 years old in the USA and Canada (1)
- Globally 0.8/1000 under 5 years old
- Considerable regional variations are present due to the difference in biological, environmental, and socioeconomic factors.

Prevalence

- In 2000, it was estimated worldwide that 1.4 million children were blind (2,3).
- Worldwide, underprivileged societies have higher prevalence of childhood blindness.

RISK FACTORS

- Poverty
- Prenatal:
  - Family history of hereditary eye diseases
  - Maternal infection during pregnancy (rubella, toxoplasmosis, CMV, HSV, and syphilis)
  - Prenatal drug use
  - Premature birth (one of the major causes in developed countries)
- Perinatal and neonatal:
  - Hypoxia/ischemia
  - Infection
  - Nonaccidental trauma
- Childhood:
  - Nutrition: Vitamin A deficiency
  - Infection
  - Trauma: nonaccidental and accidental
  - Systemic and neurological diseases

Genetics

Genetic eye disease and the ocular manifestations of systemic genetic disease are one of the leading causes of childhood blindness.

GENERAL PREVENTION

- Public health education on preventable childhood eye disease. Worldwide 50% of childhood blindness is avoidable (4).
- Genetic counseling for families with known genetic eye diseases
- Prenatal care:
  - Maternal nutrition and infectious disease immunization and monitoring
  - Avoid exposure to teratogens
  - Decrease premature birth rate
  - Prenatal ultrasound for congenital ocular anomalies (5)
- Perinatal and neonatal:
  - Neonatal prophylactic topical antibiotics
  - Early diagnosis and management of retinopathy of prematurity
  - Early diagnosis and treatment of cataract and glaucoma
- Childhood: Trauma and infectious disease prevention

PATHOPHYSIOLOGY

Blindness results both from the organic disruption of the visual system (including eye and brain) from congenital anomaly or disease and from deprivation of visual development (amblyopia) and potentially from cortical visual impairment.

ETIOLOGY

- Whole globe: Microphthalmia, anophthalmia
- Glaucoma
- Cornea:
  - Congenital opacities
  - Scarring due to infectious disease and vitamin A deficiency is a major cause in underdeveloped countries.
- Lens:
  - Cataract
  - Ectopia lentis
- Uvea:
  - Aniridia
  - Uveitis
  - Coloboma
- Retina:
  - Retinopathy of prematurity
  - Retinal dystrophy
  - Oculocutaneous albinism
  - Retinoblastoma
  - Macular hypoplasia
  - Retinal detachment or dysplasia
- Optic nerve:
  - Hypoplasia
  - Atrophy
  - Neuropathy
- Cortical:
  - Anatomical anomalies
  - Infection
  - Neurodegenerative diseases
  - Hypoxic–ischemic encephalopathy
  - Tumor
  - Trauma: Accidental of nonaccidental
- Other: Nystagmus, high refractive error

COMMONLY ASSOCIATED CONDITIONS

- Infectious diseases: Rubella, toxoplasmosis, cytomegalovirus, herpes, syphilis
- Congenital anterior segment anomalies, glaucoma and cataract in syndromes
- Retinal dystrophy associated with syndromes
- Optic nerve anomalies associated with midline facial and brain anomalies
- Metabolic, storage diseases and neurologic diseases may be associated with blindness.

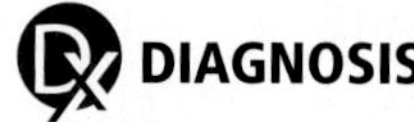

DIAGNOSIS

HISTORY

- Family history of infancy blindness and congenital ocular disease
- Maternal prenatal exposure to infection or teratogen
- Birth history
- Other known associated anomalies or developmental delay

PHYSICAL EXAM

- Ocular signs in infant:
  - Constant deviation of one eye
  - Nystagmus
  - Wandering eye movements
  - Lack of response to familiar faces
  - Staring at bright lights
  - Eye poking/gouging (oculodigital sign)
  - Absence of dampening on vestibular induced nystagmus
  - Absence of eye-popping reflex of infancy
- Systemic examination for anomalies and infections (toxoplasmosis, rubella, CMV, HSV, congenital syphilis)

- Ocular findings:
  - Corneal opacity, abnormal size
  - Lens opacity
  - Retinal findings:
    - Macular scars: Toxoplasmosis
    - Macular hypoplasia: Albinism, aniridia
    - Coloboma
    - Retinopathy of prematurity
  - Optic nerve hypoplasia, congenital optic atrophy, and other anomalies

DIAGNOSTIC TESTS & INTERPRETATION

Lab

Based on suspected etiology

Imaging

- Consider brain MRI in cases of blindness due to optic nerve anomalies or in the absence of ocular disease that explains visual loss.
- Ultrasound to assess ocular anatomy in cases of media opacity.

Diagnostic Procedures/Other

- Examination under anesthesia as needed
- Electrophysiology testing in cases of blindness without significant ocular finding or if retinal pathology suspected

Pathological Findings

Depends on cause of blindness

DIFFERENTIAL DIAGNOSIS

- Delayed visual maturation
- Developmental delay
- Functional/hysterical visual loss

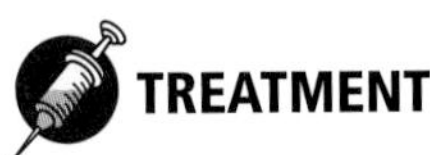

TREATMENT

MEDICATION

As appropriate for underlying disorder

ADDITIONAL TREATMENT

General Measures

- Correct refractive error
- Amblyopia treatment
- Safety glasses if poorly seeing eye <20/60
- Low vision intervention including low vision aids, mobility training, and individualized education plan

Issues for Referral

- Genetic counseling
- Consult infectious disease specialists for blindness due to infectious etiology
- Consult pediatric/genetic specialist when blindness is associated with systemic diseases

SURGERY/OTHER PROCEDURES

- Cataract extraction
- Glaucoma surgery
- Retinopathy of prematurity treatment: Laser or vitreoretinal surgery
- Strabismus surgery

IN-PATIENT CONSIDERATIONS

Admission Criteria

Admission only indicated if underlying disease warrants

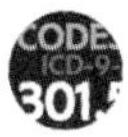

ONGOING CARE

FOLLOW-UP RECOMMENDATIONS

- Close cooperation with neonatologists, geneticist, pediatricians, and school
- Ongoing low vision and educational assessment

Patient Monitoring

- Annual eye exam to monitor the condition and the child/family progress and adaptation. More frequent if it is indicated
- Provide information and recommendation for social service and school.

PATIENT EDUCATION

- Genetic counseling
- Low vision intervention
- Family support network – National Federation of the Blind (NFB) (http://www.nfb.org), American Council of the Blind (ACB) (http://www.acb.org/resources/parents.html), and National Association for Parents with Visual Impairments (http://www.spedex.com/napvi/)

PROGNOSIS

Depends on etiology and access to treatment/intervention

REFERENCES

1. Munoz B, We, SK. Blindness and visual impairment in the Americas and the Caribbean. *Br J Ophthalmol* 2002;86:498–504.
2. Vision for Children. A global overview of blindness, childhood and VISION 2020: The right to sight. World Health Organization (WHO) and the International Agency for the Prevention of Blindness (IAPB). www.v2020.org.
3. Resnikoff S, Pascolini D, Etya'ale D, et al. Global data on visual impairment in the year 2020. *Bull World Health Organ* 2004;82:844–851.
4. Gilbert C, Foster A. Childhood blindness in the context of VISION 2020: The right to sight. *Bull World Health Organ* 2001;79:227–232.
5. Bault JP, Quarello E. Retinal coloboma: Prenatal diagnosis using a new technique, the 'virtual fetal eyeground'. *Ultrasound Obstet Gynecol* 2009; 33(4):495–496.

CODES

ICD9

- 368.00 Amblyopia, unspecified
- 369.00 Blindness of both eyes, impairment level not further specified
- 369.9 Unspecified visual loss

CLINICAL PEARLS

- Review prenatal, birth, medical, and family history.
- Complete eye examination is essential.
- The presence of nystagmus should evoke a search for ocular abnormalities. The absence of nystagmus should evoke a search for cortical/brain etiologies.
- In underdeveloped countries always consider possible infectious etiology, trauma, and vitamin deficiency as possible causes of blindness.
- Genetic consult for blindness associated with other anomalies and syndromes.
- Early low vision intervention.

BRANCH RETINAL VEIN OCCLUSION (BRVO)

Kamalesh J. Ramaiya
Gaurav K. Shah

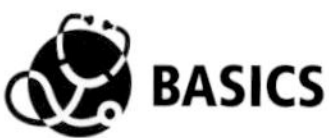

BASICS

DESCRIPTION

- An obstruction of blood flow through a branch retinal vein at an arterio-venous crossing site (1)[C]. It commonly presents with a variable level of painless decreased, blurred, or distorted vision.
  - Can be classified as one of two clinical subtypes: ischemic or nonischemic, which differ in their presentation, clinical course, and prognosis.

Geriatric Considerations

The overwhelming majority of branch retinal vein occlusions (BRVO) occur in middle aged to older individuals, especially those over 50 years of age.

Pediatric Considerations

Pediatric cases of BRVO are rare. Many cases of BRVO in young patients have a definable underlying etiology such as a hypercoagulable state; however, BRVO have been reported in otherwise healthy children.

Pregnancy Considerations

Venous occlusive disease in the setting of uncomplicated pregnancy and the absence of a hypercoagulable state is rare but has been described typically as a papillophlebitis that resolves spontaneously.

EPIDEMIOLOGY

Incidence

- Retinal vein occlusions are the most frequently encountered retinal vascular disorder second to diabetic retinopathy. BRVO are more common than central retinal vein occlusions (CRVO).
  - The 15-year cumulative incidence is 1.8% as per the Beaver Dam Eye Study.
  - Affects approximately 95,000 people in the USA per year.
  - Most commonly encountered in the fifth or sixth decades of life, but can occur at all ages.
  - Males and females are equally affected.

Prevalence

- Prevalence increases with increasing age.
- Overall prevalence is 0.6–1.6%.

RISK FACTORS

- BRVO has been strongly associated with systemic hypertension (65–75%). Other risk factors include a history of cardiovascular disease, diabetes mellitus, obesity, hyperlipidemia, and hyperviscosity syndromes.
- Unlike with CRVO, the association of glaucoma with BRVO is unclear.

PATHOPHYSIOLOGY

- The exact mechanism of pathogenesis is unknown.
- The occlusion is thought to occur because of a mechanical obstruction at the level of an arterio-venous crossing site in the retina, but this has been debated.
- Factors predisposing to this location include the close approximation of the branch retinal vein and artery which share a common adventitial sheath.
- The classical components of Virchow's triad (alterations in normal blood flow, endothelial cell injury, and hypercoagulability) are thought to be the cause of the veno-occlusive pathology.
- Stagnant blood flow results in hypoxia and damage to the capillary endothelium causing leakage of blood constituents.
- An increase in levels of vascular endothelial growth factor (VEGF) after the veno-occlusive event has been demonstrated at the molecular level.
- Vision loss can be due to secondary macular edema, macular ischemia, or neovascularization and its sequelae.

ETIOLOGY

- Most age-related BRVO are associated systemic hypertension and atherosclerotic disease.
- Vein occlusion in a younger patient necessitates further workup for a hypercoagulable state or other less common etiology.

COMMONLY ASSOCIATED CONDITIONS

- Systemic hypertension
- Diabetes mellitus
- Hyperlipidemia

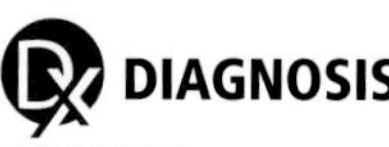

DIAGNOSIS

HISTORY

- A targeted history should be elicited from the patient, specifically inquiring about the risk factors listed above.
  - Symptoms vary on presentation, and mild cases may be asymptomatic. However, most will present with gradual or sudden vision loss and distortion of vision. Those presenting after development of neovascular disease may complain of pain, redness, and epiphora.

PHYSICAL EXAM

- A complete ocular examination including gonioscopy and dilated funduscopy at the initial and follow-up visits should be performed in all patients suspected of having BRVO.
  - Clinically this condition presents with localized flame-shaped intraretinal hemorrhages in a sectoral vascular distribution of the retina. Dilated and tortuous retinal vessels may be present distal to the occlusion. Microaneurysms, cotton wool spots, and retinal edema may also be present. Collateral vessels crossing the horizontal raphe, vascular sheathing, and macular retinal pigment epithelial changes may occur late in the course of the disease.
  - BRVO most commonly affects the superotemporal vein (44–60%), followed by the inferotemporal quadrant (22–43%), and rarely the nasal quadrants.
- Occasionally BRVO occurs after the development of neovascularization, including as a vitreous hemorrhage. Rubeosis (anterior segment neovascularization) from BRVO is very rare.

DIAGNOSTIC TESTS & INTERPRETATION

Lab

- Laboratory testing is not needed to make the diagnosis.
- No further workup is necessary in older (>50 years) individuals with known vascular disease; however, routine cardiovascular examination by a primary care physician is warranted to ensure that underlying systemic conditions are appropriately managed.
- All individuals under the age of 50 without a preexisting underlying etiology require a workup for a systemic cause.
  - This may initially include CBC, chemistry profile, fasting glucose and/or glucose tolerance testing, hemoglobin A1c, and lipid profile.
  - In addition, testing for a hypercoagulable state may include homocysteine, protein C, protein S, antithrombin III, anticardiolipin antibodies, antiphospholipid antibodies, lupus anticoagulant (DRVVT), ANA, SPEP, activated protein C resistance, factor VIIIc, factor V leiden, and prothrombin variant 20210 A.

Imaging

- Fluorescein angiography shows a delay in venous filling in the area of the occlusion, relative to the unaffected retina. Microaneurysms and leakage in the affected area may also be present. BRVO of the ischemic variety show >5 disk areas of retinal capillary nonperfusion.
- Optical coherence tomography (OCT) is useful in assessing for and following macular edema.

Diagnostic Procedures/Other

Perimetry has also been advocated by some to be useful in following patients with BRVO as visual acuity alone may not be a true indicator of visual function due to eccentric fixation.

Pathological Findings

- Early BRVO may demonstrate intraretinal edema, retinal hemorrhages, disk swelling, and cytoid bodies.
- Old BRVO may show disorganization of the retinal layers (especially inner), retinal hemosiderin deposits, and preretinal fibrosis and neovascular membranes.

DIFFERENTIAL DIAGNOSIS

- Diabetic retinopathy
- Hypertensive retinopathy
- Retinal vasculitis
- Retinal arteriolar macroaneurysm
- Radiation retinopathy

TREATMENT

MEDICATION

First Line

- Management of retinal vein occlusion typically involves treatment of macular edema and/or neovascular complications resulting from the initial event.
- Historically, medical management of BRVO had been limited to panretinal and/or macular grid laser photocoagulation (see the Surgery section below) (2)[A].
- Recent studies have demonstrated efficacy of intravitreally administered drugs in improving macular edema and improving and/or stabilizing visual acuity in patients with BRVO (3)[B].
  - Avastin (bevacizumab) is a humanized monoclonal antibody against VEGF that is injected into the vitreous cavity. It has been FDA approved for intravenous use in the management of certain cancers and has been successfully utilized intravitreally for BRVO.
  - Lucentis (ranibizumab) is also an anti-VEGF antibody approved for ophthalmic use that is injected into the vitreous cavity. Recent studies including the BRVO trial have shown its efficacy for BRVO (4)[A].
  - Ozurdex (dexamethasone, 0.7 mg) is a slow release implant that is injected into the vitreous cavity.

Second Line

- Kenalog (triamcinolone) is a steroid suspension that can be injected intravitreally or into the subtenon's space. It is not approved for ophthalmic use, but has been shown to reduce macular edema from BRVO in the short term. Although long-term efficacy has not been demonstrated, it is occasionally utilized as second line therapy (5)[A].
- Other medications are presently under investigation for use in vein occlusions.
  - VEGF-Trap is a fusion protein which binds to the VEGF-A and placental growth factor. Clinical trials are presently underway to determine its efficacy in vein occlusions.
  - Combination treatments of the above medical therapies and surgical therapies (see below) are also being studied.

ADDITIONAL TREATMENT

Issues for Referral

Feedback to the patient's primary physician is important for optimization of the patient's comorbid systemic medical conditions such as systemic hypertension.

SURGERY/OTHER PROCEDURES

- Macular grid laser photocoagulation is indicated for persistent macular edema (>3 months duration) in patients with visual acuity 20/40 or less, and lack of capillary nonperfusion on fluorescein angiography. This was shown to be effective per the Branch Vein Occlusion Study (BVOS).
- Panretinal laser photocoagulation (PRP) remains the mainstay of treatment for neovascular disease resulting from BRVO, as per the results of the BVOS. It should be noted that prophylactic PRP has not shown to be of benefit in preventing neovascularization.
- Pars plana vitrectomy with or without internal limiting membrane peeling, arteriovenous sheathotomy, and laser induced chorioretinal anastomoses are all surgical procedures that have shown mixed results in terms of efficacy, but are sometimes utilized in refractory cases of BRVO (6)[C].

ONGOING CARE

FOLLOW-UP RECOMMENDATIONS

After the initial event, patients should be followed monthly for the first 3 months, and then every 3 months for the first year.

Patient Monitoring

OCT, visual fields, and fluorescein angiography may be useful adjunctive tests to follow this condition.

PROGNOSIS

- The overall visual prognosis is relatively good with approximately 50% of patients having a final visual acuity of 20/40 or better and 20–25% of patients having a final visual acuity of 20/200 or worse.
- However, the visual prognosis for any given patient is difficult to predict as conversion from the nonischemic to the ischemic subtype is not unusual.
- Factors influencing the visual outcome of BRVO include size and location of the affected area, presence of macular edema, presence of macular nonperfusion, retinal neovascularization, and vitreous hemorrhage.

COMPLICATIONS

- Vision loss due to a variety of reasons:
  - Macular ischemia
  - Macular edema
  - Neovascular disease
- Complications secondary to comorbid systemic vascular disease or a hypercoagulable state

REFERENCES

1. Staurenghi G, Lonati C, Aschero M, et al. Arteriovenous crossing as a risk factor in branch retinal vein occlusion. *Am J Ophthalmol* 1994; 117(2):211–213.
2. The Branch Vein Occlusion Study Group. Argon laser photocoagulation for macular edema in branch vein occlusion. *Am J Ophthalmol* 1984;98(3):271–282.
3. McIntosh RL, Mohamed Q, Saw SM, et al. Interventions for branch retinal vein occlusion: an evidence-based systematic review. *Ophthalmology* 2007;114(5):835–854.
4. Campochiaro PA, Heier JS, Feiner L, et al. for The BRAVO Investigators. Ranibizumab for macular edema following Branch Retinal Vein Occlusion six-month primary end point results of a phase III study. *Ophthalmology* 2010;117:1102–1112.
5. Scott IU, Ip MS, Vanveldhuisen PC, et al. A randomized trial comparing the efficacy and safety of intravitreal triamcinolone with standard care to treat vision loss associated with macular edema secondary to branch retinal vein occlusion: The standard care vs corticosteroid for retinal vein occlusion (score) study report 6. *Arch Ophthalmology* 2009;127(9):1115–1128.
6. Cahill MT, Fekrat S. Arteriovenous sheathotomy for branch retinal vein occlusion. *Ophthalmol Clin North Am* 2002;15(4):417–423.

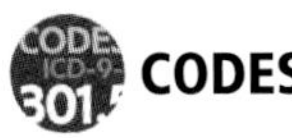

CODES

ICD9

- 362.35 Central retinal vein occlusion
- 362.30 Retinal vascular occlusion, unspecified
- 362.36 Venous tributary (branch) occlusion of retina

CLINICAL PEARLS

- The characteristic findings on clinical examination are multiple, diffuse intraretinal hemorrhages in a sectoral vascular distribution of the retina, usually superotemporally.
- A thorough search for an underlying systemic etiology must be performed in younger patients presenting with this condition.
- Patients with persistent macular edema of <3 months duration, 20/40 or worse vision, and demonstrated macular perfusion on FA should receive macular grid laser photocoagulation.
- Panretinal photocoagulation is the primary therapy after the development of neovascularization.
- Newer intravitreal therapies for managing secondary macular edema are emerging.

BROWN SYNDROME

Colleen J. Christian

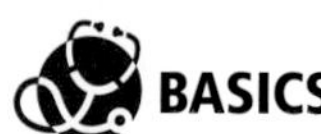

BASICS

DESCRIPTION

Ocular motility disorder characterized by an inability to actively or passively elevate the eye in adduction

EPIDEMIOLOGY

Incidence

Occurs in 1 of 450 strabismus cases

Prevalence

Unknown

RISK FACTORS

- Trauma to superior oblique muscle or trochlea
- Juvenile idiopathic or rheumatoid arthritis

Genetics

Autosomal dominant inheritance has been observed rarely.

PATHOPHYSIOLOGY

Restricted elevation when adducting caused by either an abnormal superior oblique muscle or tendon, or mechanical limitation at the trochlea.

ETIOLOGY

- Congenital: A tight or inelastic superior oblique tendon
- Acquired:
  - Due to trauma either to the superior oblique muscle/tendon, or to the trochlea
  - Inflammation, in particular juvenile idiopathic and adult rheumatoid arthritis (1)[A], (2)[A]

COMMONLY ASSOCIATED CONDITIONS

- Juvenile idiopathic or adult rheumatoid arthritis
- Trauma
- No other consistent systemic or strabismus associations (3)[A]

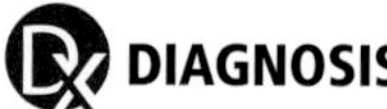

DIAGNOSIS

HISTORY

- Unusual eye movement in upgaze in adduction: May not be noticed by parents until later in childhood:
  - Acquired: Can be diplopic in upgaze and occasionally in contralateral gaze
  - Pain or sensation of a "click" on attempted elevation in adduction
  - Inflammatory causes may note supranasal orbital pain, swelling, and tenderness.
- History of arthritis or joint pain
- History of trauma

PHYSICAL EXAM

- Limited elevation in adduction can range from minimal to severe.
- Elevation in abduction is normal.
- Face-turn away from the involved eye or chin-up position to avoid associated diplopia.
- Hypotropia in primary or in gaze away from the involved eye.
- Amblyopia can occur but is rare.
- With acquired, an audible or palpable superior nasal click may be found on attempted elevation in adduction.
- Swelling and tenderness occur in the trochlear space.
- Full dilated eye examination is performed with refraction.
- Uveitis associated with arthritis is checked.

DIAGNOSTIC TESTS & INTERPRETATION

Lab

Initial lab tests

If acquired, testing for possible arthritis is performed (ANA, rheumatoid factor, erythrocyte sedimentation rate, complete blood count with differential, urinalysis) (see the Pediatric Uveitis chapter).

Follow-up & special considerations

Even if initial testing for arthritis is negative, continue follow-up as it may appear after Brown syndrome occurs.

Imaging

MRI scan can show enhancement of the superior oblique/trochlear region in acquired cases, but is not necessary to make the diagnosis (4)[A].

Diagnostic Procedures/Other

- Positive forced duction testing
- Ultrasound of trochlear area may be useful in acquired cases.

DIFFERENTIAL DIAGNOSIS

- Double elevator palsy (see the chapter on this)
- Primary inferior oblique palsy
- Orbital fracture, tumor, or hemorrhage
- Absent/anomalous muscles as in craniosynostosis syndromes

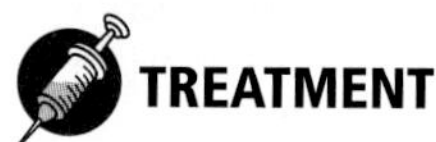

TREATMENT

MEDICATION

First Line

- In acquired nontraumatic cases:
  - In patients with associated juvenile idiopathic or rheumatoid arthritis, treatment of the underlying condition often results in resolution of Brown syndrome.
  - In patients with no associated condition, anti-inflammatory medication such as oral ibuprofen can be used.
  - If inflammation persists, oral nonsteroidal anti-inflammatory drugs can be used.

Second Line

If inflammation persists, oral corticosteroids or local steroid injections in the area of the trochlea may be helpful.

ADDITIONAL TREATMENT

General Measures

Treatment of Brown syndrome is necessary when a hypotropia in primary gaze or a cosmetically significant head turn is present. Many patients do not require treatment as they are comfortable visually, do not have an adaptive head position, and learn to avoid the involved position.

Issues for Referral

Rheumatology consultation may be helpful in acquired cases.

COMPLEMENTARY & ALTERNATIVE THERAPIES

None proven or indicated

SURGERY/OTHER PROCEDURES

- Indications for surgery include the presence of significant head position or a hypotropia in primary gaze.
- The goals of surgery are to allow a more normal head position and to lessen diplopia in the largest possible field of gaze.
- Surgical treatment is to release superior oblique restriction without causing further symptoms, such as a hypotropia due to overaction of the inferior oblique.
- Surgical procedures include:
  - Superior oblique tenotomy or tenectomy
  - Superior oblique tenotomy with:
    - Split tendon lengthening
    - Suture bridge placement
    - Silicone tendon expander placement
- Goal with the above procedures in addition to tenotomy is to lessen postoperative superior oblique weakness (5)[A], (6)[A].

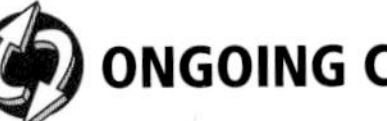

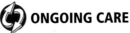

ONGOING CARE

FOLLOW-UP RECOMMENDATIONS

As needed for monitoring of amblyopia and further diplopia or unusual head position

Patient Monitoring

Visual acuity and overall function

PROGNOSIS

- Congenital:
  - Many patients do not require intervention as their related symptoms are not significant.
  - Face turn or hypotropia can be corrected with surgery but long-term follow-up is needed to rule out amblyopia or consecutive inferior oblique overaction.
- Acquired:
  - When associated with inflammatory disease, often resolves with systemic treatment
  - Can resolve spontaneously in acquired nontraumatic cases

REFERENCES

1. Wilson ME, Eustis HS Jr, Parks MM. Brown's syndrome. *Surv Ophthalmol* 1989;34(3):153–172.
2. Kaban TJ, Smith K, Orton RB, et al. Natural history of presumed congenital Brown syndrome. *Arch Ophthalmol* 1993;111(7):943–946.
3. Wang FM, Wertenbaker C, Behrens MM, et al. Acquired Brown's syndrome in children with juvenile rheumatoid arthritis. *Ophthalmology* 1984;91(1):23–26.
4. Bhola R, Rosenbaum AL, Ortube MC, et al. High-resolution magnetic resonance imaging demonstrates varied anatomic abnormalities in Brown syndrome. *J AAPOS* 2005;9(5):438–448.
5. Suh DW, Oystreck DT, Hunter DG. Long-term results of an intraoperative adjustable superior oblique tendon suture spacer using nonabsorbable suture for Brown syndrome. *J AAPOS* 2003;7(4):274–278.
6. Sprunger DT, von Noorden GK, Helveston EM. Surgical results in Brown syndrome. *J Pediatr Ophthalmol Strabismus* 1991;28(3):164–167.

CODES

ICD9

- 378.9 Unspecified disorder of eye movements
- 378.60 Mechanical strabismus, unspecified
- 378.61 Brown's (tendon) sheath syndrome

CLINICAL PEARLS

- Diagnosis made on physical exam by noting inability to elevate eye in adduction, but full elevation in abduction. Look for hypotropia in primary gaze, or adaptive head position.
- Can be congenital or acquired.
- Congenital can be asymptomatic and may not require treatment.
- Acquired may resolve spontaneously or improve with systemic medication.
- Surgical goal is to release superior oblique restriction, but can lead to further symptoms of hypertropia in the involved eye.

BULLOUS KERATOPATHY

Harminder S. Dua
Dalia G. Said
Ammar Miri

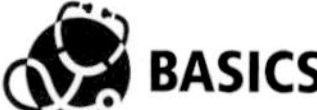

BASICS

DESCRIPTION

A condition in which corneal endothelial failure leads to chronic edema resulting in the formation of epithelial bullae or vesicles. These bullae often rupture causing episodes of severe pain.

EPIDEMIOLOGY

Incidence

The postcataract surgery reported incidence of bullous keratopathy (BK) ranges from 0.06% to 2%. It was 0.06% with posterior chamber implants, 1.2% with anterior chamber implants, and 1.5% with iris fixated lens after 1 year. The incidence increases in the setting of vitreous loss, iris fixated or closed loop anterior chamber lens, and in patients with underlying endothelial dysfunction. However, since the advent of viscoelastic substances to protect the endothelium and the improvement in lens design the incidence has been decreasing.

RISK FACTORS

- Complicated cataract surgery with vitreous loss
- Fuchs endothelial dystrophy (FED)

GENERAL PREVENTION

- Use of retentive-dispersive viscoelastic during anterior segment procedures to protect the endothelium especially when operating in eyes with endothelial dystrophies
- Minimizing phaco power and time during cataract surgery
- Adequate control of postoperative inflammation and intraocular pressure

PATHOPHYSIOLOGY

- When some of the endothelial cells are damaged or lost the remaining cells rearrange to cover the area occupied by the damaged cells. This causes the cells to enlarge (polymegathism) and assume irregular shapes (pleomorphism). With increasing loss, the endothelial pump eventually fails to deturgesce the cornea and the stroma starts to swell. In FED new basement membrane (Descemet's) is laid down by dystrophic endothelial cells. This is thickened, wavy, and differs in density and surface characteristics from the original Descemet's resulting in a silver beaten appearance. Eventually fluid accumulates between the basal epithelial cells clinically manifesting as epithelial edema. Fluid vesicles may coalesce to form epithelial and subepithelial bullae stretching the nerve endings causing pain, which can be severe when the bullae rupture exposing the subepithelial nerve plexus.
- Edema also causes separation of stromal lamellae. Visual loss is more due to epithelial rather than stromal edema. At night the cornea becomes more edematous due to lack of evaporative loss of fluid and poor endothelial cell metabolism. This results in the classic symptom of misty vision on waking, which clears with the passage of time. The time taken for improvement is related to the functional capacity of the residual endothelium.

ETIOLOGY

- Corneal endothelial dystrophies such as FED and posterior polymorphous dystrophy
- Glaucoma: End stage of acute primary and secondary glaucoma (absolute glaucoma)
- Chronic keratouveitis
- Corneal graft failure:
  - Primary endothelial failure
  - Endothelial rejection
  - Endothelial cell loss over time
  - Detached endothelial graft
- Endothelial trauma:
  - Latrogenic: Complicated cataract surgery, glaucoma filtering surgery, anterior chamber phakic and pseudophakic implants, irrigating solution toxicity, instrument-related injury, Descemet's membrane detachment or tear

Pediatric Considerations

- Birth injury to the cornea during forceps delivery can cause loss of endothelial cells with corneal edema at birth or at any time later on.
- Congenital hereditary endothelial dystrophy (CHED)
- Congenital glaucoma

DIAGNOSIS

HISTORY

- Reduced vision and mistiness typically in the morning which clears after a few hours. The duration to clearing increases as the endothelial failure proceeds eventually leading to permanent visual loss.
- Ocular surface irritation or gritty sensation associated with corneal epithelial irregularity
- Repeated episodes of severe pain photophobia and lacrimation

PHYSICAL EXAM

- Externally, the lids may be edematous with a narrow palpebral aperture. The cornea appears dull and lusterless.
- Slit lamp examination:
  - Corneal epithelium – superficial punctate keratitis and surface irregularity due to intact and ruptured epithelial bullae. On fluorescein staining the intact vesicles present as negatively staining dark dots and the ruptured bullae as green dots when visualized with cobalt blue light.
  - Stromal edema – manifests as a sectorial or generalized increase in corneal thickness and intrastromal clear fluid clefts.
  - Superficial or deep corneal vessels may be seen in longstanding cases.
  - Irregularity of Descemet's membrane is seen as folds or corrugations.
- Features of the underlying disease may be seen such as silver beaten appearance and guttata in FED; pigment dusting and old keratic precipitates in chronic uveitis and iris atrophy or a dilated fixed pupil of absolute glaucoma.
- The intraocular pressure (IOP) may be elevated, normal or low. In the presence of excessive corneal edema, IOP measured by Goldman's applanation tonometer or the Tonopen can be misleading and "finger palpation" of the eye ball may be required to assess IOP.

DIAGNOSTIC TESTS & INTERPRETATION

Imaging

- Specular microscopy will demonstrate the reduction of endothelial count with pleomorphism and polymegathism.
- In vivo confocal microscopy: Shows bullae within the basal layers of the epithelium, diffuse bright reflections at Bowman's zone with the absence of nerves, diffuse increased light reflections due to stromal edema alternating with dark bands representing that lacunae can be seen primarily in the anterior stroma. These findings are from BK in FED.

Diagnostic Procedures/Other

Pachymetry: Corneal thickness $>590\ \mu$m in a pseudophakic eye may be associated with irreversible corneal edema

Pathological Findings

- Epithelium: Intracellular epithelial edema with formation of vesicles.
  - Elongated fibrocyte like cells above Bowman's zone
  - Attrition of sub-basal nerve plexus
- Stroma: Thickening, collagen degradation, and keratocyte depletion.
  - Aberrant stromal nerves
  - Superficial and deep vascularization at times
- Endothelium: Cell loss and features of associated of FED if present – guttata and Descemet's membrane thickening.

DIFFERENTIAL DIAGNOSIS

- Certain acute conditions may present with features resembling BK:
  - Acute hydrops in keratoconus
  - Endothelial detachment or tear secondary to trauma or surgery.
  - Acute primary or secondary glaucoma
  - Disciform keratitis

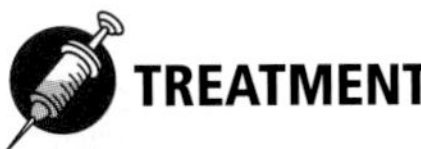

TREATMENT

MEDICATION

First Line

- Hypertonic sodium chloride (5%) drops or ointment 2–4 times especially in the first half of the day
- Warm air (from a hair dryer) blown across the open eye(s)
- Reduction of intraocular pressure with medication

Second Line

Extended wear hydrophilic contact lens can reduce the pain and may improve the vision slightly by reducing surface irregularities. However, proper lens fitting is an issue as a loose lens can cause further damage to the epithelium and a tight lens can cause hypoxia leading to further edema and anterior uveitis (toxic lens syndrome).

SURGERY/OTHER PROCEDURES

- The definitive treatment for BK is an endothelial or penetrating keratoplasty (1)[B]. This should be considered in all eyes with visual potential
- In eyes with no visual potential or when graft material is not readily available and relief from symptoms is warranted, one or a combination of the following can be tried:
  - Anterior stromal puncture (ASP): Over areas of bullae induces subepithelial scarring which allows the epithelium to adhere securely. It leaves behind small scars which can interfere with vision.
  - Phototherapeutic keratectomy (PTK) with the excimer laser (2,3)[B]
  - Amniotic membrane transplant (AMT): The loose bullous epithelium is removed and a circular disk of amnion, 9–11 mm in diameter, is glued or sutured to the corneal surface. New epithelium from the limbus migrates on the amnion (graft), which becomes incorporated into the anterior corneal stroma (2)[B].
  - Historically, conjunctival flaps have been proved to be useful in treating several ocular surface epithelial conditions including BK.
- Retrobulbar alcohol, enucleation, or evisceration: In patients with no visual potential as in end-stage rubeotic glaucoma, these measures may be considered to relieve pain and other symptoms.

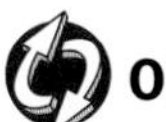

ONGOING CARE

COMPLICATIONS

- Corneal ulceration
- Secondary bacterial infection
- Corneal hypoesthesia
- Scarring and vascularization

REFERENCES

1. Dapena I, Ham L, Melles GR. Endothelial keratoplasty: DSEK/DSAEK or DMEK – the thinner the better? *Curr Opin Ophthalmol* 2009;20: 299–307.
2. Said DG, Nubile M, Alomar T, et al. Histologic features of transplanted amniotic membrane: implications for corneal wound healing. *Ophthalmology* 2009;116:1287–1295.
3. Vyas S, Rathi V. Combined phototherapeutic keratectomy and amniotic membrane grafts for symptomatic bullous keratopathy. *Cornea* 2009; 28:1028–1031.

ADDITIONAL READING

- Price MO, Price FW Jr. Endothelial keratoplasty – a review. *Clin Experiment Ophthalmol* 2010;38: 128–140.

CODES

ICD9

371.23 Bullous keratopathy

CLINICAL PEARLS

- Endothelial dysfunction from any cause can lead to BK.
- Early morning mist vision, clearing as the day progresses, is an early symptom of endothelial dysfunction and corneal edema. This can progress on to BK when vision is permanently impaired.
- Ocular surface pain of varying degrees is the most compelling symptom of BK.
- Slit lamp examination and pachymetry help in making the correct diagnosis.
- Penetrating or endothelial keratoplasty is the definitive treatment in patients with good visual potential, for restoration of sight and relief from pain.
- Other measures such as ASP, PTK, AMT, and conjunctival flaps help to provide relief from pain but do not restore sight or address the underlying endothelial dysfunction. They may be considered as temporizing measures until a keratoplasty can be performed.
- The sick epithelium is vulnerable to infection, which often supervenes. A bandage contact lens, though alleviates pain, can increase the risk of infection.

CANALICULITIS

Edward H. Bedrossian Jr.

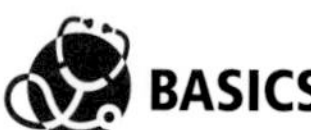

BASICS

DESCRIPTION
Acute or chronic isolated inflammation of the canalicular system

EPIDEMIOLOGY
Incidence
- 6:1 female:male
- 93% lower canaliculus

Prevalence
- Rare, varies with populations
- More common in adults

RISK FACTORS
- Canalicular plugs
- Recurrent conjunctivitis
- Dacryocystitis

GENERAL PREVENTION
- Ocular hygiene
- Avoid intracanalicular plugs

PATHOPHYSIOLOGY
Canalicular obstruction with subsequent infection and inflammation of the canalicular system

ETIOLOGY
- *Streptococcus/staphylococcus* species
- *Actinomyces/propionibacterium*
- Mixed organisms

COMMONLY ASSOCIATED CONDITIONS
- Chronic conjunctivitis
- Recurrent dacryocystitis
- History of dry eyes

DIAGNOSIS

HISTORY
- Epiphora
- Localized pain and swelling at or medial to punctum
- Mucopurulent discharge

PHYSICAL EXAM
- Purulent material at punctum
- Edematous dilated punctum
- Tender erythematous canaliculus
- Mild to severe swelling of the canaliculus
- Slit-lamp exam shows dilated punctum with discharge and tender canaliculus.

DIAGNOSTIC TESTS & INTERPRETATION
Lab
Initial lab tests
- Culture and sensitivity
- Fungal cultures

Follow-up & special considerations
Curettage of the infected canaliculus with a small chalazion curette

Imaging
Follow-up & special considerations
Dacryocystogram (DCG) to rule out dacryoliths or lacrimal sac foreign bodies if problem extends beyond the canaliculus

Diagnostic Procedures/Other
- Canalicular probing with recovery of concretions is diagnostic
- Intracanalicular plug may also be found

Pathological Findings
Concretions with or without pathologic organisms

DIFFERENTIAL DIAGNOSIS
- Dacryocystitis
- Chalazion
- Mucopurulent conjunctivitis

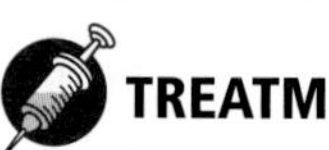

TREATMENT

MEDICATION
First Line
- Penicillin eyedrop 100,000 units/mL q.i.d. for 2 weeks. This must be formulated by the pharmacy each week and placed in a brown ultraviolet protected bottle.
- Alternative: Sodium sulfacetamide 10% 1ggt q.i.d. for 2 weeks (if penicillin eyedrops are not available).
- Warm compresses q.i.d.

Second Line
Surgery, see below

ADDITIONAL TREATMENT

General Measures

Broad spectrum antibiotic eye drops q.i.d. for 1 week postoperative canaliculotomy

Issues for Referral

Patients should follow up with ophthalmologist in 1 week, 1 month, then p.r.n.

SURGERY/OTHER PROCEDURES

- Removal of all concretions from the involved canaliculus is essential for cure. An incision into the horizontal canaliculus from the conjunctival surface, leaving the punctum intact, provides excellent exposure for removal of canaliculitis.
- The canaliculotomy is left open.

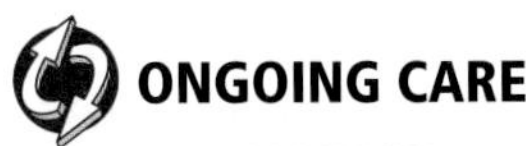

ONGOING CARE

PATIENT EDUCATION

Canaliculoplasty is safe and effective in the treatment of lacrimal canaliculitis.

PROGNOSIS

Nearly 100% cure, if all concretions are removed.

COMPLICATIONS

- Recurrence, if all concretions are not removed
- Rarely patient may have tearing from obstruction and scarring of canaliculus

ADDITIONAL READING

- Zaldivar RA, Bradley EA, Primary canaliculitis. *Ophthal Plast Reconstr Surg* 2009;25(6):481–484.
- Ahn HB, Seo JW, Roh MS, et al. Canaliculitis with a papilloma-like mass caused by a temporary punctal plug. *Ophthal Plast Reconstr Surg* 2009;25(5): 413–414.
- Lin SC, Kao SC, Tsai CC, et al. Clinical characteristics and factors assositaed the outcome of lacrimal canaliculitis. *Acta Ophthalmol* 2010. [Epub ahead of print].
- Anand S.Hollingworth K, Kumar V, et al. Canaliculitis: The incidence of long-term epiphora following canaliculotomy. *Orbit* 2004;23(10):19–26.

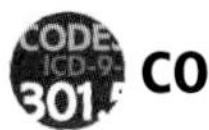

CODES

ICD9

- 375.30 Dacryocystitis, unspecified
- 375.31 Acute canaliculitis, lacrimal
- 375.41 Chronic canaliculitis

CLINICAL PEARLS

- More common in lower canaliculus
- Complete removal of concretions (canaliculolithes) necessary for cure
- Must be considered in the differential diagnosis of chronic conjunctivitis

CAROTID CAVERNOUS FISTULA

Behin Barahimi
Ann P. Murchison
Jurij R. Bilyk

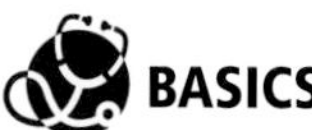

BASICS

DESCRIPTION

A carotid/cavernous sinus fistula (CCF) is an abnormal communication between an artery and the venous plexus within the cavernous sinus (CS). This can occur spontaneously or secondary to trauma. Fistulas are broadly categorized based on the flow rate (high or low) and more specifically by the feeder vessel(s) (Tables 1 and 2).

Genetics

The genetics associated with collagen vascular diseases, pseudoxanthoma elasticum, and connective tissue diseases would apply in appropriate cases. However, the majority of cases are secondary to hypertension and trauma.

GENERAL PREVENTION

Minimizing risk factors associated with hypertension and atherosclerosis would presumably be beneficial in decreasing the risk of some forms of CCF.

Table 1 A simplified schema of CCF, based on clinical findings (1)[C]

Type	Characteristics	Clinical features
High flow	• Usually direct fistulas (Barrow type A) • 70–80% are due to trauma resulting in basilar skull fracture, with a resultant tear in the internal carotid artery • Spontaneous lesions are secondary to aneurysm or atherosclerotic damage • Iatrogenic: Endovascular procedures (including carotid endarterectomy), skull base surgery	• Usually dramatic external signs • Most common in young males • May result in permanent visual loss and neurologic injury • Requires closure
Low flow	• Usually indirect fistulas (Barrow type B, C, or D) • Also called "dural-sinus fistula" • Typically fed by a smaller caliber branch of the internal or external carotid artery, or both (e.g., meningeal arteries, ascending pharyngeal artery, etc.)	• Typically subtle, more chronic signs • More common in females >50 years of age • Associated with hypertension, atherosclerosis, and connective tissue diseases • May close spontaneously

Table 2 The Barrow classification of CCF

Type	Arterial feeder
A	ICA
B	Branches of the ICA
C	Branches of the ECA
D	Branches of both ICA and ECA

ICA = internal carotid artery; ECA = external carotid artery.

EPIDEMIOLOGY

Incidence

Specific numbers are not known but overall it is a rare entity.

Prevalence

Not known

RISK FACTORS

- Hypertension
- Atherosclerosis
- Collagen vascular disease
- Connective tissue disease (Ehlers–Danlos)
- Pregnancy
- History of carotid artery aneurysm
- History of trauma

PATHOPHYSIOLOGY

CCF alters the flow dynamics of the skull base. The superior ophthalmic vein (SOV) provides almost exclusive venous drainage of the orbit into the CS. In addition, the venous plexus of the CS communicates with the contralateral CS and the deep cortical veins within the brain. An abnormal communication between an intracranial artery and the venous plexus of the CS creates flow problems in the surrounding anatomy, potentially causing damage intraorbitally and intracranially.

ETIOLOGY

See above

COMMONLY ASSOCIATED CONDITIONS

See the Risk Factors section

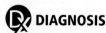

DIAGNOSIS

HISTORY

- Presenting symptoms vary widely and depend of the amount of blood flow through the fistula. High-flow fistulas can present with marked proptosis, diplopia, and decreased vision. Low-flow fistulas may only have mild conjunctival injection.
- The patient may have a recent or distant history of trauma, which may or may not have affected the head.
- Complaints of a dull retrobulbar ache or "whooshing" sound in the head may be present.
- In lower flow lesions, the patient's only complaint may be of a unilateral or, less frequently, bilateral red eye of varying duration, from days to months. Patients may have seen multiple physicians and carry a variety of misdiagnoses, including conjunctivitis, allergic reaction, dry eye, etc. (1)[C].
- Some patients may elicit a history of unilateral glaucoma, often diagnosed at the time of the red eye.
- Double vision. Since the abducens nerve is the most vulnerable cranial nerve within the CS, patients may complain of horizontal, binocular diplopia that is gaze dependent. Vertical diplopia is less common.
- The patient may complain of a bulging eye if proptosis is present.
- Neurologic symptoms (weakness, slurred speech, sensory deficits) are ominous signs of possible posterior cortical venous drainage.

PHYSICAL EXAM

- Decreased vision, dyschromatopsia, and afferent pupillary defect: Usually secondary to vascular compromise of the optic nerve or retina
- Asymmetrically elevated intraocular pressure: Secondary to decreased episcleral venous outflow into a congested orbit
- Conjunctival injection: As the CS becomes arterialized with blood from the feeding vessel(s), the venous outflow of the orbit becomes congested, causing the conjunctival vessels to become dilated and tortuous. At the slit lamp, "corkscrewing" of the conjunctival vessels extending to the limbus may be present.
- Proptosis: As orbital venous congestion develops, the globe becomes anteriorly displaced
- Diplopia: See the History section
- Bruit: A supraorbital bruit may be auscultated in higher flow lesions
- Optic nerve edema
- Central or branch retinal vein occlusion, secondary to venous stasis. Arterial occlusion is less common
- Angle-closure glaucoma from forward rotation of the iris-lens diaphragm (2)[C]

DIAGNOSTIC TESTS & INTERPRETATION

Lab

Initial lab tests

There are no diagnostic lab tests.

Imaging

Initial approach

- Orbital color Doppler ultrasonography: A noninvasive method to detect an enlarged SOV with reversal of flow and an arteriolized wave form. The sensitivity and specificity of this test is unknown, but is probably more reliable in higher flow states.
- CT/CTA: In cases where trauma is involved, this is usually the first imaging study done. Typical findings include an enlarged superior ophthalmic vein (SOV), thickened extraocular muscles and an enlarged CS. The sensitivity of CTA is dependent on the caliber of the fistula.
- MRI/MRA: Similar findings as in CT. MRI may also show slow flow or thrombus formation within the SOV.

- Angiography: This is the gold standard, can diagnose small arterial feeders, and allows simultaneous management by embolization. It is important to perform angiography of the entire cranial arterial system ("six vessel" angiography: Bilateral internal and external carotid arteries as well as vertebral arteries). This modality will also assess any posterior cortical venous outflow. Arteriography alone can be therapeutic for indirect dural fistulas in 20–50% of cases (2)[C].

Follow-up & special considerations

If no posterior cortical venous outflow is present and visual function is not at risk, many patients with low-flow fistulas may be managed conservatively.

DIFFERENTIAL DIAGNOSIS

- Thyroid eye disease
- Idiopathic orbital inflammatory syndrome
- Spheno-orbital mass
- Conjunctivitis
- Episcleritis
- Tolosa-Hunt syndrome (2)[C]

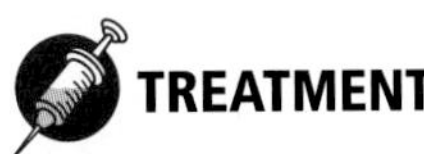

TREATMENT

MEDICATION

First Line

Glaucoma: Treated with topical medications including beta-blocker, alpha agonist, carbonic anhydrase inhibitor, or prostaglandin. An oral carbonic anhydrase inhibitor may also be utilized.

Second Line

- Systemic management of hypertension and hypercholesterolemia
- Exposure keratopathy: Treated with aggressive lubrication or tarsorrhaphy

ADDITIONAL TREATMENT

General Measures

Low-flow fistulas with few clinical manifestations can be observed and may close spontaneously. Carotid massage is an effective measure for the closure of low-flow lesions. The patient is instructed to always use the contralateral hand to perform the massage to minimize the risk of permanent ischemic injury to the brain.

Issues for Referral

- Because of the ocular manifestations, it is common for an ophthalmologist to make the initial diagnosis. All CCFs should be referred to a neurosurgeon or interventional neuroradiologist for angiography and treatment. In appropriate cases where the SOV can be used to approach the CS, an orbital specialist may also be involved.
- Timing of referral is important. Chronic symptomatology is less urgent than more acute manifestations. In acute lesions, the possibility of posterior cortical venous outflow with the attendant risk of hemorrhagic stroke must be considered.

SURGERY/OTHER PROCEDURES

- An endovascular approach using either the arterial or venous system, with embolization of the fistula using a number of materials. These procedures are technically difficult and often require a multidisciplinary approach (3)[C]. An SOV approach through a lid crease incision often requires an orbital surgeon experienced in this procedure.
- Other treatments for CCFs include craniotomy, conventional radiation therapy, stereotactic radiosurgery (3)[C].

IN-PATIENT CONSIDERATIONS

Initial Stabilization

- For trauma patients follow standard protocols.
- Following embolization, the patient should be monitored for an acute exacerbation of orbital signs, which may occur after acute closure of the SOV.

Admission Criteria

Most patients who undergo angiography or endovascular treatment are admitted for 24 h of observation.

IV Fluids

Hydration is necessary to clear the intravenous dye load of angiography.

Nursing

- Management of the angiography cut-down site
- Frequent neurologic checks to rule out cerebral vasospasm
- Observation for any worsening of orbital signs

Discharge Criteria

- Visual function is stable and intraocular pressure is normalizing
- Cut-down site is stable
- No new neurologic signs occur

ONGOING CARE

FOLLOW-UP RECOMMENDATIONS

Patients with CCFs should be seen regularly by their ophthalmologist to have a complete eye exam with monitoring of intraocular pressure, since CCFs can reopen or develop new feeder vessels.

DIET

No specific dietary recommendations

PATIENT EDUCATION

Return with any new recurrent ocular or neurologic symptoms

PROGNOSIS

- Initially, the prognosis for visual function is guarded and dependent on the dynamics of the CCF.
- With successful closure of the CCF, long-term prognosis is good.

COMPLICATIONS

- Loss of vision
- Ocular ischemia, including neovascular glaucoma
- Permanent neurologic sequelae, including stroke
- Death is more often associated with high-flow, direct fistulas.

REFERENCES

1. Chaudhry IA, Elkhamry SM, Al-Rashed W, et al. Carotid cavernous fistula: Ophthalmological implications. *Middle East Afr J Ophthalmol* 2009;16(2):57–63.
2. Miller NR. Diagnosis and management of dural carotid-cavernous sinus fistulas. *Neurosurg Focus* 2007;E 23(5):13.
3. Gemmete JJ, Ansari SA, Gandhi DM. Endovascular techniques for treatment of carotid-cavernous fistula. *J Neuro-Ophthalmol* 2009;29:62–71.

ADDITIONAL READING

- Mendicino ME, Simon DJ, Newman NJ. The ophthalmology of intracranial vascular abnormalities. *Am J Ophthalmol* 1998;125: 527–544.
- Goldberg RA, Goldey SH, Duckwiler G, et al. Management of cavernous sinus dural fistulas. *Arch Ophthalmol* 1996;114:707–714.
- Kirsh M, Henkes H, Liebig T, et al. Endovascular management of dural carotid-cavernous sinus fistulas in 141 patients. *Neuroradiology* 2006;48:486–490.
- Feiner L, Bennett J, Volpe NJ. Cavernous sinus fistulas: Carotid cavernous fistulas and dural arteriorvenous malformations. *Neuro-ophthalmology* 2003;3:415–420.

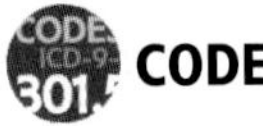

CODES

ICD9

- 365.63 Glaucoma with vascular disorder
- 376.22 Exophthalmic ophthalmoplegia
- 747.6 Intracranial arteriovenous malformation

CLINICAL PEARLS

- Indirect, low-flow fistulas can be difficult to diagnose clinically. In chronic cases where there is no threat to the vision close observation is acceptable, as spontaneous resolution may occur.
- Permanent visual loss may occur from CCFs.
- Posterior cortical venous outflow in CCF increases the risk of hemorrhagic stroke.
- CCFs can recanalize even after surgical intervention.
- Resolution of orbital signs after successful closure of CCF may take weeks to months to resolve (2)[C].

CATARACTS

Robert S. Bailey, Jr.

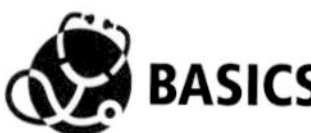

BASICS

DESCRIPTION
Any opacity of the lens.

EPIDEMIOLOGY

Incidence
- Most common cause of blindness in the world
- Account for approximately 50% of low-vision cases in adults over age 40 in the USA
- Number of individuals with cataracts in the USA will increase by 50% by 2020.

Prevalence
- Some evidence of lens opacity found in 96% of those over 60 years of age
- Visually significant cataracts in 5% at age 65 and 50% for persons older than 75 in the USA

RISK FACTORS
- Exposure to higher intensity of incident or reflected ultraviolet light especially ultraviolet-B (UV-B)
- High-energy radiation
- Exposure to high levels of oxygen
- Smoking and tobacco chewing

Genetics
- Family history is a risk factor for aging-related cataracts.
- Specific genes have not been identified.

GENERAL PREVENTION
- Smoking cessation
- Brimmed hats and UV-B blocking sunglasses
- No recommendations for the use of nutritional supplements to prevent or delay cataract progression can be made at this time
- Use of alternate medication in patients taking long-term inhaled or oral corticosteroids
- Behavior modification to reduce risk of developing type 2 diabetes

PATHOPHYSIOLOGY
- Anatomic location:
  - Nuclear
  - Cortical
  - Posterior subcapsular
  - Mixed
  - Other:
    - Capsular (polar)
    - Anterior subcapsular
    - Lens epithelial decompensation
    - Retrodots
    - Advanced
- Studies have shown that cataracts progress over time.

ETIOLOGY
- Age related—Most common
- Congenital and juvenile:
  - Part of systemic syndrome
  - Isolated
  - AD
  - AR
  - X-linked
- Traumatic
- Associated with primary ocular disease:
  - Uveitis
  - Glaucoma
  - Retinal detachment
  - Retinal degeneration
  - Sclerocornea
  - Microphthalmos
  - Intraocular tumor
  - Norrie's disease
  - Persistent hyperplastic primary vitreous (PHPV)
  - Retinopathy of prematurity
  - Aniridia
  - High myopia
- Associated with systemic disease:
  - Metabolic disorders:
    - Diabetes
    - Galactosemia
    - Hypoparathyroidism/hypocalcemia
    - Lowe's syndrome
    - Wilson's disease
  - Renal disease:
    - Alport's disease
  - Cutaneous disease:
    - Atopic dermatitis
  - Connective tissue/skeletal disorders:
    - Myotonic dystrophy
    - Marfan's syndrome
  - Central nervous system:
    - Bilateral acoustic neuroma
  - Down's syndrome
- Environmental exposure:
  - Ionizing radiation:
    - X-ray
    - Ultraviolet
    - Infrared
    - Microwave
  - Pharmaceuticals:
    - Steroids
    - Miotics
    - Antipsychotics (e.g., phenothiazines)
  - Electric
  - Infectious:
    - Rubella
  - Postsurgical:
    - Glaucoma
    - Pars plana vitrectomy
- Other:
  - Ectopic lentis
  - Lenticonus and lentiglobus

DIAGNOSIS

HISTORY
- Progressive visual loss affecting one or both eyes
- Emphasize functional difficulties related to the patient's activities of daily living
- Glare and reduced color perception
- Type of cataract determines symptoms.
- Medications—Flomax or other alpha-1 blockers associated with intraoperative floppy iris syndrome
- Systemic diseases
- Trauma
- Other ocular disease affecting vision
- Visual function prior to cataract development

PHYSICAL EXAM
- Complete ocular exam:
  - Distance and near vision
  - Pupillary examination
  - Refraction to obtain best corrected visual acuity
  - Measurement of intraocular pressure
  - Fundus exam concentrating on macula
- Slit lamp exam:
  - Cornea:
    - Clarity or localized opacities
    - Endothelial function—guttata
  - Anterior chamber depth
  - Iris:
    - Pupillary dilation
    - Posterior synechiae
  - Cataract types:
    - Nuclear
    - Posterior subcapsular
    - Cortical
  - Abnormalities of lens position
  - Zonular instability—phacodonesis
  - Pseudoexfoliation

DIAGNOSTIC TESTS & INTERPRETATION

Lab
Glare testing in patients with glare complaint and good visual acuity (1)[A]

Imaging

Initial approach
- B-scan ultrasonography if fundus obscured to rule out posterior segment disease
- A-scan or laser partial coherence optical biometry measurement of axial length
- Endothelial cell count or pachymetry if endothelial disease present
- Keratometry readings
- Corneal topography
- Fluorescein angiography
- Optical coherence tomography may be helpful to diagnose subtle macular pathology.

Follow-up & special considerations
- Latest generation lens calculation formulas should be used in the intraocular lens (IOL) selection process.

C

TREATMENT

MEDICATION

Mydriasis may be used successfully in some patients if they desire nonsurgical treatment or are not surgical candidates.

ADDITIONAL TREATMENT

General Measures

Correct refractive error if surgery not indicated

SURGERY/OTHER PROCEDURES

- Surgical indications:
  - To improve visual function
  - Surgical therapy for ocular disease (lens-related glaucoma or uveitis)
  - To aid with management of ocular disease
  - Extracapsular cataract extraction most commonly by phacoemulsification (ultrasonic technique) is a preferred method to remove a cataract
- Anesthesia techniques:
  - General
  - Local (regional):
    - Retrobulbar
    - Peribulbar
    - Sub-Tenon's
    - Topical with or without intracameral
- Technical elements of successful cataract procedure:
  - Temporal, appropriately sized clear-corneal incision with sutureless architecture
  - Use of an ophthalmic viscosurgical device (OVD) to provide protection of corneal endothelium, manipulate tissue, and maintain working space
  - Continuous circular capsulorrhexis sized to overlap the IOL edge
  - Hydrodissection of lens
  - Nuclear disassembly and emulsification technique for lens removal
  - Irrigation and aspiration of remaining cortex
  - Capsular bag fixation of the foldable posterior chamber IOL
  - Removal of the OVD to minimize postoperative IOP elevation
  - Assurance of watertight incision using sutures if necessary
- Recent IOL developments:
  - Aspheric optic IOLs improve functional vision and quality of vision by improving contrast sensitivity, decreasing haloes, and improving optical quality.
  - Toric IOLs reduce spectacle dependence in patients with corneal astigmatism.
  - Monovision and presbyopia-correcting IOLs are strategies used to reduce spectacle dependence after cataract surgery—patient selection critical.
  - Presbyopia-correcting IOLs:
    - Multifocal
    - Accommodative

IN-PATIENT CONSIDERATIONS

- Nearly all cataract surgery is performed in an outpatient setting either in a hospital-based outpatient surgical facility or in a freestanding ambulatory surgery center.
- Inpatient surgery may be necessary if the need arises for complex ocular care, multiple procedures, and general medical and nursing care, or if there are multiple ocular conditions.

ONGOING CARE

FOLLOW-UP RECOMMENDATIONS

- Use of 5% solution of povidone iodine in the conjunctival sac prior to surgery has been proven to reduce risk of endophthalmitis (2)[A]
- Postoperative regimens of topical antibiotics, corticosteroids, and NSAIDs vary from surgeon to surgeon.

Patient Monitoring

- First postoperative exam within 24–48 h
- Final refractive visit between 1 and 4 weeks after small-incision surgery and 6–12 weeks after sutured large-incision cataract surgery
- Posterior capsule opacification (PCO) incidence varies but may be up to 50% by 2 years post surgery.
  - Nd:Yag laser capsulotomy effective in restoring visual function in patients with significant PCO

PROGNOSIS

- Cataract surgery has been shown to have a significant positive impact on vision-dependent function and health-related quality of life.
- Reduced risk of falls and hip fractures following cataract surgery
- 85–90% of all patients achieve 20/40 or better best-corrected visual acuity after surgery.
- 95% without ocular comorbidities achieve 20/40 or better visual acuity.
- Ocular comorbidities that may affect outcome of surgery:
  - Amblyopia
  - AMD
  - Diabetic retinopathy
  - Fuch's corneal dystrophy
  - Glaucoma
  - Pseudoexfoliation syndrome
  - Uveitis
- High-risk ocular characteristics that increase risk of surgical complication:
  - Previous eye surgery:
    - Prior refractive surgery alters corneal curvature and makes IOL calculation difficult (3)[A].
  - Very long (high myopia) and very short eyes
  - Small pupils or eyes with posterior synechiae
  - Scarred or cloudy corneas
  - Zonular weakness
  - Prior ocular trauma
  - Systemic use of alpha-1A adrenergic antagonists (Flowmax)

COMPLICATIONS

- PCO most common event post surgery
- Sight threatening complications:
  - Endophthalmitis
  - Suprachoroidal hemorrhage
  - Cystoid macular edema
  - Retinal detachment
  - Corneal edema
  - IOL dislocation
- Intraoperative events:
  - Posterior capsule rupture
  - Vitreous loss
- Complications of IOLs:
  - Incorrect power
  - IOL malposition
  - Uveitis–glaucoma–hyphema syndrome

REFERENCES

1. Pfoff D, Werner J. Effect of cataract surgery on contrast sensitivity and glare in patients with 20/50 or better Snellen acuity. *J Cataract Refract Surg* 1994;20:620–625.
2. Ciulla T, Starr M, Masket S. Bacterial endophthalmitis prophylaxis for cataract surgery: An evidence-based update. *Ophthalmology* 2002;109:13–24.
3. Latkany R, Chokshi A, Speaker M, et al. Intraocular lens calculations after refractive surgery. *J Cataract Refract Surg* 2005;31:562–570.

ADDITIONAL READING

- Masket S, Chang D, Lane SS, et al. *Cataract in the adult eye: Preferred practice patterns.* San Francisco: AAO, 2006
- Congdon N, Chang M, et al. Cataract: Clinical types. In: *Duane's clinical ophthalmology.* Tasman W, Jaeger EA, eds. Philadelphia: Lippincott, Williams and Wilkins, 2009;1:73.
- Acquired Cataract in Ehlers J, Shah C (eds). *The Wills Eye Manual* 13.1.2008

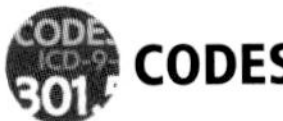

CODES

ICD9

- 366.04 Nuclear nonsenile cataract
- 366.9 Unspecified cataract
- 743.31 Congenital capsular and subcapsular cataract

CLINICAL PEARLS

- Cataracts are the most common cause of world blindness and will become more prevalent with an aging population in the USA.
- Smoking cessation and reduction of UV-B exposure have been shown to slow cataract progression.
- Modern cataract surgery is a very successful operation with 95% of patients achieving 20/40 vision or better after surgery in patients with no other ocular disease.

CAVERNOUS HEMANGIOMA OF THE ORBIT

Katherine G. Gold

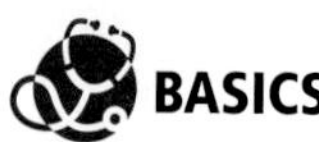

BASICS

DESCRIPTION

- Cavernous hemangioma of the orbit is a benign proliferation of vascular channels which induces progressive ectasia.
  - This may also occur in the central nervous system, liver, and thyroid
- It is also known as cavernoma

EPIDEMIOLOGY

Incidence

- Estimated 4–12% of orbital tumors – the most common orbital tumor in adults
- Rarely occurs in infants or children
- Female > male

PATHOPHYSIOLOGY

Although histologically benign, damage is through compression of the optic nerve, extraocular muscles, and the globe itself.

ETIOLOGY

Hamartomatous benign vascular growth

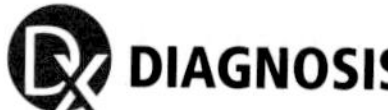

DIAGNOSIS

HISTORY

- Painless, progressive proptosis
- Hyperopic shift in refraction
- Pressure sensation
- Diplopia
- If advanced, vision loss due to optic neuropathy
- Often discovered on imaging for other reasons, i.e., headache

PHYSICAL EXAM

- Hertel exophthalmometry for baseline and comparison
- Resistance to retropulsion
- Dilated episcleral vessels
- Choroidal folds on funduscopic exam due to compression of globe
- Evaluate for compressive optic neuropathy:
  - Relative afferent pupillary defect
  - Vision loss
  - Color testing
  - Visual field testing
  - Optic nerve edema or atrophy

DIAGNOSTIC TESTS & INTERPRETATION

Diagnostic Procedures/Other

Imaging of orbits – CT/MRI

DIFFERENTIAL DIAGNOSIS

- Thyroid eye disease
- Orbital tumor – schwannoma, hemangiopericytoma, solitary fibrous tumors
- Carotid–cavernous fistula
- Optic nerve meningioma or glioma

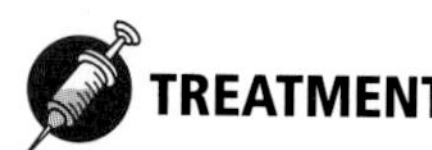

TREATMENT

- Surgical resection (orbitotomy) if compression of optic nerve, extraocular muscles, or the globe is evident. Surgery may also be indicated for severe proptosis or for pathologic diagnosis if the identity of the mass is in question. Surgical resection is usually uncomplicated unless located at the orbital apex.

ADDITIONAL TREATMENT

General Measures

If exposure keratopathy develops due to lagophthalmos, treat with lubrication and follow carefully to ensure stability or resolution.

SURGERY/OTHER PROCEDURES

As mentioned above

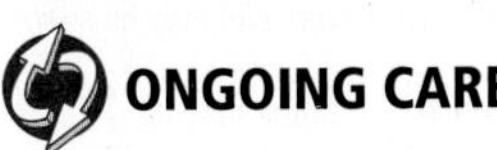

ONGOING CARE

FOLLOW-UP RECOMMENDATIONS

- Ophthalmologist
- Oculoplastic/orbital specialist
- If extends extraorbitally, may require neurosurgical or otolaryngological consult

PATIENT EDUCATION

For patients who are being observed, they must be aware of need for swift evaluation if a change in vision were to occur

PROGNOSIS

- Vast majority who are observed remain stable over time
- Majority with indications for surgery do well after resection – no risk of recurrence

COMPLICATIONS

Visual loss

ADDITIONAL READING

- Cheng JW, Wei RL, Cai JP, et al. Transconjunctival orbitotomy for orbital cavernous hemangiomas. *Can J Ophthalmol* 2008;43(2):234–238.
- Scheuerle AF, Steiner HH, Kolling G, et al. Treatment and long-term outcome of patients with orbital cavernomas. *Am J Ophthalmol* 2004;138(2): 237–244.
- Weir RE, Evans S, Hajdu SD, et al. The convex retina: Optical coherence tomography in hypermetropic shift, without choroidal folds, from intraconal cavernous haemangioma. *Orbit* 2009;28(6): 398–400.

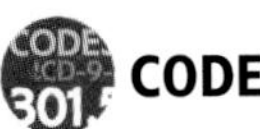

CODES

ICD9

- 224.1 Orbital tumor, benign
- 228.09 Hemangioma of other sites

C

CAVERNOUS HEMANGIOMA OF THE RETINA

Gary Shienbaum

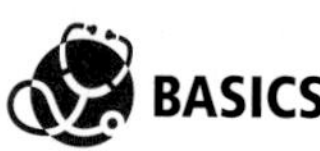

BASICS

DESCRIPTION

Rare, congenital retinal vascular hamartoma

EPIDEMIOLOGY

Incidence

Very rare, and cannot be accurately specified as many patients are asymptomatic and do not seek ophthalmic care.

Prevalence

Very rare

RISK FACTORS

Family history

Genetics

- Sporadic and autosomal dominant forms are recognized.
- Neuro-oculo-cutaneous phacomatosis:
  - Autosomal dominant with high penetrance and variable expressivity
  - Also referred to as:
    - Familial cavernous malformations of the central nervous systems (CNS) and retina
    - Cavernoma multiplex
  - Multiple cavernous hemangiomas more likely in familial cases
  - Familial cerebral cavernous malformations (CCM) have been mapped to three loci: 7q21-q22 (CCM1), 7p15-p13 (CCM2), and 3q25.2-q27 (CCM3).

GENERAL PREVENTION

None

ETIOLOGY

This is a genetic condition.

COMMONLY ASSOCIATED CONDITIONS

- Cavernous hemangiomas of the CNS
- Cutaneous vascular hamartomas

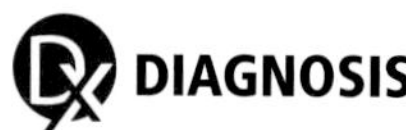

DIAGNOSIS

HISTORY

- Decreased visual acuity and floaters; however, patients are frequently asymptomatic
- Seizures, headaches, intracranial hemorrhage, and progressive focal neurologic deficits can be observed in cases involving the CNS (as part of the above neuro-oculo-cutaneous phacomatosis).

PHYSICAL EXAM

- Grape-like clusters of saccular dilatations filled with dark (venous) blood arising from the inner retina or optic nerve surface
- Overlying gliosis/fibrosis
- Associated epiretinal membranes
- Enlarged feeding or draining vessels characteristically absent
- Typically unilateral

DIAGNOSTIC TESTS & INTERPRETATION

Imaging

- Fluorescein angiography is very helpful in confirming the diagnosis
  - Characteristically patients have delayed filling
  - Plasma/fluorescein-erythrocyte level may be seen within saccules
  - Characteristic absence of leakage may be observed
- Neuroimaging (MRI brain is the preferred imaging modality)

Pathological Findings

Sessile tumor composed of multiple, dilated, thin collagenous walled vascular spaces lined by nonfenestrated endothelium with surface gliosis

DIFFERENTIAL DIAGNOSIS

- Retinal telangiectasis (e.g., coats disease)
- Retinal hemangioblastoma
- Racemose angioma

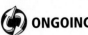

TREATMENT

MEDICATION
- Normally no treatment required
- Laser photocoagulation and/or vitrectomy used in select cases of vitreous hemorrhage

ONGOING CARE

FOLLOW-UP RECOMMENDATIONS
- Ophthalmologist
- Neurological/neurosurgical consultation
- Dermatologic consultation

PATIENT EDUCATION
- Screening required for systemic and familial involvement.
  - Detailed family history, ophthalmologic, neurologic (including neuroimaging studies), and dermatologic examinations
  - First-degree relatives should be screened if diagnosis of neuro-oculo-cutaneous phacomatosis suggestive by patient examination or family history

PROGNOSIS
- Visual loss is uncommon. Most patients are asymptomatic
- Nonprogressive; may undergo spontaneous thrombosis
- No treatment is required

COMPLICATIONS
- Vitreous hemorrhage
- Decreased visual acuity secondary to macular location
- Epiretinal membrane formation
- Intracranial hemorrhage secondary to cavernous hemangioma of the CNS

ADDITIONAL READING

- Gass JDM. Cavernous hemangioma of the retina: A neuro-oculo-cutaneous syndrome. *Am J Ophthalmol* 1971;71:799–814.
- Goldberg RE, Pheasant TR, Shields JA. Cavernous hemangioma of the retina: A four-generation pedigree with neurocutaneous manifestations and an example of bilateral retinal involvement. *Arch Ophthalmol* 1979;97:2321–2324.
- Dobyns WB, Michels VV, Groover RV, et al. Familial cavernous malformations of the central nervous system and retina. *Ann Neurol* 1987;21:578–583.
- Pancurak J, Goldberg MF, Frenkel M, et al. Cavernous hemangioma of the retina: Genetic and central nervous system involvement. *Retina* 1985;5:215–220.
- Sarraf D, Payne AM, Kitchen ND, et al. Familial cavernous hemangioma: An expanding ocular spectrum. *Arch Ophthalmol* 2000;118:969–973.
- Singh AD, Rundle PA, Rennie I. Retinal vascular tumors. *Ophthalmol Clin N Am* 2005;18:167–176.
- Kitzmann AS, Pulido JS, Ferber MJ, et al. A splice mutation in CCM1/KRIT1 is associated with retinal and cerebral cavernous hemangioma. *Ophthalmic Genet* 2006;27:157–159.

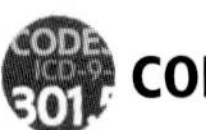

CODES

ICD9
- 228.03 Hemangioma of retina
- 757.32 Vascular hamartomas
- 759.6 Other congenital hamartoses, not elsewhere classified

CLINICAL PEARLS

- The "grape-like" cluster seen with fluorescein angiography with classic fluorescein and erythrocyte levels is typical of this disease.

CAVERNOUS SINUS SYNDROME/ORBITAL APEX SYNDROME

Robert J. Granadier

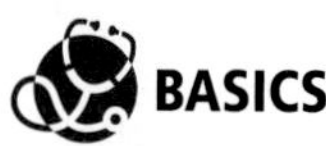

BASICS

DESCRIPTION

- Orbital apex syndrome: A constellation of findings including combined motor and sensory deficit of the eye and orbit secondary to multiple etiologies: Pathology involving the oculomotor nerve (III), trochlear nerve (IV), abducens nerve, (VI), and the first division of the trigeminal nerve (V1) in association with decreased optic nerve (II) function (1)[B]
- Cavernous sinus syndrome: orbital apex syndrome plus second branch of trigeminal nerve (V2) without optic nerve involvement
- Superior orbital fissure syndrome: cavernous sinus syndrome minus optic neuropathy

EPIDEMIOLOGY

Incidence

- Rare
- Positive correlation between the number of cranial nerves involved and presence of cavernous sinus syndrome (2)[B]

RISK FACTORS

- Diabetes
- Immunosuppression
- Cancer
- Trauma
- Sinus surgery

PATHOPHYSIOLOGY

Mass, inflammation, or vascular lesions in the region of the cavernous sinus, superior orbital fissure, or orbital apex causing dysfunction of the nerves in that area by direct compression, inflammation, or ischemia.

ETIOLOGY

- Inflammatory
- Infectious
- Neoplastic
- Traumatic/iatrogenic
- Vascular

COMMONLY ASSOCIATED CONDITIONS

- Infectious
- Fungal: aspergillosis, mucormycosis
- Bacterial: Staph, Strep, mycobacterium TB
- Inflammatory: sarcoidosis, systemic lupus erythematosus (SLE), giant cell arteritis, Wegener's granulomatosis, idiopathic orbital pseudotumor (Tolosa–Hunt syndrome)
- Local neoplastic: meningioma, nasopharyngeal carcinoma, pituitary adenoma, squamous cell Ca
- Metastatic neoplastic: lung, breast, renal cell, malignant melanoma
- Vascular: carotid cavernous aneurysm or fistula, cavernous sinus thrombosis (septic or aseptic)
- Iatrogenic: endoscopic sinus surgery
- Trauma: penetrating injury, orbital fracture, foreign body

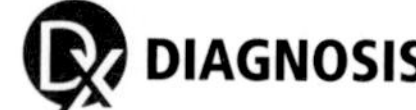

DIAGNOSIS

HISTORY

- Binocular double vision
- Reduced vision
- ±Pain
- ±Proptosis

PHYSICAL EXAM

- Best corrected visual acuity
- Decreased pupil reactivity with afferent pupillary defect
- Color vision/brightness
- Cranial nerve examination
- Decreased extraocular motility (multiple patterns)
- Oculomotor and abducens nerve most frequently involved
- Decreased sensation face, periorbital skin, cornea
- Orbital examination: lid position, resistance keratopathy associated with neurotrophic cornea (severe cases may require tarsorrhaphy.)

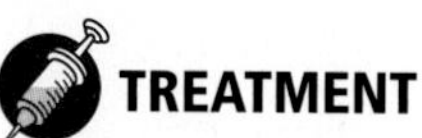

TREATMENT

ADDITIONAL TREATMENT

Issues for Referral

- Infectious disease: referral for inpatient internal medicine and infectious disease management
- Intraorbital mass with intracranial pathology refer to neurosurgery or oculoplastic surgery for biopsy, endocrinology for glucocorticoid management/replacement, infectious disease as necessary
- Inflammatory referral to rheumatology/immunology for treatment and ongoing care

Additional Therapies

Possible radiation therapy (RT), stereotactic RT.

COMPLEMENTARY & ALTERNATIVE THERAPIES

Immunosuppression for inflammatory lesions including steroids, methotrexate, azathioprine (Imuran), tumor necrosis factor alpha therapies (3)[B], (4)[C].

SURGERY/OTHER PROCEDURES

- Surgical biopsy may be required for definitive diagnosis of underlying etiology (5)[B].
- Aggressive surgical debridement required for treatment of orbital mucormycosis
- Exenteration (surgical removal of all orbital contents) may be required if patient is at risk for cavernous sinus thrombosis secondary to greater than 50% risk of death associated with septic cavernous sinus thrombosis.

IN-PATIENT CONSIDERATIONS

Initial Stabilization

- Diabetes: mucormycosis—intensive care medical stabilization of blood sugar and ketoacidosis, and initial antifungal therapy prior to any surgical management
- Septic cavernous thrombosis requires emergent inpatient management

Admission Criteria

- Evidence of sinus disease in diabetic patient consistent with fungal sinusitis
- Signs of sepsis, or infection, ketoacidosis, hyperosmolar states, hyperglycemia

Discharge Criteria

Ability to treat with outpatient therapy, oral antibiotic, or antifungal therapies

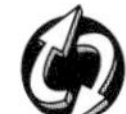

ONGOING CARE

FOLLOW-UP RECOMMENDATIONS

- In patients with infectious disease within 1 week of discharge with infectious disease and orbital surgeon or neuro-ophthalmology.
- In patients with inflammatory lesions 1 week with rheumatology, orbital surgeon or neuro-ophthalmology

Patient Monitoring

Monitor vision, corneal sensation, proptosis, and pattern of extraocular motility dysfunction

DIET

As per medical consultants

PATIENT EDUCATION

Patients with reduced vision and decreased corneal sensation must be educated to be aware of increased redness, swelling, and discharge as signs and symptoms of corneal decompensation, secondary to exposure, and possible infection with the ultimate risk of perforation and permanent visual loss or in extreme cases loss of eye.

PROGNOSIS

Related to underlying etiology

COMPLICATIONS

- Visual loss secondary to optic atrophy
- Orbital scarring with restrictive extraocular muscle dysfunction and diplopia.
- Retinal (macular) ischemia secondary to steal phenomenon in carotid–cavernous (CC) fistula

REFERENCES

1. Yeh S, Foroozon R. Orbital apex syndrome. *Curr Opin Ophthalmol* 2004;15:490–498.
2. Lin CC, Tsai JJ. Relationship between the number of involved cranial nerves and the percentage of lesions located in the cavernous sinus. *Eur Ophthalmol* 2003;49:98–102.
3. Bray WH, Giangiacomo J, Ide CH. Orbital apex syndrome. *Surv Ophthalmol* 1987;32:136–140.
4. Wilson WW, Shergy WJ, Haik BG. Infliximab in the treatment of recalcitrant idiopathic orbital inflammation. *Ophthal Plast Reconstr Surg* 2004;20(5):381–383.
5. Schick U, Hassler W. Neurosurgical management of orbital inflammations and infections. *Acta Neurolo (Wein)* 2004;146:571–580.
6. Barahimi B, Murchison AP, Bilyk JR. Forget me not. *Surv Ophthalmol* 2010;55:467–480.

CODES

ICD9

- 376.11 Orbital granuloma
- 377.9 Unspecified disorder of optic nerve and visual pathways
- 437.6 Nonpyogenic thrombosis of intracranial venous sinus

CLINICAL PEARLS

- 6th Nerve palsy with Horner's syndrome localizes to the anterior cavernous sinus.
- Divisional 3rd nerve palsy localizes to anterior cavernous sinus/orbital apex.
- Any diabetic must rule out mucormycosis

CAVERNOUS SINUS THROMBOSIS

Behin Barahimi
Ann P. Murchison
Jurij R. Bilyk

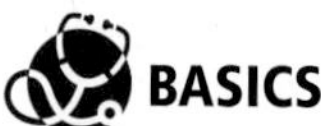

BASICS

DESCRIPTION

- Cavernous sinus thrombosis (CST) is a potentially life-threatening condition.
- The etiology of CST can either be septic, aseptic, or vascular.
- Septic CST is an infectious thrombophlebitis that develops as a sequela of head and neck infections. The most common sources include the paranasal sinuses (ethmoid and sphenoid), periodontal abscesses, parapharyngeal abscesses, facial infections (furuncles, boils), and middle ear infections (1)[C], (4)[C].
- In the pre-antibiotic era, septic CST was universally fatal. With current treatment mortality has been reduced to 30% (1)[C], (2)[C].
- Aseptic CST can occur from hypercoagulable states or direct injury from trauma or surgery.
- CST may also occur from a cavernous sinus arteriovenous fistula, typically fed by branches of the internal or external carotid arteries, or both.

EPIDEMIOLOGY

- The most common etiology of CST is vascular from a cavernous sinus fistula.
- CST is rare and there are no data on incidence.

RISK FACTORS

- Most patients presenting with bacterial septic CST are otherwise healthy individuals.
- In aseptic CST, risk factors include genetic or acquired prothrombotic conditions such as polycythemia, sickle-cell anemia, leukemia, antiphospholipid syndrome, Factor V Leiden, malignancy, oral contraceptives, and pregnancy.
- CST from a fistula typically occurs in two patient groups: Those with a history of head or neck trauma (typically younger males) and older patients with vasculopathic risk factors.

Genetics

- No specific genetic cause of CST is known.
- Genetic causes of hypercoagulable and immunosuppressed states apply when indicated.

GENERAL PREVENTION

- Prompt treatment of head and neck infections
- Genetic/hematologic testing in patients with family history of hypercoagulable conditions
- Control of vasculopathic risk factors
- Avoidance of head and neck trauma

PATHOPHYSIOLOGY

- Septic CST: The venous anatomy of the face is directly connected with the valveless veins of the skull base (orbit, pterygopalatine fossa, cavernous sinus), which then openly communicates with the deeper central venous sinuses. This facilitates infectious spread from superficial structures into the deeper venous plexuses (1)[C].
- Aseptic CST: Deformation of the sinus wall or turbulent flow within the sinus from trauma or surgery on adjacent tissue can cause thrombus formation (3)[C]. In hypercoagulable states, an error in the clotting cascade can prompt thrombosis.
- CST secondary to cavernous sinus fistula: An abnormal communication forms between the cavernous sinus and either the intracavernous internal carotid artery or a smaller caliber intracranial arterial branch. Thrombus may form because of the turbulent flow in the cavernous sinus or from spontaneous closure of the fistula (5)[C].

ETIOLOGY

- Head and neck infections
- Hypercoagulable states
- Vasculopathic
- Head and neck trauma
- Iatrogenic

COMMONLY ASSOCIATED CONDITIONS

See etiology

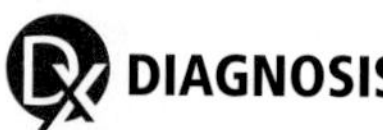

DIAGNOSIS

HISTORY

- The most common presenting symptom is headache. Focal neurologic deficits may be present. In cases of septic CST there is usually a history of a recent head or neck infection.
- Paranasal sinus infections have nonspecific symptoms. Ask directed questions about nasal congestion, purulent nasal discharge, a history of chronic sinusitis, and recurrent headaches
- Symptoms of other head and neck sources should be sought: Toothache, recent dental work, ear pain, sore throat, and facial furuncles
- Any predisposing immunosuppressive conditions, including diabetes, ketoacidosis, malignancy, chemotherapy, and primary or acquired immunodeficiency states
- History of hypercoagulability in the patient or family members
- Recent or distant head trauma

PHYSICAL EXAM

- For septic CST, highly variable and frequently indistinguishable from orbital cellulitis
- External ophthalmoplegia may or may not be present and may manifest from several etiologies
- Orbital congestion from decreased venous egress from the superior ophthalmic vein (SOV) into the cavernous sinus may cause a mechanical ophthalmoplegia
- Orbital inflammation from orbital cellulitis may result in external ophthalmoplegia.
- Cranial nerve paresis of III, IV, V_1, V_2, VI may be present from direct involvement of the cavernous sinus or orbital apex.
- Trigeminal dysfunction is highly atypical in pure orbital cellulitis. If present, this finding raises the possibility of septic CST.
- Bilateral orbital cellulitis is very uncommon. Conversely, sequential bilateral septic CST manifesting as bilateral orbital congestion is common. Therefore, "bilateral orbital cellulitis" should immediately raise the suspicion of septic CST (4)[C].
- Dental caries/abscess
- Pharyngeal erythema, edema, or abscess
- Signs of middle ear infection
- Facial cellulitis, furuncle, or boil
- Signs of orbital congestion and possible cellulitis are often present: Eyelid edema and erythema, exophthalmos (proptosis), chemosis, external ophthalmoplegia, afferent pupillary defect, optic nerve swelling, retinal venous congestion or tortuosity (see also section on orbital cellulitis)

DIAGNOSTIC TESTS & INTERPRETATION

Lab

Initial lab tests for suspected septic CST

- Complete blood count with differential
- Coagulation profiles (PT/PTT/INR)
- Blood cultures
- Culture of the inciting infectious nidus
- Lumbar puncture: If signs of meningitis

Follow-up & special considerations

Suspected septic CST is a medical emergency. Admit for immediate intravenous antibiotic therapy and further workup.

Imaging

Initial approach

- Detecting CST on imaging is difficult and clinical suspicion often guides the radiologist in finding the subtle changes. The first study obtained is usually a CT scan, as it is readily available. Frequently, indirect signs of CST are more readily identifiable. Any enlargement of the SOV, unilaterally or bilaterally, raises the suspicion of CST. With contrast injection, a heterogeneous filling of the venous plexus within the cavernous sinus is suggestive of CST.
- Imaging is also important in identifying occult sources of infection such as ethmoid and sphenoid sinusitis, mastoiditis from middle ear infection, odontogenic abscess, and parapharyngeal abscess.
- MRI may be a useful adjunct to CT.
- Septic CST is frequently a clinical diagnosis. Neuroimaging is helpful for confirmation of the diagnosis and identification of an occult infectious nidus; however, because of the lack of absolute sensitivity, it should never be used exclusively to rule out the possibility of septic CST.
- In CST from a fistula, initial orbital color Doppler may show reversal of flow in the SOV.
- If CST from a cavernous sinus fistula is suspected, a six-vessel (both internal and external carotid arteries, both vertebral arteries) arteriogram is recommended for elucidation of abnormal flow and to assess for the presence of posterior cortical venous outflow, which increases the risk for hemorrhagic stroke (5)[C].

Follow-up & special considerations

- Close clinical follow-up is mandated.
- If the neurologic/ophthalmologic exams deteriorate, repeat imaging should be performed to rule out progression of CST to intracranial abscess formation, meningitis, or hemorrhagic stroke.

Diagnostic Procedures/Other

Lumbar puncture if signs of meningitis are present.

Pathological Findings

- Pathologic specimens are rarely taken from the cavernous sinus.
- Culture of infectious nidus: Bacteria are the most common cause with *Staphylococcus aureus* in 69% and *Streptococcus* sp in 17%. Fungal infections with *Mucor* and *Aspergillus* sp also occur (1)[C].

DIFFERENTIAL DIAGNOSIS
- Orbital cellulitis
- Carotid cavernous fistula
- Dural sinus fistula
- Orbital apex syndrome
- Idiopathic orbital inflammatory syndrome
- Idiopathic granulomatous cavernous sinus inflammation (Tolosa-Hunt syndrome)

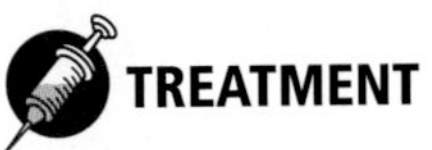

TREATMENT

MEDICATION

First Line
- Septic CST: Broad-spectrum intravenous antibiotics with a third generation cephalosporin and vancomycin are started initially (1)[C]. The antibiotic regimen is tailored once a specific pathogen has been identified. Since antibiotic sensitivity takes several days, potential resistance should be covered during empiric therapy.
- If fungal organisms are suspected, systemic antifungal therapy should be started empirically.
- Aseptic CST: Anticoagulation should be initiated in hypercoagulable states. Hemorrhagic stroke is a risk regardless of anticoagulation (2)[C], (3)[C].
- If a cavernous sinus arteriovenous malformation is suspected, anticoagulation should be avoided and angiography should be performed.

Second Line
- Septic CST: Anticoagulation may be offered to the patient based on indirect evidence.
- Anticoagulation has been shown to have some benefit in the treatment of aseptic central venous sinus thrombosis.
- Two retrospective studies have concluded that there may be some benefit in decreasing morbidity and mortality.
- Hemorrhagic stroke is a risk of septic CST, with or without anticoagulation (1)[C].

ADDITIONAL TREATMENT

General Measures
All patients suspected of CST need admission.

Issues for Referral
Consult infectious disease, otolaryngology, ophthalmology, neurosurgery, and hematology when clinically indicated.

Additional Therapies
- Corticosteroids are necessary if pituitary insufficiency develops to prevent adrenal crisis.
- The use of corticosteroids to decrease edema caused by inflammation is controversial.

SURGERY/OTHER PROCEDURES
- The need for surgical intervention is dependent on the cause of CST.
- Septic CST: Drain source of infection
- Cavernous sinus fistula:
  - Arteriography for diagnosis and possible intra-arterial closure
  - A transvenous approach through the SOV may be helpful in selected cases (5)[C].

IN-PATIENT CONSIDERATIONS

Initial Stabilization
- Septic CST: Admit to ICU, close neurologic monitoring, intravenous antibiotic, and possible anticoagulation
- Cavernous sinus fistula with thrombosis: Admission for arteriography
- Aseptic CST: Admission for neurologic monitoring and anticoagulation

Admission Criteria
All suspected patients need admission.

IV Fluids
Hydration is important in all cases of CST.

Nursing
Close neurologic monitoring is needed.

Discharge Criteria
- Septic CST: Treatment and resolution of underlying cause, transition to oral antibiotics, and stable neurologic exam
- Aseptic CST: Stable neurologic exam with therapeutic oral anticoagulation
- CST secondary to fistula: Evidence of fistula closure either spontaneously or from intervention

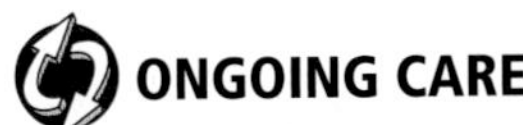

ONGOING CARE

FOLLOW-UP RECOMMENDATIONS
- Septic CST: Depending on cause of infection follow-up with ophthalmology, oral surgery, or otolaryngology. Continue oral antibiotics for at least 14 days and possibly up to 6 weeks. Anticoagulation, if used, should be continued for a minimum of 2 weeks and up to 6 weeks (1)[C].
- Aseptic CST: Follow-up with hematology and internal medicine for therapeutic anticoagulation
- Instruct patients to contact health care providers if new or worsening symptoms develop.

Patient Monitoring
- Septic CST: Once underlying infection has resolved no continuous monitoring is necessary beyond 3 months unless cranial neuropathies persist.
- Within the first 3 months, there is a theoretical risk of recurrent infection from bacterial sequestration within the thrombus.
- A residual cranial neuropathy should be followed conservatively for at least 6 months to allow for improvement.
- Aseptic CST: Need lifelong monitoring to ensure anticoagulations remain therapeutic
- CST from fistula: Monitor for 3–6 months to assure that a fistula does not reform

DIET
Dietary restriction depends on the antibiotic and anticoagulation used.

PATIENT EDUCATION
- Obtain genetic/hematologic testing if there is a family history of thrombotic events.
- If there is a history of CST, contact health care provider immediately if new or recurrent neurologic symptoms develop.

PROGNOSIS
- Septic CST has a guarded prognosis, with an estimated mortality of 30%.
- 50% of patients who survive will be left with permanent neurologic sequelae (1)[C].
- Patients with CST secondary to fistula do well if the fistula is successfully closed.

COMPLICATIONS
- For all forms of CST:
  - Cranial nerve palsy, including optic neuropathy with visual loss
  - Pituitary insufficiency
  - Hemorrhagic infarction
  - Death
- For septic CST:
  - Intracranial infections: Meningitis, encephalitis, and empyema formation

REFERENCES

1. Barahimi B, Murchison AP, Bilyk JR. Forget me not. *Surv Ophthalmol* 2010;26(4):295–297.
2. Stam J. Thrombosis of the cerebral veins and sinuses. *New Engl J Med* 2005;352:1791–1798.
3. Fisher C, et al. Cerebral venous sinus thrombosis in the emergency department: A retrospective analysis of 17 case and review of literature. *J Emerg Med* 2010;38(2):140–147.
4. Pavlovich P, Looi A, Rootman J. Septic thrombosis of cavernous sinus: Two different mechanisms. *Orbit* 2006;25:39–43.
5. Chaudhry IA, et al. Carotid cavernous fistula: Ophthalmological implications. *Middle East Afr J Ophthalmol* 2009;16(2):57–63.

ADDITIONAL READING

- Southwick FS, Richardson EP, Jr, Swartz MN. Septic thrombosis of the dural venous sinus. *Medicine(Baltimore)* 1986;65:82–106.
- Bhatia K, Jones NS. Septic cavernous sinus thrombosis secondary to sinusitis: are anticoagulants indicated? A review of the literature. *J Laryngol Otol* 2002;116:667–676.
- Diaz JM, Schiffman JS, Urban ES, et al. Superior sagittal sinus thrombosis and pulmonary embolism: a syndrome rediscovered. *Acta Neurol Scand* 1992;86:390–396.
- Einhaupl KM, Villringer A, Meister W, et al. Heparin treatment in sinus venous thrombosis. *Lancet* 1991;338:597–600.
- Stam J, Canhao P, Fal cao F, et al. Anticoagulation for cerebral sinus thrombosis (Cochrane Review). *The Cochrane Library* Issue 3, 2004.
- Levine SR, Twyman RE, Gilman S. The role of anticoagulation in cavernous sinus thrombosis. *Neurology* 1988;38(4):517–522.

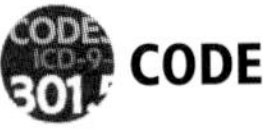

CODES

ICD9
- 325 Phlebitis and thrombophlebitis of intracranial venous sinuses
- 376.01 Orbital Cellulitis
- 995.92 Sepsis

CLINICAL PEARLS
- Septic CST is a rare but potentially lethal condition that may initially present with subtle symptoms and radiographic findings. Early diagnosis and treatment decrease potential morbidity and mortality
- In the cases of septic CST where the external exam is normal, be suspicious for paranasal sinus, periodontal, or parapharyngeal infections
- Isolated aseptic CST from hypercoagulability is rare. Usually, CST is seen in conjunction with thrombosis in the larger central venous sinuses (2)[C]
- CST and SOV thrombosis occur in the setting of cavernous sinus fistula. Arteriography is needed for definitive diagnosis and management

CENTRAL AND BRANCH RETINAL ARTERY OCCLUSION

John B. Davies

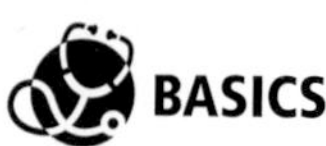

BASICS

DESCRIPTION

- The central retinal artery exits the optic nerve to provide blood supply to the inner retinal layers.
- Occlusion of either the central retinal artery or one of its branches leads to acute, painless, monocular vision loss.

RISK FACTORS

- Hypertension
- Diabetes mellitus
- Carotid artery atherosclerosis
- Cardiac valve disease
- Hypercoagulable states

PATHOPHYSIOLOGY

Loss of perfusion leads to retinal ischemia and infarction in the associated vascular territory.

ETIOLOGY

- Embolus.
  - Types of emboli:
  - Cholesterol emboli (hollenhorst plaque) – yellow and refractile
  - Platelet-fibrin emboli – chalky white
  - Calcium emboli (often from cardiac valves)
  - Fat emboli
  - Cardiac myxoma
  - Septic emboli (from endocarditis)
  - Talc emboli (intravenous drug users)
- Intravascular thrombosis: For CRAO, usually it occurs at the lamina cribrosa of the optic nerve.
- Vasculitis. Giant cell arteritis accounts for 1–2% of cases of CRAO.
- Other collagen vascular disease includes systemic lupus erythematosus, polyarteritis nodosa, Wegener's granulomatosis.
- Vasospasm
- Dissecting aneurysm
- Trauma
- Hypercoagulable states: Antiphospholipid antibody syndrome, oral contraceptive use, polycythemia
- Syphilis
- Behçet's syndrome
- Sickle cell anemia

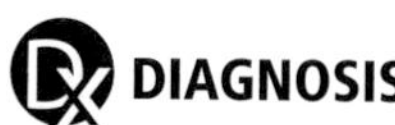

DIAGNOSIS

HISTORY

- Acute, painless, monocular vision loss
- BRAO may present with loss of vision, a scotoma, visual field deficit, or may be asymptomatic.
- CRAO typically causes profound vision loss.
- There are chances of possible history of preceding transient vision loss.
- In patients over 50 years old, headache, jaw claudication, scalp tenderness, or fatigue may suggest giant cell arteritis.

PHYSICAL EXAM

- Blood pressure
- Listen for carotid bruit and cardiac murmurs
- For BRAO, visual acuity depends on the location of the obstruction, and may be normal.
- Approximately 90% of eyes with CRAO have visual acuity between count fingers and light perception (1).
- Approximately 25% of eyes with CRAO have a patent cilioretinal artery, which arises from the choroidal circulation. This may lead to macular sparing and resultant preservation of some visual function (2).
- Relative afferent pupillary defect is often present, especially with CRAO.
- For CRAO: Whitening and opacification of the inner retina in the posterior pole with a cherry red spot in the central macula
- For BRAO: Whitening and opacification of the inner retina in the vascular territory affected. Cotton wool spots may also be seen
- Embolic material may be present in retinal arterioles.
- Retinal vessels may appear poorly perfused, with "boxcarring" of the blood column.

DIAGNOSTIC TESTS & INTERPRETATION

Lab

- Complete blood count with platelets
- Erythrocyte sedimentation rate
- C-reactive protein
- Fibrinogen
- Lipid profile
- Fasting blood sugar
- Other tests in certain situations:
  - Prothrombin time/activated partial thromboplastin time
  - Rapid plasmin reagin
  - Fluorescent treponemal antibody absorbed
  - Antinuclear antibody
  - Rheumatoid factor
  - Serum protein electrophoresis
  - Hemoglobin electrophoresis
  - Antiphospholipid antibodies
  - Homocysteine
  - Hypercoagulable work-up in select situations

Imaging
Fluorescein angiography may reveal delayed arteriolar filling or delayed arteriovenous transit time.

Diagnostic Procedures/Other
- Carotid ultrasound
- Echocardiogram (consider trans-esophageal study)
- Electrocardiography
- Temporal artery biopsy if giant cell arteritis is suspected
- Visual field testing

DIFFERENTIAL DIAGNOSIS
Ophthalmic artery occlusion: Suspect if there is associated optic disc edema and in cases of light perception vision or worse.

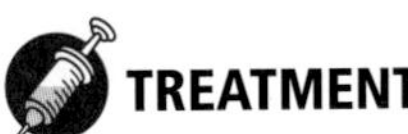

TREATMENT

MEDICATION
First Line
- In general, treatment options for CRAO and BRAO are limited.
- Medication is prescribed to decrease intraocular pressure: Either topical drops or oral acetazolamide.
- If giant cell arteritis is suspected, systemic steroids is immediately started to decrease the risk of second eye involvement.
  - Oral prednisone 1 mg/kg per day or intravenous methylprednisolone 250 mg per 6 h

Second Line
Consider aspirin

ADDITIONAL TREATMENT
Issues for Referral
Patients are referred to a primary care provider for complete medical evaluation and for vascular risk factor management.

SURGERY/OTHER PROCEDURES
- Anterior chamber paracentesis
- Ocular massage: In an attempt to dislodge embolus and move it downstream
- The role of thrombolytic agents in the management of CRAO is not clear (4).

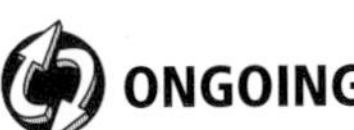

ONGOING CARE

FOLLOW-UP RECOMMENDATIONS
- Repeat eye examination in 1–4 weeks.
  - Assess for development of neovascularization of the iris. This may occur in approximately 20% of eyes with CRAO, usually after 4–5 weeks (3).
- Neovascularization of the optic disc or retina also occurs, although more rarely.
  - If neovascularization develops, proceed with retinal panretinal photocoagulation.
  - Consider intravitreal pharmacotherapy with antivascular endothelial growth factor agents.

Patient Monitoring
Monitor for worsening vision, development of eye pain (which could arise from neovascular glaucoma), and any visual changes in the contralateral eye.

PROGNOSIS
- Long-term visual prognosis for CRAO is poor.
- For BRAO, many eyes will recover visual acuity to the level of 20/40 or better.

COMPLICATIONS
- Neovascular glaucoma
- Other complications may occur from ocular neovascularization, such as vitreous hemorrhage.

REFERENCES

1. Brown GC, Magargal LE. Central retinal artery obstruction and visual acuity. *Ophthalmology* 1982;89:14–19.
2. Brown GC, Shields JA. Cilioretinal arteries and retinal arterial occlusion. *Arch Ophthalmol* 1979;97:84–92.
3. Duker JS, et al. A prospective study of acute central retinal artery obstruction. The incidence of secondary ocular neovascularization. *Arch Ophthalmol* 1991;109:339–342.
4. Biousse V. Thrombolysis for acute central retinal artery occlusion: is it time? *Am J Ophthalmol* 2009;148:172–173.

CODES

ICD9
- 362.30 Retinal vascular occlusion, unspecified
- 362.31 Central retinal artery occlusion
- 362.32 Retinal arterial branch occlusion

CENTRAL CORNEAL ULCERS

Rajesh K. Rajpal
Gitanjali B. Baveja

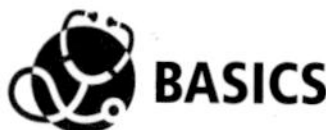

BASICS

DESCRIPTION

- Local epithelial defect with degradation or inflammation of underlying tissue
- Synonyms: Corneal infiltrate, infectious or noninfectious keratitis

EPIDEMIOLOGY

Incidence

Bacterial keratitis

- 30,000 cases annually in the United States
- 10–30 cases per 100,000 of contact lens wearers per year (United States)

Prevalence

- Varies greatly geographically
- Secondary variable is etiology

RISK FACTORS

- Contact lens use
- Compromised host factors: Ocular surface disease
- Inadequate eyelid closure or apposition
- Corneal hypoesthesia
- Systemic autoimmune diseases (less likely to be central)

GENERAL PREVENTION

- Contact lens hygiene
- Preventing compromise of epithelium
- Sufficient lubrication
- Surgical correction of eyelid abnormalities
- Control of acute inflammatory state in autoimmune diseases

PATHOPHYSIOLOGY

- Breakdown of epithelium
- Marked inflammatory response: Leukocyte infiltration (usually neutrophils)
- Degradation of extracellular matrix: Prolonged activation of plasmin, matrix metalloproteinase secretion

ETIOLOGY

- Infectious: Bacterial, fungal, viral, acanthamoeba
- Noninfectious/sterile: Neurotrophic, autoimmune related, corneal exposure (inadequate eyelid closure)

COMMONLY ASSOCIATED CONDITIONS

- Infectious ulcer: Contact lens abuse/overwear, trauma
- Neurotrophic keratitis: VII nerve palsy, herpes simplex, herpes zoster
- Sterile ulcer: Rheumatoid arthritis, systemic lupus erythematosus, Wegener's granulomatosis, Sjögren's syndrome
- Exposure keratopathy: Thyroid orbitopathy

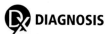

DIAGNOSIS

HISTORY

- Elicit comprehensive history of contact lens wear if applicable including extended vs daily wear, storage/disinfecting methods, swimming with lenses, exposure to any source of water, including tap water, lake, pond, etc.
- Recent trauma to the ocular surface including acid/alkali burn
- History of dry eyes
- Comprehensive review of systems (especially autoimmune diseases)

PHYSICAL EXAM

- Eyelid examination to determine adequate closure, apposition, trichiasis
- Conjunctival injection
- Tear film insufficiency
- Epithelial loss (fluorescein staining)
- Density and size of stromal infiltrate
- Thinning of stromal tissue
- Anterior chamber cell and flare
- Hypopyon

DIAGNOSTIC TESTS & INTERPRETATION

Lab

Initial lab tests

- Corneal cultures: Scrapings obtained from border of infiltrate and placed on specific culture media
- Can use Kimura spatula or moistened calcium alginate swab
- Blood agar: Aerobic bacteria (*S. aureus*, *S. epidermidis*, *S. pneumoniae*, *P. aeruginosa*), saprophytic fungi, *Nocardia*
- Chocolate agar: Aerobic and facultative bacteria (*N. gonorrhea*, *H. influenzae*, *Bartonella*)
- Thioglycollate broth: Aerobic, facultative, anaerobic bacteria
- Thayer–Martin agar: *Neisseria*
- Lowenstein–Jensen agar: *Mycobacteria*, *Nocardia*
- Nonnutrient agar with *E. coli* overlay: *Acanthamoeba*

Follow-up & special considerations

- Central ulcers should be cultured prior to starting topical antibiotics.
- Also culture if ulcer is nonresponsive to topical antibiotics

Imaging

Slit lamp photography can document size and density of infiltrate.

Diagnostic Procedures/Other

- Special stains include gram stain (bacteria), Giemsa stain (*Chlamydia*, *Acanthamoeba*, Acid fast stain (*Mycobacteria*), Calcofluor white (*Acanthamoeba*)
- Corneal biopsy if unresponsive to treatment
- Confocal microscopy (*Acanthamoeba*)

DIFFERENTIAL DIAGNOSIS

- Gram positive: *S. aureus, Coagulase Negative Staph, Streptococcus pneumoniae, Streptococcus viridians, Corynebacterium diphtheriae. Propionibacterium, Mycobacterium, Bacillus cereus*
- Gram negative: *Pseudomonas, Serratia, Proteus mirabilis, H. influenzae, Moraxella, Neisseria*
- Fungal: *Candida, Fusarium, Aspergillus, Curvularia, Mucor, Rhizopus*
- *Acanthamoeba*
- Neurotrophic keratitis
- Herpes simplex keratitis
- Exposure keratopathy
- Autoimmune diseases (primarily *peripheral* corneal ulcer): Rheumatoid arthritis, Systemic Lupus Erythematosis (SLE), Wegener's granulomatosis, collagen vascular diseases

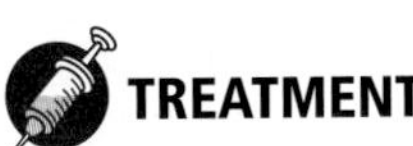

TREATMENT

MEDICATION

First Line

- 4th-generation fluoroquinolone: 1 drop every 15 min for the 1st hour, then per hour around the clock
- 4th generation: Moxifloxacin, gatifloxacin, besifloxacin
- Others: Ciprofloxacin, levofloxacin 1.5%
- For severe or nonresponsive infiltrate: Fortified topical antibiotics can be prepared by the pharmacy.
- Fortified vancomycin 25–50 mg/mL combined with fortified tobramycin/gentamicin 9–14 mg/mL or combined with fortified ceftazidime 50 mg/mL
- Regimen can be modified according to culture results/susceptibility testing.

Second Line

- If unresponsive and culture negative consider *acanthamoeba*, fungal keratitis, atypical organisms.
- *Acanthamoeba*: Topical ophthalmic Neosporin, PHMB, hexamidine, chlorhexidine
- *Fungal keratitis*: Topical natamycin 5%, amphotericin B, imidazoles (voriconazole, itraconazole, ketoconazole, clotrimazole, fluconazole)
- *Nontuberous mycobacteria*: Amikacin/clarithromycin 20–40 mg/mL
- *Nocardia*: Amikacin 20–40 mg/mL

ADDITIONAL TREATMENT

General Measures

- Cycloplegic agent helps with pain and prevents synechiae: Homatropine 5% b.i.d., isopto-hyoscine 0.25% t.i.d., atropine 1% q.i.d.
- Topical ointment or gel at bedtime: Ciloxan/erythromycin/bacitracin ointment, azithromycin (viscous drop)

Issues for Referral

Refer to cornea specialist if:

- Unable to culture
- Unresponsive to treatment (24–48 h)
- Progressive lesion
- Atypical infiltrate

Additional Therapies

- Systemic antibiotics for *Neisseria*
- Systemic antifungals for *Acanthamoeba*

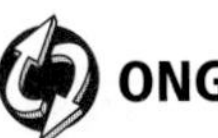

ONGOING CARE

FOLLOW-UP RECOMMENDATIONS

- Daily follow-up until lesion is stabilized
- Criteria of stabilization: Healing of overlying epithelium, resolution of hypopyon, decrease in density of infiltrate, no further thinning of cornea, improvement in visual acuity, symptomatic improvement

ADDITIONAL READING

- Baum J, Barza M. The evolution of antibiotic therapy for bacterial conjunctivitis and keratitis. *Cornea* 2000;19(5):659–672.
- Charukamnoetkanok P, Pineda R. Controversies in management of bacterial keratitis. *Int Ophthalmol Clin* 2005;45(4):199–210.
- Loh AR, Hong K, Lee S, Mannis M, Acharya NR. Practice patterns in the management of fungal corneal ulcers. *Cornea* 2009;28(8):856–859.
- Acharya NR, Srinivasan M, Mascarenhas J, et al. The steroid controversy in bacterial keratitis. *Arch Ophthalmol* 2009;127(9):1231.
- Kaye S, Tuft S, Neal T, et al. Bacterial susceptibility to topical antimicrobials and clinical outcome in bacterial keratitis. *Invest Ophthal Visual Sci* 2010;51(1):362–368.

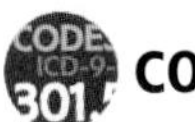

CODES

ICD9

- 370.00 Corneal ulcer, unspecified
- 370.03 Central corneal ulcer

CENTRAL RETINAL VEIN OCCLUSION (CRVO)

Kamalesh J. Ramaiya
Gaurav K. Shah

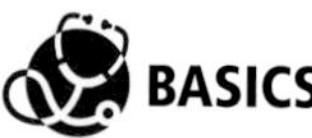

BASICS

DESCRIPTION

- An obstruction of blood flow through the central retinal vein. It commonly presents with a variable level of decreased or blurred vision.
  - Can be classified as one of two clinical subtypes, i.e. ischemic or nonischemic, which differ in their presentation, clinical course, and prognosis (1)[C]

Geriatric Considerations

The overwhelming majority of central retinal vein occlusions (CRVOs) occur in older individuals, with over 90% of patients >50 years of age.

Pediatric Considerations

Pediatric cases of CRVO are rare. Most cases of CRVO in patients younger than 30 years have a definable underlying etiology such as a hypercoagulable state; however, CRVOs have been reported in otherwise healthy children.

Pregnancy Considerations

Venous occlusive disease in the setting of uncomplicated pregnancy and the absence of a hypercoagulable state is rare but has been described, typically as a papillophlebitis that resolves spontaneously. Recent studies have shown higher rates of spontaneous miscarriages in women with a history of CRVO (28%), compared to the general US population (15%). CRVO has also been described in the setting of pre-eclampsia, a disorder seen in up to 5% of pregnancies.

EPIDEMIOLOGY

Incidence

- Second to diabetic retinopathy, retinal vein occlusions are the most frequently encountered retinal vascular disorder. Branch retinal vein occlusions (BRVO, see a separate chapter on this) are more common than CRVOs.
  - Occurs in 2–8 per 1000 persons
  - The 15-year cumulative incidence is 0.5% as per the Beaver Dam Eye Study
  - Most commonly encountered in the 60- to 70-year-old age group, but can occur at all ages
  - Males and females are equally affected
  - There is a 5–10% risk of the fellow eye becoming involved in 5 years

Prevalence

- Affects an estimated 2.5 million people worldwide.
  - Prevalence is approximately 0.8 per 1000 persons.

RISK FACTORS

- CRVO has been associated with primary open angle glaucoma, systemic hypertension, diabetes mellitus, oral contraceptive use, vasculitis, blood dyscrasias, clotting disorders, autoimmune disorders, and trauma.
- Increasing levels of physical activity, moderate alcohol consumption, and exogenous estrogens (in women) have been shown to be protective.

PATHOPHYSIOLOGY

- The exact mechanism of pathogenesis is unknown.
- The occlusion is thought to occur at the level of the lamina cribrosa of the optic nerve secondary to a thrombotic event, though this has been questioned (2)[C].
- Factors predisposing to this location include the close approximation of the central retinal vein and artery which share a common adventitial sheath, and hemodynamic changes secondary to atherosclerosis of the central retinal artery.
- Stagnant blood flow results in hypoxia and damage to the capillary endothelium causing leakage of blood constituents.
- The veno-occlusive event causes an increase in levels of vascular endothelial growth factor (VEGF).
- Vision loss can be due to secondary macular edema, macular ischemia, or neovascularization and its sequelae.

ETIOLOGY

- Most age-related CRVOs are associated with hypertensive or diabetic vasculopathy or increased intraocular pressure.
- Vein occlusion in a younger patient necessitates further workup for a hypercoagulable state or other less common etiology.

COMMONLY ASSOCIATED CONDITIONS

- Systemic vasculopathy is often a comorbidity.
  - Diabetes is present in 5–10%
  - Hypertension is seen in >50% of patients

DIAGNOSIS

HISTORY

- A targeted history should be elicited from the patient, specifically inquiring about the risk factors listed above.
  - Symptoms vary on presentation, and mild cases may be asymptomatic. However, most will present with gradual or sudden vision loss, blurring of vision, and photophobia. Those presenting after development of neovascular disease may complain of pain, redness, and epiphora.

PHYSICAL EXAM

- A complete ocular examination including gonioscopy and dilated funduscopy at the initial and follow-up visits should be performed in all patients suspected of having CRVO.
  - Clinically, this condition presents with diffuse flame-shaped intraretinal hemorrhages in all four quadrants of the retina ("Blood and Thunder" appearance). Dilated and tortuous retinal vessels may be present, as well as disk edema, cotton wool spots, and retinal edema. Optociliary shunt vessels, optic atrophy, and macular retinal pigment epithelial changes may occur late in the course of the disease.
- Occasionally CRVO will present after the development of neovascularization, which manifests itself as vitreous hemorrhage, rubeosis (anterior segment neovascularization), or neovascular glaucoma.
- Signs of an ischemic CRVO include poor visual acuity (<20/200), a diminished B-wave on ERG, >10 disk areas of nonperfusion on fluorescein angiography, and the presence of an afferent papillary defect.

DIAGNOSTIC TESTS & INTERPRETATION

Lab

- Laboratory testing is not needed to make the diagnosis.
- No further workup is necessary in older (>50 years) individuals with known vascular disease.
- All individuals under the age of 50 without a preexisting underlying etiology require a workup for a systemic cause.
  - This may initially include CBC, chemistry profile, fasting glucose and/or glucose tolerance testing, hemoglobin A1c, and lipid profile.
  - In addition, testing for a hypercoagulable state may include homocysteine, protein C, protein S, antithrombin III, anticardiolipin antibodies, antiphospholipid antibodies, lupus anticoagulant (DRVVT), ANA, SPEP, activated protein C resistance, factor VIIIc, factor V leiden, and prothrombin variant 20210A.

Imaging

- Fluorescein angiography shows a delayed arterio–venous transit time as well as diffuse capillary leakage. Ischemic CRVOs will show >10 disk areas of retinal capillary nonperfusion.
- Optical coherence tomography (OCT) is useful in assessing the presence of macular edema.

Diagnostic Procedures/Other

- Electroretinography shows a decreased B-wave (negative ERG), decreased bright flash, more pronounced in the ischemic variant.
- Perimetry can also be useful in determining the ischemic subtype of the vein occlusion.

Pathological Findings

- Early CRVOs may demonstrate intraretinal edema, retinal hemorrhages, disk swelling, and cystoid macular edema.
- Old CRVOs may show disorganization of the retinal layers (especially inner), retinal hemosiderin deposits, and preretinal fibrosis and neovascular membranes.

DIFFERENTIAL DIAGNOSIS

- Ocular ischemic syndrome
- Diabetic retinopathy
- Hypertensive retinopathy
- Hyperviscosity syndrome
- Anterior ischemic optic neuropathy
- Papilledema
- Retinal vasculitis
- Radiation retinopathy

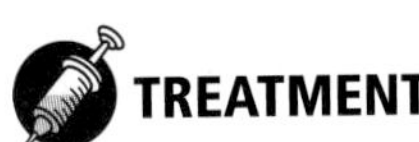

TREATMENT

MEDICATION

First Line

- Management of retinal vein occlusion typically involves treatment of neovascular complications and macular edema resulting from the initial event.
- Historically, medical management of CRVO has been limited and primary therapy was panretinal laser photocoagulation (PRP) for neovascular complications (see the Surgery section below) (3)[A].
- Recent studies have demonstrated efficacy of intravitreally administered drugs in improving macular edema and improving and/or stabilizing visual acuity in patients with CRVO.
  - Avastin (bevacizumab) is a humanized monoclonal antibody against VEGF that is injected into the vitreous cavity. It has been FDA approved for intravenous use in the management of certain cancers; however, it has been successfully utilized intravitreally for CRVO.
  - Lucentis (ranibizumab) is also an anti-VEGF antibody approved for ophthalmic use that is injected into the vitreous cavity. Recent studies including the CRUISE trial have shown its efficacy for CRVO (4)[A].
  - Kenalog (triamcinolone) is a steroid suspension that can be injected intravitreally or into the subtenon's space. Though not approved for ophthalmic use, its efficacy in improving macular edema has been demonstrated in the SCORE trial (5)[A].
  - Ozurdex (dexamethasone, 0.7 mg) is a slow release implant that is injected into the vitreous cavity.

Second Line

- Other medications are presently under investigation for use in vein occlusions.
  - VEGF-trap is a fusion protein which binds to the VEGF-A and placental growth factor. Clinical trials are presently underway to determine its efficacy in vein occlusions.
  - Combination treatments of the above medical therapies and surgical therapies (see below) are also being studied.

ADDITIONAL TREATMENT

Issues for Referral

Coordination of care with the patient's primary physician is important for optimization of the patient's comorbid systemic medical conditions such as hypertension.

SURGERY/OTHER PROCEDURES

- PRP remains the mainstay of treatment for neovascular disease resulting from CRVO, as per the results of the central vein occlusion study (CVOS). It should be noted that prophylactic PRP has not shown to be of benefit in preventing neovascularization.
  - If neovascular glaucoma is present a combination of treatments with anti-VEGF agents and panretinal photocoagulation may be of benefit (6)[C].
- Pars plana vitrectomy with or without internal limiting membrane peeling, endovascular administration of tissue plasminogen activator, radial optic neurotomy, and laser-induced chorioretinal anastomoses, are all surgical procedures that have shown mixed results in terms of efficacy, but are sometimes utilized in refractory cases of CRVO.

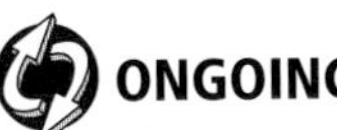

ONGOING CARE

FOLLOW-UP RECOMMENDATIONS

- After the initial event, patients should be followed monthly for the first 3 months, then every 3 months for the first year.
  - A dilated fundus examination and gonioscopy should be performed at each follow-up visit.

Patient Monitoring

OCT, visual fields, and fluorescein angiography may be useful adjunctive tests to follow this condition.

PROGNOSIS

- As shown in the CVOS, initial visual acuity is strongly correlated with final visual outcome.
- Many nonischemic CRVOs will spontaneously resolve and have lower rates of vision loss.
  - 10% of patients eventually develop neovascularization.
- The overall prognosis is worse in patients with an ischemic CRVO.
  - <15% will have a visual acuity better than 20/400 after 1 year
  - 40% of patients eventually develop neovascularization

COMPLICATIONS

- Vision loss due to a variety of reasons:
  - Macular ischemia
  - Macular edema
  - Neovascular disease, including glaucoma
- Complications secondary to comorbid systemic vascular disease or a hypercoagulable state

REFERENCES

1. Haymore JG, Mejico LJ. Retinal vascular occlusion syndromes. *Int Ophthalmol Clin* 2009;49(3):63–78.
2. Hayreh SS. Pathogenesis of occlusion of the central retinal vessels. *Am J Ophthalmol* 1971;72(5): 998–1011.
3. The Central Vein Occlusion Study Group. Natural history and clinical management of central retinal vein occlusion. *Arch Ophthalmol* 1997;115(4): 486–491.
4. Brown DM, Campochiaro PA, Singh RP, et al. Ranibizumab for macular edema following central retinal vein occlusion six-month primary end point results of a phase III study. The CRUISE investigators. *Ophthalmology* 2010, in press.
5. Ip MS, Scott IU, Vanveldhuisen PC, et al. A randomized trial comparing the efficacy and safety of intravitreal triamcinolone with observation to treat vision loss associated with macular edema secondary to central retinal vein occlusion: The standard care vs corticosteroid for retinal vein occlusion (score) study report 5. *Arch Ophthalmology* 2009;127(9):1101–1114.
6. Gheith M, Siam G, de Barros D, Garg SJ, Moster M. Role of intravitreal bevacizumab (Avastin®) in neovascular glaucoma. *J Ocul Pharmacol Ther* 2007;23(5):487–491.

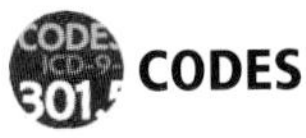

CODES

ICD9

362.35 Central retinal vein occlusion

CLINICAL PEARLS

- The characteristic findings on clinical examination are multiple, diffuse intraretinal hemorrhages throughout the retina.
- A thorough search for an underlying systemic etiology must be performed in younger patients presenting with this condition.
- Panretinal photocoagulation is the primary therapy after the development of neovascularization.
- Newer intravitreal therapies for managing secondary macular edema are emerging.

C

CENTRAL SEROUS CHORIORETINOPATHY

Gary Brown

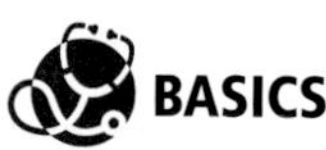

BASICS

DESCRIPTION

- Central serous chorioretinopathy, also called central serous retinopathy or idiopathic central serous retinopathy, is an ocular condition characterized by:
  - Serous retinal detachment, typically seen in the macular region
  - One or more retinal pigment epithelial detachments, which are generally less than 300 microns across, are responsible for the leakage of plasma into the subretinal space.
  - Signs and symptoms are limited to the eye.
  - Rarely, bullous central serous chorioretinopathy can be associated with a large serous retinal detachment with shifting subretinal fluid. Retinal pigment epithelial leaks in this variant are typically greater than 500 microns across.

EPIDEMIOLOGY

Incidence

- Men outnumber women by a factor of 6:1.
- The mean annual age-adjusted incidence per 100,000 for men is 9.9 (95% confidence interval [CI], 7.4–12.4).
- The mean annual age-adjusted incidences per 100,000 for women is 1.7 (95% CI, 0.7–2.7).
- Approximately two-third of fellow eyes followed for 10 years demonstrate some evidence, (although often asymptomatic) of central serous chorioretinopathy.
- The entity is most typically encountered in patients aged 25–50 years.
- Recurrence:
  - Approximately 30% of cases will experience a recurrence
  - The median time of recurrence is 1.3 years
  - Recurrences have been seen from 3 months to 18 years

RISK FACTORS

- Use of corticosteroids
- Type "A" personality profile
- Cushing's disease

Genetics

No genetic or hereditary association has routinely been described.

GENERAL PREVENTION

- Since central serous chorioretinopathy appears to be associated with the classic type A personality profile, patients should at least be informed of the association.
- Patients should be cautioned about the association of glucocorticosteroid use and central serous chorioretinopathy.

PATHOPHYSIOLOGY

A retinal pigment epithelial detachment, or other leak at the retinal pigment epithelium level, facilitates the leakage of plasma into the subretinal space.

ETIOLOGY

- Plasma from the choroid travels through damaged retinal pigment epithelium and into the subretinal space.
- The cause of the leak is uncertain, although glucocorticosteroids have been implicated in select cases.
- An association with *Helicobacter pylori* was noted in one paper, but this association needs confirmation.

COMMONLY ASSOCIATED CONDITIONS

- Central serous chorioretinopathy is often associated with a "type A" personality profile
- Recent use of glucocorticosteroids

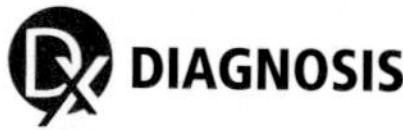

DIAGNOSIS

- A serous detachment of the sensory retina is seen in the macular region with ophthalmoscopy.
- Subretinal precipitates can be seen on the underside of the retina in select cases.
- The presence of subretinal and/or intraretinal blood rules out the diagnosis of central serous chorioretinopathy.
- The anterior segment is uninvolved.
- Intravenous fluorescein angiography discloses one or more leaks at the level of the pigment epithelium. The leaks are often difficult to see ophthalmoscopically.
- Leaks can occur superiorly to the posterior pole view. Thus, the fluorescein angiographic photographer should take at least 1 frame in this region.

HISTORY

- Patients most often complain about a gray or black spot centrally
- Micropsia is also often present
- Metamorphopsia is present in two-third of affected eyes
- A history of severe stress (losing a loved one, a house, or a job) may be present
- The use of some form of corticosteroid (oral, injected, or topical) may be present

PHYSICAL EXAM

- Ophthalmoscopic examination demonstrates a serous detachment of the sensory retina, most often involving the central macular retina.
- Subretinal precipitates may be seen on the underside of the detached sensory retina.
- Retinal or subretinal blood is not seen with this entity. If blood is present, consider neovascular macular degeneration.

DIAGNOSTIC TESTS & INTERPRETATION

Diagnostic Procedures/Other

- Intravenous fluorescein angiography typically demonstrates a focal area of hyperfluorescence corresponding to a retinal pigment epithelial detachment leaking plasma into the subretinal space.
  - A "smokestack" pattern of leakage can be seen as the fluorescein dye rises within the subretinal space in 20% of cases.
  - Fluorescein leakage may be sufficient to produce hyperfluorescence throughout the entire retinal detachment.
  - In more chronic cases, one or more linear streaks of "guttering", characterized by retinal pigment changes can be seen. This occurs secondary to chronic subretinal fluid tracking inferiorly.
- Optical coherence tomography generally reveals a retinal pigment epithelial detachment associated with a larger area of overlying serous retinal detachment.

Pathological Findings

A serous, sensory retinal detachment associated with a smaller retinal pigment epithelial detachment.

DIFFERENTIAL DIAGNOSIS

- Entities in the differential diagnosis for central serous chorioretinopathy include those which can produce serous detachment of the sensory retina in the posterior pole.
  - Neovascular macular degeneration, age-related or from other causes
  - Polypoidal choroidal vasculopathy
  - Subretinal or intraretinal fluid associated with a congenital pit of the optic nerve head
  - Shallow rhegmatogenous retinal detachment
  - Severe hypertensive retinopathy with serous retinal detachment due to hypertensive choroidopathy
  - Posterior retinal detachment with macular hole
  - Posterior retinal detachment with high myopia and posterior retinal break
  - Harada's disease
  - Nanophthalmos with serous retinal detachment
  - Serous retinal detachment associated with choroidal metastasis
  - Serous retinal detachment associated with choroidal melanoma
- Among patients with a diagnosis of Cushing's disease, 5% of patients have one or more episodes of documented central serous chorioretinopathy. The cases seem to occur during episodes of hypercortisolism.

TREATMENT

ADDITIONAL TREATMENT

General Measures

- Approximately 85% of cases demonstrate spontaneous reabsorption of the subretinal fluid within 4 months.
- Laser photocoagulation can be considered in those cases in which the subretinal fluid has not reabsorbed within 3–4 months.
  - Laser photocoagulation results in reabsorption of the subretinal fluid 2 months earlier than no therapy, although the visual results are similar with treatment and without treatment in a Level A randomized, clinical trial by Robertson and Ilstrup.
  - Light laser photocoagulation using 100–200 micron spot sizes can be applied to the leaking retinal pigment epithelial detachment(s).
  - Follow-up by Yap and Robertson at 11–15 years disclosed that none of 6 eyes treated with laser photocoagulation had a recurrence, while 17/32 (53%) eyes that did not undergo laser therapy had at least 1 recurrence.
  - Remember that the laser scars can enlarge considerably over a decade or more, resulting in late vision loss.
- In instances in which the leak is closer than 750 microns from the center of the foveal avascular zone, half fluence photodynamic therapy can be utilized.
- Intravitreal bevacizumab has also been shown to be of therapeutic benefit (Level B non-randomized clinical trial, Artunay et al.).

SURGERY/OTHER PROCEDURES

Surgery has not been shown to be of benefit.

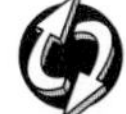

ONGOING CARE

FOLLOW-UP RECOMMENDATIONS

- Ophthalmologist
- Low vision if vision is decreased in both eyes.
- Annual visits if stable.

PROGNOSIS

- Wang et al. noted that over 90% of eyes regain vision of 20/30 or better by 6 months.
- Although most retina specialists treat leaks at the level of the retinal pigment epithelium if the serous retinal detachment is still present at 3–4 months, a long-term prospective clinical trial with Level I evidence (type 1 error <0.05, and type 2 error <0.20) does not exist.
- At 10 years, persistence of a retinal pigment epithelial detachment, persistent subretinal fluid, and recurrences resulted in a greater chance of having vision less than 20/40.

COMPLICATIONS

It is questionable whether laser therapy results in a higher incidence of subsequent choroidal neovascularization.

ADDITIONAL READING

- Kitzmann AS, Pulido JS, Diehl NN, et al. The incidence of central serous chorioretinopathy in Olmsted County, Minnesota, 1980–2002. *Ophthalmology* 2008 Jan;115(1):169–173.
- Bouzas EA, Scott MH, Mastorakos G, et al. Central serous chorioretinopathy in endogenous hypercortisolism. *Arch Ophthalmol*. 1993;111: 1229–1233.
- Robertson DM, Ilstrup D. Direct, indirect, and sham laser photocoagulation in the management of central serous chorioretinopathy. *Am J Ophthalmol* 1983;95:457–466.
- Yap EY, Robertson DM. The long-term outcome of central serous chorioretinopathy. *Arch Ophthalmol* 1996;114(6):689–692.
- Lim JW, Kim MU. The efficacy of intravitreal bevacizumab for idiopathic central serous chorioretinopathy. *Graefes Arch Clin Exp Ophthalmol*. 2011;249(7):969–974.
- Gemenetzi M, De Salvo G, Lotery AJ. Central serous chorioretinopathy: An update on pathogenesis and treatment. *Eye (Lond)*. 2010;24(12):1743–1756.
- Artunay O, Yuzbasioglu E, Rasier R, et al. Intravitreal bevacizumab in treatment of idiopathic persistent central serous chorioretinopathy: A prospective, controlled clinical study. *Curr Eye Res*. 2010;35: 91–98.
- Loo RH, Scott IU, Flynn HW Jr, et al. Factors associated with reduced visual acuity during long-term follow-up of patients with idiopathic central serous chorioretinopathy. *Retina* 2002; 22(1):19–24.
- Wang M, Munch IC, Hasler PW, et al. Central serous chorioretinopathy. *Acta Ophthalmologica* 2008; 86:126–145.

CODES

ICD9

362.41 Central serous retinopathy

CLINICAL PEARLS

- Be certain to look at the optic nerve with slit-lamp biomicroscopy to rule out the possibility of a serous, macular retinal detachment occurring secondary to a congenital pit of the optic disc. Pits of the optic disc can be missed with indirect ophthalmoscopy.
- If any retinal blood and/or subretinal blood is present, the most probable diagnosis is choroidal neovascularization.
- Chronic central serous retinopathy may eventually lead to neovascular age-related macular degeneration years later.
- Consider early, aggressive laser therapy to the larger retinal pigment epithelial leaks seen in association with bullous central serous chorioretinopathy.

CHALAZION

Edward H. Bedrossian Jr

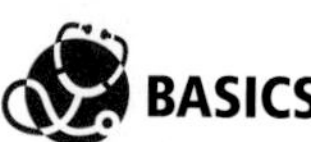

BASICS

DESCRIPTION
A chalazion, or internal hordeolum, is a localized inflammatory papule of the posterior eyelid due to obstruction of the meibomian (sebaceous) glands. In contrast, an external hordeolum or stye, is an inflammatory lesion of the anterior eyelid due to obstruction of the glands of Moll (sweat gland) and Zeis (sebaceous).

EPIDEMIOLOGY
Incidence
Most common eyelid lesion

RISK FACTORS
- Poor lid hygiene
- Acne Rosacea
- Dry eye syndrome

GENERAL PREVENTION
- Good lid hygiene
- Treatment of rosacea (oral tetracycline)
- Treatment of dry eye syndrome

PATHOPHYSIOLOGY
Obstruction of the meibomian gland orifice prevents normal egress of sebaceous holocrine secretion at the lid margin, eliciting a lipogranulomatous foreign body reaction.

ETIOLOGY
Obstruction of the meibomian glands either from the bacteria (*S. aureus*, Strep) and/or from the associated inflammation.

COMMONLY ASSOCIATED CONDITIONS
- Chronic bacterial blepharitis
- Chronic allergic blepharoconjunctivitis
- Chronic keratitis sicca
- Acne Rosacea
- Lid malposition
- Lid trauma

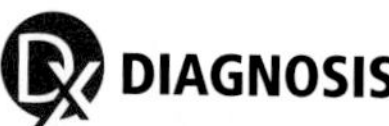

DIAGNOSIS

HISTORY
- Tender swelling, erythema (acute)
- Non tender eyelid lump (chronic)
- Exposure to dusty environment
- Blurred vision (possible induced astigmatism)

PHYSICAL EXAM
- Eyelid swelling and erythema (acute, subacute)
- Localized eyelid tenderness
- Well-defined subcutaneous lid nodule (chronic)
- Blocked meibomian gland orifices
- Associated blepharitis or acne rosacea

DIAGNOSTIC TESTS & INTERPRETATION
Imaging
CT scan orbit if suspect orbital cellulitis

Diagnostic Procedures/Other
Biopsy recurrent lesions to rule out meibomian gland carcinoma

Pathological Findings
Zonal granulomatous inflammatory reaction. Central clear space, surrounded by histiocytes and Langhans' multinucleated giant cells, surrounded by PMNs, leukocytes, plasma cells, and eosinophils. Asteroid bodies and Schaumann bodies may also be present.

DIFFERENTIAL DIAGNOSIS
- Meibomian gland (sebaceous cell) carcinoma
- Preseptal cellulites
- Adenovirus conjunctivitis
- Pyogenic granuloma

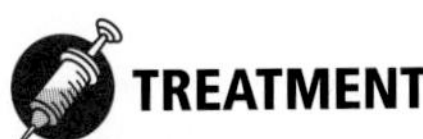

TREATMENT

MEDICATION

First Line

- Warm compresses q.i.d × 2 weeks (10 min each)
- Sulfacetamide 10% 1gtt. q.i.d × 2 weeks or prednisolone 0.2%/sulfacetamide 10%, if no contraindication to topical steroids
- Alternative: Bacitracin or erythromycin ointment b.i.d

Second Line

- Surgical incision and curettage
- Triamcinolone acetonide intralesional injections

ADDITIONAL TREATMENT

General Measures

Biopsy recurrent lesions

Issues for Referral

- Recurrent lesion
- Suspect meibomian gland carcinoma
- Treatment of acne rosacea

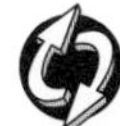

ONGOING CARE

FOLLOW-UP RECOMMENDATIONS

Every 2 weeks as outpatient to monitor progress.

PROGNOSIS

Excellent.

COMPLICATIONS

- Entropion
- Lid scar

ADDITIONAL READING

- Bagheri A, Hasani HR, Karimian F, et al. Effect of chalazion excision on refractive error and corneal topography. *Eur J Ophthalmol* 2009;19(4):521–6.
- Goawalla A, Lee V. Prospective randomized treatment study comparing three treatment options for chalazia: Triamcinolone acetonide injections, incision and curettage and treatment with hot compresses. *Clin Experiment Ophthalmol* 2007; 35(8):706–12.
- Ben Simon GJ, Huang L, Nakra T, et al. Intralesional triamcinolone acetonide injection for primary and recurrent chalazia: Is it effective? *Ophthalmology* 2005;112(5):913–7.

CODES

ICD9

- 373.2 Chalazion
- 373.12 Hordeolum internum

CLINICAL PEARLS

- Most common inflammatory lid lesion
- Recurrent chalazia need biopsy to rule out meibomian gland carcinoma

C

CHEMICAL BURNS

Harminder S. Dua
Dalia G. Said

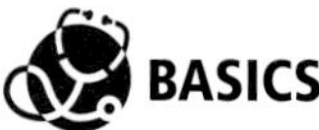

BASICS

DESCRIPTION

Injury that follows exposure of the ocular surface or adnexa to solid, liquid, or gaseous form of corrosive substances such as acids and alkalis or irritants such as oxidants, solvents, reducing agents, and alkylating agents.

EPIDEMIOLOGY

Incidence

- Chemical burn to the eye represents 7–10% of eye injuries.
- Burns to the face are reported to involve at least 1 eye in 15–20% of cases.
- Chemical burns are largely accidental, 73.9% being work related. In a smaller proportion they result from an assault.
- It is more common in men than women, related to increased occupational and industrial exposure in men.
- The incidence ratio of acid burn to alkali burn ranges from 1:1 to 1:4.

RISK FACTORS

- Certain occupations: Ocular chemical burn is reported to account for 3–4% of occupational injuries.
- Noncompliance with health and safety regulations, e.g., inadequate or inappropriate use of protective eye wear and clothing

GENERAL PREVENTION

Safety goggles with side shields should be worn when working with chemicals or caustics or helmets with safety goggles for workers with occupational exposure to chemicals. Appropriate masks or breathing apparatus should be used when working with noxious fumes or gases.

PATHOPHYSIOLOGY

- The severity of the burn depends on the nature of the substance and the duration of exposure. Alkalis cause more damage than acids.
- Tissue damage occurs through denaturation and coagulation of the cellular proteins as well as vascular ischemia.
- The high pH (hydroxyl ion content) of alkaline agents causes saponification of the fatty elements of cell membranes with cell disruption and death. Cations react with carboxyl groups of stromal collagen and the interfibrillary glycosaminoglycans resulting in hydration with thickening and shortening of stromal collagen and hydrolysis of glycosaminoglycans. Loss of glycosaminoglycans renders the collagen susceptible to enzymatic digestion and degradation. Alkalis, especially ammonia and sodium hydroxide, penetrate tissue rapidly and are more likely to damage deeper structures within the anterior chamber.
- Acids penetrate tissue less readily (except hydrofluoric acid). The hydrogen ion causes damage by pH change and the anion causes protein precipitation and denaturation, which in turn retards penetration of acid.
- Chemical penetration into the anterior chamber lowers aqueous ascorbate and glucose. Low ascorbate concentrations are related to subsequent retarded collagen synthesis.

ETIOLOGY

Chemical burns can be caused by acids, bases, oxidants, solvents, reducing agents, and alkylating agents. They can also be caused by chemical weapons such as mustard gas or urticants such as phosgene oxide.

DIAGNOSIS

HISTORY

- History is the key to diagnosis. Nature of the chemical can be ascertained if a sample is available.
  – pH testing of the conjunctival sac using a pH paper strip will help differentiate acids from alkalis.
- Symptoms: Pain, photophobia, lacrimation, and visual impairment. Blepharospasm may supervene.

PHYSICAL EXAM

- Besides the eye(s), the surrounding skin of the face and scalp or further afield may also be involved and occasionally injury to the oral mucosa and respiratory and gastrointestinal tracts related to inhalation or ingestion of chemicals can threaten life.
- Clinical manifestations are described in three stages (1): Immediate effects of the injury, extending from onset to 1 week postinjury; Intermediate, representing the host healing response from the end of week 1 to week 3; and Late, representing changes associated with repair, regeneration, or lack thereof.
  – Ocular surface epithelium: There may a central corneal abrasion with an intact limbus or the limbus may be partially or totally involved. Varying areas of the conjunctiva too may be involved. Limbal and conjunctival involvement is more common in the inferior half. Fluorescein staining is helpful in determining the extent of abrasion.
  – Limbus ischemia: Presents as sectors of blanched or pale limbus with associated necrosis and hemorrhage. Injured blood vessels appear as dark columns of blood with no visible flow.
  – Corneal stroma: May be hazy or opaque and thick with folds or striae secondary to endothelial involvement. Corneal sensations may be impaired.
  – Anterior chamber: The iris may show injection, hemorrhage, necrosis, and pigment dispersion. The pupil response may be sluggish or absent. The lens may be intumescent and ciliary body damage can manifest as hypotony. Clogging of the trabecular meshwork with inflammatory debris can result in raised pressure.
- In the intermediate stage, if some limbal or conjunctival epithelium survives, re-epithelization commences. The cornea may be covered by corneal or conjunctival epithelium. If no epithelium survives, the ocular surface is covered by a centripetally advancing fibrovascular pannus. Recanalization of some of the damaged blood vessels may lead to further hemorrhages. Inflammatory cell infiltration occurs and can later lead to stromal melts and ulceration.
- In the late stage of moderate to severe burns, the cornea is covered by a fibrovascular pannus. Superficial and deep vascularization, stromal ulceration, persistent epithelial defects can lead to a descemetocele and perforation. Loss of nerves may lead to a neurotrophic state with repeated healing and breakdown of the surface.
  – Conjunctival repair may lead to symblepharon, subepithelial fibrosis with progressive contracture leading to forniceal shortening and lid margin deformities such entropion, trichiasis, and lagophthalmos with exposure. Tear film abnormalities due to loss of goblet cells (mucin) and obstruction of orifices of the lacrimal or accessory lacrimal ductules (aqueous) may manifest. This can lead to keratinization of the cornea and conjunctiva. Cicatricial stenosis or occlusion of the lacrimal puncta may occur and offset a "dry eye" state.
  – Retrocorneal or cyclitic membranes and fibrosis of the ciliary body can lead to persistent hypotony and phthisis. On the other hand, scarring in the drainage angle and peripheral anterior synechiae can lead to intractable glaucoma.
- Secondary infection can occur at any stage.

DIAGNOSTIC TESTS & INTERPRETATION

Diagnostic Procedures/Other

- Eyes with chemical burns must be graded at the first opportunity. Dua's classification indicating the number of clock hours of limbal involvement and percentage of conjunctival involvement is recommended (2).
- Clinical appearances can be deceiving and change rapidly.
  – Total corneal and limbal epithelial loss can be associated with a clear cornea.
  – A clear cornea with a good view of the iris can rapidly become hazy or opaque.
  – An initially "stable" cornea may develop stromal thinning or melting within hours, especially after the first week.
  – Intraocular pressure (IOP) can be difficult to measure with the Goldman tonometer or Tonopen. An irregular and thick cornea can produce erratic readings. Digital palpation may be the only reliable method in some cases.
  – Secondary infection may have an atypical presentation.

TREATMENT

MEDICATION

First Line

- Check pH of conjunctival sac with a pH filter paper strip. Instill a topical anesthetic agent. Keep eye(s) open with a speculum, keep room lights dim, and perform copious irrigation with normal saline, balanced salt solution, or Ringer's lactate. Use approximately 1–2 L over 30–40 min delivered through an intravenous tube with free flow.
  - Recheck pH. If around 7, stop irrigation and examine conjunctival sac right up to fornices by double everting the upper lid. Remove any particulate matter and excise devitalized tissue.
  - Recheck pH after a 20-min interval. Chemicals may leach out of tissues and alter pH. If less or greater than 7, recommence irrigation.

Second Line

- Lubrication: Preservative-free artificial tear drops and ointment
- Anti-inflammatory: Steroid drops. Be wary of steroid use in the presence of melting.
- Antibiotics: drops or ointment
- Ascorbate: 10% drops 2–4 times a day. Can cause pronounced stinging and may not be tolerated. Oral tablets 2 g q.i.d.
- Sodium citrate: a potent inhibitor of polymorphonuclear proteases. 10% drops, 4–6 times a day. Oral doxycycline (protease inhibitor) 50 mg twice a day
- Atropine 1% or cyclopentolate 1% b.i.d. Avoid phenylephrine as it can exacerbate ischemia by vasoconstriction.
- IOP lowering: drops, e.g., timolol 0.25% twice a day if needed. Oral acetazolamide tablets 250 mg q.i.d. may be preferable especially if there is marked pigment dispersion and AC inflammation.
- Pain management: according to severity

ADDITIONAL TREATMENT

General Measures

- Punctal plugs: if tear film is inadequate
- Lid taping: to reduce exposure and in the presence of stromal melts
- Conformer ring: to limit or avoid symblepharon formation

Issues for Referral

- Most chemical burns are mild and can be managed in the primary care setting.
- Severe burns with extensive limbal and anterior chamber involvement should be referred to a specialist center.

Additional Therapies

- Autologous serum drops: 20–100%, 4 to 6 times a day
- Acetylcysteine 20%, fibronectin, epidermal growth factor, sodium or calcium EDTA (0.2 mol) subconjunctival heparin and others have been tried

SURGERY/OTHER PROCEDURES

- Valve shunts or cycloablation to control pressure. The latter can increase intraocular inflammation
- Lens extraction if lens is swollen and causing pupil block
- Mucus membrane and amniotic membrane graft to cornea and conjunctiva
- Lid surgery to address entropion, ectropion, trichiasis, or lagophthalmos
- Sequential sector conjunctival epitheliectomy (SSCE) to prevent conjunctival epithelium from migrating on to the cornea in partial corneal burns or to remove conjunctival epithelium that has already encroached on to the cornea
- Auto or allo limbal transplants (in cases with total stem cell deficiency). Avoid use of autolimbal or living related donor tissue in the early to intermediate stages as the risk of losing the transplanted tissue in the ongoing inflammatory reaction is high.
- Transplant of ex vivo expanded sheets of limbal or oral mucosal cells
- Corneal graft procedures should be considered only after the cornea is repopulated with limbus derived epithelial cells. Some form of immunosuppression is usually required postoperatively.

ONGOING CARE

PROGNOSIS

- The more superficial the burn, the better the prognosis.
- 12 clock hours of limbus involvement with 100% conjunctival involvement (grade VI) [Dua's classification] has the worst prognosis.

COMPLICATIONS

- Lid deformities
- Dry eyes
- Extensive symblepharon
- Limbal stem cell deficiency
- Corneal vascularization and scarring
- Secondary infection
- Glaucoma or phthisis
- Cataract
- Disorganization of anterior segment
- Severe visual impairment including loss of eye

REFERENCES

1. McCulley JP. Chemical injuries. In: *The Cornea: Scientific Foundation and Clinical Practice*. Smolin G, Thoft RA, eds. Boston, MA: Little, Brown & Co., 1987:527–542.
2. Dua HS, King AJ, Joseph A. New classification of ocular surface burns. *Br J Ophthalmol* 2001;85: 1379–1383.

CODES

ICD9

- 940.2 Alkaline chemical burn of cornea and conjunctival sac
- 940.3 Acid chemical burn of cornea and conjunctival sac

CLINICAL PEARLS

- Early elimination of the injurious agent is the key to success.
- Documentation of epithelial and limbal involvement by photographs or diagrams and grading of burns is useful to monitor progress.
- Any epithelial (conjunctival) cover of the cornea is better than no epithelial cover.
- IOP monitoring may be difficult but is very important.
- Steroid drops help to control inflammation but may exacerbate melting.

CHIASMAL DISORDERS

Rod Foroozan

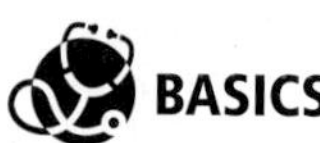

BASICS

DESCRIPTION

- The optic chiasm is formed by the confluence of the intracranial optic nerves, is 12–18 mm in diameter, lies 10 mm above the sella turcica of the sphenoid bone, and contains the decussation of nasal nerve fibers from each optic nerve. Visual loss is often the initial symptom of a disorder involving the optic chiasm (1). Nearly 25% of all brain tumors occur in the area of the optic chiasm.

EPIDEMIOLOGY

Incidence

- Unknown for all chiasmal disorders
- It is difficult to measure all pituitary adenomas because many of them are asymptomatic. Pituitary tumors have been estimated to occur in 5 per 100,000 based on neurosurgical series.

Prevalence

- Prevalence of visual loss in patients with pituitary tumors varies widely (30–90%) depending on the source of the report.

RISK FACTORS

- Underlying risk factors for certain disorders involving the optic chiasm such as radiation therapy or genetic syndromes predisposing to tumor formation (neurofibromatosis and multiple endocrine neoplasia)

Genetics

- Genetic predisposition for certain types of disorders affecting the optic chiasm including multiple sclerosis and sarcoidosis

GENERAL PREVENTION

None

PATHOPHYSIOLOGY

- Typically compressive lesions around the sella turcica. The optic chiasm may also be directly affected by infiltration or inflammation. The crossing nasal retinal fibers are predisposed to compression resulting in temporal visual field loss.

ETIOLOGY

Conditions involving the optic chiasm can be broadly categorized as those that are intrinsic to the chiasm and those that are extrinsic (1,2). These include:

- Congenital
- Traumatic
- Iatrogenic (herniation of optic chiasm after surgery)
- Intrinsic tumors (glioma)
- Ischemia
- Inflammation
- Infection
- Extrinsic mass lesions (most common)
  - Pituitary adenoma
  - Craniopharyngioma
  - Meningioma

COMMONLY ASSOCIATED CONDITIONS

- Hormonal abnormalities associated with pituitary dysfunction

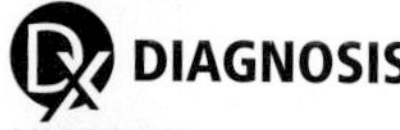

DIAGNOSIS

HISTORY

- Hormonal dysfunction with galactorrhea, amenorrhea, decreased libido, and infertility
- Visual complaints, such as nonspecific visual blurring, double vision, visual field loss and decreased acuity, are the most common symptoms.
- Less commonly there may be
  - Photophobia
  - Loss of stereopsis
  - Abnormalities in motion perception (Pulfrich phenomenon)
  - Diplopia from compression of adjacent cranial nerves (III, IV, VI) within the cavernous sinus
- Headache and facial pain with cranial nerve V involvement. Headache may be abrupt and severe in patients with rapid expansion of a sellar lesion (see below).
- Diplopia from hemifield slide – variable vertical or horizontal diplopia that occurs due to disruption of latent heterophorias as images formed on corresponding portions of each retina fall into the affected nasal retina and are not detected
- Postfixation blindness (visual information from beyond the point of fixation falls into the affected temporal visual fields and is not seen)
- Oscillopsia from see-saw nystagmus (rare)

PHYSICAL EXAM

- Visual acuity and color vision are often normal early on in chiasmal dysfunction. As progression occurs, central vision may become affected.
- There may be a relative afferent pupillary defect with asymmetric involvement. The pupils may be sluggish with the progression of the deficit.
- Visual field loss is often the most important finding suggestive of a chiasmal syndrome and defects may include:
  - Bitemporal hemianopia/quadrantanopia
  - Unilateral central defect with contralateral hemianopia (junctional scotoma – which appears to be due to incomplete compression of the optic chiasm rather than due to the existence of Wilbrand's knee – an anterior loop of nasal fibers at the junction of the optic nerves and the chiasm) (3)[B] or temporal visual field loss
  - Homonymous hemianopia (from an optic tract syndrome)
- Pattern of visual field loss from a compressive lesion is dependent on the anatomic position of the optic chiasm (prefixed, normal, or postfixed) in relation to the sella turcica and the compressive lesion (4)[B].
- Optic disc pallor develops, primarily involving the papillomacular bundle and nasal retinal fibers, in a band (bow-tie) pattern that spares the inferior and superior portions of the optic disc. Pallor may take weeks to develop and the absence of optic disc pallor should not preclude an evaluation for a chiasmal disorder, especially with acute visual loss.
- See-saw nystagmus (rare) may occur in congenital achiasma or with the involvement of the brainstem and interstitial nucleus of Cajal.

DIAGNOSTIC TESTS & INTERPRETATION

Lab

Initial lab tests

- Hormonal levels (including prolactin) are typically performed for compressive lesions that may involve the pituitary gland or stalk.

Follow-Up & Special Considerations

- Following prolactin levels over time may be an important indicator as to the treatment efficacy of a prolactinoma.

Imaging

Initial approach

- Neuroimaging with CT or MRI. Imaging with MRI is generally better for assessing soft tissue, including the chiasm. Imaging should typically include contrast and should be targeted toward the sella.

Follow-up & special considerations

- MRI may show a heterogeneous signal with variable signal intensities suggestive of blood within a preexisting mass lesion (most commonly a pituitary adenoma) including within the optic chiasm (chiasmal cavernoma). When bleeding occurs acutely it may cause rapid expansion of a mass within or around the sella causing chiasmal compression and/or involvement of surrounding cranial nerves III, IV, V, and VI in the cavernous sinus.
- Rapid expansion of other intrasellar or parasellar lesions (such as expansion of a paranasal sinus mucocele) may cause similar symptoms.
- Pituitary apoplexy may cause shock and death, especially with the ensuing hypocortisolemia that may occur as the pituitary gland becomes necrotic.
- Symptoms of pituitary apoplexy include:
  - Visual loss
  - Severe headache
  - Vomiting
  - Meningismus
  - Diplopia
- Pituitary apoplexy in the peripartum period (Sheehan syndrome) occurs with hypotension and hemorrhage that frequently accompany this period.
- Stimulatory agents, such as thyroid-stimulating hormone and gonadotropin-releasing hormone, have been thought to cause an increase in metabolic needs of an adenoma, leading to necrosis.
- Corticosteroid replacement therapy may be life saving in patients with pituitary apoplexy.

Diagnostic Procedures/Other

- Imaging of the retinal nerve fiber layer (including with optical coherence tomography) has shown decreased nerve fiber layer thickness, particularly nasally and temporally, in patients with chiasmal dysfunction (5)[C].

Pathological Findings

- Pathological findings depend on the cause of the chiasmal syndrome (for example granulomatosis inflammation from sarcoidosis).
- Chronically, optic nerve atrophy and thinning of the optic chiasm may be seen with any cause of a chiasmal syndrome.
- Pituitary adenomas are typically benign but can show high rates of mitoses in more aggressive and invasive tumors.

DIFFERENTIAL DIAGNOSIS

- Some optic neuropathies such as hereditary optic neuropathy (particularly dominant optic atrophy) and toxic optic neuropathy can cause visual field loss with cecocentral scotomas that can be difficult to distinguish from bitemporal visual field defects of a chiasmal syndrome.
- Congenitally anomalous optic discs (especially tilted optic discs) can cause temporal visual field loss; often these defects cross the vertical meridian.
- Retinopathy preferentially affecting the nasal retina

TREATMENT

MEDICATION

First Line

- Corticosteroids are used for acute pituitary compromise such as in pituitary apoplexy.
- Corticosteroids are typically used for inflammatory chiasmal syndromes, including those caused by multiple sclerosis (6)[C].
- Dopaminergic agents; including bromocriptine and cabergoline, may cause marked shrinkage of pituitary adenomas, primarily prolactin secreting tumors.

ALERT

Chiamsal dysfunction may be a marker of a potentially life threatening condition such as pituitary apoplexy

CONSIDERATIONS

Pediatric Considerations

Compressive lesions involving the optic chiasm are often related to gliomas involving adjacent structures like the hypothalamus

Pregnancy Considerations

Compressive lesions involving the sella such as pituitary adenomas, meningiomas, and aneurysms may grow rapidly during pregnancy, causing acute symptoms including bilateral visual loss. Hemorrhage within a pituitary adenoma and pituitary apoplexy is common in the peurperium

ADDITIONAL TREATMENT

Issues for Referral

- Patients with sellar tumors are typically sent for endocrinologic evaluation.
- Neurosurgical referral to remove or biopsy of the compressive lesion
- Radiation oncology for consideration of radiation therapy depending on specifics of lesion or for patients who cannot undergo surgery

SURGERY/OTHER PROCEDURES

- Neurosurgery (including transsphenoidal and craniotomy) to remove compressive mass lesions involving the optic chiasm
- MRA/CTA and less often catheter arteriography may be necessary to exclude sellar or parasellar aneurysms

IN-PATIENT CONSIDERATIONS

Initial Stabilization

- It may be required for acute visual loss related to pituitary apoplexy.
- Corticosteroids may need to be instituted to avoid hypocortisolemia in pituitary apoplexy.
- Acute visual loss from chiasmal compression of any cause may require emergent neurosurgical intervention.

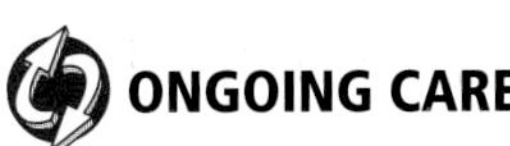

ONGOING CARE

FOLLOW-UP RECOMMENDATIONS

- Serial eye examinations and visual field testing

Patient Monitoring

- Patients should report new onset visual loss or worsening of visual field defects.

DIET

- No specific dietary needs for most patients with a chiasmal disorder
- Some patients with hormonal dysfunction may require alterations in diet.

PROGNOSIS

- It may depend on the causative lesion, duration of chiasmal involvement, and severity of visual loss.
- Measurement of retinal nerve fiber layer thickness may be predictive of visual outcome.

COMPLICATIONS

- Pituitary apoplexy can be life threatening.
- It may lead to hormonal dysfunction requiring therapy.
- Some other complications are persistent visual loss related to compressive effects of tumor or iatrogenic related to intraoperative manipulation or other factors related to surgery, including postoperative empty sella with herniation of the optic chiasm.
- Persistent diplopia may be evidenced.
- Side effects related to radiation therapy including radiation optic neuropathy and neuromyotonia may also occur.

ADDITIONAL READING

- Levin LA. Topical diagnosis of chiasmal and retrochiasmal disorders *Walsh & Hoyt's clinical neuro-ophthalmology*. In: Miller NR, Newman NJ, (eds), 6th ed. Lippincott Williams & Wilkins, 2005:503–573.
- Burde RM, Savino PJ, Trobe JD (eds). Chiasmal disorders. *Clinical decisions in neuro-ophthamology*, 2nd ed. St. Louis: Mosby, 2002:59–82.

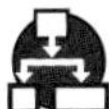

See Also (Topic, Algorithm, Electronic Media Element)

Table 1 Common causes of chiasmal syndromes

Congenital	Traumatic	Iatrogenic	Intrinsic lesions	Extrinsic lesions
Albinism	Motor vehicle accident	Radiation	Glioma	Pituitary adenoma
Achiasmatism	Skull fracture	Surgical injury	Demyelination	Craniopharyngioma
		Fat packing [34]	Chiasmal inflammation/infiltration (sarcoidosis [35]/leukemia and lymphoma)	Meningioma
		Empty sella	Ganglioglioma [36]	Aneurysm
		Dopamine agonists	Cavernoma [37]	Mucocele
			Histiocytosis	Lymphocytic hypophysitis [39]
			Ischemia [38]	Hydrocephalus [40]
				Arachnoid cyst
				Epithelial cyst
				Dysgerminoma
				Metastasis

REFERENCES

1. Blieden L, Foroozan R. Disorders of the optic chiasm. *Expert Rev Ophthalmol* 2009;4:649–659.
2. Foroozan R. Chiasmal syndrome. *Curr Opin Ophthalmol* 2003;14:325–331.
3. Lee JH, Tobias S, Kwon JT, Sade B, Kosmorsky G. Wilbrand's knee: Does it exist? *Surg Neurol* 2006;66:11–17.
4. Kosmorsky GS, Dupps WJ, Drake RL. Nonuniform pressure generation in the optic chiasm may explain bitemporal hemianopsia. *Ophthalmology* 2008;115:560–565.
5. Danesh-Meyer HV, Carroll SC, Foroozan R, et al. Relationship between retinal nerve fiber and visual field sensitivity as measured by optical coherence tomography in chiasmal compression. *Invest Ophthalmol Vis Sci* 2006;4827–4835.
6. Kawaski A, Purvin VA. Idiopathic chiasmal neuritis: Clinical features and prognosis. *Arch Ophthalmol* 2009;127:76–81.

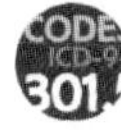

CODES

ICD9

- 377.51 Disorders of optic chiasm associated with pituitary neoplasms and disorders
- 377.52 Disorders of optic chiasm associated with other neoplasms
- 377.54 Disorders of optic chiasm associated with inflammatory disorders

CLINICAL PEARLS

- Visual field loss is often the most important clue to the diagnosis of a chiasmal syndrome.
- Chiasmal dysfunction may be the initial manifestation of a life-threatening disorder such as pituitary apoplexy.
- Evaluation and management of chiasmal disorders typically begins with neuroimaging and involves a multidisciplinary approach, including endocrinologic evaluation.

CHILD ABUSE

Brian Forbes
Anne Jensen
Gil Binenbaum

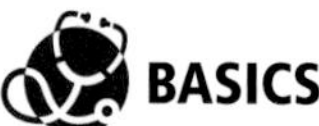

BASICS

DESCRIPTION

- ***Child abuse and neglect*** as defined by the Child Abuse Prevention and Treatment Act (CAPTA) is any act or failure to act on the part of a parent or caretaker, which results in death or serious physical or emotional harm. It includes sexual abuse or exploitation. State-specific guidelines are based on this definition. (1)
- ***Child neglect*** involves the omission of fundamental resources and support, including food, clothing, supervision, shelter, medical care, and education.
- ***Shaken Baby Syndrome (SBS),*** a subset of ***abusive head trauma***, refers to a constellation of findings (retinal hemorrhage, subdural or subarachnoid hemorrhage, and brain injury, with or without fractures, usually with minimal apparent external trauma) thought to arise from repetitive acceleration–deceleration forces, with or without head impact. (2).

EPIDEMIOLOGY

Incidence

- In 2008, there were 3.3 million referrals in the US to child protection services alleging abuse or neglect of 6 million children. Of the 63% investigated, 772,000 cases were confirmed.
- About 2,000 deaths annually result from child maltreatment. (1)
- Over 80% of all offenses and over 70% of all child fatalities in 2008 were caused by parents of the victim. (1)

RISK FACTORS

- **Age**: Almost 33% of all victims in 2008 were under 4 years old. Younger children are at much greater risk, with 22% of all cases and over 40% of all fatalities occurring in children under 1 year of age. (1)
- **Gender**: Risk for victimization is essentially equal between both boys and girls except for sexual abuse where girl victims predominate. (1)
- **Race**: Though almost half of all victims are Caucasian, African American children, Native American children, and children of mixed ethnicity are most at risk per 1,000 children of the same race. (1)

GENERAL PREVENTION

Parental education upon discharge from the hospital, in the form of videos, pamphlets, and signed contracts regarding the risks associated with shaking as well as suggestions for coping with a crying child are thought to decrease rates of SBS.

PATHOPHYSIOLOGY

- **Rotational acceleration**: Leads to axonal injury and tearing of bridging veins. This leads to the formation of subdural hematoma (SDH), subarachnoid hemorrhage (SAH), and cerebral edema. (3)
- **Tractional ocular injury:** The typical pattern of retinal hemorrhage in SBS coincides with areas of maximal vitreoretinal adhesion: Vessels, macula, and peripheral retina. Vigorous repeated acceleration–deceleration produces translational movement of the vitreous, which can lead to characteristic macular tractional retinoschisis with or without surrounding retinal folds. (6) Trauma may also occur to orbital tissues.

ETIOLOGY

- SBS involves an act of shaking so violent that observers would easily recognize it as dangerous. The injuries from this type of trauma are distinct from injuries sustained from short falls. Seizures, coughing, and vaccinations do not simulate these injury patterns. (2)
- In infants the most common catalyst for abuse is crying or issues around feeding. In toddlers, toilet training is a common inciting event.

COMMONLY ASSOCIATED CONDITIONS

- Caretaker substance/domestic abuse
- Neglect and failure to thrive
- Poverty
- Sexual abuse
- Mental/physical/behavioral disability
- Chronic medical conditions

DIAGNOSIS

- Approximately 85% of SBS cases involve retinal hemorrhage, which in two-thirds are too numerous to count, multilayered, and extending to the ora serrata.
- Initial presentation will vary widely based on the type of abuse that has occurred. Suspect abuse with unexplained delay in seeking medical care.
- Physicians are required by law to report all suspected cases of child abuse and/or neglect. Abuse need not be proven by the reporting physician.

HISTORY

- A detailed history including a specific timeline should be recorded to assess plausibility of injuries. (2)
- A diagnosis of abuse is suggested by a clinical history that is changing or incongruent with the current presentation.
- Evaluation of developmental history is especially pertinent.

PHYSICAL EXAM

- **General:** Complete exam should be performed. Any external evidence of injury should be well-documented with forensic photographs, labeled with patient name and date. (2)
- **Funduscopic:** *A dilated eye examination* should be performed by a trained ophthalmologist, preferably within 24 hours but no later than 72 hours when abusive head injury is suspected or a child sustains and unexplained acute life threatening event (ALTE). Care should be taken to view the peripheral retina. *Hemorrhages,* present in 50–80% of SBS cases, may be preretinal, subretinal, or within the retina itself. Thorough *documentation* of the number, type, asymmetry/unilaterality, extent, and pattern of hemorrhage should be carefully recorded. These patterns can be used to narrow the differential diagnosis. *Retinoschisis*, with blood accumulation between retinal layers, with/without an associated hypopigmented circumlinear retinal pleat or fold at its edge is strongly suggestive of abuse. Blood in the retinoschisis cavity may leak into the vitreous over several days and require surgical intervention for vitreous hemorrhage. Therefore, patients with retinoschisis should be assessed serially.
- **Other ocular injuries:** Signs of direct ocular trauma, such as bruising, hyphema, lens dislocation, and so on, should raise the suspicion of abuse in the absence of a plausible history of accidental trauma.
- **Sexually Transmitted Infections** (4)
  - Ocular manifestations of sexually transmitted diseases may represent a congenitally acquired infection or a "red flag" for sexual abuse. Incubation after perinatal transmission may be delayed, especially for chlamydia.
  - Some genital infections may rarely be transmitted to the eye by infected secretions on contaminated fingers.
  - Syphilis uniquely travels to the eye through the bloodstream and always indicates sexual transmission.
  - Infections associated with ocular manifestations include *Chlamydia trachomatis, Phthirus pubis,* syphilis, gonorrhea, *HIV*, and herpes simplex virus (usually nonsexual transmission).

DIAGNOSTIC TESTS & INTERPRETATION

Lab

Diagnostic tests should be performed at the discretion of the primary care provider or child abuse pediatrician.

Imaging

- **Radiographic findings:** Skeletal survey, including all bones (not a babygram), should be performed to evaluate for rib, skull, and long bone fractures, particularly in children less than 2 years old. Neuroimaging (CT or MRI) may reveal subdural hematoma, skull fractures, axonal injury, and edema. Subdural hemorrhages involving bilateral convexities, posterior interhemispheric fissure, or posterior fossa are particularly worrisome as signs of abuse in the absence of a clear history of accidental trauma. (3)
- **Retinal photography:** Retinal imaging is not a necessary component of a thorough work-up. A diagram with detailed written descriptions is acceptable. When available, fundus photos can be useful for documentation. Photography should not replace the clinical examination.

Pathological Findings

- Pathological brain findings include hemorrhage, cerebral edema, cerebral contusions, and diffuse axonal injury, atrophy, or infarction. (2)
- Postmortem, a full autopsy must be performed with *en bloc* removal and evaluation of the eyes and orbital tissues.

DIFFERENTIAL DIAGNOSIS

Nonabuse causes of retinal hemorrhage are almost always few in number and confined to the posterior pole, or are associated with abnormal laboratory findings, physical examination findings, or historical information that readily makes the diagnosis.

- Retinal hemorrhage
  - Shaken baby syndrome
  - Hypertension
  - Coagulopathy/leukemia
  - Meningitis/sepsis/endocarditis
  - Vasculitis
  - Cerebral aneurysm
  - Anemia
  - Hypoxia/hypotension
  - Papilledema (peripapillary hemorrhages)
  - Glutaric aciduria type 1, Osteogenesis imperfecta
  - Retinopathy of prematurity
  - Extracorporeal membrane oxygenation
  - Hypo- or hypernatremia
  - Birth
  - Vitamin K deficiency
  - Carbon monoxide poisoning
  - Drowning

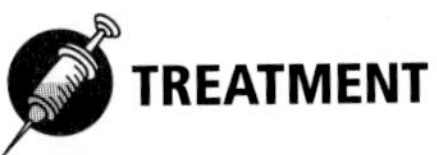

TREATMENT

ADDITIONAL TREATMENT

General Measures

- ***Hospitalization*** may be indicated for protection and diagnosis.
- ***Reporting*** suspected cases to child protective services in a timely manner is crucial.
- ***Multidisciplinary treatment plan*** is needed to address medical, social, and psychological needs of the patient and family, including family counseling and mental health therapy.
- ***Removal*** of the child from the current home or social situation is a matter determined by child protective service agencies.
- **State laws require medical staff to report *suspected* cases to a child protective service.** (1)

SURGERY/OTHER PROCEDURES

Retinal hemorrhages generally resolve without intervention. Vitrectomy should be considered in young patients when the risk of amblyopia arises secondary to prolonged visual axis obstruction. (6)

IN-PATIENT CONSIDERATIONS

Initial Stabilization

- Should address acute respiratory or neurological decompensation, though notably some victims will present with little or no external signs of trauma and nonspecific symptoms
- Systemic stabilization takes priority over eye examination.

Admission Criteria

The American Academy of Pediatrics recommends that in communities without specialized crisis intervention centers, all children who present with concern for abuse be hospitalized until they are medically stable and safe placement options are identified.

Discharge Criteria

Patient may be discharged when medically stable to safe care as identified by child protective services.

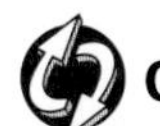

ONGOING CARE

FOLLOW-UP RECOMMENDATIONS

- Retinal hemorrhages generally resolve without intervention. Close monitoring may be required to ensure appropriate management of amblyopia, refractive changes, optic atrophy, and central visual impairment.
- Serial fundus exams may be necessary as blood accumulation within a retinoschisis cavity may leak out into the vitreous over the course of several days and obstruct the visual axis.
- Skeletal surveys should be repeated 2 weeks after presentation to identify callus around areas of previously undetectable fractures.

PATIENT EDUCATION

- Patient education should include strategies for coping with a crying child, as well as information regarding the danger of violent shaking even in the absence of impact.
- Discuss family stressors, especially with families caring for a disabled child.

PROGNOSIS

- Overall reported mortality rates in SBS range between 15–38%. (2)
- Younger age at injury is associated with poorer prognosis, with the highest mortality rates in children under 2 years old. This effect may in part be due to some disruption of normal development.
- Severity of injury is also a strong predictor of poor outcomes, as lower Glasgow Coma Scale scores and longer periods of unconsciousness are associated with subsequent cognitive, motor, and behavioral deficits.
- Long term deficits may include cortical visual impairment, spasticity, seizure disorders, microcephaly, chronic subdural fluid collections, cerebral atrophy, and encephalomalacia. (2)
- There is a direct relationship between the severities of brain and eye injury. (5)
- More common mechanisms of permanent vision loss in abusive head injury include occipital cortical damage, optic atrophy, and less commonly, retinal detachment.

COMPLICATIONS

- Death
- Developmental delay
- Cerebral palsy
- Seizures
- Central visual impairment
- Optic atrophy
- Amblyopia
- Myopia

REFERENCES

1. US Department of Health and Human Services Administration for Children, Youth and Families, Children's Bureau). Child Maltreatment 2008. (2010)
2. American Academy of Pediatrics: Committee on Child Abuse and Neglect. Shaken baby syndrome: Rotational cranial injuries- technical report. *Pediatrics* 2001;108(1):206–210.
3. Sato Y. Imaging of nonaccidental head injury. *Pediatric Radiology* 2009;39(s2):s230–s235.
4. Morad Y, Kim YM, Armstrong DC, et al. Correlation between retinal abnormalities and intracranial abnormalities in the shaken baby syndrome. *Am J Ophthalmol* 2002;134(3):354–359.
5. Deschenes J, Seamone C, Baines M. The ocular manifestations of sexually transmitted diseases. *Can J Ophthalmol* 1990;25(4):177–185.

ADDITIONAL READING

- American Academy of Pediatrics, www.aap.org
- Healthy Children, HealthyChildren.org
- US Department HHS, Child Maltreatment 2008.

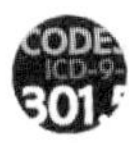

CODES

ICD9

- 995.55 Shaken baby syndrome
- 995.59 Other child abuse and neglect
- 362.81 Retinal hemorrhage

CLINICAL PEARLS

- Suspected child abuse warrants immediate reporting to local child protection services for further investigation.
- Hospitalization is warranted to ensure proper diagnosis, medical stabilization, and that safe placement has been identified.
- Retinal hemorrhage identified by an experienced ophthalmologist on fundus examination should be documented with specific mention of number, type, side symmetry/asymmetry, location, and pattern.
- In young children, serial ophthalmologic examination is warranted to evaluate the visual axis, as this population is especially vulnerable to amblyopia.
- The most common causes of permanent vision loss in the abused child are cortical visual impairment and optic atrophy.

CHOROIDAL EFFUSION/DETACHMENT

Kristina Pao

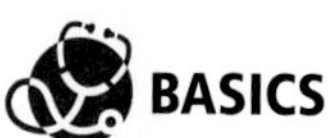

BASICS

DESCRIPTION

- Choroidal effusion is the accumulation of fluid (serous) or blood (hemorrhagic) into the suprachoroidal potential space due to increased intramural pressure.
- Often occur after trauma, perioperatively, postoperatively, or spontaneously (rare)

EPIDEMIOLOGY

Incidence

- Frequency varies between 0.05–6%
- No racial or sexual predilection
- Hemorrhagic choroidal detachments are more common in the elderly

RISK FACTORS

- Serous choroidal effusion: Nanophthalmos, uveal effusion syndrome, carotid-cavernous fistula, primary or metastatic tumor, scleritis, Vogt-Koyanagi-Harada syndrome, globe hypotony, trauma, inflammation, iatrogenic (i.e., isoniazid)
- Hemorrhagic choroidal effusion: Older age, arteriosclerosis, uncontrolled glaucoma, previous eye surgery, myopia, history of choroidal hemorrhage in fellow eye, sickle cell disease, systemic hypertension
- Intraoperative or postoperative: Wound leak, perforation of sclera from superior rectus, bridle suture, cyclodialysis cleft, leakage from filtering bleb, laser photocoagulation or cryotherapy

GENERAL PREVENTION

See "Risk Factors".

PATHOPHYSIOLOGY

- Pressure within the suprachoroidal space is dependent upon intraocular pressure, intracapillary blood pressure, and oncotic pressure.
- Choroidal effusions result from increased vascular permeability leading to the exudation of large serum proteins into the suprachoroidal space leading to choroid edema.

ETIOLOGY

Choroidal effusion is commonly caused by hypotony of any etiology, trauma, and rarely occur spontaneously.

COMMONLY ASSOCIATED CONDITIONS

- Trauma
- Perioperatively or postoperatively following cataract and glaucoma surgery

DIAGNOSIS

- Signs of recent surgery or trauma: Filtering bleb, intraocular lens, photocoagulation, cyclodialysis cleft
  - Perform Seidel test
  - Perform gonioscopy
- Smooth, bullous, orange elevation of retina and choroid on funduscopic examination
  - Bullous elevation often extends 360 degrees around the periphery in a lobular configuration
- Serous choroidal effusion is often asymptomatic or noted with painless decrease in vision
- Often associated with low intraocular pressure (IOP <6 mm Hg), shallow anterior chamber with mild cell and flare
- Hemorrhagic choroidal effusion is often sudden, severely painful loss of vision associated with a red eye
- Often associated with elevated intraocular pressure, shallow anterior chamber with mild cell and flare

HISTORY

- Past ocular history
  - Recent surgery, ocular trauma, corneal ulcer, laser therapy, IOP-lowering medications?
- Recent Valsalva, straining, coughing?
- Use of aspirin or anticoagulants?

PHYSICAL EXAM

- Scalp and cutaneous examination
  - Look for alopecia and vitiligo to rule-out Vogt-Koyanagi-Harada syndrome

DIAGNOSTIC TESTS & INTERPRETATION

Diagnostic Procedures/Other

- B-scan may demonstrate domed-shaped lesions, choroidal thickening, and low-medium internal reflectivity.
  - Helps to differentiate between serous and hemorrhagic choroidal effusion
  - Helps to determine if hemorrhage is mobile or coagulated
  - May note large degree of fluid accumulation resulting in retina-to-retinal contact centrally known as kissing choroidals
- Transillumination is present in serous choroidal detachment, but also in nonpigmented choroidal tumors.
  - Hemorrhagic choroidal effusions do not transilluminate

- CT scan shows a semilunar or ring-shaped lesion of variable attenuation.
- MR demonstrates crescentic or ring-shaped area of hyperintensity on both T1-weighted and T2-weighted images.
  - Helps to differentiate between choroidal effusion and choroidal melanoma, which is hyperintense on T1-weighted images and hypointense on T2-weighted images
  - May be difficult to differentiate between subacute choroidal hematomas from choroidal effusion

Pathological Findings

Accumulation of serous or serosanguineous material in the suprachoroidal potential space.

DIFFERENTIAL DIAGNOSIS

- Malignant glaucoma
- Choroidal melanoma
- Aphakic pupillary block
- Pseudophakic pupillary block
- Exudative retinal detachment
- Postoperative retinal detachment
- Tractional retinal detachment
- Rhegmatogenous retinal detachment
- Melanoma of the ciliary body
- Vogt-Koyanagi-Harada syndrome
- Uveal effusion syndrome
- Wegener's granulomatosis
- Anterior and posterior scleritis
- Carotid-cavernous or dural-sinus fistula

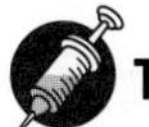

TREATMENT

ADDITIONAL TREATMENT

General Measures

- Topical corticosteroids
- Topical cycloplegics
- Intraocular pressure-lowering medication (topical and systemic)
- Oral steroids if inflammation implicated
- Parasympathomimetics are contraindicated

SURGERY/OTHER PROCEDURES

- Posterior sclerotomy if choroidal detachment persists greater than 1 week
- Anterior chamber paracentesis to drain suprachoroidal fluid
- Injection of viscoelastics if anterior chamber is flattened

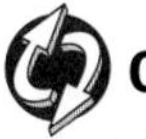

ONGOING CARE

FOLLOW-UP RECOMMENDATIONS

Ophthalmologist

PROGNOSIS

- No mortality
- Prognosis dependent on cause of choroidal effusion
- Loss of useful vision in 40%
- Worse prognosis with hemorrhagic detachment

COMPLICATIONS

- Loss of useful vision
- Phthisis
- Retinal detachment
- Cataract formation
- Cyclitic pupillary membranes
- Corneal endothelial damage
- Peripheral anterior synechiae
- Intractable secondary glaucoma

C

ADDITIONAL READING

- Mafee MF, Linder B, Peyman GA, et al. Choroidal hematoma and effusion: Evaluation with MR imaging. *Radiology* 1988;168:781–6.

CODES

ICD9

- 363.70 Choroidal detachment, unspecified
- 363.71 Serous choroidal detachment
- 363.72 Hemorrhagic choroidal detachment

CHOROIDAL FOLDS

Kamalesh J. Ramaiya
Gaurav K. Shah

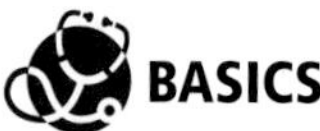

BASICS

DESCRIPTION

- Parallel striae that may be oriented in a horizontal, vertical, or oblique fashion at the posterior pole. (1)[C]
- Not a condition, but rather a clinical finding that may be idiopathic or secondary to another underlying ocular or orbital etiology

EPIDEMIOLOGY

Unknown

RISK FACTORS

See Etiology.

PATHOPHYSIOLOGY

- Wrinkling of the retinal pigment epithelium, Bruch's membrane, and the inner choroid layers
- The lighter colored peaks of the folds are thought to be created by stretching and thinning of the overlying retinal pigment epithelium (RPE), and the darker troughs represent compression of the RPE. However, histopathologic studies have challenged this notion.
- Thought to occur because of an imbalance between the contractile and stretching forces affecting the eye wall (2)[B]
  - Intraocular forces: For example, hypotony
  - External forces: For example, orbital mass lesions, papilledema (increased cerebrospinal fluid pressure transmitted to the eye wall)
  - Direct tractional effect: For example, choroidal neovascular membranes

ETIOLOGY

- Most often, choroidal folds are idiopathic. However, a secondary etiology may be present.
- Ocular conditions
  - Choroidal nevi and tumors
  - Choroidal neovascularization
  - Choroidal inflammation
  - Choroidal detachment or effusions.
  - Central serous chorioretinopathy
  - Hypotony
  - Posterior scleritis
  - Vogt-Koyanagi-Harada syndrome
  - Hyperopia
  - Scleral buckle
- Optic neuropathies
  - Papilledema
  - Optic nerve tumors
- Orbital conditions
  - Orbital tumors
  - Orbital inflammation
  - Thyroid orbitopathy
- Increased intracranial pressure (ICP)
  - Has been shown to cause choroidal folds, independent of the presence of papilledema

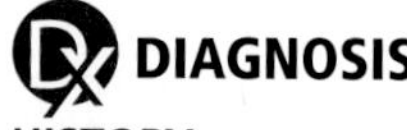

DIAGNOSIS

HISTORY

May be asymptomatic, however, patients may complain of a variety of visual disturbances including blurring of vision or metamorphopsia

PHYSICAL EXAM

- Choroidal folds are a clinical finding seen on dilated funduscopy of the posterior pole. They appear as parallel lines of lighter (yellow) colored peaks alternating with darker (orange) colored troughs.
- A thorough external, anterior, and posterior segment examination, along with measurement of intraocular pressure, should be performed on all patients with choroidal folds, as this may provide clues to an underlying etiology.

DIAGNOSTIC TESTS & INTERPRETATION

Imaging

- Fluorescein angiography (FA) can be useful in demonstrating choroidal folds.
  - A characteristic dark-light alternating pattern of hypo- and hyper- fluorescence is seen, which represents compression and stretching of the RPE, respectively.
  - This test can help differentiate choroidal folds from retinal folds, as the latter will not show alterations in background fluorescence.
  - FA may also help to elucidate an underlying etiology.
- Optical coherence tomography has also been demonstrated to be a useful imaging modality for this condition, especially for differentiating choroidal folds from retinal folds and chorioretinal folds. (3)[C]
- Fundus autofluorescence may also demonstrate characteristics. (4)[C]

Diagnostic Procedures/Other

- Orbital imaging may be indicated in patients with choroidal folds to determine an underlying etiology. This may include:
  - B-Scan ultrasonography of the eye and orbit
  - CT of the orbits and brain
  - MRI of the orbits and brain (5)[C]

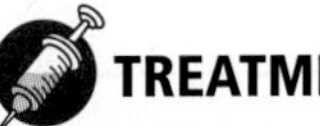

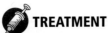

TREATMENT

MEDICATION

- Treatment of choroidal folds is targeted toward the underlying etiology.
- Asymptomatic, idiopathic choroidal folds may be observed.

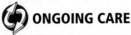

ONGOING CARE

FOLLOW-UP RECOMMENDATIONS

Serial fundus examinations

REFERENCES

1. Machemer R. Choroidal folds. *Am J Ophthalmol* 1979;87:252.
2. DelPriore LV. Stiffness of retinal and choroidal tissue: A surface wrinkling analysis of epiretinal membrane and choroidal Folds. *Am J Ophthalmol* 2006;142:435–440.
3. Giuseppe G, Distefano MG. Optical coherence tomography of chorioretinal and choroidal folds. *Acta Ophthalmol Scand* 2007;85:333–336.
4. Fine HF, Cunningham ET, Kim E, et al. Autofluorescence imaging findings in long-standing chorioretinal folds. *Retin Cases Brief Rep.* 2009;3(2):137–139.
5. Shields JA, Shields CL, Rashid RC. Clinicopathologic correlation of choroidal folds: Secondary to massive cranioorbital hemangiopericytoma. *Ophthal Plast Reconstr Surg* 1992;9:62–68.

CODES

ICD9

743.54 Congenital folds and cysts of posterior segment

CLINICAL PEARLS

- Although choroidal folds may be idiopathic, a search for an underlying etiology should be performed.

CHOROIDAL HEMANGIOMA

Arman Mashayekhi
Carol L. Shields

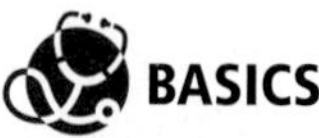

BASICS

DESCRIPTION

Benign vascular hamartomatous tumors of the choroid. Present in 2 forms based on extent of choroidal involvement:

- Circumscribed choroidal hemangioma (CCH): Solitary tumor with no systemic associations
- Diffuse choroidal hemangioma (DCH): Usually in association with Sturge-Weber syndrome (SW syndrome) (encephalofacial angiomatosis)

EPIDEMIOLOGY

Incidence

- CCH is a rare tumor.
  - Only 200 patients with CCH were diagnosed on the Oncology Service at Wills Eye Institute between 1974 and 2000 compared with more than 10,000 patients with choroidal melanoma in the same time period.
- DCH is a very rare tumor.
  - Half of patients with SW syndrome have DCH.

RISK FACTORS

Genetics

- There is no known genetic predisposing factor for CCH.
- SW syndrome is entirely sporadic but several somatic mutations have been described in association with this condition.

COMMONLY ASSOCIATED CONDITIONS

- CCH is a sporadic condition with no associated ocular or systemic conditions.
- DCH is a manifestation of SW syndrome. Other features of this syndrome include:
  - Cutaneous nevus flammeus in the distribution of the first or second branches of the trigeminal nerve (Port-wine stain)
  - Leptomeningeal hemangioma ipsilateral to the cutaneous nevus flammeus
  - Seizure (80%)
  - Hemiparesis/hemiplegia
  - Mental retardation
  - Ocular features:
    - Eyelid nevus flammeus (95–100%)
    - Prominent episcleral vessels (70%)
    - Glaucoma (70%)
    - Diffuse choroidal hemangioma (DCH) (50%)

DIAGNOSIS

HISTORY

- Both CCH and DCH presents with painless visual loss or metamorphopsia (1)[B].
  - CCH usually causes symptoms in the third to sixth decades of life.
  - DCH generally becomes symptomatic earlier in life (First or second decades).

PHYSICAL EXAM

- CCH presents as a circumscribed, round, orange–red elevated choroidal mass. Other typical features include:
  - Unilateral
  - Posterior to equator
  - Serous retinal detachment (RD) (common)
  - Overlying retinal pigment epithelial (RPE) changes (atrophy, hyperplasia, fibrous metaplasia, lipofuscin clumps)
  - Overlying retinal edema (cystoid macular edema in sub- or peri-foveal tumors)
  - Lipid exudation is rare
- DCH presents as diffuse orange thickening of the choroid referred to as the "tomato catsup" fundus
  - Other ocular features of SW syndrome are present (see "Commonly associated conditions")
  - Extensive serous RD and RPE alterations are common
  - Neovascular glaucoma secondary to long-standing RD can develop

DIAGNOSTIC TESTS & INTERPRETATION

Lab

Initial lab tests

- Angiography: Both fluorescein angiography (FA) and indocyanine green angiography (ICGA) are helpful in establishing the diagnosis of CCH.
  - Fluorescein angiography: Lacy hyperfluorescence in prearterial or early arterial phase followed by late staining and leakage.
  - Indocyanine green angiography: Early intense hyperfluorescence followed by dye washout in late frames (tumor hypofluorescence with surrounding rim of hyperfluorescence).
- Ultrasonography
  - CCH: Solid dome-shaped tumor on B-scan with acoustic features similar to adjacent normal choroid. A-scan shows high internal reflectivity.
  - DCH: Acoustic features are similar to CCH but choroidal thickening is more diffuse.
- Optical coherence tomography (OCT) is a useful tool for detection of associated retinal changes such as retinal edema, retinal atrophy, or minimal serous RD.

Follow-up & special considerations

- Ultrasonography and OCT are the most useful tests for monitoring of tumor and retinal status after treatment.
  - Absorption of subretinal or intraretinal fluid is the earliest evidence of response to treatment.

Pathological Findings

- Both CCH and DCH are composed of small to large, thin-walled vessels lined by flat endothelium and separated by thin intervascular connective tissue septa.
  - Overlying RPE alterations include fibrous and osseous metaplasia.
  - Overlying retina usually shows variable degrees of edema and photoreceptor degeneration.

DIFFERENTIAL DIAGNOSIS

- The diagnosis of CCH can be challenging. The main differential diagnosis includes:
  - Amelanotic choroidal melanoma
  - Choroidal metastasis
  - Retinal detachment
  - Central serous chorioretinopathy
  - Posterior scleritis
  - Age-related macular degeneration

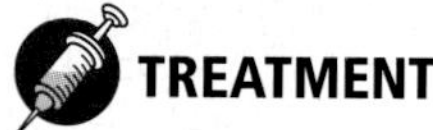

TREATMENT

MEDICATION

There are no known medical treatments available for CCH or DCH.

ADDITIONAL TREATMENT

General Measures

- CCH and DCHs that affect or threaten central vision should be treated before irreversible RPE or retinal damage develops.
- Long delay between onset of symptoms and treatment is associated with a worse visual prognosis.
- In advanced cases with long-standing extensive serous retinal detachment, treatment may prevent development of neovascular glaucoma.
- Observation is the recommended management for asymptomatic CCH or DCH.
  - In a large series from Oncology Service at Wills Eye Institute, 43% of patients were initially observed without treatment.
- The endpoint of treatment should be resolution of intra- or subretinal fluid and not complete tumor regression.

Additional Therapies

- Photodynamic therapy (PDT) with verteporfin is the treatment of choice for CCH and has been used successfully for treatment of DCH (2)[B], (3)[B].
  - Depending on the size of the tumor, one or more spots are necessary to adequately cover the tumor.
  - Successful treatment with PDT leads to absorption of subretinal or intraretinal fluid and variable degrees of tumor regression within the first 3 months after treatment.
  - Can be repeated if there is recurrence of serous RD or macular edema
  - The most common complication of PDT is choroidal atrophy in the area of treatment.
    - The risk of choroidal atrophy can be reduced by using a single spot, non-overlapping spots, lower laser power and by avoiding treatment of surrounding normal choroid.
- Low-dose (20 Gy in 10 fractions) or standard dose (40 Gy in 20 fractions) external beam radiotherapy (EBRT) is the most commonly used method for management of DCH and can be used for treatment of CCH when other treatment methods are not available or are not possible due to hazy media or bullous retinal detachment.
- Plaque radiotherapy (20–40 Gy) has been used successfully for management of CCH.
  - Due to success and excellent safety profile of PDT, currently plaque radiotherapy is reserved for tumors that have failed or are not good candidates for PDT (hazy media, bullous RD) (4)[B].
- Laser photocoagulation and transpupillary thermotherapy are more destructive than PDT and their use is limited to treatment of extrafoveal CCHs when PDT is not available or possible.
  - Laser photocoagulation although initially successful in resolution of subretinal fluid, is associated with high rates of recurrent subretinal fluid.

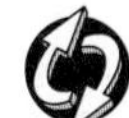

ONGOING CARE

FOLLOW-UP RECOMMENDATIONS

Patient Monitoring

All patients with untreated or treated CCH or DCH need to be monitored regularly for development of new or recurrent subretinal fluid.

PATIENT EDUCATION

- Patients should report any new symptoms such as blurred vision, light flashes, or visual field defect.
  - Amsler grid can be useful for self-monitoring of the central vision.

PROGNOSIS

- Long delay between onset of symptoms (caused by subfoveal fluid or cystoid macular edema) and treatment, is associated with a worse final visual outcome.
- Subfoveal CCHs lead to overlying RPE and photoreceptor damage at the fovea and are associated with poor long-term visual prognosis.

COMPLICATIONS

Neovascular glaucoma is the end result of long-standing extensive serous RD in eyes with CCH or DCH and may require enucleation in some cases.

Pregnancy Considerations

There are several reports of women with CCH presenting with serous RD and decreased vision during the second or third trimesters of pregnancy. Spontaneous resolution of serous RD has been noted in some of these patients following delivery.

REFERENCES

1. Shields CL, Honavar SG, Shields JA, et al. Circumscribed choroidal hemangioma: Clinical manifestations and factors predictive of visual outcome in 200 consecutive cases. *Ophthalmology* 2001;108:2237–48.
2. Schmidt-Erfurth UM, Michels S, et al. Photodynamic therapy for symptomatic choroidal hemangioma: Visual and anatomic results. *Ophthalmology* 2002;109:2284–94.
3. Boixadera A, García-Arumí J, Martínez-Castillo V, et al. Prospective clinical trial evaluating the efficacy of photodynamic therapy for symptomatic circumscribed choroidal hemangioma. *Ophthalmology* 2009;116:100–105.
4. Chao AN, Shields CL, Shields JA, et al. Plaque radiotherapy for choroidal hemangioma with total retinal detachment and iris neovascularization. *Retina* 2001;21:682–4.

ADDITIONAL READING

- Mashayekhi A, Shields CL. Circumscribed choroidal hemangioma. *Curr Opin Ophthalmol* 2003;14: 142–9.
- Shields JA, Shields CL, Materin MA, et al. Changing concepts in management of circumscribed choroidal hemangioma: The 2003 J. Howard Stokes Lecture, Part 1. *Ophthalmic Surg Lasers Imaging* 2004; 35:383–94.

See Also (Topic, Algorithm, Electronic Media Element)

- www.fighteyecancer.com
- www.eyecancerinfo.com

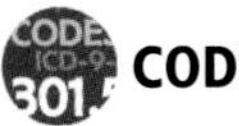

CODES

ICD9

- 228.09 Hemangioma of other sites
- 759.6 Other congenital hamartoses, not elsewhere classified

CLINICAL PEARLS

- CCH should be considered in the differential diagnosis of patients diagnosed with chronic central serous chorioretinopathy.
- Asymptomatic choroidal hemangiomas can be observed without treatment.
- Photodynamic therapy is the treatment of choice for circumscribed choroidal hemangioma.

CHOROIDAL MELANOMA

Carol L. Shields
Jerry A. Shields

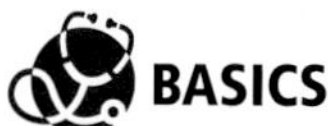

BASICS

DESCRIPTION

- Most common primary intraocular malignancy
- Melanoma occurs in the uvea with iris involvement in 4%, ciliary body involvement in 6%, and choroidal involvement in 90%.
- Choroidal melanoma appears as a pigmented (55%), nonpigmented (15%), or mixed pigmented (30%) mass
- Median choroidal melanoma basal dimension is 11 mm (range 2–33 mm).
- Median choroidal melanoma thickness is 5 mm (range 1–23 mm).
- Assumes a configuration of dome-shape (75%), mushroom shape (19%), or flat [diffuse] (6%).
- Often associated with subretinal fluid, orange pigment, and occasionally subretinal or vitreous hemorrhage.

ALERT

Any pigmented lesion in the ocular fundus should be critically evaluated for possible choroidal melanoma.

Geriatric Considerations

Choroidal melanoma occurs at a median age of 55 years.

Pediatric Considerations

Uveal melanoma most often occurs in adults but 1% of patients are children <20 years.

Pregnancy Considerations

Uveal melanoma in pregnant patients show same risks for metastasis as those that are not pregnant.

EPIDEMIOLOGY

Incidence

Choroidal melanoma incidence in the US is 4–6 per million Caucasian population and 8 per 10 million African American population.

Prevalence

Most authorities believe that there are approximately 2,500 new cases per year in the US.

RISK FACTORS

- Caucasian blue-eyed patients with tendency for sunburn
- Oculodermal melanocytosis (Nevus of Ota)
- Choroidal nevus especially those with:
  - Thickness ≥2 mm
  - Subretinal fluid
  - Symptoms
  - Orange pigment
  - Margin of tumor ≤3 mm to disc
  - Ultrasound hollow
  - Drusen absent
  - Halo absent

Genetics

- No systemic hereditary tendency
- Genetic studies of uveal melanoma disclose that chromosome 3 monosomy and duplication of 8q are the most important factors related to poor prognosis.

GENERAL PREVENTION

- Avoidance of chronic sunlight exposure
- Avoidance of arc welding

PATHOPHYSIOLOGY

Choroidal melanoma arises from preexisting nevus, ocular melanocytosis, or de novo.

ETIOLOGY

No proven cause.

COMMONLY ASSOCIATED CONDITIONS

Oculodermal melanocytosis is found in 3% of eyes with melanoma.

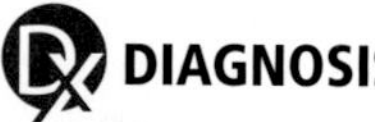

DIAGNOSIS

HISTORY

- Decrease in visual acuity
- Flashes
- Floaters
- No symptoms in some cases.

PHYSICAL EXAM

- Tumor color is brown (55%), yellow (15%), or mixed brown–yellow (30%).
- Tumor quadrant can be macula (5%), inferior (20%), temporal (29%), superior (22%), nasal (21%), and diffuse (3%).
- Median proximity to disc is 3 mm.
- Median proximity to foveola is 3 mm.

DIAGNOSTIC TESTS & INTERPRETATION

Lab

Initial lab tests

Liver function tests, chest x-ray, liver MRI, and sometimes liver PET scan to evaluate for systemic metastasis.

Follow-up & special considerations

The above tests are repeated once or twice yearly.

Imaging

Initial approach

- Systemic imaging as listed above.
- Ocular imaging with fundus photography, ultrasonography, fluorescein angiography, indocyanine green angiography, autofluorescence, optical coherence tomography, and occasionally visual fields.

Follow-up & special considerations

The imaging is repeated as needed on each ophthalmic visit.

Diagnostic Procedures/Other

Fine needle aspiration biopsy to confirm the melanoma cytologically as well as to evaluate the malignancy for cytogenetic abnormalities.

Pathological Findings

- Variably pigmented nodular or flat mass of the choroid
- 3 histopathologic types include:
  - Spindle cell type – slender cells with thin elongated nucleus and nucleolus
  - Epithelioid cell type – large cells with prominent nucleus
  - Mixed spindle and epithelioid cell type

DIFFERENTIAL DIAGNOSIS

- Choroidal nevus
- Peripheral exudative hemorrhagic chorioretinopathy
- Congenital hypertrophy of the RPE
- RPE hemorrhagic detachment
- Choroidal hemangioma
- Choroidal metastasis
- Scleritis
- Uveal effusion
- Retinal detachment

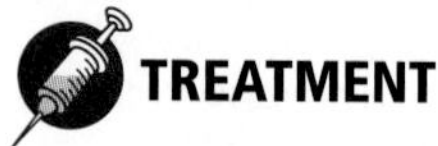

TREATMENT

MEDICATION

- There are no medications for this tumor.
- For metastatic disease, some consider chemotherapy, immunotherapy, vaccination, protein kinase inhibition, and other therapies.

ADDITIONAL TREATMENT

General Measures

- Treatment is based on tumor location, size, associated features, patient age, and general health and status of the opposite eye and includes enucleation, plaque radiotherapy, proton beam radiotherapy, surgical excision (resection), and thermotherapy
- Plaque radiotherapy or proton beam radiotherapy is the most common conservative therapy
- Enucleation is employed for large tumors

Issues for Referral

All patients with choroidal melanoma should be referred to an experienced center of excellence for treatment.

Additional Therapies

Thermotherapy or photodynamic therapy is offered for consolidation of the scar.

SURGERY/OTHER PROCEDURES
- Enucleation for large melanoma over 8 mm thickness or those with extrascleral extension, glaucoma, or encircling the optic disc
- Plaque radiotherapy or proton beam radiotherapy for medium melanoma of 3–8 mm thickness or small melanoma of ≤3 mm thickness. Both treatments are delivered over approximately 5 days and provide excellent local tumor control of 98%, but can lead to vision loss from radiation maculopathy and/or papillopathy.
- Local resection to microsurgically remove the tumor from the eye and leave the eye intact
- Laser therapy using transpupillary thermotherapy to treat small melanoma or consolidate larger tumors following radiotherapy

IN-PATIENT CONSIDERATIONS
Initial Stabilization
Treatment of choroidal melanoma is outpatient.

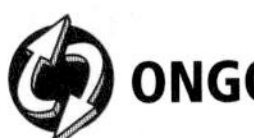

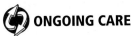

ONGOING CARE

FOLLOW-UP RECOMMENDATIONS
Patients should be examined every 4 months for the first 3 years and thereafter every 6 months for life for local recurrence in the eye and systemic metastasis.

PATIENT EDUCATION
- www.fighteyecancer.com
- www.eyecancer.info
- www.eyetumor.org
- www.eyecancerbook.com
- www.etrf.org
- www.choroidmelanoma.com

PROGNOSIS
- Metastasis by general size @ 10 years is:
  - Small (0–3 mm thickness) – 12% metastasis
  - Medium(3–8 mm thickness) – 25% metastasis
  - Large (≥8 mm thickness) – 50% metastasis
- Metastasis by specific size at 10 years is:
  - 0–1 mm is 5%
  - 1–2 mm is 10%
  - 2–3 mm is 15%
  - 3–4 mm is 20%
  - 4–5 mm is 25%
  - 5–6 mm is 30%
  - 6–7 mm is 35%
  - 7–8 mm is 40%
  - 8–9 mm is 45%
  - 9–10 mm is 50%
  - ≥10 mm is 55%
- Visual prognosis following enucleation is complete and following plaque radiotherapy depends on tumor thickness and location. Approximately 70% of patients have 20/200 visual acuity after plaque radiotherapy by 5 years.

COMPLICATIONS
- If enucleation, sunken socket, poor prosthesis motility, socket infection, socket conjunctivitis
- If plaque radiotherapy, complications are loss of vision from radiation retinopathy, papillopathy, cataract, or glaucoma, neovascular glaucoma, and loss of eye

ADDITIONAL READING

- Shields CL. The hunt for the secrets of uveal melanoma. Perspective. Editorial. *J Clin Exp Ophthalmol* 2008;36:277–80.
- Shields CL. To find small ocular melanoma. A mnemonic to identify choroidal melanoma in its early stages. In: Rapuano C, (ed), *Yearbook of ophthalmology* St Louis: Mosby, 2005;267–272.
- Weis E, Shah CP, Lajous M, et al. The association of host susceptibility factors and uveal melanoma. A meta-analysis. *Arch Ophthalmol* 2006;124:54–60.
- Shah CP, Weis E, Lajous M, et al. Blue light exposure and uveal melanoma. Correspondence. *Ophthalmology* 2006;113:1062.
- Shields CL, Furuta M, Berman EL, et al. Choroidal nevus transformation into melanoma. Analysis of 2514 consecutive cases. *Arch Ophthalmol* 2009; 127(8):981–7.
- Shields CL, Furuta M, Thangappan A, et al. Metastasis of uveal melanoma millimeter-by-millimeter in 8033 consecutive eyes. *Arch Ophthalmol* 2009;127(8):989–98.
- Shields JA, Shields CL. *Intraocular Tumors: A Text and Atlas*. Philadelphia: Saunders, 1992.
- Shields JA, Shields CL. *Atlas of Intraocular Tumors*. Philadelphia: Lippincott Williams and Wilkins, 2008.
- Sagoo MS, Shields CL, Mashayekhi A, et al. Plaque radiotherapy for choroidal melanoma encircling the optic disc (circumpapillary choroidal melanoma. *Arch Ophthalmol* 2007;125:1202–9.
- Shields CL, Bianciotto C, Pirondini C, et al. Autofluorescence of choroidal melanoma in 51 cases. *Br J Ophthalmol* 2008;92:617–22.

CODES

ICD9
190.6 Malignant neoplasm of choroid

CLINICAL PEARLS
- Remember "to find small ocular melanoma – using helpful hints daily" to recall TFSOM – UHHD that represents thickness >2 mm, fluid, symptoms, orange pigment, margin near disc, ultrasound hollow, halo absent, drusen absent. Any small lesion with these features should be evaluated for melanoma by an experienced consultant.

C

CHOROIDAL NEOVASCULARIZATION

J. Arch McNamara

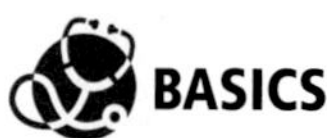

BASICS

DESCRIPTION

- Choroidal neovascularization (CNV) is the development of new blood vessels from the choroid layer through a dehiscence or disturbance in Bruch's membrane into the subretinal space.
- Choroidal neovascularization is often accompanied by fibroblasts. The resulting fibrovascular complex is unstable and can frequently leak serous fluid, hemorrhage, and result in a disciform scar.
- Multiple disorders that affect the retinal pigment epithelium (RPE)-Bruch's membrane-choriocapillaris complex can cause choroidal neovascularization.
  - Over 40 disease processes are associated with choroidal neovascularization with age-related macular degeneration (AMD), angioid streaks, pathologic myopia, ocular histoplasmosis syndrome, and blunt trauma being the commonest.

EPIDEMIOLOGY

Incidence

- Varies by underlying diagnosis
  - Choroidal neovascularization associated with age-related macular degeneration is the leading cause of permanent visual loss in people over 65 years of age in developed countries.
    - Advanced AMD affects 25–30 million people worldwide and 1.75 million in the US.

Prevalence

- Varies by underlying diagnosis
  - In AMD, the prevalence of choroidal neovascularization is primarily influenced by advancing age.

RISK FACTORS

- Varies by underlying diagnosis
  - In AMD, advancing age is an obvious risk factor. Other factors include strong family history of AMD, race (more common in whites and Hispanics than blacks), cigarette smoking, hypertension, hyperlipidemia, abdominal obesity, reduced physical activity, and high dietary fat intake.

Genetics

- Varies by underlying diagnosis
  - AMD –and its most severe complication, choroidal neovascularization– is recognized as resulting from a convergence of multiple risk factors. Family history is a consistent risk factor. Twin studies support a genetic basis for the disease with both early and late-onset findings (CNV) being approximately twice as high in monozygotic as dizygotic twins.
    - Genome-wide linkage analyses have identified a number of chromosomal loci linked to AMD.

GENERAL PREVENTION

- Avoid modifiable risk factors
- Nutritional supplementation has been shown to reduce the risk of progression of AMD to its more severe "wet" form in which there is development of CNV.
  - The Age-related Eye Disease Study (AREDS) recommended the following: 500 mg vitamin C, 400 IU vitamin E, 15 mg beta-carotene, 80 mg zinc as zinc oxide, 2 mg copper as cupric oxide (the latter to prevent copper deficiency anemia associated with high levels of zinc intake).
    - AREDS II, currently underway, is assessing supplementation with micronutrients lutein, zeaxanthin, and omega-3 fatty acids (DHA and EPA).

PATHOPHYSIOLOGY

- Any disturbance of Bruch's membrane, such as blunt trauma, an infectious process, or the non-neovascular abnormalities of AMD (drusen, RPE atrophy) can allow buds of neovascular tissue from the choriocapillaris to perforate the outer aspect of Bruch's membrane.
  - Once the stage is set for CNV, proangiogenic factors including vascular endothelial growth factor (VEGF), advanced glycosylation end-products (AGEs), platelet-derived growth factor (PDGF), and pigment epithelium-derived factor facilitate continued growth of CNV.

ETIOLOGY

Degenerative, infectious, traumatic, and genetically-determined disruptions of Bruch's membrane

COMMONLY ASSOCIATED CONDITIONS

Age-related macular degeneration, angioid streaks, pathologic myopia, ocular histoplasmosis syndrome, blunt trauma/choroidal rupture, and multifocal choroiditis.

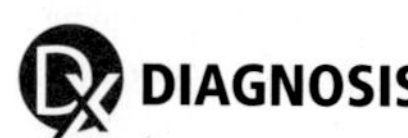

DIAGNOSIS

HISTORY

Sudden onset of decreased vision with metamorphopsia, and paracentral scotoma

PHYSICAL EXAM

Elevation of the RPE, serous subretinal fluid, intraretinal lipid, subretinal or less commonly intraretinal hemorrhage, RPE detachment, RPE rip, gray–green CNV lesion seen through retina.

DIAGNOSTIC TESTS & INTERPRETATION

Imaging

Initial approach

- Fluorescein angiography
  - Various patterns may be seen including a classic CNV and occult CNV
  - Blood may block CNV

Follow-up & special considerations

Treatment can be monitored with serial fluorescein angiography and optical coherence tomography.

Diagnostic Procedures/Other

- Optical coherence tomography (OCT)
  - CNV appears as increased reflectivity deep to the retina
    - Secondary findings on OCT include RPE detachment, subretinal fluid, and intraretinal edema.

Pathological Findings

- New blood vessel growth from the choroid through Bruch's membrane into the subretinal space
  - In AMD, 3 growth patterns of CNV have been identified based upon the relationship of the CNV to the RPE
    - Type 1: CNV beneath the RPE
    - Type 2: CNV through RPE into subretinal space
    - Combined pattern of type 1 & 2

DIFFERENTIAL DIAGNOSIS

Retinal arteriolar macroaneurysm, central serous chorioretinopathy, Best's disease, adult vitelliform dystrophy, polypoidal choroidal vasculopathy, posterior scleritis, multifocal choroiditis/inflammatory conditions, and choroidal hemangioma.

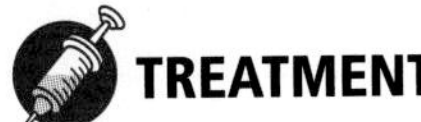

TREATMENT

MEDICATION

First Line

- In AMD, anti-VEGF drugs have become the standard of care in treating CNV. Ranibizumab and bevacizumab are the most frequently used.
- CNV outside the central macula (extrafoveal), especially when associated with disorders other that AMD (such as blunt trauma) may be treated with laser photocoagulation (thermal laser).

Second Line

- Photodynamic therapy (PDT - administration of a photosensitizing drug, verteporfin, followed by application of laser at the appropriate wavelength)
  - The use of PDT has been largely supplanted by anti-VEGF therapy but still has a place in the management of CNV.

ADDITIONAL TREATMENT

General Measures

Low vision evaluation and prescription of aids, especially when CNV is bilateral.

Issues for Referral

New onset of decreased vision.

SURGERY/OTHER PROCEDURES

- Vitrectomy for evacuation of submacular hemorrhage from a ruptured CNV membrane may be considered.
  - Vitrectomy for removal of CNV membranes is not useful in AMD patients, especially since anti-VEGF agents have become available.
    - Vitrectomy for removal of CNV membranes where the etiology is trauma or inflammation can still be considered.

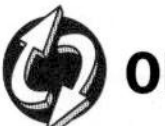

ONGOING CARE

FOLLOW-UP RECOMMENDATIONS

CNV may recur, so patients should be followed until complete stabilization has occurred.

Patient Monitoring

Amsler grid

DIET

AMD patients should eat a balanced diet low in high dietary fat and consider eating fish twice a week.

PROGNOSIS

Prognosis depends on location of CNV and whether or not hemorrhaging from the CNV has occurred.

COMPLICATIONS

Rarely massive subretinal hemorrhage can lead to a hemorrhagic retinal detachment and loss of all vision.

ADDITIONAL READING

- Do DV. Antiangiogenic approaches to age-related macular degeneration in the future. *Ophthalmology* 2009;116(10 Suppl):S24–26.
- Bressler NM. Antiangiogenic approaches to age-related macular degeneration in the future. *Ophthalmology* 2009;116(10 Suppl):S15–23.
- Cohen SY. Anti-VEGF drugs as the 2009 first-line therapy for choroidal neovascularization in pathologic myopia. *Retina* 2009;29(8):1062–1026.

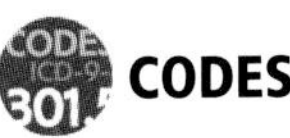

CODES

ICD9

362.16 Retinal neovascularization nos

CHOROIDAL NEVUS

Carol L. Shields
Jerry A. Shields

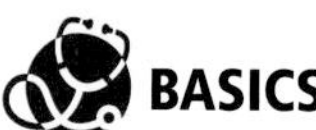

BASICS

DESCRIPTION

- Most common intraocular tumor
- Can occur within the eye in the uveal tissue including the iris, ciliary body, or choroid
- Appears as a pigmented (80%) or nonpigmented (20%) mass
- Generally measures about 2 mm in diameter and 1.5 mm in thickness
- Can produce overlying changes in the retinal pigment epithelium (RPE) such as RPE hyperplasia, atrophy, and drusen

ALERT
Choroidal nevus is a benign mass in the ocular fundus, but the patient should be evaluated to rule out simulating choroidal melanoma.

Geriatric Considerations

Choroidal nevus can occur in all ages.

Pediatric Considerations

Choroidal nevus can be present in children but often without drusen.

Pregnancy Considerations

There are no pregnancy considerations.

EPIDEMIOLOGY

Incidence

- Far more common in Caucasians than non-Caucasians
- Believed to be equivalent between male and female, although some studies show more common in females.
- Most authorities believe that the prevalence is approximately 7% of Caucasian adults.
- In population-based studies, choroidal nevus prevalence has varied including
  - 1.9% of persons over age 13 years
  - 3.1% of persons over age 30 years
  - 6.5% of persons over age 49 years

Prevalence

- It is believed that choroidal nevus is present at birth but is recognized later in life after it acquires pigmentation or the patient cooperates for a dilated examination
- Age of onset:
  - Young (≤20 years) in 2%
  - Middle adult (20–50 years) in 23%
  - Older adult (>50 years in) 75%

RISK FACTORS

Caucasian blue-eyes

Genetics

No hereditary tendency

GENERAL PREVENTION

There is no method for prevention of choroidal nevus.

PATHOPHYSIOLOGY

No known cause

ETIOLOGY

No known cause

COMMONLY ASSOCIATED CONDITIONS

- Ocular and oculodermal melanocytosis classically show diffuse pigmentation of the uvea (and choroid) consistent with a large flat nevus.
- Neurofibromatosis type 1 can manifest diffuse multifocal nevi.

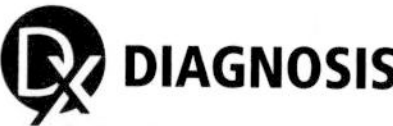

DIAGNOSIS

HISTORY

- Decrease in visual acuity in 10%
- Flashes or floaters in 1%
- Visual field defect in 5%
- No symptoms in 84%

PHYSICAL EXAM

- Color is brown (80%) or yellow (20%)
- Location is subfoveolar (10%) or extrafoveolar (90%)
- Sector quadrant is macula (25%), inferior (20%), temporal (20%), superior (15%), nasal (20%)
- Anteroposterior quadrant macula (25%), macula to equator (70%), equator to ora serrata (5%)

DIAGNOSTIC TESTS & INTERPRETATION

Lab

Initial lab tests
No blood laboratory tests needed

Follow-Up & Special Considerations
No systemic follow-up as this is localized to the eye.

Imaging

Initial approach

- Ophthalmic Imaging includes: Fundus photography, ultrasonography, optical coherence tomography, fluorescein angiography, indocyanine green angiography, autofluorescence, and occasionally visual fields
  - Ophthalmoscopy – dilated eye examination with indirect ophthalmoscopy and tumor measurement
  - Fundus photography – to confirm the location and size of the tumor and its effects on the surrounding fundus
  - Ultrasonography – imaging of the globe using sound waves to detect intraocular mass or retinal detachment to resolution of 0.5 mm
  - Optical coherence tomography – imaging of the retina cross section to 8 micrometer resolution using light reflection to visualize the overlying retina to evaluate for subretinal fluid, photoreceptor loss, intraretinal edema, pigment epithelial detachment, choroidal neovascularization
  - Fluorescein angiography – imaging of the retina and choroidal vasculature to evaluate for RPE atrophy or hyperplasia, choroidal neovascular membrane, and intrinsic choroidal tumor blood flow
  - Indocyanine green angiography – imaging of the choroidal vasculature to evaluate for intrinsic tumor blood supply as well as choroidal neovascular membrane
  - Autofluorescence – photographic imaging technique to evaluate for intrinsic RPE, choroidal, and scleral autofluorescence using special filters to detect emitted wavelengths of light after stimulation with light
  - Visual fields – o evaluate for focal or diffuse loss of peripheral or central vision

Follow-up & special considerations
At each visit, some or all of the above tests are performed.

Diagnostic Procedures/Other

If suspicious, a fine needle aspiration biopsy for cytology or cytogenetics can be performed.

Pathological Findings

- Variably pigmented placoid choroidal lesion
- Involves outer choroid and usually spares the choriocapillaris
- Typically <2 mm thickness
- 4 histopathologic types include
  - Plump polyhedral cells with round to ovoid small uniform nuclei
  - Slender spindle cells with thin basophilic nuclei
  - Plump fusiform and dendritic cells
  - Balloon cells, found in 4% of nevi and have foamy cytoplasm

DIFFERENTIAL DIAGNOSIS

- Choroidal melanoma
- Congenital hypertrophy of the RPE
- RPE hyperplasia
- Choroidal metastasis from skin melanoma
- Subretinal hemorrhage
- Choroidal hemorrhage
- Peripheral exudative hemorrhagic chorioretinopathy
- Age related macular degeneration

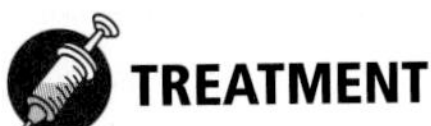

TREATMENT

MEDICATION

There are no medications

ADDITIONAL TREATMENT

General Measures

- Observation on 3–6 month basis depending on risk factors
- Fundus photography to confirm appearance
- Ultrasonography to measure thickness
- Optical coherence tomography to confirm the features of the overlying retina
- Autofluorescence to evaluate for status of the RPE

Issues for Referral

- If risk factors present, then referral advised. Nevi with <3 risk factors could be observed. Nevi with >3 factors should be considered for treatment as they might represent melanoma. Risk factors include:
  - To – thickness >2 mm
  - Find – subretinal fluid
  - Small – symptoms
  - Ocular – Orange pigment
  - Melanoma – Margin within 3 mm of disc
  - Using Helpful – Ultrasound Hollow
  - Hints – Halo absent
  - Daily – Drusen absent

SURGERY/OTHER PROCEDURES

- If subretinal fluid into the fovea, consider laser photocoagulation or photodynamic therapy to the leaks detected on fluorescein angiography. Consideration for intravitreal bevacizumab to reduce subfoveal fluid can be made
- If documented growth of the mass, this could represent transformation into melanoma and plaque radiotherapy, thermotherapy, enucleation, or a combination of the above should be considered

IN-PATIENT CONSIDERATIONS

This is not managed as inpatient.

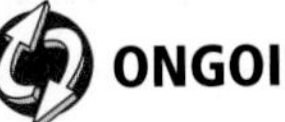

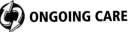

ONGOING CARE

FOLLOW-UP RECOMMENDATIONS

Patient Monitoring

Monitor in 3 months to document stability, then twice yearly for life.

PATIENT EDUCATION

- www.fighteyecancer.com
- www.eyecancer.info
- www.eyetumor.info
- www.eyecancerbook.com
- www.etrf.org
- www.choroidmelanoma.com

PROGNOSIS

- Systemic – If stable nevus with no growth then systemic prognosis excellent
- Visual prognosis depends on tumor location:
  - If the nevus is extrafoveal, then vision likely to be good
  - If the nevus is subfoveal, then 26% risk for loss of at least 3 lines of visual acuity

COMPLICATIONS

- Loss of vision
- Transformation into melanoma

ADDITIONAL READING

- Ganley JP, Comstock GW. Benign nevi and malignant melanomas of the choroid. *Am J Ophthalmol* 1973;76:19–25.
- Sumich P, Mitchell P, Wang JJ. Choroidal nevi in a white population: The Blue Mountains Eye Study. *Arch Ophthalmol* 1998;116:645–50.
- Thiagalingam S, Wang JJ, Mitchell P. Absence of change in choroidal nevi across 5 years in an older population. *Arch Ophthalmol* 2004;122:89–93.
- Shields CL, Mashayekhi A, Materin MA, et al. Optical coherence tomography of choroidal nevus in 120 patients. *Retina* 2005;25:243–52.
- Shields CL, Shields JA, Kiratli H, et al. Risk factors for growth and metastasis of small choroidal melanocytic lesions. *Ophthalmology* 1995;102: 1351–61.
- Shields CL, Cater JC, Shields JA, et al. Combination of clinical factors predictive of growth of small choroidal melanocytic tumors. *Arch Ophthalmol* 2000;118:360–4.
- Shields CL, Furuta M, Mashayekhi A, et al. Visual acuity in 3422 consecutive eyes with choroidal nevus. *Arch Ophthalmol* 2007;125:1501–7.
- Shields CL, Furuta M, Mashayekhi A, et al. Clinical spectrum of choroidal nevi based on age at presentation in 3422 consecutive eyes. *Ophthalmology* 2008;115:546–52.
- Collaborative Ocular Melanoma Study Group. Factors predictive of growth and treatment of small choroidal melanoma: COMS report no. 5. *Arch Ophthalmol* 1997;115:1537–44.
- Shields JA, Shields CL. *Atlas of Intraocular Tumors*. Philadelphia: Lippincott Williams and Wilkins, 2008:59–67.
- Shields JA, Shields CL. *Intraocular Tumors: A Text and Atlas*. Philadelphia: Saunders, 1992:85–100.

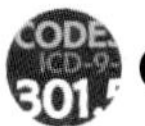

CODES

ICD9

224.6 Benign neoplasm of choroid

CLINICAL PEARLS

- Choroidal nevus is benign and should be monitored twice yearly.
- Choroidal nevus should be evaluated for clinical risk factors to ascertain whether or not it might show features of simulating malignant melanoma.
- Risk factors include:
  - Thickness >2 mm
  - Subretinal fluid
  - Symptoms
  - Orange pigment
  - Margin within 3 mm of disc
  - Ultrasound hollow
  - Drusen absent
  - Halo absent

CHOROIDAL RUPTURE

Raza M. Shah

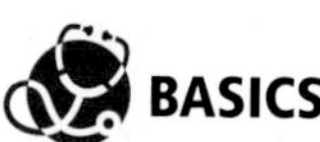

BASICS

DESCRIPTION

Choroidal ruptures are breaks in the choroid, the Bruch membrane, and the retinal pigment epithelium (RPE), and are the result of blunt ocular trauma.

Pediatric Considerations

Traumatic choroidal rupture in children can occur in all ages following blunt injury.

Pregnancy Considerations

Choroidal rupture may occur at the time of delivery, particularly when forceps are used.

EPIDEMIOLOGY

Incidence

- Blunt ocular trauma is the most common type of eye injury. Approximately 5–10% of these patients develop a choroidal rupture.
- Most eyes have a single rupture, but up to 25% of eyes have multiple ruptures.
- About 80% of ruptures occur temporal to the disc, and 66% involve the macula.

Prevalence

Rare (approximately 1/10,000), except in patients with a history of ocular trauma.

RISK FACTORS

- Ocular trauma
- More common in eyes with angioid streaks following minor ocular trauma

Genetics

Currently, no genes have been mapped indicating a predilection for eyes sustaining choroidal ruptures.

GENERAL PREVENTION

- Protective eyewear (e.g., polycarbonate lenses) during any contact sports and activities exposing eyes to possible trauma
- When Bruch's membrane is abnormal, minor trauma can result in extensive choroidal rupture.
- High-risk patients should be advised of the hazards associated with blunt ocular trauma related to contact sports and other activities.

PATHOPHYSIOLOGY

- After blunt trauma, the eye undergoes mechanical compression and then sudden expansion. Because of its tensile strength, the sclera can resist this insult; the retina is also protected because of its elasticity. The Bruch membrane does not have enough elasticity or tensile strength; therefore, it breaks.
- Concurrently, the small capillaries in the choriocapillaris are damaged, leading to subretinal or sub-RPE hemorrhage. The larger choroidal vessels are usually spared. Hemorrhage along with retinal edema may obscure the choroidal rupture during the acute phases. As the blood clears, a white, curvilinear, crescent-shaped streak concentric to the optic nerve is seen.
- Classified as:
  - Direct, occurring at the site of impact, most commonly anterior and parallel to the limbus; or
  - Indirect, occurring away from the site of impact, usually in the posterior pole concentric to the optic disc or through the fovea

ETIOLOGY

Choroidal rupture occurs most commonly as a result of trauma, usually in young males.

COMMONLY ASSOCIATED CONDITIONS

Choroidal neovascularization (CNV) may occur. (1)[B]

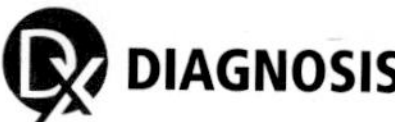

DIAGNOSIS

HISTORY

- Choroidal ruptures typically present after an episode of blunt trauma to the globe
- Also commonly associated with patients having a history of previous angioid streaks
- Patients complain of new onset decreased vision and/or a paracentral or central scotoma

PHYSICAL EXAM

- A thorough search for other signs of trauma to the, head, orbit, ocular adnexa, and eye (2)[C]
- Ophthalmologic findings may include:
  - Subretinal hemorrhage, which may obscure rupture of Bruch's membrane
  - White subretinal streak(s) concentric to the optic nerve in areas of previous subretinal hemorrhage.
  - The nerve fiber layer usually intact
  - Chorioretinal membranes
  - Macular hole, retinal tears, retinal dialysis, and retinal detachment may occur

DIAGNOSTIC TESTS & INTERPRETATION

Lab

None generally necessary as it is a clinical diagnosis.

Imaging

Initial approach

- Fluorescein angiography (FA) often is helpful in confirming the presence, location, and extent of choroidal ruptures.
  - FA demonstrates a hypofluorescent curvilinear streak early followed by hyperfluorescence in the late phase.
- Indocyanine green angiography (IGGA) is useful in localizing ruptures obscured by hemorrhage.
- CT scan of the head to assess possibility of intraocular foreign body, ruptured globe or other head injury not previously detected
- B scan of globe and orbit

Follow-up & special considerations

Serial examinations may be necessary to establish a diagnosis of choroidal rupture

DIFFERENTIAL DIAGNOSIS

- Chorioretinal scars – may be related to old infectious process such as toxoplasmosis or histoplasmosis
- Angioid Streaks – red or brown irregular lesions that radiate from the optic nerve
- Exudative Age-Related Macular Degeneration (ARMD)
- Valsalva retinopathy

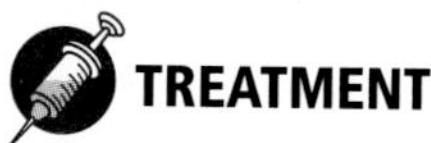

TREATMENT

MEDICATION

- There is no treatment for choroidal ruptures, but a careful examination is important to exclude other ocular injuries associated with blunt ocular trauma, such as commotio retinae, retinal dialysis, hyphema, angle recession, and traumatic iritis.
- Inflammation of the anterior segment can be treated with topical steroids and cycloplegics.
- CNV is a common sequelae of choroidal ruptures. CNV may be treated as needed, with anti-VEGF therapy showing the most promise. (3)[C]

ADDITIONAL TREATMENT

Issues for Referral

Vitreoretinal specialists should be consulted in instances of suspected choroidal rupture.

SURGERY/OTHER PROCEDURES

- If CNV is extrafoveal, it may be treated with laser photocoagulation. Recurrences are rare.
- Prior to anti-VEGF therapy, pars plana vitrectomy with membrane extraction was considered for subfoveal or juxtafoveal CNV.

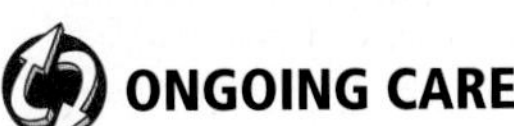

ONGOING CARE

FOLLOW-UP RECOMMENDATIONS

Patients will need close monitoring until the disease is brought under control. Patients may need follow-up with other specialists.

Patient Monitoring

Patients should be followed closely.

PATIENT EDUCATION

Teach patients to monitor each eye using an Amsler grid and a near card.

PROGNOSIS

- A prognostic indicator of the patient's eventual vision is the location of the rupture in relation to the fovea. In patients with:
  - Subfoveal rupture, the vision tends to remain poor
  - Extrafoveal rupture, the vision may remain excellent until and unless CNV develops
  - Contusion maculopathy, the visual potential is limited
- Most do not reach a final visual acuity of 20/40 or better
- If rupture does not involve the fovea, good vision is expected.

COMPLICATIONS

- CNV is the most common late complication of choroidal ruptures.
- Retinal detachment is occasionally found in anterior choroidal ruptures.
- A variety of visual field defects have been observed.

REFERENCES

1. Ament CS, Zacks DN, Lane AM, et al. Predictors of visual outcome and choroidal neovascular membrane formation after traumatic choroidal rupture. *Arch Ophthalmol* 2006;124(7):957–66. (B)
2. Dubinski W, Sharma S. Choroidal rupture. *Can Fam Phys* 2006;52:1071–1079. (C)
3. Liang F, Puche N, Soubrane G, et al. Intravitreal ranibizumab for choroidal neovascularization related to traumatic Bruch's membrane rupture. *Graefes Arch Clin Exp Ophthalmol* 2009; 247(9):1285–8. (C)

ADDITIONAL READING

- Lambert S, Hutchinson, A. Pediatric ocular trauma. *Pediatric Ophthalmology: Current Thought and a Practical Guide*. In: Edward Wilson, Richard A. Saunders, Rupal H. Trivedi, (eds). Germany: Springer-Verlag Berlin Heidelberg, 2009.
- Pendergast S. Choroidal ruptures. *Roy and Fraunfelder's Current Ocular Therapy*. In: Frederick Roy, Frederick T. Fraunfelder, Frederick W. Fraunfelder, (eds). China: Saunders Elsevier, 2008.
- Engelbrecht N, Sternberg P Jr. Choroid. *Ocular Trauma: Principles and Practice*. In: Ferenc Kuhn, Dante J. Pieramici. (eds). New York: Thieme: 2002.

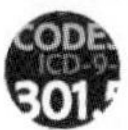

CODES

ICD9

- 363.61 Choroidal hemorrhage, unspecified
- 363.63 Choroidal rupture

CLINICAL PEARLS

- Early identification of a transfoveal choroidal rupture helps assist in providing the patient with a more realistic prediction regarding visual outcomes.
- CNV associated with choroidal rupture, may involute spontaneously, leaving a relatively small scotoma.

CHOROIDEREMIA

Jared D. Peterson

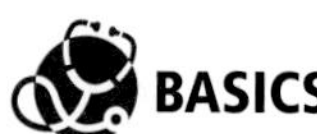

BASICS

DESCRIPTION

Choroideremia (CHM) is a progressive, X-linked condition that results in slow degeneration of the retinal pigment epithelium (RPE), choroid, and photoreceptors.

Pediatric Considerations

Although many patients with choroideremia may not present with symptoms until their early teens, others develop nyctalopia in the first decade.

EPIDEMIOLOGY

Prevalence

Estimated to be around 1:50,000

RISK FACTORS

- Male gender with family history of choroideremia
  - Although extremely rare, female carriers can manifest signs and symptoms of CHM, but it is usually mild.

Genetics

X-linked recessive

PATHOPHYSIOLOGY

- The CHM gene, located on the X chromosome (Xq21.2), codes for a component of rab geranylgeranyltransferase (GGTase), otherwise known as Rab escort protein (REP), an important component of RPE cell function.
- Strunnikova et al. studied monocytes and primary skin fibroblasts from CHM individuals. Monocytes showed impaired phagocytosis and intracellular vesicle transport, decreased lysosomal acidification, and hampered rates of proteolytic degradation compared to controls. Fibroblasts showed decreased secretion of several cytokines/growth factors (1).
- The RPE serves multiple functions including phagocytosis/degradation of shed outer photoreceptor segments, as well as processing/transport of Vitamin A and other nutrients. Altered lysosomal function and cell trafficking may contribute to the RPE degeneration seen in CHM patients.

ETIOLOGY

Multiple types of mutations including full deletions, partial deletions, nonsense mutations, and splice site mutations have been reported (over 100 different mutations have been described overall (2)). All mutations are thought to lead to complete loss of REP-1.

DIAGNOSIS

HISTORY

- Affected males usually present with trouble with night vision (nyctalopia). Some males may not develop any symptoms until their teen years, whereas others develop nyctalopia during the first decade.
- Nyctalopia is followed by gradual loss of peripheral vision.

PHYSICAL EXAM

- The visual field loss starts as annular scotomas which progresses to concentric field loss.
  - By 40 years of age, affected males will typically have a severely impaired peripheral visual field at or near the level of legal blindness.
- Central visual acuity is usually good until age 60 years or greater (3).
- Funduscopic findings include pigmentary stippling and areas of RPE and choroidal atrophy in the equatorial fundus that eventually progress to involve the peripheral retina and posterior pole.
- In advanced stages, the RPE and choroid loss is so severe that the only apparent retinal vasculature being apparent is in the far periphery, the macula, and around the optic disc. The underlying sclera is visible through the areas of atrophy.

DIAGNOSTIC TESTS & INTERPRETATION

Lab

- CHM is a clinical diagnosis. However, genetic testing is valuable.
  - Duplication/deletion analysis, sequence analysis, and targeted mutation analysis are available.
  - If the above mentioned tests fail to identify a mutation, reverse transcriptase PCR, northern blot analysis, protein truncation testing, and immunoblot analysis are available (primarily as research tools only).
    - Immunoblot analysis is used to detect anti-REP-1 antibody. Because all CHM gene mutations are thought to result in absence of REP-1, most cases can be diagnosed by this method 2.

Imaging

Initial approach

- To establish extent of disease and to obtain a baseline for monitoring, obtain the following:
  - Dilated ophthalmologic examination
  - Goldmann visual field testing
  - Electroretinography (ERG)
    - In the early stages, patients may have a nonspecific rod-cone degenerative pattern which eventually becomes non-recordable. Carriers typically have normal ERG studies.

Follow-up & special considerations

Annual exams, along with ERG and visual field testing, may be helpful to follow disease progression.

Diagnostic Procedures/Other

Fluorescein angiography may show large areas of capillary non-perfusion/loss.

Pathological Findings

- Earlier reports suggested choroidal atrophy was the primary event that led to secondary loss of RPE and photoreceptors (4)
- More recent reports suggest independent degeneration of the retina, RPE, and choriocapillaris (5)
- Focal choroidal T-lymphocyte infiltration and retinal gliosis occur, suggesting inflammation may play a role (5)

DIFFERENTIAL DIAGNOSIS

- CHM may be difficult to distinguished from:
  - Retinitis Pigmentosa
  - Diffuse Choriocapillaris Atrophy
  - Gyrate Atrophy of the retina and choroid
  - Usher Syndrome Type I
  - Kearns-Sayre Syndrome

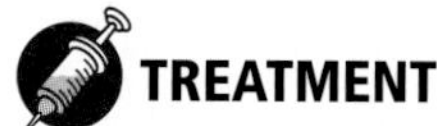

TREATMENT

ADDITIONAL TREATMENT

General Measures

In the future, gene therapy may be effective in delaying progression of CHM. Using a recombinant adenovirus, Anand et al. were able to successfully deliver human cDNA coding for REP-1 to CHM-affected lymphocytes and fibroblasts. It is still uncertain whether or not delivery of REP-1 to retinal cells in CHM patients would stop or slow the progression of CHM, but this was an important first step in gene therapy development for CHM (bib6).

Issues for Referral

- As patient symptoms progress and peripheral and central vision worsen, patients may benefit from referral to a specialist in low vision services to help them learn to optimize residual vision.
- As vision declines, patients may have to cope with multiple social difficulties which may include job loss, loss of independence, and depression. Patients may benefit from referral to appropriate professionals to enable them to better cope with these issues.

Additional Therapies

Precautions from UV exposure may be beneficial, thus affected individuals should wear UV-blocking sunglasses when outdoors (7).

SURGERY/OTHER PROCEDURES

Nearly one-third of affected males are found to have posterior subcapsular cataracts that can be removed as needed.

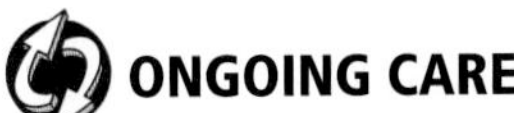

ONGOING CARE

FOLLOW-UP RECOMMENDATIONS

- Patients should be examined periodically, and be monitored for progression with ERG and peripheral visual field analysis.
- Refer for low vision services as indicated.

DIET

- Lutein supplementation (20 mg daily) may be helpful, but this data is weak (8).
- Omega-3 fatty acids, fresh fruit, dark green leafy vegetables, and antioxidant supplements may be beneficial (7).

PATIENT EDUCATION

- Patients and their families should undergo genetic counseling to educate them regarding the X-linked recessive nature of transmission of CHM:
  - A mother of more than 1 affected male is an obligate carrier (A proband with no family history of CHM may have a de novo mutation, and it is appropriate to examine the retina of the mother to look for signs of carrier status.)
  - A carrier mother has a 50% chance of passing on the CHM gene mutation to each offspring; each male child has a 50% chance of having CHM and each female child has a 50% chance of being a CHM carrier.
  - The father of an affected male does not have CHM nor would be a CHM carrier.
  - All daughters of an affected male will receive the abnormal gene and will be CHM carriers, however, it is impossible for an affected male to pass the disease on to his sons.
  - Prenatal testing for at-risk pregnancies is possible using cells obtained from amniocentesis or chorionic villous sampling, however, the disease-causing allele of an affected family member must be identified *prior to* prenatal testing.

PROGNOSIS

- Most affected males will have severely reduced peripheral vision by age 40 years.
- Visual acuity in affected males is typically preserved until later in life, but is also eventually lost, resulting in blindness.
- Most carrier females are asymptomatic, but a small percentage will demonstrate symptoms and exam findings of CHM (typically much more mild than affected males).

COMPLICATIONS

Blindness as disease progresses

REFERENCES

1. Strunnikova NV, Barb J, Sergeev YV, et al. Loss-of-function mutations in Rab escort protein 1 (REP-1) affect intracellular transport in fibroblasts and monocytes in choroideremia patients. *PLoS ONE* 2009;4(12):e8402.
2. MacDonald IM, Mah DY, Ho YK, et al. A practical diagnostic test for choroideremia. *Ophthalmology* 1998;105(9):1637–40.
3. Roberts MF, Fishman GA, Roberts DK, et al. Retrospective, longitudinal, and cross sectional study of visual acuity impairment in choroideraemia. *Br J Ophthalmol* 2002;86(6): 658–62.
4. McCulloch JC. The pathologic findings in two cases of choroideremia. *Trans Am Acad Ophthalmol Otolaryngol* 1950;56:565–72.
5. MacDonald IM, Russel L, Chan CC. Choroideremia: New findings from ocular pathology and review of recent literature. *Surv Ophthalmol* 2009;54(3): 401–07.
6. Anand V, Barral DC, Zeng Y, et al. Gene therapy for choroideremia: In vitro rescue mediated by recombinant adenovirus. *Vision Research* 2000;43:919–26.
7. MacDonald IM, Meltzer MR, Smaoui N, et al. Choroideremia. In: Pagon RA, Bird TC, Dolan CR, Stephens K (eds). GeneReviews, Univ. Of Washington: Seattle, 1993–2003, May 2008 update.
8. Duncan JL, Aleman TS, Gardner LM, et al. Macular pigment and lutein supplementation in choroideremia. *Exp. Eye Res* 2002;74:371–81.

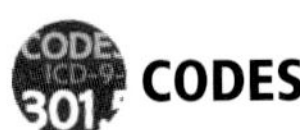

CODES

ICD9

363.55 Choroideremia

CLINICAL PEARLS

- Choroideremia should be considered in patients who present with a history of nyctalopia, peripheral visual field loss, a genetic transmittance pattern consistent with an X-linked recessive disorder, and a characteristic funduscopic appearance of extensive RPE/choroidal atrophy.
- By approximately age 40 years, many affected males will have severely reduced peripheral vision with relative sparing of central acuity into the seventh decade.
- Most female carriers are asymptomatic, but a small number of female carriers may present with symptoms ranging from nyctalopia to visual field loss and with funduscopic findings of peripheral RPE changes and macular RPE mottling.

CHRONIC IRIDOCYCLITIS

Riz Somani
Matthew Tennant

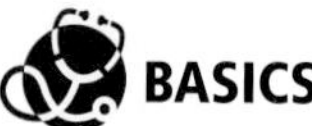

BASICS

DESCRIPTION
- Chronic iridocyclitis typically has an insidious onset and lasts longer than 6 weeks
- Diagnosis may be delayed as it is often asymptomatic
- Bilateral involvement is common

EPIDEMIOLOGY
Incidence
Idiopathic chronic iridocyclitis: 1 case per 300,000 population (1)

Prevalence
Idiopathic chronic iridocyclitis uveitis: 1 case per 14,000 population (1)

RISK FACTORS
Chronic systemic diseases associated with iridocyclitis.

Genetics
Increased prevalence with HLA-A2, *DR8*, *DR11*, *DR12*, *DQA1*0401*, **0501*, **0601*, and *DPB1*0201* in association with early onset pauciarticular juvenile arthritis (2)

GENERAL PREVENTION
Patients at risk of developing chronic iridocyclitis should be routinely screened.

PATHOPHYSIOLOGY
Hallmark is infiltration of leukocytes out of microvasculature and into surrounding inflamed tissue.

ETIOLOGY
- Juvenile idiopathic arthritis (JIA)
- Sarcoidosis
- Fuchs heterochromic iridocyclitis
- Tuberculosis
- Syphilis
- Postsurgical uveitis
- Herpes simplex/zoster
- Ankylosing spondylitis
- Inflammatory bowel disease
- Behçet's disease

DIAGNOSIS

HISTORY
- Many patients are asymptomatic until they develop complications such as cataract and/or band keratopathy
- Questions to ask:
  - Onset and duration of symptoms – usual gradual onset with duration >6 weeks
  - Past episodes/recurrences and response to treatment
  - Review of systems- presence or absence of rash, joint pain, GI symptoms (e.g., bloody diarrhea)

PHYSICAL EXAM
- Red eye with episcleral injection, although, absence of episcleral injection is common
- Aqueous cell and flare
- Keratic precipitates – cellular deposits on corneal endothelium composed of epithelioid cells, lymphocytes, and polymorphs
- Characteristics and distribution provide clues to etiology
  - Fuchs heterochromic iridocyclitis – stellate KP diffusely over entire endothelium
  - Granulomatous disease – Mutton fat KP (large, greasy) usually more inferiorly
  - Iris nodules
  - Koeppe nodules – at pupillary border
  - Busacca – anterior iris stroma
  - Rarely iris crystals
  - Posterior synechiae
  - Peripheral anterior synechiae
  - Granulomatous deposits (Berlin nodules) on trabecular meshwork
  - Band keratopathy – from chronic inflammation
  - Cystoid macular edema
  - Elevated intraocular pressure from trabeculitis or PAS
  - Hypotony can develop in longstanding iridocyclitis

DIAGNOSTIC TESTS & INTERPRETATION
Lab
Initial lab tests
- Screening tests should be tailored to causes of chronic iridocyclitis
- CBC
- JIA – antinuclear antibodies, rheumatoid factor, x-ray of affected joints, HLA typing
- Sarcoidosis – angioconverting enzyme assay (ACE), lysozyme, chest x-ray
- TB – PPD skin test, chest x-ray, QuantiFERON gold
- Syphilis enzyme immunoassay
- HLA typing: Ankylosing spondylitis, inflammatory bowel disease

Follow-Up & Special Considerations
Patients with pauciarticular arthritis should have slit-lamp assessments every 3–4 months for the first 5 years of arthritis onset (3).

Imaging
- Chest x-ray or CT Scan – for TB, sarcoidosis
  - x-ray of affected joints in JIA
  - Gallium scan if indicated- sarcoidosis

Diagnostic Procedures/Other
Anterior chamber tap for PCR testing may be performed to rule out toxoplasmosis, HSV, VZV, TB if no other systemic disease is identified.

DIFFERENTIAL DIAGNOSIS
See "Etiology."

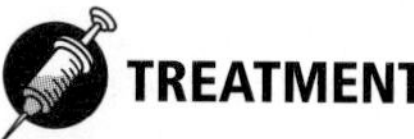

TREATMENT

MEDICATION
First Line
- Topical steroid (prednisolone acetate 1%) frequency varies depending on severity
  - Cycloplegic (scopolamine 0.25% b.i.d or Cyclogyl 1% b.i.d for significant synechiae and/or inflammation)
  - Topical glaucoma therapy if IOP elevated

Second Line
Periocular/subtenons steroid (Triamcinolone acetonide 40 mg) or intravitreal steroid (2–4 mg). Triesence (preservative-free Triamcinolone)

ADDITIONAL TREATMENT
General Measures
- Local therapy for monocular disease – subtenons or intravitreal Kenalog/Triesence
- For bilateral disease consider systemic steroid treatment
- Consider corticosteroid sparing agent if inflammation is not controlled within 6 weeks of therapy initiation

Issues for Referral
- Patients with ocular sarcoidosis should be referred to a Pulmonologist
  - Pediatric patients with chronic iridocyclitis need a Rheumatology evaluation
  - Co-manage systemic steroid sparing agents with Rheumatology

Additional Therapies

- Steroid sparing agents for long term immunosuppression – delayed onset of action – typically 8–12 weeks (4)
  - Immunosuppressive agents requires routine blood work for potential side effects and should be co-managed with a Rheumatologist
  - Antimetabolites – Azathioprine (Imuran), Methotrexate, and Mycophenolate mofetil (CellCept)
  - T-cell inhibitors – Cyclosporine and Tacrolimus
  - Alkylating agents – Cyclophosphamide (Cytoxan) and Chlorambucil (Leukeran)
  - Biologics
  - IL-2 inhibitors – Daclizumab
  - Anti-TNF alpha – Infliximab, Etanercept (Enbrel)
  - Recombinant interferon alpha
  - Antilymphocytic – Rituximab

SURGERY/OTHER PROCEDURES

- Cataract surgery can reactivate or worsen iridocyclitis. Preoperative treatment with systemic steroids 4 days prior to cataract surgery is recommended (5).
  - Ideally uveitis should be inactive for at least 3 months prior to cataract surgery.
  - When medical management of glaucoma fails, consider surgery with tube-shunt.
  - Conventional glaucoma filtration surgery tends to fail in the setting of uveitis.
  - Pars plana vitrectomy with membrane peel when epiretinal membrane present.

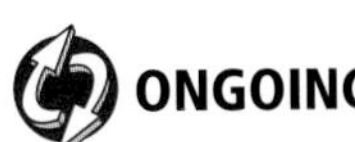

ONGOING CARE

FOLLOW-UP RECOMMENDATIONS

Patient Monitoring

- JIA is often asymptomatic and requires ongoing uveitis screening
  - If the child is <7 years old and ANA positive, screening eye examination every 3–4 months for 4 years, then every 6 months for 3 years, then annually
  - If the child is <7 years old and ANA negative, screening eye exam every 6 months for 4 years, then annually
  - If the child is >7 years old regardless of ANA status, screening eye exam every 6 months for 4 years, then annually

PATIENT EDUCATION

Return immediately if iritis recurs, as early treatment reduces complications.

PROGNOSIS

- Remissions and exacerbations of inflammatory activity are common
  - Reduction in vision can occur secondary to delayed presentation and complications of prolonged iridocyclitis

COMPLICATIONS

- Cataract
- Band keratopathy
- Glaucoma
- Cystoid macular edema
  - Posterior synechiae

REFERENCES

1. Paivonsalo-Hietanen T, Tuominen J, Vaahtoranta-Lehtonen H, et al. Incidence and prevalence of different uveitis entities in Finland. *Acta Ophthalmol Scand* 1997;75(1):76–81.
2. Albert ED, Scholz S. Juvenile arthritis: Genetic update. *Baillieres Clin Rheumatol* 1998;12(2): 209–18.
3. Southwood TR, Ryder CA. Ophthalmological screening in juvenile arthritis: Should the frequency of screening be based on the risk of developing chronic iridocyclitis? *Br J Rheumatol* 1992;31(9): 633–4.
4. Jabs DA, Rosenbaum JT, Foster CS, et al. Guidelines for the use of immunosuppressive drugs in patients with ocular inflammatory disorders: Recommendations of an expert panel. *Am J Ophthalmol* 2000;130:492–513.
5. Levy-Clarke GA, Nussenblatt RB, Smith JA. Management of chronic pediatric uveitis. *Curr Opin Ophthalmol* 2005;16:281–288.

ADDITIONAL READING

- Nussenblatt RB, Whiteup SM. *Uveitis fundamentals and clinical practice*. 3rd ed. Philadelphia, PA, 2004.
- Kanski JJ, Pavesio CE, Tuft SJ. *Ocular inflammatory disease*. Philadelphia, PA, 2006.
- Ehlers JP, Chirag PS (eds). *The Wills eye manual*. 5th ed. Baltimore, MD, 2008.

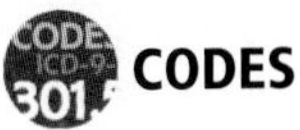

CODES

ICD9

- 364.10 Chronic iridocyclitis, unspecified
- 364.11 Chronic iridocyclitis in diseases classified elsewhere

CLINICAL PEARLS

- Chronic iridocyclitis is most commonly associated with juvenile idiopathic arthritis.
- All children with pauciarticular arthritis should be screened for iridocyclitis every 3–4 months for first 5 years after arthritis onset.
- Systemic treatment is often required to control intraocular inflammation.
- Ocular complications from chronic iridocyclitis are common requiring surgical intervention.
- When possible, ocular inflammation should be controlled for 3 months prior to attempting intraocular surgery.

CHRONIC PROGRESSIVE EXTERNAL OPHTHALMOPLEGIA (CPEO)

Raed Behbehani

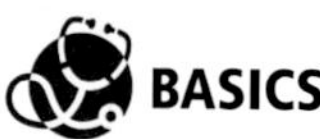

BASICS

DESCRIPTION

- Chronic Progressive External Ophthalmoplegia (CPEO) is a frequent manifestation of mitochondrial cytopathies, a group of disorders characterized by dysfunction of the mitochondria due to mutations in mitochondrial DNA (mtDNA) or in nuclear genomes that code for mitochondrial components.
- CPEO is not a nosologic entity and is only a sign in the clinical spectrum of mitochondrial cytopathies, in which the heart, central nervous system, and endocrine disturbances can occur.
- Kearns-Sayers syndrome (KSS) is a clinical phenotype of mitochondrial cytopathy defined as CPEO and pigmentary retinopathy before the age of 20 years and at least one of the following: Complete heart block, high CSF protein (>1 mg/mL), cerebellar ataxia, and endocrine disturbances.

ALERT

Cardiac conduction defects can be lethal and should be ruled out in patients with suspected CPEO, especially KSS.

EPIDEMIOLOGY

Incidence

CPEO typically have an onset in childhood or early adolescence but they can occur at any age.

RISK FACTORS

Genetics

- Most cases of CPEO are due to **sporadic** single mutations in the mitochondrial DNA occurring during the maternal oocyte stage, which is propagated to all future mtDNA during embryogenesis. These single large mutations cause large gene rearrangements in mitochondrial DNA (1).
- **Autosomal dominant** and **autosomal recessive** forms of inheritance (nuclear inheritance) are less frequent and some nuclear genes have been implicated including TP, ANTI, Twinkle, POLG1, POLG2, and OPA1 (2).
- Cells have multiple mitochondria, which can have different variations in mutant and wild-type mtDNA. This condition is referred to as **heteroplasmy** and occurs because of the non-random nature of mtDNA replication.
- When a certain tissue reaches a certain ratio of mutant versus wild-type mitochondria, a disease will present itself (**threshold expression).**
- Tissues high in energy demand such as the heart, central nervous system, skeletal muscles have low tissue-specific threshold of expression.

PATHOPHYSIOLOGY

- The mitochondria is responsible for production of ATP by oxidative phosphorylation, the detoxification of reactive oxygen species, regulation of cell apoptosis, and other functions such iron metabolism, fatty acid oxidation, and amino acid biosynthesis.
- The protein complexes carrying out oxidative phosphorylation are partly encoded by mitochondrial genome (complex I, III, IV, ATP synthetase) and complex II is encoded exclusively by nuclear genome.
- The majority of mitochondrial proteins are encoded by nuclear genome and are transported into the mitochondria. Therefore, nuclear gene mutation can result in mitochondrial dysfunction.

COMMONLY ASSOCIATED CONDITIONS

- Mitochondrial encephalopathy with lactic acidosis and stroke-like episodes (MELAS)
  - A phenotype characterized by the triad of 1) stroke-like episodes before the age of 40, 2) encephalopathy with seizures or dementia and, 3) lactic acidosis and/or ragged red fibers
  - 79% of patients with MELAS will have homonymous hemianopsia due involvement of the retrochiasmal visual pathways in the occipital and parietal lobes.
- Mitochondrial neurogastrointestinal encephalomyopathy (MNGIE)
  - Autosomal recessive CPEO in association with peripheral neuropathy, leukoencephalopathy and gastrointestinal symptoms (nausea, vomiting, diarrhea)
- Myelonic epilepsy with ragged-red fibers (MERRF)
- Progressive myoclonic epilepsy, ataxia, optic atrophy, and/or dementia

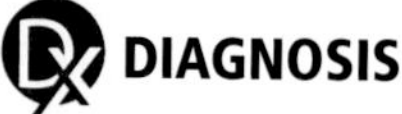

DIAGNOSIS

HISTORY

- Progressive ptosis.
- Muscle weakness (limbs)
- Decreased vision and night blindness.
- Hearing loss
- Imbalance
- Short stature/skeletal abnormalities
- Seizures or stroke-like episodes.
- Absence of family history does not exclude CPEO

PHYSICAL EXAM

- Ptosis
- Symmetric ophthalmoplegia sparing the pupils
- Facial/limb weakness
- Pigmentary (salt-pepper) retinopathy in KSS
- Ataxia
- Deafness

DIAGNOSTIC TESTS & INTERPRETATION

Lab

Initial lab tests

- Blood
  - Routine blood tests (CBC and electrolytes) and endocrine work up (Hb A1c, TSH, thyroxine)
  - Serum creatinine kinase and resting lactate can be elevated
  - Acetylcholine receptor antibodies to rule out myasthenia gravis
- CSF
  - High CSF protein in KSS (>1 mg/mL) and high lactate in MELAS
  - Electrocardiography to rule out cardiac conduction defects and cardiac hypertrophy are essential in all cases of suspected CPEO

Follow-Up & Special Considerations

- Electroretinography (ERG)
  - In pigmentary retinopathy in KSS, ERG can be normal or show rod, cone, or mixed rod-cone dysfunction.

Imaging

- Neuroimaging of the orbit and brain is recommended to rule out other causes of ophthalmoplegia.
  - MRI of the orbits: Thin extraocular muscles
  - MRI of the brain: White matter and basal ganglia hyperintensities (KSS), cortical and cerebellar atrophy (3)
  - MR spectroscopy: Large lactate peaks within the stroke-like lesions (MELAS)

Diagnostic Procedures/Other

- Skeletal muscle biopsy
  - The gold standard test for diagnosis
  - Staining with Gomori Trichrome stain will show ragged-red fibers in 50% of cases of CPEO.
  - Biochemical stains for mitochondrial respiratory chain (I,II,IV) to show defects in oxidative phosphorylation enzymes
  - Polymerase chain reaction (PCR) has been recently used to detect mutations in swabbed buccal cells.

Pathological Findings

- Ragged-red fibers are classic histological hallmarks of CPEO and represent large accumulation of enlarged mitochondria beneath the sarcolemma.
- Transmission electron microscopy can show paracrystalline ("parking-lot") inclusions inside the abnormal mitochondria.

DIFFERENTIAL DIAGNOSIS

- Myogenic ptosis
  - Congenital fibrosis syndrome
  - Congenital myopathy (Myotonic dystrophy)
  - Oculopharyngeal dystropy
- Neuromuscular disease
  - Myasthenia Gravis

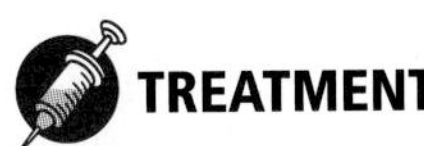

TREATMENT

MEDICATION

First Line

- There is no known effective treatment for CPEO and treatment is mainly symptomatic.
  - Surgical treatment of severe ptosis can be beneficial in patients with CPEO. Lid surgery should be done with care since Bell's phenomenon is often weak, which can result in exposure keratopathy.
  - Strabismus surgery can be offered to patients suffering from diplopia.

Second Line

- Treatment of endocrine disturbances such as hyperglycemia with anti-hyperglycemic agents
- Cardiac conduction defects should be treated with pacemakers.
- Seizures can be treated with anti-epileptics.
- Cochlear implant can be offered to patients with neurosensory deafness.

ADDITIONAL TREATMENT

Issues for Referral

Cardiac and endocrinological manifestations can be serious and should be managed by specialists.

COMPLEMENTARY & ALTERNATIVE THERAPIES

Non-proven measures such as the supplementation of vitamins (vitamin C, thiamine, B12, vitamin E), cofactors (Coenzyme q10) can be provided and they are not toxic in their usual doses. (4)

SURGERY/OTHER PROCEDURES

Ptosis/strabismus surgery.

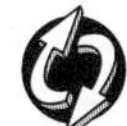

ONGOING CARE

PATIENT EDUCATION

- Avoidance of mitochondrial stressors (tobacco, excessive alcohol intake) is a nonspecific, yet prudent recommendation.
- Genetic counseling
  - Most cases of CPEO are due to sporadic mutations with only 4% risk of transmission from mother to child.
  - Men and women with nuclear DNA mutations need to be counseled about the risk of transmission depending on the mode of inheritance.
  - Men with mitochondrial mutations need to be reassured that they cannot transmit the disease to their offspring.

PROGNOSIS

Course: Chronic, slowly progressive.

COMPLICATIONS

- Cardiac conduction defects
- Endocrine disturbances

REFERENCES

1. Cardaioli E, da Pozzo P, Malfatti E, et al. Chronic progressive external ophthalmoplegia: A new heteroplasmic tRNA Leu (CUN) mutation of mitochondrial DNA. *J Neuro Sci* 2008;272:106–9.
2. Ammati-Bonneau P, Valentino ML, Reynier P, et al. OPA1 mutations induce mitochondrial DNA instability and optic atrophy 'plus' phenotype. *Brain* 2008;131:338–51.
3. Barragán-Campos HM, Vallée JN, Lô D, et al. Brain magnetic resonance imaging findings in patients with mitochondrial cytopathies. *Arch Neurol* 2005;62:737–42.
4. Rotig A, Appelkvist EL, Geromel V, et al. Quinine-responsive multiple respiratory chain dysfunction due to widespread coenzyme q10 deficiency. *Lancet* 2000;356:391–5.

ADDITIONAL READING

- Fraser JA, Biousse V, Newman NJ. The Neuro-ophthalmology of mitochondrial disease. *Surv Ophthalmol* 2010;55(4):299–334.

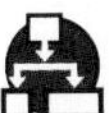

See Also (Topic, Algorithm, Electronic Media Element)

- The United Mitochondrial disease foundation. www.umdf.org

CODES

ICD9

378.72 Progressive external ophthalmoplegia

CLINICAL PEARLS

- Bilateral symmetric ptosis can precede ophthalmoplegia by many years and can the only initial sign of CPEO.
- Patients with CPEO do not usually complain of diplopia despite limitation of ocular movement since the ophthalmoplegia is often quite symmetric.
- Mitochondrial cytopathies have a wide spectrum of clinical manifestations involving many organs and significant overlap between different phenotypes can occur.

CICATRICIAL PEMPHIGOID (CP)/MUCOUS MEMBRANE PEMPHIGOID (MMP)

Nicole R. Fram

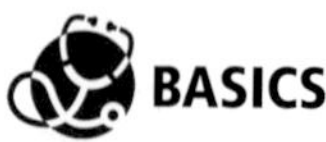

BASICS

DESCRIPTION

- Mucous membrane pemphigoid (MMP) or cicatricial pemphigoid (CP) encompasses a number of systemic autoimmune diseases that involve cicatrization or scarring of mucous membranes and the skin. Traditionally, when there is primarily ocular involvement the term ocular cicatrizing pemphigoid (OCP) is used (1).
  - Extraocular mucosal involvement: Oral (up to >60%), nasal mucosa, sinuses, pharynx, larynx, esophagus, bowel, anus, urethra, and genitals.

EPIDEMIOLOGY

Incidence

- 1/15,000–1/16,000 (possibly an underestimation as these are advanced cases at the time of diagnosis) (2)
- Mean age of onset sixth to seventh decade (2)
- 2:1 female:male ratio (2)

RISK FACTORS

- Increased incidence of autoimmune disease such as rheumatoid arthritis (17%) (2)
- Mean duration of symptoms to diagnosis is 2.8 years.

Genetics

Increased frequency in HLA-DR4 and HLA-Dqw3 (3).

PATHOPHYSIOLOGY

- Systemic autoimmune disease where circulating antibodies bind to antigens of the basement membrane zone (BMZ), activating a complement cascade, recruitment of inflammatory cells and hydrolytic enzymes leading to digestion of the lamina lucida and activation of fibroblasts with eventual scar tissue formation (1,4)
- Linear deposition of antibodies IgG, IgA, or C3 along the epithelial BMZ

ETIOLOGY

- Idiopathic autoimmune disease
- "Pseudopemphigoid": Medication induced (see Differential Diagnosis)

COMMONLY ASSOCIATED CONDITIONS

- Cicatrizing conjunctivitis
- Skin involvement
- Desquamative gingivitis
- Esophageal or laryngeal involvement may be fatal if adhesions and/or strictures develop.

DIAGNOSIS

HISTORY

- Targeted history of onset, duration, location, quality of symptoms, associated conditions, and oral/topical medications. Early ocular symptoms include redness, foreign body sensation, burning, tearing, and mucus discharge.
- **Review of systems (ROS):**
  - **Skin/Mucocutaneous:** Rash on face, scalp, or extremities (flat erythematous plaques) or inguinal area (small vesicobullous lesions), oral ulcers, bleeding gums (desquamative gingivitis)
  - **ENT:** New onset sinus disease, epistaxis (nose bleeds)
  - **Respiratory:** Hoarseness or dysphonia (laryngeal/vocal cords), laryngeal adhesions, and strictures causing difficulty breathing (tracheostomy)
  - **Gastrointestinal:** Dysphagia, heartburn
  - **Genitourinary:** Genital ulcers

PHYSICAL EXAM

Classic signs include:

- In early disease, nonspecific papillary conjunctivitis, conjunctival vesicles and ulcers, fine ("lacy") subepithelial scarring on tarsal conjunctiva, shrinkage of inferior fornix, and symblepharon formation, trichiasis, corneal scarring. In later disease, obliteration of fornix and lacrimal gland ductules, and keratinization of ocular surface.
- Stages (Foster/Mondino)[2,5]
  - Stage I: Subepithelial fibrosis
  - Stage II: Fornix
    - a) 0–25%
    - b) 25–50%
    - c) 50–75%
    - d) 75–100%
  - Stage III: Symblepharon
    - a) 0–25%
    - b) 25–50%
    - c) 50–75%
    - d) >75% involvement of symblepharon
  - Stage IV: Ankyloblepharon & keratinization
- **External exam:** Rashes and oral ulcers
- **Eyelids:** Keratinization of lid margin, trichiasis, distichiasis, scarring of meibomian glands, entropion, lagophthalmos, and ankyloblepharon
- **Conjunctiva/Sclera:** Papillary conjunctivitis, conjunctival vesicles, and ulcers, subepithelial conjunctival fibrosis (use red-free broad beam on slit-lamp), limbitis, shrinkage of inferior/superior fornix, symblepharon, obliteration of lacrimal gland ductules (late), keratinization (late)
- **Cornea:** Punctate epithelial keratitis, epithelial defect, corneal ulcer, neovascularization or scarring, keratinization, perforation
- Remainder of anterior and posterior segment examination typically unremarkable

DIAGNOSTIC TESTS & INTERPRETATION

Lab

Direct immunofluorescence (DIF) microscopy or immunoperoxidase.

- Sensitivity DIF alone: 52% (5)
- Sensitivity DIF and immunoperoxidase: 83% (5)
- Specimen incubated with fluorescein labeled anti-human immunoglobulins directed at IgA, IgG, IgM, IgD, IgE, C3, C4, and fibrinogen

Diagnostic Procedures/Other

- **Gold Standard:** Conjunctival biopsy
  - Choose an area of inflamed conjunctiva adjacent to limbus in interpalpebral fissure. Do not perform biopsy in fornix–can promote symblepharon formation
  - Place topical anesthetic drop and apply cotton swab soaked with 4% lidocaine over the intended area for conjunctival biopsy. Inject 0.5 cc of 2% lidocaine with epinephrine subconjunctivally and excise 1.5 × 1.5 mm area of conjunctiva for biopsy. Must be processed fresh (no formalin) (1)

Pathological Findings

- A line of homogenous linear fluorescence at the BMZ
- Eosinophils may be found on conjunctival scrapings

DIFFERENTIAL DIAGNOSIS

Cicatrizing conjunctivitis (1)

- Infectious conjunctivitis:
  - Bacterial (*Corynebacterium diphtheriae*, Beta-hemolytic streptococcus, *Neisseria gonorrhea*)
  - Viral (Adenovirus (8&19), Herpes Simplex Conjunctivitis)
  - Chlamydia (Trachoma, *Lymphogranuloma venereum*)
- Medication Induced: "Pseudopemphigoid"
  - Systemic: Practolol, D-penicillinamine
  - Topical: Epinephrine, Echothiophate iodide, Pilocarpine, Idoxuridine
- Dermatobullous:
  - Toxic Epidermal Necrolysis
  - Dermatitis Herpetiformis
  - Epidermolysis bullosa
  - Pemphigus vulgaris
  - Linear IgA
  - Porphyria cutanea tarda
- Autoimmune
  - Graft—versus–host disease
  - OCP
  - Sjögren's syndrome
  - Stevens-Johnson Syndrome
  - Systemic lupus erythematosus

- Trauma
  - Chemical/thermal burn
  - Conjunctival surgery
  - Radiation
- Other
  - Atopic Keratoconjunctivitis
  - Rosacea blepharoconjunctivitis
  - Ligneous conjunctivitis
  - Sarcoidosis
  - Paraneoplastic ocular cicatricial pemphigoid (POCP)

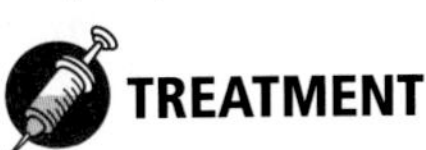

TREATMENT

Overall Approach to Treatment (1)

- Address systemic findings and consult Internal Medicine and/or Dermatology depending on comorbidities
- Initiate systemic treatment with immunosuppressives and consult Rheumatology or Hematology/Oncology for dosage/patient monitoring
- Management of local eyelid and ocular surface disease

MEDICATION

- Begin systemic chemotherapy when conjunctival/oral mucosa biopsy proven or overwhelming clinical suspicion with documented progression of conjunctival scarring and/or symblepharon
- Prior to initiation of any systemic therapy, obtain baseline CBC, liver enzymes, Basic Metabolic panel, Hepatitis panel, Urinalysis, pregnancy test, or sperm banking (if applicable).

First Line

- **Mild Disease: Dapsone,** a sulfone derivative, for early, active but non-progressive disease
- Least effective treatment. Should discontinue if no result after 4 weeks and switch to cyclophosphamide

ALERT
Dapsone should not be used in patients with sulfa allergy. Prior to initiation, **test for G6PD deficiency** (severe hemolytic anemia with dapsone). Side effects include nausea, abdominal pain, hepatitis, and peripheral neuropathy.

- **Moderate to severe disease: Cyclophosphamide** ± oral corticosteroids while waiting for cyclophosphamide to take effect. Must taper oral steroids over 1–2 months due to adverse side effects (bone loss, GI bleeding, hyperglycemia, adrenal suppression). Oral prednisone alone is not appropriate treatment for OCP and can confound overall therapeutic goal secondary to leukocytosis.
- Therapeutic treatment goal is a WBC count between 3,000–4,000. Typical starting dose is 75 mg PO q daily. Patients should drink large amounts of water to minimize bladder side effects. Treatment should be continued for at least 9 months before tapering. Consult Rheumatology or Hematology/Oncology for assistance with dosage and monitoring (1).

ALERT
Cyclophosphamide side effects include anemia, alopecia, anovulation, azoospermia, hemorrhagic cystitis (bone marrow suppression), bladder cancer.

Second Line

Methotrexate, Mycophenolate, Azathioprine, Cyclosporin A, IVIG, Biologics (see additional reading).

ADDITIONAL TREATMENT

General Measures

Treatment of local eyelid disease:

- **Trichiasis/Distichiasis:** Epilation with electrolysis or permanent surgical removal
- **Keratinization of the eyelid margin:** Keratinization can lead to colonization of bacteria and subsequent microbial keratitis. Topical Vitamin A (all-*trans*retinoic acid) ointment 0.01% to the eyelids q.h.s–q.i.d will reduce keratinization

COMPLEMENTARY & ALTERNATIVE THERAPIES

- Treatment of blepharitis/meibomian gland dysfunction; consider oral doxycycline, topical antibiotics, lid hygiene)
- Punctal occlusion if Schirmer testing without anesthesia <2 mm

SURGERY/OTHER PROCEDURES

- **Fornix reconstruction/Lagophthalmos:** Can perform eyelid procedure and/or mucous membrane graft (buccal)/amniotic membrane graft if eye is quiet and on patient is on systemic immunosuppression
- **Entropion:** Only perform when eye is quiet and patient is on systemic immunosuppression
- **Corneal transplantation/Permanent Keratoprosthesis:** For successful corneal transplantation, disease should be quiet and the patient should be on systemic therapy. Further, patient must have adequate tear production with functioning stem cells for re-epithelialization. Permanent keratoprosthesis may be considered in patients with adequate tear production and stem cell deficiency.

ALERT
Any surgical procedure may trigger acute exacerbation of disease. Therefore, all procedures (eyelid, conjunctival, cataract, or corneal) should be performed while patient is quiet and on systemic immunosuppression.

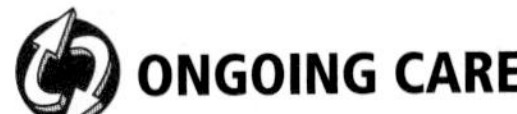

ONGOING CARE

FOLLOW-UP RECOMMENDATIONS

Patient Monitoring

- Monitor with regular exams and anterior segment photographs for progression
- Serial bacterial conjunctival cultures to evaluate overpopulation/colonization with bacteria that may lead to microbial keratitis

PROGNOSIS

Depends on stage of disease at presentation. High clinical suspicion, early diagnosis, and appropriate therapy can reduce morbidity.

REFERENCES

1. Holsclaw DS. Ocular cicatricial pemphigoid. *Int Ophthalmol Clin* 1998;38:89–106. [A]
2. Foster CS. Cicatricial pemphigoid. *Trans Am Ophthalmol Soc* 1986;84:527–663. [A]
3. Zaltas MM, Ahmed AR, Foster CS. Association of HLA-DR4 with ocular cicatricial phemphigoid. *Curr Eye Res* 1989;8:184. [A]
4. Mondino BJ, Brown SI. Ocular cicatricial pemphigoid. *Ophthalmology* 1981;88:95–100. [A]
5. Power WJ, Neves RA, Rodriguez A, Dutt JE, Foster CS. Increasing the diagnostic yield of conjunctival biopsy in patients with suspected ocular cicatricial pemphigoid. *Ophthalmology* 1995;102(8): 1158–63. [A]

ADDITIONAL READING

- Roat MI, Sossi G, Lo CY, et al. Hyperproliferation of conjunctival fibrobroblasts from patients with cicatricial pemphigoid. *Arch Ophthalmol* 1989;107: 1064–1067. [A]
- Saw VPJ, Dart JKG, Rauz S, et al. Immunosuppressive therapy for ocular mucous membrane pemphigoid strategies and outcomes. *Ophthalmology* 2008;115(2):253–261. [A]
- Sami N, Letko E, Androudi S, Daoud Y, Foster CS, Ahmed AR. Intravenous immunoglobulin therapy in patients with ocular cicatricial pemphigoid: A long-term follow-up. *Ophthalmology* 2004; 111:1380–1382. [A]

See Also (Topic, Algorithm, Electronic Media Element)

- Conjunctivitis

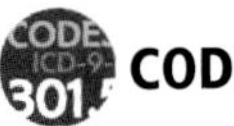

CODES

ICD9

- 372.63 Symblepharon
- 694.60 Benign mucous membrane pemphigoid without mention of ocular involvement
- 694.61 Benign mucous membrane pemphigoid with ocular involvement

CLINICAL PEARLS

- Early signs: Papillary conjunctivitis, trichiasis, subepithelial scarring of tarsal conjunctiva, fornix foreshortening, and corneal scarring
- Later signs: Symblepharon, entropion, lagophthalmos, keratinization, and ankyloblepharon

CLINICALLY SIGNIFICANT DIABETIC MACULAR EDEMA (CSME)

Mimi Liu

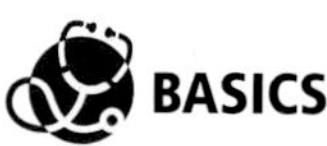

BASICS

DESCRIPTION

- The Early Treatment Diabetic Retinopathy Study (EDTRS) defined CSME as one of the 3 following criteria:
  - 1) Any retinal thickening within 500 microns of the center of the fovea
  - 2) Hard exudates within 500 microns of the center of the fovea, which has adjacent retinal thickening
  - 3) Retinal thickening at least 1 disc area in size, any part of which is within 1 disc diameter of the center of the fovea
- CSME may be focal or diffuse:
  - Focal CSME is caused primarily by focal leakage from individual microaneurysms or small clusters of microaneurysms and dilated retinal capillaries.
  - Diffuse CSME is characterized by generalized leakage from the posterior retinal capillary bed due to a generalized breakdown of the inner blood-retinal barrier.

EPIDEMIOLOGY

Incidence

- CSME is the leading cause of visual loss in diabetic patients.
- Up to 4% of all patients with diabetes will develop CSME during their lifetime.

The Wisconsin Epidemiologic Study of Diabetic Retinopathy (WESDR) showed that the 4 year incidence of CSME was 4.3%, 5.1%, and 1.3% in type I, insulin-treated type II, and non-insulin-treated type II patients respectively. The 10-year incidence was 20.1%, 25.4%, and 13.9% respectively. The 25 year incidence of CSME in type I diabetes was 17% (1).

Prevalence

Approximately 500,000 Americans have CSME.

RISK FACTORS

- Duration of diabetes
- Poor glycemic, blood pressure, and blood lipid control
- In adult onset diabetes, the use of insulin is a risk factor
- Proteinuria and nephropathy
- Level of diabetic retinopathy (CSME occurs in 3% mild non-proliferative diabetic retinopathy (NPDR) versus in 71% of patients with proliferative diabetic retinopathy (PDR)

Pregnancy Considerations

- Diabetic retinopathy and clinically significant diabetic macular edema (CSME) may accelerate during pregnancy. Consider a dilated eye examination and optimization of glucose control prior to pregnancy
- Dilated exam is recommended during the first trimester, then every 1–3 months thereafter, depending on the severity of the retinopathy. Retinopathy usually returns to baseline at 9–12 months postpartum

Genetics

Although there is a higher incidence of diabetic retinopathy in certain ethnic groups, diet and lifestyle factors outweigh these risks.

GENERAL PREVENTION

- Diabetic control – Glycosylated hemoglobin [HbA1c] should be less than 7%
- Control of systemic hypertension
- Normalization of triglycerides and lipids
- Regular exercise

PATHOPHYSIOLOGY

- Chronic hyperglycemia causes breakdown of the blood retinal barrier by a number of metabolic and cellular alterations:
  - Accumulation of polyols and advanced glycosylation end products
  - Overproduction of reactive oxygen intermediates
  - Pathologic activation of protein kinase C
  - Increased expression of multiple cytokines (VEGF, PDGF, TNF-a, and others)
  - Thickening of the basement membrane, loss of pericytes, and increased leukostasis
  - Diabetics are thought to be in a chronic state of subclinical inflammation

ETIOLOGY

- Chronic hyperglycemia
- Vitreomacular traction may contribute to the development of CSME.

DIAGNOSIS

HISTORY

- Duration and control of diabetes
- Insulin dependent?
- History of hypertension or hyperlipidemia?
- Renal insufficiency?

PHYSICAL EXAM

- CSME is a clinical diagnosis
- Macular thickening is visualized by slit-lamp biomicroscopy (contact lens exam may aid in diagnosis)
- Note the severity of diabetic retinopathy
- Note presence of vitreomacular interface abnormalities

DIAGNOSTIC TESTS & INTERPRETATION

Lab

Evaluation of Hb A1C, blood pressure and blood lipids, and renal function (BUN and creatinine).

Imaging

Initial approach

- Fluorescein angiography is not required for the diagnosis of CSME.
- Fluorescein angiography is obtained for the
- following reasons:
  - To rule out central macular ischemia
  - To identify the leaking microaneurysms
  - To identify areas of diffuse capillary leakage
  - To identify areas of capillary nonperfusion elsewhere in the macula
- Color stereo fundus photographs are useful to monitor long-term retinal changes.
- Optical coherence tomography is very helpful to rule out macular pucker/epiretinal membrane, vitreomacular traction, and to monitor response to therapy.

Follow-up & special considerations

- Close follow-up (every 1–3 months) while actively treating CSME.
- Continued monitoring is critical as CSME is frequently a chronic process.
- Regular communication and coordination of care with primary care provider and/or endocrinologist.

Pathological Findings
- Thickening of the basement membrane, loss of pericytes, and decreased cellularity of endothelium
- Accumulation of fluid can be extracellular or intracellular (Muller cells)

DIFFERENTIAL DIAGNOSIS
- Exudative ARMD
- Retinal vein occlusions
- Hypertensive retinopathy
- Cystoid macular edema, Irvine-Gass
- Uveitis
- Macular pucker
- Radiation retinopathy

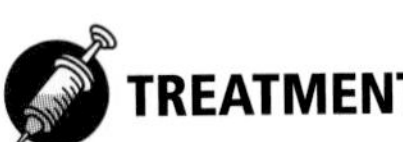

TREATMENT

MEDICATION
First Line
- Control of blood glucose, blood pressure, and lipids
- Focal laser photocoagulation

Second Line
- As of the summer of 2010, none of the following are FDA approved treatments for CSME.
- Intravitreal anti-VEGF agents (ranibizumab, bevacizumab) alone or in combination with laser treatment may be superior to laser alone (2)[A], (3)[A].
- Intravitreal steroids may be a useful adjunct but when used alone are inferior to focal laser (4)[A]. However, among patients with poor visual acuity at baseline (approximately 20/200 or worse), intravitreal triamcinolone 4 mg was associated with better visual acuity outcomes than photocoagulation (4)[A].
- Periocular steroids may be used in cases of severe CSME, but is less effective than intravitreal steroids.
- Various sustained release steroid implants (Retisert, Iluvien, Posurdex, I-vation) are in clinical trials.
- Additional pharmacotherapy agents are currently under investigation.
  - Aflibercept (VEGF Trap-Eye) is a recombinant fusion protein active against all VEGF-A isoforms and placental growth factor.
  - Sirolimus (rapamycin) is a macrolide antifungal with anti-VEGF activity.

ADDITIONAL TREATMENT
Issues for Referral
Consider referral to a vitreoretinal specialist, especially if there is diffuse CSME or CSME with vitreomacular interface abnormalities.

Additional Therapies
Fenofibrate, a fibric acid derivative with lipid modifying effects, may reduce the need for laser treatment for CSME in diabetic patients.

SURGERY/OTHER PROCEDURES
- Consider vitrectomy with membrane peeling for CSME (without refractory to laser and pharmacotherapy
- Membrane peeling (both epiretinal membrane and internal limiting membrane) may benefit patients with CSME and taut posterior hyaloid and/or macular pucker (5)[B].

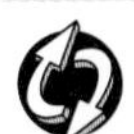

ONGOING CARE

FOLLOW-UP RECOMMENDATIONS
Dilated eye exam every 3–4 months for severe NPDR and PDR.

DIET
ADA diet

PROGNOSIS
- 24% of patients with CSME will develop moderate visual loss (doubling of the visual angle) in 3 years.
- Focal laser photocoagulation reduces the risk of vision loss by 50%.
- Newer therapies and combination therapies may further improve visual outcome in patients with CSME.

REFERENCES

1. Klein R, Knudtson MD, Lee KE, et al. The Wisconsin Epidemiologic Study of Diabetic Retinopathy XXIII: The twenty-five-year incidence of macular edema in persons with type 1 diabetes. *Ophthalmology* 2009;116:497–503.
2. Elman MJ, Aiello LP, Beck RW, et al. Randomized trial evaluating ranibizumab plus prompt or deferred laser or triamcinolone plus prompt laser for diabetic macular edema. *Ophthalmology* 2010;117(6):1064–1077.e35.
3. The Diabetic Retinopathy Clinical Research Network. Randomized trial evaluating ranibizumab plus prompt or deferred laser or triamcinolone plus prompt laser for diabetic macular edema. *Ophthalmology* 2010 Apr 22. Epub ahead of print.
4. Beck RW, Edwards AR, Aiello LP, et al. Diabetic retinopathy clinical research network three-year follow-up of a randomized trial comparing focal/grid photocoagulation and intravitreal triamcinolone for diabetic macular edema. *Arch Ophthalmol* 2009;127:245–51.
5. Diabetic Retinopathy Clinical Research Network. Vitrectomy outcomes in eyes with diabetic macular edema and vitreomacular traction. *Ophthalmology* 2010;117(6):1087–1093.e3.

ADDITIONAL READING

- Early Treatment Diabetic Retinopathy Study research group. Photocoagulation for diabetic macular edema. Early treatment diabetic retinopathy study report number 1. *Arch Ophthalmology* 1985;103: 1796–806.
- Schwartz SG, Flynn HW Jr, Scott IU. Pharmacotherapy for diabetic retinopathy. *Expert Opin Pharmacother* 2009;10(7):1123–31.
- Keech AC, Mitchell P, Summanen PA, et al. Effect of fenofibrate on the need for laser treatment for diabetic retinopathy (FIELD study): A randomized controlled trial. *Lancet* 2007;370:1687–97.

CODES

ICD9
- 250.50 Diabetes mellitus with ophthalmic manifestations, type ii or unspecified type, not stated as uncontrolled
- 362.01 Background diabetic retinopathy
- 362.83 Retinal edema

CLINICAL PEARLS
- Strict control of blood glucose, blood pressure, and lipids are essential in the prevention and management of CSME and diabetic retinopathy.
- Focal/grid laser photocoagulation remains the standard of care for CSME.
- Numerous pharmacological therapies are in clinical trials and may offer improved outcomes in patients with CSME.

COLOBOMA

Irina Belinsky
Jonathan H. Salvin

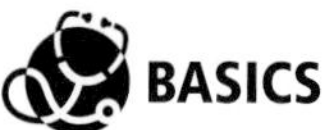

BASICS

DESCRIPTION

- Congenital coloboma (plural: "colobomata") is a defect manifesting as a cleft or gap due to the incomplete closure of the fetal (choroidal) fissure:
  - Unilateral or bilateral, typically located in the inferonasal quadrant
  - Isolated or associated with other intraocular anomalies or multisystem anomalies

EPIDEMIOLOGY

- 2.6 per 10,000 births in the USA (1)[C]

RISK FACTORS

- Microphthalmia:
  - Numerous genetic defects, chromosomal aberrations, systemic syndromes
  - Possibly teratogens, such as thalidomide and alcohol
  - Prenatal vitamin A deficiency has also been implicated

Genetics

- Key coloboma-associated disease genes include *Sonic hedgehog* (*SHH*), *PAX6, MAF1, CHX10, OTX2, CHD7* (*CHARGE syndrome*), *GDF6, CRYAA*, and *DPD*:
  - 15% cases are isolated, 58% occur in conjunction with other congenital anomalies, and 27% as part of a well-defined multisystem syndrome (5)[C].
  - Isolated forms are most often sporadic, but can be autosomal dominant, autosomal recessive, or X-linked recessive (least common).
  - Most common multisystem syndrome is CHARGE (MIM 214800) (6)[C].
  - Syndromic forms can be autosomal dominant (i.e., Papillorenal syndrome, *PAX2, isolated optic nerve "coloboma"*), autosomal recessive (i.e., Meckel–Gruber syndrome, *MKS1*), X-linked recessive (i.e., Lenz microphthalmia syndrome, *BCOR*), or X-linked dominant (i.e., Goltz focal dermal hypoplasia).

GENERAL PREVENTION

- Genetic counseling and/or prenatal testing (if gene mutation or syndrome known in family):
  - Avoidance of in utero exposures to teratogens

PATHOPHYSIOLOGY

- Failure of the fetal fissure to close during the 5th to 7th week of gestation:
  - Primary defect is a failure of closure of the retinal pigmented epithelium resulting in the failure of neural crest differentiation of underlying choroid, and dysplastic differentiation of overlying sensory retina (intercalary membrane), or a complete absence of overlying iris.
  - Timing of the defect may explain the associations with specific systemic malformations.

ETIOLOGY

- Multiple genetic mutations and chromosomal defects have been identified:
  - Infection or teratogen exposure in utero
  - Intrauterine vitamin A deficiency
  - Idiopathic

COMMONLY ASSOCIATED CONDITIONS

- Microphthalmia with or without cyst:
  - Visual field defect (superior scotoma)
  - Nystagmus
  - Lens notch may be present due to deficient zonules in the area of ciliary body coloboma (there is no true lens coloboma).
  - Other systemic malformations (6)[C]

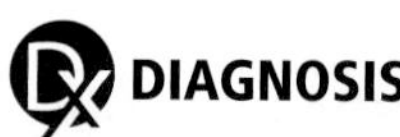

DIAGNOSIS

HISTORY

- Detailed family history of coloboma or related congenital ocular disease (family members may have asymptomatic coloboma) pregnancy and birth history, known exposure to infection or teratogen in utero:
  - Other known associated systemic anomalies
  - May have history of leukocoria

PHYSICAL EXAM

- Vision assessment.
- Slit-lamp exam and indirect ophthalmoscopy (with general anesthesia as needed):
  - Iris coloboma will appear as a pupil notch in the inferonasal quadrant ("keyhole" pupil). It may have mild forms with absent collarette or deficient iris stroma in the same quadrant.
  - Chorioretinal coloboma appears as a sharply demarcated, white, excavation in the fundus. It may have overlying retinal vessels or hyperpigmented edges.
  - Strabismus and nystagmus assessment
  - Assess visual fields for superior scotoma
  - Perform accurate refraction, as risk of amblyopia is high
  - Assess for retinal detachment
  - Assess for the presence of foveal reflex when macula involved
  - Thorough systemic examination for other anomalies
  - Full dilated exam and careful iris slit lamp of family members

DIAGNOSTIC TESTS & INTERPRETATION

Lab

Initial lab tests

- Karyotype and microarray if systemic abnormalities not in keeping with a recognizable syndrome
- Specific genetic analysis based on the clinical diagnosis of systemic syndrome

Follow-up & special considerations

- Genetics consult

Imaging

Initial approach

- Ultrasound to confirm coloboma and assess for the presence of orbital cyst if not clinically apparent:
  - A scan for axial length and possible microphthalmia
  - Brain MRI to assess for CNS pathology especially if bilateral optic nerve involvement

Follow-up & special considerations

- Radiographs, echocardiogram, and audiology evaluation as indicated in some cases:
  - Examine every 6 months for retinal detachment (NOTE: Breaks will be in intercalary membrane within coloboma)

Diagnostic Procedures/Other

- Genetic counseling and molecular genetic testing as appropriate and available

Pathological Findings

- Defective, dysplastic, or absent segment of ocular tissue:
  - Overlying retina is dysplastic and gliotic with rosettes sometimes present. RPE at the edge of defect is hyperplastic (2)[C]

DIFFERENTIAL DIAGNOSIS

- Morning glory disk anomaly (may be considered a form of optic nerve coloboma):
  - Optic nerve pits (may be considered a form of optic nerve coloboma)
  - Optic nerve hypoplasia
  - Optic nerve staphyloma
  - In papillorenal syndrome, the abnormal optic nerve is not truly colobomatous but larger with an enlarged cup.
  - The term "macular coloboma" has been used to describe a geographic defect of the macula as seen in Leber congential amaurosis or infections such as toxoplasmosis or amniocentesis needle injury. This is an incorrect use of the term coloboma (i.e., fetal fissure not involved).
  - Upper and eyelid coloboma are not defects of the fetal fissure.

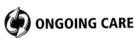

TREATMENT

MEDICATION
- None for the primary disorder but may need treatment for systemic involvement

ADDITIONAL TREATMENT
General Measures
- Maximization of visual prognosis with amblyopia therapy as indicated

Issues for Referral
- Genetic counseling, especially if family history or genetic mutation detected:
  - Pediatric specialist consultation if systemic abnormalities present
  - Retina surgery for detachment
  - Ocularist referral if severe microphthalmia to consider prosthetic shell

Additional Therapies
COMPLEMENTARY & ALTERNATIVE THERAPIES
- None proven or indicated

SURGERY/OTHER PROCEDURES
- Retinal detachment, cataract, strabismus, nystagmus surgeries as needed

IN-PATIENT CONSIDERATIONS
Initial Stabilization
- Inpatient care required for systemic associations only

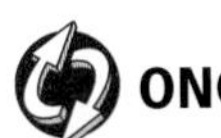

ONGOING CARE

FOLLOW-UP RECOMMENDATIONS
- Periodic dilated fundoscopy by an ophthalmologist for retinal detachment):
  - As needed for amblyopia monitoring and treatment
  - Low vision support
  - As needed for any systemic involvement, if present

Patient Monitoring
- School performance, mental and physical development:
  - Visual function and acuity
  - Development of systemic signs and symptoms, especially if known syndrome

PATIENT EDUCATION
- Genetic counseling:
  - Low vision intervention (importance of safety glasses and goggles, teaching compensation for visual field limitations, ameliorating photophobia with tinted glasses or brimmed hat, etc.)
  - Special assistance in school as needed
  - Support group: http://health.groups.yahoo.com/group/Coloboma_Moms/
  - The CHARGE Family Support Group: http://www.chargesyndrome.org.uk/
  - International Children's Anophthalmia and Microphthalmia Network: http://www.anophthalmia.org/index.shtml

PROGNOSIS
- Visual prognosis varies greatly with defect, which can range from a small iris coloboma without visual consequences to a large chorioretinal coloboma with microphthalmia and cyst and profound visual impairment.
- Prognosis is worse if fovea or dysplastic optic nerve is absent:
  - Overall patient prognosis also varies with any associated systemic involvement

COMPLICATIONS
- Amblyopia secondary to sensory strabismus or anisometropia:
  - Retinal detachment
  - Cataract
  - Secondary glaucoma especially if coexistent microphthalmia (uncommon)
  - Chorioretinal neovascularization (occurs most often at the superotemporal edge of coloboma, very rare)

REFERENCES

1. Porges Y, Gershoni-Baruch R, Leibu R, et al. Hereditary microphthalmia with colobomatous cyst. *Am J Ophthalmol* 1992;114:30–34.
2. Onwochei BC, Simon JW, Bateman JB, et al. Ocular colobomata: Major review. *Surv Ophthalmol* 2000;45:175–194.
3. Chang L, Blain D, Bertuzzi S, et al. Uveal coloboma: Clinical and basic science update. *Curr Opin Ophthalmol* 2006;17:447–470.
4. Gregory-Evans CY, Williams MJ, Halford S, et al. Ocular coloboma: A reassessment in the age of molecular neuroscience. *J Med Genet* 2004;41: 881–891.
5. Bermejo E, Martinez-Frias ML. Congenital eye malformations: Clinical-epidemiological analysis of 1,124,654 consecutive births in Spain. *J Med Genet* 1998;75:497–504.
6. Blake KD, Prasad C. CHARGE syndrome: Review. *Orphanet J Rare Dis* 2006;1:34.

ADDITIONAL READING

- www.genetests.org
- www.chargesyndrome.org

CODES

ICD9
- 743.10 Microphthalmos, unspecified
- 743.49 Other congenital anomalies of anterior segment
- 743.59 Other congenital anomalies of posterior segment

CLINICAL PEARLS

- May be associated with multisystem anomalies and syndromes
- Most common intracoular malformation in microphthalmia
- Diagnosis of coloboma by an ophthalmologist should prompt a careful family history, ocular examination of parents and siblings, and systemic evaluation of patient.
- A genetic evaluation is warranted in all cases with multisystem involvement.
- Patient should have an ocular and systemic follow-up twice a year.
- The most common syndrome among patients with coloboma is CHARGE syndrome.

COLOBOMA: EYELID, IRIS, OPTIC NERVE, RETINA

Hyung Cho
Assumpta Madu

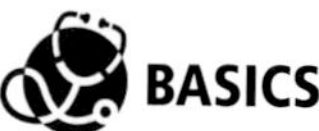

BASICS

DESCRIPTION

- A developmental abnormality caused by failure of complete closure of the embryonic fissure during the fifth week of gestation
- A hole in one of the structures of the eye, such as the eyelid, iris, retina, choroid, or optic nerve
- Coloboma derived from Greek, meaning "curtailed" or "mutilated"

EPIDEMIOLOGY

Incidence

- 0.5–0.7 per 10,000 births
- May be unilateral or bilateral with approximately equal frequency

RISK FACTORS

Genetics

- Most cases are sporadic, some are autosomal dominant or recessive
- Mutation in the PAX2 gene on chromosome 10 has been noted in 50% of cases.
  - PAX2 gene expressed in primitive cells of the kidney, ureter, eye, ear, and CNS

GENERAL PREVENTION

Genetic Counseling

PATHOPHYSIOLOGY

Incomplete or abnormal coaptation of the proximal end of the embryonic fissure.

ETIOLOGY

- The iris, retina, and choroid are absent in areas affected
- Usually located inferiorly, because the embryonic fissure is located inferonasally in the developing eye.

COMMONLY ASSOCIATED CONDITIONS

- Eyelid coloboma
  - Goldenhar syndrome (upper lid)
    - Developmental malformation of the first and second branchial arches associated with epibulbar dermoids, auricular appendages, malformations of the auricle, and hemifacial microsomia
  - Treacher Collins syndrome (lower lid)
    - Downward slanting eyes, micrognathia (small lower jaw), conductive hearing loss, underdeveloped zygoma, drooping part of the lateral lower eyelids, and malformed or absent ears
- Iris/optic nerve coloboma:
  - Basal encephalocele
    - Results from failure of the surface ectoderm to separate from the neuroectoderm causing a defect in the skull floor with herniation of brain tissue along the cribriform plate or the sphenoid bone
  - Renal coloboma syndrome
    - Autosomal dominant syndrome characterized by hypodysplastic kidneys and optic nerve abnormalities
  - Trisomy 13
    - Patau syndrome: Heart and kidney defects
  - Sturge Weber
    - Phakomatosis associated with port-wine stain of the face, glaucoma, seizures, mental retardation
  - Wolf-Hirschhorn syndrome
    - Mental retardation, microcephaly, seizures, cleft lip/palate
  - Klinefelter syndrome
    - XXY, most common sex chromosome disorder, small testicles and reduced fertility
- Chorioretinal coloboma $\pm$ iris or optic nerve coloboma
  - CHARGE syndrome
    - Colobomas, Heart defects, choanal Atresia, Retardation of Growth and Ear abnormalities
  - Joubert syndrome
    - Agenesis of the cerebellar vermis leading to ataxia, hyperpnea, and hypotonia
  - Lenz microphthalmia
    - Microphthalmia, cataract, nystagmus, and glaucoma
  - Walker-Warburg syndrome
    - Congenital muscular dystrophy, brain and eye abnormalities
  - Focal dermal hypoplasia
    - Skin, skeletal system, eye and face abnormalities
  - Aicardi syndrome
    - Absence of corpus callosum, infantile spasms, distinctive chorioretinal lacunae
  - Linear sebaceous nevus syndrome
    - Eye, nervous system, and skin abnormalities
  - Noonan syndrome
    - Dwarfism, congenital heart defect, impaired blood clotting

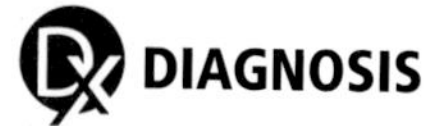

DIAGNOSIS

HISTORY

- Patients are usually asymptomatic unless the optic nerve or macula are involved or if there are secondary effects:
  - Patients with eyelid colobomas may complain of dry eye due to exposure
  - Patients with iris colobomas may have photophobia
  - Blurry vision due to refractive error
  - Visual field defects

PHYSICAL EXAM

- Ophthalmoscopy usually suffices to make the diagnosis
- Iris coloboma
  - Typical inferonasal keyhole-shaped defect
  - Lens may be flattened at the pole corresponding to the coloboma owing to the missing zonule
- Optic nerve coloboma
  - Microphthalmia
  - Inferiorly decentered, white-colored excavation, with minimal peripapillary pigmentary changes
  - Nystagmus if significant visual deprivation
  - Leukocoria
  - Astigmatism or myopia
  - Serous retinal detachment
- Chorioretinal coloboma
  - A white area (sclera) is visible in the inferior fundus to a variable extent depending on the size of the defect
  - Margins well defined
  - Rhegmatogenous retinal detachment
  - Often a pigmented border marking the transition from the coloboma to the normal retina or choroid

DIAGNOSTIC TESTS & INTERPRETATION

Imaging

- Eyelid coloboma
  - CT scan of the orbits and skull is indicated in patients with Treacher Collins syndrome to document and assess craniofacial structures
- Optic nerve coloboma
  - Axial CT scan shows a crater-like excavation of the posterior globe at its junction with the optic nerve
  - Coronal T1-weighted MRI confirms the intracranial portion of the optic nerve is reduced in size
  - CT and MRI delineates the anatomy of the skeletal defect and the associated cerebral abnormalities in basal encephaloceles

Diagnostic Procedures/Other
- Slit-lamp examination
- Chromosome analysis, especially if other organ system involvement
- B-scan ultrasound to evaluate for posterior cyst
- Renal ultrasound in syndromes with kidney involvement (CHARGE, renal coloboma, Patau)

Pathological Findings
- Optic nerve coloboma
  - Intrascleral smooth muscle strands oriented concentrically around the distal optic nerve
  - Heterotopic adipose tissue also present within and adjacent to some optic disc colobomas

DIFFERENTIAL DIAGNOSIS
- Iris coloboma
  - Ectopia lentis et pupillae
  - Iridocorneal endothelium syndrome (ICE)
  - Traumatic iris tear
  - Aniridia
- Optic nerve coloboma
  - Morning glory disc
  - Glaucomatous cupping
  - Optic nerve pit or staphyloma
  - Anterior segment dysgenesis
  - Retinopathy of prematurity (ROP)
  - Coats disease
  - Retinoblastoma
- Chorioretinal coloboma
  - Chorioretinal scar (e.g., ocular toxoplasmosis)
  - Degenerative myopia
  - Trauma

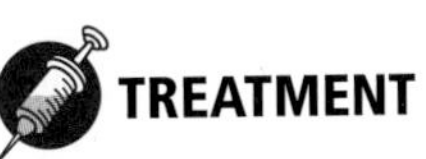

TREATMENT

ADDITIONAL TREATMENT
General Measures
- There are no medical or surgical treatments for colobomas
- Iris coloboma
  - Cosmetic contact lenses and sunglasses
  - Fully correct refractive error in both eyes with glasses if lenticular astigmatism
- Optic nerve coloboma
  - Scleral shell or orbital expander if microphthalmic
  - Amblyopia may be treated with patching
- Chorioretinal coloboma
  - No treatment is necessary unless retinal detachment or choroidal neovascularization occurs

SURGERY/OTHER PROCEDURES
- Correct strabismus if present
- Monitor and treat for retinal detachment
- Internal drainage through the hole in the intercalary membrane (extracolobomatous inner retinal layers that are extended centrally over coloboma) is performed and laser photocoagulation is placed around the margins of the coloboma.

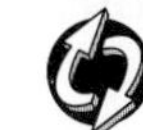

ONGOING CARE

FOLLOW-UP RECOMMENDATIONS
- Ophthalmologist
- Pediatrician/Internist

PATIENT EDUCATION
- http://www.rnib.org.uk/eyehealth/eyeconditions/conditionsac/Pages/coloboma.aspx

PROGNOSIS
- Mild or severe depending on the extent and location of the gap or cleft
- Excellent visual prognosis if isolated iris coloboma
- In optic nerve colobomas, visual acuity may be mildly to severely decreased, and is difficult to predict from the appearance of the disc.

COMPLICATIONS
- Amblyopia
- Refractive error
- Glaucoma
- Retinal detachment
- Choroidal neovascularization

ADDITIONAL READING

- Steahly LP. Retinochoroidal coloboma: varieties of clinical presentations. *Ann Ophthalmol* 1990; 22(1):9–14.
- Berk AT, Yaman A, Saatci AO. Ocular and systemic findings associated with optic disc colobomas. *J Pediatr Ophthalmol Strabismus*. 2003;40(5): 272–278.
- McMain K, Blake K, Smith I, et al. Ocular features of CHARGE syndrome. *J AAPOS*. 2008;12(5):460–465.

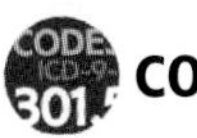

CODES

ICD9
- 377.23 Coloboma of optic disc
- 743.46 Other specified congenital anomalies of iris and ciliary body
- 743.62 Congenital deformities of eyelids

CLINICAL PEARLS

- Colobomas arise from a defect in the closure of the embryonic fissure during the fifth week of gestation.
- Visual potential depends on the extent of the retinal, optic nerve, and other organ systems involved.
- Association between coloboma, heart defects, choanal atresia, mental retardation, and genitourinary or ear anomalies (CHARGE).
- There are no medical or surgical treatments for colobomas

COMMOTIO RETINAE (BERLIN'S EDEMA)

J. Luigi Borrillo

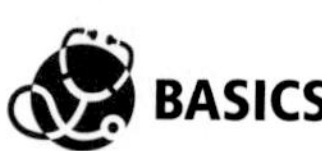

BASICS

DESCRIPTION

Contusive injury resulting in confluent areas of opacified, whitened retina.

EPIDEMIOLOGY

Incidence

Blunt ocular trauma annually affects approximately 4.9 per 1,000 individuals.

Prevalence

- Sports-related injury tends to affect younger male patients
- May affect individuals performing household projects or work-related activity

RISK FACTORS

Activities that carry potential for eye trauma such as high impact or contact sports.

GENERAL PREVENTION

- Use of protective eyewear that meets American National Standards Institute (ANSI) Z87.1 safety standard for work-related activities
- Use of protective sport specific eyewear that meet American Society for Testing and Materials (ASTM) standards

PATHOPHYSIOLOGY

Disruption of outer retina with shearing of photoreceptors due to coup and countercoup forces.

ETIOLOGY

Blunt ocular trauma.

COMMONLY ASSOCIATED CONDITIONS

- Subconjunctival hemorrhage
- Eyelid ecchymosis
- Hyphema
- Traumatic iritis
- Angle recession
- Orbital fracture
- Choroidal rupture
- Traumatic macular hole

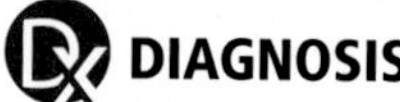

DIAGNOSIS

- Ophthalmic features of commotion retinae include:
  - Opacified, whitish minimally edematous retina
  - Undisturbed retinal vessels
  - Sometimes associated with sparse retinal hemorrhages or pre-retinal bleeding
  - Variable visual acuity (20/20 – 20/400) depending on affected area

HISTORY

Blunt ocular trauma.

PHYSICAL EXAM

- Complete ophthalmic examination
  - Dilated fundus examination with scleral depression

DIAGNOSTIC TESTS & INTERPRETATION

Diagnostic Procedures/Other

- Color fundus photography
- Optical coherence tomogram (OCT) may demonstrate hyper-reflective lesion representing disruption at level of photoreceptors and retinal pigment epithelium if affecting macula.

Pathological Findings

Photoreceptor outer segments demonstrate shearing injury or fragmentation on electron microscopy.

DIFFERENTIAL DIAGNOSIS

- White without pressure
- Shallow retinal detachment
- Branch/central retinal artery occlusion

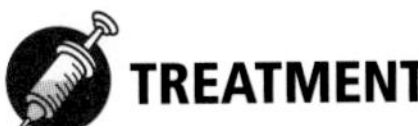

TREATMENT

ADDITIONAL TREATMENT

General Measures

Observation. Condition usually resolves without intervention.

SURGERY/OTHER PROCEDURES

Not indicated.

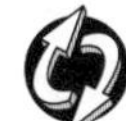

ONGOING CARE

FOLLOW-UP RECOMMENDATIONS

Ophthalmologist evaluation in 1–2 weeks.

PATIENT EDUCATION

Patients instructed to call immediately with signs/symptoms of retinal tear and/or retinal detachment.

PROGNOSIS

Favorable. Usually resolves without sequela.

COMPLICATIONS

- Retinal tear and/or detachment
- Possible permanent visual loss
- Macular hole development

ADDITIONAL READING

- Meyer CH, Rodrigues EB, Mennel S. Acute commotio retinae determined by cross-sectional optical coherence tomography. *Eur J Ophthalmol* 2003;13(9–10):816–818.
- Gass JD. Stereoscopic Atlas of Macular Diseases Diagnosis and Treatment1997:739–741.
- Sony P, Venkatesh P, Gadaginamath S, et al. Optical coherence tomography findings in commotio retina. *Clin Experiment Ophthalmol* 2006;34(6):621–623.

CODES

ICD9

921.3 Contusion of eyeball

CLINICAL PEARLS

- Whitened retina due to blunt trauma
- Resolves without treatment
- May be associated with visual loss

CONE DYSTROPHY

Jared D. Peterson
Julie Rosenthal

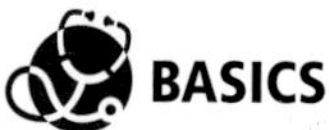

BASICS

DESCRIPTION

- A progressive degeneration that results in the triad of central vision loss, photophobia, and dyschromatopsia (color vision problems) due to the selective degeneration of cones.
- Cone dystrophy is a heterogeneous disorder both in clinical features and in underlying molecular genetics. The spectrum of cone disorders can be categorized as: (1)
  - "Cone Dysfunction Syndromes" that present shortly after birth or during infancy and are stationary (non-progressive). Achromatopsia occurs in 1:30,000, and these infants present with photophobia, poor vision, and pendular nystagmus.
  - Cone dystrophies can present anytime during childhood to early adulthood and are progressive.
    - "Cone-Rod Dystrophies" involve both the rods and cones at an early age, which results in both central vision problems as well as poor night vision.
    - "Cone Dystrophy" refers to conditions in which the cones are primarily affected. (Of note, many of these patients also have rod dysfunction, but this is less prominent.)

EPIDEMIOLOGY

Prevalence

1/40,000

RISK FACTORS

Family history of cone dystrophy.

Genetics

Most cases of cone dystrophy are sporadic, but autosomal dominant, autosomal recessive, and X-linked recessive inheritance patterns have been reported. Autosomal dominant is the most common inherited form.

PATHOPHYSIOLOGY

- Cone degeneration is thought to be the primary event. Subjective visual loss, and decreased visual acuity occur before any ophthalmoscopic changes can be seen.
- There are 3 major subtypes of cones, all of which are affected, therefore color defects will be present along all color axes, sometimes progressing to complete color vision loss over time.
- Varying degrees of rod degeneration can occur over time in some patients.

ETIOLOGY

Several affected genes and their chromosomal loci have been identified, including COD2 (Xq27), RCD1 (6a25-q26), RCD2 (17p12-p13), GUCA1 A, RPGR, CNGA3, and CNGB3 (1).

COMMONLY ASSOCIATED CONDITIONS

- There are several inherited systemic conditions that have cone-rod dystrophy as a component:
  - Neurofibromatosis I
  - Amelogenesis
  - Spinocerebellar Ataxia type 7
  - Pierre-Marie Ataxia
  - Trichomegaly
  - Bardet-Biedl Syndrome
  - Alstrom Syndrome

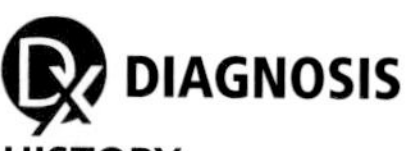

DIAGNOSIS

HISTORY

- Cone dystrophy causes photophobia, loss of visual acuity, and color vision abnormalities
- Symptoms typically occur before age 20 years
- Color vision problems are usually noted early in the course of the disease, in contrast to other macular dystrophies
- Earlier onset of symptoms is associated with more severe disease
- Nyctalopia in the setting of photophobia and visual acuity/color vision loss points more toward a Cone-Rod Dystrophy

PHYSICAL EXAM

- Funduscopic examination
  - May be normal in many cases as cone dysfunction occurs before any ophthalmoscopic changes can be seen
  - Quite variable, ranging from subtle macular granularity to a well-demarcated, circular, depigmented area of macular atrophy (bull's-eye maculopathy)
  - Optic discs may have temporal pallor
- Visual acuity can range from 20/20 to counting fingers
- Color vision testing with the Hardy-Rand-Rittler plates and/or the Farnsworth-Munsell 100-Hue test will reveal varying degrees of abnormality

DIAGNOSTIC TESTS & INTERPRETATION

Imaging

Initial approach

- Electroretinogram (ERG)
  - One of the most important diagnostic tests, as deficits on the ERG occur before changes on ophthalmoscopy are noted
  - Patients should undergo full-field and multifocal ERG
  - The characteristic finding is markedly abnormal photopic (cone) responses with normal to slightly abnormal scotopic (rod) responses
  - Selective diminution of the photopic 'B' wave along with decreased amplitude of the 30 Hz flicker may be seen
- Optical Coherence Tomography (OCT) may show transverse photoreceptor loss with disruption/focal loss of the inner segment-outer segment junction
- Fundus autofluorescence shows foveolar hyper-autofluorescence as a nonspecific manifestation in some patients (2)
- Fluorescein angiography can demonstrate early hyperfluorescence
- Visual field testing may show full peripheral fileds, but often have bilateral central scotomas

Follow-up & special considerations

Of note, a study of a large family with AD cone dystrophy found that no single test or finding was adequate to make the diagnosis. Thus, a constellation of history, physical examination, and diagnostic tests should be used, especially in more mildly affected individuals (3).

Pathological Findings

- There are few studies in the literature.
  - One study of a 69-year-old male with X-linked cone-rod dystrophy due to a mutation in RPGR showed focally absent RPE in the macula with the remaining RPE showing abnormal pigmentation (hypo- or hyper-). Cones and rods were absent in the perifovea, whereas the remaining retina showed some cone loss but near-normal rod numbers. All photoreceptors had shortened outer segments (4).

DIFFERENTIAL DIAGNOSIS

- Includes Stargardt's Disease, hereditary optic atrophies, and toxic maculopathy
- Must differentiate from cone-rod dystrophies, which present with similar symptoms, but also has severe rod dysfunction (nyctalopia)

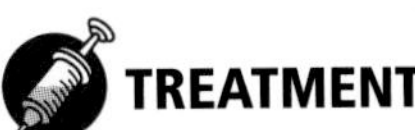

TREATMENT

ADDITIONAL TREATMENT

General Measures

Red contact lenses have been shown to alleviate. In one study, 23 out of 23 subjects showed immediate resolution of light aversion and experienced dramatic improvement in visual function (5).

Issues for Referral

- Patients may benefit from referral to a low vision specialist.
- As vision declines, patients may have to cope with multiple social difficulties, which may include loss of employment, loss of independence, depression, and so on. Patients may benefit from referral to appropriate professionals to enable them to better cope with these issues.

Additional Therapies

- Stem cell therapy
  - Parameswaran et al. (6) recently successfully programmed differentiated mouse fibroblast cells to a pluripotent state from which they were successfully reprogrammed using different developmental cues into cones, ganglion cells, and rods.
- Photoreceptor transplantation
  - Replacement of defective photoreceptor cells through transplantation of developing photoreceptors has restored vision in blind mice (7).

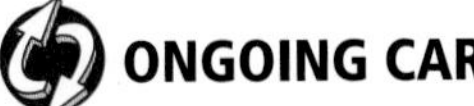

ONGOING CARE

FOLLOW-UP RECOMMENDATIONS

- Patients should be followed periodically to monitor changes in vision, color vision, and rod function (ERG).
- Refer for low vision services as indicated.

PATIENT EDUCATION

Genetic counseling on the suspected mode of inheritance, if any, can be helpful to patients in providing knowledge of the likelihood that other family members may be affected

PROGNOSIS

- Variable. Some patients will experience severe vision loss.
- Earlier onset of symptoms portends a more severe manifestation of the disease.
- The later the onset of symptoms, the better the prognosis.

COMPLICATIONS

Blindness, loss of color vision.

REFERENCES

1. Michaelides M, Hardcastle A, Hunt DM, et al. Progressive cone and cone-rod dystrophies: Phenotypes and underlying molecular genetic basis. *Surv Ophthalmol* 2006;51(3):232–58.
2. Wang NK, Chou CL, Lima LH, et al. Fundus autofluorescence in cone dystrophy. *Doc Ophthalmol* 2009;119(2):141–44.
3. Small KW, Gehrs K. Clinical study of a large family with autosomal dominant progressive cone degeneration. *Am J Ophthalmol* 1996;121:1–12.
4. Demirci FY, Gupta N, Radak AL, et al. Histopathologic study of X-linked cone-rod dystrophy (CORDX1) caused by a mutation in the RPGR exon ORF15. *Am J Ophthalmol* 2005;139(2): 386–88.
5. Park WL, Sunness JS. Red contact lenses for alleviation of photophobia in patients with cone disorders. *Am J Ophthalmol* 2004;137:774–75.
6. Parameswaran S, Balasubramanian S, Babai N, et al. Induced pluripotent stem cells generate both retinal ganglion cells and photoreceptors: Therapeutic implications in degenerative changes in glaucoma and age-related macular degeneration. *Stem Cells* 2010;28(4):695–703.
7. MacLaren RE, Pearson RA, MacNeil A, et al. Retinal repair by transplantation of photoreceptor precursors. *Nature* 2006;444:203–07.

C

ADDITIONAL READING

- Michaelides M, Hunt DM, Moore AT. The cone dysfunction syndromes. *Br J Ophthalmol* 2004;88: 291–97.

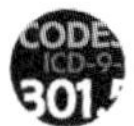

CODES

ICD9

- 362.75 Other dystrophies primarily involving the sensory retina
- 368.13 Visual discomfort
- 368.41 Scotoma involving central area

CLINICAL PEARLS

- Consider this diagnosis in patients with decreased visual acuity with seemingly normal retinal exams.
- Unlike what the name implies, color vision is not usually the presenting compliant of these patients.
- Symptoms usually begin before age 20 years and include photophobia, decreased visual acuity, and impaired color vision.
- Presence of poor night vision (nyctalopia) in addition to the above should prompt consideration of a combined cone-rod disorder.
- ERG is the most important diagnostic test as it shows selective defects in the cone system with normal (or only slightly abnormal) rod system defects.

CONGENITAL AND INFANTILE GLAUCOMA

Andrea Knellinger Sawchyn
Daniel T. Weaver
Alex V. Levin

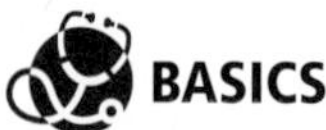

BASICS

DESCRIPTION

- Trabeculodysgenesis with aqueous outflow obstruction resulting in increased intraocular pressure detected at birth or by age 3–4 years
- Differentiated from secondary forms of childhood glaucoma that may be associated with: Persistent fetal vasculature, Peters anomaly, Axenfeld-Rieger spectrum, aniridia, retinopathy of prematurity, Marfan syndrome, and microspherophakia.
- Differentiated from acquired forms of pediatric glaucoma, such as aphakic or pseudophakic glaucoma, infectious, uveitic, or trauma-related glaucoma.
- Unilateral (25%) or bilateral (75%)

EPIDEMIOLOGY

Incidence

- Variable depending on country
- In some Middle Eastern countries: 1 per 4 to 10,000
- In the US, 0.38 per 100,000 (1)[C]

Prevalence

- In the US, 1.46 per 100,000 (1)[C]

RISK FACTORS

- 3:2 Males:Females
- Family history

Genetics

- 10% are autosomal recessive with variable penetrance and expressivity; autosomal dominant forms are less common.
- Four loci have been identified (2)[C]:
  - GLC3A (2p21), due to mutations in the cytochrome P450, family 1, subfamily B, polypeptide 1 (CYP1B1) gene
  - GLC3B (1p36), gene not yet identified
  - GLC3C (14q24.3), gene not yet identified
  - GLC3D, due to mutations in the latent transforming growth factor binding protein 2 (LTBP2) gene
  - Digenic with mutations in CYP1B1 and FKHL7/FOXC1/forkhead transcription factor
- Mutations in the myocillin (MYOC) gene have been identified in some cases of infantile glaucoma (autosomal dominant)
- Other loci are thought to exist but have not yet been characterized (2)[C]

GENERAL PREVENTION

- No known modes of prevention, other than genetic counseling. Prenatal testing only available if mutation known.

PATHOPHYSIOLOGY

- There are several theories of pathogenesis:
  - Barkan's membrane covering the trabecular meshwork (may not be true)
  - Anterior insertion of the ciliary body (due to arrest in the normal migration of the uvea) may contribute to narrowing or collapse of Schlemm's canal
  - Absent Schlemm's canal
  - Anomalous trabecular meshwork development (neural crestopathy)

ETIOLOGY

- May result from genetic or teratogenic interference with neural crest cell formation, migration, and final differentiation during fetal development.

COMMONLY ASSOCIATED CONDITIONS

- Congenital glaucoma may be associated with many systemic syndromes including Sturge-Weber syndrome, Lowe syndrome, congenital rubella, Kniest skeletal dysplasia, Robinow syndrome, and others as well as with chromosomal abnormalities.

DIAGNOSIS

HISTORY

- Classic triad:
  - Epiphora
  - Photophobia
  - Blepharospasm
- Large or asymmetric eyes
- Iris heterochromia may be present
- Cloudy cornea(s)
- Rapid myopic shift

PHYSICAL EXAM

- Exam under anesthesia or sedation may be needed to detect the following signs:
  - Long axial length by A-scan
  - Large corneal diameter (>12 mm for full term infants)
  - Hand held slit-lamp examination may reveal cloudy corneas or Haab's striae (breaks in Descemet's membrane, usually horizontal)
  - Cycloplegic streak retinoscopy may be useful in detecting progressive myopia or rapid loss of hyperopia
  - Tonometry should be obtained at anesthesia induction with the Tonopen or Perkins tonometer. Normal infant IOP is 10–15 mm Hg; IOP in congenital glaucoma typically 25–35 mm Hg
  - Gonioscopy may reveal an anterior iris insertion and indistinct trabecular meshwork.
  - Ophthalmoscopy will reveal optic nerve cupping, which is usually concentric with healthy surrounding disc tissue until late stages (sloping, notching, and hemorrhage are uncommon). May be reversible.
- In the office, assess the following:
  - Visual acuity
  - Pupils (assess for afferent pupillary defect)

ALERT

Beware of falsely high (hypercarbia, speculum, pressure from anesthetic mask, 2–5 minutes after intubation, ketamine) or falsely low (corneal epithelial edema, halothane, hypocarbia) IOP

DIAGNOSTIC TESTS & INTERPRETATION

Imaging

- Optic disc photos
- Consider hand held optical coherence tomography (OCT)

Diagnostic Procedures/Other

- Visual field (once the child is old enough to complete this test reliably; the age will vary depending on the child)

Pathological Findings

- Haab's striae: Breaks in Descemet's membrane
- Variable amounts of goniodysgenesis including collagenous tissue in the trabecular meshwork or juxtacanalicular tissue, mucopolysaccharides in the juxtacanalicular tissue, +/– absence of Schlemm's canal (3)[C]
- Optic cupping with posterior bowing of the lamina cribosa.

DIFFERENTIAL DIAGNOSIS

- Differential of tearing:
  - Nasolacrimal duct obstruction
  - Conjunctivitis
  - Corneal epithelial defect
  - Uveitis
  - Trichiasis or foreign body
  - Blepharitis
- Differential of Haab's striae:
  - Birth trauma (forceps injury)
  - Covert or overt trauma
  - Syphilis
  - Descemet folds
- Differential of corneal clouding:
  - Congenital hereditary endothelial or stromal corneal dystrophy
  - Keratitis
  - Metabolic disorders
  - Infection
  - Peters anomaly
  - Sclerocornea
- Differential of enlarged cornea:
  - X-linked recessive megalocornea
  - Phakomatoses
- Differential of buphthalmos:
  - Exorbitism
  - High myopia
- Differential of optic nerve cupping:
  - Physiologic cupping
  - Optic nerve pit
  - Optic nerve coloboma

TREATMENT

MEDICATION

First Line

- Medications can be used as a temporizing measure to lower the intraocular pressure and clear the cornea prior to proceeding with angle surgery and may also be used as adjunctive treatment following surgical management.
- Topical beta-blockers (e.g., timolol 0.25%, levobunolol 0.25%, betaxolol)
- Topical carbonic anhydrase inhibitors (e.g., dorzolamide, brinzolamide)
- Prostaglandin analogues (e.g., latanoprost, travoprost, and bimatoprost)

ALERT

Use of alpha$_2$-agonists (e.g., iopidine, brimonidine) in children <1 year of age is not recommended due to potential central nervous system depression.

Second Line

- Oral carbonic anhydrase inhibitors (e.g., acetazolamide 15–30 mg/kg per day, divided into 3–4 doses)

ADDITIONAL TREATMENT

General Measures

- Spectacles for refractive error
- Treat ambylopia and strabismus
- Tinted (or transition) lenses may help with photophobia

ALERT

Amblyopia is the most common cause of visual loss in congenital/infantile glaucoma. Correction of refractive error (especially astigmatism and anisometropia) is critical in preventing the development of amblyopia. Frequent cycloplegic refraction (q 4–6 months) is often necessary with rapid IOP changes.

Issues for Referral

- Consider a genetics consultation for counseling, molecular testing, and identification of systemic syndromes.
- Consider a low vision referral if indicated.

SURGERY/OTHER PROCEDURES

- Procedures of choice:
  - Goniotomy is the mainstay of initial surgical treatment. Approximately 80% of children are cured with goniotomy.
  - Trabeculotomy +/− trabeculectomy is an alternative in the setting of a cloudy cornea and is preferred as the initial choice by some surgeons.
- If angle surgery fails: (4)[B]
  - Tube shunt
  - Trabeculectomy+/−Mitomycin-C (lifelong risks must be considered)
  - Transcleral or endoscopic cyclophotocoagulation in advanced cases that have failed medical and surgical treatment.

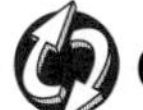

ONGOING CARE

FOLLOW-UP RECOMMENDATIONS

- All patients require lifelong follow up.
- Patients should be monitored closely during the first 4–6 weeks postoperatively to monitor for corneal clearing, reversal of optic nerve cupping, and IOP reduction.
- During the first few years of life, office visits and exams under anesthesia should be completed every 3–4 months depending on disease severity.
- Remember awake examinations to screen for amblyopia.

PATIENT MONITORING

- Repeat examination under anesthesia every 3 months for the first year of life periodically including measurements and imaging to assess disease control.
- Regular reexamination during early childhood including measurements and imaging should be completed to assess disease control.
- Visual fields should be repeated at least annually once reliable tests can be obtained.

PATIENT EDUCATION

- The Pediatric Glaucoma and Cataract Family Association www.pgcfa.org
- American Association for Pediatric Ophthalmology and Strabismus www.aapos.org

PROGNOSIS

- The prognosis is variable depending on age at presentation and timing of surgery. The prognosis for congenital glaucoma is worse than the infantile presentation.
- Patients who undergo angle surgery between 2–12 months of age tend to achieve better IOP control than those who undergo surgery before or after this age range.
- Intraocular pressure control can be achieved in approximately 80% of cases, including those on medications.
- 40% of affected patients may maintain a visual acuity of 20/40 or better (5)[C]

COMPLICATIONS

- Glaucomatous visual field loss
- Decreased visual acuity
- Blindness
- Anisometropia
- Astigmatism
- Myopia
- Amblyopia
- Cataract
- Corneal scarring
- Phthisis bulbi
- Intractable pain

REFERENCES

1. Aponte EP, Diehl N, Mohney BG. Incidence and clinical characteristics of childhood glaucoma: A population based study. *Arch Ophthalmol* 2010;128:478–482.
2. Narooie-Nejad M, Chitsazian F, Khoramian Tusi B, et al. Genotyping results of Iranian PCG families suggests one or more PCG loci other than GCL3A, GCL3B, and GLC3C exist. *Mol Vis* 2009;15: 2155–2161.
3. Hollander DA, Sarfarazi M, Soilov I, et al. Genotype and phenotype correlations in congenital glaucoma: CYP1B1 mutations, goniodysgenesis, and clinical characteristics. *Am J Ophthalmol* 2006;142:993–1004.
4. Tanimoto SA, Brandt JD. Options in pediatric glaucoma after angle surgery has failed. *Curr Opin Ophthalmol* 2006;17:132–137.
5. Biglan AW. Glaucoma in children: Are we making progress? *J AAPOS* 2006;10:7–21.

ADDITIONAL READING

- Papdopoulos M, Khaw PT. Advances in the management of paediatric glaucoma. *Eye* 2007;21:1319–1325.

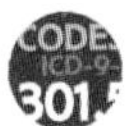

CODES

ICD9

- 365.14 Glaucoma of childhood
- 743.20 Glaucoma of childhood
- 743.22 Buphthalmos associated with other ocular anomalies

CLINICAL PEARLS

- Buphthalmos, corneal clouding, blepharospasm, epiphora, and photophobia occurring in the first 3–4 years of life should alert the clinician to the potential diagnosis of congenital/infantile glaucoma.
- Rapid myopic shift or asymmetric myopia in the infant and young child should lead the examiner to consider the diagnosis of congenital glaucoma.
- Amblyopia is the most common cause of visual loss.
- Definitive management is surgical.

CONGENITAL AND PEDIATRIC CATARACTS

Harold P. Koller
Christopher M. Fecarotta

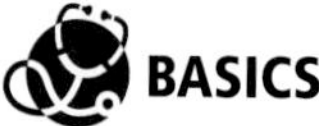

BASICS

DESCRIPTION

- Any opacity of the crystalline lens is called a cataract
- Can be congenital or developmental
- Isolated or associated with anterior ocular segment dysgenesis
- With or without systemic disease
- Multitude of morphology including anterior polar, lamellar, nuclear, posterior lenticonus, persistent fetal circulation with vascularized plaque, anterior lenticonus, pulverulent, cerulean, sutural, total, and others
  - Known cause or inherited in approximately 60–70% of cases

EPIDEMIOLOGY

Incidence

In the US, the incidence is estimated to be 1.2–6 cases per 10, 000.

RISK FACTORS

- Intrauterine infections
- Metabolic conditions
- Family history
- Trauma including birth trauma
- Some genetic syndromes
- Steroids
- Uveitis

Genetics

- The most common mode of transmission is autosomal dominant with variable penetrance.
- Multiple genes are identified that, when mutated, can result in cataracts. Multiple additional loci are known without mapped genes.
- Can also be autosomal recessive or X-linked recessive

GENERAL PREVENTION

- Maternal vaccination can prevent certain infections that cause cataracts in newborns, but otherwise prevention is limited.
- Prenatal ultrasound is unreliable.
- Genetic testing not currently useful due to large number of possible genes but genetic counseling may be helpful in family planning.
- Prevention of visual loss by early identification. All children born to a parent with known heritable cataract should be examined by an eye doctor in the first 2 days of life and followed serially thereafter.

PATHOPHYSIOLOGY

Depends on the cause, but generally involves a loss of lens clarity in a specific region of the lens based on the time of intrauterine insult or the specific mutated gene.

ETIOLOGY

- Most commonly idiopathic
- Most common known cause is genetic and many isolated otherwise idiopathic cataracts may prove later to be heritable
- Other etiologies: Chronic corticosteroid use, genetic syndromes, metabolic disorders, and intrauterine infections are the most common

COMMONLY ASSOCIATED CONDITIONS

- Intrauterine infection
  - Rubella, varicella, toxoplasmosis, herpes simplex, bacterial, or fungal endophthalmitis, cytomegalovirus.
- Metabolic disorders
  - Galactosemia, hypocalcemia, hypoglycemia, diabetes mellitus, mannosidosis, hyperferritinemia
- Chromosomal
  - Trisomy 21, Turner syndrome, trisomy 13, trisomy 18, Cri du chat syndrome and many others
- Renal disease
  - Lowe syndrome, Alport syndrome, Hallermann-Streiff-Francois syndrome
- Drug induced
  - Corticosteroids, chlorpromazine
- Other
  - Microphthalmia, aniridia, retinitis pigmentosa, persistent fetal vasculature, retinopathy of prematurity, endophthalmitis

DIAGNOSIS

HISTORY

- History of parents seeing an abnormal pupillary reflex (leukokoria) directly or in a photograph
- History of condition known to be associated with pediatric cataracts
- Strabismus
- Nystagmus
- Cataract alone does not cause an afferent pupillary defect.

PHYSICAL EXAM

- Visual assessment of each eye individually
- Cycloplegic refraction
- Slit-lamp biomicroscopy
- Determination of the cataract's visual significance by quality of retinoscopy reflex, fundus view, and when possible, visual acuity
- Examination of the optic nerve and retina
- If unable to visualize the retina, B-scan ultrasonography is necessary to rule out persistent fetal vasculature, retinal detachment, and retinoblastoma
- The size, location, density, and visual acuity are all considered in determination of therapy

DIAGNOSTIC TESTS & INTERPRETATION

Lab

Initial lab tests

- TORCH titers in bilateral congenital cases with systemic indicators
- Consider galactokinase levels to rule out galactosemia in bilateral cases
- Other tests as suggested by systemic or ocular examination

Follow-up & special considerations

Referral to geneticist if a systemic syndrome is suspected

DIFFERENTIAL DIAGNOSIS

- Leukokoria
  - Retinoblastoma, toxocariasis, Coats disease, persistent fetal vasculature, retinal astrocytoma, retinochoroidal coloboma, retinal detachment, myelinated nerve fibers, uveitis, incontinentia pigmenti, toxoplasmosis

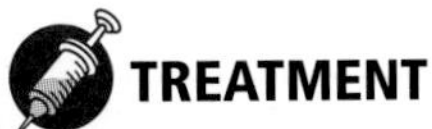

TREATMENT

MEDICATION
- If the cataract is central but less than 3 mm, occlusion therapy over the opposite eye combined with mydriatic drops (2.5% phenylephrine) can be an effective therapy.
- A unilateral punctuate cataract often requires careful monitoring only.

ADDITIONAL TREATMENT
General Measures
- If systemic disease is uncovered, referral to the appropriate pediatric subspecialist should be made.
- Referral to geneticist if a systemic syndrome is suspected
- Postoperative refractive correction and occlusion therapy are essential for visual rehabilitation.

SURGERY/OTHER PROCEDURES
- Larger, denser central cataracts that are more visually significant require surgery
- Pediatric cataracts are usually removed using mechanical aspiration techniques rather than phacoemulsification.
- Primary posterior capsulotomy and anterior vitrectomy are indicated in any child not old enough to perform postoperative YAG laser.
- Placing the IOL in the capsular bag is best, but if that is not possible then sulcus fixation is acceptable.
- Use of intraocular lens implants in children under 1–2 years of age is controversial.
- Contact lenses (usually silicone elastomer and rigid gas permeable lenses) or glasses in unilateral or bilateral cases are acceptable alternatives to IOL implantation. Contact lens is the standard of care for children <1 year old.

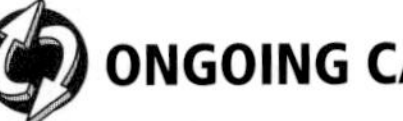

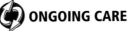

ONGOING CARE

FOLLOW-UP RECOMMENDATIONS
Amblyopia therapy is carried out in the standard manner depending on the density of visual loss.

PATIENT EDUCATION
The Pediatric Glaucoma and Cataract Family Association: http://www.pgcfa.org.

PROGNOSIS
Depends on the presence of concomitant ocular disease, age of onset, length of time of visual axis occlusion, and density of amblyopia.

COMPLICATIONS
- Most common complications are posterior capsule/anterior vitreous face opacification and aphakic/pseudophakic glaucoma.
- Other complications include hyphema, iris incarceration in the incision, pupillary distortion, vitreous hemorrhage, retinal hemorrhages, retinal detachment, intraocular lens subluxation, and endophthalmitis.
- Later complications including aphakic or pseudophakic glaucoma can arise years later in up to 30% of cases. Highest risk if microphthalmia, nuclear cataract or persistent fetal circulation. Average time of onset is 8 years postoperatively. Minimum annual IOP measurement even if sedation/anesthesia required
- Toxic anterior segment syndrome (TASS) causing postoperative corneal edema must be prevented with careful instrument and solution sterilization.

ADDITIONAL READING

- Taylor D, Hoyt CS. Pediatric ophthalmology and strabismus, 3rd ed. Philadelphia, PA: Elsevier Limited, 2005:441–457.
- Wright KW. Lens abnormalities: Chapter 27 in pediatric ophthalmology and strabismus. In: Wright KW, Spiegel PH (eds), 2nd ed. New York: Springer-Verlag, 2003:450–480.
- Tesser RA, Hess DB, Buckly EG. Pediatric cataracts and lens anomalies, Chapter 13 in Harley's Pediatric Ophthalmology. In: Nelson LB, Olitsky SE (eds), 5th ed. Philadelphia: Lippincott Williams & Wilkins, 2005:255–284.
- Parks MM, Johnson DA, Reed GW. Long-term visual results and complications in children with aphakia. A function of cataract type. *Ophthalmology* 1993;100(6):826–840; disc p 840–1.
- Awner S, Buckley EG, DeVaro JM, et al. Unilateral pseudophakia in children under 4 years. *J Pediatr Ophthalmol Strabismus* 1996;33(4):230–236.
- Huang Y, Dai Y, Wu X, et al. Toxic anterior segment syndrome after pediatric cataract surgery. *J AAPOS* 2010;14(5):444–446.

C

CODES

ICD9
- 366.00 Nonsenile cataract, unspecified
- 743.30 Congenital cataract, unspecified
- 743.39 Other congenital cataract and lens anomalies

CLINICAL PEARLS

- Congenital and pediatric cataracts can be caused by ocular developmental dysgenesis, intrauterine infections, metabolic syndromes, gene mutation, or as part of a multisystem syndrome.
- Work-up for systemic disease or referral to a pediatric genetics specialist should be considered as suggested by ocular and systemic evaluation.
- Determination of a cataract being visually significant determines necessity for and method of treatment.
- After cataract surgery, patients should be followed closely for development of amblyopia, glaucoma, and other complications.

CONGENITAL HYPERPIGMENTED ABNORMALITIES OF THE FUNDUS

Ahmara V. Gibbons
Alex V. Levin

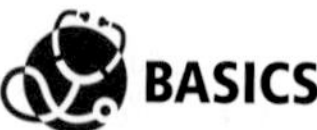

BASICS

DESCRIPTION

- Congenital hyperpigmented lesions of the fundus are differentiated based on appearance, pattern, and distribution in the ocular fundus and are present at birth.
- Includes: Grouped pigmentation (bear tracks), congenital hypertrophy of retinal pigmented epithelium (CHRPE), combined hamartoma of the retina, choroidal nevi, melanocytoma, chorioretinal scar (usually associated with hypopigmentation)

EPIDEMIOLOGY

- Grouped pigmentation: 1.2/100 (3)[C]
- Congenital hypertrophy of Retinal pigmented epithelium (CHRPE): 5 per 1,000 (3)[C]
- Combined hamartoma of the retina: Precise frequency in the general population is unknown (3)[C]
- Choroidal nevi: 10–13 per 100 (4)[B]
- Melanocytoma: Frequency in population is generally unknown (4)[B]
- Chorioretinal scar due to *in* utero toxoplasmosis: 1 in 10,000 live births (3)[C]

RISK FACTORS

- CHRPE: Family history of Gardner syndrome (adenomatous polyposis coli)
- Combined hamartoma of the retina and RPE: Family history of neurofibromatosis 2

Genetics

- CHRPE lesions associated with mutations in the adenosis polyposis coli gene (APC, 5q21, autosomal dominant) if bilateral or >2 in one eye
- Combined hamartoma of the retina and RPE is associated with mutations in the gene for NF2 (22q12.2, autosomal dominant)

GENERAL PREVENTION

Genetic counseling (1,3) [B,C]

PATHOPHYSIOLOGY

- Hyperpigmentation arises either from the neuroectodermal derived RPE or from melanocytes (neural crest) in the choroid
  - Grouped pigmentation, CHRPE, and combined hamartoma arise from RPE
  - Choroidal nevi arise from melanocytes in the choroid
  - Melanocytoma is a benign optic nerve tumor of melanocytes with abundant melanin
- Migration and distribution of pigment containing cells may be dysfunctional during fetal development
- Pigment-containing cells may be altered genetically and by systemic and external stimuli (e.g., trauma, infection)

ETIOLOGY

- Mutated or abnormal genes (1,3)[B,C]
- Inflammatory/infectious conditions causing chorioretinal scar
- Idiopathic

COMMONLY ASSOCIATED CONDITIONS

- CHRPE: Gardner Syndrome and Turcot Syndrome (adenomatous polyposis coli, tumors of the brain and spinal cord)
  Combined hamartoma of the retina and RPE is associated with iris hamartoma: Manifestations of NF2 include acoustic neuromas, meningiomas of the optic nerve, and presenile posterior polar cataracts.
- Melanocytomas can be associated with iris melanocytomas, pupillary disfunction and corectopia, and secondary glaucoma (from spontaneous necrosis with the resultant pigment dispersion) (1,5)[B,C]
- Chorioretinal scar can be a manifestation of intrauterine infection, which may also affect central nervous system

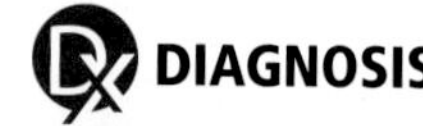

DIAGNOSIS

HISTORY

- History of prenatal infections (2)[C]
- Family history of colon cancer, NF2
- History of sarcomas, neurofibromas (1,2)[B,C] History about seizures, learning disabilities, and mental retardation
- For chorioretinal scars inquire about maternal history of ingestion of contaminated raw or undercooked beef, lamb, or pork, blood transfusions, organ transplants, or exposure to cats.

PHYSICAL EXAM

Full ocular examination including visual acuity, visual field testing (if age permits), and dilated funduscopic exam (3,4)[C,B].

DIAGNOSTIC TESTS & INTERPRETATION

Lab

Initial lab tests

None indicated

Follow-up & special considerations

- Genetic consult if genetic syndrome (2)[C]
- Choroidal nevi and melanocytoma require serial follow-ups (4)[B] and photo imaging for risk of malignant potential or advancement of disease.
- Colonoscopy beginning at the age of 8 years if Gardner syndrome
- Serial audiology if NF2

Imaging

Initial approach

- If combined hamartoma associated with NF2, MRI of brain
  - B-Scan and OCT may be used to evaluate hyperpigmented lesions

Diagnostic Procedures/Other

Molecular genetic testing as appropriate and available (2)[C].

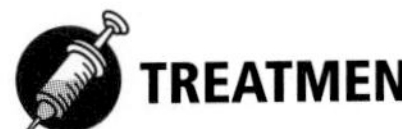

TREATMENT

MEDICATION

None

ADDITIONAL TREATMENT

General Measures

Amblyopia therapy as indicated (1)[B]

Issues for Referral

- If Gardner syndrome suspected: Gastroenterology (2)[C]
- If NF2 suspected: Otorhinolaryngology and Neurosurgery (2)[C]
- Activation of toxoplasmosis chorioretinal scar: Consider Infectious Disease consultation
- Progression of choroidal nevus or melanocytoma require referral to an Ocular Oncologist

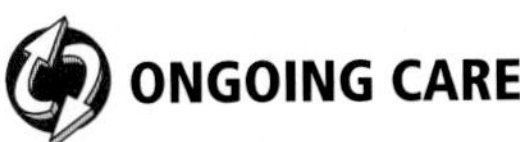

ONGOING CARE

FOLLOW-UP RECOMMENDATIONS

Choroidal nevi and melanocytoma: Photo documentation and serial examination (4)[B]

Patient Monitoring

- Visual acuity
- Photo documentation of tumor growth for potential malignant transformation

PATIENT EDUCATION

- Genetic counseling
- Visual acuity and low vision intervention as indicated
  - Report concerns regarding hearing or neurologic change if NF2

REFERENCES

1. Ellis FD. Selected pigmented fundus lesions of children. *J AAPOS* 2005;9(4):306–314.
2. Lee DA, Higginbotham EJ. *Clinical guide to comprehensive ophthalmology.* New York: Thieme New York, 1999:478–485.
3. Taylor D. *Paediatric ophthalmology.* Oxford: Blackwell Science Ltd, 1990:122–143, 153–154, 587–598, 614–620.
4. Shields CL, Furuta M, Mashayekhi A, et al. Clinical spectrum of choroidal nevi based on age at presentation in 3422 consecutive eyes. *Ophthamology* 2008;115(3):546.e2–552.e2.
5. Yanoff M, Duker JS. *Ophthalmology,* 3rd ed. New York, NY: Mosby, 2008:511–516, 552–554, 935–936.

ADDITIONAL READING

For more on Chorioretinal scars, see chapter Hypopigmented Lesions of the Fundus.

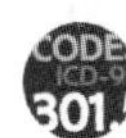

CODES

ICD9

- 224.0 Benign neoplasm of eyeball, except conjunctiva, cornea, retina, and choroid
- 224.6 Benign neoplasm of choroid
- 361.30 Retinal defect, unspecified

CLINICAL PEARLS

- If bilateral or multiple unilateral CHRPE, consider Gardner syndrome and inquire about family history of colon cancer. Consider colonoscopy.
- If combined hamartomas of the retina and RPE, consider NF2.
- If choroidal nevi or melanocytoma, there is an extremely low chance of malignant transformation, however these lesions should be observed with photodocumentation and serial examinations.
- In patients with chorioretinal scaring inquire about intrauterine infections, particularly *Toxoplasma gondii* exposure.

C

CONGENITAL HYPERTROPHY OF THE RETINAL PIGMENTED EPITHELIUM (CHRPE)

Hermann D. Schubert

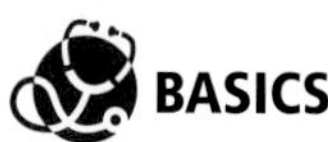

BASICS

DESCRIPTION

- Congenital hamartias/hamartomas: Placoid melanocytic lesions of the retinal pigment epithelium, solitary, grouped, or multiple in one or both eyes, the latter maybe associated with familial adenomatous polyposis (FAP) and – historically – Gardner or Turcot syndrome (1).
- **Solitary** lesions: Flat, well demarcated round, oval, or geographic with smooth or scalloped margins. The color is gray brown or jet black with a surrounding halo of depigmentation and/or central depigmented lacunae which bare the underlying choroidal vessels. The depigmentation may progress to involve the entire lesion (1). The usual size is 1–2 disc diameters (DD), however, can occupy one entire quadrant of the fundus. Slow concentric enlargement has been noted and seems to be the rule (2) The most common location is superotemporal and equatorial. Macular involvement is rare. There are few, if any, systemic associations. (3).
- **Grouped** lesions: Flat, well demarcated round, oval, or geographic smaller black spots (0.1–0.5 DD) arranged in groups reminiscent of "bear tracks". These are usually found in one sector, however can involve a large area of the fundus. Smaller lesions are found more posteriorly, larger ones are located peripherally. Bilateral involvement does occur. Cutaneous sectorial pigmentations, the lines of Blaschko, may be seen, suggesting patterns of pigmentary mosaicism in both eye and skin. There are no systemic associations (1–3).
- **Multiple** small ovoid hyperplastic lesions associated with familial adenomatous polyposis (FAP): Slightly raised, oval, with irregular borders and fishtail – shaped areas of depigmentation at one or both poles of the lesion. The lesions have a meridional orientation and haphazard distribution. Retinal invasion and glial, capillary and pigment epithelial proliferation and hypertrophy are typical. More than 4 widely spaced small (<0.5 DD) lesions per eye and bilateral involvement are suggestive of FAP (4).

EPIDEMIOLOGY

Incidence

Stevenson described 3 cases in 2,400 examinations in 1891.

Prevalence

- The prevalence of CHRPE was found to be 1.2% in the optometric population in 2007.
- Familial adenomatous polyposis occurs in approximately 1 of 13–18,000 live births.
- 70–80% of patients with FAP have pigmented ocular fundus lesions.

RISK FACTORS

Multiple small ovoid "typical" lesions, more than 4, and involving both eyes.

Genetics

- **Solitary** and **grouped** lesions can be familial
- **Multiple** lesions may indicate a mutation in the adenomatous polyposis coli (APC) gene in which case the inheritance pattern is autosomal dominant.
- The APC gene is a tumor suppressor gene, affecting cell cycle, cell adhesion, and migration.
- Germline truncating mutation in the APC gene causes the disease by not inhibiting tumorigenesis.
- The APC gene is located on the long arm of chromosome 5 (5q21).
- The APC gene encodes for a 312-kDa protein, 2,843 amino acids long.
- CHRPE lesions help to predict the mutation site on the APC gene; mutations between codons 543 and 1309 are associated with a high incidence of CHRPE.
- More than 700 of disease-causing APC mutations have been reported. An updated database is available at http://www.cancer-genetics.org.

COMMONLY ASSOCIATED CONDITIONS

- **Solitary** and **grouped** lesions are restricted to the eye (3)
- **Multiple** bilateral ocular lesions: Familial adenomatous polyposis (FAP), and/or attenuated FAP, if fewer than 100 adenomas in a more proximal colonic location are present
- Extracolonic manifestations: Dental anomalies, osteomas of mandible skull and orbits, fibromas, lipomas, epidermal and sebaceous cysts, adrenal, thyroid, bladder tumors, sarcomas, and hepatoblastomas
- Gardner syndrome (historic term): FAP and prominent extracolonic manifestations (see above)
- Turcot Syndrome (historic term): FAP and brain tumors, that is, medulloblastomas, astrocytomas, ependymomas (4)

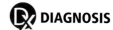

DIAGNOSIS

HISTORY

- Solitary and grouped lesions rarely have systemic implications (1–3).
- Multiple and bilateral lesions may be markers of FAP and must not be missed. The family health history is a "21st century genetic tool" inquiring about gastrointestinal polyps or other tumors and, about
- Abdominal pain, rectal bleeding, diarrhea, mucous discharge in any family member.
- In patients with FAP, hundreds of adenomatous colorectal polyps variably develop around puberty to 30 years of age. Patients with polyps develop symptoms 10 years after onset of polyposis by which time (35–40 years of age) carcinomatous transformations is present in a majority of cases.

PHYSICAL EXAM

- Ophthalmoscopy, looking for placoid solitary, grouped and multiple melanocytic lesions of the pigmented epithelium
  - Characteristic widely spaced meridionally oriented hyperplastic lesions, bilateral involvement, and more than 4 lesions are reason to suspect FAP (4)

DIAGNOSTIC TESTS & INTERPRETATION

Lab

Initial lab tests

- Fundus photography is used to document the size, color, and appearance of the lesions. Growth, depigmentation with age, as well as the rare (case report) malignant change have been documented.
- Fluorescein angiography: Capillary leakage, capillary nonperfusion
- Visual Field testing: Relative or absolute scotomas in large and old solitary lesions

Follow-up & special considerations

Solitary CHRPE grows in size in 46–83% over 3 or more years follow-up (2).

Imaging
All lesions of CHRPE show reduced autofluorescence, since they contain mostly melanin and little lipofuscin.

Diagnostic Procedures/Other
If FAP is suspected, annual flexible sigmoidoscopy should be performed starting at age 10 years. Depending on the polyp burden, endoscopy of the stomach, duodenum, and periampullary region should be performed every 6 months to 4 years.

Pathological Findings
- Solitary and grouped lesions are composed of a single layer of enlarged pigmented cells which contain macromelanosomes and little lipofuscin. The basement membrane may be thickened and there maybe degeneration and atrophy of the overlying outer retina. Halos and lacunae correspond to areas of neuroepithelial atrophy. The lesions are flat and have no mass, resembling "hamartias."
- Multiple lesions associated with familial polyposis may be similar to grouped lesions, however, more often show hypertrophy and hyperplasia of plump retinal pigment epithelial cells, retinal invasion as well as retinal vascular changes. Lesions are multilayered and have thickness, resembling "hamartomas" (5).

DIFFERENTIAL DIAGNOSIS
- Malignant melanoma
- Reactive retinal pigment epithelial hyperplasia
- Pigment epithelial adenoma/adenocarcinoma
- Albinotic nevi of the RPE
- Black sunburst lesion of sickle cell retinopathy
- Choroidal nevi

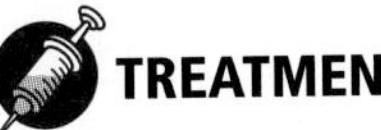

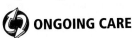

TREATMENT

ADDITIONAL TREATMENT
Issues for Referral
Gastrointestinal evaluation, APC gene testing.

SURGERY/OTHER PROCEDURES
- Solitary and grouped pigmentations of the RPE: None
- Multiple, bilateral, associated with FAP: Flexible sigmoidoscopy, colonoscopy, subtotal colectomy

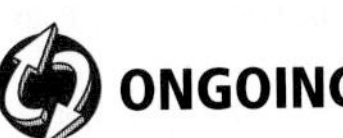

ONGOING CARE

FOLLOW-UP RECOMMENDATIONS
Patients with multiple CHRPE and a diagnosis of FAP: Annual colonoscopy.

PROGNOSIS
Solitary and grouped CHRPE typically enlarge. Retinal atrophy can contribute to visual field defects.

COMPLICATIONS
Carcinomatous transformation

REFERENCES

1. Gass JDM. Focal congenital anomalies of the retinal pigment epithelium. *Eye* 1989;3:1.
2. Shields CL, Mashayekhi A, Ho T, et al. Solitary congenital hypertrophy of the retinal pigment epithelium. *Ophthalmology* 2003;110:1968.
3. Shields JA, Shields CL, Shah PG, et al. Lack of association among typical congenital hypertrophy of the retinal pigment epithelium, adenomatous polyposis, and Gardner syndrome. *Ophthalmology* 1992;99:1709.
4. Romania A, Zakov ZN, McGannon E, et al. Congenital hypertrophy of the retinal pigment epithelium in familial adenomatous polyposis. *Ophthalmology* 1989;96:879.
5. Kasner L, Traboulsi EI, Delacruz Z, et al. A histopathologic study of the pigmented fundus lesions in familial adenomatous polyposis. *Retina* 1992;12:35.

ADDITIONAL READING

- Galiatsatos P, Foulkes WD. Familial adenomatous polyposis. *Am J Gastroenterol* 2006;101:385.
- Meyer CH, Rodrigues EB, Mennel S, et al. Grouped congenital hypertrophy of the retinal pigment epithelium follows developmental patterns of pigmentary mosaicism. *Ophthalmology* 2005; 112:841.

CODES

ICD9
- 190.5 Malignant neoplasm of retina
- 361.30 Retinal defect, unspecified
- 362.89 Other retinal disorders

CLINICAL PEARLS

- Patients with solitary lesions need to be informed that slow growth of the lesion is the rule, whereas transformation to adenocarcinoma is extremely rare.
- Patients with grouped lesions should check their skin for the lines of Blaschko.
- Patients with bilateral and more than 4 (multiple) small hyperplastic haphazardly spaced lesions should be investigated for familial adenomatous polyposis, Gardner (extracolonic, mesodermal) and Turcot (neuroectodermal, brain tumor) Syndromes. Family health history, indirect ophthalmoscopy, flexible sigmoidoscopy/colonoscopy, APC genetic testing should be done, in this order.

CONGENITAL HYPOPIGMENTED RETINAL LESIONS

Avni Badami
Alex V. Levin

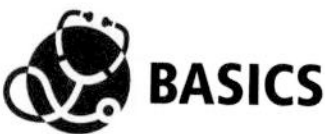

BASICS

DESCRIPTION

- Lesions characterized by reduced or absent pigment in or absence of the retinal pigmented epithelium or choroid present at birth.
- Includes, but is not limited to: Tumors (retinoblastoma, astrocytic hamartoma of tuberous sclerosis, congenital benign gliotic tumors), infections (cytomegalovirus, toxoplasmosis, varicella), retinal dystrophies (torpedo maculopathy, Leber congenital amaurosis), and congenital abnormalities (coloboma, Aicardi syndrome)

ALERT
Retinoblastoma should be considered in the differential diagnosis of any white retinal lesion in infancy.

RISK FACTORS

- Family history of retinoblastoma or tuberous sclerosis
- Congenital infections: Cytomegalovirus (CMV), toxoplasmosis, varicella
- Chromosomal aberration
- Parental consanguinity leading to autosomal recessive disease

Genetics

- Retinoblastoma is an autosomal dominant disease associated with loss of heterozygosity of the RB1 gene (13q14).
- Tuberous sclerosis is autosomal dominant (associated with TSC1 or TSC2 gene mutations)
- Coloboma-CHARGE syndrome (CHD7, SEMA3E, CHX10, OTX2, SHH genes and others, del22q11.2 and other chromosomal aberrations. Multiple systemic syndromes associated with coloboma
- Isolated coloboma can be either autosomal dominant or autosomal recessive.
- Aicardi syndrome-X-linked dominant inheritance
- Leber congenital amaurosis- autosomal recessive (GUCY2D, RPE65, RDH12, AIPL1, LRAT, RPGRIP1, SPATA7, CRX, CRB1, RPGR1P1, CEP290, IMPDH1 and other genes)

GENERAL PREVENTION

- For conditions with genetic associations, genetic counseling, and/or prenatal testing (if mutated gene is known or congenital abnormalities are identified in family members)
- For infections:
  - Toxoplasmosis-pregnant women should not eat undercooked meat and avoid exposure to cat litter. With confirmed maternal infection, systemic treatment may prevent infection of fetus.
  - Varicella-women should be vaccinated no later than 1 month before pregnancy. If a nonimmunized previously noninfected mother is exposed to varicella virus, consider administration of prophylactic treatment with varicella zoster immune globulin (VZIG) or acyclovir or valacyclovir to prevent fetal infection.
  - Cytomegalovirus-good hygiene is essential to prevent maternal infection. If mother becomes infected, consider treatment with CMV immune globulin to protect fetus.

PATHOPHYSIOLOGY

- Hypopigmented retinal epithelium due to a wide range of disease processes; cell may contain a low amount of melanin or there may be a complete absence of RPE.
- In coloboma, a failure of complete closure of the choroid fissure results in a gap in the choroid and overlying dysplastic retina (intercalary membrane).
- Infections result in RPE destruction.
- Retinoblastoma and astrocytic hamartoma are neoplastic processes.

ETIOLOGY

- Genetic mutation (two-hit mechanism in retinoblastoma and astrocytic hamartoma)
- Cytomegalovirus, *Toxoplasma gondii* spread through the placenta in utero.

COMMONLY ASSOCIATED CONDITIONS

- Retinoblastoma may also affect pineal gland or bone marrow, later secondary tumors especially if radiated.
- Astrocytic hamartoma of tuberous sclerosis
  - may have seizures, skin lesions, subependymal periventricular tubers, developmental delay
- Prenatal varicella
  - Microphthalmia, optic atrophy, cataracts, cicatricial skin lesions, atrophy/hypoplastic lesions of limbs
- Cytomegalovirus
  - Jaundice, thrombocytopenia/purpura/
- Petechia, hepatosplenomegaly, porencephalic cyst
- Toxoplasmosis
  - Intracranial calcifications, uveitis, hydrocephalus
- Coloboma
  - Systemic abnormalities (e.g., **C**oloboma + **H**eart + **A**tresia choanae + **R**etardation + **G**enitourinary + **E**ar defines full expression of CHARGE syndrome)
- Aicardi syndrome
  - Central nervous system malformation (absent corpus callosum), seizures, developmental delay, skeletal abnormalities
- Leber congenital amaurosis
  - Renal disease, deafness, developmental delay

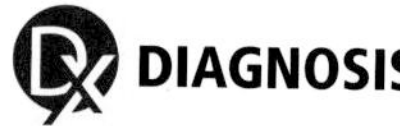

DIAGNOSIS

HISTORY

- Family history of retinoblastoma, tuberous sclerosis, coloboma, Aicardi syndrome, or Leber congenital amaurosis
- History of prior fetal loss with infection or Aicardi (male fetuses)
  - Known exposure to infection in utero
  - Other known associated anomalies

PHYSICAL EXAM

- Complete ophthalmologic and systemic exam
- In retinoblastoma, Tumors may be endophytic or exophytic, unilateral or bilateral, single or multiple, may have vitreous seeding, or rarely inflammatory involvement of anterior segment or orbit
- Coloboma may also affect iris and/or optic nerve, retinal detachment caused by breaks in dysplastic retina within coloboma.
- Astrocytic hamartoma in infancy presents with gray–white and translucent with a smooth surface, in retina or optic nerve.
- Toxoplasmosis chorioretinal scars are large and up to 5 optic disc diameters in size. Uni or multifocal, preferential involvement of macula, hyperpigmented margins
- Chorioretinal scars of congenital varicella are similar to those of toxoplasmosis.
- Leber congenital amaurosis examination in infancy can have yellow–white "macular coloboma", may or may not have other signs of retinal dystrophy, poor vision.
- In Aicardi syndrome, hypopigmented lacunar lesions are multiple, bilateral, and characterized by pigmented borders with preferential involvement of posterior pole.
- Cytomegalovirus lesions are usually necrotic/inflammatory macular lesions (maculitis) in one or both eyes.

DIAGNOSTIC TESTS & INTERPRETATION

Lab

Initial lab tests

- Karyotype for congenital abnormalities
- Gene analysis based on diagnosis
- Serology test for toxoplasmosis, varicella, cytomegalovirus

Follow-up & special considerations

- Consult genetics counselor if genetic disorder
- Low vision support, as needed
- Evaluation of family members if genetic disease

Imaging

Initial approach

- Ultrasound to confirm tumor in retinoblastoma (calcification)
- MRI or CT to confirm diagnosis of retinoblastoma, tuberous sclerosis, Aicardi, congenital infection

Follow-up & special considerations

For progressive conditions, continue to monitor patients.

Diagnostic Procedures/Other

- Bone marrow test or lumbar puncture if retinoblastoma
- Electroretinogram to assess for Leber's amaurosis (ERG severely reduced or isoelectric)

Pathological Findings

- See Retinoblastoma chapter
- Cytomegalovirus infections: Retinal necrosis and edema with nuclear viral inclusions
- Astrocytic hamartomas of tuberous sclerosis: Elongated fibrous astrocytes with interlacing cytoplasmic processes in the nerve fiber layer of retina (1)
- Toxoplasmosis: Tachyzoites appear as crescent shapes and stain well with Giemsa or Wright stain.
- Leber congenital amaurosis: Underdeveloped and hypomelanized retinal pigmented epithelium and photoreceptors
- Aicardi syndrome: Thinned out RPE and decreased number and size of vessels

DIFFERENTIAL DIAGNOSIS

Astrocytic hamartoma of tuberous sclerosis.

- Retinoblastoma
- Coloboma
- Cytomegalovirus
- Toxoplasmosis
- Varicella
- Leber congenital amaurosis
- Aicardi syndrome
- Astrocytic hamartoma of tuberous sclerosis
- Torpedo maculopathy

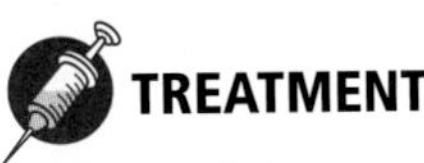

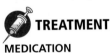

TREATMENT

MEDICATION

- For active congenital toxoplasmosis lesions (overlying vitreitis, active retinitis): Systemic pyrimethamine, sulfadiazine, trisulfapyrimidine, folinic acid
- For cytomegalovirus retinitis usually no treatment is needed – self-limiting, if infant immune system normal
- For varicella lesions – no treatment needed (inactive scars)
- Chemotherapy for retinoblastoma (see chapter Retina Retinoblastoma)

ADDITIONAL TREATMENT

General Measures

Low vision early intervention.

Issues for Referral

- Genetic consultation
- Oncology for retinoblastoma
- Enucleation may be indicated in retinoblastoma patients followed by ocularist.

Additional Therapies

- See Retinoblastoma chapter
- Seizure management in Aicardi

COMPLEMENTARY & ALTERNATIVE THERAPIES

None known.

SURGERY/OTHER PROCEDURES

- Surgery for retinal detachment in coloboma patients.
- Enucleation for some retinoblastoma patients.

IN-PATIENT CONSIDERATIONS

Initial Stabilization

See Retinoblastoma chapter.

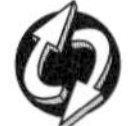

ONGOING CARE

FOLLOW-UP RECOMMENDATIONS

- Long-term follow-up is recommended for all retinoblastoma patients (see Retinoblastoma chapter).
- Low vision support and intervention
- Monitor coloboma every 6–12 months for detachment
- Monitor toxoplasmosis for activation of lesions

PATIENT EDUCATION

- http://www.tsalliance.org/
- http://www.aicardisyndrome.org/site/
- http://www.blindness.org/
- http://www.ffb.ca/

PROGNOSIS

- Retinoblastoma has variable prognosis depending on size and extent of tumor.
- Ocular lesions of tuberous sclerosis usually not visually significant
- Leber congenital amaurosis usually blindness but gene therapy now becoming available for certain gene mutations
- Aicardi syndrome usually complicated by cortical visual impairment
- Toxoplasmosis may or may not reactivate, poor vision if fovea involved
- CMV maculitis self-limited
- Varicella lesions rarely progress.
- Coloboma may be asymptomatic or visually devastating.

COMPLICATIONS

- Retinoblastoma; death, visual loss
- Coloboma: Retinal detachment
- Toxoplasmosis: Reactivation

REFERENCE

1. Shields JR, Eagle RC, Shields CL, et al. Aggressive retinal astrocytomas in four patients with tuberous sclerosis complex. *Trans Am Ophthalmol Soc* 2004;102:139–148.

ADDITIONAL READING

- Shah PK, Narendran V, Kalpana N. Aicardi syndrome: The importance of an ophthalmologist in its diagnosis. *Indian J Ophthalmol* 2009;57(3): 234–6.
- Verloes A. Updated diagnostic criteria for CHARGE syndrome: A proposal. *Am J Med Genet A* 2005;133A(3):306–8.
- Villard O, Filisetti D, Roch-Deries F, et al. Comparison of enzyme-linked immunosorbent assay, immunoblotting, and PCR for diagnosis of toxoplasmic chorioretinitis. *J Clin Microbiol* 2003;41(8):3537–41.
- Wilson ME, Saunders RA, Trivedi RH, eds. *Pediatric ophthalmology: Current thought and a practical guide*. Germany: Springer-Verlag Berlin Heidelberg, 2009.

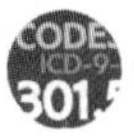

CODES

ICD9

- 190.5 Malignant neoplasm of retina
- 743.56 Other retinal changes, congenital
- 759.6 Other congenital hamartoses, not elsewhere classified

CLINICAL PEARLS

- Always consider retinoblastoma in the differential diagnosis of a hypopigmented retinal lesion and refer urgently if suspected.
- Tuberous sclerosis should be considered in any infant presenting with seizures or cardiac lesions.
- Always check family history for background of diseases causing congenital hypopigmentary lesions.
- Consider known associated conditions when assessing an infant with retinal hypopigmentary lesions.

CONGENITAL PIT OF THE OPTIC DISC

Paul S. Baker

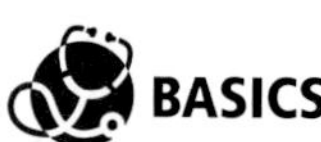

BASICS

DESCRIPTION

A rare, usually unilateral, congenital excavation of the optic nerve head that can be associated with a serous macular detachment.

EPIDEMIOLOGY

Prevalence

- Approximately 1 in 10,000 eyes
- Men and women affected equally

RISK FACTORS

No risk factors have been conclusively identified.

Genetics

Most cases are sporadic, but a few reports of autosomal dominant pattern of inheritance.

PATHOPHYSIOLOGY

- Optic disc originates from the optic cup when the optic vesicle invaginates and forms an embryonic fissure (or groove).
- Optic pits may develop due to failure of the superior edge of the embryonic fissure to close completely.
- Two-layered maculopathy consisting of a primary inner retinal layer schisis and a secondary outer layer detachment
- Mechanism of macular detachment.
  - Previously proposed that cerebrospinal fluid leaked through optic pit into subretinal space subarachnoid space
  - Widely accepted that liquefied vitreous fluid leaks through optic pit into subretinal space
  - One alternative theory suggests direct communication between optic pit and retina, causing schisis-like separation with a secondary accumulation of subretinal fluid.
  - Vitreomacular or vitreopapillary traction may play a role in fluid entry into retina from optic pit.

COMMONLY ASSOCIATED CONDITIONS

Rarely associated with basal encephalocele.

DIAGNOSIS

HISTORY

- Asymptomatic if isolated. Usually an incidental finding on examination
- If serous macular detachment, may notice blurred vision, distortion, blind spot, or micropsia
- When symptomatic for subretinal fluid, most eyes present with visual acuity between 20/40 to 20/60 (1)[B].

PHYSICAL EXAM

- Small, round, hypopigmented, grayish, excavated depression in the optic nerve head
- Bilateral in 10–15% of cases
- 70% located on temporal side of disc, 20% located centrally (2)[B].
- More commonly seen in larger optic discs
- Adjacent peripapillary chorioretinal atrophy
- White or gray membrane overlying pit
- Visual field defects: Arcuate scotoma is most common
- Serous retinal detachment extending from the disc to the macula
  - Estimated 40–50% of pits
  - More commonly when pit is large and located in temporal region of disc
  - Rare with small pits and located more centrally
  - Most confined between superior and inferior arcades in macula and are contiguous with optic disc, sometimes through a small isthmus of subretinal fluid
  - Serous detachments are generally low (<1 mm in height) and contain cystic regions.

Pediatric Considerations

Watch for amblyopia in children, especially in eyes with serous macular detachment.

DIAGNOSTIC TESTS & INTERPRETATION

Imaging

- Baseline visual field testing
- Optical coherence tomography
  - Typically shows schisis-like separation between inner and outer retina and subretinal fluid
- Fluorescein angiography
  - Unremarkable with no dye accumulation in area of serous detachment, but may have late hyperfluorescence of the optic pit
  - Rule out choroidal neovascular membrane or central serous chorioretinopathy

DIFFERENTIAL DIAGNOSIS

- Acquired pit (pseudopit): Can be seen in low-tension and primary open-angle glaucoma
- Optic disc anomalies such as scleral crescent
- Tilted disc syndrome
- Circumpapillary staphyloma
- Central serous chorioretinopathy and subretinal neovascular membrane in setting of serous macular detachment

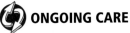

TREATMENT

SURGERY/OTHER PROCEDURES

- Laser photocoagulation
  - One or several rows of light laser burns between the area of serous retinal detachment and the optic disc
  - Several studies reported successful resolution of serous detachment, but this outcome did not always translate into improved visual outcome (3)[B].
- Macular buckling
  - Converts posterior hyaloid traction from an inward to an outward vector, which leads to reattachment of the macula
- Posterior vitrectomy, internal tamponade, and photocoagulation (4,5)[B]
  - Most encouraging long-term visual outcomes
  - Induction of posterior vitreous detachment helps relieve vitreous traction

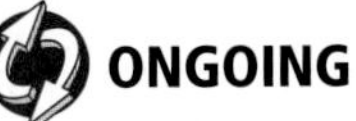

ONGOING CARE

FOLLOW-UP RECOMMENDATIONS

- Isolated optic pits
  - Yearly dilated fundus examination and visual field testing if indicated
  - Amsler grid
- Optic pits with serous macular detachment
  - Reexamine 3–4 weeks after treatment to check for fluid resorption
  - Watch for amblyopia in children

PROGNOSIS

- Optic nerve head pits are stationary, but associated retinal complications such as serous macular detachment can be progressive.
- In a series by Brown et al, mean visual acuity at 5 years was 20/80 (2)[B].
- In a study by Sobol et al, most patients lost 3 or more lines of vision within the first 6 months of presentation. With long-term followup, only 20% of patients maintained visual acuities better than 20/200 (1)[B].
- Spontaneous macular reattachment can occur in rare instances, especially in eyes undergoing posterior vitreous separation.

COMPLICATIONS

Serous retinal detachment in macula.

REFERENCES

1. Sobol WM, Blodi CF, Folk JC, et al. Long-term visual outcome in patients with optic nerve pit and serous retinal detachment of the macula. *Ophthalmology* 1990;97:1539–1542.
2. Brown GC, Shields JA, Goldberg RE. Congenital pits of the optic nerve head. II. Clinical studies in humans. *Ophthalmology* 1980;87:51–65.
3. Theodossiadis G. Evolution of congenital pit of the optic disc with macular detachment in photocoagulated and nonphotocoagulated eyes. *Am J Ophthalmol* 1977;84:620–631.
4. Schatz H, McDonald HR. Treatment of sensory retinal detachment associated with optic nerve pit or coloboma. *Ophthalmology* 1988;95:178–186.
5. Johnson TM, Johnson MW. Pathogenic implications of subretinal gas migration through pits and atypical colobomas of the optic nerve. *Arch Ophthalmol* 2004;122(12):1793–1800.

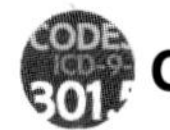

CODES

ICD9

- 363.71 Serous choroidal detachment
- 743.57 Specified congenital anomalies of optic disc

CLINICAL PEARLS

- Any change in appearance of the optic pit over time indicates that the lesion may be an acquired notch of the neuroretinal rim secondary to a glaucoma.

CONJUNCTIVAL AND CORNEAL FOREIGN BODIES

Melissa B. Daluvoy
Christopher J. Rapuano

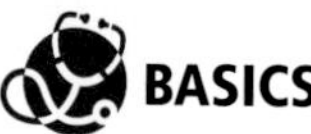

BASICS

DESCRIPTION

- Foreign material on or in the cornea or conjunctiva
  - Most commonly metallic or organic material

EPIDEMIOLOGY

Incidence

- One of the most common causes of emergent ophthalmic visits:
  - Peak incidence in second decade
  - More common in males

RISK FACTORS

- Use of power tools/machinery:
  - Windy weather

GENERAL PREVENTION

Use of safety glasses

PATHOPHYSIOLOGY

Small foreign material becomes imbedded in conjunctiva, corneal epithelium, or stroma.

ETIOLOGY

Often work related

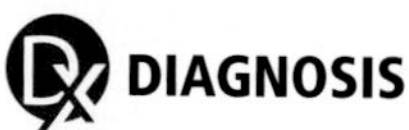

DIAGNOSIS

HISTORY

- The patient may have pain, foreign body (FB) sensation (both relieved with topical anesthetic), photophobia, tearing, and redness
- May or may not have a known history of trauma
- Important to know mechanism of injury including the material and velocity of the FB

ALERT

Be highly suspicious for intraocular foreign body (IOFB) or scleral laceration with high-velocity injuries (e.g., metal on metal).

PHYSICAL EXAM

- Signs can include normal or decreased visual acuity (VA), eyelid edema, conjunctival injection, anterior chamber reaction, corneal edema, and/or infiltrate.
- Always check VA.
- Meticulous slit lamp biomicroscopy examination is performed to assess the location, size, and depth of the FB.
- Metallic foreign bodies can leave a residual rust ring.
- A long-standing FB can lead to infection, inflammation, and necrosis of surrounding tissue.
- Check anterior chamber for inflammation as a result of traumatic iritis.
- Always look for signs of IOFB. Gonioscopy examination is performed if appropriate to check the angle for FB.
- Clues for IOFB or occult lacerations include:
  - Chemosis
  - Subconjunctival or anterior chamber hemorrhage
  - Poor VA
  - Afferent pupillary defect
  - Irregular pupil
  - Iris transillumination defects
  - Abnormally deep or shallow anterior chamber
  - Hypotony
  - Vitreous hemorrhage
  - Traumatic cataract
- Fluorescein staining may highlight conjunctival or corneal defects and may indicate an FB under the upper lid.
- If no signs of a globe rupture, evert the upper lid and sweep the fornices to search for foreign bodies.
- Dilated fundus exam to look for IOFB

DIAGNOSTIC TESTS & INTERPRETATION

Lab

Corneal or conjunctival cultures should be performed if the surrounding tissue appears infected.

Imaging

An anterior segment ultrasound biomicroscopy, gentle B-scan ultrasound, or orbital CT scan (1 mm coronal and axial cuts) can be helpful to rule out IOFB. MRI should be avoided if there is a possibility the FB contains metal.

Diagnostic Procedures/Other

A positive Seidel test at the slit lamp proves that the anterior chamber has been entered.

DIFFERENTIAL DIAGNOSIS

- Conjunctival, corneal, scleral laceration
- IOFB
- Corneal abrasion
- Ruptured globe
- Dry eyes

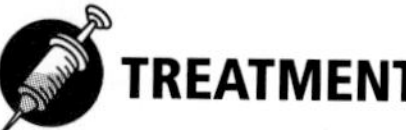

TREATMENT

MEDICATION

First Line

Conjunctival FB (after FB removal):

- Topical antibiotic ointment or drops q.i.d. for 5–7 days is recommended.

Corneal FB (after FB removal):

- Topical antibiotic ointment or drops q.i.d. for 7 days is prescribed. The author recommends a topical fluoroquinolone

Second Line

- Cycloplegics can be added for anterior chamber inflammation.
- Oral NSAIDS can be used for pain control; topical NSAIDS can also be used for pain management but are avoided by the author due to small risk of corneal thinning.

ALERT

Under no circumstances should topical anesthetics be given or prescribed to the patient for pain control.

ADDITIONAL TREATMENT

General Measures

Removal of FB:

- Apply topical anesthetic
- A lid speculum can be used
- Multiple superficial fragments can often be removed with copious irrigation.
- Small foreign bodies in the conjunctiva or cornea can be removed with a moistened cotton tip applicator or jeweler forceps.
- A special hockey stick-shaped FB spud is often helpful to remove corneal FBs.
- FBs that are small, inert, and not easily accessible can be left without harm – they may surface later and be more easily removed.

ALERT

Carefully assessment of the depth of the FB prior to removal is done. Extension into the anterior chamber mandates removal under sterile conditions and may require closure with glue or sutures.

- Metallic corneal FBs often leave a rust ring that can be removed using a small ophthalmic drill. Deep remaining rust is safer to leave behind.
- Insect hairs are common ocular FBs that can incite a profound inflammatory response. Removal of the FB should be attempted and treated with topical steroids and antibiotics.
- Measure the final epithelial defect to monitor healing.

Issues for Referral

- Suspicion for intraocular FB or ruptured globe
- Suspicion for infection

Additional Therapies

Pressure patching has been recommended but has not been proven to expedite healing and can mask infections; therefore, the author does not recommend patching.

SURGERY/OTHER PROCEDURES

Evaluation in the operating room is required if there is a high suspicion for an occult laceration/rupture.

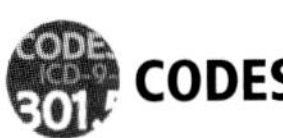

ONGOING CARE

FOLLOW-UP RECOMMENDATIONS

- Follow-up in 48–72 h after conjunctival FB removal
- Follow-up visits every 24–48 h until the epithelial defect heals after corneal FB removal

Patient Monitoring

Routine dilated fundus exams, intraocular pressure checks, and gonioscopy should be performed after injury.

PATIENT EDUCATION

Patients who engage in high-risk professions, sports, or hobbies should always use protective eyewear.

PROGNOSIS

Usually very good with full recovery for small FB injuries

COMPLICATIONS

- Infection
- Inflammation
- Scarring

ADDITIONAL READING

- Turner A, Rabiu M. Patching for corneal abrasion. *Cochrane Database Syst Rev* 2006:CD004764.
- Gumus K, Karakucuk S, Mirza E. Corneal injury from a metallic foreign body: An occupational hazard. *Eye & Contact Lens* 2007;33:259–260.
- Kah TA, Salowi MA, Tagal JMet al. Occult open globe injury in a patient with a corneal foreign body: A case report. *Cornea* 2009;28:1164–1166.
- Jayamanne DGR, Bell RWD. Non-penetrating corneal foreign body injuries: Factors affecting delay in rehabilitation of patients. *J Accid Emerg Med* 1994;11:195–197.
- Wong BWC, Lai JS, Law RW, et al. In vivo confocal microscopy of corneal insect foreign body. *Cornea* 2003;22:56–58.
- Ehlers JP, Shah CP. *The Wills eye manual*. Philadelphia: Lippincott Williams & Wilkins, 2008:17–19.

CODES

ICD9

- 360.60 Foreign body, intraocular, unspecified
- 930.0 Corneal foreign body
- 930.1 Foreign body in conjunctival sac

C

CONJUNCTIVAL AND CORNEAL LACERATIONS

Melissa B. Daluvoy
Christopher J. Rapuano

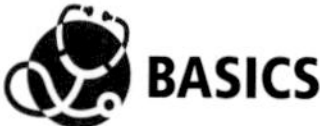

BASICS

DESCRIPTION

- A tear or cut in the conjunctiva and/or cornea
- Corneal lacerations can be full or with partial thickness

EPIDEMIOLOGY

Incidence

- Exact incidence is unknown
- It is more common in young males

RISK FACTORS

Hazardous occupations, sports, or hobbies without the use of protective eyewear

GENERAL PREVENTION

Use of protective eyewear

ETIOLOGY

Can occur following blunt or sharp penetrating trauma

COMMONLY ASSOCIATED CONDITIONS

There should always be a high index of suspicion for an intraocular foreign body (IOFB) and/or occult scleral lacerations.

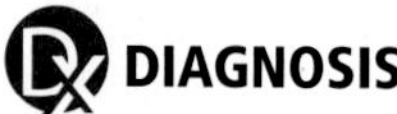

DIAGNOSIS

HISTORY

Details of the traumatic event and mechanism of injury

ALERT

Be highly suspicious for IOFB or ruptured globe with high-velocity injuries (e.g., metal on metal; BB gun injuries):

- Symptoms include pain, foreign body (FB) sensation, redness, and photophobia.
- Determine the last time the patient ate; this may influence time of surgical repair if required.
- Obtain complete history of previous ocular surgeries.

PHYSICAL EXAM

- Avoid pressure to the eye.
- Check visual acuity (VA); do not check intraocular pressure if you suspect there is a full thickness laceration.
- Diligent slit lamp examination is performed to learn the size and extent of the laceration and any entrapment or loss of intraocular contents; it is done without applying any pressure to the globe.
- Fluorescein staining may highlight subtle conjunctival or corneal defects.
- Clues for full thickness lacerations include:
  - Chemosis
  - Subconjunctival or anterior chamber hemorrhage
  - Poor VA
  - Afferent pupillary defect
  - Irregular pupil
  - Abnormally deep or shallow anterior chamber
  - Hypotony
  - Vitreous hemorrhage
  - Traumatic cataract
- A positive Seidel test confirms full thickness laceration. Apply concentrated fluorescein to site of interest and watch for green (dye diluted by aqueous) stream of dye under the blue light.
- Always examine both eyes carefully.
- For conjunctival lacerations, perform a gentle but thorough examination using topical anesthesia and a sterile cotton tip applicator to rule out scleral laceration and/or subconjunctival FB.
- If possible perform a dilated fundus exam to look for the possibility of IOFB.

Pediatric Considerations

Pediatric patients often give a poor history and are difficult to examine and may require examination under anesthesia.

DIAGNOSTIC TESTS & INTERPRETATION

Imaging

- An orbital CT scan (1 mm axial and coronal cuts) may be helpful to rule out IOFB. MRI should be avoided if there is a possibility that the FB contains metal.
- An expert may be able to perform a gentle B-scan ultrasound to identify an IOFB.

ALERT

A normal CT scan does not rule out an occult laceration/ruptured globe; therefore, if there is clinical suspicion, a high standard of care mandates surgical exploration.

DIFFERENTIAL DIAGNOSIS

- Corneal abrasion
- Corneal or conjunctival FB
- Ruptured globe/scleral laceration
- IOFB

TREATMENT

MEDICATION

First Line

Conjunctival lacerations:

- Conjunctival lacerations without scleral involvement can be treated with topical antibiotic ointments.
  - Consider polysporin, bacitracin, or erythromycin ointment q.i.d.

Corneal lacerations:

- Partial thickness corneal lacerations can be treated with an ophthalmic ointment and fluoroquinolones drops.
- Full thickness corneal lacerations should be treated with a 7- to 10-day course of systemic antibiotics perioperatively:
  - For example, moxifloxacin 400 mg per day or cefazolin 1 g IV per 8 h or vancomycin 1 g IV per 12 h (pediatric patients: cefazolin 25–50 mg/kg per day is divided into t.i.d. dosing and gentamicin 2 mg/kg IV per 8 h)
- Subconjunctival, intravitreal, or intracameral antibiotics can also be considered at the time of surgery.
  - Subconjunctival: 0.05 mL of cefazolin (25–50 mg/mL) or vancomycin (25 mg/mL) and gentamicin (40 mg/mL)
  - Intraocular: 0.1 m of ceftazidime (2 mg/0.1 mL) or amikacin (0.4 mg/0.1 mL) and vancomycin (1 mg/0.1 mL)
- Topical antibiotics can be initiated once the wound is closed (fluoroquinolones or fortified antibiotics).
- Antiemetics and pain medications should be given before and after surgical repair to prevent vomiting or straining that can raise intraocular pressure and prolapse intraocular contents.

Second Line

- Cycloplegics can be added for inflammation and/or iris damage.
- Topical steroids should be used cautiously on a case-by-case basis.

ADDITIONAL TREATMENT

General Measures

Conjunctival lacerations:

- Conjunctival lacerations <1 cm and those in the fornix can often be observed without repair.
- Large lacerations can be closed using interrupted or running 8–0 Vicryl sutures and using caution not to incorporate folds of conjunctiva or Tenon's capsule.
- Exploration is warranted if there is concern for an underlying scleral laceration or muscle involvement.

Corneal lacerations:

- Small self-sealing or slowly leaking lacerations may be treated with a combination of aqueous suppressants, cyanoacrylate tissue adhesive, a bandage soft contact lens and topical fluoroquinolones.
- Partial thickness corneal lacerations with associated wound gape should be surgically approximated to prevent excessive scarring and irregularity especially when in the visual axis.
- Large full thickness corneal lacerations require urgent repair in the OR.
- While waiting for repair, keep the eye covered with a firm shield to prevent eye rubbing.
- Administer a tetanus shot if appropriate.
- Nothing to eat or drink 6–8 h prior to surgical repair

Issues for Referral

Full thickness corneal lacerations need urgent repair by a qualified ophthalmologist.

SURGERY/OTHER PROCEDURES

- Full thickness corneal lacerations should be repaired in the operating room preferably under general anesthesia.
- A comprehensive informed consent should be signed prior to surgery.

ALERT

The anesthesiologist should be made aware of the open globe status which may influence which medications they use for induction.

- Take care during the prep and drape not to apply undue pressure to the globe.
- The goal of the primary repair is to restore integrity of the globe.
- Traumatic cataracts and iris damage are usually addressed at a later date under a more controlled setting.
- Regardless of the extent of injury and loss of intraocular contents, primary enucleation is *rarely* performed.

ALERT

The patient should be warned of the risks of sympathetic ophthalmia (SO) which can occur anytime after the trauma and cause loss of vision to the uninjured eye.

Tips for repair:

- Find identifiable land marks (e.g., limbus or distinct area of laceration) and begin wound apposition there.
- Reposit any protruding uveal tissue unless it appears necrotic, infected, or epithelialized. Use of a viscoelastic agent may help with this process.
- If vitreous is present, it is important to perform manual or automated vitrectomy to remove any vitreous traction to the wound.
- Continue placing sutures until water-tight closure is achieved.
- If scleral involvement is suspected a conjunctival peritomy should be performed and any lacerations repaired as far posteriorly as possible.
- Suture recommendations: 10–0 nylon in the cornea; 9–0 nylon at the limbus; 8–0 nylon in the sclera; 8–0 Vicryl for conjunctival closure.

IN-PATIENT CONSIDERATIONS

Initial Stabilization

A patient with a full thickness laceration requiring repair should be admitted and treated with systemic antibiotics until surgery can be performed ideally within 24 h.

Discharge Criteria

Once primary repair is complete

ONGOING CARE

FOLLOW-UP RECOMMENDATIONS

- Most patients can be followed on an out-patient basis with close follow-up for signs of infection, endophthalmitis, and SO.
- The patient should wear a shield or protective eyewear at all times until the wound is secure.
- Dilated fundus exam or Bscan should be performed in the early postoperative period to evaluate the posterior pole for retinal tears, detachment, choroidal effusions, or hemorrhages.

Pediatric Considerations

Children <8 years old are at high risk of amblyopia and may require prompt intervention to restore vision and/or patching to prevent irreversible amblyopia.

PATIENT EDUCATION

- Patients should always use protective eyewear when engaging in high-risk occupations, sports, or hobbies.
- If vision is severely affected in the injured eye, the patient may experience difficulty with depth perception and should gradually return to activities where depth perception is crucial.

PROGNOSIS

- Prognosis depends on the severity of the injury.
- Poor VA on presentation and delay in presentation tend to have worse prognoses.
- Some injuries will require multiple surgeries (e.g., cataract removal, lens implantation; repair of retinal detachment; iris repair) to restore vision.
- Injuries contaminated with organic material are at a higher risk of infections.

COMPLICATIONS

- Endophthalmitis (2–7%)
- Cataract (27–65%)
- Glaucoma
- Retinal detachment
- Iris damage
- SO
- Missed FB
- Missed scleral laceration
- Conjunctival cysts

ADDITIONAL READING

- Segev F, Assia EI, Harizman N, et al. Corneal laceration by sharp objects in children seven years of age and younger. *Cornea* 2007;26:319–323.
- Arey ML, Mootha VV, Whittemore AR, et al. Computed tomography in the diagnosis of occult open-globe injuries. *Ophthalmology* 2007; 114:1448–1452.
- Essex RW, Yi Q, Charles PG, et al. Post-traumatic endophthalmitis. *Ophthalmology* 2004;111: 2015–2022.
- Ehlers JP, Shah CP. *The Wills eye manual*. Philadelphia: Lippincott Williams & Wilkins, 2008:24–25, 35–36.

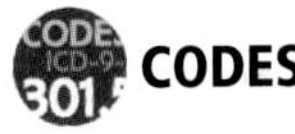

CODES

ICD9

- 871.0 Ocular laceration without prolapse of intraocular tissue
- 918.1 Superficial injury of cornea
- 918.2 Superficial injury of conjunctiva

CLINICAL PEARLS

- Always have a high clinical suspicion for underlying scleral laceration or IOFB.
- In full thickness lacerations the immediate goal is restoration of the integrity of the globe in a complete and timely fashion to prevent loss of intraocular contents, infection, and other ocular complications.

CONJUNCTIVAL LYMPHOMA

Carol L. Shields
Jerry A. Shields

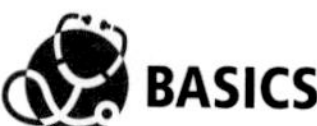

BASICS

DESCRIPTION

- Lymphoid tumors comprise a spectrum of neoplasia from benign hyperplasia to malignant lymphoma, based on microscopic features and immunophenotypic findings. Lymphoma, in general, is classified into 2 major groups, including those of lymph node or splenic origin (nodal) and those that originate at other sites without lymph nodes (extranodal). It has been found that approximately one-fourth to half of lymphomas are extranodal.
- The most common extranodal sites for lymphoma include stomach, tonsils/adenoids, skin, small intestine, and these represent more than 50% of extranodal lymphomas.
- Ocular lymphoma represents only 2% of extranodal lymphoma and the ocular sites include conjunctiva, orbit, eyelid, uvea, vitreous, and retina.
- Ocular lymphoma can be related to the eventual development of systemic lymphoma.

ALERT

A painless, pink conjunctival mass could represent lymphoma and could be the first sign of a life-threatening malignant lymphoma.

Geriatric Considerations

Most conjunctival lymphoma occurs in mid adults or older adults.

Pediatric Considerations

It is rare to find conjunctival lymphoma in children.

Pregnancy Considerations

No relationship to pregnancy.

EPIDEMIOLOGY

Prevalence

- In a large cohort of 1,643 patients with conjunctival tumors from the Wills Eye Institute Ocular Oncology Service, the most common tumors included melanocytic in 53%, epithelial in 11%, lymphoid in 8%, and simulating conditions in 13%.
- The 3 most common conjunctival malignancies include squamous cell carcinoma, lymphoma, and melanoma.

RISK FACTORS

Immunosuppressed patients from organ transplant or human immunodeficiency virus are generally at risk for lymphoma.

Genetics

Most conjunctival lymphoma is of the mucosal associate lymphoid tissue (MALT) type. This represents 8% of all lymphoma and tends to occur in mucous membranes like the intestines and the conjunctival. MALT lymphoma can show t(11;18)(q21;q21) chromosomal translocation giving rise to a AP12-MLT fusion gene. Other genetic alterations are found at the locus 1p22 and 18q21.

GENERAL PREVENTION

PATHOPHYSIOLOGY

- There is some evidence that conjunctival lymphoma might be related to chronic infection with *Helicobacter pylori*, *Chlamydia psittaci*, or no infection at all. Data from the US tend to show *H. pylori* as the cause, data from Italy report *C. psittaci*, and data from Scandinavia show no organisms.
- It is believed that the chronic infection leads to multiple mutational events that eventuate in lymphoma.
- Patients with chronic immune stimulation like those with autoimmune diseases like Sjögren's syndrome and Hashimoto's thyroiditis are at risk for lymphoma.

ETIOLOGY

The exact etiology is not known but it is speculated that chronic infection or immune stimulation can lead to malignant degeneration of the chronic inflammatory cells into lymphoma.

COMMONLY ASSOCIATED CONDITIONS

Most conjunctival lymphoma is unassociated with systemic disease but the patient should be checked for immune deregulatory diseases like HIV, immune suppression with medications, and autoimmune conditions.

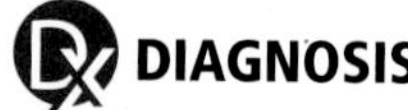

DIAGNOSIS

HISTORY

In a review of 117 consecutive cases of conjunctival lymphoid tumors from the Wills Eye Institute Ocular Oncology Service, the main findings noted by the patient included a mass in 30%, irritation in 29%, blepharoptosis in 8%, epiphora in 7%, blurred vision in 5%, proptosis in 3%, diplopia in 3%, and no symptoms in 15%.

PHYSICAL EXAM

- Data from the Wills Eye Institute Ocular Oncology Service has revealed the following findings listed below.
- Tumor location at limbus in 7%, midbulbar in 42%, fornix in 44%, tarsus in 0%, and caruncle or plica semilunaris in 7%.
- Tumor quadrant location was superior in 41%, temporal in 10%, inferior in 21%, nasal in 14%, and multiple sites in 13%.
- Additional lymphoma was found in the eyelid in 3%, orbit in 15%, uvea in 4%, retina in 0%, and vitreous in 1%.
- Systemic lymphoma was present in 31% and absent in 69%.

DIAGNOSTIC TESTS & INTERPRETATION

Lab

Initial lab tests

CBC to rule out leukemia.

Follow-up & special considerations

Repeat CBC as necessary.

Imaging

Initial approach

- Orbital magnetic resonance imaging (MRI) is preferred over computed tomography (CT) because of superior soft tissue resolution.
- Evaluate for orbital invasion
- Evaluate for systemic lymphoma and most oncologists prefer yearly abdominal MRI and physical examination.

Follow-up & special considerations

Repeat above testing annually for life because it may be 30 years before systemic involvement is apparent.

Diagnostic Procedures/Other

- Complete surgical excision is preferred if possible. Cryotherapy to the surrounding margins is often performed to ensure complete removal.
- If the tumor is enwrapping anatomic sites then an incisional biopsy would be preferred to protect the normal tissue. This would be followed by therapy with chemotherapy, monoclonal antibodies, or radiotherapy.

Pathological Findings

- There is a range of findings from reactive lymphoid hyperplasia, atypical lymphoid hyperplasia, to frank malignant lymphoma.
  - Reactive lymphoid hyperplasia is composed of diffuse densely cellular polymorphous infiltrate of small bland lymphocytes with reactive germinal centers.
  - Atypical lymphoid hyperplasia is an indeterminate lesion with diffuse small lymphocytes with some atypia and no frank cytological malignancy.
  - Lymphoma shows malignant lymphocytes often with mitotic activity in monotonous sheets of tumor.

DIFFERENTIAL DIAGNOSIS

- Conjunctivitis
- Conjunctival allergy
- Conjunctival melanoma
- Conjunctival squamous cell carcinoma
- Conjunctival amyloidosis
- Conjunctival sarcoidosis

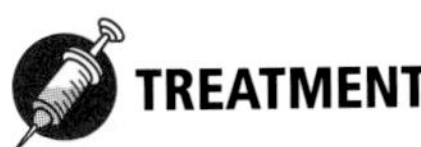

TREATMENT

MEDICATION

First Line

- Chemotherapy
- Rituximab monoclonal antibody to CD 20 cells
- Many patients use antibiotics for 1 month even if the above agents are used.

Second Line

Interferon alpha 2B injection is another alternative.

ADDITIONAL TREATMENT

General Measures

Radiotherapy with external beam, stereotactic, CyberKnife, or other methods. The usual dose is 2,500 cGy–4,000 cGy. This malignancy is radiosensitive and responds within 1–2 months of treatment.

Additional Therapies

Antibiotics using Prevpac (lansoprazole, amoxicillin, clarithromycin) or doxycycline.

SURGERY/OTHER PROCEDURES

- Complete excision is warranted if the tumor is not enwrapping normal anatomic structures. Otherwise, incisional biopsy is employed.
- The surgical approach depends on the location of the mass. If the mass is relatively small and involves only one quadrant of the eye, then the mass can be unroofed with elevation of the conjunctival epithelium and the stromal mass carefully dissected and removed. Surround cryotherapy is warranted. The spared epithelium is then reposited into normal position and closed with Vicryl.
- If the mass is large and involves multiple quadrants on the surface of the eye then an incisional biopsy is performed with unroofing the tumor and taking a biopsy and then replacing the roof down to the conjunctival bed and suturing with Vicryl sutures.

ONGOING CARE

FOLLOW-UP RECOMMENDATIONS

- Conjunctival inspection of both eyes for recurrent lymphoma or new lymphoma
- Orbital and systemic magnetic resonance imaging for evaluation of local orbital disease and to search for systemic lymphoma

Patient Monitoring

Patient should be evaluated minimum twice yearly by ophthalmologist or ocular oncologist.

PATIENT EDUCATION

- www.fighteyecancer.com
- www.eyecancer.info
- www.eyetumor.org
- www.eyecancerbook.com
- www.etrf.org
- www.choroidmelanoma.com

PROGNOSIS

- The following results were obtained from the Wills Eye Institute Ocular Oncology Service.
- If the conjunctival lymphoma was unilateral, the risk for eventual systemic lymphoma was 17%.
- If the conjunctival lymphoma was bilateral, the risk for eventual systemic lymphoma was 47%.
- Overall, in patients who had no systemic lymphoma at presentation but only had conjunctival lymphoma, systemic lymphoma was eventually found in 7% at 1 year, 15% at 5 years, and 28% at 10 years.
- In that group, <1% died of systemic lymphoma by approximately 3 years average follow-up.

COMPLICATIONS

Following surgery, the patient might have dysmotility, blepharoptosis, double vision, and loss of vision.

ADDITIONAL READING

- Shields CL, Shields JA, Carvalho C, et al. Conjunctival lymphoid tumors: Clinical analysis of 117 cases and relationship to systemic lymphoma. *Ophthalmology* 2001;108:979–84.
- Shields CL, Demirci H, Karatza E, et al. Clinical survey of 1643 melanocytic and nonmelanocytic tumors of the conjunctiva. *Ophthalmology* 2004;111:1747–54.
- Shields JA, Shields CL. Eyelid, Conjunctival, and Orbital Tumors. *An atlas and textbook*, 2nd ed. Philadelphia: Lippincott Williams and Wilkins, 2008:383–391.

CODES

ICD9

- 190.3 Malignant neoplasm of conjunctiva
- 200.50 Primary central nervous system lymphoma, unspecified site, extranodal and solid organ sites

CLINICAL PEARLS

- If possible, complete resection of a conjunctival lymphoma should be attempted.
- Systemic monitoring for life should be used for affected patients to rule out systemic lymphoma.

CONJUNCTIVAL MELANOMA

Carol L. Shields
Jerry A. Shields

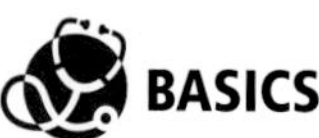

BASICS

DESCRIPTION

- Malignant tumor arising within the conjunctiva, the mucous membrane that lines the surface of the eye
- Classically pigmented but can be completely nonpigmented and appear pink
- Has prominent blood vessels feeding the tumor and within the tumor
- Tends to occur in mid to older adults and grows slowly over many months or years
- Can be unifocal or multifocal
- Painless, despite the eye appearing red and irritated
- Often manifests surrounding flat conjunctival pigment known as primary acquired melanosis that can predispose to future melanomas
- Can erode into the eye or grow deep in the orbit
- Risk for metastasis and eventual death from this cancer is approximately 25%
- Patients with this malignancy should be managed at by physicians familiar with this disease

ALERT

Any patient with a pigmented conjunctival mass should be evaluated by an ophthalmologist familiar with conjunctival tumors, particularly melanoma.

Geriatric Considerations

Most patients with conjunctival melanoma are >60 years old.

Pediatric Considerations

<1% of conjunctival melanomas occur in children.

Pregnancy Considerations

Pregnancy has not been shown to affect outcome.

EPIDEMIOLOGY

Incidence

- Race
  - 5 per 10 million white population
  - 1 per 10 million black population
- Sex
  - 3 per 10 million female population
  - 5 per 10 million male population
- Age
  - 0.8 per 10 million <40 years old
  - 4 per 10 million 40–59 years old
  - 18 per 10 million >60 years old

Prevalence

This tumor predominantly occurs in the older Caucasian population.

RISK FACTORS

- Conjunctival nevus–<1% evolve into melanoma
- Conjunctival primary acquired melanosis (PAM) – 9–32% evolve into melanoma
  - If the PAM shows severe atypia, the risk for transformation into melanoma is 13–90%.
  - The greater the extent of PAM, the greater the risk for melanoma.

Genetics

- There is no single genetic abnormality commonly expressed by conjunctival melanoma.
- It is anticipated that the genetic abnormalities found with cutaneous melanoma and uveal melanoma might differ from conjunctival melanoma.

GENERAL PREVENTION

Several studies have implied that the risk for conjunctival melanoma is increasing similar to cutaneous melanoma. These studies have suggested that sun exposure could be the cause, so avoidance of excessive sun exposure could be a factor in prevention of this malignancy.

PATHOPHYSIOLOGY

The development of conjunctival melanoma is multistep, multigenetic process.

ETIOLOGY

Sunlight exposure has been postulated as a possible etiology.

COMMONLY ASSOCIATED CONDITIONS

- Lentigo maligna of the periocular cutaneous region. It is a flat pigmentation of the skin that carries 20% risk for the development of cutaneous melanoma. This condition is similar to conjunctival PAM that leads to conjunctival melanoma. Often the 2 conditions occur in the same region.
- Neurofibromatosis carries slight association.

DIAGNOSIS

HISTORY

Painless brown mass on the eye that is slow growing.

PHYSICAL EXAM

- Pigmented brown in 80%
- Nonpigmented pink in 20%
- Can occur at all sites on conjunctiva including limbus, bulbus, fornix, palpebrum, caruncle
- Size can range from<1 mm to huge, covering the entire globe at 40 mm or more
- Larger tumors have greater risks for intraocular, orbital, and lymphatic spread
- Mass has smooth reflective surface with nodular appearance and dilated feeder blood vessels
- A wreath of dilated conjunctival vessels often encircles the mass.

DIAGNOSTIC TESTS & INTERPRETATION

Lab

Initial lab tests

CBC.

Follow-up & special considerations

- Slit-lamp examination essential
- Large detailed conjunctival drawing with high magnification
- Note all areas of thickened tissue compatible with melanoma
- Note all areas of precancerous primary acquired melanosis
- Flip upper and lower eyelid to evaluate tarsal and forniceal conjunctiva
- Palpate behind orbital rim for deeper nodules

Imaging

Initial approach

- Photography of entire anterior segment of the eye, including tarsal conjunctiva
- Anterior segment optical coherence tomography if intrascleral or intraocular extension considered
- Magnetic resonance imaging if orbital extension considered

Follow-up & special considerations

Sentinel lymph node biopsy to ascertain metastasis to regional lymph nodes.

Diagnostic Procedures/Other

- Fine needle aspiration biopsy of lymph node if palpable
- No need to needle biopsy conjunctival tumor as the best treatment is complete resection.
- Do not perform incisional biopsy as this could seed the tumor.

Pathological Findings

- 4 types of atypical melanocytes within melanoma include small polyhedral spindle, balloon, round epithelioid cells with eosinophilic cytoplasm.
- Growth in sheets or nests of cells deep to the epithelium within the substantia propria

DIFFERENTIAL DIAGNOSIS

- Conjunctival nevus
- Conjunctival primary acquired melanosis
- Conjunctival racial melanosis
- Conjunctival squamous cell carcinoma
- Oculodermal melanocytosis
- Extraocular extension of uveal melanoma
- Conjunctival metastasis from cutaneous melanoma
- Ochronosis
- Conjunctival arygyrosis (silver staining)

TREATMENT

MEDICATION

Surgical excision is first line therapy. If medications are used, they only follow surgery after complete healing and might include topical mitomycin C, 5 fluorouracil, or interferon to resolve residual flat melanosis.

ADDITIONAL TREATMENT

General Measures

- Any patient with conjunctival primary acquired melanosis or nevus should be followed by a competent ophthalmologist familiar with those conditions as well as melanoma and understanding that those conditions could lead to melanoma.
- If melanosis is extensive (>2 clock hours) or evolving, then surgical resection, cryotherapy and alcohol epitheliectomy should be performed.

SURGERY/OTHER PROCEDURES

- The goal of the "no touch" surgical technique is critical for complete excision, clean margins, and avoidance of tumor shedding.
- There is no role for incisional biopsy.
- Therapeutic steps are listed below:
  - Removal of corneal component with controlled absolute alcohol application followed by careful excision of corneal epithelium
  - Removal of conjunctival component with complete wide surgical resection using operating microscope to achieve tumor free margins and without touching or directly manipulating the tumor (no touch technique)
  - Cryotherapy to all surrounding conjunctival margins
  - Excision or cryotherapy to all surrounding primary acquired melanosis
  - Closure of tissue primarily or by using transpositional flap, free conjunctival graft, or amniotic membrane transplantation
  - Plaque radiotherapy for intrascleral involvement
  - Orbital exenteration for orbital involvement

ONGOING CARE

FOLLOW-UP RECOMMENDATIONS

- Follow closely after surgery every 3 months and if stable for 1 year without recurrence, then monitor twice yearly.
- If residual or recurrent melanoma, then surgical resection should be performed.
- If residual or recurrent melanosis, then surgical resection or cryotherapy should be performed.

Patient Monitoring

- Ophthalmic examination with photographic documentation at each visit
- Systemic evaluation for metastasis to lymph nodes, lung, and brain

PATIENT EDUCATION

- www.eyecancer.info
- www.eyetumor.org
- www.fighteyecancer.com
- www.eyecancerbook.com
- www.etrf.org
- www.choroidmelanoma.com

PROGNOSIS

- Systemic – Metastasis occurs in 16% by 5 years, 26% by 10 years, and 32% by 15 years.
- Ocular – melanoma recurrence or new tumor occurs in 26% by 5 years, 51% by 10 years, and 65% by 15 years. Exenteration is necessary in % by 5 years, 16% by 10 years, and 32% by 15 years.
- Visual – Following treatment, vision is 20/20–20/50 in 70%, 20/60–20/100 in 6%, and 20/200 or worse (including exenteration) in approximately 24%.

COMPLICATIONS

- Vision loss
- Dry eye
- Surgical pterygium
- Symblepharon
- Ptosis
- Conjunctival scarring
- Diplopia

ADDITIONAL READING

- Shields CL, Shields JA. Tumors of the conjunctiva and cornea. *Surv Ophthalmol* 2004;49:3–24.
- Grossniklaus HE, Green WR, Luckenbach M, et al. Conjunctival lesions in adults: A clinical and histopathologic review. *Cornea* 1987;6:78–116.
- Shields CL, Demirci H, Karatza EC, et al. Clinical survey of 1643 melanocytic and nonmelanocytic conjunctival tumors. *Ophthalmology* 2004;111: 1747–1754.
- Shields CL, Fasiudden A, Mashayekhi A, et al. Conjunctival nevi: Clinical features and natural course in 410 consecutive patients. *Arch Ophthalmol* 2004;122:167–175.
- Folberg R, McLean IW, Zimmerman LE. Primary acquired melanosis of the conjunctiva. *Hum Pathol* 1985;16:136–143.
- Shields JA, Shields CL, Mashayekhi A, et al. Primary acquired melanosis of the conjunctiva. Risks for progression to melanoma in 311 eyes. The 2006 Lorenz E. Zimmerman Lecture. *Ophthalmology* 2008;115(3):51–19.
- Shields CL, Shields JA, Gunduz K, et al. Conjunctival melanoma: Risk factors for recurrence, exenteration, metastasis, and death in 150 consecutive patients. *Arch Ophthalmol* 2000;118:1497–1507.
- Seregard S. Conjunctival melanoma. *Surv Ophthalmol* 1998;42:321–350.
- Yu GP, Hu DN, McCormick S, et al. Conjunctival melanoma: Is it increasing in the United States? *Am J Ophthalmol* 2003;135:800–6.
- Shields JA, Shields CL, De Potter P. Surgical management of conjunctival tumors. The 1994 Lynn B. McMahan Lecture. *Arch Ophthalmol* 1997;115: 808–15.
- Shields JA, Shields CL. Conjunctival melanocytic lesions. In: Eyelid, Conjunctival, and Orbital Tumors. *An atlas and textbook*. Philadelphia: Lippincott Williams and Wilkins Co, 2008:307–347.
- Shields JA, Shields CL. Surgical management of conjunctival tumors. In: Eyelid, Conjunctival, and Orbital Tumors. *An atlas and textbook*. Philadelphia: Lippincott Williams and Wilkins Co, 2008:437–445.

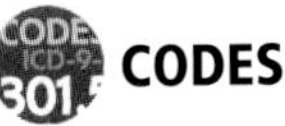

CODES

ICD9

- 190.3 Malignant neoplasm of conjunctiva
- 232.1 Carcinoma in situ of eyelid, including canthus
- 372.55 Conjunctival pigmentations

CLINICAL PEARLS

- Any pigmented conjunctival mass should be examined by a qualified ophthalmologist for features of melanoma.

C

CONJUNCTIVAL NEVUS

Britt J. Parvus
Carol L. Shields

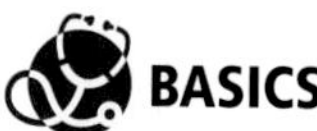

BASICS

DESCRIPTION

- Most common conjunctival tumor
- Represents 28% of all conjunctival tumors and over 50% of all melanocytic conjunctival tumors
- Can be melanotic (~80%) or amelanotic (~20%)
- Can be congenital (present at birth or within the first 6 months of life) or acquired
- If acquired, usually clinically visible by the first or second decade of life
- Can become more pigmented over time, especially during hormonal changes, such as puberty and pregnancy

Pediatric Considerations

- An increase in size may be seen in young children.
- Increased pigmentation may be seen during puberty.

Pregnancy Considerations

Increased pigmentation may be seen during pregnancy in cutaneous nevi, but this has not been well documented in conjunctival nevi.

EPIDEMIOLOGY

Occurrence is most common in Caucasians (89%); less frequently seen in African Americans (6%) and Asians, Hispanics, or Indians (5%).

RISK FACTORS

Ethnicity: Non-Hispanic whites.

GENERAL PREVENTION

Most conjunctival nevi occur at the nasal and temporal limbus in the sun exposed regions of the eye. Avoidance of sun exposure might reduce conjunctival nevus development, but more importantly, avoidance of sun exposure might reduce transformation of conjunctival nevus into melanoma.

COMMONLY ASSOCIATED CONDITIONS

- Generally sporadic without systemic associations
- Rare association with the Carney complex and the dysplastic nevus syndrome

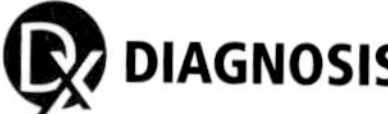

DIAGNOSIS

HISTORY

Patients may be asymptomatic (10%) or may report noticing a "spot" on the eye (88%), inflammation (3%), or rarely pain (<1%) (1)[C].

PHYSICAL EXAM

- Usually presents as a discrete, variably pigmented, slightly elevated conjunctival mass.
- The mass is within the conjunctiva and moves with conjunctival displacement.
- Nevus typically occurs on the bulbar conjunctiva (~70%), most commonly in the interpalpebral zone (~85%) (1,2)[C].
- May be pigmented (51%), partially pigmented (28%), or completely amelanotic (21%) (2)[C].
- Multiple, intralesional clear cysts can be seen on slit-lamp biomicroscopy (1,2)[C].
- If located on the bulbar conjunctiva, conjunctival nevi typically abruptly stop at the limbus and do not involve the cornea (1)[C].
- In the bulbar conjunctiva, temporal (46%) or nasal (44%) location is more common than superior (6%) or inferior (%5) location (1)[C].

DIAGNOSTIC TESTS & INTERPRETATION

Imaging

Initial approach

- Slit-lamp photography
- Anterior segment optical coherence tomography to document cysts

Follow-up & special considerations

Serial photography every 6–12 months to rule out growth/malignant transformation.

Diagnostic Procedures/Other

Anterior segment optical coherence tomography.

Pathological Findings

- Diffuse infiltration or distinct nests of benign melanocytes near the basal layer of the epithelium
- Most often classified as junctional (small nest of melanocytes in the basal layer of the epithelium), compound (cell migration into the underlying stroma), or subepithelial/deep (cell migration entirely into the stroma)
- Caveat: In general, the melanoma-specific antigen (HMB-45) shows a positive reaction with conjunctival nevus and melanoma and can therefore not be used reliably to differentiate the two conjunctival lesions.

DIFFERENTIAL DIAGNOSIS

- Primary acquired melanosis
- Racial melanosis
- Secondary melanosis
- Malignant melanoma (melanotic & amelanotic)
- If amelanotic
  - Inflamed pinguecula
  - Conjunctival cyst
  - Allergic conjunctivitis
  - Foreign body granuloma
  - Episcleritis
  - Squamous epithelial neoplasia
  - Papilloma
  - Lymphoma
  - Lymphangioma

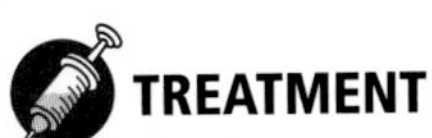

TREATMENT

MEDICATION

None available

ADDITIONAL TREATMENT

General Measures

Initial management for a small, typical conjunctival nevus is periodic observation with photographic documentation (2)[C].

Issues for Referral

- Any diagnostic uncertainty
- When surgical excision is considered

SURGERY/OTHER PROCEDURES

- Excisional biopsy using the "no touch" technique whereby the tumor is never manipulated should be used. This is approached using a dry ocular surface without balanced salt solution. The cornea is dried and absolute alcohol on a Weck sponge is precisely applied to the limbus immediately adjacent to the nevus without spillage to other sites. The corneal epithelium is removed. The conjunctival mass is removed with Westcott scissors and a 3–4 mm margin. After removal, cryotherapy is applied to the remaining conjunctival margins. Closure is done with absorbable sutures.
- Consider complete excisional biopsy if
  - Suspicious changes
  - Documented growth
  - Location in the forniceal or tarsal conjunctiva
  - Limbal location with corneal involvement
  - Feeder vessels
  - Intrinsic vessels
  - Larger lesion without cysts
  - Family history of conjunctival or cutaneous melanoma
  - Distinct onset in middle age or later life
  - Recurrence of a previously excised lesion
  - Ocular irritation
  - Cosmetic concern
  - Cancerophobia
- In general, incisional biopsies are contraindicated in lesions that can be resected entirely in one procedure.

IN-PATIENT CONSIDERATIONS

- None required
- Outpatient surgery and management

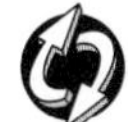

ONGOING CARE

FOLLOW-UP RECOMMENDATIONS

Annual ophthalmologic examinations if lesion is typical and nonsuspicious in appearance.

Patient Monitoring

Slit-lamp photography and anterior segment optical coherence tomography every 6–12 months to monitor stability.

DIET

No dietary restrictions.

PATIENT EDUCATION

- See related websites.
- Avoid excessive sun exposure.

PROGNOSIS

Excellent in most cases.

COMPLICATIONS

Irritation and/or dry eye occasionally seen after excisional biopsy.

REFERENCES

1. Shields CL, Fasiudden A, Mashayekhi A, et al. Conjunctival nevi: Clinical features and natural course in 410 consecutive patients. *Arch Ophthalmol* 2004;122:167–175.
2. Levecq L, DePotter P, Jamart J. Conjunctival nevi: Clinical features and therapeutic outcomes. *Ophthalmology* 2010;117:35–40.

ADDITIONAL READING

- Shields CL, Demirci H, Ekaterina K, et al. Clinical survey of 1643 melanocytic and nonmelanocytic conjunctival tumors. *Ophthalmology* 2004;111: 1747–1754.
- Shields JA, Shields CL. Tumors of the conjunctiva. In *Eyelid, conjunctival, and orbital tumors: an atlas and textbook*. Philadelphia: Lippincott Williams & Wilkins, 2008:308–319.
- www.fighteyecancer.com
- www.eyecancerinfo.com
- www.malignantmelanomainfo.com
- www.etrf.org

CODES

ICD9

- 190.3 Malignant neoplasm of conjunctiva
- 224.0 Benign neoplasm of eyeball, except conjunctiva, cornea, retina, and choroid
- 224.3 Benign neoplasm of conjunctiva

CLINICAL PEARLS

- Locations in the forniceal conjunctiva, tarsal/palpebral conjunctiva, or cornea should raise suspicion that the lesion is an early conjunctival melanoma (1,2)[C].
- Conjunctival nevi may exhibit minor gradual changes in pigmentation (7–13%) and size (5–8%) (1,2)[C].

CONJUNCTIVAL PRIMARY ACQUIRED MELANOSIS

Carol L. Shields
Jerry A. Shields

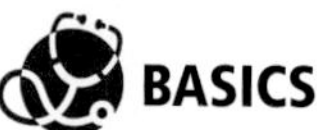

BASICS

DESCRIPTION

- Primary acquired melanosis (PAM) is an acquired flat pigmentation of the conjunctiva.
- Slowly progressive
- Generally without excessive vascularity
- Can affect the limbus, bulbar, forniceal, plical, caruncular, and tarsal conjunctiva
- Unilateral and nonhereditary
- Risk for development of conjunctival melanoma

ALERT
Any patient with a new onset flat pigmented conjunctival lesion should be examined to evaluate for primary acquired melanosis, a known precursor to melanoma.

Geriatric Considerations
Generally a disease of middle aged or older individuals.

Pediatric Considerations
This condition is rarely found in children.

Pregnancy Considerations
This condition is rarely seen during pregnancy.

RISK FACTORS
None clearly identified but patients at highest risk are those of:

- Caucasian race
- Older age
- Excessive sunlight exposure

GENERAL PREVENTION
Avoid excess sunlight exposure.

PATHOPHYSIOLOGY

- Begins as a flat area of pigmentation on the conjunctival surface. Histopathology shows it arising in the basal epithelial layers. As it progresses, the atypical cells involve the mid portion and then superficial portion of the conjunctival epithelium. With time, the anaplastic cells can grow through the basement membrane into the stroma and be classified then as microscopically invasive melanoma.
- Slowly and progressively enlarging pigmented conjunctival tumor

COMMONLY ASSOCIATED CONDITIONS
Lentigo maligna of eyelid skin that carries a 20% risk for cutaneous melanoma.

DIAGNOSIS

HISTORY

- Most patients note an area of pigmentation that slowly evolves and grows over time.
- Based on an analysis of 311 eyes with PAM by Shields and associates, the patient demographics include:
  - Female in 44%, male in 38%
  - Caucasian in 96%, African American in 1%, Hispanic in 2%, and Asian in <1%
  - Unilateral in 87%, bilateral in 13%
  - Eye color brown in 58%, blue in 35%, green in 5%
  - Mean patient age 56 years (range 15–90)
- Patient symptoms include:
  - Spot stable on eye in 29%
  - Spot growing on eye in 16%
  - Ocular redness in 1%
  - No symptom in 55%

PHYSICAL EXAM

- Ocular examination, based on analysis of 311 eyes shows:
- Number (mean) of PAM per eye 2 (1–7)
- Quadrant location superior in 37%, temporal in 57%, inferior in 45%, nasal in 42%
- Anatomic location of PAM in cornea in 23%, limbal conjunctiva in 55%, fornix in 13%, palpebra in 12%, caruncle in 11%
- Extent (mean) of PAM in clock hours of 3

DIAGNOSTIC TESTS & INTERPRETATION

Lab

Initial lab tests

- None other than ocular exam
- If there is associated melanoma then the patient should have lymph node evaluation and chest x-ray.

Follow-up & special considerations
Careful follow-up is warranted for evolution of PAM into melanoma. Based on clinical studies, untreated PAM evolves into melanoma in 0% of those with minimal or no atypia and 13% of those with severe atypia. Based on pathology studies, PAM evolves into melanoma in 0% of those with no atypia, 46% if any atypia, and 75–90% of those with severe atypia.

Imaging

Initial approach
For PAM alone, anterior segment optical coherence tomography might be beneficial to demonstrate the lack of deep involvement.

Follow-up & special considerations
If there is conversion to melanoma then imaging with MRI is warranted.

Diagnostic Procedures/Other

- Some authorities prefer no manipulation of the conjunctiva prior to surgical treatment in the operating room.
- Other authorities wish to have superficial scraping of the conjunctival for cytologic documentation.

Pathological Findings

- Pathology reveals 2 basic types of PAM, those without atypia and those with atypia.
- PAM without atypia is defined as pigmentation of the conjunctival epithelium, usually the basal layer, with benign melanocytic hyperplasia.
- PAM with atypia is defined as the presence of atypical melanocytic hyperplasia in a mild, moderate, or severe form with gradually extension from the basal portion of the epithelium to the more superficial portion in a pagetoid fashion.

DIFFERENTIAL DIAGNOSIS

- Racial melanosis (also referred to as complexion related melanosis)
- Conjunctival nevus
- Conjunctival melanoma
- Secondary conjunctival pigmentation from medications (argyrosis), exposure, trauma (shrapnel injury)

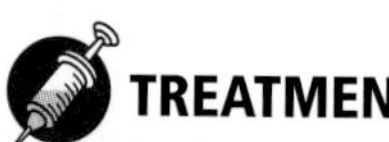

TREATMENT

MEDICATION

First Line

- First line therapy for PAM requires biopsy proof of the condition. Our first choice is to biopsy and provide cryotherapy to all sites of pigmentation. If the PAM is completely resectable, then that would be our first choice. Closure of all wounds is advised following therapy.
- Regarding medications, Mitomycin C (MMC) 0.02% or 0.04% can be given 4 times daily for 1–2 weeks then 1–2 weeks of drop-free recovery. This can be repeated as need be. MMC can effectively reduce the pigmentation and can be used as a primary or adjuvant therapy.
- 5 Fluorouracil and interferon have been used to treat PAM.

Second Line
If there is extensive PAM with multiple recurrences, consideration for custom fit plaque radiotherapy in a conformer design can effectively treat the entire surface of the eye in a fairly homogeneous fashion.

ADDITIONAL TREATMENT
General Measures
Topical lubricants are given to help heal the ocular surface following surgery, cryotherapy, or topical chemotherapy.

Issues for Referral
All patients with PAM should be managed by consultants familiar with this condition as this precancerous disease carries a strong risk for life-threatening melanoma.

SURGERY/OTHER PROCEDURES
- Surgery is usually the main initial procedure for PAM. The treatment strategy depends on the extent of tumor and the presence or history of previous melanoma. Patients are discharged the same day following therapy.
- If PAM is <1 clock hour, its significance remains debatable and most would observe it.
- PAM is 4–5 clock hours or less, consideration is given for complete resection followed by cryotherapy of the remaining conjunctival margins and closure with absorbable sutures.
- If PAM is >5 clock hours then wide resection of the suspicious areas is performed with heavy double freeze thaw cryotherapy to all residual areas of pigmentation. This can be used for PAM involving the entire ocular surface, except the cornea.
- If cornea PAM, then epithelial removal following topical absolute alcohol with microscopic monitoring is performed.
- If recurrent extensive PAM, then topical MMC is considered.
- If there is a history of conjunctival or cutaneous melanoma, then complete treatment is encouraged to the point that the patient shows no conjunctival pigmentation at all.

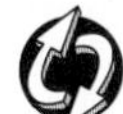

ONGOING CARE

FOLLOW-UP RECOMMENDATIONS
Return visits initially every 3–4 months and after stability documented, then every 6 months for life.

Patient Monitoring
Monitor the ocular surface for PAM using slit-lamp biomicroscopy.

PATIENT EDUCATION
If the patient notices recurrent pigmentation, then return visit is justified.

PROGNOSIS
- Excellent if there is no transformation into melanoma
- Guarded if there is transformation into melanoma

COMPLICATIONS
- Dry eye
- Symblepharon
- Blepharoptosis
- Diplopia
- Limbal stem cell loss
- Conjunctival overgrowth onto cornea
- Chronic pain
- Loss of the eye

ADDITIONAL READING

- Shields JA, Shields CL, Mashayekhi A, et al. Primary acquired melanosis of the conjunctiva. Risks for progression to melanoma in 311 eyes. The 2006 Lorenz E. Zimmerman Lecture. *Ophthalmology* 2008;115(3):511–519.
- Shields CL, Shields JA. Conjunctival primary acquired melanosis and melanoma. Tales, fairy tales and facts. *Ophthal Plast Reconstr Surg* 2009;25:167–72.
- Folberg R, McLean IW, Primary acquired melanosis and melanoma of the conjunctiva: Terminology, classification, and biologic behavior. *Hum Pathol* 1986;76:307–8.
- Shields JA, Shields CL. *Eyelid, Conjunctival and orbital tumors: An atlas and text*, 2nd ed. Philadelphia: Lippincott, Williams and Wilkins, 2008.

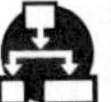

See Also (Topic, Algorithm, Electronic Media Element)

- www.fighteyecancer.com
- www.eyecancer.info
- www.eyetumor.org
- www.eyecancerbook.com
- www.etrf.org
- www.choroidmelanoma.com

CODES

ICD9
- 190.3 Malignant neoplasm of conjunctiva
- 372.55 Conjunctival pigmentations

CLINICAL PEARLS

- Any patient with PAM of more than 1 clock hour should have consultation by an experienced examiner.
- If a patient with previous skin or conjunctival melanoma shows evidence of PAM, then eradication of PAM is warranted.

CONJUNCTIVITIS, ACUTE BACTERIAL

Robert Sambursky

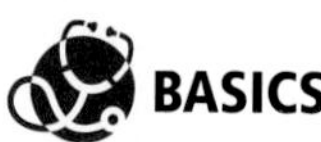

BASICS

DESCRIPTION

Acute conjunctivitis defines an inflammation of the conjunctiva, or the mucous membrane lining the inner surface of the eyelids and the outer surface of the eyeball extending over the sclera. Bacterial conjunctivitis is a very common condition.

EPIDEMIOLOGY

- Affects both children and adults of all ages
- No sex predominance

Incidence

- Acute conjunctivitis comprises about 1–2% of a primary care office visits.
- 1 in 8 schoolchildren has an episode of acute infective conjunctivitis every year.
- There are approximately 6 million cases of conjunctivitis annually.

Prevalence

Bacteria are responsible for about 50–75% of all cases of acute conjunctivitis in young children.

RISK FACTORS

- Bacterial conjunctivitis occurs in otherwise healthy individuals.
- Risk factors include exposure to infected individuals, sinusitis, and immunodeficiency states.

Genetics

No genetic predisposition

GENERAL PREVENTION

Isolation of contagious patients for 24–48 h after initiation of antibiotic therapy

PATHOPHYSIOLOGY

Inflammation of the conjunctiva, or the mucous membrane lining the inner surface of the eyelids, and outer surface of the eyeball extending over the sclera

ETIOLOGY

- Acute bacterial conjunctivitis:
  - *Staphylococcus aureus, Haemophilus influenzae, Streptococcus pneumonia, Moraxella catarrhalis, Staphylococcus epidermidis:*
    - *H. influenzae* and *S. pneumonia* are most common in children.
    - *S. aureus* are most common in adults.
- Hyperacute bacterial conjunctivitis:
  - *Neisseria gonorrhea*
- Chronic bacterial conjunctivitis:
  - *Chlamydia*

COMMONLY ASSOCIATED CONDITIONS

- Otitis media:
  - Frequently caused by *H. influenzae*

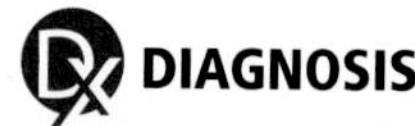

DIAGNOSIS

There is considerable overlap in clinical signs and symptoms between viral and bacterial conjunctivitis; clinical accuracy of 50%. Four clinical factors were independently associated with negative cultures: 1) age ≥6 years, 2) presentation during April through November, 3) watery or no discharge, 4) no glued eye in the morning. A child who presented with all four clinical factors would have a negative culture 92% of the time, whereas a child who presented with none of these factors would have a negative culture 12% of the time (2)[B].

HISTORY

- More commonly associated with a bilateral > unilateral red eye
- Eyelash matting
- Purulent yellow-green discharge
- Copious discharge associated with hyperacute bacterial conjunctivitis
- History of sexual activity associated with hyperacute and chronic conjunctivitis
- Exposure to a sick contact

PHYSICAL EXAM

- Palpebral papillary reaction
- Follicles develop with *Chlamydia*.
- Only 10% have associated a preauricular lymphadenopathy.
- Moraxella species, *Chlamydia*, and *N. gonorrhea*

DIAGNOSTIC TESTS & INTERPRETATION

Lab

Initial lab tests

- Cell culture:
  - "Gold Standard"; Not routinely performed
  - Blood agar and chocolate agar
  - Recommended for patients not responding to therapy, immune compromised patients, contact lens wearers, in the setting of an outbreak, sexual active person with copious discharge
  - Copious discharge suggests *N. gonorrhea*; requires culture on chocolate agar.
- Gram stain (1–5)[A]:
  - Copious discharge suggests *N. gonorrhea*; intracellular diplococci are suggestive.
- Polymerase chain reaction:
  - Usually a send-out test; expensive
  - Not FDA cleared
  - Available for confirmation of *Chlamydia* and *N. gonorrhea*

Follow-up & special considerations

- Follow-up in 5–7 days
- 70% of patients with confirmed ocular chlamydia have a coexistent chlamydia genital infection.
- Follow-up should be in 5–7 days. *N. gonorrhea* needs daily follow-up in the first 3 days.
  - High risk of corneal ulceration with perforation

Diagnostic Procedures/Other

Immunoassay to rule out adenovirus

DIFFERENTIAL DIAGNOSIS

Acute viral conjunctivitis (HSV and adenovirus), allergic conjunctivitis, episcleritis/scleritis, blepharitis, infectious or inflammatory keratitis, uveitis, and angle closure glaucoma

TREATMENT

MEDICATION

- A meta-analysis of antibiotics versus placebo for acute bacterial conjunctivitis was published in a Cochrane review in 2006. 5 randomized trials including a total of 1034 participants were analyzed and it was determined that clinical recovery with antibiotics was faster in the first 2–5 days after presentation (relative risk of clinical cure 1.24; 6 patients needed treatment in order to achieve one more clinical cure than with placebo) (1,3)[A].
- 6–10 days after presentation the benefit of antibiotics was less (relative risk of clinical cure 1.11; 13 patients needed treatment) (1,3)[A].
- The benefit of topical antibiotics versus placebo was greater on microbiological cure than on clinical cure. At 2–5 days after presentation the relative risk of microbiological cure was 1.77; at 6 to 10 days the relative risk was 1.56 (1,3)[A].
- Delayed therapy for 3 days is an option but forces isolation of contagious persons.

First Line

- Acute bacterial conjunctivitis:
  - Polytrim 1 drop every 4–6 h for 7 days
  - Fluoroquinolone 1 drop every 4–6 h for 7 days
    - i.e., moxifloxacin, gatifloxacinlevofloxacin, besifloxacin
- Hyperacute bacterial conjunctivitis:
  - Ceftriaxone 1 g intramuscularly (i.m.) in a single dose for presumed *N. gonorrhea*
  - If corneal involvement exists, treat with ceftriaxone 1 g intravenously (i.v.) every 12–24 h
  - Topical fluoroquinolone q.i.d. without corneal involvement and q1–2h with corneal involvement
  - In penicillin-allergic patients, consider an oral fluoroquinolone (e.g., ciprofloxacin 500 mg p.o., for 5 days.

Second Line

- Azithromycin 1 drop twice daily for 2 days and then once daily for 3 additional days
- Older generation medications suffer from high rates of antibiotic resistance.
- Medications such as topical Tobramycin and Gentamycin may be associated with corneal toxicity. Other antibiotics such as Sulfa and Neomycin are associated with increased rates of allergic reactions and should be avoided.

ADDITIONAL TREATMENT

General Measures

- Supportive care:
  - Refrigerated preservative-free artificial tears
  - Frequent hand washing
  - Limit sharing of towels and linens

Issues for Referral

- Severe eye pain or headache, photophobia, decreased vision acuity, trauma, or contact lens use
- Mid-dilated fixed pupil, hazy cornea
- No improvement after 7 days of antibiotic treatment

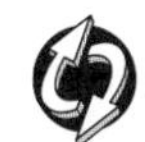

ONGOING CARE

FOLLOW-UP RECOMMENDATIONS

Follow-up is recommended for patients who develop reduced vision, pain, light sensitivity or if symptoms persist beyond 7 days.

PATIENT EDUCATION

Educate patients on contagiousness.

PROGNOSIS

Self-limiting; most patients recover spontaneously.

COMPLICATIONS

Complications are rare.

ADDITIONAL READING

- O'Brien TP, Jeng BH, McDonald M, et al. Acute conjunctivitis: Truth and misconceptions. *Curr Med Res Opin* 2009;25:1953–1961.
- Høvding G. Acute bacterial conjunctivitis. *Acta Ophthalmol* 2008;86:5–17.
- Meltzer JA, Kunkov S, Crain EF. Identifying children at low risk for bacterial conjunctivitis. *Arch Pediatr Adolesc Med* 2010;164:263–267.
- Oliver GF, Wilson GA, Everts RJ. Acute infective conjunctivitis: evidence review and management advice for New Zealand practitioners. *N Z Med J* 2009;122:69–75.
- Tarabishy AB, Jeng BH. Bacterial conjunctivitis: A review for internists. *Cleve Clin J Med* 2008;75: 507–512.
- American Academy of Ophthalmology. Conjunctivitis Preferred Practice Patterns 2008.

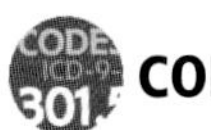

CODES

ICD9

- 372.00 Acute conjunctivitis, unspecified
- 372.03 Other mucopurulent conjunctivitis
- 372.30 Conjunctivitis, unspecified

CLINICAL PEARLS

- Consider more serious eye disease if there is a unilateral red eye, reduced visual acuity, severe pain, significant photophobia, contact lens wear, or recent ocular surgery or trauma. Purulent discharge is associated with bacterial conjunctivitis.
- Negative cultures are associated with: 1) age ≥6 years, 2) presentation during April through November, 3) watery or no discharge, and 4) no glued eye in the morning.
- Antibiotic treatment of bacterial conjunctivitis reduces the duration of clinical illness by 0.5–1.5 days and hastens microbiological cure.

CONJUNCTIVITIS, ACUTE VIRAL

Robert Sambursky

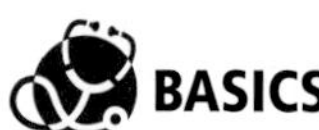

BASICS

DESCRIPTION

Acute conjunctivitis defines an inflammation of the conjunctiva, or the mucous membrane lining the inner surface of the eyelids and outer surface of the eyeball extending over the sclera. Viral conjunctivitis is a very common condition and adenovirus is the most frequent cause of conjunctivitis worldwide.

EPIDEMIOLOGY

- Affects both children and adults of all ages
- No sex predominance

Incidence

- Acute conjunctivitis comprises about 1–2% of a primary care office visits.
- There are approximately 6 million cases of conjunctivitis annually.

Prevalence

20–70% of acute conjunctivitis is viral.

RISK FACTORS

- <5% of the US population shows natural immunity against adenovirus.
- Adenovirus can live on inanimate surfaces for 5 weeks:
  - Overcrowding or close quarters
  - Urban setting
  - Exposure to a sick contact

Genetics

No genetic predisposition

GENERAL PREVENTION

- Isolation of contagious patients:
  - Adenoviral conjunctivitis shows close contact and intrafamilial spread of 20–40%.

PATHOPHYSIOLOGY

Inflammation of the conjunctiva, or the mucous membrane lining the inner surface of the eyelids, and outer surface of the eyeball extending over the sclera

ETIOLOGY

- Viral conjunctivitis represents 20–70% of all acute conjunctivitis.
  - Adenovirus accounts for 65–90% of viral conjunctivitis.
    - Presents as 1 of 4 clinical conditions: Epidemic keratoconjunctivitis (EKC), acute hemorrhagic conjunctivitis (AHC), pharyngoconjunctival fever (PCF), and nonspecific follicular conjunctivitis (NFC)
  - Herpes simplex virus (HSV) accounts for 1.3–21% of viral conjunctivitis.
    - These cases occur without associated skin vesicles or keratitis.
  - Other less common viruses include *Molluscum contagiosum*, varicella-zoster virus (VZV), coxsackie virus, enterovirus, echovirus, Epstein-Barr virus, human immunodeficiency virus, and cytomegalovirus.

COMMONLY ASSOCIATED CONDITIONS

- Adenovirus may be associated with viral prodrome followed by adenopathy, fever, pharyngitis, or an upper respiratory tract infection.
- HSV and VZV may be associated with a vesicular skin rash and/or keratitis.

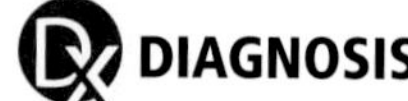

DIAGNOSIS

HISTORY

- More commonly associated with a bilateral red eye
- Starts in one eye and then moves to the other several days later
- Watery to mucoid discharge
- Recent upper respiratory symptoms
- Exposure to a sick contact

PHYSICAL EXAM

- Injection
- Palpebral follicular reaction
- Microhemorrhages
- Pseudomembranes
- Superficial punctuate keratopathy
- Subepithelial infiltrates:
  - Only occurs after 7–10 days
- Pre-auricular lymphadenopathy:
  - Only present in 30–50%

DIAGNOSTIC TESTS & INTERPRETATION

Lab

- Point of care immunoassay for adenovirus with a sensitivity of 88–89% and a specificity of 91–94% (1)[A]:
  - 10 min in office test
  - Detects viable and nonviable virus fragments
  - Antigen levels diminish after 7 days
- Viral cell culture (3)[A]:
  - May take 3–21 days to grow
  - "Gold Standard"
  - Only detects live virus
- Polymerase chain reaction (3)[A]:
  - Usually a send-out test; expensive
  - Not FDA cleared
  - Detects both viable and nonviable viral fragments

Diagnostic Procedures/Other

Serological tests for HSV IgM and IgG

DIFFERENTIAL DIAGNOSIS

Acute bacterial conjunctivitis, allergic conjunctivitis, episcleritis/scleritis, blepharitis, dry eyes, infectious or inflammatory keratitis, uveitis, and angle closure glaucoma

TREATMENT

MEDICATION

First Line

- Adenoviral conjunctivitis has no FDA approved antiviral agents.
  - Refrigerated preservative-free artificial tears every 2 h
  - Topical antihistamines twice daily for significant itching
  - Topical ganciclovir gel:
    - Small, randomized, controlled, masked series of 18 patients showed decreased duration of disease (4)[A].
- HSV should be treated with topical antiviral:
  - Topical ganciclovir gel 0.15% 5 times per day (4)[B]
  - Trifluridine 1% (Viroptic) drops 5 times per day (4)[B]

Second Line

- Topical steroids may be considered in the presence of pseudomembranes or subepithelial infiltrates.
  - Steroids should be avoided except in severe disease because of associated increased viral replication and prolonged infectivity.
    - Consider loteprednol twice to 4 times daily or a steroid ointment such as fluorometholone 0.1% or dexamethasone/tobramycin 4 times daily.

ADDITIONAL TREATMENT

General Measures

- Supportive care:
  - Refrigerated preservative-free artificial tears
  - Frequent hand washing
  - Limit sharing of towels and linens
  - Home disinfection

Issues for Referral

- After 7–10 days patients may develop subepithelial infiltrates (corneal deposits).
  - Manifest as reduced vision or photosensitivity

Additional Therapies

Analytical laboratory studies and anecdotal support for povidone iodine therapy exist.

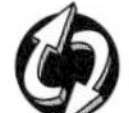

ONGOING CARE

FOLLOW-UP RECOMMENDATIONS

Follow-up is recommended for patients who develop reduced vision, light sensitivity, or if symptoms persist beyond 10 days.

PATIENT EDUCATION

- Educate patients on extreme contagiousness.
- Educate patients on the ineffectiveness of topical antibiotics.

PROGNOSIS

- Most patients recover spontaneously.
- 20–50% of patients with EKC develop SEIs or chronic dry eyes.

COMPLICATIONS

- Corneal subepithelial infiltrates (inflammatory deposits)
- Chronic dry eye
- Conjunctival scarring
- Chronic epiphora (tearing)

ADDITIONAL READING

- American Academy of Ophthalmology. Conjunctivitis Preferred Practice Patterns. 2008.
- Udeh BL, Schneider JE, Ohsfeldt RL. Cost effectiveness of a point-of-care test for adenoviral conjunctivitis. *Am J Med Sci* 2008;336:254–264.
- Sambursky R, Tauber S, Schirra F, et al. The RPS adeno detector for diagnosing adenoviral conjunctivitis. *Ophthalmology* 2006;113: 1758–1764.
- Rietveld RP, van Weert HC, ter Riet G, et al. Diagnostic impact of signs and symptoms in acute infectious conjunctivitis: Systematic literature search. *BMJ* 2003;327:789.
- O'Brien TP, Jeng BH, McDonald M, et al. Acute conjunctivitis: truth and misconceptions. *Curr Med Res Opin* 2009;25:1953–1961.
- Colin J. Ganciclovir ophthalmic gel, 0.15%: A valuable tool for treating ocular herpes. *Clin Ophthalmol* 2007;1:441–453.

CODES

ICD9

- 077.3 Other adenoviral conjunctivitis
- 077.99 Unspecified diseases of conjunctiva due to viruses
- 372.00 Acute conjunctivitis, unspecified

CLINICAL PEARLS

- A 50% clinical accuracy was found compared to laboratory diagnosis.
- HSV may present with EKC that is indistinguishable from adenovirus.

CONTACT LENS COMPLICATIONS

Brett Levinson

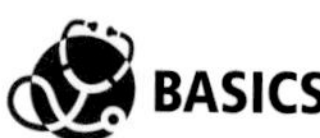

BASICS

DESCRIPTION

Complications from contact lens use can occur in any patient who wears contact lenses. Problems associated with contact lens use include infection (most commonly bacterial but rarely fungal or amoebal), allergic, overwear (corneal hypoxia and neovascularization), toxicity (from multipurpose cleaning solutions or improper use of hydrogen peroxide solutions), and corneal warpage (seen most commonly with rigid gas permeable lenses).

ALERT

While rare, always ask about exposure to fresh water from lakes or streams while wearing contacts, or cleaning contacts with tap water (especially from wells) as this is a risk factor for *Acanthamoeba* keratitis.

Pediatric Considerations

Teenagers are prone to improper use of contact lenses, including wearing contacts for extended periods of time, not changing contacts as directed, and wearing their contacts despite having red or painful eyes.

EPIDEMIOLOGY

Complications more commonly occur in patients who improperly clean or store their contacts, or who wear contacts with a low-oxygen permeability (Dk), or wear contact lenses overnight and/or for many days continuously.

Incidence

- Incidence of bacterial keratitis is estimated to be between 0.04 and 0.21%. The incidence is much higher in patients wearing contact lenses overnight and for extended periods of time without changing their lenses.
- Fungal and amoebal keratitis are rare, but rates can be higher when associated with epidemic outbreaks from contaminated water or from contact lens solutions.
- Incidence of giant papillary conjunctivitis (GPC) varies based on the types of lens, but has been reported at 4.6% for silicone hydrogel lenses.

Prevalence

As most contact lens problems are acute, prevalence generally equals incidence.

ALERT

There have been 2 major outbreaks of infectious keratitis related to multipurpose solutions (MPS). ReNu with MoistureLoc was linked to fungal (*Fusarium*) keratitis, and Complete was linked to *Acanthamoebal* keratitis. The incidence of infectious keratitis can increase sporadically, and practitioners should be aware if an outbreak of infectious keratitis has been reported.

RISK FACTORS

- Use of a contact lens with a low permeability for oxygen (Dk), especially if worn continuously
- Improper storage and disinfection of contact lenses
- Exposure to fresh water lakes and streams, or tap water (especially well water)
- Dry eyes
- Atopy
- Use of an MPS
  - Solutions which are intended to clean, disinfect, and store contacts are considered multipurpose solutions. Recent outbreaks of infectious keratitis have highlighted the fact that many contact lens wears improperly use their MPS, increasing the risk of infection.
  - Also, as these solutions are designed to be antimicrobial, they can cause toxicity to the corneal epithelium. This problem is more pronounced in people with risk factors for dry eyes.

GENERAL PREVENTION

- Avoidance of overnight and extended wear of contact lenses
- Following the manufacturers' recommended replacement, schedule for the particular contact lenses
- Use of daily disposable contact lenses (contacts designed to be worn once and then disposed)
- Avoidance of multipurpose solutions:
  - If multipurpose solutions are used, rub contact lenses with a solution prior to storage. Do not "top off" the solution in the contact lens case – dispose the old solution in the contact lens case and use a new solution from the bottle. Change the contact lens cases frequently.
- Use of hydrogen peroxide disinfection systems decreases the risk of complication by providing better disinfection of the contacts, and having less residual toxicity than multipurpose solutions (after complete neutralization of the hydrogen peroxide solution).
  - Hydrogen peroxide solutions can never be placed directly in the eye; otherwise a severe toxic keratitis will occur.
  - Use of 1-day disposable contacts reduces the overall risk of contact lens complications

PATHOPHYSIOLOGY

- Contact lenses can decrease the transmission of oxygen to the ocular surface, leading to hypoxia, neovascularization, and conjunctivalization of the cornea.
- Improperly cleaned contact lenses can increase the risk of infection.
- Toxicity from multipurpose solutions can damage the epithelial cells of the cornea, causing a keratitis.
- GPC is an immune reaction in the tarsal conjunctiva to the contact lens material, or to deposit on the contact lens material, or a combination of both.

ETIOLOGY

- Contact lens overuse and misuse
- Improper cleaning of contact lenses
- Toxicity from multipurpose solutions
- Inadequate disinfection of contacts from multipurpose solutions

COMMONLY ASSOCIATED CONDITIONS

- Dry eye
- Blepharitis
- Atopy

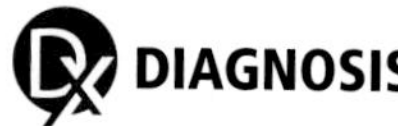

DIAGNOSIS

HISTORY

- History of contact lens use, especially with planned replacement lenses (lenses worn for more than 1 day at a time)
- History of multipurpose solution use
- Red, painful eyes
- Photophobia
- Conjunctival discharge (often clear and intermittent)
- History of frequent "eye infections"
  - Patients with a history of contact lens overwear often report a history of frequent red eyes, previously diagnosed or believed to be infections, but often represent a contact lenses-related condition
  - Severe pain out of proportion to clinical findings should raise suspicion for *Acanthamoeba*.

PHYSICAL EXAM

- Bacterial infection:
  - Dense, white corneal infiltrate with overlying epithelial defect
  - Corneal edema surrounding infiltrate
  - Conjunctival redness
  - Inflammation in anterior chamber (cell and flare seen in slit lamp)
  - Layered white blood cells (hypopyon) may be seen in the anterior chamber
- Fungal infections:
  - "Fluffy" corneal infiltrate, often with multiple, smaller, "satellite" lesions
  - May or may not have an associated epithelial defect
- Amoebal infections:
  - Diffuse epithelial irregularity and edema
  - Visible corneal nerves (radial keratoneuritis)
  - Ring-shaped corneal infiltrate – this is a late sign.
- Contact lens overwear:
  - Conjunctival redness
  - Diffuse punctate keratitis
  - May have subepithelial infiltrates – fine, white opacities in the anterior stroma with negative fluorescein staining
  - May have corneal neovascularization, old stromal scars, and other signs of previous episodes of contact lens overwear
- Multipurpose solution toxicity (or use of nonneutralized hydrogen peroxide solution):
  - Diffuse punctate keratitis
- Giant papillary conjunctivitis:
  - Large papillae on the tarsal conjunctiva (seen with upper lid eversion)
  - Conjunctival hyperemia

DIAGNOSTIC TESTS & INTERPRETATION

Imaging
- Corneal topography can be used to diagnose and monitor corneal warpage.
- Specular microscopy can be useful to see intrastromal amoebal cysts.

Diagnostic Procedures/Other
- For suspected bacterial, fungal, or amoebal infections, the cornea can be cultured to determine the infectious organism and get the antimicrobial sensitivities. A gram stain can also be useful in determining if the bacteria are gram positive or negative, or possibly fungal hyphae may be seen.
  - Amoeba can sometimes be cultured on specialized culture plates or seen with specular microscopy.

Pathological Findings
- Bacteria (gram positive or negative) or hyphae may be seen on gram staining.
- Bacteria, fungi, or amoeba may grow on the appropriate culture media.

DIFFERENTIAL DIAGNOSIS
- Viral conjunctivitis
- Herpetic keratitis
- Chronic dry eye
- Corneal scarring from old contact lens infection or inflammation
- Thygeson's keratitis

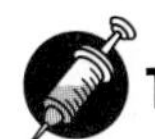

TREATMENT

MEDICATION

First Line
- For bacterial keratitis – fluoroquinolones (moxifloxacin, gatifloxacin, besifloxacin) eyedrops or a broad spectrum (combination eyedrop such as polymixin B/trimethoprim) is dosed frequently (1 drop every hour after an initial loading dose on 1 drop every 5 min for 15 min)
- For fungal keratitis – natacyn (natamycin) eyedrops 1 drop per h
  - If drops can be administered to patients around the clock, this is preferred. If cannot, consider a broad spectrum ophthalmic ointment at night time such as ciloxan or polysporin.
  - For *Acanthamoeba* keratitis – brolene (propamidine) and baquacil (PHMB) eyedrops
  - For GPC – mild topical steroid drops, such as alrex or FML (for short-term use). Topical antihistamines and mast cell stabilizers, such as pataday, are useful for chronic use.

Second Line
- For bacterial keratitis – fortified antibiotics made in a compounding pharmacy or in the in-patient hospital pharmacy. Use fortified vancomycin or ancef, to cover gram-positive bacteria, in conjunction with fortified tobramycin or gentamicin to cover gram-negative bacteria. For suspected pseudomonas, add fortified ceftazidime.
- For fungal keratitis – fortified amphotericin B or fortified voriconazole
  - For *Acanthamoeba* – chlorhexidine, neomycin, and miconazole eyedrops

ADDITIONAL TREATMENT

General Measures
- The use of 1-day disposable contact lenses is often very effective in the treatment for GPC.
  - A brief cessation of contact lens use is also often beneficial in GPC.
  - For corneal warpage from rigid gas permeable lenses, the contact lens use should be discontinued, and the lens should be refit, or changed to a soft lens.

Issues for Referral
Any corneal infection not resolving or getting worse on first-line therapy should be referred to a corneal specialist.

Additional Therapies
Avelox 400 mg per 24 h by mouth may be considered as adjunctive therapy for bacterial corneal ulcers, as it has a high penetration through the blood–retina barrier in the inflamed eye.

SURGERY/OTHER PROCEDURES
- In rare cases, for bacterial, fungal, or amoebal corneal infections not responding to hourly fortified antibiotics, antifungal or antiamoebal therapy, a corneal transplant can be considered.
  - There is a risk of recurrence of the infection in the corneal transplant.

IN-PATIENT CONSIDERATIONS

Initial Stabilization
If patients are admitted to the hospital, administer a loading dose of fortified eyedrops.

Admission Criteria
In select cases, patients may be admitted for round-the-clock eyedrops for severe corneal infections.

Nursing
Patients need to be admitted to a ward where nurses can administer drops every 30–60 min.

Discharge Criteria
Patients can be discharged when the corneal ulcer has resolved or significantly resolved.

ONGOING CARE

FOLLOW-UP RECOMMENDATIONS
For bacterial, fungal, and amoebal corneal infections, the patient should be seen every day for a few days, until the condition is stabilized.

Patient Monitoring
After the contact lens complication is resolved, it is important to maintain routine eye care to monitor the contact lens use, and monitor for risk factors for further contact lens problems.

PATIENT EDUCATION
Proper contact lens care and usage

PROGNOSIS
- Good for most problems from contact lens overwear
- Good for most small and peripheral corneal infections
- Central, large corneal infections can cause decreased vision
- GPC can be chronic and difficult to treat

COMPLICATIONS
- Central bacterial or fungal infections can lead to vision loss and possibly the need for a corneal transplant.
- Use of topical steroid eyedrops on active bacterial, fungal, or amoebal infections can significantly prolong the infection and worsen the clinical course.

ADDITIONAL READING

- Chang DC, Grant GB, O'Donnell K, et al. Multistate outbreak of fusarium keratitis associated with use of a contact lens solution. *JAMA* 2006;296:956.
- Foulks GN. Prolonging contact lens wear and making contact lens wear safer. *Am J Ophthalmol* 2006;141(2):369–373.
- Levinson BA, Hammersmith KM, Cohen EJ. Fungal keratitis in contact lens wearers. In: Tasman W, Jaeger EA, ed. *Duane's Ophthalmology.* Lippincott Williams & Wilkins, 2010.
- Levinson BA, Rutzen AR. New antimicrobials in ophthalmology. *Ophthalmol Clin North Am* 2005;18(4):493–509.
- Suchecki JK, Donshik P, Ehlers WH. Contact lens complications. *Ophthalmol Clin North Am* 2003;16(3):471–484.

CODES

ICD9
- 370.00 Corneal ulcer, unspecified
- 371.82 Corneal disorder due to contact lens
- 372.30 Conjunctivitis, unspecified

CLINICAL PEARLS
- It is critical to obtain a thorough history of the contact lens use, including wear time (hours/day or any overnight wear), the exact brand and type of the contact lens and the type of solution used to clean and/or store the contact lens and the frequency of replacement of the lens
- Be very cautious in the use of topical steroids. Steroids should only be used if infectious etiologies have been ruled out or fully treated.

CONVERGENCE INSUFFICIENCY

Judith B. Lavrich

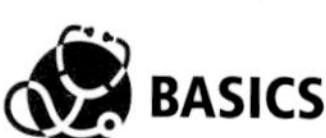

BASICS

DESCRIPTION

The inability to converge the eyes smoothly and effectively from distance to near and/or the inability of maintain the convergent near point.

EPIDEMIOLOGY

Prevalence

Reports vary from 1–25% of the population.

RISK FACTORS

Like many strabismic conditions, symptoms are aggravated by stress, illness, or lack of sleep.

Genetics

No specific gene or locus known, although there are complex genetic influences on fusional amplitudes, version amplitudes, and convergence/accommodation (AC/A) ratio.

GENERAL PREVENTION

Avoidance of near tasks prevents symptoms but there is no prevention for the disorder.

PATHOPHYSIOLOGY

- Ineffective muscular action on attempted convergence results in an inability to maintain proper binocular alignment on visual objects as they approach from distance to near. This causes an exophoria or intermittent exotropia at near.
- The increased convergence effort and/or the increased accommodative effort facilitated in the attempt to maintain ocular alignment causes a variety of symptoms ranging from mild to severe.
- Particularly distressing is when the divergent strabismus causes binocular diplopia at near.
- Symptoms result from sustained effort to increase fusional convergence.

ETIOLOGY

- Our current understanding suggests an innervational etiology because of the dramatic response to treatment both in the patient's subjective improvement and the objective measurements of near point of convergence and fusional convergence amplitudes.
- The symptoms of convergence insufficiency are directly related with reading or other near vision tasks.

COMMONLY ASSOCIATED CONDITIONS

Closed head trauma and lesions in the pretectal area or the dorsal midbrain have been associated with acquired convergence insufficiency.

DIAGNOSIS

HISTORY

- **Headaches** – occurring during reading or after long periods of reading but may not be associated with reading at all. Frequently located in the frontal or periocular area. Can potentiate other underlying headaches such as migraines.
- **Asthenopia** – can manifest as tired, strained eyes or eyes that hurt or feel sore with near work. Some patients describe a pulling or pressure sensation around the eyes.
- **Difficulty with reading/near tasks** – patients describe intermittent blurriness of the words, print moving on the page, frequently losing their place, lack of concentration, or difficulty with comprehension. Increased time at the near task usually increases symptoms. Some patients will not describe symptoms at near because of their strong avoidance of near tasks.
- **Diplopia** – can present as 2 distinct images or an overlap of images. Many patients will have difficulty deciphering the double images and will complain of blur. Some patients will close one eye to read to relieve the diplopia.

PHYSICAL EXAM

- Complete eye examination including cycloplegic refraction to rule out other causes of symptoms (e.g., papilledema due to increased intracranial pressure causing headaches, high hyperopia causing convergence spasm)
- Measure near point of convergence. Have the patient fixate on a near target as the target is slowly moved toward the patient's eyes. The eyes will converge until a point is reached when the eyes will deviate from a convergent position to a divergent position. The point prior to the divergent deviation is the near point of convergence. In a normal child this point should be 4 cm or closer to their nose.
- Assess the ability to converge. Look for increased effort with convergence manifesting as a slow and/or jerking movement rather than a smooth consistent movement seen in normal convergence.
- Look for inability to maintain near fixation.
- Measure fusional amplitudes. Look for low fusional convergence amplitudes. Have the patient fixate on a line of Snellen letters and add base-out prism in a slow, gradual manner. Diplopia will occur when fusion is no longer possible. The amount of prism added is the measurement of fusional convergence.
- Assess for strabismus at near by alternate cover test. Most commonly, exodeviations at near including exophoria, intermittent exotropia, or a constant exotropia.
  - Lack of a strabismus at near or even a mild esophoria has been observed.
  - Some patients will have a reduced stereoacuity.

DIAGNOSTIC TESTS & INTERPRETATION

Imaging

Initial approach

No initial imaging necessary if accommodation and pupillary reflexes are intact.

Follow-up & special considerations

Consider neuroimaging if symptoms and clinical measurements fail to improve with orthoptic therapy or if other neurologic indicators present or severe recalcitrant headaches especially if vomiting or waking from sleep or other constitutional symptoms (e.g., weight loss).

DIFFERENTIAL DIAGNOSIS

- Patients with high-uncorrected hyperopia will make little or no effort to accommodate as the demand outweighs their accommodative ability.
- Some myopic patients have little need to accommodate to maintain clear vision at near.
- First-time bifocal wearers will get relief of their sustained accommodative convergence by the bifocal segment which can initiate an exophoria and other symptoms of convergence insufficiency.
- Accommodative insufficiency can be associated with convergence insufficiency. These patients usually have more severe symptoms and can be less responsive to treatment. Causes include febrile illness, viral encephalopathy, closed head trauma, and anticholinergic drugs.
- Convergence paralysis is a distinct clinical entity. The patient is unable to converge but maintains normal adduction and manifests diplopia at near. Normal accommodation and pupillary reflexes are present on attempted convergence. Results most commonly from head trauma but can be seen with encephalitis, midbrain lesion, and other intracranial pathology.
- Headaches can be from a wide variety of causes including brain tumor, migraine, and convergence spasm.

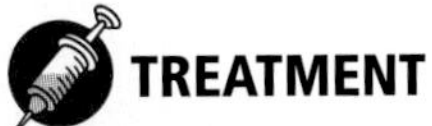

TREATMENT

MEDICATION

First Line

- Orthoptic therapy/computer orthoptics – There is recent strong and persuasive evidence to support its use for treatment for convergence insufficiency. (1)[A] The patient performs vergence/accommodative therapy with a series of exercises using lenses, prisms, and stereograms. Recently, computerized orthoptics programs are used to perform similar exercises.
- Pencil push-ups/accommodative target – have been used as a mainstay of treatment. Despite their widespread use, very limited studies have evaluated their effectiveness. (2) [B] In this exercise, the patient is instructed to maintain single vision as a target (commonly the letters on a pencil are used for fixation) is moved toward their eyes. The patient then sustains the closest fixation possible before diplopia occurs.

Second Line

Base-in prism reading glasses – have been shown to decrease symptoms of convergence insufficiency in the presbyopic population. (3)[A]

ADDITIONAL TREATMENT

Additional Therapies

- Bifocal glasses (plus lenses) can be used to reduce symptoms as they magnify the print and lessen the need for accommodation and its related convergence. This therapy may worsen the convergence insufficiency in some patients due to lack of accommodative demand.
- Over-minus glasses (glasses with excessive myopic correction for the patient) can be used to stimulate accommodation and its related convergence. This may intensify the symptoms in some patients.

SURGERY/OTHER PROCEDURES

Eye muscle surgery (typically unilateral or bilateral medial rectus resection) should be reserved for only the most protracted cases. The decision to proceed with surgery should be made only after all nonsurgical treatment efforts have failed.

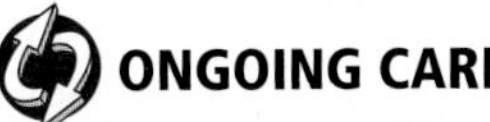

ONGOING CARE

FOLLOW-UP RECOMMENDATIONS

Nonsurgical therapy will need to be continued until symptoms are controlled and convergence is well maintained at the near point.

Patient Monitoring

- Improvement in symptoms at near tasks, especially reading
- Reduction of headaches with near tasks
- Resolution of diplopia at near

PATIENT EDUCATION

- Inform the patient that the symptoms will reoccur with time and therapy may need to be restarted periodically.
- During the presbyopic years it may be difficult to differentiate if the symptoms at near are secondary to the normal loss of accommodation or the recurrence of the convergence insufficiency.

PROGNOSIS

Excellent prognosis with reduction or elimination of symptoms with treatment.

REFERENCES

1. Scheiman M, Rouse M, Kulp MT, et al. Treatment of convergence insufficiency in childhood: A current perspective. *Optom Vis Sci* 2009;86:420–428.
2. Gallaway M, Scheiman M, Malhotra K. The effectiveness of pencil pushups treatment for convergence insufficiency: A pilot study. *Optom Vis Sci* 2002;79:265–267.
3. Teitelbaum B, Pang Y, Krall J. Effectiveness of base in prism for presbyopes with convergence insufficiency. *Optom Vis Sci* 2009;86:153–156.

ADDITIONAL READING

- Lavrich JB. Convergence insufficiency and its current treatment. *Cur Opin Ophthalmol* 2010;21(5): 356–360.
- Bartiss MJ. Convergence insufficiency. Emedicine.medscape.com2010;1–9.
- American Association of Pediatric Ophthalmology and Strabismus Website search Convergence Insufficiencyhttp://www.aapos.org/faq_list/convergence_insufficiency.

C

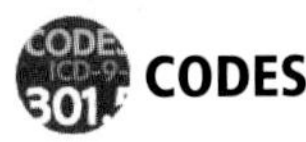

CODES

ICD9

- 368.2 Diplopia
- 368.13 Visual discomfort
- 378.83 Convergence insufficiency or palsy

CLINICAL PEARLS

- On intake, patients should be asked about any problems they may have with reading. All patients with significant reading difficulties should have a comprehensive eye examination to rule out strabismus and refractive errors, and identify convergence insufficiency.
- Perform an alternate cover test at near on any patient with reading difficulties to assess for strabismus.
- Measure near point of convergence on any patient with reading difficulties to look for a remote near point.

CORNEAL ABRASION

Benjamin H. Bloom

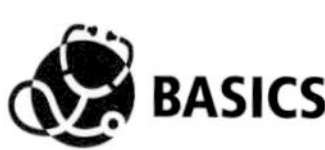

BASICS

DESCRIPTION

- A corneal epithelial defect from several possible causes:
  - Traumatic (most common)
  - Nontraumatic

RISK FACTORS

- Related to trauma:
  - Athletes without suitable eye protection
  - Contact lens wearers
  - Industrial workers without suitable eye protection:
    - Machine operators
    - Construction trades
    - Welders
- Poor adhesion of epithelium to basement membrane/Bowman's layer:
  - Previous injury to Bowman's layer:
    - Trauma involving the subepithelium
    - Previous ocular surgery, especially refractive surgery
  - Recurrent corneal erosion from organic matter:
    - Fingernail
    - Tree branch
  - Corneal dystrophy, especially epithelial and anterior membrane:
    - Map-dot-fingerprint dystrophy (Cogan's microcystic) (most common)
    - Reis–Bucklers, Meesmann's dystrophy (much less common)
    - Stromal and endothelial dystrophies have also been described (rare)

Genetics

- Dominant inheritance in many of the corneal dystrophies:
  - Cogan's: Dominant with variable penetrance
  - Reis–Bucklers' autosomal dominant

GENERAL PREVENTION

- Industrial or agricultural workers should wear safety glasses or goggles as appropriate.
- Athletes should consider wearing eye protectors.
- Eyelids should be taped closed in patients undergoing general anesthesia.

PATHOPHYSIOLOGY

Previous injury to Bowman's layer or certain corneal dystrophies can cause recurrent corneal abrasion months after the initial trauma due to poor adhesion between the epithelium and basement membrane (1)[B].

ETIOLOGY

- Blunt or penetrating trauma:
  - Retained conjunctival foreign body
  - Paper cut
  - Defective contact lens
  - Vigorous eye rubbing from unrelated ocular irritation, such as allergic conjunctivitis

COMMONLY ASSOCIATED CONDITIONS

- Eyelid, ocular, orbital trauma:
  - Eyelid laceration
  - Hyphema/microhyphema
  - Orbital fracture

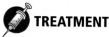

DIAGNOSIS

HISTORY

- Patients almost always can describe the exact time and circumstances of the event that caused the abrasion. If they cannot and the time of onset is vague and the pain seemed to occur spontaneously, you should question a traumatic Dx and be more suspicious of an infectious etiology, e.g., herpes simplex (H. simplex).
  - Severe pain
  - Redness
  - Foreign body sensation
  - Photophobia
  - Pain on blinking
  - Tearing
  - Pain worsens with blinking and improves with lids closed
  - Visual acuity may be decreased
- Recurrent corneal abrasion patients frequently have a history of prior corneal abrasion(s) in that same eye:
  - May have had multiple previous episodes of corneal abrasion in the same eye
  - Symptoms frequently occur upon awakening as the eyelids are opened.
  - Abrasion may be caused by minimal trauma such as eye rubbing.

PHYSICAL EXAM

- Fluorescein, viewed under cobalt blue light, stains basement membrane revealing the area of absent epithelium:
  - Abrasions usually irregular in shape; should measure and diagram to chart progress
  - Should not flood the eye with fluorescein. This can cause "pooling" and give the impression of staining where none exists
- A drop of topical anesthetic greatly aids patient comfort and cooperation during the exam. However, do not send the patient home with a prescription for topical anesthetic. This impedes healing.
- Vertical staining lines on the cornea are highly suggestive of a foreign body on the tarsal conjunctiva of the upper lid. Be sure to evert the lid with a cotton stick or with a lid everter.
- Examine both eyes for dystrophic changes, such as map-like lines, microcysts or fingerprint lines. The fellow eye may provide a valuable clue of anterior membrane dystrophy.
- The underlying stroma should be clear. A whitish infiltrate is a sign of infection.
- Examine the eye carefully for other evidence of ocular trauma.
- If the eye was examined over 24 h after the trauma, the abrasion may have healed and the diagnosis of corneal abrasion may only be presumed.

DIFFERENTIAL DIAGNOSIS

- Conjunctival laceration
- Corneal or conjunctival foreign body
- Traumatic iritis
- Infectious keratitis or conjunctivitis:
  - H. simplex
  - Epidemic keratoconjunctivitis (pink eye)

TREATMENT

MEDICATION

First Line

- Topical antibiotic drops [e.g., polymyxin B/trimethoprim (polytrim), aminoglycoside, or fluoroquinolone] q.i.d.
  - Drops have the advantage of allowing better vision during healing.
- Topical antibiotic ointment (e.g., erythromycin, bacitracin, aminoglycoside, or fluoroquinolone) q.i.d.
  - Ointments have the advantage of better lubrication so as to decrease the pain that occurs during blinking.
- The dose of either of the above may be increased to per 2 h if infection is a concern.
- Short-acting cycloplegics (e.g., tropicamide or cyclopentolate) may be used if there is photophobia or if traumatic iritis is a concern.

- Topical NSAID drops (e.g., diclofenac or ketorolac) will help decrease pain. Steroids and slow healing should be avoided.
- When treating recurrent abrasions/erosions hypertonic 5% NaCl drops and/or ointment (e.g., Muro 128) q.i.d. increases the adhesion of the epithelium to the basement membrane. Should be continued for 6 months and, on occasion, indefinitely.
- Recurrent erosions are also helped by artificial tears (e.g., systane) and/or artificial tear ointment (e.g., systane PM) after the epithelium has healed. These lubricate the ocular surface to help prevent recurrence.

Second Line

- Sulfonamides have the disadvantage of serious ocular adverse reactions (e.g., Stevens–Johnson syndrome) (rare).
- Chloramphenicol is widely used in Europe but there have been a few reported cases, which some consider questionable, of blood dyscrasias. The eyedrop form has the disadvantage of requiring refrigeration.
- Fusidic acid viscous solution (fucithalmic) is widely used in Canada and Europe. Advantages are the high efficacy with gram positives, especially staph, and the b.i.d. dosage. A disadvantage is the weak efficacy with gram negatives.

ADDITIONAL TREATMENT

General Measures

Pressure patching is not necessary for small abrasions but can help healing and comfort if the abrasion is large. If the patient is more comfortable with the eye closed, then patch. If you do not know how to apply a proper pressure patch, it is better not to patch at all. A loose gauze pad over an open eye may abrade the cornea further and prevent healing or may even make the abrasion larger. If there is a suspicion of infection, i.e., if a whitish corneal infiltrate is seen or if plant matter or a fingernail was the cause of injury, then patching may worsen the infection and should not be used. If the patient is a contact lens wearer, the abrasion should be assumed to be infected and patching should not be done. The contact lens should not be worn until the cornea is healed (2)[A], (3)[A].

Issues for Referral

- Cases with noninfected abrasions and no other ocular trauma usually heal quickly and need not be referred.
- Cases with infection or which show poor or no response to the above treatment should be referred.

Additional Therapies

- Bandage contact lens
- Epithelial debridement and diamond burr polishing of Bowman's layer (4)[B]
- Anterior stromal puncture
- Alcohol delamination/debridement

SURGERY/OTHER PROCEDURES

- Anterior stromal puncture by the Nd:YAG laser
- Excimer laser phototherapeutic keratectomy

ONGOING CARE

FOLLOW-UP RECOMMENDATIONS

- Patients should be seen daily for signs that the epithelial defect is improving. Document size of defect at every visit.
- When healing progress is certain, you may extend exam interval to 2–3 days.
- When epithelial defect is completely closed, you may extend exam interval to 3–5 days. Discontinue antibiotic. Continue NSAID and/or cycloplegic as necessary. Instruct all patients about the possibility of recurrent abrasions.
- Discharge when the epithelial surface is restored to normal. If this is a recurrent erosion, continue artificial tears and/or ointment and hypertonic saline drops and/or ointment as above. Follow-up for recurrent erosions may be extended and patients may become familiar with the symptoms of a recurrence. They should be instructed to return immediately if a recurrence is suspected.

COMPLICATIONS

Untreated corneal abrasions can progress to bacterial keratitis and corneal ulceration. All patients should be informed of this possibility and the need for immediate management if this occurs.

REFERENCES

1. Ramamurthi S, Rahman MQ, Dutton GN, et al. Pathogenesis, clinical features and management of recurrent corneal erosions. *Eye (Lond)* 2006;20(6):635–644.
2. Turner A, Rabiu M. Patching for corneal abrasion. *Cochrane Database Syst Rev* 2006;(2):CD004764.
3. Watson SL, Barker NH. Interventions for recurrent corneal erosions. *Cochrane Database Syst Rev* 2007;(4):CD001861.
4. Aldave AJ, Kamal KM, Vo RC, et al. Epithelial debridement and Bowman's layer polishing for visually significant epithelial irregularity and recurrent corneal erosions. *Cornea* 2009;28(10):1085–1090.

ADDITIONAL READING

- Das S, Seitz B. Recurrent corneal erosion syndrome. *Surv Ophthalmol* 2008;53(1):3–15.
- Ewald M, Hammersmith KM. Review of diagnosis and management of recurrent erosion syndrome. *Curr Opin Ophthalmol* 2009;20(4):287–291.
- Fraser S. Corneal abrasion. *Clin Ophthalmol* 2010;4:387–390.

CODES

ICD9

- 371.42 Recurrent erosion of cornea
- 371.82 Corneal disorder due to contact lens
- 918.1 Superficial injury of cornea

CLINICAL PEARLS

- Lack of definite history of trauma can be a tip-off for an infectious Dx.
- Vertical scratches on the cornea are a tip-off for a conjunctival foreign body under the lid.
- Remember to examine both eyes. This helps discover corneal dystrophies.
- Patching not necessary for small abrasions
- White infiltrates indicate infection and should be promptly referred to an ophthalmologist.

CORNEAL TRANSPLANT COMPLICATIONS

Irving M. Raber

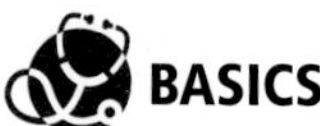

BASICS

DESCRIPTION

- Cadaveric corneal transplantation
- Penetrating keratoplasty
- Lamellar keratoplasty
- Anterior
- Posterior
- Descemet's stripping endothelial keratoplasty
- Descemet's membrane endothelial keratoplasty

EPIDEMIOLOGY

Incidence

Complications are dependent on preoperative status of eye, skill of surgeon, intraoperative circumstances, and postoperative variables including medications and trauma.

RISK FACTORS

- Corneal neovascularization
- Glaucoma (1)
- Active corneal infection:
  - Bacterial
  - Fungal
  - Herpes simplex
  - *Acanthamoeba*
- Lens status:
  - Cataract
  - Intraocular lens
  - Posterior capsule
- Anterior segment disorganization:
  - Peripheral anterior synechiae
  - Pupil/iris distortion
- Corneal hypesthesia
- Ocular surface abnormalities:
  - Dry eyes
  - Blepharitis
  - Trichiasis
  - Exposure
  - Toxic medicamentosa
  - Limbal stem cell deficiency
  - Chemical burn
  - Aniridia
- Steroid responsiveness
- Corneal dystrophy

Genetics

As related to various corneal dystrophies

GENERAL PREVENTION

- Control of intraocular pressure:
  - Pre-op
  - Intra-op
    - Intravenous mannitol
    - Avoid external pressure
  - Post-op
- Meticulous surgical technique
- Anticipate problems
- Use of favorable donor tissue
- Preferable to operate on a quiet, noninfected eye

PATHOPHYSIOLOGY

- Corneal opacification:
  - Edema
  - Scarring
  - Surface breakdown
  - Infection
- Glaucomatous optic neuropathy
- Cataract
- Anterior segment disorganization

ETIOLOGY

- Intraoperative difficulties:
  - Positive pressure
  - Vitreous loss
  - Choroidal effusion/hemorrhage
  - Hyphema
- Immune rejection
- Endothelial failure
- Poor wound apposition/healing
- Elevated intraocular pressure
- Infection:
  - Corneal ulceration
  - Crystalline keratopathy
  - Endophthalmitis
  - Lamellar interface infection

COMMONLY ASSOCIATED CONDITIONS

- Glaucoma
- Complicated cataract surgery
- Ocular surface abnormalities

DIAGNOSIS

HISTORY

- Acute:
  - Blurred vision
  - Redness
  - Photophobia
  - Pain
  - Discharge
  - Lid swelling
  - Trauma
- Chronic:
  - Blurred vision
  - Monocular diplopia
  - Halos/glare
  - Pain/irritation
  - Redness

PHYSICAL EXAM

- Conjunctival injection/ciliary flush
- Corneal transplant edema
- Corneal transplant subepithelial infiltrates
- Corneal infiltrate/crystalline accumulation
- Corneal surface breakdown
- Corneal epithelial dendrite/geographic ulcer
- Lamellar interface haze/opacification
- Detached posterior lamellar graft (2)
- Secondary anterior chamber/detached Descemet's membrane in deep anterior lamellar keratoplasty
- Anterior chamber reaction
- Keratic precipitates/endothelial rejection line
- Exposed sutures
- Wound leak/dehiscence
- Elevated intraocular pressure (3)
- Hypotony
- Cataract
- Recurrent corneal dystrophy
- Expanding curvilinear ridge on endothelium (epithelial downgrowth)
- Refractive error:
  - High cylinder (4)
    - Regular/irregular astigmatism
  - High sphere
- Retinal/choroidal detachment
- Macular edema/pucker

DIAGNOSTIC TESTS & INTERPRETATION

Imaging

- When intraocular visualization obscured by corneal opacification
  - B scan ultrasonography
  - Ultrasound biomicroscopy
  - Optical coherence tomography
- Serial pachymetry to monitor endothelial cell function
- Serial specular microscopy to monitor endothelial cell status

Diagnostic Procedures/Other

- When suspect infection:
  - Corneal scrapings for cultures and smears
- Rigid contact lens refraction – if results in significant improvement in vision compared to spectacle correction it confirms irregular astigmatism as a source of reduced vision.

Pathological Findings

- Corneal edema
- Corneal scarring
- Corneal vascularization
- Corneal ulceration
- Corneal thinning
- Corneal inflammation
- Organisms on gram and/or various fungal stains
- Endothelial cell atrophy
- Recurrent corneal dystrophy (Bowman's membrane, stromal, endothelial, keratoconus)

DIFFERENTIAL DIAGNOSIS

- Immune rejection vs nonimmunological endothelial failure
- Immune rejection vs herpes simplex keratouveitis
- Infectious vs noninfectious corneal ulcer/ infiltrate/ulceration
- Immune rejection vs epithelial downgrowth
- Glaucoma vs steroid responder
- Regular vs irregular astigmatism

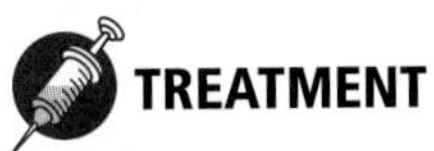

TREATMENT

MEDICATION

First Line

- Immune rejection:
  - Topical steroid
  - Topical cyclosporine
  - Topical cycloplegia
- Infection:
  - Topical antimicrobial therapy
  - Topical cycloplegia
- Noninfectious epithelial breakdown:
  - Topical lubrication, preferably preservative free
  - Reduce use of toxic topical medications
  - Punctal occlusion
- Glaucoma:
  - Topical antiglaucoma medication
  - Reduced topical steroid
- Astigmatism/anisometropia:
  - Spectacle correction
- Contact lens correction

Second Line

- Immune rejection:
  - Subconjunctival steroid
  - Oral steroid
  - Oral cyclosporine, tacrolimus
- Infection:
  - Oral antimicrobial therapy
- Noninfectious epithelial breakdown:
  - Bandage contact lens
  - Oral omega 3 fatty acid supplementation
  - Oral doxycycline
- Glaucoma:
  - Oral carbonic anhydrase inhibitor

SURGERY/OTHER PROCEDURES

- Repeat keratoplasty for graft rejection/failure/ scarring
- Permanent keratoprosthesis for repeat graft rejection/failure
- Glaucoma surgery for uncontrolled intraocular pressure
- Tarsorrhaphy, amniotic membrane transplantation, conjunctival flap, limbal stem cell transplant for persistent epithelial defect
- Refractive surgery (incisional astigmatic keratotomy $\pm$ compression sutures, wedge resection, excimer laser photorefractive keratectomy, lasik, intraocular lens, conductive keratoplasty) for high residual refractive error/anisometropia

ONGOING CARE

FOLLOW-UP RECOMMENDATIONS

Frequency of follow-up visits predicated by severity of the complication and integrity of the globe, i.e., daily for initial treatment of severe infection

Patient Monitoring

- Visual acuity
- Corneal clarity
- Intraocular pressure

PATIENT EDUCATION

Need to seek prompt evaluation at first signs of rejection/infection, i.e., blurred vision, pain, redness, photophobia, discharge, lid swelling.

PROGNOSIS

Depends upon original diagnosis and severity of complication. Ultimate visual recovery related to status of posterior segment

COMPLICATIONS

Pediatric Considerations

- Children are more difficult to follow which leads to delayed diagnosis of complications. Repeated examinations under anesthesia are frequently necessary.
- High incidence of immune rejection occurs.
- Congenital corneal clouding frequently associated with anterior chamber abnormalities is present that increases risk for complications and reduces success rate of corneal transplantation.
- Amblyopia appears.

ADDITIONAL READING

- Rumelt S, Bersudsky V, Blum-Hareuveni T, et al. Preexisting and postoperative glaucoma in repeated corneal transplantation. *Cornea* 2002;2(18): 759–765.
- Shih CY, Ritterband DC, Rubino S, et al. Visually significant and nonsignificant complications arising from Descemet stripping automated endothelial keratoplasty. *Am J Ophthalmol* 2009;148(6): 837–843.
- Karadaq O, Kugu S, Erdogan G, et al. Incidence of and risk factors for increased intraocular pressure after penetrating keratoplasty. *Cornea* 2010;29(3): 278–282.
- Bartels MC, van Rooij J, Geerards AJ, et al. Comparison of complication rates and postoperative astigmatism between nylon and mersilene sutures for corneal transplants in patients with Fuchs endothelial dystrophy. *Cornea* 2006;25(5):533–539.
- Michaeli A, Markovich A, Rootman DS. Corneal transplants for the treatment of congenital corneal opacities. *J Pediatr Ophthalmol Strabismus* 2005; 42(1):34–44.

CODES

ICD9

- V42.5 Cornea replaced by transplant
- 370.8 Other forms of keratitis
- 996.89 Complications of other specified transplanted organ

COTTON WOOL SPOTS

James F. Vander

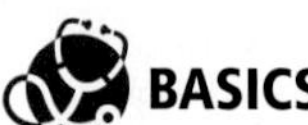

BASICS

DESCRIPTION
- Localized area of superficial retinal whitening
- Generally smaller than 1/2 disc area
- Primary importance is as a marker of underlying disease, usually systemic.

EPIDEMIOLOGY
Unknown.

RISK FACTORS
- Diabetes
- Systemic hypertension
- Atherosclerotic peripheral vascular disease
- Collagen vascular disease
- Other systemic abnormalities (see Differential Diagnosis)

PATHOPHYSIOLOGY
Occlusion of precapillary retinal arterioles.

ETIOLOGY
Damming of axoplasmic flow caused by small vessel obstruction.

COMMONLY ASSOCIATED CONDITIONS
- Diabetes
- Systemic hypertension
- Atherosclerotic peripheral vascular disease

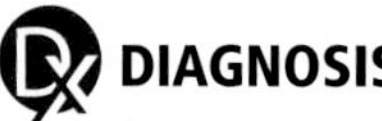

DIAGNOSIS

HISTORY
- Cotton wool spots alone rarely cause symptoms unless very close to center of macula.
- Vision loss if associated with other features of retinal vascular disease such as macular edema or bleeding

PHYSICAL EXAM
- Discrete area of superficial retinal whitening
- Retinal hemorrhages, edema, exudation, neovascularization are often associated

DIAGNOSTIC TESTS & INTERPRETATION

Lab

Initial lab tests
- CBC with differential
- Fasting blood sugar
- Hemoglobin A1C
- Lipid panel
- Sedimentation rate
- C-reactive protein

Follow-up & special considerations
- If initial work-up is negative, additional testing is essential given that nearly all patients end up with some underlying systemic abnormality identified.
  - Further blood work to include infectious causes, with guidance based on history and review of systems (RPR, FTA, Lyme, HIV, Leptospirosis, Rocky Mountain spotted fever, Onchocerciasis), inflammatory/autoimmune, hematologic, protein electrophoresis, pancreatic enzymes, and blood cultures.

Imaging

Initial approach

Intravenous fluorescein angiography – will confirm diagnosis and possibly identify additional aspects of retinal vascular disease such as vasculitis or microaneurysms.

Follow-up & special considerations

Consider cardiac ultrasound, chest x-ray, and carotid ultrasound.

Diagnostic Procedures/Other
In elderly patients, temporal artery biopsy.

Pathological Findings
- Cytoid bodies – nerve fiber layer, eosinophilic cellular appearing structures with "pseudonuclei" (1,[C]).
  - On electron microscopy – accumulation of axoplasm with mitochondria and neurofilaments. The "pseudonuclei" is likely accumulation of lipid.

DIFFERENTIAL DIAGNOSIS
- Myelinated nerve fiber layer
- Central or branch retinal artery obstruction
- Retinal hamartoma
- Nematode

Differential for Underlying Illness: (2[B])
- Systemic hypertension
- Diabetes mellitus
- Collagen vascular diseases
  - Systemic lupus erythematosus
  - Dermatomyositis
  - Scleroderma
  - Giant cell arteritis
- Cardiac valvular disease
  - Mitral valve prolapse
  - Rheumatic heart disease
  - Endocarditis
- AIDS
- Leukemia
- Trauma (Purtscher's retinopathy)
- Radiation retinopathy
- Central/branch retinal vein occlusion
- Systemic malignancy
- Leptospirosis
- Rocky Mountain spotted fever
- Altitude retinopathy
- Severe anemia
- Acute blood loss
- Ocular ischemic syndrome (carotid disease)
- Dysproteinemias
- Septicemia
- Aortic arch syndrome
- Intravenous drug abuse
- Acute pancreatitis
- Onchocerciasis
- Interferon toxicity

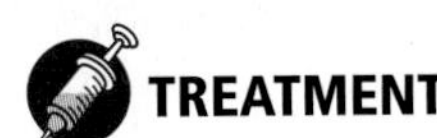

TREATMENT

ADDITIONAL TREATMENT

General Measures
Treat underlying systemic disease.

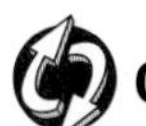

ONGOING CARE

FOLLOW-UP RECOMMENDATIONS
Ensure follow up with primary physician until underlying diagnosis achieved.

Patient Monitoring
- Reexamine 1–2 months to ensure resolution or development of other findings
- Patient to monitor vision and report changes if they occur

PROGNOSIS
- Visual prognosis generally good
- Prognosis systemically dependent on underlying cause

REFERENCES

1. Wolter JR. Pathology of a cotton-wool spot. *Am J Ophthalmol* 1959;48:473–485.
2. Brown GC, Brown MM, Hiller T, et al. Cotton wool spots. *Retina* 1985;5:206–214.

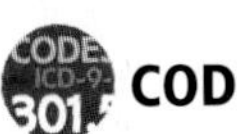

CODES

ICD9
362.83 Retinal edema

CRANIOSYNOSTOSES

Brian J. Forbes
Kathleen Romero
Alex V. Levin

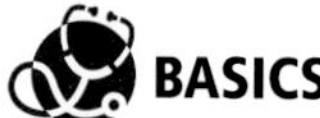

BASICS

DESCRIPTION

- Craniofacial syndromes are divided into craniosynostoses and clefting syndromes.
- *Craniosynostosis* describes premature sutural fusion. *Craniostenosis* is the result.
- Simple craniosynostosis refers to premature closure of a single suture. Compound craniosynostosis involves 2 or more sutures.
- In primary synostosis, the most common type, cranial sutures are fused prematurely because of genetic factors. In secondary craniosynostosis, premature sutural fusion is secondary to another known disorder/process (1).

EPIDEMIOLOGY

Prevalence

- Crouzon syndrome: 16.5 per million live births and accounts for 4.8% of all craniosynostosis, making it the most common craniosynostosis syndrome.
- Apert syndrome: Estimated of 1 per 160,000 live births, approximately 4.5% of all craniosynostosis.
- Other craniofacial disorders are less common.

RISK FACTORS

No known risk factors other than genetic.

Genetics

- Crouzon syndrome: Autosomal dominant, variable expression. 25% are spontaneous mutations (no family history), although affected parents may be missed if mild. Mutations in fibroblast growth factor receptor genes: FGFR2 (10q26) or FGFR3 (4p16) gene. Associated with advanced paternal age (2).
- Apert syndrome: Autosomal dominant, FGFR2 gene. Most patients have 1 of 2 specific mutations in exon IIIa. Associated with advanced paternal age. (3)
- Pfeiffer syndrome: Autosomal dominant, complete penetrance and variable expression, FGFR2 and FGFR1 (8p11.2) (4).
- Saethre-Chotzen: Autosomal dominant, high penetrance and variable expression, basic helix—loop—helix transcription factor called TWIST1 (7p21–22) or FGFR3. Advanced maternal age is a risk factor for new mutations (5).
- Treacher Collins syndrome (mandibulofacial dysotosis): Autosomal dominant, variable expression. Positive family history in approximately 40% of patients, TCOF1 gene (5q32–33.1). Advanced paternal age is a risk factor for new spontaneous mutations.
- Goldenhar syndrome (oculo-auricular-vertebral spectrum): Most cases sporadic, autosomal recessive and autosomal dominant, estimated recurrence in first-degree relatives approximately 2%. Several loci described including 5p15.33-pter (dominant), 8q11 (dominant), 11q12–13 (dominant), 14q22 (dominant or recessive) and 22q11.2 (dominant). The SALL1 gene (16q12.1) has been mutated in some sporadic cases.

PATHOPHYSIOLOGY

Virchow first described how premature closure of one cranial suture promotes growth parallel to that suture and inhibits growth perpendicular to it (1).

ETIOLOGY

There are 3 classic theories: Primary dysgenesis with secondary cranial base abnormalities, primary cranial base malformation with secondary obliteration of the cranial sutures, primary defect in the mesenchymal blastema producing both an abnormal cranial base and craniosynostosis.

DIAGNOSIS

HISTORY

- Family history and examination of parents and siblings may be helpful.
- History of associated syndromic abnormalities may help direct diagnosis (e.g., hearing loss, developmental delay, acanthosis nigricans, upper airway obstruction, hydrocephalus, syndactyly).

PHYSICAL EXAM

- Visual function 90% of vision loss is secondary to amblyopia, and 10% is secondary to structural abnormalities of the globe or visual pathways.
- Position/shape/integrity of the lids, palpebral fissures, and canthi. Examine for trichiasis, entropion, ectropion, colobomas, distichiasis, ptosis, epicanthal folds, symblepharon, and ankyloblepharon. Vertical and horizontal fissure length, upper and lower lid crease position, and marginal reflex distance are important points of information, when obtainable. Ptosis (especially Saethre-Chotzen).
- Characteristic downslanting lower lid coloboma with sharp upswing medially in Treacher-Collins. Horizontal lid shortening on forced closure (e.g., crying).
- Evaluate for exorbitism and corneal exposure.
- Evaluation of the optic nerves papilledema.
- Telecanthus is measured by the intercanthal distance. In infants, generally <20 mm; in older children <24 mm; in adults, <30 mm.
- Hypertelorism is technically measured by the distance between the bony medial orbital walls. Mustarde Index: ratio of the intercanthal distance to the interpupillary distance. Normal$\leq$0.50. Values greater than this represent telecanthus and a possible underlying hypertelorism.
- Assess for caruncle abnormalities in Goldenhar
- Strabismus and refractive error common. Amblyopia common. Most common strabismus is exotropia slightly more than esotropia. Vertical deviations and A- or V-patterns can occur alone or in combination with the horizontal deviation. Dissociated vertical deviation, pseudo-overacting inferior oblique muscles.
- May have nasolacrimal duct anomalies/obstruction/dysfunction
- Rare associated anterior segment or retinal abnormalities other than optic nerve malformations (frontonasal dysplasia)
- Systemic malformations: Syndactyly (Apert), large great toe and thumb (Pfeiffer), hearing loss, external ear malformations, midfacial hypoplasia, protruding tongue, acanthosis nigricans (Apert), dental malocclusion, and palatal abnormalities

DIAGNOSTIC TESTS & INTERPRETATION

Lab

Molecular genetic testing

Imaging

Initial approach

- The use of ancillary testing is on a case-by-case basis
- Skeletal survey if skeletal dysplasia also suspected
- Magnetic resonance imaging (MRI) of the brain
- Computerized tomography (CT) with 3-dimensional reconstruction of the skull and face
- Dental Panorex radiography

Follow-up & special considerations

- Follow up is largely dictated by the severity of ophthalmic findings.
- Requires multidisciplinary team, which may include genetics, plastic surgery, neurosurgery, oral surgery, orthodontics, ophthalmology, otolaryngology, pediatrics, psychiatry, nutrition, speech therapy, and social work.
- Ongoing concern of corneal exposure, may be worse with older age, especially if exorbitism or lower lid coloboma.

- Risk in first decade of amblyopia. Monitor visual function.
- Ophthalmology may be asked to attend craniofacial surgical interventions for prophylactic probing of nasolacrimal system, monitoring of eye pressure, or optic nerve concerns.
- Monitor for papilledema or optic nerve compression.

DIFFERENTIAL DIAGNOSIS

The differential diagnosis can often be easily limited to a few syndromes and further delineated by a genetic workup.

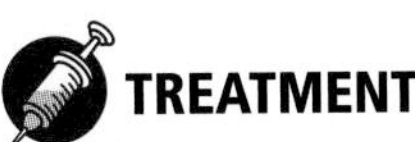

TREATMENT

ADDITIONAL TREATMENT

General Measures

Immediate ophthalmic consultation is usually obtained to evaluate for corneal exposure, orbital dystopia, extraocular muscle dysfunction lid abnormalities, and papilledema.

SURGERY/OTHER PROCEDURES

- Maximize multidisciplinary procedures under anesthesia
- Initial craniofacial surgery usually aimed at relieving increased intracranial pressure and allowing for brain growth (e.g., strip craniectomy). Later surgery to reposition orbits (orbital advancement) often requires periosteal elevation and dissection of orbital contents from the orbital walls. Orbital walls fractured approximately 15 mm anterior to the orbital apex as needed for particular syndrome repairs, allowing the orbit to be shifted in any desired direction. Later surgery designed for further reconstruction to improve appearance.
- Ophthalmology may be needed during or after craniofacial surgery. Postoperative concerns include chemosis, exposure, optic nerve impingement, papilledema, extraocular muscle dysfunction, and lid malposition.
- The variety and types of surgical repairs for the ophthalmic surgical problems generally follow the basic tenets that govern their use in patients who do not have craniofacial problems. Tarsorrhaphy or lid reconstruction may be needed for corneal exposure.
- If nasolacrimal probing/intubation indicated, pathway may be very anomalous and intranasal anatomy crowded, nasal endoscopy may be helpful. Preoperative evaluation to ensure no anterior encephalocele with brain in nasopharynx (frontonasal dysplasia).
- Strabismus surgery complicated by absent/anomalous extraocular muscles. Preoperative plan may be assisted by ultrasound, CT, and MRI. Intraoperative exploration using limbal incision recommended. Preoperative assessment often cannot predict muscle patterns. Reoperation frequent. May not be able to normalize alignment in all fields of gaze.

IN-PATIENT CONSIDERATIONS

Initial Stabilization

- The initial ophthalmic evaluation should be accomplished as soon as possible after the diagnosis of any craniofacial abnormality is made, preferably before any surgical intervention.
- The most common initial concern, especially in the multiple craniosynostoses (e.g., Apert, Crouzon, clover-leaf deformity) is maintenance of an adequate airway.

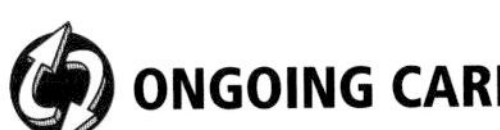

ONGOING CARE

FOLLOW-UP RECOMMENDATIONS

Ongoing monitoring is essential to evaluate for corneal exposure (which may increase with age), vision abnormalities, papilledema, and ocular misalignment.

REFERENCES

1. Virchow R. Über den Crestinismus, Manenlick in franken, and über pathologische Schadelformen. *Ver Phys Med (Warsburg)* 1851;2:230.
2. Preston RA, Post JC, Keats BJ, et al. A gene for Crouzon craniofacial dysostosis maps to the long arm of chromosome 10. *Nat Genet* 1994;7:149.
3. Park WJ, Theda C, Maestri NE, et al. Analysis of phenotypic features and FGFR2 mutations in Apert syndrome. *Am J Hum Genet* 1995;57:321.
4. Schell B, Hehr A, Feldman GJ, et al. Mutations in FGFR1 and FGFR2 cause familial and sporadic Pfeiffer's syndrome. *Hum Med Genet* 1995;4:323.
5. Reid C, McMorrow LE, McDonald-McGinn DM, et al. Saethre-Chotzen syndrome with familial translocation at chromosome 7, p. 22. *Am J Med Genet* 1993;47:637.

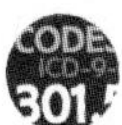

CODES

ICD9

- 755.55 Acrocephalosyndactyly
- 756.0 Congenital anomalies of skull and face bones

CLINICAL PEARLS

- Multidisciplinary team approach is essential.
- Early ophthalmic consultation is needed to assess for corneal exposure, papilledema, and risk factors for amblyopia such as refractive error and strabismus.
- In the repair of ocular and adnexal deformities, the concept of timing underscores the importance of the interaction of the clinicians who comprise the craniofacial team. Preservation and development of vision are the primary goals of the ophthalmologist and may require early and persistent intervention.
- Nasolacrimal surgery may be challenging due to anatomic abnormalities.
- Abnormal eye muscle anatomy is a frequent challenge during strabismus surgery. Alignment in all fields of gaze may not be possible.

CROHN'S DISEASE & UC

Douglas M. Wisner

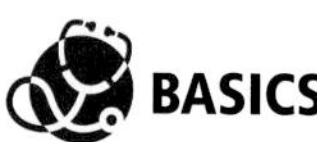

BASICS

DESCRIPTION

- Inflammatory bowel disease (IBD) is an idiopathic inflammatory disease of the intestinal tract that is associated with a number of extra-intestinal manifestations. IBD can be classified as Crohn's disease (CD) or ulcerative colitis (UC) based on the pathologic location of the diseased areas within the gut. Ocular manifestations of IBD are variable and can be evident as inflammation in all of the ocular tissues. The most common ocular associations include non-granulomatous anterior uveitis (e.g., iritis), episcleritis, scleritis, keratitis, retinal vasculitis, and posterior uveitis.
- Unless indicated, CD and UC will be discussed as part of the same clinical spectrum (IBD) in regard to the eye.

EPIDEMIOLOGY

Prevalence

- IBD has a prevalence of 70–150 cases per 100,000 persons.
- 3.5–11.8% of patients with IBD will have ocular inflammation at some point.
- Ophthalmic manifestations are infrequently the presenting complaint leading to a diagnosis of IBD.
- UC appears to have less associated ocular inflammation than CD.
- Episcleritis is the most common extra-intestinal manifestation of IBD (up to 29%) and is reported to be closely correlated to disease activity, but is not often seen by clinicians due to its relatively asymptomatic nature.
- Anterior uveitis is the most common extra intestinal manifestation of IBD seen by clinicians and is more common in women (1).
- Approximately 2% of all uveitis cases are reported to be secondary to IBD (2).

RISK FACTORS

- Active intestinal IBD is associated with, but not required for, ocular manifestations.
- Presence of other extra-intestinal manifestations, such as arthritis or erythema nodosum, are associated with a higher risk of ocular involvement (3).
- Genetic (see below)

Genetics

- IBD is familial but displays non-Mendelian inheritance and variable expressivity, likely reflecting a multifactorial genetic influence.
- HLA-B27 is present in approximately 8% of the Caucasian population and is associated with higher rates of acute anterior uveitis in general.
- Patients with IBD and HLA-B27 are at increased risk for ocular disease manifestations than IBD patients without HLA-B27 positivity.
  - 50% of patients with IBD and anterior uveitis will be HLA-B27 positive.
  - Ocular inflammation in IBD is also strongly associated with HLA-B58 and HLA-DRB10103 (3).

GENERAL PREVENTION

Control of IBD flares and chronic disease activity.

PATHOPHYSIOLOGY

An imbalance of inflammatory mediators leads to nonspecific inflammatory infiltrates in affected tissues, resulting in edema, local destruction, and tissue dysfunction.

ETIOLOGY

- Idiopathic
  - IBD is generally thought to be secondary to an environmental trigger in genetically predisposed individuals that results in a pro-inflammatory response.

COMMONLY ASSOCIATED CONDITIONS

- HLA-B27 arthropathies
- Malabsorption syndromes
- Chronic anemia
- Osteoporosis
- Colon cancer
- Primary sclerosing cholangitis
- Erythema nodosum
- Depression

DIAGNOSIS

HISTORY

- Episcleritis
  - Epibulbar injection, foreign body sensation. No pain or blurred vision
- Anterior uveitis
  - Aching pain, photophobia, blurred vision
- Scleritis
  - Deep boring pain, ocular tenderness, headache, photophobia, blurred vision
- Keratitis
  - Sharp, superficial pain, photophobia. No other source of keratitis by history (contact lenses, trauma)
- Retinal vasculitis/posterior uveitis
  - Aching pain, blurred vision. No infectious source (prior surgery, trauma, endogenous)

PHYSICAL EXAM

Slit-lamp examination

- Episcleritis
  - Epibulbar injection that blanches with 2.5% phenylephrine. No anterior chamber cell and flare
- Anterior uveitis
  - Ciliary flush (vascular injection adjacent to the limbus), anterior chamber cell and flare
- Scleritis
  - Diffuse or nodular epibulbar injection (not conjunctival, usually does not blanch with phenylephrine 2.5%), severe tenderness to ocular palpation, anterior chamber cell and flare. Occasionally can be necrotizing and painless. Posterior scleritis can lead to an exudative retinal detachment
- Keratitis
  - Conjunctival injection, corneal epithelial defect, corneal stromal infiltrates, anterior chamber cell and flare
- Retinal vasculitis/posterior uveitis
  - Posterior chamber cell, vitreous snowballs or snowbanks, retinal vascular sheathing, macular edema

DIAGNOSTIC TESTS & INTERPRETATION

Lab

No lab tests are useful in the diagnosis of ocular manifestations in IBD.

Imaging

- If posterior scleritis is suspected, B-scan ultrasound of the eye may demonstrate a T-sign, caused by posterior peribulbar edema.
- If retinal vasculitis is suspected, a fluorescein angiogram preformed by a retina specialist may be useful.

DIFFERENTIAL DIAGNOSIS

- Infectious or allergic conjunctivitis
- Idiopathic anterior uveitis, episcleritis, scleritis, posterior uveitis, retinal vasculitis or optic neuritis; or one of the above associated with an alternate systemic inflammatory condition (sarcoidosis, tuberculosis, etc.)
- Infectious keratitis

TREATMENT

MEDICATION

First Line

- Episcleritis
  - Artificial tears 1 drop q.i.d escalating to prednisolone acetate 1% 1drop q.i.d if needed
- Anterior uveitis
  - Prednisolone acetate 1% 1 drop every hour, taper as inflammation is controlled. Scopolamine 0.25% or cyclopentolate 1% 1 drop twice a day for cycloplegia and synechiae prevention
- Scleritis
  - Oral NSAIDs (ibuprofen 800 mg PO t.i.d or indomethacin 25 mg PO t.i.d).
  - Topical steroids are generally not effective and may predispose to scleral thinning.
- Keratitis
  - Epithelium intact – prednisolone acetate 1% frequency dependent on severity
  - Epithelial loss – prednisolone acetate 1%, topical antibiotics, and possibly oral steroids
- Posterior uveitis/retinal vasculitis
  - Oral steroids, intravitreal or sub-tenons steroid

Second Line

- Anterior uveitis, scleritis, keratitis, posterior uveitis, and retinal vasculitis.
  - Oral steroids (4)[C]
  - Azathioprine, cyclosporine, methotrexate
  - Anti-TNF agents (5)[C]

Pregnancy Considerations

Patients who are pregnant should practice punctual occlusion when instilling topical eye drops to minimize systemic effects. Immunosuppressive therapy should be used with extreme caution in pregnant patients.

ADDITIONAL TREATMENT

Issues for Referral

Referral to a comprehensive ophthalmologist should be strongly considered for all suspected ophthalmic manifestations of IBD.

SURGERY/OTHER PROCEDURES

Intravitreal or sub-Tenons steroid injection may be considered by a retinal specialist for recalcitrant ocular inflammation.

IN-PATIENT CONSIDERATIONS

Patients with IBD associated ocular inflammation do not usually require hospital admission.

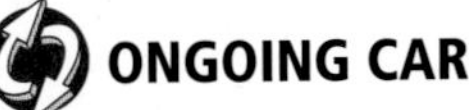

ONGOING CARE

FOLLOW-UP RECOMMENDATIONS

- Patients with ocular manifestations of IBD should be seen by an ophthalmologist until the inflammation is resolved.
- There is no evidence supporting screening patients with IBD for ocular manifestations.

Patient Monitoring

- Patients with uveitis and/or with long-term high dose oral corticosteroid therapy are at risk for developing cataracts (a reversible cause of visual loss) and glaucoma (a nonreversible cause of visual loss).
- There are no evidence-based recommendations regarding glaucoma screening in patients on long-term oral corticosteroids. The risk of developing glaucoma increases with treatment duration (especially >1 year), treatment dose, and pre-treatment morbidity (age, preexisting glaucoma or ocular hypertension and connective tissue disorders) (6)[C].

PATIENT EDUCATION

- Crohn's and Colitis Foundation of America – Patient fact sheet on eye diseases
  - http://www.ccfa.org/frameviewer/?url=/media/pdf/FactSheets/eyes.pdf
- A family history of IBD is an independent risk factor for the development of idiopathic uveitis, scleritis, and keratitis (7).

PROGNOSIS

- Good
  - Most patients with ocular manifestations of IBD are treatment-responsive at some level and maintain their visual acuity.

COMPLICATIONS

- Glaucoma and cataracts secondary to long-term oral/topical steroids or prolonged intraocular inflammation
- Macular edema secondary to inflammation
- Phthisis bulbi in a chronically inflamed eye

REFERENCES

1. Bernstein CN, Blanchard JF, Rawsthorne P, et al. The prevalence of extraintestinal diseases in inflammatory bowel disease: A population-based study. *Am J Gastroenterol* 2001;96(4):1116–1122.
2. McCannel CA, Holland GN, Helm CJ, et al. Causes of uveitis in the general practice of ophthalmology. *Am J Ophthalmol* 1996;121:35–46.
3. Orchard TR, Chua CN, Ahmad T, et al. Uveitis and erythema nodosum in inflammatory bowel disease: Clinical features and the role of HLA genes. *Gastroenterology* 2002;123(3):714–718.
4. Ghanchi FD, Rembacken BJ. Inflammatory bowel disease and the eye. *Surv Ophthalmol* 2003; 48:663–676.
5. Barrie B, Regueiro M. Biologic therapy in the management of extraintestinal manifestations of inflammatory bowel disease. *Inflamm Bowel Dis* 2007;13:1424–1429.
6. Chadhas V, Cruikshank I, Swingler R, et al. Advanced glaucomatous visual loss and oral corticosteroids. *BMJ* 2008;337:670.
7. Lin P, Tessler HH, Goldstein DA. Family history of inflammatory bowel disease in patients with idiopathic ocular inflammation. *Am J Ophthalmol* 2006;141(6):1097–1104.

C

ADDITIONAL READING

- Latkanky PA, Jabs DA. Ocular manifestations of inflammatory bowel disease. In: Bayless TM, Hanauer SB, eds. *Advanced therapy of inflammatory bowel disease*. Hamilton, Ontario: BC Decker Inc., 2001:275–277.

CODES

ICD9

- 555.9 Regional enteritis of unspecified site
- 556.8 Other ulcerative colitis
- 558.9 Other and unspecified noninfectious gastroenteritis and colitis

CLINICAL PEARLS

- Anterior uveitis is the most common clinically encountered ocular manifestation of IBD.
- Treatment with topical or systemic corticosteroids is usually effective in controlling ocular inflammation secondary to IBD.
- Infection must be ruled out before starting topical ocular steroid drops.
- Glaucoma and cataract are long-term complications of inflammation and/or topical or systemic steroid therapy.

CROUZON SYNDROME

Deepak P. Grover

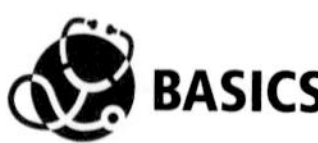

BASICS

DESCRIPTION

- Crouzon syndrome, a craniosynostosis disorder, is characterized by premature closure of calvarial and cranial base sutures, as well as those of the orbit and maxillary complex.
- Distinctive malformations of the skull and facial region are its hallmark.

EPIDEMIOLOGY

Incidence

1 case per 60,000 live births.

Prevalence

1 case per 25,000 population.

RISK FACTORS

Genetics

- It may be transmitted as an autosomal dominant disorder with complete penetrance and variable expressivity, or appear as a new mutation. Crouzon syndrome has no race or sex predilection.
- Caused by mutations in the fibroblast growth factor receptor-2 (*FGFR2*) gene, which is mapped to chromosome locus 10q25–10q26.
- 50% of incidents are not inherited and are the result of new mutations.

GENERAL PREVENTION

Genetic counseling.

PATHOPHYSIOLOGY

Premature closure of cranial sutures, most commonly the coronal and sagittal sutures, results in abnormal skull growth of the orbits and maxillary complex. The degree of deformity is dictated by the order and rate of suture fusion. Growth perpendicular to a fused suture is restricted promoting compensatory growth at the remaining open sutures (1)[B].

ETIOLOGY

See "Genetics."

COMMONLY ASSOCIATED CONDITIONS

- Acanthosis nigricans is the main dermatologic manifestation of Crouzon syndrome.
  - Characterized by thickened, velvety, light-brown to black markings on the neck, under the arms, or in the groin
  - Detectable after infancy

DIAGNOSIS

HISTORY

- Craniofacial abnormalities are often present at birth and may progress with time.
- Headaches and loss of vision secondary to elevated intracranial pressure
- Decreased mental function
- Visual disturbance secondary to excessive exposure of cornea or conjunctiva leading to ocular redness and irritation or burning sensation
- Unexplained loss of visual acuity or double vision
- Hearing loss secondary to ear canal stenosis or atresia

PHYSICAL EXAM

- **Common ophthalmic features**
  - Proptosis secondary to shallow orbits
  - Divergent strabismus or exotropia
  - Ocular hypertelorism
  - Exposure keratitis or conjunctivitis
- **Common facial features**
  - Midfacial hypoplasia secondary to small, underdeveloped maxilla
  - Beaked nose
  - Short upper lip
  - Relative mandibular prognathism secondary to protrusion of the lower jaw
- **Other manifestations**
  - Upper airway obstruction
  - Obstructive sleep apnea which can often present in infancy
  - Papilledema or optic atrophy secondary to elevated intracranial pressure
  - Progressive hydrocephalus
  - Chronic tonsillar herniation
  - Hearing loss secondary to recurrent ear infections
  - Crowding of the upper teeth
  - V-shaped maxillary dental arch
  - Narrow, high, or cleft palate
  - Bifid uvula
  - Cervical vertebral body fusions

DIAGNOSTIC TESTS & INTERPRETATION

Lab

- Molecular analysis for *FGFR2* mutation
  - Although the mutation is present in more than 50% of patients with Crouzon syndrome, it may also be present in Apert syndrome, Pfeiffer syndrome, and Jackson-Weiss syndrome.
  - All patients with associated acanthosis nigricans have an Ala391Glu mutation within the transmembrane region of the *FGFR3* gene.

Imaging

Initial approach

- Skull radiography – to show synostosis, craniofacial deformities, digital markings on skull, widening of hypophyseal fossa, small paranasal sinuses, maxillary hypoplasia, and shallow orbits
- Spine radiography – to show fusion of the vertebral bodies and posterior elements
- Limb radiography – to demonstrate subluxation of the radial head
- CT head/orbits with 3-dimensional reconstruction – to define pathologic anatomy
- MRI brain – to show corpus callosum agenesis and optic atrophy

Follow-up & special considerations

Genetics evaluation.

Diagnostic Procedures/Other

- Laryngologic examination with audiography
- Sleep study to evaluate for obstructive apnea
- Ophthalmologic examination
- General physical examination with ECG
- Psychiatric examination and psychological testing
- EEG – low-voltage, increased convulsive excitability

Pathological Findings

- Immunohistochemical analysis of cranial sutures, performed with labeled anti-*FGFR2* antibodies, demonstrates that sutures obtain lower levels of *FGFR2* activity in both stenosed and nonstenosed sutures.
- Histological features of acanthosis nigricans demonstrate hyperkeratosis, acanthosis, and papillomatosis. There are increased pigment cells in the upper dermis of the basal layer.

DIFFERENTIAL DIAGNOSIS

- **Apert syndrome**
  - Craniosynostosis combined with syndactyly of the hands and feet involving second, third, and fourth digits
- **Pfeiffer syndrome**
  - Craniosynostosis combined with broad thumbs and great toes, complex cardiovascular malformations and variable partial soft tissue syndactyly of the hands and feet.
- **Carpenter syndrome**
  - Craniosynostosis combined with craniofacial dysmorphism, finger and toe abnormalities, heart defects, growth and mental retardation.
- **Saethre-Chotzen syndrome**
  - Craniosynostosis combined with low-set frontal hair line, deviated nasal septum, variable facial asymmetry and partial cutaneous syndactyly

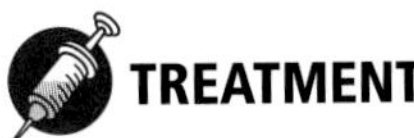

TREATMENT

ADDITIONAL TREATMENT

General Measures

- Early detection and management of amblyopia and refractive error
- Nasal continuous positive airway pressure device to relieve obstructive sleep apnea
- Nasopharyngeal airway as a better tolerated treatment modality in the management for obstructive sleep apnea (2)[B]
- Speech management

Issues for Referral

- Neurosurgeon
- Neuroradiologist
- Neurologist
- Ophthalmologist
- Oromaxillofacial surgeon
- Genetic specialist
- Psychiatrist
- Stomatologist
- Laryngologist

SURGERY/OTHER PROCEDURES

- Craniofacial and neurosurgical intervention with the goal to stage reconstruction to correlate with facial growth patterns, visceral function, and psychosocial development (1)[B].
  - In the first year of life, it is preferable to release the synostotic sutures of the skull to allow adequate cranial volume to promote brain growth and expansion. This can be performed with fronto-orbital advancement with cranial decompression.
  - Subsequent development of midfacial hypoplasia may be repaired with the Le Fort III osteotomy, monobloc frontofacial advancement or bipartition osteotomy.
    - Endoscopy before midface advancement is recommended to identify airway obstruction that may interfere with respiratory improvement after midface advancement (3)[B].
  - Early craniectomy with frontal bone advancement may be needed to prevent or treat increased intracranial pressure secondary to multiple suture synostoses and fused synchondroses.
  - Skull reshaping may be repeated as the child grows.

IN-PATIENT CONSIDERATIONS

Initial Stabilization

- Admit for surgical intervention
  - Shunting procedures for hydrocephalus
  - Tracheostomy for airway compromise

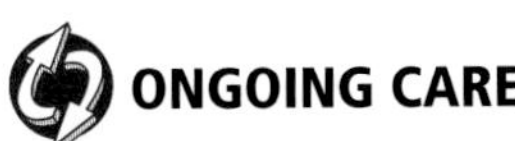

ONGOING CARE

FOLLOW-UP RECOMMENDATIONS

Ophthalmology and neurology for long-term monitoring.

Patient Monitoring

Monitor postoperative complications.

DIET

No special diet is required.

PROGNOSIS

- Depends on the severity of the malformation
- Patients usually have a normal lifespan

COMPLICATIONS

- Brain compression and mental retardation may result in severely affected individuals unless relieved by early craniectomy.
- Upper airway obstruction can lead to acute respiratory distress.
- Increased intracranial pressure and optic atrophy may occur secondary to a disproportion between craniostenosis and growing brain matter.
- Postoperative complications
  - Postoperative hydrocephalus and elevated intracranial pressure
  - Cerebrospinal fluid leak
  - Respiratory distress
  - Wound infections, extradural abscess, frontal bone osteomyelitis, periorbital abscess
  - Blindness, diplopia, facial nerve palsy

REFERENCES

1. Bowling E, Burnstein F. Crouzon syndrome. *Optometry* 2006;77:217–222.
2. Ahmed J, Marucci D, Cochrane L, et al. The role of the nasopharyngeal airway for obstructive sleep apnea in syndromic craniosynostosis. *J Craniofac Surg* 2008;19(3):659–663.
3. Bannink N, Nout E, Wolvius EB, et al. Obstructive sleep apnea in children with syndromic craniosynostosis: Long-term respiratory outcome of midface advancement. *Int J Oral Maxillofac Surg* 2010;39(2):115–121.

CODES

ICD9

- 378.10 Exotropia, unspecified
- 743.66 Specified congenital anomalies of orbit
- 756.0 Congenital anomalies of skull and face bones

CLINICAL PEARLS

- Unlike some other forms of craniosynostosis, there are no digital abnormalities with Crouzon syndrome.
- Surgical intervention for craniofacial reconstruction is staged to correlate with facial growth patterns, visceral function, and psychosocial development.
- Close monitoring of neurological and respiratory complications is fundamental for an overall good prognosis.

CRYSTALLINE KERATOPATHY

Michel J. Belliveau
Jacky Y.T. Yeung
Stephanie Baxter

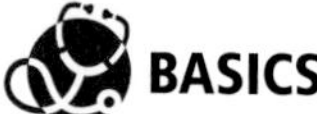

BASICS

DESCRIPTION

- There are 2 broad categories of crystalline keratopathy:
  - Infectious type
  - Deposition type
- When discussing crystalline keratopathy, it is generally accepted that one is referring to the infectious type, unless otherwise stated.
  - Synonym: Infectious crystalline keratopathy (ICK)
- Branching, crystalline corneal opacity caused by interlamellar colonization by microorganisms without significant adjacent stromal inflammation

EPIDEMIOLOGY

Incidence

Unknown, uncommon

RISK FACTORS

- Corneal graft
- Chronic topical steroid use
- Refractive surgery
- Contact lens wear
- Topical anesthetic abuse
- Acanthamoeba keratitis (co-infection)
- Prior herpes simplex virus (HSV) keratitis
- Systemic immunosuppression

GENERAL PREVENTION

- Prudent steroid use
- Routine follow-up

PATHOPHYSIOLOGY

Implantation and colonization of interlamellar spaces by microorganisms. The organisms are typically nonvirulent bacterial and fungal species. Extracellular matrix secretion and biofilm formation mask the antigenic stimuli and likely contribute to the characteristically scarce inflammatory response, in conjunction with the anti-inflammatory effects of steroids.

ETIOLOGY

- *Streptococcus viridans* (α-hemolytic)
- Candida sp
- Nontuberculous mycobacteria
- Other gram-positive and gram-negative bacteria may be polymicrobial

COMMONLY ASSOCIATED CONDITIONS

Corneal transplantation

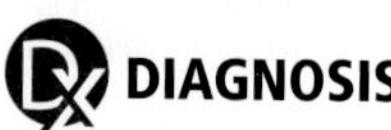

DIAGNOSIS

HISTORY

Typically insidious onset of vision loss and/or identification of a corneal opacity in the setting of known risk factors

PHYSICAL EXAM

- White, branching, crystalline opacity in the anterior stroma
- Lack of significant inflammation
- Slow expansion
- Rarely keratic precipitates or anterior chamber cells if posterior location

DIAGNOSTIC TESTS & INTERPRETATION

Lab

Initial lab tests

- Corneal scraping
  - Send for culture and sensitivity
- Lamellar biopsy
  - Send for culture and sensitivity and histopathology
- Consider lipid profile (Schnyder's crystalline dystrophy) and protein electrophoresis (monoclonal gammopathies)

Follow-up & special considerations

- Routine culture growth often unsuccessful:
  - May require specific nutrient (pyridoxal) for viridans streptococci (1)
  - Lowenstein–Jensen agar for isolation of nontuberculous mycobacteria
- If cystinosis is suspected, examine conjunctival biopsy, WBCs, or bone marrow for cystine crystals.
- If Bietti crystalline corneoretinal dystrophy is suspected, do visual fields and electroretinography.

Imaging

- Anterior segment photography
- Corneal optical coherence tomography, laser confocal microscopy

Diagnostic Procedures/Other

- Ocular evaluation:
  - Polymerase chain reaction of corneal scrapings
- Systemic evaluation:
  - CBC and differential
  - Protein electrophoresis
  - Lipid profile
  - Uric acid
  - Bone marrow aspiration

Pathological Findings

ICK – anterior stroma shows distended interlamellar spaces filled with microorganisms and without significant adjacent inflammation

DIFFERENTIAL DIAGNOSIS

- Infectious keratitis:
  - Bacterial – ICK
  - Fungal
  - Viral
  - Protozoan – *Acanthamoeba*
- Deposition:
  - Acquired immunoprotein keratopathies – multiple myeloma, essential cryobulinemia, and other monoclonal gammopathies
  - Lipid keratopathies – Schnyder's crystalline dystrophy, Tangier disease, familial lipoprotein disorders
  - Drugs deposition – ciprofloxacin, chrysiasis, chloroquine, chlorpromazine
  - Errors of protein metabolism – cystinosis, tyrosinemia, hyperuricemia, gout
  - Miscellaneous dystrophies and metabolic abnormalities – posterior crystalline corneal dystrophy, Bietti crystalline corneoretinal dystrophy, calcium deposition, porphyria, oxalosis

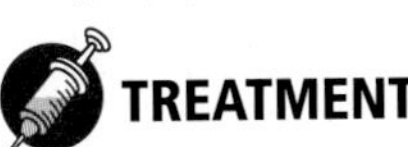

TREATMENT

MEDICATION

First Line

- Tailor treatment is performed according to specific organism if known.
- Duration of treatment often requires weeks to months with slow taper.
- Bacterial:
  - Depending on severity of disease, consider broad spectrum fluoroquinolones (e.g., gatifloxacin, moxifloxacin) as initial therapy
- May also add/replace with:
  - Gram +ve: cefazolin 50 mg/mL or vancomycin 25–50 mg/mL 1gtt per 1 h
  - Gram –ve: gentamicin or tobramycin 14 mg/ml 1gtt per 1 h
  - See the chapter on Bacterial Keratitis.
- Fungal:
  - Amphotericin B 0.15% or voriconazole 0.5–1% per 1 to 2 h drops for Candida
  - See the chapter on Fungal Keratitis.

Second Line

May consider systemic antibacterial or antifungal agents if refractory to topical treatment

ADDITIONAL TREATMENT

General Measures

Suspend immunosuppressive medication (e.g., topical steroids) if possible

Additional Therapies

Possible Nd:YAG laser for crystal disruption of ICK (2)

SURGERY/OTHER PROCEDURES

- Early surgical debridement and culture are advised, especially for post-LASIK patients.
- Full thickness or partial thickness anterior lamellar keratoplasty may be required for severe and/or refractory cases.

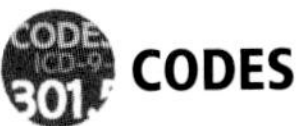

ONGOING CARE

FOLLOW-UP RECOMMENDATIONS

- Long-term follow-up required for treatment failure:
  - Corneal graft follow-up: Possible rejection or recurrence

PROGNOSIS

Guarded due to chronic, recurrent nature of most crystalline keratopathies

COMPLICATIONS

Failure or rejection of corneal graft

REFERENCES

1. Ormerod LD, Ruoff KL, Meisler DM, et al. Infectious crystalline keratopathy. Role of nutritionally variant streptococci and other bacterial factors. *Ophthalmology* 1991;98:159–169.
2. Masselos K, Tsang HH, Ooi JL, et al. Laser corneal biofilm disruption for infectious crystalline keratopathy. *Clin Experiment Ophthalmol* 2009; 37(2):177–180.

ADDITIONAL READING

- Bron AJ. Inherited dystrophies and developmental anomalies of the cornea, In: Tasman W, Jaeger EA, eds. *Duane's ophthalmology, foundations of clinical ophthalmology*, Lippincott Williams & Wilkins, 2010;3: chapter 63.
- Grimmett MR. Hematologic disorders. In: Krachmer J, Mannis M, Holland E, eds. *Cornea: Fundamentals and medical aspects of cornea and external disease*, Mosby, 2004;1.
- Kaiser-Kupfer MI, Gazzo MA, Datiles MB, et al. A randomized placebo-controlled trial of cysteamine eye drops in nephropathic cystinosis. *Arch Ophthalmol* 1990;108:689.

CODES

ICD9

- 371.00 Corneal opacity, unspecified
- 371.49 Other corneal degenerations

CLINICAL PEARLS

- ICK is the most common presentation of crystalline keratopathy, and it is very uncommon.
- ICK is often slow to resolve and requires treatment for a prolonged period of time.
- Deposition crystalline keratopathy may be the initial presentation of cystinosis or multiple myeloma.

CYSTOID MACULAR EDEMA

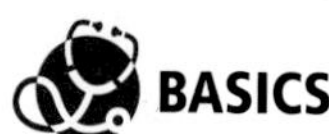

BASICS

DESCRIPTION
- Accumulation of fluid within and under the perifoveal region causing decreased acuity.
- Changes are often visible on clinical examination but sometimes may only be evident on fluorescein angiography (FA) or optical coherence tomography (OCT).
- Cystoid macular edema (CME) is a final common pathway of various retinal disorders. The most common cause is postoperative CME.

EPIDEMIOLOGY
Incidence
- CME may be detected by FA in up to 20% of uncomplicated cataract surgery cases.
- Clinically significant CME (vision worse than 20/40) occurs in up to 2.4% of patients after uncomplicated phacoemulsification (1).

RISK FACTORS
- Complicated cataract surgery (vitreous incarceration, iris trauma, long-operative times, prior history of intraocular inflammation)
- Diabetes
- Other retinal vascular disease
- Intraocular inflammation
- Macular pucker
- Preoperative use of topical prostaglandin agonists

Genetics
Unknown

GENERAL PREVENTION
- Postoperative topical steroids and nonsteroidal anti-inflammatory drugs (NSAIDs)
- Consider preoperative topical NSAIDs

PATHOPHYSIOLOGY
Not completely understood. Theories of contributing factors include UV light exposure, mechanical vitreous traction, and inflammation leading to vascular instability/breakdown of the blood aqueous barrier.

ETIOLOGY
- May occur after any type of ocular surgery, including laser.
- Uveitis, retinal vasculitis
- Diabetic retinopathy
- Exudative age-related macular degeneration
- Retinal vein occlusions
- Retinitis pigmentosa
- Retinal telangiectasis (Coats' disease)
- Venous or arterial macroaneurysms
- Drugs (tamoxifen, niacin, betaxolol, epinephrine, dipivefrin, prostaglandin agonists)
- Macular pucker, vitreomacular traction
- Radiation retinopathy
- Other (intraocular tumor, systemic hypertension, serous and rhegmatogenous retinal detachments)
- Optic nerve head abnormalities (optic pit, coloboma, diabetic papillopathy)
- Pseudo-CME (no leakage seen in: Nicotinic acid retinopathy, docetaxel, X-linked retinoschisis, and Goldmann-Favre disease)

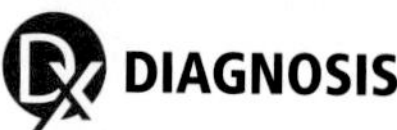

DIAGNOSIS

HISTORY
- Recent intraocular surgery or lasers?
- History of diabetes, uveitis, radiation, hypertension?
- Medication history: Does it include tamoxifen, niacin, betaxolol, epinephrine, dipivefrin, prostaglandin agonists, docetaxel?
- Any family history of CME?

PHYSICAL EXAM
- Foveal thickening
- Cystic spaces in the perifoveal area
- Evaluate for signs of retinal vascular disease (diabetic retinopathy, retinal vascular occlusion, retinal telangiectasis, or macroaneurysm)
- Evaluate for signs of intraocular inflammation
- Evaluate for occult retinal detachment and intraocular tumors

DIAGNOSTIC TESTS & INTERPRETATION
Lab
- None for post-op CME
- If clinical suspicion is present for uveitis, hypertension, retinal venous occlusion, or undiagnosed diabetes, laboratory studies may be indicated.

Imaging
Initial approach
- OCT: Increased foveal thickness, cystic spaces in outer plexiform layer, and subretinal fluid
- Fluorescein angiogram: Most cases of pseudophakic CME will show late intraretinal pooling of dye in a petaloid fashion, as well as hyperfluorescence of the optic nerve.
- Causes of CME without leakage on FA include nicotinic acid retinopathy, docetaxel, X-linked retinoschisis, and Goldmann-Favre disease.

Follow-up & special considerations
- OCT is helpful for monitoring response to treatment and for evaluating CME caused by an epiretinal membrane or vitreomacular traction.

Pathological Findings
May be intracellular (Muller cells) or extracellular accumulation of fluid.

DIFFERENTIAL DIAGNOSIS
- Diabetic macular edema
- Retinal venous occlusions
- Macular pucker
- Exudative AMD
- Chronic retinal detachment
- Other (intraocular tumor, systemic hypertension, serous and rhegmatogenous retinal detachments)
- Optic nerve head abnormalities (optic pit, coloboma, diabetic papillopathy)
- Pseudo-CME (no leakage seen in: Nicotinic acid retinopathy, docetaxel, X-linked retinoschisis, and Goldmann-Favre disease)
  – See Algorithm.

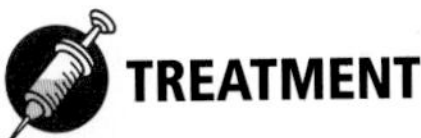

TREATMENT

MEDICATION

First Line

- Treatment outlined below focuses on post-op CME.
- 70% of post-cataract CME resolves spontaneously within 6 months.
- Treat if symptomatic with decreased vision or metamorphopsia.
- Trial of topical steroids (prednisolone 1% q.i.d, or difluprednate q.i.d) and topical NSAIDs (diclofenac 0.1% t.i.d, ketorolac 0.4% t.i.d, nepafenac t.i.d (2)[C], or bromfenac 0.09% b.i.d). Use in combination for 4–6 weeks.
- Consider stopping prostaglandin agonists and other exacerbating medications.

Second Line

- Periocular steroids (triamcinolone 40 mg) or intravitreal steroids (triamcinolone 4 mg)
- Intravitreal anti-VEGF agents (bevacizumab 1.25 mg) (3)[B]
- Steroids and anti-VEGF may be used simultaneously or sequentially while continuing topical therapy (4)[C].
- Repeat treatments may be necessary at 1 (for bevacizumab) to 3 months (for depot steroids) intervals.

ADDITIONAL TREATMENT

Issues for Referral

Consider referral to a vitreoretinal specialist if CME is not responsive to topical treatment, or if there are coexisting conditions such as DME, uveitis, retinal vascular occlusions, and others.

Additional Therapies

- Acetazolamide 250–500 mg b.i.d may be beneficial in post-op CME.
- Oral acetazolamide 250–500 mg b.i.d for CME associated with retinitis pigmentosa
- Intravitreal ranibizumab 0.5 mg may be useful for CME associated with retinitis pigmentosa (5)[C].

SURGERY/OTHER PROCEDURES

- Nd:YAG vitreolysis may be helpful in eyes with vitreous to cataract wound.
- Focal and/or grid laser is useful in CME predominantly related to diabetic macular edema and retinal vein occlusions.
- Vitrectomy and membrane peel

Useful in diffuse DME, macular pucker, vitreomacular traction, and in cases of post-op CME unresponsive to other treatment modalities.

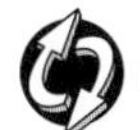

ONGOING CARE

FOLLOW-UP RECOMMENDATIONS

Patient Monitoring

- Every 4–6 weeks until CME resolves, then as needed
- Ocular steroids may cause acceleration of cataract formation and may increase the intraocular pressure.

PROGNOSIS

Usually good for post-op CME.

REFERENCES

1. Henderson BA, Kim JY, Ament CS, et al. Clinical pseudophakic cystoid macular edema. Risk factors for development and duration after treatment. *J Cataract Refract Surg* 2007;33(9):1550–1558.
2. Hariprasad SM, Akduman L, Clever JA, et al. Treatment of cystoid macular edema with the new-generation NSAID nepafenac 0.1%. *Clin Ophthalmol* 2009;3:147–154.
3. Arevalo JF, Maia M, Garcia-Amaris RA, et al. Intravitreal bevacizumab for refractory pseudophakic cystoid macular edema: The Pan-American Collaborative Retina Study Group results. *Ophthalmology* 2009;116:1481–1487.
4. Warren KA, Bahrani H, Fox JE. NSAIDs in combination therapy for the treatment of chronic pseudophakic cystoid macular edema. *Retina* 2010;30:260–266.
5. Artunay O, Yuzbasioglu E, Rasier R, et al. Intravitreal ranibizumab in the treatment of cystoid macular edema associated with retinitis pigmentosa. *J Ocul Pharmacol Ther* 2009;25: 545–550.

ADDITIONAL READING

- Benitah NR, Arroyo JG. Pseudophakic cystoid macular edema. *Int Ophthalmol Clin* 2010 Winter;50:139–153.
- Johnson MW. Etiology and treatment of macular edema. *Am J Ophthalmol* 2009;147:11–21.

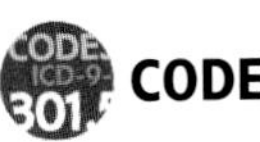

CODES

ICD9

- 362.18 Retinal vasculitis
- 362.53 Cystoid macular degeneration of retina
- 364.3 Unspecified iridocyclitis

CLINICAL PEARLS

- CME is the final pathway for a variety of prevalent retinal disorders.
- Post-op CME is often subclinical and self-limited.
- Symptomatic post-op CME are treated with a step-wise approach using topical therapy first.
- Second line therapy includes subtenon's steroid injection, or intravitreal steroid, and/or anti-VEGF in combination with topical treatment.

CYTOMEGALOVIRUS (CMV) RETINITIS

Amro Ali
Steven T. Bailey

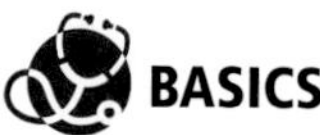

BASICS

DESCRIPTION
- Cytomegalovirus (CMV) retinitis is a full thickness retinal necrosis resulting in progressive vision loss.
- CMV is an ubiquitous herpes virus.
- Retinitis occurs in immunosuppressed hosts, typically those infected with human immunodeficiency virus (HIV) and a CD4+ count <50 cells/mL.
- Leading cause of acquired immunodeficiency syndrome (AIDS) related blindness
- Treated with immune reconstitution with highly active anti-retroviral therapy (HAART) and anti-CMV medications

EPIDEMIOLOGY
Incidence
- AIDS patients pre-HAART era: 30% lifetime probability
- HAART era: Reduced incidence by 75–80%
- Much less common in non-HIV immunosuppressed individuals

RISK FACTORS
- HIV+ with CD4 <50 cells/mL
- HIV-associated microvasculopathy
- Organ transplant recipients
- Steroid treatment
- Systemic chemotherapy
- Malignancies, that is, leukemia, lymphoma

GENERAL PREVENTION
- Safe sex practice
- Avoid contact with bodily fluids
- Ophthalmic examination with dilated fundus examination for high risk individuals

PATHOPHYSIOLOGY
- CMV transmission: Transplacental, contact with bodily fluids, blood transfusion, organ transplant
- Immunosuppressed host susceptible to primary infection or reactivation of latent infection
- CMV reaches eye through the bloodstream
- All layers of retina infected resulting in full thickness retinal necrosis
- Untreated retinitis slowly progressively enlarges over weeks to months
- Rhegmatogenous retinal detachment may develop in 15–40% of eyes

ETIOLOGY
Cytomegalovirus beta-herpes virus.

COMMONLY ASSOCIATED CONDITIONS
- CMV pneumonitis
- CMV colitis and esophagitis
- CMV transverse myelitis and meningoencephalitis
- Congenital CMV infection

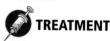

DIAGNOSIS

HISTORY
- May be asymptomatic
- Decreased central or peripheral vision
- New onset of floaters
- AIDS with CD4+ count <50 cell/mL
- Leukemia, lymphoma, and aplastic anemia
- Organ transplant recipient
- Systemic immunosuppression chemotherapy

PHYSICAL EXAM
- Visual acuity: Decreased or normal
- Confrontation to visual fields: Decreased or normal
- Afferent papillary defect may be present
- Typically minimal anterior and/or vitreous inflammation
- Fulminant retinitis with retinal edema, retinal hemorrhage, and vasculitis
- Indolent/granular retinitis with faint grainy retinal opacification
- Zone I: Within 3000 microns from fovea
- Zone II: Peripheral to zone 1 to vortex veins
- Zone III: Peripheral to zone 2 to ora serrata

DIAGNOSTIC TESTS & INTERPRETATION
Lab
- HIV Serology (if unknown)
- CD4+ T-lymphocyte count
- HIV ribonucleic acid (RNA) blood level

Imaging
Initial approach
Fundus photography

Follow-up & special considerations
Serial fundus photographs are useful to evaluate for disease progression.

Diagnostic Procedures/Other
If clinical diagnosis unclear, polymerase chain reaction (PCR) of vitreous or aqueous humor samples can detect CMV.

DIFFERENTIAL DIAGNOSIS
- Acute retinal necrosis (HSV or VZV)
- Progressive out retinal necrosis (VZV)
- HIV-associated retinopathy
- Syphilis
- Toxoplasmosis
- Endophthalmitis
- Tuberculosis

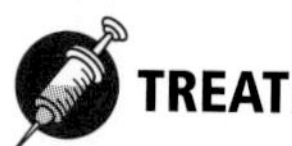

TREATMENT

MEDICATION
First Line
- HAART naïve with Zone I disease: Intravitreal ganciclovir implant 4.5 mg with oral valganciclovir (1) (see dose below)
- Heart naïve with Zone II/III disease: Valganciclovir oral 900 mg b.i.d for 3 weeks followed by maintenance dose of 900 mg per day (2)
- HAART experienced with Zone 1 disease: Ganciclovir implant with oral Valganciclovir
- HAART experienced with Zone II/III disease: Oral Valganciclovir +/− ganciclovir implant
- Zone I disease: May also consider intravitreal ganciclovir injection 2 mg/0.1 mL twice weekly or foscarnet 2.4 mg/0.1 mL twice weekly until ganciclovir implant available
- Valganciclovir toxicities: Renal toxicity, neutropenia, anemia, thrombocytopenia
- Initiate HAART or alter HAART if ineffective
- If HAART naïve, consider treatment of CMV retinitis prior to HAART to limit immune recovery uveitis

Second Line

- Ganciclovir: Induction dose 5 mg/kg IV b.i.d for 14–21 days. Oral maintenance dose: 1000 mg PO t.i.d. Intravenous (IV) maintenance dose: 5 mg/kg IV daily or 6 mg/kg IV 5 days/week
- Ganciclovir toxicities: Renal toxicity, neutropenia, anemia, thrombocytopenia
- Foscarnet: Induction dose: 90 mg/kg IV b.i.d for 14–21 days. Maintenance dose: 90 mg/kg IV daily.
- Foscarnet toxicities: Renal impairment, neutropenia, anemia, electrolyte imbalances
- Cidofovir: Induction dose: 5 mg/kg IV weekly for 2 weeks. Maintenance dose: 5 mg/kg IV every 2 weeks
- Cidofovir toxicities: Nephrotoxicity, ocular hypotony, and iritis

ADDITIONAL TREATMENT

Issues for Referral

- Retina specialist for evaluation and treatment of suspected CMV retinitis
- Infectious disease specialist to evaluate for other end-organ CMV related disease and/or other opportunistic infections
- General internist, oncologist, or hematologist for non-HIV related CMV retinitis

Additional Therapies

Low vision evaluation for those with substantial vision loss.

SURGERY/OTHER PROCEDURES

- Surgical insertion of ganciclovir sustained release implant – lasts 6–10 months
- Surgical repair of retinal detachment may include vitrectomy, scleral buckle, and silicone oil or gas endotamponade.

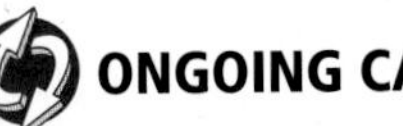

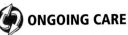

ONGOING CARE

FOLLOW-UP RECOMMENDATIONS

- Those on HAART with CD4+ counts >100–150 cells/mL for 3–6 months may discontinue the anti-CMV drugs (3)
- Reactivation of CMV retinitis may present with appearance of a new lesion or expansion of previously inactive border.
- Reactivation is treated with re-induction with anti-CMV medications and possible adjustment in HAART to establish immune recovery.
- Evaluate for ganciclovir resistance if treatment response is inadequate.

Patient Monitoring

Frequent dilated fundus examinations dependent on extend of CMV retinitis and degree of immune recovery.

PATIENT EDUCATION

- Symptoms of CMV retinitis: Floaters, photophobia, central or peripheral vision loss
- Appropriate medication use and side effect profile

PROGNOSIS

Dependent on ability of immune recovery – much less likely to lose significant vision in HAART era.

COMPLICATIONS

- Vision loss
- Retinal detachment
- Immune recovery uveitis may result in: Macular edema, epiretinal membrane, neovascularization of the retina, and cataract

REFERENCES

1. Jabs DA. AIDS and ophthalmology, 2008. *Arch Ophthalmol* 2008;126(8):1143–1146.
2. Patil AJ, Sharma A, Kenney MC, et al. Valganciclovir in the treatment of cytomegalovirus retinitis in HIV-infected patients. *Clin Ophthalmol* 2010;4: 11–119.
3. Holland GN. AIDS and ophthalmology: The first quarter century. *Am J Ophthalmol* 2008;145: 397–408.

ADDITIONAL READING

- Foscarnet-Ganciclovir Cytomegalovirus Retinitis Trial. 4. Visual outcomes. Studies of Ocular Complications of AIDS Research Group in collaboration with the AIDS Clinical Trials Group. *Ophthalmology* 1994;101(7):1250–1261.
- Jabs DA. Ocular manifestations of HIV infection. *Trans Am Ophthalmol Soc* 1995;93:623–683.
- Martin DF, Kuppermann BD, Wolitz RA, et al. Oral ganciclovir for patients with cytomegalovirus retinitis treated with ganciclovir implant: Roche ganciclovir study group. *N Engl J Med* 1999;340(14):1063–1070.
- Martin DF, Sierra-Madero J, Walmsley S, et al. A controlled trial of valganciclovir as induction therapy for cytomegalovirus retinitis. *N Engl J Med* 2002;346(15):1119–1126.

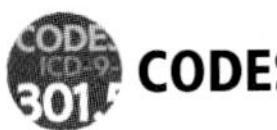

CODES

ICD9

- 053.29 Herpes zoster with other ophthalmic complications
- 078.5 Cytomegaloviral disease
- 363.13 Disseminated choroiditis and chorioretinitis, generalized

CLINICAL PEARLS

- Retinitis with paucity of anterior and vitreous inflammation
- Slowly progressive
- Immunosuppressed hosts, typically AIDS patients with CD4+ count <50 cells/mL
- Zone I treated with intravitreal ganciclovir, oral Valganciclovir, and HAART
- Zone II/III treated with oral Valganciclovir and HAART

DACRYOCELE

Rudolph S. Wagner

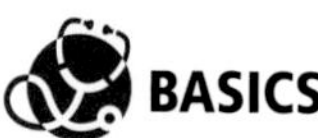

BASICS

DESCRIPTION

- Distended lacrimal sac usually in neonates or very early infancy
- With or without associated intranasal cyst
- Also known as dacryocele, lacrimal sac mucocele, dacryocystocele, or amniotocele

EPIDEMIOLOGY

Incidence

Incidence unknown

Prevalence

0.1% of infants with congenital nasolacrimal duct obstruction (NLD) (1)[A]

RISK FACTORS

Unknown

Genetics

- Usually sporadic
- Familial cases have been reported

GENERAL PREVENTION

- Can be detected by prenatal ultrasound (2)[A]
  - No preventive measures identified

PATHOPHYSIOLOGY

Congenital distal membranous blockage of nasolacrimal duct at inferior meatus intranasally causing lacrimal sac distension and obstruction of the entrance to the sac by the common canaliculus at valve of Rosenmüller. Antegrade and retrograde discharge of accumulated secretions prevented.

ETIOLOGY

Congenital membrane or valve (Hasner) obstruction related to canalization failure or persistence of embryologic membrane.

COMMONLY ASSOCIATED CONDITIONS

- Dacryocystitis
- Pre-septal cellulitis
- Congenital NLD obstruction
  - Cystic bulging of the mucosa of the distal nasolacrimal duct into the nasal cavity
  - May cause nasal airway obstruction and respiratory distress

DIAGNOSIS

HISTORY

- Distended mass with bluish discoloration below the medial canthal tendon within the medial aspect of the lower lid, presenting in a neonate unilaterally or bilaterally
- May be history of overlying progressive erythema and swelling (if infected)
- May be history of difficulty breast feeding on mother's breasts ipsilateral to dacryocele (e.g., right breast of woman feeding child with a right dacryocele) due to compression of contralateral patent nares against nipple

PHYSICAL EXAM

- Palpable mass
  - Distended and firm
  - May be tender
  - Non-moveable
  - Medial lower eyelid displaced superiorly
  - May be signs of NLD obstruction or dacryocystitis
  - Mucoid discharge may be expressed from puncta or nasal cavity on compression of mass
  - Conduct full eye examination with attention to possible secondary periorbital/orbital cellulitis, globe displacement, strabismus, amblyopia, or induced astigmatism

DIAGNOSTIC TESTS & INTERPRETATION

Lab

Initial lab tests

- CBC with differential and blood culture if dacryocystitis or cellulitis suspected
- Consider additional cultures (rule out sepsis) including urine and cerebrospinal fluid if infection present and child showing systemic signs

Follow-up & special considerations

Monitor for infection

Imaging

Initial approach

- In the presence of signs and symptoms of nasal airway obstruction
  - CT or MRI to demonstrate endonasal cyst occasionally indicated (4)[A]

Follow-up & special considerations

Consider otorhinolaryngology consult to evaluate nasal cysts

Diagnostic Procedures/Other

Endoscopic identification of nasal cysts at time of surgery (when indicated)

Pathological Findings

Membranous intranasal cyst wall at inferior meatus with ciliated respiratory epithelium on nasal side and stratified columnar epithelium on side of NLD

DIFFERENTIAL DIAGNOSIS

- Other masses in medial canthal area
  - Capillary hemangioma (not present at birth, rubbery and soft to palpation, and possible reddish surface component)
  - Dermoid or epidermoid cyst (moveable subcutaneous mass, typically superonasal, no blue discoloration, rarely infected)
  - Encephaloceles (typically present above medial canthal ligament, usually with hypertelorism)

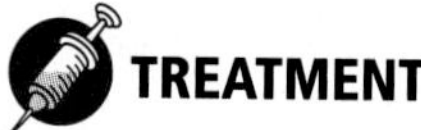

TREATMENT

MEDICATION

- Decompression by firm but careful digital massage (if successful, immediate decompression of mass occurs)
  - If dacryocystitis and/or cellulitis present, some recommend warm compresses and systemic antibiotics but in this age group risk for systemic infection is high and surgery should be considered

ADDITIONAL TREATMENT

General Measures

Monitor and treat subsequent NLD obstruction if present

Issues for Referral

Consider otorhinolaryngology consult to evaluate nasal cysts

COMPLEMENTARY & ALTERNATIVE THERAPIES
None known

SURGERY/OTHER PROCEDURES
- Probing and irrigation with or without nasal endoscopy if nonresponse to medical therapy, airway obstruction, or infection
  - If not infected, gentile probing through puncta into proximal lacrimal sac by common canaliculus in cases resistant to digital message
- Probing under general anesthesia is the mainstay of surgical therapy
  - Nasal endoscopy useful to visualize nasal cyst and to guide probe
  - Nasal mucocele can be marsupialized under endoscopic guidance (5)[A]
  - In office awake nasal endoscopy has been performed but is technically challenging (6)[B]

IN-PATIENT CONSIDERATIONS
Admission Criteria
- Advised if dacryocystitis/periorbital cellulitis especially if signs of systemic infection for intravenous antibiotics prior to surgery
- Some recommend an additional intravenous day of antibiotics after surgery

Discharge Criteria
- Reduction or resolution of cystic mass and infection
  - No evidence of nasal airway compromise

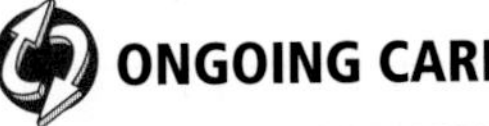

ONGOING CARE

FOLLOW-UP RECOMMENDATIONS
As needed if cystic mass recurs

Patient Monitoring
- Care givers to observe for recurrence of cystic mass
  - Monitor for breathing difficulty
  - Monitor for signs of infection
  - May have residual NLD obstruction

PATIENT EDUCATION
- Parents instructed to gently digitally massage inferior medial canthal area where cyst was present for a few days to possibly prevent reformation of dacryocele
  - Parents educated as to signs of infection and urgent need for returning to care in that circumstance

PROGNOSIS
- 99% complete recovery and resolution of signs and symptoms with surgery including nasal endoscopy
- Success less for probing without endoscopy (approximately 70–80%)
  - May develop signs and symptoms to typical nasolacrimal duct obstruction in the future

COMPLICATIONS
- Development of fistulous tract through skin over distended dacryocele (NOTE: Do not drain dacryocele through skin)
- Chronic nasolacrimal duct obstruction
- Pre-septal cellulitis
  - Sepsis/meningitis
  - May be transient excavation of infraorbital bone that is palpable after cyst decompressed

REFERENCES

1. Wong RK, VanderVeen DK. Presentation and management of congenital dacryocystocele. *Pediatrics* 2008;122:e1108–e1112.
2. Mackenzie PJ, Dolman PJ, Stokes J, et al. Dacryocele diagnosed prenatally. *Br J Ophthalmol* 2008;92:437–438.
3. Mansour AM, Cheng KP, Mumma JV, et al. Congenital dacryocele. A collaborative review. *Ophthalmology* 1991;98:1744–1751.
4. Paysse EA, Coats DK, Bernsetin JM, et al. Management and complications of congenital dacryocele with concurrent intranasal mucocele. *J AAPOS* 2000;4:46–53.
5. Levin AV, Wygnanski-Jaffe T, Forte V, et al. Nasal endoscopy in the treatment of congenital lacrimal sac mucoceles. *Int J Pediatr Otorhinolaryngol* 2003;67:255–261.
6. Hain M, Bawnik Y, Warman M, et al. Neonatal dacryocele with endonasal cyst: Revisiting the management. *Am J Otolaryngol* 2011;32(2): 152–155.

ADDITIONAL READING

- http://www.pediatrics.org/cgi/content/full/122/5/e1108

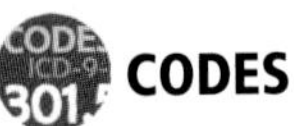

CODES

ICD9
375.43 Lacrimal mucocele

CLINICAL PEARLS

- Try to decompress the dacryocele with gentle but firm massage (this may help to avoid a surgical procedure)
- Ask the mother if she has observed her baby having breathing difficulty while she is breast feeding. This may suggest the presence of an intranasal mucocele.
- Consider the use of nasal endoscopy when probing
- Secondary dacryocystitis/periorbital cellulitis in a neonate should be considered an urgent concern with a risk for systemic spread

DACRYOCYSTITIS

Katherine Gold
Jacqueline R. Carrasco

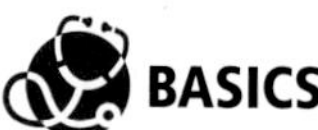

BASICS

DESCRIPTION

- Dacryocystitis is an inflammatory condition of the lacrimal sac, usually infectious in nature
- May occur as sequelae of nasolacrimal duct obstruction (NLDO), and it may lead to recurrent episodes
- May be chronic, acute, or congenital

RISK FACTORS

- Structural predispositions:
  - Brachycephalic head
  - Narrow face with flat nose

GENERAL PREVENTION

There is no preventive counseling prior to a first episode. Once an episode of dacryocystitis has occurred, undergoing a dacryocystorhinostomy (DCR) procedure in certain cases may help to prevent future recurrences.

PATHOPHYSIOLOGY

The surfaces of the lacrimal passages are normally colonized with bacteria. When blockage occurs for any reason, and tears do not flow normally through the system, dacryocystitis can result.

ETIOLOGY

- Structural midface abnormalities
- Ethmoidal inflammation
- Obstruction, including nasal fractures, impacted punctal plugs, lacrimal sac tumors, or cysts
- Bacterial: *Staphylococcus epidermidis*, *Staphylococcus aureus*, *Streptococci*, and *Pneumococci*, as well as gram-negative bacteria and anaerobes.

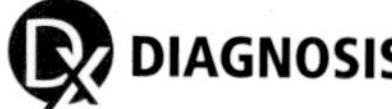

DIAGNOSIS

HISTORY

- Acute, chronic, or congenital forms
- Pain, redness, swelling over medial canthal region
- Epiphora

PHYSICAL EXAM

- Tenderness to palpation over lacrimal sac region
- Firm nodule inferior to medial canthus
- Purulent discharge from puncta
- May have drainage through dacryocutaneous fistula, which may close spontaneously
- A secondary orbital cellulitis may result in an afferent pupillary defect, limited extraocular movement

DIAGNOSTIC TESTS & INTERPRETATION

Diagnostic Procedures/Other

- Usually a clinical diagnosis
- If an inflammatory etiology is suspected: ANA, ANCA, ACE, CBC
- If unresponsive to empiric therapy, may obtain cultures of discharge or blood cultures
- CT scan to evaluate for structural abnormalities and other obstructive causes, not always necessary.
- Dacryocystography and dacryoscintigraphy may be used to help define the lacrimal system anatomy.
- Jones dye test (I or II)
- Endoscopy to evaluate anatomy by direct visualization

DIFFERENTIAL DIAGNOSIS

- Canaliculitis
- Encephalocele
- Lacrimal sac tumor

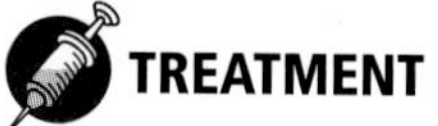

TREATMENT

ADDITIONAL TREATMENT

General Measures

- Oral antibiotics
- Warm compresses
- Topical antibiotic ophthalmic drops and/or ophthalmic ointment
- IV antibiotics for severe cases, or concern for orbital cellulitis

SURGERY/OTHER PROCEDURES

Usually a DCR – external or endonasal – must be done to avoid recurrence once the initial infection has resolved with antibiotic therapy. Although endonasal DCR avoids external scars, there are no recent randomized prospective trials with direct comparison of efficacy. A Cochrane Review found mixed data and paucity of randomized controlled trials (1)[B]. A comparison of external DCR with endonasal laser-assisted (endocanalicular) DCR found similar efficacy (92.4 vs. 94.2% respectively) (2)[B]. Routine biopsy of lacrimal sac at time of DCR is controversial. A recent large retrospective review suggests biopsy in atypical or suspicious cases (3)[C].

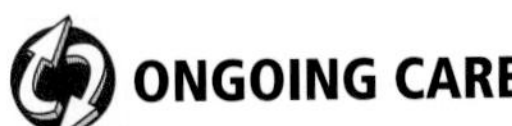

ONGOING CARE

FOLLOW-UP RECOMMENDATIONS

- Ophthalmologist
- Oculoplastic surgeon

Patient Monitoring

See "Follow-up"

PROGNOSIS

Excellent

COMPLICATIONS

- Orbital cellulitis
- If severe infection, may lead to sepsis and rarely death

REFERENCES

1. Anijeet D, Dolan L, Macewen CJ. Endonasal versus external dacryocystorhinostomy for nasolacrimal duct obstruction. *Cochrane Database Syst Rev* 2011;1:CD007097.
2. Ajalloueyan M, Fartookzadeh M, Parhizgar H. Use of laser for dacryocystorhinostomy. *Arch Otolaryngol Head Neck Surg* 2007;133:340–343.
3. Salour H, Hatami MM, Parvin M, et al. Clinicopathological study of lacrimal sac specimens obtained during DCR. *Orbit* 2010;29(5):250–253.

ADDITIONAL READING

- Barrett RV, Meyer DR. Acquired lacrimal sac fistula after incision and drainage for dacryocystitis: A multicenter study. *Ophthal Plast Reconstr Surg* 2009;25(6):455–457.
- Bharathi MJ, Ramakrishnan R, Maneksha V, et al. Comparative bacteriology of acute and chronic dacryocystitis. *Eye (Lond)* 2008;22(7):953–960.
- Vicinanzo MG, McGwin G, Boyle M, et al. The consequence of premature silicone stent loss after external dacryocystorhinostomy. *Ophthalmology* 2008;115(7):1241–1244.

CODES

ICD9

- 375.30 Dacryocystitis, unspecified
- 375.32 Acute dacryocystitis
- 375.42 Chronic dacryocystitis

CLINICAL PEARLS

- A mass below the medial canthal tendon indicates infectious etiology, whereas a mass above the medial canthal tendon may indicate a slowly enlarging mass, such as a tumor of the lacrimal sac.
- Chronic conjunctivitis of unknown etiology may be due to chronic, undiagnosed dacryocystitis. A diagnostic probing/irrigation should be performed to rule out underlying NLDO and dacryocystitis.
- Once a patient has had an episode of dacryocystitis, they are at risk for future attacks if a DCR is not performed.

DELLEN

Robert Eyck Fintelmann

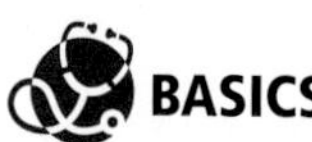

BASICS

DESCRIPTION
- Small, saucer-like excavation at the corneal margin
- Most often form an ellipse; 2 × 1.5 mm parallel to the limbus
- Associated with adjacent elevation of paralimbal tissue

EPIDEMIOLOGY
Incidence
- 9% after trabeculectomy (1)[C]
- Up to 19% after muscle surgery (2)[C]

RISK FACTORS
Any process causing elevation of the perilimbal tissue

PATHOPHYSIOLOGY
Localized dehydration of the cornea secondary to a localized break in the precorneal oily tear film layer

ETIOLOGY
Elevation of paralimbal tissue leads to a change in the tear film probably by affecting lid function

COMMONLY ASSOCIATED CONDITIONS
- Episcleritis
- Pinguecula
- Pterygium
- Subconjunctival injection
- Glaucoma surgery with creation of a filtering bleb
- Subconjunctival hemorrhage
- Limbal malignancy
- Paralytic lagophthalmus

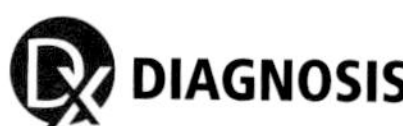

DIAGNOSIS

HISTORY
- Recent surgery
- Any change in the appearance of the eye

PHYSICAL EXAM
- Apparent corneal thinning evident on slit lamp exam (3)[C]
- Steep wall on the corneal side, sloping wall on the limbal side
- May or may not stain with fluorescein
- Cornea can appear markedly thinned (may resemble a descemetocele without a bulge)

DIFFERENTIAL DIAGNOSIS
- Peripheral ulcerative keratitis
- Corneal ulcer
- Terrien's marginal degeneration

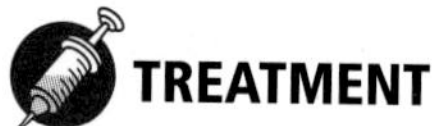

TREATMENT

MEDICATION
First Line
- Artificial tears, 1 drop q.i.d (3)[C]
- Ointment (antibiotic or tear) q.h.s (3)[C]

Second Line
Topical antibiotic, 1 drop q.i.d (2)[C]

ADDITIONAL TREATMENT
General Measures
- Patching of the involved eye for a day (3)[C]
- Treatment of the cause for the tissue elevation

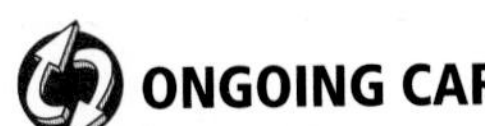

ONGOING CARE

FOLLOW-UP RECOMMENDATIONS

Should be seen in a week

PROGNOSIS

- If treated, resolves without sequelae
- May leave scar if present for a prolonged period of time

COMPLICATIONS

- Rarely, severe thinning may occur (4)[C]
- May need surgical intervention (4)[C]

REFERENCES

1. Fresina M, Campos EC. Corneal 'dellen' as a complication of strabismus surgery. *Eye* 2009; 23(1):161–163.
2. Soong HK, Quigley HA. Dellen associated with filtering blebs. *Arch Ophthalmol* 1983;101: 385–387.
3. Baum JL, Mishima S, Boruchoff SA. On the nature of dellen. *Arch Ophthalmol* 1968;79:657–662.
4. Insler MS, Tauber S, Packer A. Descemetocele formation in a patient with a postoperative corneal dellen. *Cornea* 1989;8:129–130.

ADDITIONAL READING

- Fuchs E. Ueber Dellen in der Hornhaut. *Albrecht v Graefes Arch Ophthal* 1911;78:82–92.

CODES

ICD9

371.41 Senile corneal changes

CLINICAL PEARLS

- Dellen may occur when elevated limbal tissue is present
- Dellen do not represent true loss of tissue
- Dellen usually respond rapidly to patching and lubrication

DERMATOCHALASIS

Edward H. Bedrossian Jr

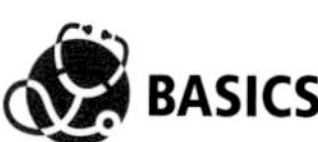

BASICS

DESCRIPTION

- Dermatochalasis refers to excess eyelid skin associated with the aging process.
- Blepharochalasis is a rare eyelid disorder that often presents in childhood, characterized by recurrent episodes of idiopathic painless edema of the upper and occasionally lower eyelids.
- Steatoblepharon describes the herniation of orbital fat.

EPIDEMIOLOGY

Incidence

- Data unavailable
- Frequently occurs by the age of 40 years and progresses with age.
- May develop by age 20 years in those with family history.

Prevalence

Data unavailable

RISK FACTORS

- Advancing age
- Smoking
- Sun exposure
- Facial trauma
- Positive family history of dermatochalasis

Genetics

Unknown

GENERAL PREVENTION

- Avoid smoking
- Avoid eyelid rubbing
- UV protection-hat, sunglasses, and sunscreen advised

PATHOPHYSIOLOGY

- Consistent with normal aging changes of the skin
- Loss of elastic and reticular fibers of the dermis, thinning of the epidermis with resultant skin redundancy

ETIOLOGY

- Age
- Family tendency
- Chronic manipulation of eyelids

COMMONLY ASSOCIATED CONDITIONS

- Blepharoptosis
- Herniated orbital fat
- Eyelid laxity
- Dry eye syndrome
- Chronic blepharitis
- Chronic dermatitis
- Thyroid eye disease
- Chronic renal insufficiency

DIAGNOSIS

HISTORY

- Excess skin of the upper lids and/or lower lids
- Brow ache
- Ocular fatigue when reading
- Difficulty applying eye make-up

PHYSICAL EXAM

- Brow ptosis
- Horizontal forehead creases
- Excess upper eyelid skin
- Excess lower eyelid skin
- Descent of retro- orbicularis oculi fat (ROOF)
- Descent of suborbicularis oculi fat (SOOF)
- Herniated orbital fat
- Prominent bony orbital rim
- Low or absent eyelid crease
- Prominent nasojugal fold
- Prominent nasolabial fold

DIAGNOSTIC TESTS & INTERPRETATION

Lab

Initial lab tests

- In most cases, none is needed
- Tensilon test, if associated with ptosis
- Schirmer test, for tear function
- Visual field, for functional defect(surgery)
- Pre-op external photography
- Serum TSH if thyroid disease is suspected
- C1-esterase inhibitor, if hereditary angioedema is suspected

Follow-up & special considerations

- If positive tensilon test, need to rule out Myasthenia Gravis
- If low tear film, conservative skin excision is advised to avoid lid lagophthalmos.
- If superior visual field loss, surgery is functional and may be covered by insurance.
- External pre-op photography is essential for documentation.

Imaging

Initial approach

- In most cases, none needed.
- CT scan or MRI of orbit and midbrain if associated third nerve palsy or proptosis

Follow-up & special considerations

Treat underlying condition if present

Pathological Findings

- Atrophy of eyelid skin, actinic elastosis, and basophilic degeneration of dermal collagen
- Attenuation of orbital septum

DIFFERENTIAL DIAGNOSIS

- Blepharoptosis
- Blepharochalasis
- Floppy eyelid syndrome
- Prolapsed lacrimal gland
- Entropion

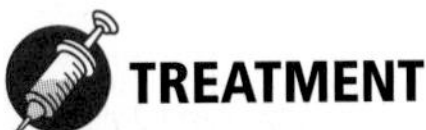

TREATMENT

MEDICATION

First Line

- Skin care products (Retin-A, Alpha-Hydroxy Acids)
- If blepharitis, consider lid hygiene, topical antibiotics, and topical steroids.
- If dry eye, consider appropriate topical lubricant and/or punctual occlusion.

Second Line

- Fractional CO_2 laser treatment
- Infra-brow botulinum toxin injections

ADDITIONAL TREATMENT

Issues for Referral

- Underlying eyelid ptosis
- Dry eye syndrome
- Corneal pathology
- Brow ptosis requiring brow lift
- Laxity of lower lid requiring lid tightening procedure
- Prolapsed lacrimal gland

COMPLEMENTARY & ALTERNATIVE THERAPIES

- Vitamin supplements
- Fish oil and alpha omega–3 supplements

SURGERY/OTHER PROCEDURES

- The upper and lower lid blepharoplasty has undergone numerous refinements in recent years. These refinements include techniques to elevate and re-inflate descended and deflated tissues, as well as ethnic considerations. The technique is essentially the same whether surgery is for functional or cosmetic reasons.
- Primary treatment is surgical

IN-PATIENT CONSIDERATIONS

Initial Stabilization

Most are outpatient

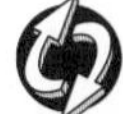

ONGOING CARE

FOLLOW-UP RECOMMENDATIONS

Slit-lamp evaluation for corneal health

Patient Monitoring

1 day, 1 week, 1 month post-op, and as needed.

DIET

- Low salt diet
- Fruits, berries,
- Leafy green vegetables
- Fish (salmon, sardines)

PATIENT EDUCATION

See risk factors

PROGNOSIS

Excellent in most cases

COMPLICATIONS

- Undercorrection
- Overcorrection (lagophthalmos)
- Exposure keratopathy
- Hollow superior sulcus (excess fat removal)
- Asymmetry of lid crease, fold or arch
- Medial canthal web
- Brow ptosis
- Blepharoptosis
- Complete loss of vision

ADDITIONAL READING

- Ancona D, Katz BE. A prospective study of the improvement in periorbital wrinkles and eyebrow elevation with a novel fractional CO2 laser-the fractional eye lift. *J Drugs Dermatol* 2010;9(1): 16–21.
- Grant D Gilliland, Md Dermatochalasis Emedicine ophthalmology from WebbMD emedicine.medscape.com/article/1212294-printup Feb 25 2010.
- Korn BS, Kikkawa DO, Cohen SR. Transcutaneous lower eyelid blepharoplasty with orbitomalar suspension: Retrospective review of 212 consecutive cases. *Plast Reconstr Surg* 2010;125(1):315–323.
- Mack WP. Complications in periocular rejuvenation. *Facial Plast Surg Clin North Am* 2010;18(3): 435–456.

CODES

ICD9

- 374.34 Blepharochalasis
- 374.87 Dermatochalasis

CLINICAL PEARLS

- Determine and address the patient's main concern. Treatment is surgical if symptoms warrant treatment
- The patient needs to understand the true risks and have realistic expectations before surgery is undertaken
- Thorough preoperative evaluation and meticulous surgical technique are necessary to obtain satisfactory results

DEVIC'S DISEASE/NEUROMYELITIS OPTICA

Sarkis M. Nazarian

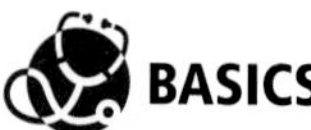

BASICS

DESCRIPTION

Neuromyelitis Optica (NMO) or Devic's disease is an autoimmune relapsing demyelinating disease of the CNS that has been thought to be a variant of multiple sclerosis (MS). It manifests with severe optic neuritis, often bilateral, and transverse myelitis, usually sparing the brain and the brainstem. Recovery of vision can occur in a few weeks, though myelitis takes months to recover. NMO was found to be a distinct entity from MS when an autoantibody, NMO-IgG, to the aquaporin-4 channel protein (AQP4), a water channel protein important in the regulation of cell fluid balance in the CNS, was discovered in 2004 (1)[A].

EPIDEMIOLOGY

Incidence

The incidence is unknown but rare.

Prevalence

Prevalence in the Caribbean is about 1:100,000. It is very uncommon in White patients in Europe and North America, and makes up <1% of demyelinating diseases in that group. It is most common in Japan, where it may represent one-third of all demyelinating diseases.

RISK FACTORS

Women have 4–9 times the risk than men, and median onset is in the thirties, a decade later than MS.

Genetics

No genetic influence has been discovered.

GENERAL PREVENTION

No primary preventive measures are known, but immunomodulatory therapies discussed below are used for secondary prevention.

PATHOPHYSIOLOGY

Autoantibodies targeting the aquaporin-4 channel activate complement and cause inflammation, resulting in demyelination and extensive tissue necrosis.

ETIOLOGY

The etiology of NMO is idiopathic, but post-infectious cases linked to syphilis, HIV, Chlamydia, varicella, CMV, and EBV have been reported.

COMMONLY ASSOCIATED CONDITIONS

No other conditions are known to be associated with NMO.

DIAGNOSIS

HISTORY

Following a viral-type prodrome, sudden, painful, complete loss of vision in one eye occurs, often followed by similar symptoms in the other eye. Paraplegia due to multilevel spinal cord involvement is a less common presentation. Patients often have concurrent fever, headache, severe muscle spasms, and anorexia.

PHYSICAL EXAM

- Visual loss presents as central and peripheral visual loss and achromatopsia.
- The usual pattern of spinal cord involvement is transverse myelitis, or complete spinal dysfunction with paraparesis or quadriparesis (depending on location of lesion), and bowel and bladder dysfunction.
- Hemisection (Brown-Sequard) or central cord syndromes (loss of function in upper extremities, with preservation of lower extremities) have been reported.
- Severe, painful flexor spasms of the trunk and extremities are common.

DIAGNOSTIC TESTS & INTERPRETATION

Lab

Initial lab tests

IgG test for aquaporin-4 antibody is positive in 80% of cases.

Follow-up & special considerations

Optical coherence tomography (OCT) findings in NMO parallel central and peripheral vision defects.

Imaging

Initial approach

- MRI of the brain, optic nerves, and appropriate portions of the spinal cord are mandatory for the correct diagnosis.
- The earlier diagnostic requirement that the initial brain MRI be normal has been dropped in the revised criteria (2)[A]. Brain MRI is atypical and does not meet diagnostic criteria for MS.
- Brain lesions are ovoid and concentrated in the cerebellum, brainstem, and in periventricular regions.
- MRI lesions in the spinal cord typically cause expansion of the cord, and extend over more than 3 spinal segments.

Follow-up & special considerations

Follow-up imaging is dependent on the development of new symptoms.

Diagnostic Procedures/Other

Lumbar puncture is useful in differentiating NMO from MS; 50 or more WBC/mm^3 or 5 or more neutrophils/mm^3 is considered diagnostic. Oligoclonal bands are generally absent.

Pathological Findings

The hallmark of NMO distinction from MS is the severe inflammatory demyelination seen in spinal cord lesions, with neutrophil, eosinophil and macrophage predominance, severe edema, and patchy necrosis involving both the white and gray matter. Perivascular complement activation and immunoglobulin deposition suggest an antibody-mediated response. It is postulated that NMO antibody to aquaporin-4 channels is a component of this antibody-mediated inflammation.

DIFFERENTIAL DIAGNOSIS

- Demyelinating optic neuritis
- Recurrent/relapsing optic neuritis
- Relapsing inflammatory optic neuropathy
- Multiple sclerosis and variant forms
- Acute transverse myelitis
- Tropical spastic paraparesis
- Neurosarcoidosis
- Systemic lupus erythematosus
- Neuro-Behçet's disease
- Neurosyphilis
- HIV-related myelopathy

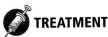

TREATMENT

MEDICATION

First Line

- High-dose intravenous corticosteroids (e.g., methylprednisolone 1 g/d for 5 days). Patients who do not respond can be treated with plasmapheresis (7 exchanges of 55 mL/kg every other day).
- Early treatment has been found to be more effective.

Second Line

- Prevention of relapsing disease (more than 1 attack), especially in patients with positive NMO serology, requires immunosuppressive therapy.
- The most standard approach is a combination of oral prednisone (1 mg/kg/d) and azathioprine (2–3 mg/kg/d), with the prednisone being tapered as azathioprine exerts its effect (reduction in WBC and MCV, mean corpuscular volume).
- Rituximab, a murine monoclonal CD-20 positive B-cell depleting agent, has been used, based on the theory that NMO is a humorally-mediated disease, and small studies have shown success.
- Other agents, such as mycophenolate mofetil, mitoxantrone, methotrexate, and cyclophosphamide, have been used, although no studies have been conducted.

ADDITIONAL TREATMENT

General Measures

No specific measures other than medication treatment are available.

Issues for Referral

Since NMO is potentially a relapsing disease, even patients with full recovery need to be followed on a regular basis.

Additional Therapies

Rehabilitation, such as physical or occupational therapy, is indicated for patients with spinal cord involvement.

COMPLEMENTARY & ALTERNATIVE THERAPIES

No specific therapies have been used.

SURGERY/OTHER PROCEDURES

No surgical procedures available.

IN-PATIENT CONSIDERATIONS

Initial Stabilization

Patients with severe myelopathy need to be admitted to hospital, and if they have a high cervical lesion that interferes with respiration, may need to be intubated and artificially ventilated.

Admission Criteria

Severe visual loss, paraparesis or quadriparesis

IV Fluids

As needed for hydration.

Nursing

Ventilator care, management of paralysis, and bladder and bowel care are the mainstay of nursing care.

Discharge Criteria

Patients can be discharged as they finish their treatments; often, transfer to a rehabilitation facility will be necessary.

ONGOING CARE

FOLLOW-UP RECOMMENDATIONS

Patients with spinal cord involvement will need rehabilitation by physical and occupational therapy.

Patient Monitoring

Follow-up visits with an ophthalmologist or neurologist usually will occur on a quarterly basis.

DIET

No specific diet needed

PATIENT EDUCATION

Patients need to be educated on all the possible visual, motor, and sensory manifestations of a relapse and advised to seek immediate medical attention if any occur.

PROGNOSIS

The mortality rate can be as high as 20–25%, and median survival has been found to be 8 years from date of diagnosis. The mortality rates are highest in patients of African origin.

COMPLICATIONS

Permanent neurologic defects are common, with only partial remission of symptoms, after each attack.

REFERENCES

1. Lennon VA, Wingerchuk DM, Kryzer TJ, et al. A serum autoantibody marker of neuromyelitis optica: Distinction from multiple sclerosis. *Lancet* 2004;354(9451):2106–2112.
2. Wingerchuk DM, Lennon VA, Pittock SJ, et al. Revised diagnostic criteria for neuromyelitis optica. *Neurology* 2006;66:1485–1489.

ADDITIONAL READING

- Hazin R, Khan F, Bhatti MT. Neuromyelitis optica: Current concepts and prospects for future management. *Curr Opin Ophthalmol* 2009;20: 434–439.
- Nandhagopal R, Al-Asmi A, Gujjar AR. Neuromyelitis optica: An overview. *Postgrad Med J* 2010;86:153–159.
- Wingerchuk DM. Diagnosis and treatment of neuromyelitis optica. *Neurologist* 2007;13(1):2–11.

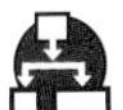

See Also (Topic, Algorithm, Electronic Media Element)

- Multiple Sclerosis, Optic Neuritis

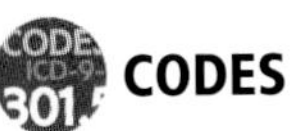

CODES

ICD9

341.0 Neuromyelitis optica

CLINICAL PEARLS

- NMO morbidity, unlike MS, is entirely due to optic nerve and spinal cord involvement, and lesions in other CNS areas do not cause much problems.
- NMO is much more severe disease than MS, with high mortality, especially in patients with high cervical lesions and those of African descent.

DIABETIC PAPILLOPATHY

David B. Auerbach

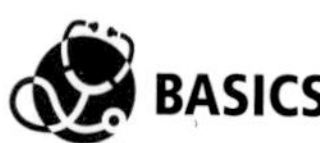

BASICS

DESCRIPTION

An uncommon unilateral or bilateral swelling of the optic disc seen in diabetics of all ages. The optic disc edema is transient and usually resolves over the course of a few months. Impairment of optic nerve function is usually mild. It is important to differentiate between diabetic papillopathy and proliferative diabetic retinopathy with neovascularization on the optic disc.

EPIDEMIOLOGY

Incidence

- Although more common in juvenile diabetics, diabetic papillopathy has been reported in patients as old as 79 years.
- Sexes are equally affected.

RISK FACTORS

- Poor glucose control
- Duration of diabetes

GENERAL PREVENTION

All diabetics should be counseled on the importance of strict blood glucose control.

PATHOPHYSIOLOGY

- The pathophysiology of disc swelling is unclear.
- Some consider this as being a vasculopathy of the superficial layers of the disc capillaries.

COMMONLY ASSOCIATED CONDITIONS

- Diabetic retinopathy
- Macular edema

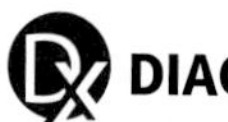

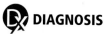

DIAGNOSIS

HISTORY

- Painless decrease in vision
- Visual field defect (most common is an enlarged blind spot)

PHYSICAL EXAM

- Visual acuity can be normal
- Minimal or no afferent pupillary defect
- Dyschromatopsia is mild or absent
- Enlarged blind spot or mild arcuate defect on visual field
- Hyperemic swelling of the optic disc with dilated, radially oriented superficial telangiectatic vessels (1)[A]
- Background diabetic retinopathy
- Macular edema
- Small optic disc ratio in fellow eye if only one eye affected

DIAGNOSTIC TESTS & INTERPRETATION

Lab

- May have an elevated Hb A1c
- Blood pressure
- CBC
- ANA
- ACE
- Lyme titer
- RPR
- ESR

Imaging

MRI brain and orbits with and without gadolinium to rule out demyelination and/or a compressive lesion.

Diagnostic Procedures/Other

Intravenous fluorescein angiography (IVFA). Follow up IVFA can show capillary nonperfusion and rule out neovascularization.

Pathological Findings

- IVFA shows focal or diffuse optic disc hyperfluorescence
- Leakage from telangiectatic vessels
- Need to differentiate this disc swelling from disc neovascularization where fluorescein is leaked into the vitreous in the latter (2)[A].

DIFFERENTIAL DIAGNOSIS

- NAION
- Papilledema
- Hypertensive retinopathy
- Proliferative diabetic retinopathy
- Optic Neuritis (Papillitis)
- Inflammatory optic neuropathies

TREATMENT

MEDICATION
- No medication for treatment
- Self-limited
- May require laser photocoagulation for diabetic retinopathy and/or macular edema

ADDITIONAL TREATMENT
General Measures
May need retinal photocoagulation after the disc edema has resolved to treat diabetic retinopathy and/or macular edema

Issues for Referral
Follow up with neuro-ophthalmologist or retinal specialist 2 weeks after initial diagnosis is made

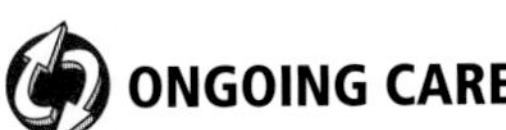

ONGOING CARE

FOLLOW-UP RECOMMENDATIONS
Patient Monitoring
- Every 2–3 weeks to look for resolution of edema and assess optic nerve function (color vision, visual field, and pupillary exam)
- Need to confirm there is no proliferative diabetic retinopathy
- Need to reconsider the diagnosis if severe optic nerve dysfunction noted at presentation (this remains a diagnosis of exclusion).

DIET
Diabetic diet

PATIENT EDUCATION
The importance of strict blood glucose control must be stressed.

PROGNOSIS
Good clinical outcome, however, there may be mild permanent visual field defects and morbidity from associated macular edema.

REFERENCES

1. Regillo CD, Brown GC, Savino PJ, et al. Diabetic papillopathy. *Arch Ophthalmol* 1995;113: 889–895.
2. Stransky TJ. Diabetic papillopathy and proliferative retinopathy. *Graefe's Arch Clin Exp Ophthalmol* 1986;224:46–50.

ADDITIONAL READING

- Appen RE, Chandra SR, Klein MD, et al. Diabetic papillopathy. *Am J Ophthalmol* 1980;90:203–209.
- Bayraktar Z, Alacali N, Bayraktar S. Diabetic papillopathy in type II diabetic patients. *Retina* 2002;22:752–758.

CODES

ICD9
- 250.50 Diabetes mellitus with ophthalmic manifestations, type ii or unspecified type, not stated as uncontrolled
- 377.00 Papilledema, unspecified
- 377.31 Optic papillitis

CLINICAL PEARLS

- Must differentiate disc edema from neovascularization
- With disc edema, dilated capillaries are within the nerve and retina. Vessels are radially oriented and leak fluorescein into the disc and retina.
- With neovascularization, vessels are usually peripheral, have a random course, and leak fluorescein into the vitreous obscuring the vessels.
- Must differentiate from papilledema when bilateral.

DISSOCIATED STRABISMUS

Harold Koller

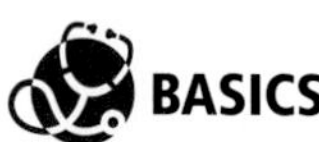

BASICS

DESCRIPTION

- Dissociated strabismus is an ocular deviation in which refixation of the deviated eye does not elicit an opposing deviation of the other eye (i.e., it is not a true tropia)
- Due to 3 recognizable components – vertical, horizontal, and torsional – a more appropriate designation of the condition is *dissociated strabismus complex* (DSC). DSC is characterized by slow elevation, abduction, and extorsion of a non-fixing eye.
- DSC can be subdivided into dissociated vertical deviation (DVD), dissociated horizontal deviation (DHD), and dissociated torsional deviation (DTD), and may have features of one or more simultaneously.
- DCS is usually comitant in all fields of gaze.

EPIDEMIOLOGY

Incidence

DVD found in 45–92% of patients with congenital/infantile esotropia.

Prevalence

Unknown

RISK FACTORS

- Congenital/infantile esotropia
- Monofixation syndrome
- Latent or manifest-latent nystagmus
- Amblyopia

Genetics

Unknown

GENERAL PREVENTION

Maintenance of alignment and correction of refractive error and amblyopia helps to promote bifoveal fixation without dissociated deviation.

PATHOPHYSIOLOGY

Generally unknown. DVD violates Hering's law of yolk muscles. Covering one eye induces the dissociated deviation with no associated opposite deviation of the fellow eye when the dissociated eye refixates. Helveston believed that DSC resulted from maldeveloped supranuclear centers. Guyton suggested that DVD may be secondary to a cycloversion/vertical vergence produced to dampen a cyclovertical nystagmus that occurs in patients with an early onset defect of binocular function.

ETIOLOGY

Unknown

COMMONLY ASSOCIATED CONDITIONS

- Congenital/infantile esotropia
- Monofixation syndrome
- Latent or manifest-latent nystagmus
- Amblyopia

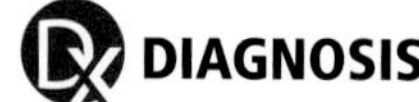

DIAGNOSIS

HISTORY

- Parents notice the eyes drifting out or up or both; often to different degrees and at different times. May be more frequent when child is ill or tired.
- It should be looked for in any case of congenital/infantile esotropia or latent or manifest-latent nystagmus.

PHYSICAL EXAM

- Deviations can be small and well controlled on one visit and large and manifest spontaneously on the next visit. The eye may be "up" one time and "out" the next time.
- The non-fixing eye is elevated, abducted, and extorted. Diplopia is not present. Bi-fixation is absent.
- The degree of each component of DSC can be documented using a +4 to +1 designation separately, with +4 being the most severe. Alternatively, use the prism cover–uncover test.
- Use the cover–uncover test or the cross-cover test. In a true hypertropia, the opposite eye is lower when the hypertropic eye is uncovered. The absence of upward refixation movements in either eye on alternate cover testing can distinguish DVD from a true hypertropia. In a true DVD, the opposite eye is never hypotropic unless the DVD is present with a true hypertropia simultaneously.

- Any of the components of DSC can be present at any examination (DHD, DTD) as well as nystagmus.
- In DVD, binocular involvement but asymmetry is the rule, with expected variability.
- DSC often coexists with true inferior oblique overaction, with or without, a "V"-pattern. DVD can simulate inferior oblique overaction by becoming manifest in adduction as the nose interrupts fixation. True vertical or horizontal deviations can also be confused with any other component of DSC.
- Prolonged patch or cover may encourage the dissociated deviation to appear
  - Complete ocular examination including cycloplegic refraction
  - Worth 4-dot test, Bagolini striate glasses, and Titmus or Randot stereo tests to rule out monofixation

DIFFERENTIAL DIAGNOSIS

- Inferior oblique overaction
  - True hypertropia
  - True exotropia
  - True cyclotorsion

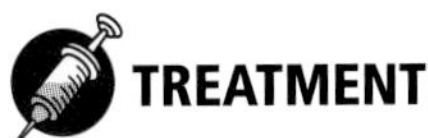

TREATMENT

MEDICATION

Atropine is ineffective for DSC; use only for moderate to mild associated amblyopia.

ADDITIONAL TREATMENT

General Measures

Correct refractive error and amblyopia to encourage fixation with affected eye.

SURGERY/OTHER PROCEDURES

There is no total surgical cure for any component of DSC. Options include:

- For DVD, large recessions of the superior rectus. If asymmetry exists, do unequal recessions
- For DVD, anterior transposition of the inferior oblique, especially if inferior oblique overaction exists
- For DVD, resection of the inferior oblique (less often performed)
- For DVD, Faden suture of the superior rectus
- For DHD, recession of the lateral rectus
  - Correction of associated strabismus (e.g., infantile esotropia)

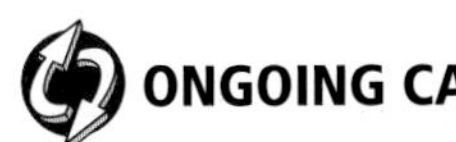

ONGOING CARE

FOLLOW-UP RECOMMENDATIONS

Monitor for amblyopia, recurrent deviation, and coexisting tropias.

PATIENT EDUCATION

Keep parents and family informed about the limitations of treatment including the diagnosis, treatment plan, and prognosis.

PROGNOSIS

Variable with recurrences possible. No full cure is available.

COMPLICATIONS

- Amblyopia
- Complications of strabismus surgery

ADDITIONAL READING

- Wright KW. *Complex strabismus. Pediatric Ophthalmology and Strabismus*, 2nd ed. Wright KW, Spiegel PH, (Eds). New York: Spinger-Verlag, 2003:450–480.
- Olitsky SE, Nelson LB. Strabismus disorders. *Harley's Pediatric Ophthalmology*, 5th ed. Nelson LB, Olitsky SE, (Eds). Philadelphia: Lippincott, Williams & Wilkins, 2005:255–284.
- Wilson ME. *Dissociated deviations. Strabismus Surgery, Basic and Advanced Strategies Ophthalmic Monographs 17*, Plager DA (Ed). New York: Oxford University Press, 2004.

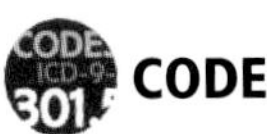

CODES

ICD9

378.9 Unspecified disorder of eye movements

CLINICAL PEARLS

- The 3 components of the DSC may all be present simultaneously or in different proportions at different times during subsequent examinations.
- Recurrence is common
- Correction of DSC in one eye may "uncover" DSC in the other eye.
- Deviations may be asymmetric between the two eyes.

DOMINANT OPTIC ATROPHY

Louis C. Blumenfeld

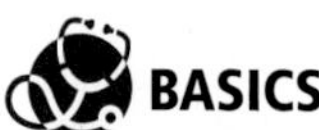

BASICS

DESCRIPTION

- Most common hereditary form of optic atrophy causing vision loss within the first decade of life. Vision loss tends to be insidious with slow progression described.
  - May be referred to as Kjer type optic atrophy
  - Vision is typically reduced to between 20/70–20/100, but range can be from 20/20 to counting fingers

EPIDEMIOLOGY

Prevalence

- 1:50,000 worldwide
- Most prevalent in Denmark 1:10,000

RISK FACTORS

Positive family history

Genetics

- Autosomal dominance inheritance pattern with incomplete penetrance and variable clinical expression
- OPA1 gene, chromosome 3q28 most commonly involved. Other loci include OPA3 (10q13.2), OPA4 (18q12.2), and OPA5 (22q12.1-q13.1)

PATHOPHYSIOLOGY

- Primary retinal ganglion cell degeneration
- The OPA1 gene on chromosome 3 produces a protein that is essential for maintaining the shape and structure of mitochondria. It is also involved in cellular apoptosis and maintenance of mitochondrial DNA. OPA 1 is also involved in oxidative phosphorylation.
- Mutations in the OPA1 gene lead to overall mitochondrial dysfunction and increased cell death (apoptosis). This leads to primary retinal ganglion cell degeneration and subsequent optic atrophy.

ETIOLOGY

Inherited mutation usually involving OPA1 gene of chromosome 3.

COMMONLY ASSOCIATED CONDITIONS

- Majority of patients are otherwise completely healthy.
- Recent studies suggest that up to 20% of OPA1 mutational carriers may have other extraocular neurological complications (1)
  - Bilateral sensorineural deafness beginning in late childhood and early adulthood
  - Ataxia
  - Myopathy
  - Peripheral neuropathy
  - Progressive external ophthalmoplegia
  - Spastic multiple sclerosis-like illness
  - Mental retardation

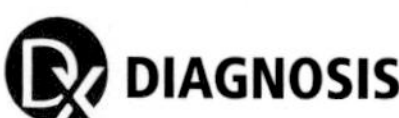

DIAGNOSIS

HISTORY

- Vision loss is often insidious and may be found incidentally on routine examination in some children
- Mild photophobia may be present
- May have positive family history

PHYSICAL EXAM

- Decreased visual acuity (typically 20/70–20/100, range 20/20 – counting fingers)
  - Decreased color vision (blue–yellow defect (tritanopia) most common, but other color defects may be present)
  - Variable degree of optic atrophy (may range from mild temporal pallor to complete atrophy (2)
  - Characteristic focal temporal excavation of optic discs is present in some patients.

DIAGNOSTIC TESTS & INTERPRETATION

Lab

Initial lab tests

Genetic testing of OPA1 gene sequence is available. This detects mutations in 70–90% of familial cases and 50% of simplex cases.

Follow-up & special considerations

- Auditory testing – auditory brainstem responses, auditory evoked potentials
- Glucose tolerance test may be appropriate.
- Blue cone ERG may help distinguish from congenital tritanopia.

Imaging

MRI with attention to the optic nerves and chiasm may be necessary to rule out compressive lesion if diagnosis is questionable.

Diagnostic Procedures/Other

- Visual field testing is appropriate if the child is of appropriate maturity to reliably do this test. Most children are not able to respond reliably to this test below the age of 10 years. Static perimetry may be more sensitive than kinetic perimetry.
- Electroretinography – markedly reduced negative component with normal positive component
- Visual evoked potentials – decreased amplitude

Pathological Findings

Ganglion cell loss, primarily in the macula, and papillomacular bundle.

DIFFERENTIAL DIAGNOSIS
- Leber hereditary optic neuropathy
- Toxic deafness optic neuropathies
- Deafness-dystonia-optic neuronopathy syndrome
- Wolfram syndrome (AKA DIDMOAD) – Diabetes insipidus, Diabetes mellitus, optic atrophy
- Congenital tritanopia
- Optic atrophy secondary to retinal dystrophy
- Idiopathic intracranial hypertension
- Intracranial tumor

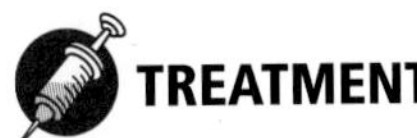

TREATMENT

MEDICATION
No medical therapy is available

ADDITIONAL TREATMENT

General Measures
Symptomatic treatment with low vision aids

Issues for Referral
- Audiology referral may be appropriate to detect associated hearing loss
- Low vision evaluation

COMPLEMENTARY & ALTERNATIVE THERAPIES
There are no known effective complementary or alternative therapies. Stem cell treatment (outside of US) has been proposed and tried without proven efficacy.

SURGERY/OTHER PROCEDURES
No known surgical procedures.

IN-PATIENT CONSIDERATIONS
Generally, does not require hospitalization.

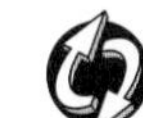

ONGOING CARE

FOLLOW-UP RECOMMENDATIONS
Yearly ophthalmic evaluations

Patient Monitoring
- Visual field testing
- Monitor for possible sensorineural hearing loss
- Neurologic evaluation based on symptoms

PATIENT EDUCATION
Genetic counseling

PROGNOSIS
- Children seem to function better than expected for their given visual deficits
- Vision tends to remain stable or decrease imperceptibly beyond mid-teens

REFERENCES

1. Yu-Wai-Man P, Griffiths PG, Gorman GS, et al. Multi-system neurological disease is common in patients with OPA1 mutations. *Brain* 2010;133(3):771–786.
2. Hoyt CS. Dominant optic atrophy: A spectre of disability. *Ophthalmology* 1980;87:245.

ADDITIONAL READING

- Newman NJ. Hereditary optic neuropathies: From the mitochondria to the optic nerve. *Am J Ophthalmol* 2005;140:517–523.

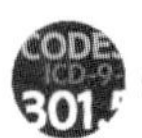

CODES

ICD9
377.16 Hereditary optic atrophy

DOUBLE ELEVATOR PALSY

Colleen J. Christian

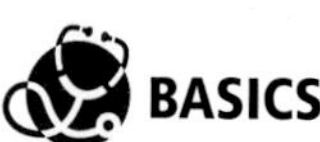

BASICS

DESCRIPTION

- An inability to elevate the eye in all fields of gaze often resulting in a large hypotropia, with associated ptosis
- Also called monocular elevation deficiency

EPIDEMIOLOGY

Incidence

Very rare

Prevalence

Unknown

RISK FACTORS

None Known

Genetics

No known genetic association (although monocular elevation deficit may also be seen in Congenital cranial dysinnervation disorders and some craniosynostosis syndromes)

PATHOPHYSIOLOGY

Neurologic (cranial nerve, nuclear, or supranuclear deficits and mechanical restriction (or both) can contribute.

ETIOLOGY

- Classified into 3 subgroups with different underlying mechanisms:
  - Primary inferior rectus restriction
  - Primary paresis or of the superior rectus
  - Supranuclear deficit (1)[A]

COMMONLY ASSOCIATED CONDITIONS

- Marcus Gunn jaw-winking ptosis is seen in 25% of patients
- Hypotropia
- Ptosis
- Chin lift (2)[A]

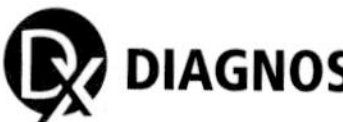

DIAGNOSIS

HISTORY

Family notices limited elevation and ptosis of the involved eye, along with an abnormal chin up head position.

PHYSICAL EXAM

- Reduced elevation of the eye in all positions of gaze
- When fixing with the non-paretic/restricted eye, the involved eye is hypotropic and the lid becomes ptotic.
- Fixation with the involved eye results in a hypertropia of the non-paretic eye (which is often of greater magnitude than the baseline hypotropia) and often, resolution of the ptosis.
- Many patients present with a large chin up position, used to maintain binocular vision.
- Full ocular examination including dilated retinal examination and refraction.
- Evaluate visual acuity for amblyopia.

DIAGNOSTIC TESTS & INTERPRETATION

Lab

None

Imaging

Can be helpful in differential diagnosis, but is not necessary if clinical diagnosis is clear.

Diagnostic Procedures/Other

- Forced duction testing is necessary to establish etiology and best surgical approach.
- If positive, indicates inferior rectus restricted.
- If negative, indicates no inferior rectus restriction.
- Assessment of Bell's phenomenon:
  - When present, cause is likely supranuclear
  - When absent, consider inferior rectus restriction (3)[A]

DIFFERENTIAL DIAGNOSIS

- Brown's syndrome
- Orbital blowout fracture
- Thyroid ophthalmopathy
- Orbital fibrosis syndrome
- Congenital cranial dysinnervation disorders
- Anomalous/absent muscles (as in craniosynostosis syndrome)
- Superior orbital tumor or hemorrhage
- Parinaud syndrome
  - Hydrocephalus
  - Abnormality in the midbrain region of the quadrigeminal plate
- Cranial Nerve III palsy (4)[A]

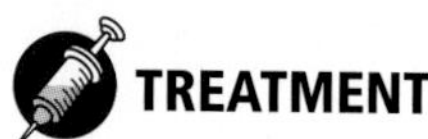

TREATMENT

MEDICATION

None

ADDITIONAL TREATMENT

General Measures

- Correct refractive error
- Treat amblyopia

Issues for Referral

- Consider neurology consult if concern about intracranial cause
- Consider endocrinology consult if concern about thyroid eye disease

Additional Therapies

Ptosis surgery should not be done until final alignment is established (5)[A]

COMPLEMENTARY & ALTERNATIVE THERAPIES
None

SURGERY/OTHER PROCEDURES
- Surgery is indicated for relief of strabismus and/or limiting head position.
- Some patients are orthophoric in primary and do not require surgery.
- Forced duction
  - If positive, include inferior rectus recession in surgical plan
  - If negative:
    - And large hypotropia present, a transposition procedure should be done, moving all or a portion of the medial and lateral rectus muscles to the superior rectus insertion
    - With a smaller hypotropia, resection of the superior rectus and recession of the inferior rectus can be done (5)[A], (6)[A], (7)[A]

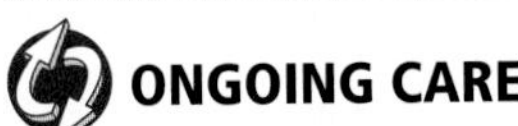

ONGOING CARE

FOLLOW-UP RECOMMENDATIONS
More frequently in young children to rule out amblyopia.

Patient Monitoring
- For visual acuity to rule out amblyopia
- For recurrent strabismus and diplopia, or head position

PATIENT EDUCATION
Importance of regular follow-up to monitor for amblyopia

PROGNOSIS
- Reoperation frequently needed
- Good visual outcome with refractive correction and treatment of amblyopia

COMPLICATIONS
- Recurrent strabismus
- Persistent/recurrent true ptosis
- Amblyopia

REFERENCES

1. Cadera W, Bloom JN, Karlik S. An MRI study of double elevator palsy. *Ophthalmology* 1997;32: 250–253.
2. Mims JK 3rd. "Double elevator palsy" eye supraducts during stage II general anesthesia supporting hypothesis of (supra) nuclear etiology. *Binocul Vis Strabismus Q* 2005;20:199–204.
3. Zafar SN, Khan A, Azad N, et al. Ptosis associated with monocular elevation deficiency. *J Pak Med Assoc* 2009;59:522–524.
4. Mets HS. Double elevator palsy. *J Pediatr Ophthalmol Strabismus* 1991;18:31–35.
5. Foster RS. Vertical muscle transposition augmented with lateral fixation. *J AAPOS* 1997;1(1):20–30.
6. Knapp P. The surgical treatment of double-elevator paralysis. *Trans Am Ophthalmol Soc* 1969;67: 304–323.
7. Burke JP, Ruben JB, Scott WE. Vertical transposition of the horizontal recti (Knapp procedure) for the treatment of double elevator palsy: Effectiveness and long-term stability. *Br J Ophthalmol* 1992; 76(12):734–737.

CODES

ICD9
- 374.30 Ptosis of eyelid, unspecified
- 378.31 Hypertropia

CLINICAL PEARLS
- Diagnosis made by presence of complete inability to elevate the eye in all fields of gaze.
- Patients may develop large chin up position to allow binocular vision.
- Forced duction testing results help determine etiology and best surgical plan.

D

DOWN SYNDROME

Donelson Manley

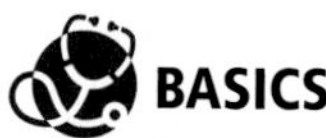

BASICS

DESCRIPTION
- Down syndrome is a chromosomal disorder caused by the presence of all or part of an extra 21st chromosome and is named after John Langdon Down who described it in 1866.
- It is also called Trisomy 21.

EPIDEMIOLOGY
Incidence
- Down syndrome occurs worldwide in all ethnic groups and economic classes.
- In 2006, the Centers for Disease Control and Prevention estimated the rate as 1 per 733 live births in the US (5,529 new cases per year).

RISK FACTORS
- Advanced maternal age. At maternal age 20–24 years, the probability is 1 in 1,562, at age 35–39 years, the probability is 1 in 214, and above 45 years the probability is 1 in 19.
- 8% of children with Down syndrome are born to women under the age of 35 reflecting the fertility in this group.
- Paternal age over 42 years also increases the risk.

Genetics
Chromosomal abnormality characterized by the presence of an extra copy of genetic material on the 21st chromosome. If whole, it is Trisomy 21, which is caused by a meiotic nondisjunction event.

GENERAL PREVENTION
Screening can be performed during pregnancy and includes amniocentesis, chorionic villus sampling, or percutaneous umbilical cord blood sampling.

COMMONLY ASSOCIATED CONDITIONS
- Males are usually infertile exhibiting defects in spermatogenesis and females have significantly lower rates of conception.
- Hematologic malignancies
- Thyroid disorders
- Gastrointestinal disorders
- Epilepsy
- Alzheimer's disease tends to develop at an earlier age, often before age 50 years, and shortens the life expectancy.

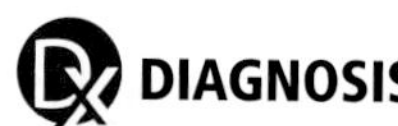

DIAGNOSIS

HISTORY
Maternal and paternal age

PHYSICAL EXAM
- Small chin (microgenia)
- Round face
- Protruding or oversized tongue (macroglossia) associated with a small oral cavity
- Short neck
- Brushfield spots (white or grayish/brown) in the periphery of the iris
- Epicanthal eyelid folds causing an almond shaped appearance
- Upward slanting palpebral fissures
- Shorter limbs
- A single palmar fold
- Poor muscle tone (hypotonia)
- Mental retardation
- Speech delay
- Short stature
- Strabismus
- Cataracts
- Increased obesity with age

DIAGNOSTIC TESTS & INTERPRETATION
Diagnostic Procedures/Other
- Prenatal diagnosis possible if gene mutation known
- Albinism is a clinical diagnosis that can be confirmed in some cases with DNA testing
- Optical coherence testing (OCT) demonstrates macular hypoplasia
- Multichannel visual evoked potentials demonstrate excessive decussation of retinal ganglion cell axons at the chiasm in most cases
- Molecular genetic testing may determine the specific mutations and thus helps identify the subtype of oculocutaneous albinism
- Tests for OCA1, OCA2, and OA1 are available clinically
- Tests for other genes only for research purposes

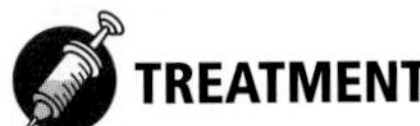

TREATMENT

ADDITIONAL TREATMENT

General Measures

Medical and surgical treatment as indicated for any associated conditions.

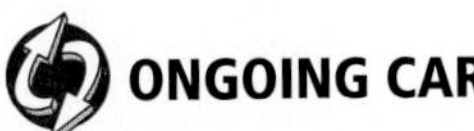

ONGOING CARE

FOLLOW-UP RECOMMENDATIONS

Childhood intervention, vocational training, a supportive environment, and medical treatment can improve the development of children with Down syndrome and improve the quality of life. Cognitive ability can be improved with education.

PATIENT EDUCATION

National Down Syndrome Society (NDSS): www.ndss.org

PROGNOSIS

- The life expectancy of people with Down syndrome has increased in recent years.
- In 1980 it was 25 years. In 2002 it was 49 years. The causes of death have changed. Those who survive into their 40s and 50s often develop chronic neurodegenerative disease (Alzheimer's).

ADDITIONAL READING

- Center for Disease Control and Prevention (CDC). Improved national prevalence estimates for 18 selected major birth defects, United States, 1999–2001. *MMWR Morb Mortal Wkly Rep* 2006;54(51):1301–1305.
- Huether CA, Ivanovich J, Goodwin BS, et al. Maternal age specific risk estimates for Down syndrome among live births in whites and other races from Ohio and metropolitan Atlanta, 1970–1989. *J Med Genet* 1998;35(6):482–490.
- National Down Syndrome Center. http://www.ndsccenter.org/resources/package.

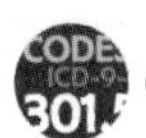

CODES

ICD9

- 379.99 Other ill-defined disorders of eye
- 743.69 Other congenital anomalies of eyelids, lacrimal system, and orbit
- 758.0 Down's syndrome

CLINICAL PEARLS

- Risk factors for Down syndrome include advanced maternal and paternal age.
- Ophthalmic features of Down syndrome include Brushfield spots, or grayish brown spots on the peripheral iris, and cataracts.
- The life expectancy has increased in recent years.

DRY EYE SYNDROME

Melvin I. Roat

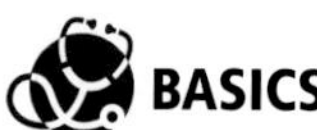

BASICS

DESCRIPTION
- Multifactorial disease characterized by an abnormal tear film that is inadequate to support the health of the ocular surface
- Types
  - Aqueous tear-deficient
  - Evaporative
  - Exposure
- Isolated ocular disease
  - Primary aqueous tear production deficient
  - Secondary aqueous tear production deficient (e.g., surgery, radiation)
  - Lacrimal ducts not transporting tears (e.g., chemical injury, mucous membrane pemphigoid, Stevens-Johnson syndrome)
  - Seborrheic blepharitis
  - Meibomian gland dysfunction
  - Primary lagophthalmos
  - Secondary abnormal lid closure (e.g., chemosis, conjunctivochalasis, ectropion, post blepharoplasty)
  - Eyelid or cheek scar (burn, chemical, thermal, radiation, trauma, surgical)
  - Loss of corneal sensation (e.g., herpes simplex virus, varicella zoster virus)
- Associated ocular manifestation of a systemic disease
- Synonym(s). Dry Eyes, Keratoconjunctivitis Sicca, Keratitis Sicca

EPIDEMIOLOGY

Incidence
22% over 10 years

Prevalence
- 17% of females, 12% of males
- 8% in subjects <60 years, 19% >80 years

RISK FACTORS
- Age, female
- Ocular surgery (cataract, corneal transplant, LASIK)
- Diabetes, contact lens use

PATHOPHYSIOLOGY
Desiccation of the ocular surface leads to squamous metaplasia with loss of goblet cells, enlargement and increased cytoplasmic/nuclear ratio of superficial epithelial cells, keratinization and secondary inflammation.

ETIOLOGY
- Aqueous tear-deficient
  - **insufficient volume** of tears to keep conjunctiva and cornea moist, relative to the **volume of tears lost** by evaporation and via puncta
- Evaporative
  - **insufficient duration of coating** by tears to keep conjunctiva and cornea moist, relative to the **speed that tears are lost** by evaporation and via the puncta
- Exposure
  - **insufficient area** of the conjunctiva and cornea **coated by tears**

COMMONLY ASSOCIATED CONDITIONS
- Aqueous tear-deficient
  - Gland not producing tears
    - Sjögren's syndrome
    - Drugs, (e.g., beta blockers, antihistamine)
    - HIV
    - Graft—versus–host disease
    - Sarcoidosis
    - Familial dysautonomia
    - Xerophthalmia
  - Ducts not transporting tears
    - Mucous membrane pemphigoid
    - Stevens-Johnson syndrome
  - Insufficient hormonal stimulation
    - Menopause
    - BCP
    - Pregnancy
    - Androgen deficient?
  - Insufficient neural stimulation
    - Stroke
    - Neurotrophic keratitis
    - Radiation
    - Surgery
- Evaporative
  - Androgen deficient
  - Drugs, for example, Accutane
  - Ectodermal dysplasia
  - Meibomian gland dysfunction associated with acne rosacea
- Exposure
  - Neurologic
    - Unconscious
    - Parkinson's disease (slow blink rate or incomplete)
    - Seventh nerve palsy; Bell's palsy, acoustic neuroma, surgical, traumatic, congenital (Goldenhar syndrome), CVA
  - Loss of corneal sensation
    - Radiation
    - Fifth cranial nerve palsy; CVA, Trauma, surgery, tumor
  - Muscular
    - Botulinum toxin
  - Endocrine
    - Thyroid (i.e., Grave's disease)

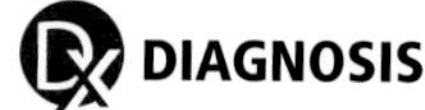

DIAGNOSIS

HISTORY
- Itching, burning, gritty, foreign body sensation, sharp stabbing pain
- Ache, pressure behind the eye, eyes pulling, tired eyes, eye strain
- Photophobia
- Hard to open eyes upon awakening
- Blurring with prolonged visual effort (e.g., reading, watching TV, computer, driving)
- Inability to tear in response to irritants or emotions
- Intermittent flood of tears, tearing while reading
- Decreased contact lens tolerance
  - Chronic, usually worsening over years
  - Waxing and waning course
  - Seasonal: Often worse in the winter, better in the spring and fall
  - Worse toward the end of the day and with blowing air (e.g., fans, A/C), low humidity (e.g., blue sky days, airplanes, malls, offices), fumes, vapors, or smoky areas
  - Better with high humidity days (e.g., cool rainy days, foggy days), high humidity environments (e.g., shower, kitchen, basement)
  - Bilateral, asymmetrical

PHYSICAL EXAM
- ALL TYPES:
  - Conjunctival hyperemia in the exposure zone
  - Conjunctivochalasis
  - Superficial punctate keratitis in the exposure zone
  - Corneal epithelial defect
  - Filamentary keratitis
  - Lusterless cornea
- Aqueous tear-deficient:
  - Poor tear meniscus
  - Mucous in tear film
  - Enlarged lacrimal gland
- Evaporative:
  - Meibomian gland inspissation
  - Acne rosacea (i.e., rhinophyma, pustules, telangiectatic vessels of the nose, chin, and cheeks)
  - Seborrheic blepharitis
  - Seborrheic dermatitis
  - Blood vessels crossing the gray line
  - Foam in tear lake or lid margin
  - Debris in tear film
- Exposure
  - Poor blink rate
  - Incomplete blink
  - Facial weakness

DIAGNOSTIC TESTS & INTERPRETATION

Diagnostic Procedures/Other

- Schirmer Test I (Whatman filter paper #41, 0.5 × 35 mm, lateral or medial third, not center, no topical anesthesia, i.e., a standardized tear stimulus, repeated at least 3 times, 5.5 mm = 85% true positive, 15% false positive)
- Tear breakup test (TBUT) (instill a small volume of highly concentrated fluorescein-made by wetting a fluorescein strip with saline and shaking the strip to remove any excess moisture, after several blinks to distribute fluorescein throughout the tear film, the patient stares and the length of time until the first dry spot develops is determined, normal is >10 seconds)
- Rose Bengal 1% (stains desiccated epithelium, traumatized cells, and mucous. Van Bijsterveld score: 1+ sparsely scattered, 2+ densely scattered, 3+ confluent; determined at nasal, temporal conjunctiva & cornea, then sum scores; a total ≥4 is abnormal)

Pathological Findings

- Schirmer Test I <5.5 mm on repeated testing is consistent with Aqueous tear-deficient dry eye
- Tear breakup test <10 seconds on repeated testing is consistent with evaporative dry eye
- Aqueous tear-deficient dry eye (i.e., Schirmer Test I <5.5 mm) and dry mouth needs a further work-up for Sjögren's Syndrome
- Van Bijsterveld score of ≥4 is consistent with dry eyes of any type

DIFFERENTIAL DIAGNOSIS

- Allergic conjunctivitis
- Corneal foreign body
- Conjunctival foreign body
- Trichiasis

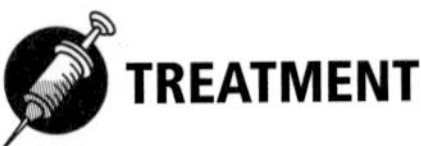

TREATMENT

MEDICATION

First Line

- Supplemental moisture
  - Artificial tear drops (usually more viscous formulations for evaporative dry eye, usually less viscous formulations for Aqueous tear-deficient), gels, sprays
- Preserving moisture
  - Artificial tear ointment, h.s ± during day
  - Humidifier

Second Line

- Seborrheic blepharitis
  - Eyelid margin scrubs
  - Culture eyelid margin then antibiotic
- Meibomian gland dysfunction
  - Warm compresses (gel filled)
  - Eyelash scrubs contraindicated
  - Doxycycline
  - Omega-3 supplements
- Exposure
  - Moisture chamber h.s
  - Lid taping h.s
- All types of dry eye
  - Cyclosporin A eye drops
  - Autologous serum eye drops
  - Secretagogue
    - Pilocarpine or cevimeline tablets
  - Consider changing to non-drying systemic medications

Pediatric Considerations

Doxycycline, tetracycline, and derivatives should not be used in children <8 years of age.

Pregnancy Considerations

Doxycycline, tetracycline, and derivatives should not be used in pregnant or nursing mothers.

ADDITIONAL TREATMENT

General Measures

- Stay hydrated
- Blink often while reading, watching TV, on the computer or driving
- Avoid drying or irritating environments

Issues for Referral

Patients with signs and symptoms of Sjögren's syndrome should be evaluated by a rheumatologist.

SURGERY/OTHER PROCEDURES

- First line
  - Preserving moisture
    - Punctal plugs
    - Punctal occlusion
- Second line
  - Exposure
    - Eye lid spring
    - Eye lid gold weight
    - Tarsorrhaphy
    - Lid lengthening
    - Conjunctival flap
    - Hypoglossal transposition

ONGOING CARE

FOLLOW-UP RECOMMENDATIONS

Patient Monitoring

- It can take 2 weeks to know if a new artificial tear, warm compresses or plugs are helping
- It can take 4 weeks to know that doxycycline or cyclosporin A drops are helping

DIET

- Stay hydrated
- A diet high in Omega 3 fatty acids

PROGNOSIS

Excellent, for most patients dry eyes are easily controlled

COMPLICATIONS

- Secondary bacterial conjunctivitis
- Filamentary keratitis
- Secondary bacterial keratitis – rare
- Persistent corneal epithelial defects – very rare
- Calcific band keratopathy– very rare
- Keratinization – very rare
- Corneal perforation—very, very rare
  - Spontaneous
  - After cataract
- Psychological-social-economic
- Multiple serious systemic complications are with Sjögren's Syndrome (see . . .)

ADDITIONAL READING

- Moss SE, Klein R, Klein BE. Incidence of dry eye in an older population. *Arch Ophthalmol* 2004;122: 369–373.
- Graham JE, Moore JE, Goodall EA, et al. Concordance between common dry eye diagnostic tests. *Br J Ophthalmol* 2009;93(1):66–72.
- Perry HD, Solomon R, Donnenfeld ED, et al. Evaluation of topical cyclosporine for the treatment of dry eye disease. *Arch Ophthalmol* 2008;126: 1046–1050[A].
- Vogel R, Crockett RS, Oden N, et al. Demonstration of efficacy in the treatment of dry eye disease with 0.18% sodium hyaluronate ophthalmic solution (Vismed, Rejena). *Am J Ophthalmol* 2010;149: 594–601.
- Jackson WB. Management of dysfunctional tear syndrome: A Canadian consensus. *Can J Ophthalmol* 2009;44:385–394.

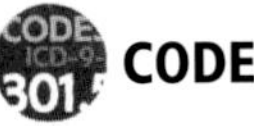

CODES

ICD9

- 373.02 Squamous blepharitis
- 373.12 Hordeolum internum
- 375.15 Tear film insufficiency, unspecified

CLINICAL PEARLS

- All artificial tears are formulated differently, patients will need direction.
- There are different types of dry eye that have different mechanisms and treatments.
- It is important to check for Sjögren's Syndrome, ask about a dry mouth.

DUANE SYNDROME

Leonard B. Nelson
Rizwan A. Alvi
Scott Olitsky

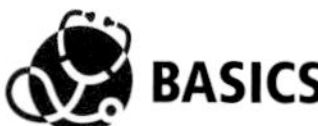

BASICS

DESCRIPTION

- A congenital eye movement disorder characterized primarily by abduction deficiency, associated with globe retraction and palpebral fissure narrowing on attempted adduction as well as possible adduction limitation.
- Type I. Marked limitation or complete absence of abduction, normal or only slightly restricted adduction.
- Type II. Limitation or absence of adduction with exotropia of the affected eye. Normal or slightly limited abduction.
- Type III. Severe limitation of both abduction and adduction.

EPIDEMIOLOGY

Incidence

- Found in approximately 1% of individuals with strabismus
  - More frequently
  - More common in females
  - Bilateral less frequent

Prevalence

Unknown

RISK FACTORS

- Thalidomide ingestion during first trimester
- Associated with some specific syndromes

Genetics

- Two genes known to be causative when mutated: CPAH (carboxypeptidase, 8q12–13, DURS1) and CHN1 (alpha2 chimerin, 2q31–32, DURS2). Both autosomal dominant. DURS2 80% type 1 Duane and 20% type 3
- DURS1 can also be involved in contiguous gene deletion syndrome: branchio-oto-renal syndrome overexpression, 80% type 1, 20% type 3
- Other loci noted based on chromosomal aberrations: del4q27–31, 22pter-q11 (marker chromosome), trisomy 8, del1q42.13–43 (with abnormal cerebellum)
- Duane + radial ray (Okihiro syndrome) +/– hearing/heart/renal/absent thumbs due to mutations in SALL4 (20q13.2). Autosomal dominant. Also causes IVIC syndrome = thrombocytopenia + radial ray defect + hearing loss
- Duane + anal abnormalities + renal + ear + thumb abnormalities and occasional cataract, coloboma, optic atrophy, limbal dermoid (Town Brocks syndrome) due to mutation in SALL1 (16q12.1). Autosomal dominant

GENERAL PREVENTION

None

PATHOPHYSIOLOGY

- Various theories include structural and innervational anomalies of the extraocular muscles as well as absence or hypoplasia of the sixth nerve nucleus.
- Up and down shoots and globe retraction due to coinnervation of the horizontal and vertical rectus muscles or, for the former, slippage of the lateral rectus muscle above or below the eye, commonly referred to as a "leash phenomenon."

ETIOLOGY

- Considered as one of the congenital cranial dysinnervation disorders (CCDD)
- Embryologic field defect involving branchial arches particularly when associated with Klippel-Feil anomaly, oculo-auriculo-vertebral spectrum (e.g., Goldenhar), hearing loss, and Wildervanck syndrome.

COMMONLY ASSOCIATED CONDITIONS

- Congenital labyrinthine hearing loss
- Amblyopia
- Anomalous head position (face turn) Strabismus in primary position

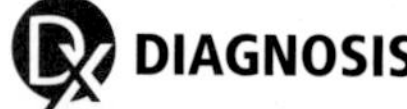

DIAGNOSIS

HISTORY

Child presents with an eye that does not appear to abduct and history of possible esotropia.

PHYSICAL EXAM

- Absence of abduction with possible limitation of adduction, retraction of globe in attempted adduction, and up and down shooting or both in adduction
- Full ocular examination with attention in particular to amblyopia and possible face turn
- Ocular anomalies may include dysplasia of the iris stroma, pupillary anomalies, cataract, heterochromia, Marcus Gunn jaw winking, coloboma, crocodile tears, and microphthalmos.
- Full physical examination for associated systemic abnormalities
- Consider audiology especially if speech delay or malformation of external ears

DIAGNOSTIC TESTS & INTERPRETATION

Lab

None

Imaging

None

Follow-up & special considerations

- Cine-MRI has been used to characterize upshoot and downshoot movement
- High resolution MRI of brain may identify associated malformation or abnormalities of sixth cranial nerve and its nucleus

Diagnostic Procedures/Other

Consider audiology

Pathological Findings

Autopsy findings include hypoplasia or aplasia of sixth cranial nerve

DIFFERENTIAL DIAGNOSIS

- Sixth Nerve Palsy
- Congenital Esotropia
- Exotropia
- Orbital fracture, tumor, or restrictive infiltrative process

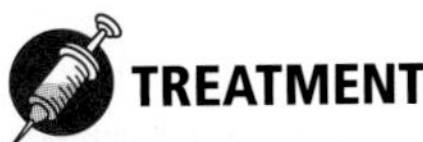

TREATMENT

MEDICATION

None

ADDITIONAL TREATMENT

General Measures

Before surgery is contemplated, coexisting significant refractive errors, anisometropia, and amblyopia should be treated.

Issues for Referral

Consider genetic consult if other malformations present or genetic testing desired.

Additional Therapies

- Occlusion or penalization therapy for amblyopia
- Glasses for refractive error

COMPLEMENTARY & ALTERNATIVE THERAPIES

None

SURGERY/OTHER PROCEDURES

- Indications for surgery include:
  - 1. Significant deviation in primary position.
  - 2. Anomalous head position.
  - 3. Large up or down shoot or retraction of the globe that is cosmetically intolerable.
- Surgery usually involves recession of the medial or lateral rectus for patients with esotropia of exotropia. Some surgeons prefer transposition surgery. The medial rectus of the involved eye is usually tight and forced duction testing is often positive because of the contracture of the muscle.
- Resection of the ipsilateral lateral rectus should almost never be performed because it will increase retraction of the globe in adduction.
- If an up or down shoot of the eye occurs, surgical options include recessing a stiff, fibrotic lateral rectus muscle, performing a Y-splitting of the muscle or placement of a posterior fixation suture to reduce the leash effect when present.
- Patients who suffer from a cosmetically noticeable retraction of the globe in attempted adduction may benefit from recession of both horizontal recti to reduce the co-contraction. This can be done in the absence of a deviation in primary gaze or adjusted to eliminate a deviation if present.

IN-PATIENT CONSIDERATIONS

None

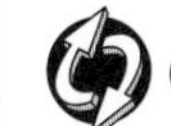

ONGOING CARE

FOLLOW-UP RECOMMENDATIONS

Follow the child for the development of amblyopia, strabismus in the primary position, or a face turn.

Patient Monitoring

Periodic for assessment of vision and alignment

PATIENT EDUCATION

- http://www.experienceproject.com/groups/Have-Duane-Syndrome/97737
- http://health.groups.yahoo.com/group/duanes/

PROGNOSIS

- Surgery can help to reduce or eliminate an associated face turn.
- Few patients show improvement in abduction following surgery and some patients undergoing medial rectus recession may have a decrease in adduction. In patients with significant co-contraction, large over-corrections can occur following medial rectus recession.
- Excellent prognosis for vision if amblyopia and refractive error addressed
- Surgical results can be very satisfactory.

COMPLICATIONS

- Recession of the medial rectus more than 6 mm may cause consecutive exotropia.
- Amblyopia

ADDITIONAL READING

- Isenberg S, Urist MJ. Clinical observations in 101 consecutive patients with Duane's retraction syndrome. *Am J Ophthalmol* 1972;84:419.
- Jampolsky A. Duane syndrome. In: Rosenbaum AL, Santiago AP, eds. *Clinical strabismus management: Principles and surgical techniques*. Philadelphia: Saunders, 1999:325–346.

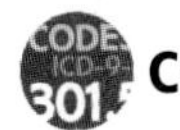

CODES

ICD9

378.71 Duane's syndrome

CLINICAL PEARLS

- Most children with Duane syndrome have no strabismus in the primary straight ahead position.
- Duane syndrome does not usually worsen with age.

D

DYSLEXIA

Michael D. Tibbetts

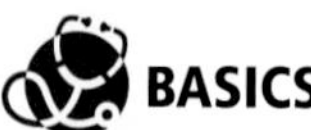

BASICS

DESCRIPTION

- Dyslexia is a primary reading disorder. It is characterized by difficulty in understanding and using alphabetic and logographic principles to acquire accurate and fluent reading skills
  - Results from a written word processing abnormality in the brain
  - Not explained by sensory deficits, cognitive deficits, lack of motivation or lack of adequate reading instruction
  - Historically termed "word blindness," but most commonly due to deficit in auditory processing of language (phonological processing) and not visual processing
  - Word reversals and skipping words result from linguistic deficiencies rather than visual or perception disorders

EPIDEMIOLOGY

Prevalence

- In a population, reading ability and reading disability occur along a continuum, with reading disability representing the lower tail of the distribution
- Depending on definition, 5–17% of children affected; boys more than girls
  - Similar rates across languages
- Approximately 80% of people with learning disabilities have dyslexia

RISK FACTORS

Genetics

- Strongly heritable (54–75%)
  - 68% concordance in identical twins and 40% of individuals with affected parent or sibling
  - Heritability greater among children whose parents have higher education level
- Polygenic inheritance
  - At least 9 associated loci

GENERAL PREVENTION

Early identification and intervention key to improving outcomes

ETIOLOGY

- Disorder within the language system, specifically phonological processing:
  - Disruption of left hemisphere posterior brain systems while performing reading tasks
  - Increased reliance on ancillary brain regions including frontal lobes and right hemisphere posterior circuits
- Vision problems can interfere with the process of learning.
- However, vision problems are not the cause of primary dyslexia or learning disabilities.

COMMONLY ASSOCIATED CONDITIONS

- Some children may have visual problems that contribute to primary reading or learning dysfunction
  - Treatable ocular conditions include:
    - Strabismus
    - Amblyopia
    - Convergence and/or focusing deficiencies
    - Refractive errors

DIAGNOSIS

HISTORY

- In young children, language delay or not attending to the sounds of words:
  - Trouble learning letters of alphabet or nursery rhymes
  - Confusing words that sound alike or mispronouncing words
- In older children, slow and laborious reading and writing
- Discrepancy between general intelligence (IQ) and standardized reading test scores

PHYSICAL EXAM

- If a child has suspected learning disabilities, child should be evaluated for medical problems which could affect the child's ability to learn
- Children with dyslexia should have hearing and visual screenings, according to national standards for all children
  - Visual screening with non-letter symbols may be necessary for testing children with dyslexia
- Children with dyslexia have the same visual function and ocular health as other children (1) [A]
  - Dyslexia is **not** caused by subtle eye or visual problems including (2)[A]:
  - Visual perceptual disorders
  - Refractive error
  - Abnormal focusing
  - Jerky eye movements,
  - Binocular dysfunction
  - Misaligned or crossed eyes
- Readers with dyslexia may have saccadic eye movements and fixations similar to beginning readers but show normal saccadic eye movements when content is corrected for ability
  - Saccadic patterns are result of reading disability but not the cause

DIAGNOSTIC TESTS & INTERPRETATION

Imaging

Currently, there is no indication for imaging in the standard evaluation of dyslexia or other learning disorders.

Diagnostic Procedures/Other

- Dyslexia as well as other learning disorders should not be diagnosed by physicians but by educators, psychologists, or neuropsychologists with specialized, comprehensive assessments.
- Standardized tests of reading including:
  - Comprehensive Test of Phonological Processing in Reading
  - Woodcock Johnson Tests for word decoding
  - Gray Oral Reading Test for fluency
- In the future, the combination of standardized neurocognitive tests, neuroimaging, genetic and familial information may improve diagnosis and allow for earlier intervention.

Pathological Findings

- Functional neuroimaging studies have revealed differences in brain function and connectivity that are characteristic of dyslexia: (3)
  - Reduced or absent activation of left temporoparietal cortex
  - Atypical activation in other regions including:
    - Left prefrontal regions associated with verbal working memory
    - Left middle and superior temporal gyri associated with receptive language
    - Left occipito-temporal regions associated with visual analysis of words and letters.
- Experimental functional neuroimaging studies have demonstrated brain plasticity associated with effective intervention for dyslexia
  - Neuroimaging studies have not revealed any differences in the brains of children who do and do not respond to treatment

DIFFERENTIAL DIAGNOSIS

- Other important reasons for reading failure on the population level include:
  - Reduced vocabulary and strategies needed for text comprehension
  - Reduced motivation to read
  - Both these reasons are often tied to socioeconomic factors at home and at school
- Attention deficit hyperactivity disorder (ADHD)
- Aphasia
- Auditory processing disorder
- Less common reasons include visual problems such as strabismus, amblyopia, and refractive errors.
- Other conditions such as convergence insufficiency and poor accommodation (both of which are rare in children under age 10 years) can interfere with the physical act of reading but not decoding and comprehension.

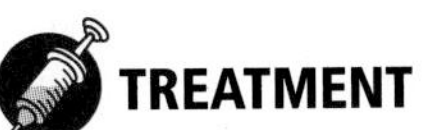

TREATMENT

ADDITIONAL TREATMENT

General Measures

- Multidisciplinary evaluation and management
- Explicit and systematic intensive instruction in small groups in phonological awareness and decoding strategies
  - Improvements more likely in younger children (ages 6–8 years) than in older children
- Providing accommodations for older children including extra time for reading, spell check computer programs, tape recorders
- Vision training is not a primary or adjunctive therapy for dyslexia (4)[B]
- Scientific evidence does **not** support the following alternative therapies for improving the long-term educational performance efficacy:
  - Eye exercises
  - Behavioral vision therapy
  - Special colored or tinted filters or lenses

Issues for Referral

- Patients with suspected learning disabilities should be referred for further educational, psychological, or other appropriate evaluation.
- If vision problem is suspected, children should be referred to an ophthalmologist with experience in assessment and treatment of children.

COMPLEMENTARY & ALTERNATIVE THERAPIES

Scientific evidence does not support alternative therapies aimed at visual training.

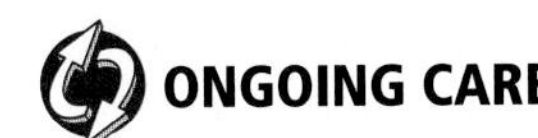

ONGOING CARE

FOLLOW-UP RECOMMENDATIONS

Multidisciplinary management by educators

PATIENT EDUCATION

- The International Dyslexia Association (http://www.interdys.org)

PROGNOSIS

- Persistent, chronic condition, not a transient developmental lag
- A student who fails to read adequately in the 1st grade has a 90% probability of reading poorly in 4th grade and a 75% probability of reading poorly in high school
- For students with dyslexia, early intervention (before the 3rd grade) is key to improving reading ability (5) [C]

REFERENCES

1. Helveston EM, Weber JC, Miller K, et al. Visual function and academic performance. *Am J Ophthalmol* 1985;99(3):346–355.
2. Polatajko HJ. Visual-ocular control of normal and learning disabled children. *Dev Med Child Neurol* 1987;29(4):477–485.
3. Shaywitz SE, Shaywitz BA, Pugh KR, et al. Functional disruption in the organization of the brain for reading in dyslexia. *Proc Natl Acad Sci U S A* 1998;95(5):2636–2641.
4. Barrett B. A critical evaluation of the evidence supporting the practice of behavioural vision therapy. *Ophthalmic Physiol Opt* 2009;29(1):4–25.
5. Schatschneider C, Torgesen JK. Using our current understanding of dyslexia to support early identification and intervention. *J Child Neurol* 2004;19(10):759–765.

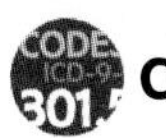

CODES

ICD9

- 368.00 Amblyopia, unspecified
- 378.9 Unspecified disorder of eye movements
- 784.61 Alexia and dyslexia

CLINICAL PEARLS

- Dyslexia is a primary reading disorder from a word processing abnormality in the brain.
- Dyslexia is not due to a visual problem.
- It is important to recognize the signs and symptoms of dyslexia early so that affected children can receive appropriate instruction and improve their long-term reading ability.

D

EALES DISEASE

P. Kumar Rao

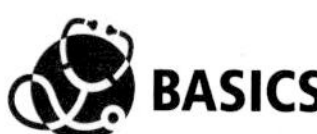

BASICS

DESCRIPTION

An idiopathic obliterative vasculopathy. The classic triad is a retinal phlebitis, associated with peripheral retinal nonperfusion and vitreous hemorrhage, typically in young adults.

EPIDEMIOLOGY

Incidence

- Most commonly reported in India and the Middle East.
- In India, it occurs in 1/250 patients with eye disease.
- It usually occurs in adults 20–30 years old.
- Prior studies suggested a higher incidence in men; however recent reports suggest a more even distribution between men and women.

RISK FACTORS

Living in areas such as India and the Middle East.

PATHOPHYSIOLOGY

A nonspecific obliterative vasculitis.

A hypersensitivity to tuberculin protein has been suggested, and tubercle bacilli have been identified in pathology specimens.

COMMONLY ASSOCIATED CONDITIONS

Myelopathy, ischemic stroke, hemiplegia, multifocal white matter abnormalities, and vestibuloauditory dysfunction have been reported.

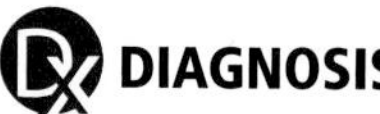

DIAGNOSIS

HISTORY

The most common symptoms include decreased vision and cobwebs or floaters.

PHYSICAL EXAM

- Retinal phlebitis appears as vascular sheathing with adjacent nerve fiber layer hemorrhages and hard exudates.
- Over half of patients will have bilateral disease.
- Anterior chamber cell and flare with keratic precipitates may be present. Vitreous debris and cells, as well as vitreous hemorrhage, can be seen.
- Cystoid macular edema may be present.
- Nonperfusion in the temporal periphery is typical and is associated with other microvascular changes such as microaneurysms, venous shunting, venous beading, hard exudates, and cotton wool spots. Neovascularization of the disc or elsewhere in the retina is present in up to 80% of patients. Neovascular glaucoma may also occur.

DIAGNOSTIC TESTS & INTERPRETATION

Lab

Initial lab tests

No specific testing can determine the diagnosis; however Eales disease is a diagnosis of exclusion and testing should be done to rule out causes of vasculitis (see Differential Diagnosis section).

Follow-up & special considerations

Lumbar puncture (not routinely needed) shows pleocytosis of CSF. In addition, MRI and CT imaging may be used to identify CNS lesions.

Imaging

Initial approach

- Fluorescein angiography (FA) is helpful to analyze presence of active vasculitis, vascular damage, and to look for areas of nonperfusion and neovascularization.
- OCT may reveal cystoid macular edema and/or epiretinal membranes.

Follow-up & special considerations

Patients should be monitored for neovascularization of the retina, iris, and anterior chamber angle. Retinal neovascularization may lead to vitreous hemorrhage. Epiretinal membranes may develop after pan-retinal photocoagulation (but may also occur without laser photocoagulation).

Diagnostic Procedures/Other

- Eales disease is diagnosis of exclusion and therefore entities in the differential diagnosis must be ruled out with appropriate history, physical exam, and ancillary testing.
- MRI testing of the CNS may reveal multifocal white matter abnormalities.

DIFFERENTIAL DIAGNOSIS

- Sickle cell disease.
- Diabetes mellitus.
- Branch retinal vein or artery occlusion.
- Retinal embolization.
- Retinopathy of prematurity.
- Familial exudative vitreoretinopathy.
- Hyperviscosity syndromes (e.g., leukemia).
- Ocular ischemic syndrome.

- Carotid–cavernous fistula.
- Multiple sclerosis.
- Toxemia of pregnancy.
- Sarcoidosis.
- Collagen-vascular disease.
- Vasculitis secondary to infection.
- Uveitis.
- Birdshot retinochoroidopathy.
- Toxoplasmosis.
- Acute retinal necrosis.
- Long-standing retinal detachment.
- Retinitis pigmentosa.
- Retinoschisis.
- Choroidal melanoma or hemangioma.
- Incontinentia pigmenti.

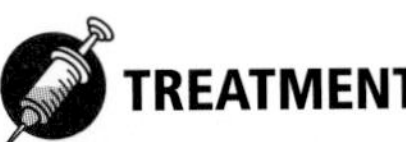

TREATMENT

ADDITIONAL TREATMENT

Issues for Referral

CNS findings warrant a referral to neurology.

COMPLEMENTARY & ALTERNATIVE THERAPIES

Thyroid extract, osteogenic hormones, androgenic hormones, and systemic steroids and antioxidant vitamins A, C, and E have been suggested. None have been proven effective in the treatment of this disease.

SURGERY/OTHER PROCEDURES

- Panretinal photocoagulation for neovascular complications is necessary.
- Vitrectomy and membrane removal may be considered for epiretinal membranes.
- Both oral steroids and intravitreal triamcinolone has been used to stabilize vascular leakage.
- Intravitreal bevacizumab has been used to induce regression of neovascularization.

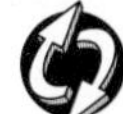

ONGOING CARE

FOLLOW-UP RECOMMENDATIONS

Patient Monitoring

Patients should been followed every 3 to 12 months, depending on the extent of nonperfusion and neovascularization.

PATIENT EDUCATION

Patients should be taught the symptoms of vitreous hemorrhage, such as sudden onset of floaters. Early detection and treatment of vitreous hemorrhage and neovascularization can allow laser photocoagulation, which may prevent the tractional complications such as retinal detachment or neovascular glaucoma.

PROGNOSIS

The majority of patients maintains 20/40 vision or better with disease stabilization.

COMPLICATIONS

Retinal neovascularization, rhegmatogenous retinal detachment, vitreous hemorrhage, and traction retinal detachment can also occur.

REFERENCES

1. Chanana B, Azad RV, Patwardhan S. Role of intravitreal bevacizumab in the management of Eales' disease. *Int Ophthalmol* 2010;30(1):57–61. E-pub Jan 23, 2009.
2. Das T, Pathengay A, Hussain N, Biswas J. Eales disease: Diagnosis and management. *Eye* 2010;24:472–482.
3. Ishaq M, Feroze AH, Shahid M, et al. Intravitreal steroids may facilitate treatment of Eales' disease (idiopathic retinal vasculitis): An interventional case series. *Eye (Lond)* 2007;21(11):1403–1405. E-pub Sept 15, 2006.
4. Therese KL, Deepa P, Therese J, Bagyalakshmi R, Biswas J, Madhavan HN. Association of mycobacteria with Eales' disease. *Ind J Med Res* 2007;126(1):56–62.

CODES

ICD9

- 362.18 Retinal vasculitis
- 379.23 Vitreous hemorrhage

CLINICAL PEARLS

- Suspect Eales disease in young men from India who have no other underlying systemic disease that could cause retinal neovascularization.

E

ECTOPIA LENTIS

Dorothy H. Hendricks

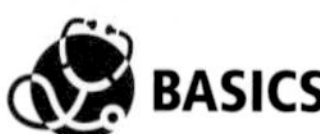

BASICS

DESCRIPTION

- Displacement of the lens.
- This may be divided into subluxed lens, which is partially displaced, and luxated or dislocated lens, which is completely displaced.
- May be an isolated anomaly, or associated with various systemic diseases or trauma.

EPIDEMIOLOGY

Incidence

- Marfan disease 4–6/100,000 births (1) and approximately 60–75% have ectopia lentis.
- Homocystinuria 1/200,000 births (1) and approximately 80–85% have ectopia lentis.

Prevalence

Unknown.

RISK FACTORS

- Trauma.
- Family history.
- Marfan syndrome
- Type 1 Ehlers–Danlos.
- Weill–Marchesani
- Homocystinuria.
- Hyperlysinemia.
- Sulfite oxidase deficiency.
- Molybdenum cofactor deficiency.
- Infantile glaucoma with buphthalmos.
- Persistent ocular fetal vasculature.
- Coloboma of ciliary body.

Genetics

- Isolated ectopia lentis can be autosomal dominant due to mutations in the fibrillin 1 gene (FBN1,15q21), the same gene involved in Marfan syndrome (1).
- An autosomal recessive form of isolated ectopia lentis is associated with mutation in ADAMTSL4 gene (1q21) (2).
- Ectopia lentis et pupillae is autosomal recessive (3), gene unknown.
- Weill–Marchesani may be autosomal dominant due to mutation in FBN1 or autosomal recessive due to mutations in ADAMTS10 (19p13.3) or ADAMTS17 (15q24) (4).
- Type 1 Ehlers Danlos is due to mutations in collagens COL5A1, COL5A2, or COL1A1.
- Homocystinuria is autosomal recessive and linked to the gene coding cystathionine beta-synthase (21q22.3) (1). Other less common disorders of cysteine metabolism may also be associated with ectopia lentis.
- Mutation in the sulfite oxidase gene (SUOX, 12q13.13) cause autosomal recessive sulfite oxidase deficiency (5).
- Hyperlysinemia is caused by mutation in the alpha-aminoadipic semialdehyde synthase gene (AASS, 7q31.3) (6).
- Virtually any form of glaucoma resulting in buphthalmus may rarely be a cause of ectopia lentis. The genetics of the underlying disorder determine the inheritance pattern. The same holds true for other rare syndromic causes of ectopia lentis and coloboma.
- Persistent ocular fetal vascular is usually not genetic (see chapter).

GENERAL PREVENTION

- Genetic counseling.
- Some recommend restricted activity or protective polycarbonate lens in patients with systemic conditions associated with ectopia lentis.
- Some forms of homocystinuria may respond to vitamin B6, methionine-restricted diet, betaine, or supplementary cysteine (1).
  - This treatment has been shown to reduce the incidence of lens dislocation.

PATHOPHYSIOLOGY

Weakening or stretching of the zonular attachments lens (1).

ETIOLOGY

- Traumatic rupture of zonules.
- Congenital zonular deficiency (e.g., ciliary body coloboma).
- Defective zonules that results in weakening.
  - Marfan—defect in fibrillin.
  - Ehlers–Danlos—defect in type V collagen.
  - Homocystinuria—zonules deficient in cysteine.

COMMONLY ASSOCIATED CONDITIONS

- Marfan syndrome: Aortic root dilation, Marfanoid habitus, pectus excavatum/carinatum, and other features.
- Ehlers–Danlos: joint laxity, "cigarette paper" scars of skin and other features.
- Weill–Marchesani: short stature, cardiac abnormalities, abnormal hands
- Homocystinuria: Developmental delay (50%), Marfanoid habitus, premature grey hair, hypercoagulability and other features.
- Hyperlysinemia: Severe developmental delay.
- Sulfite oxidase deficiency: Severe developmental delay.

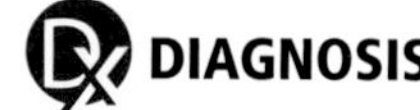

DIAGNOSIS

HISTORY

- Family history of ectopia lentis or any of the above-mentioned associated conditions.
- History of ocular trauma.

PHYSICAL EXAM

- Full ocular examination including slit lamp examination pre- and post-dilation.
- Pupil position (e.g., corectopia).
- Assess if zonules absent, broken, or stretched.
- Assess if lens edge flat, round, crenulated.
- Measurement of intraocular pressure.
- Cycloplegic refraction and assessment of vision: Can refract through aphakic (with or without pharmacologic mydriasis) or phakic visual axis for best vision.
- Full physical exam for systemic associations.

DIAGNOSTIC TESTS & INTERPRETATION

Lab

Initial lab tests

- None if history of ocular trauma (ectopia always unilateral).
- All patients without clear family history or diagnosis and no trauma should have urine/blood homocysteine levels as risk of stroke/death under general anesthesia.

Follow-up & special considerations

- Genetic consult for further work up and evaluation if warranted.
  - Consider cardiology consultation.

Imaging

Initial approach

Consider echocardiogram if considering Marfan syndrome or Weill–Marchesani.

Follow-up & special considerations

- Follow for increased movement of lens, change in vision/refraction, and amblyopia.
  - Weill–Marchesani follow for progressive shallowing of anterior chamber and secondary closed angle glaucoma.
  - Glaucoma risk also in other forms of ectopia lentis (Marfan, persistent ocular fetal circulation, trauma).

Diagnostic Procedures/Other
Molecular genetic testing as indicated.

Pathological Findings
- Fibrillinopathy: Loss of periodicity in zonules with fibrillin staining.
  - Homocystinuria and related disorders: PAS positive zonular material on lens edge and ciliary body.
  - Weill–Marchesani: Peripheral anterior synechia.

DIFFERENTIAL DIAGNOSIS
Microspherophakia.

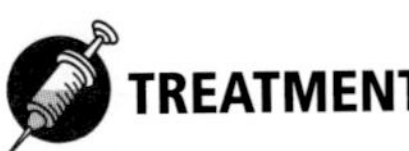

TREATMENT

MEDICATION
- Homocystinuria (see earlier).
- If lens dislocated into anterior chamber consider glaucoma treatment including mannitol to shrink vitreous, topical steroids to reduce inflammation, and short acting mydriatics with patient in supine position. After lens floats back behind pupil, then pilocarpine.
- Weill–Marchesani: Aggressive cycloplegia (e.g., atropine) may deepen anterior chamber as short-term treatment.

ADDITIONAL TREATMENT
General Measures
- Correction of refractive error (1).
  - Treatment of amblyopia if present.

Issues for Referral
- Genetic consultation.
  - Cardiology as indicated.
  - Metabolics consultation as indicated.

Additional Therapies
Massage of cornea may be needed to release lens dislocated into anterior chamber.

COMPLEMENTARY & ALTERNATIVE THERAPIES
None.

SURGERY/OTHER PROCEDURES
- Lensectomy and anterior vitrectomy.
  - Typically poor zonule support prevents lens implantation in children (1).
  - Contact lens or spectacles are then used for aphakic correction.
  - Weill–Marchesani: Early lensectomy advised if anterior chamber deepening.
  - Use of argon laser iridoplasty or YAG laser lysis of zonules has been reported.

IN-PATIENT CONSIDERATIONS
Initial Stabilization
- As needed for associated systemic diseases.
  - If lens in anterior chamber maintain supine position.

Admission Criteria
- As indicated by systemic disease.
  - Admit all patients with homocystinuria undergoing surgery night before and after surgery.

IV Fluids
Homocystinuria 1.5 × maintenance starting night before surgery and continuing through 1 night after.

Nursing
Maintain supine position and strict bed rest as long as lens in anterior chamber.

Discharge Criteria
If lens is not returned to retropupillary position by medical means, lensectomy before discharge.

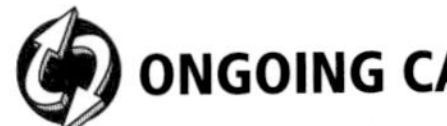

ONGOING CARE

FOLLOW-UP RECOMMENDATIONS
Routine ophthalmic examination depending on degree of dislocation and presence of other pathology including amblyopia.

Patient Monitoring
- Cardiology, metabolics, developmental services as needed.
  - Visual acuity, intraocular pressure.

DIET
Methionine-restricted diet in patients with homocystinuria.

PATIENT EDUCATION
- Genetic counseling.
- http://www.marfan.ca/ and http://www.marfan.org/marfan/.
- http://www.mdjunction.com/homocystinuria.

PROGNOSIS
- Good visual prognosis with early intervention and routine follow-up.
- Even in patients requiring lensectomy most achieve vision of 20/40 or better (1).
  - If not complicated by untreated amblyopia.

COMPLICATIONS
Amblyopia, glaucoma, retinal detachment (particularly in patients with Marfan disease), lens dislocation.

REFERENCES

1. Neely DE, Plager DA. Management of ectopia lentis in children. *Ophthalmol Clin North America* 2001;14(3):493–497.
2. Ahram D, Sato TS, Kohilan A, et al. A homozygous mutation in ADAMTSL4 causes autosomal-recessive isolated ectopia lentis. *Am J Hum Genet* 2009;84:274–278.
3. Colley A, Lloyd IC, et al. Ectopia lentis et pupillae: The genetic aspects and differential diagnosis. *J Med Genet* 1991;Nov 28(11):791–794.
4. Faivre L, Dollfus H, Lyonnet S, et al. Clinical homogeneity and genetic heterogeneity in Weill-Marchesani syndrome. *Am J Med Genet* 2003;123A:204–207.
5. Kisker C, Schindelin H, Pacheco A, et al. Molecular basis of sulfite oxidase deficiency from the structure of sulfite oxidase. *Cell* 1997;91:973–983.
6. Sacksteder KA, Biery BJ, Morrell JC, et al. Identification of the alpha-aminoadipic semialdehyde synthase gene, which is defective in familial hyperlysinemia. *Am J Hum Genet* 2000;66:1736–1743.

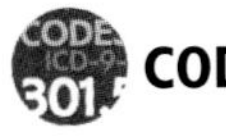

CODES

ICD9
- 743.37 Congenital ectopic lens
- 996.53 Mechanical complication of prosthetic ocular lens prosthesis

CLINICAL PEARLS

- Trauma rarely cause bilateral ectopia lentis.
- If considering surgery and diagnosis not clear, do urine and blood homocysteine measurement and ECG.
- If cannot clarify vision through phakic visual axis, consider aphakic correction with pharmacologic mydriasis as needed.

E

ECTROPION

Thaddeus S. Nowinski

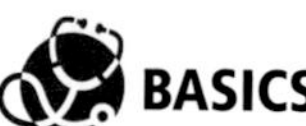

BASICS

DESCRIPTION
- Outward turning/eversion of the upper eyelid margin.
- Types:
  - Congenital.
  - Involutional (most common).
  - Paralytic.
  - Cicatricial.

EPIDEMIOLOGY
Incidence
Bells palsy—25 per 100,000.

Prevalence
Involutional ectropion—increases with age.

RISK FACTORS
- Increased skin sun sensitivity.
- Lighter iris color.
- Diabetes.
- Hypertension.
- Stroke.
- Smoking.

PATHOPHYSIOLOGY
- Involutional—horizontal eyelid laxity.
- Cicatricial—skin contracture secondary to inflammatory or infiltrative dermatitis, tumor, previous eyelid, or facial surgery
- Paralytic—Bell's palsy, herpes zoster, parotid gland surgery, surgery involving the 7th nerve.
- Allergic—contact dermatitis.

Pediatric Considerations
Congenital—Blepharophimosis, Downs, Ichthyosis, congenital eyelid eversion, facial dysmorphic syndromes.

ETIOLOGY
- Drug toxicity, eyedrops or systemic.
- Severe cellulitis.

COMMONLY ASSOCIATED CONDITIONS
- Bells—Lyme

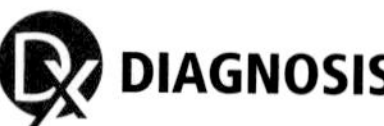

DIAGNOSIS

HISTORY
- Foreign body sensation.
- Redness.
- Tearing.
- Mucous secretion.
- 7th nerve palsy.
- Previous surgery—cosmetic, ENT, neurosurgery, MOHS.

PHYSICAL EXAM
- Outturning of eyelid margin, pull away of eyelid from globe.
- Lagophthalmos.
- Hyperemia/keratinization of conjunctival epithelium.
- Retractor disinsertion.
- Superficial punctuate keratitis.
- Horizontal eyelid laxity.
- Lacrimal punctal eversion and atresia.
- Inability to push lower eyelid up to normal position (cicatricial).
- Signs of 7th nerve palsy (paralytic)—check orbicularis squeezing tone.
- Bells Palsy—signs of herpes zoster (Ramsay Hunt), signs of sarcoid (Heerfordt's).

DIAGNOSTIC TESTS & INTERPRETATION
Lab
- Bells palsy—Lyme titers.
- Congenital eversioninclusion conjunctival swab.

DIFFERENTIAL DIAGNOSIS
- Thyroid ophthalmopathy.
- Floppy eyelid syndrome.

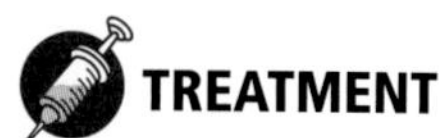

TREATMENT

MEDICATION
First Line
- Ocular lubrication.
- Artificial tears, gel, ointment.

Second Line
- Ocular antibiotic/steroid ointment to lower eyelid skin (1)[C].
- Bells palsy.
  - Corticosteroids.
  - Possible antivirals (2)[C].
- Lyme—antibiotic tx
- Herpes zoster—antiviral tx, possible corticosteroids.

ADDITIONAL TREATMENT
General Measures
- Warm compresses.
- Temporary taping of eyelid.
- Possible cyanoacrylate at lateral canthus.

Issues for Referral
Ophthalmologist for cornea monitoring 1 week.

Additional Therapies
- Cicatricial—massage.
- Palsy—massage, TENS unit.

COMPLEMENTARY & ALTERNATIVE THERAPIES

- Hyaluronic acid filler injection.

SURGERY/OTHER PROCEDURES

- Involutional—horizontal tightening, medial spindle.
- Paralytic—same, upper lid gold weight, wait months before surgical repair to allow for spontaneous improvement unless cornea threatened (3)[C].
- Cicatricial—above, full thickness skin graft, flap, or midface suspension.

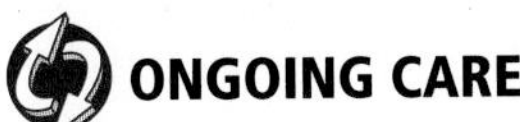

ONGOING CARE

FOLLOW-UP RECOMMENDATIONS

- Bells palsy—ophthalmologist in few days.
- Involutional ectropion—2 weeks.

PROGNOSIS

- Surgery may be needed if cornea affected or very symptomatic.
- Involutional.
- Paralytic—may resolve depending on etiology.

COMPLICATIONS

Corneal abrasion, ulcer, scarring, perforation.

REFERENCES

1. Libau J, Schulz A, Arens A, Tilkorn H, Schwipper V. Management of lower lid ectropion. *Dermatologic Surgery* 2006;32:1050–1056.
2. De Almeida J, et al. Combined corticosteroid and antiviral treatmentfor Bells palsy. A systematic review and meta-analysis. *JAMA* 2009;985–993.
3. Mehta R. Sugical treatment of facial paralysis. *Clin Exp Otorhinolaryngol* 2009;2:1–5.

ADDITIONAL READING

- Fezza J. Nonsurgical treatment of cicatricial ectropion with hyaluronic acid filler. *Plast Reconstr Surg* 2008;121:1009–1014.
- Heimmel M, Enzer Y, Hoffman R. Entropion-ectropion: The influence of axial globe projection on lower eyelid malposition. *Ophthalmic Plast Reconstr Surg* 2009;25:7–9.
- Mehta R. Surgical treatment of facial paralysis. *Clin Exp Otorhinolaryngol* 2009;2:1–5.

See Also (Topic, Algorithm, Electronic Media Element)

- www.asoprs.org
- Topic
  - Bells palsy
  - Herpes zoster
  - Lyme disease
- Figure

CODES

ICD9

- 374.10 Ectropion, unspecified
- 374.12 Mechanical ectropion
- 743.62 Congenital deformities of eyelids

CLINICAL PEARLS

- Most forms are ectropion can be treated conservatively to protect the cornea before elective surgery is considered.
- Many cases of involutional ectropion have a cicatricial component of dermatitis, which may respond to a short course of topical steroids.

EHLERS–DANLOS SYNDROME

Swathi Reddy

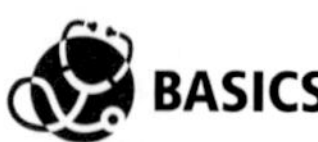

BASICS

DESCRIPTION

- Ehlers–Danlos syndrome is a group of connective tissue disorders characterized by joint hypermobility, hyperextensible skin, and fragile connective tissue.
- New classification system describes 6 types:
  - Classic type (formerly types I and II, characterized by joint hypermobility, skin laxity and fragility).
  - Hypermobility type (formerly type III, characterized by joint hypermobility).
  - Vascular type (formerly type IV, complicated by arterial or bowel rupture).
  - Kyphoscoliosis type (formerly type VI or ocular-scoliotic type, characterized by globe fragility, scoliosis, and skin and joint laxity).
  - Arthrochalasis type (formerly type VIIB, characterized by short stature, joint laxity and dislocations).
  - Dermatosparaxis type (formerly type VIIC, characterized by fragile skin with sagging and folding).
  - Tenascin-X-deficient type (characterized by joint hypermobility, hyperelastic skin, and fragile tissue).

EPIDEMIOLOGY

Prevalence

- The prevalence of Ehlers–Danlos syndrome is reported to be 1 in 5,000–10,000 individuals. However, the disease may be underdiagnosed due to milder presentations.
  - The kyphoscoliosis type affects 2% and is 1 of the less common types.

RISK FACTORS

Genetics

- Varies by type: the kyphoscoliosis and the dermatosparaxis types are autosomal recessive, and the remaining types are autosomal dominant.
- The *ADAMTS2*, *COL1A2*, *COL3A1*, *COL5A1*, *COL5A2*, *PLOD1*, and *TNXB* genes are all associated with Ehlers–Danlos.
  - These genes are responsible for the assembly and modification of collagen molecules.

GENERAL PREVENTION

Genetic counseling.

PATHOPHYSIOLOGY

Gene mutations result in deficient collagen biosynthesis, primarily of types I and III, leading to fragility of collagen-containing structures.

ETIOLOGY

The various types of Ehlers–Danlos syndrome are due to mutations in many genes coding for collagen synthesis or posttranslational modification.

DIAGNOSIS

HISTORY

- Family history.
- Muscle weakness.
- Joint pain.
- Easy bruising.
- Dental problems.
- Ocular problems.

PHYSICAL EXAM

- Skin usually white, soft, doughy, hyperextensible, fragile, and with visible underlying vessels.
- Flexible fingers and toes.
- Molluscoid pseudotumors—spongy tumors overlying scars
- Cardiac defects.
  - Mitral valve prolapse.
  - Dysautonomia.
- Abnormal wound healing.
- Increased bleeding (platelet aggregation dysfunction).
- Ocular defects.
  - Retinal hemorrhage.
  - Retinal detachment (due to stretching of collagenous sclera).
  - Keratoconus.
  - Lens subluxation.
  - Angioid streaks.
  - Dry eyes.
  - Strabismus.
  - Glaucoma.
  - Blue sclera.
  - Carotid–cavernous sinus fistula.
  - Globe rupture.
  - Myopia.
  - Posterior staphyloma.
  - Photophobia.
- Musculoskeletal features.
  - Hyperextensible joints.
    - Spontaneous dislocation.
    - Sprain.
    - Subluxation.
  - Kyphoscoliosis (convex curving of the spinal column both backwards and sideways).
  - Hallus valgus (bunion).
  - Pes planus (flat foot).
  - Genu recurvatum (hyperextension of knee).
- Functional bowel disorder.
  - Gastritis.
  - Irritable bowel syndrome.
- Nerve compression (carpal tunnel).

DIAGNOSTIC TESTS & INTERPRETATION

Lab
- No screening laboratory tests.
- Secondary laboratory testing includes the following:
  - Collagen typing.
  - Collagen gene mutation testing (see "Genetics").
  - Lysyl oxidase or hydroxylase activity.

Imaging
- No initial imaging.
- Secondary imaging may show:
  - Calcification of nodules opaque on radiographs.
  - Joint dislocation/subluxation.

Diagnostic Procedures/Other
- Echocardiography (mitral valve prolapse).
- Skin biopsy (not sensitive).

Pathological Findings
- Histology reveals whorled, sparse, and disorderly collagen.
- Irregular diameter of fibrils.

DIFFERENTIAL DIAGNOSIS
- Elastolysis.
- Loeys–Dietz syndrome.
- Pseudoxanthoma elasticum.
- Turner syndrome.
- Cartilage-hair hypoplasia syndrome.
- Muscular hypotonia.

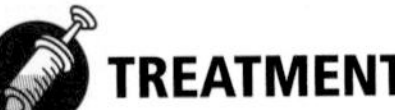

TREATMENT

MEDICATION

First Line
- Unsatisfactory medical treatments.
- Treatment is largely supportive.

Second Line
- Vitamin C—cofactor for collagen fibril synthesis.

ADDITIONAL TREATMENT

General Measures
- Care with surgery (vascular rupture and increased bleeding risk).
- Care with anesthesia (cervical spine and airway trauma).
- Avoidance of contact sports (types IV and VI) due to spontaneous vascular rupture.
- Care with pregnancy—reports of premature rupture of membranes.

Issues for Referral
- Ophthalmology.
- Dental.
- Orthopedics.

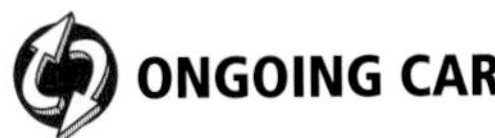

ONGOING CARE

FOLLOW-UP RECOMMENDATIONS
- Ophthalmology.
- Primary care doctor or dermatologist for periodic skin examinations.
- Orthopedics (braces, surgical repair of joints).
- Rehabilitation (physical and occupational therapy).
- Genetic counseling prior to pregnancy.

PATIENT EDUCATION
- The Ehlers–Danlos National Foundation (http://www.ednf.org).

PROGNOSIS
- Generally patients have a normal lifespan.
- Risk of large vessel or organ rupture with the vascular and kyphoscoliosis types with possible sudden death.

COMPLICATIONS
- Organ rupture (uterus or bowel).
- Vessel rupture (aortic aneurysm).
- Globe rupture.
- Arthritis.

ADDITIONAL READING

- Beighton P. Serious Ophthalmological complications in the Ehlers-Danlos syndrome. *Br J Ophthalmol* 54(4):263–268.
- Beighton P, De Paepe A, Steinmann B, Tsipouras P, Wenstrup RJ. Ehlers-Danlos Syndromes: Revised Nosology, Villefranche, 1997. *Am J Med Genet* 77:31–37.
- Pollack JS, Custer PL, Hart WM, Smith ME, Fitzpatrick MM. Ocular Complications in Ehlers-Danlos Syndrome Type IV. *Arch Opthalmol* 115:416–419.

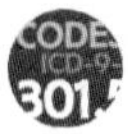

CODES

ICD9
- 361.9 Unspecified retinal detachment
- 362.81 Retinal hemorrhage
- 756.83 Ehlers-danlos syndrome

CLINICAL PEARLS
- Ehlers–Danlos is underdiagnosed because of varied presentation.
- The vascular type of Ehlers–Danlos may not present with joint hypermobility or skin hyperelasticity.
- Ehlers–Danlos syndrome is primarily a clinical diagnosis, and most individuals will not likely have any symptoms throughout their lifetime.

ENDOPHTHALMITIS

Benjamin D. Spirn

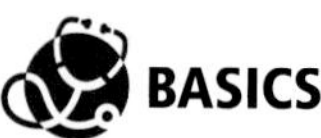

BASICS

DESCRIPTION
- Endophthalmitis is a serious intraocular inflammatory reaction marked by inflammation of intraocular fluid and tissues.
  - Infectious causes of endophthalmitis may be classified as postoperative, posttraumatic, or endogenous.
  - Noninfectious causes of endophthalmitis may clinically mimic infectious cases (e.g., sterile endophthalmitis).

EPIDEMIOLOGY
Incidence
- Varies by cause: Postoperative 75% of cases, posttraumatic 20%, endogenous 5%.
- Postoperative endophthalmitis incidence ranges from approximately 0.05–0.16% of cataract cases.

Prevalence
Endophthalmitis occurs in approximately 1500 patients in the United States per year.

RISK FACTORS
- Postoperative: Recent ocular surgery, prolonged ocular surgery, wound leak, open posterior capsule, vitreous incarceration to wound.
- Posttraumatic: recent penetrating eye trauma, intraocular foreign body, vegetable matter in wound, delayed presentation.
- Endogenous: Immunocompromised patients, indwelling catheters, intravenous drug use

GENERAL PREVENTION
- Patient's own external bacterial flora from conjunctiva and ocular adnexa are most likely culprits.
- Preoperative preparation with 5% povidone–iodine solution reduces risk from own bacteria flora.
- Intracameral injection of cefuroxime may reduce the incidence of postcataract endophthalmitis.

PATHOPHYSIOLOGY
- Initial infiltration of vitreous by infectious organism is followed by invasion of ocular tissue by polymorphonucleocytes within 24 h.
- Significant photoreceptor damage by 48 h.
- Experimental models of bacterial and fungal endophthalmitis have shown tissue damage continues to occur after organisms are able to be isolated from vitreous cavity; thus, implicating endotoxin in disease progression.

ETIOLOGY
Bacterial or fungal infection of vitreous cavity.

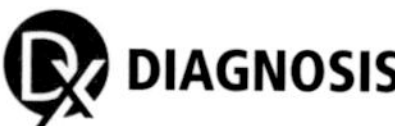

DIAGNOSIS

HISTORY
- Ocular pain.
- Loss of vision.
- Red eye.
- History of recent ocular surgery, trauma, hospitalization, IV drug use.

PHYSICAL EXAM
- Exogenous cases are typically unilateral, endogenous cases may be bilateral.
- Ocular findings may include the following:
  - Adnexal swelling.
  - Conjunctival chemosis and injection.
  - Corneal edema.
  - Hypopyon.
  - Anterior chamber fibrin.
  - Infiltrated conjunctival bleb.
  - Vitreitis.
  - Reduced view of retina.

DIAGNOSTIC TESTS & INTERPRETATION
Lab
Initial lab tests

Blood and urine cultures may be useful in suspected cases of endogenous endophthalmitis where the underlying source in not apparent.

Follow-up & special considerations
- Careful history and physical examination important for identifying source in endogenous cases.
- Consider echocardiogram to rule out endocarditis in patients with endogenous endophthalmitis.

Imaging
B-scan ultrasound to evaluate vitreous cavity for vitreitis.

Diagnostic Procedures/Other
- Vitreous tap (0.5 cc) for gram stain, culture, KOH prep, and fungal culture.
- Consider vitrectomy with vitreous tap in patients with nondiagnostic tap.

Pathological Findings
- Coagulase negative bacteria followed by *S. aureus* are the most common cause of endophthalmitis.
- Endogenous cases may also be associated with fungal infection (approx 50% of cases). *Candida albicans* and Aspergillus are the predominant species.

DIFFERENTIAL DIAGNOSIS
- Sterile endophthalmitis.
- Noninfectious posterior uveitis: Sarcoidosis, pars planitis.
- Infectious posterior uveitis: Toxoplasmosis, Toxocara, syphilis.
  - Other causes of postoperative inflammation: Sympathetic ophthalmia, Phacoanaphylactic uveitis.

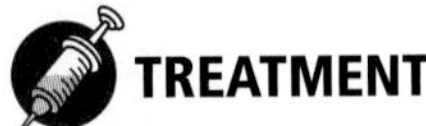

TREATMENT

MEDICATION

First Line

- Intravitreal antibiotic injections to empirically treat Gram-positive and Gram-negative bacteria.
- Intravitreal antifungal medications in patients with endogenous disease.
- Intravitreal steroid injections to reduce inflammatory response.
  - Ceftazidime 2.25 mg in 0.1 mL.
  - Vancomycin 1.0 mg in 0.1 mL.
  - Dexamethasone 0.4 mg in 0.1 mL.

Second Line

- Patients presenting with light perception vision should be treated initially with vitrectomy, vitreous tap, and intravitreal antibiotics.
- Patients who do not respond adequately to initial injection of intravitreal antibiotics with 48 h should undergo either additional injection or vitrectomy.
- Fortified topical antibiotics may be used in addition.
  - Vancomycin 50 mg/mL every hour.
  - Ceftazidime 100 mg/mL every hour.

ADDITIONAL TREATMENT

General Measures

Patients with endogenous endophthalmitis will need complete evaluation by infectious disease specialist to diagnose and treat underlying disease source (e.g., Abscess, endocarditis, sepsis).

Issues for Referral

- All patients require evaluation and treatment by an ophthalmologist/retinal specialist.
- Patients require close daily re-evaluation until stabilization is achieved.

Additional Therapies

Patient may require delayed vitrectomy to treat nonclearing vitreous debris.

SURGERY/OTHER PROCEDURES

- Initial treatment with vitreous tap and injection of intravitreal antibiotics is recommended for postop patients presenting with vision of hand-motions or better.
- Initial pars plana vitrectomy with injection of intravitreal antibiotics is recommended for postop patients presenting with vision of light perception.

IN-PATIENT CONSIDERATIONS

Initial Stabilization

- Complete history and examination.
- Complete eye exam including dilated ophthalmoscopy.

Admission Criteria

While most commonly treated in the outpatient setting, hospital admission should be considered for patients unable to care for their condition as outpatient or unable to comply with close daily observation.

Discharge Criteria

- Hospital discharge should be considered once clinical stabilization has occurred.
  - Improving vision.
  - Resolving hypopyon and vitreitis.

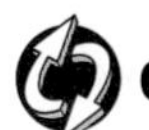

ONGOING CARE

FOLLOW-UP RECOMMENDATIONS

Patient Monitoring

Patients will require close daily observation until clinical stabilization has been achieved.

PATIENT EDUCATION

Patients should be instructed to urgently contact their physician with any sign of disease progression (e.g., worsening redness, pain, or decline in vision).

PROGNOSIS

This remains a serious ocular condition with a significant possibility of vision loss and permanent blindness. However, with prompt diagnosis and treatment, vision can be saved with promising long-term visual results.

COMPLICATIONS

- Retinal detachment.
- Phthisis.

REFERENCES

1. Endophthalmitis Vitrectomy Study Group. Results of the Endophthalmitis Vitrectomy Study. A randomized trial of immediate vitrectomy and of intravenous antibiotics for the treatment of postoperative bacterial endophthalmitis. *Arch Ophthalmol* 1995;113:1479–1496.
2. Barry P, Seal DV, Gettinby G. ESCRS Study of Prophylaxis of Postoperative Endophthalmitis after Cataract Surgery. Preliminary Report of Principal Results from a European Multicenter Study. *J Cataract Refract Surg* 2006;32:407–410.
3. Lemley CA, Han DP. Endophthalmitis: A review of current evaluation and management. *Retina* 2007;27:662–680.

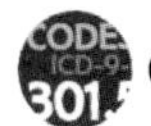

CODES

ICD9

- 360.01 Acute endophthalmitis
- 360.19 Other endophthalmitis

E

ENOPHTHALMOS

Katherine Gold
Jacqueline R. Carrasco

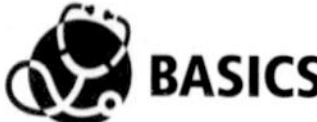

BASICS

DESCRIPTION

- Enophthalmos is a descriptive term and condition referring to the posterior recession of the normal-sized globe within the orbit.
- Acquired or congenital.

PATHOPHYSIOLOGY

- Congenital type is due to fetal/embryologic maldevelopment.
- Acquired.
  - Mechanical pull of orbital contents by fibrous contracture.
  - Enlargement of orbit or lack of support by orbital floor may cause enophthalmos with hypoglobus.

ETIOLOGY

- 3 categories: Structural abnormality, fat atrophy, and traction.
- Orbital floor fracture.
- Postsurgical (s/p decompression or mass resection).
- Scirrhous breast carcinoma metastatic to the orbit.
- Orbital fat atrophy (such as that secondary to radiation or wasting syndromes, among others).
- Silent sinus syndrome.
- Orbital venous malformation (due to bone erosion or fat atrophy).
- Duane retraction syndrome.
- Reported cases due to inflammatory conditions and after CSF shunting procedure.

COMMONLY ASSOCIATED CONDITIONS

See Etiology section.

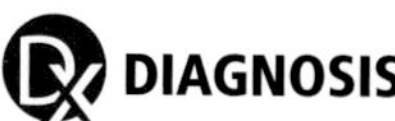

DIAGNOSIS

HISTORY

- Patient may report sinking in of eyeball, unilateral or bilateral, over time or may note a droopy lid.
- May have old photographs for comparison.

PHYSICAL EXAM

- Superior sulcus deepened.
- Narrowed palpebral fissure.
- Hertel exophthalmometry to establish baseline or chart progression, may not be helpful in diagnosis if bilateral.
- Skin changes—thinned if wasting syndrome, thickened in scirrhous carcinoma.
- Motility or sensation may be affected if the etiology is fracture.
- Check vision and for afferent papillary defect to evaluate concomitant optic neuropathy.

DIAGNOSTIC TESTS & INTERPRETATION

Diagnostic Procedures/Other

- CT scan of orbits with coronal and axial cuts.
- If concern for inflammatory cause or malignancy, MRI with and without gadolinium and fat suppression.
- May need orbitotomy for tissue biopsy.

DIFFERENTIAL DIAGNOSIS

- Pseudo-enophthalmos.
  - Contralateral exophthalmos.
  - Horner syndrome.
  - Phthisis bulbi.
  - Microphthalmos.

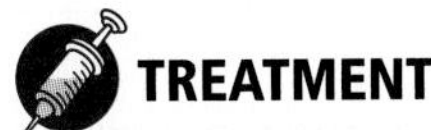

TREATMENT

ADDITIONAL TREATMENT

General Measures

- Depending on etiology.
  - Fracture repair.
  - Oncologic evaluation for treatment of metastatic carcinoma.
  - Orbital soft tissue replacement with filler material, such as porous implant, hyaluronic acid, polyacrylamide gel injection.
  - Sinus aeration with functional endoscopic sinus surgery if suspect silent sinus syndrome.

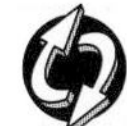

ONGOING CARE

FOLLOW-UP RECOMMENDATIONS

Patient Monitoring

- Ophthalmologist.
- Otolaryngologist for sinus pathology.

PATIENT EDUCATION

If the cause is orbital fracture or unknown, no nose-blowing or sneezing with mouth closed.

COMPLICATIONS

If chronic, may be difficult or impossible to correct fully.

ADDITIONAL READING

- Athanasiov PA, Prabhakaran VC, Selva D. Non-traumatic enophthalmos: A review. *Acta Ophthalmol* 2008;86(4):356–364.
- Bernardini FP, Rose GE, Cruz AA, Priolo E. Gross enophthalmos after cerebrospinal fluid shunting for childhood hydrocephalus: The "silent brain syndrome." *Ophthal Plast Reconstr Surg* 2009; 25(6):434–436.
- Hamedani M, Pournaras JA, Goldblum D. Diagnosis and management of enophthalmos. *Surv Ophthalmol* 2007;52(5):457–473.

CODES

ICD9

- 376.50 Enophthalmos, unspecified as to cause
- 376.51 Enophthalmos due to atrophy of orbital tissue
- 376.52 Enophthalmos due to trauma or surgery

CLINICAL PEARLS

- Enophthalmos with lid retraction may be a sign of silent sinus syndrome.

E

ENTROPION

Thaddeus S. Nowinski

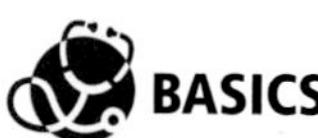

BASICS

DESCRIPTION
- Inward rotation of the eyelid margin, allowing the eyelashes and skin to abrade the globe.
- Types:
  - Congenital.
  - Involutional (most common)(1)[C].
  - Spastic.
  - Cicatricial.

EPIDEMIOLOGY
Incidence
- Involutional—increases with age.
- Spastic—temporary secondary to trauma, ocular irritation, blepharospasm.
  - Cicatricial—ocular cicatricial pemphigoid (OCP)—females > males
  - Average age 60–70 years.

Prevalence
Cicatricial—OCP—1 in 15,000–20,000.

RISK FACTORS
Genetics
OCP–associated with HLA–DQB7*301.

PATHOPHYSIOLOGY
- Increased orbicularis muscle tone and override secondary to loss of adhesions to orbital septum.
- Thinning/dehiscence of lower lid retractors.
- Horizontal laxity.
- Atrophied tarsal plates.

ETIOLOGY
- Dipivefrin, practolol, pilocarpine, timolol, echothiophate, iodide, epinephrine eye drops.
- OCP—a systemic autoimmune pemphigoid disorder that has ocular and nonocular manifestations.
  - OCP thought to be a type 2 hypersensitivity reaction, genetically predisposed.

COMMONLY ASSOCIATED CONDITIONS
- Cicatricial.
- OCP
- Stevens–Johnson (erythema multiforme major).
- Trachoma.
- Trauma.
- Chemical burns.
- Chronic topical medications.

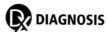

DIAGNOSIS

HISTORY
- Foreign body sensation.
- Tearing.
- Redness.

PHYSICAL EXAM
- Redness of conjunctiva.
- Inverted eyelid margin.
- Thickened muscle band of orbicularis muscle.
- Lashes abrading globe.
- Superficial punctuate keratopathy, corneal abrasion.
- Corneal scarring, thinning, or ulceration, vascularization in severe cases.
- Symblepharon—cicatricial—linear scar/fold of palpebral conjunctiva to bulbar conjunctiva, shortening of fornix.
  - Scarring of upper eyelid tarsal conjunctiva on eyelid eversion (trachoma).

DIAGNOSTIC TESTS & INTERPRETATION
Lab
Initial lab tests
- None.
- OCP—ANA.

Follow-up & special considerations
- OCP—elevated soluble CD 8 glycoprotein, elevated tumor necrosis factor.

Diagnostic Procedures/Other
Cicatricial—conjunctival biopsy.

Pathological Findings
- Cicatricial—ANA
- OCP—biopsy of conjunctiva for direct immunofluorescence studies or indirect immunofluorescence for presence of antibodies—positive in >80%.

DIFFERENTIAL DIAGNOSIS
- Epiblepharon.
- Trichiasis.
- Distichiasis.

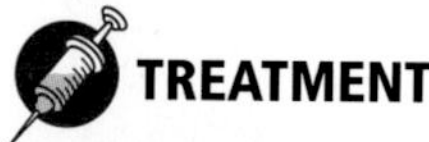

TREATMENT

MEDICATION
- Topical lubrication.
  - Frequent artificial tears, ophthalmic lubricating ointment.

ADDITIONAL TREATMENT
General Measures
Taping of lower eyelid skin to cheek.

Issues for Referral
- Decreased vision.
- Pain.

Additional Therapies

OCP—prednisone, dapsone, methotrexate, cyclophosphamide, CellCept, doxycycline (2)[C].

SURGERY/OTHER PROCEDURES

- Surgical treatment is almost always necessary, timing depends on corneal health.
- Suture repair—may be done bedside—highest recurrence rate.
- Outpatient eyelid surgery, including horizontal tightening, lower lid retractor tightening, orbicularis muscle stabilization or marginal rotation (3)[C].

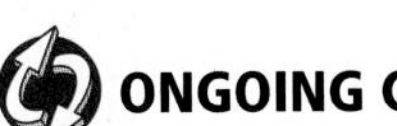

ONGOING CARE

FOLLOW-UP RECOMMENDATIONS

Ophthalmologist 1 week to monitor cornea.

Patient Monitoring

Warning signs: Pain, redness, tearing, photophobia.

PATIENT EDUCATION

Ocular cicatricial pemphigoid also be present in other mucous membranes.

PROGNOSIS

- Most patients require surgical repair.
- Ocular cicatricial pemphigoid is characterized by remissions and exacerbations and regardless of therapy can lead to loss of vision.

COMPLICATIONS

ALERT

Corneal abrasion, ulcer, scarring, perforation, loss of eye.

REFERENCES

1. Heimmel M, Enzer Y, Hoffman R. Entropion-ectropion: The influence of axial globe projection on lower eyelid malposition. *Ophthal Plast Reconstr Surg* 2009;25:7–9.
2. Neff AG, Turner M, Mutasim DF. Treatment strategies in mucous membrane pemphigoid. *Ther Clin Risk Manag* 2008;4:617–626.
3. Bieyen I, Dolman PJ. The Wies procedure for management of trichiasis or cicatricial entropion of either upper or lower eyelids2009;93:1612–1615.

ADDITIONAL READING

- Foster CS, Chang PY, Ahmed AR. Combination of rituximab and intravenous immunoglobulin for recalcitrant ocular cicatricial pemphigoid. *Ophthalmology* 2010;117:861–869.
- Hatton M, Raizman M, Foster CS. Exacerbation of undiagnosed ocular cicatricial pemphigoid after repair of involutional entropion. *Ophthal Plast Reconstr Surg* 2008;24:165–166.
- Scheepers MA, Singh R, Ng J, et al. A randomized controlled trial comparing everting sutures and a lateral tarsal strip for involutional entropion. *Ophthalmology* 2010;117:352–355.
- Shiu M, McNab A. Cicatricial entropion and trichiasis in an urban Australian population. *Clin Exp Ophthalmol* 2005;33:582–585.
- Wu AY, Thakker MM, Wladis EJ, et al. Eyelash resection procedure for severe, recurrent, or segmental cicatricial entropion. *Ophthal Plast Reconstr Surg* 2010;26:112–116.

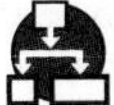

See Also (Topic, Algorithm, Electronic Media Element)

- www.asoprs.org
- Topic:
  - Trichiasis
  - Ocular cicatricial Pemphigoid
  - Trachoma
- Figure – Involutional entropion

CODES

ICD9

- 374.00 Entropion, unspecified
- 374.01 Senile entropion
- 743.62 Congenital deformities of eyelids

CLINICAL PEARLS

- Entropion if untreated may lead to corneal scarring, infection and permanent loss of vision.
- Cicatricial entropion may be associated with a severe autoimmune disorder.
- Trachoma should be suspected in appropriate patients with cicatricial entropion, especially of the upper eyelid.

EPIPHORA

Scott M. Goldstein

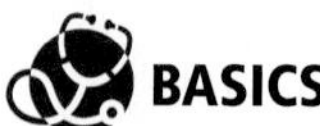

BASICS

DESCRIPTION

Epiphora, or tearing, represents an imbalance between tear production and tear drainage. The lacrimal gland and accessory tear glands produce tears while the nasolacrimal drain carries the tears form the ocular surface down into the nose. An overproduction from ocular irritation will cause tearing as will a blockage of the drainage system.

EPIDEMIOLOGY

- This can occur in patients of any age, but there is typically a bimodal distribution, in infancy and late adulthood. In infants, tearing most commonly represents a blocked tear duct, which occurs in about 5% of all babies. Fortunately, 90% of these resolve by age 1.
- In the adult population, tearing is a much more common problem, often from a dry eye. This is more common in women, especially postmenopause.

PATHOPHYSIOLOGY

- In normal patients, aqueous tears are produced by the lacrimal glands, which mix with sebaceous secretions and mucus, to lubricate the eye. The force of blinking, with a negative pressure within the tear drain on opening the lids, pulls the tears off the ocular surface down the drain and into the nose. Any imbalance along this pathway can result in tearing.
- Congenital obstruction occurs from incomplete canalization of the nasolacrimal duct during embryogenesis.
- Adults with tearing most often have a dry eye or an unstable tear film that leads to ocular irritation and secondary reflexive tearing, which is intermittently symptomatic. The imbalance can occur from associated blepharitis with poor sebaceous secretions from the eyelid or decreased aqueous tear production.
- Ocular surface irritation from trichiasis, entropion, a foreign body, keratitis, uveitis, or conjunctivitis can all cause reflexive tearing acutely.
- Lower lid laxity, with or without frank ectropion, can limit the normal tear pump mechanism.
- Acquired obstructions occur from progressive narrowing anywhere along the course of the drain. This usually results secondarily from infection, inflammation, or trauma. These patients typically have constant tearing. Certain chemotherapeutics can also cause stenosis.

ETIOLOGY

Again, a multitude of things can trigger tearing. Over production of tears occurs from irritation of the ocular surface while a blockage of the drain leads to poor drainage.

COMMONLY ASSOCIATED CONDITIONS

Blepharitis, trichiasis, entropion, ectropion, dry eye, tear drain obstruction, ocular surface inflammation, foreign body.

DIAGNOSIS

HISTORY

- Infants most commonly present with constant tearing in 1 or both eyes that starts shortly after birth and continues constantly. They often awake from naps and bedtime, which crusting on the lashes. Finally, symptoms are often worse with nasal congestion.
- In adults with dry eye, the symptoms have an insidious onset with intermittent symptoms. The tearing is typically worse with activities that require more concentration, and thus less blinking, such as reading, watching TV, using a computer, and driving. Cold, windy weather also exacerbates symptoms.
- In the adult patient with a poor tear pump or blocked drain, the symptoms are more constant.
- Patients with acquired obstruction may have a history of eye infection, dacryocystitis, or trauma to the drain system, but not always.

PHYSICAL EXAM

- Examine tear film for quality and quantity.
- Lid anatomy and position, looking specifically for misdirected lashes, entropion, ectropion, lower lid laxity. Also, they may have macerated skin in the lower lid from chronically being moist.
- Ocular surface exam looking for evidence of dry eye, foreign body, conjunctivitis, or keratitis.
- Examine tear drainage both functionally and physically with evaluation of the puncta, canaliculi, and irrigation down the nasolacrimal duct. Palpation of the lacrimal sac is important if a distal obstruction of the drain is suspected.

DIAGNOSTIC TESTS & INTERPRETATION

- Dye disappearance test: Fluorescein is applied to the conjunctival cul de sac, and the patient is observed for 5 min.
  - In a negative test (normal), the tear meniscus will become relatively unstained as the tears naturally flow down through the drainage system. Dye can sometimes be found in the nose.
  - In a positive test (abnormal), the height of the stained tear meniscus will increase owing to the obstructed lacrimal system.
  - No change in the tear meniscus can be encountered with either an obstructed drain or a dry eye where there are not enough tears to wash the dye down the drain.
- Schirmer testing of tear production. This is best done with topical anesthesia of the eye to measure basal tear secretion alone. Less then 5 mm of wetting in 5 min is considered dry. 5–10 mm is borderline and greater then 10 mm is normal.

Lab

Follow-up & special considerations

Sjögren antibodies—if the patient is a young adult or is middle aged and has a dry mouth or other rheumatologic symptoms.

Diagnostic Procedures/Other

- Dacryocystogram can be helpful in differentiating between poor tear pumping versus obstruction of the tear drain.
- Lacrimal scintigraphy can also be performed on occasion to evaluate drainage form the eye into the nose, but is rarely done in children.
- CT scan be obtained if there is a concern of a nasolacrimal cyst or dacryocele, or tumor in the lacrimal sac.
- In teenagers and adults, in office irrigation of lacrimal system at the level of the canaliculus can be used diagnostically to evaluate for obstruction within the drain system.

Pathological Findings

- Intrapalpebral punctuate staining of the cornea and conjunctiva is seen with moderate-to-severe dry eye.
- A distended lacrimal sac, which extrudes purulent debris from the puncta with manual pressure, is indicative of a chronic dacryocystitis and blocked nasolacrimal duct.

DIFFERENTIAL DIAGNOSIS

- Children (chronic) congenital obstruction of nasolacrimal duct, congenital glaucoma, epiblepharon.
- Children (acute) conjunctivitis foreign body, keratitis.
- Adult (chronic) dry eye, acquired nasolacrimal duct obstruction, ectropion, entropion, trichiasis, old facial palsy.
- Adult (acute) conjunctivitis, keratitis, uveitis, foreign body, cranial nerve 7 palsy.

Geriatric Considerations

Tearing in this age group is usually intermittent and often represents a dry eye that becomes irritated and secondarily waters.

Pediatric Considerations

In this age group, the most common diagnoses are a congenitally blocked tear duct and infection. Don't overlook infantile glaucoma, but this is relatively uncommon by comparison.

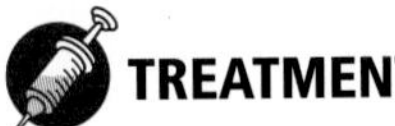

TREATMENT

MEDICATION

First Line

- Pediatric (chronic)—topical antibiotic ointment (erythromycin, bacitracin, polysporin) PRN if significant discharge and crusting.
- Adult (chronic)—artificial tears drops.
- Acute pediatric and adult epiphora—treat underlying issue such as removal of foreign body, topical antibiotics for bacterial conjunctivitis or keratitis, removal of irritating lashes with trichiasis.

Second Line

Adult (chronic)—topical cyclosporin eyedrops b.i.d., topical steroid eyedrops for short-term treatment of chronic ocular inflammation.

ADDITIONAL TREATMENT

General Measures

- Punctal occlusion if dry eye present.
- Punctoplasty for punctual stenosis.

Issues for Referral

Acute dacryocystitis, especially in infants.

COMPLEMENTARY & ALTERNATIVE THERAPIES

Pediatric tearing from congenital obstruction can be treated with daily massage over the lacrimal sac, hoping to help open the obstruction distally.

SURGERY/OTHER PROCEDURES

- Pediatric—probing and irrigation, P & I with stenting of tear drain, balloon dacryoplasty, dacryocystorhinostomy, conjunctivodacryocystorhinostomy.
- Adult (blocked tear drain)—Punctoplasty, P & I with stenting or balloon dacryoplasty, dacryocystorhinostomy, conjunctivodacryocystorhinostomy.
- Adult (lid malposition)—entropion repair, ectropion repair, horizontal lid tightening for pump failure.

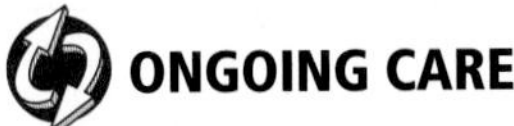

ONGOING CARE

FOLLOW-UP RECOMMENDATIONS

- Infants can be followed conservatively during the 1st year of life. If they fail to resolve by age 1 year, surgery should be scheduled at this time.
- Adults can be followed as needed depending on the severity of their symptoms. Chronic dry eye and blepharitis patients can be seen with their routine care. Lid malposition and nasolacrimal obstruction patients should be scheduled for surgery and seen postoperatively to ensure resolution.

DIET

Fish oil, flax seed, and other sources of omega-3 fatty acids can improve tear film stability in adult patients with dry eyes.

PATIENT EDUCATION

- For pediatric patients, instruct parents on proper nasolacrimal massaging technique.
- For adult patients with chronic blepharitis, daily lid scrub can be helpful usinga warm wash cloth.

PROGNOSIS

- Pediatric cases—excellent.
- Adult cases—mixed depending on underlying etiology. Chronic dry eye and blepharitis patients will tend to have intermittent chronic symptoms. Patients with nasolacrimal duct obstruction do well after DCR surgery.

REFERENCE

1. Katowitz JA, Goldstein, SM, Kherani F, Lowe J. Lacrimal drainage surgery. *Duane's Ophthalmology*, Tasman & Jaeger, eds,2005.

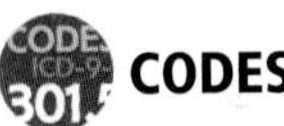

CODES

ICD9

- 375.20 Epiphora, unspecified as to cause
- 375.21 Epiphora due to excess lacrimation
- 375.22 Epiphora due to insufficient drainage

E

EPIRETINAL MEMBRANES

Magdalena F. Shuler

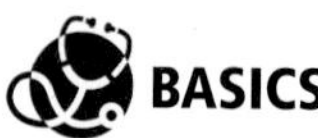

BASICS

DESCRIPTION

- Epiretinal membranes are also known as macular pucker, cellophane maculopathy, and surface wrinkling retinopathy.
- It is a thin layer of tissue found on the surface of the retina.
- It can cause distortion of the retina and lead to decreased vision.
  - It is associated with abnormal vitreous separation and sometimes presents with vitreomacular traction.

Geriatric Considerations

Epiretinal membranes (ERM) most commonly occur in the elderly population.

Pediatric Considerations

Very uncommon as a primary diagnosis. Most likely associated with other conditions that can cause macular dragging and ERM formation due to glial abnormalities/proliferation and traction.

Pregnancy Considerations

Intervention and full evaluation can usually be postponed until after the birth of the infant.

EPIDEMIOLOGY

Incidence

- ERM is a common condition that is usually benign and causes no visual symptoms and does not require surgery.
- Although bilateral in 20–30% of cases, it is often asymmetric.

Prevalence

- Most likely to be found in patients over 50 years old.
- ERMs occur in 2% of eyes in patients aged 50 years, and the prevalence increases to 20% of eyes at 75 years of age.

RISK FACTORS

- Gender (women).
- Elderly.
- History of retinal laser, ocular surgery, or trauma.
- Diabetes.
- Retinal vascular conditions.
- History of vitreous hemorrhage.
- History of intraocular inflammation.

Genetics

No genetic predisposition.

PATHOPHYSIOLOGY

- ERM forms due to an abnormal proliferation of glial cells (primarily fibrous astrocytes but also Muller cells, fibrocytes, myofibroblasts, macrophages, and hyalocytes) on the surface of the retina.
- Glial cells usually access the retinal surface following a posterior vitreous detachment (PVD) but can also migrate to the retina prior to PVD.
- Traction may result from the cells assuming myofibroblastic properties exerting traction on the retinal collagenous scaffold and ultimately leading to distortion and decreased vision.

ETIOLOGY

- Abnormal cellular proliferation on the surface of the retina causes the visual appearance of an ERM.
  - Primary idiopathic ERM occurs with no history of trauma, surgery, inflammatory disease or other ocular disease.
  - Secondary ERM occurs due to ocular inflammation, trauma, surgery, or retinovascular disease.

COMMONLY ASSOCIATED CONDITIONS

- Diabetes.
- Retinal vascular diseases.
- Ocular inflammation.

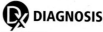

DIAGNOSIS

HISTORY

- Most are asymptomatic.
- Gradual worsening in vision.
- Monocular distortion in linear objects.
- Difficulty reading due to blurry vision.
- Diplopia or central photopsias.

PHYSICAL EXAM

- Biomicroscopic examination reveals the abnormal appearance of the surface of the retina.
- Subtle ERM may only appear like a glinting or irregular light reflex of the fovea.
- A contracting ERM can produce retinal striae due to traction on the internal limiting membrane (ILM).
- Traction results in visible tortuosity of the retinal vessels.
- Occasionally retinal hemorrhages, cotton wool spots, and commonly macular edema are visible.

DIAGNOSTIC TESTS & INTERPRETATION

Lab

Initial lab tests

No laboratory studies are needed to diagnose routine ERM.

Follow-up & special considerations

Amsler grid testing is useful in determining the symptomatic nature of the ERM.

Imaging

Initial approach

- Optical coherence tomography (OCT) can be useful to show objective evidence of retinal surface disease and underlying macular edema.
- OCT can also show abnormalities in retinal architecture such as edema and cystoid changes.
  - ERM associated with significant CME may confer a poor visual prognosis.

Follow-up & special considerations

- Asymptomatic patients can be observed.
- Counseling patients in the use of Amsler grid.
- Prompt re-evaluation for worsening of symptoms is warranted since surgical intervention prior to induced abnormalities in retinal architecture confers a better ultimate visual prognosis.

Diagnostic Procedures/Other

- Fluorescein angiography (FA) is useful to evaluate the retina for any underlying retinovascular diseases and evaluating for macular leakage.
  - Significant vascular leakage or capillary nonperfusion helps in counseling patients about decreased visual prognosis following surgery.

Pathological Findings

- Extensive cystoid macular edema confers a poor visual prognosis after surgical intervention.
- Thin and irregular photoreceptor layers can be visualized on spectral domain-OCT (SD-OCT).

DIFFERENTIAL DIAGNOSIS

- Fibrotic fronds from proliferative diabetic retinopathy or ischemic vein occlusions.
- Incomplete partial posterior vitreous detachment with adherent posterior hyaloid.

TREATMENT

MEDICATION

First Line

When associated with idiopathic edema, topical steroids, topical NSAIDs or subtenon injection of triamcinolone can be considered.

Second Line

Not usually treated with any other medications.

ADDITIONAL TREATMENT

General Measures

Presence of an ERM does not require surgical intervention unless there are significant symptoms or worsening retinal appearance on OCT.

Issues for Referral

Patients who are symptomatic should be referred to a vitreoretinal surgeon for evaluation.

Additional Therapies

Underlying associated conditions such as age-related macular degeneration and diabetes should be addressed prior to entertaining surgical intervention.

COMPLEMENTARY & ALTERNATIVE THERAPIES

- When associated with cystoid edema of the retina, primary treatment to the underlying edema can be considered.
- Current clinical trials are studying the effect of intravitreal injection causing medical vitreolysis to facilitate the release of focal vitreomacular traction. (1)[A].

SURGERY/OTHER PROCEDURES

- Vitrectomy surgery with membrane peel is recommended for patients who are symptomatic from visual distortion or with vision worse than 20/40.
- Some vitreoretinal surgeons advocate attempted removal of the ILM during ERM removal to decrease the chance for recurrent ERM formation (2)[B], (3)[B].
  - Recent advances in minimally invasive vitrectomy systems have led to quicker visual recovery and higher patient satisfaction.

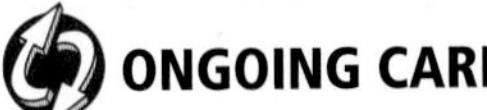

ONGOING CARE

FOLLOW-UP RECOMMENDATIONS

- Depending on underlying disease and appearance, routine follow-up is needed.
- Patients without symptoms can be observed.
- Initial timely follow-up is indicated but if no symptoms occur, follow-up can be extended.
- ERM can commonly stay dormant for many years; however acute PVD or surgery may incite contraction and cause symptoms.

Patient Monitoring

- Amsler grid monitoring is essential.
- Distortions in vision should warrant re-evaluation.

DIET

No specific diet is recommended.

PATIENT EDUCATION

- Amsler grid testing is imperative to follow the severity of distortion.
- Any new symptom should warrant re-evaluation.

PROGNOSIS

- Asymptomatic ERM that are observed and do not require intervention have an excellent visual prognosis.
- Symptomatic ERM that require surgery usually results in visual improvement with 80–90% improving 2 or more Snellen lines.
- Most patients can regain half of the vision lost due to the ERM distortion.
  - ERM surgery usually results in greatly diminished metamorphopsia, however few eyes will regain 20/20.
  - Preoperative vision is a good indicator of postoperative visual prognosis.

COMPLICATIONS

- Cataract formation: Most common.
- Peripheral retinal breaks:
  - 1–6%.
  - As high as 13.9% in recent study of 20 gauge vitrectomy (4)[C].
- Retinal detachment: 1–7%.
- Recurrent ERM: 0–5%.
- Retinal phototoxicity.
- Endophthalmitis is rare.

REFERENCES

1. MIVI TRUST Clinical Trial, Phase III study for focal VMT using microplasmin for intravitreal injection-traction release without surgical treatment, Thrombogenics. 2010
2. Shimada H, Nakashizuka H, Hattori T, Mori R, Mizutani Y, Yuzawa M. Double staining with brilliant blue G and double peeling for epiretinal membranes. *Ophthalmology* 2009 Jul; 116(7):1370-6.
3. Kwok A, Lai TY, Yuen KS. Epiretinal membrane surgery with or without internal limiting membrane peeling. *Clin Exp Ophthalmol*. 2005 Aug:33(4); 379-85.
4. Ramkissoon YD, Aslam SA, Shah SP, Wong SC, Sullivna PM. Risk of Iatrogenic Peripheral Retinal Breaks in 20-G Pars Plana Vitrectomy. *Ophthalmology* 2010 May 13 [E-pub ahead of print]

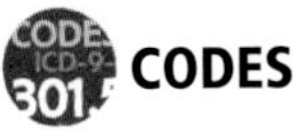

CODES

ICD9

362.56 Macular puckering of retina

CLINICAL PEARLS

- Most ERMs are asymptomatic.
- Symptomatic ERMs should be evaluated by a vitreoretinal surgeon for possible surgical intervention.

EPISCLERITIS

Vasudha A. Panday

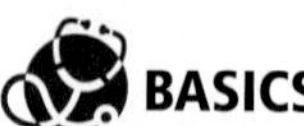

BASICS

DESCRIPTION

- An inflammatory condition, usually mild and self-limiting, although it can be recurrent.
  - Usually affects females, usually seen in young adults, up to 30% may have underlying systemic condition.
  - Simple: Intermittent episodes of inflammation that resolve in 2–3 weeks.
  - Nodular: Prolonged attacks, more painful, usually solitary nodule. Associated systemic disease more likely.

EPIDEMIOLOGY

Incidence

Difficult to determine, most patients do not seek medical attention (1).

Prevalence

Unknown.

RISK FACTORS

- Underlying systemic condition such as collagen vascular disease (rheumatoid arthritis, lupus, etc.) (1)
  - Can be associated with infection such as Lyme disease, syphilis.
  - Stress, hormonal changes may be associated.

PATHOPHYSIOLOGY

Not clearly understood, thought to be an inflammatory response to an inciting event.

ETIOLOGY

- Idiopathic
- Underlying systemic condition or infection

COMMONLY ASSOCIATED CONDITIONS

- Collagen vascular diseases
- Gout
- Herpes zoster or simplex
- Rosacea

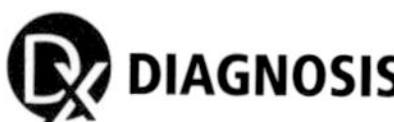

DIAGNOSIS

HISTORY

Acute onset of redness, irritation, tearing; can be diffuse or sectorial.

PHYSICAL EXAM

- Sectorial or diffuse hyperemia, or localized injected nodule over bulbar conjunctiva seen at slit-lamp examination
- Area of injection or nodule can be freely moved over sclera using cotton tip applicator after topical anesthesia.
- 10% may have associated anterior uveitis.

DIAGNOSTIC TESTS & INTERPRETATION

Lab

Initial lab tests

- Topical 2.5% phenylephrine will blanch inflamed vessels in simple episcleritis (2)[C].
- Additional systemic testing dependent on review of systems.

Follow-up & special considerations

If severe, recurrent, or nodular episcleritis, check serum uric acid, CBC with differential, ANA, RF, ESR, CXR, VDRL, and FTA-ABS.

Pathological Findings

Histopathology shows nongranulomatous inflammation with vascular dilatation and perivascular infiltrates of lymphocytes and plasma cells.

DIFFERENTIAL DIAGNOSIS

- Bacterial or viral conjunctivitis
- Scleritis
- Pingueculitis

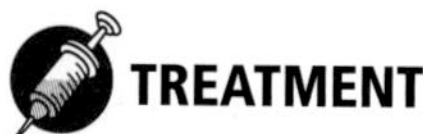

TREATMENT

MEDICATION

First Line

Artificial tears, cool compresses at least 4 times a day.

Second Line

Short course of topical antihistamine or NSAID 2–4 times a day.

ADDITIONAL TREATMENT

General Measures

- Oral NSAID for moderate to severe cases (e.g., indomethacin 75—100 mg per day) (3)[C]
  - Short course of topical steroid 4 times a day

Geriatric Considerations

Side effects of long term topical steroid use include cataract formation and glaucoma.

Pediatric Considerations

Side effects of long term topical steroid use include cataract formation and glaucoma.

Pregnancy Considerations

Topical NSAIDs and steroids are class C and of unknown safety in lactation.

Issues for Referral

Associated corneal changes, resistant to treatment, recurrent.

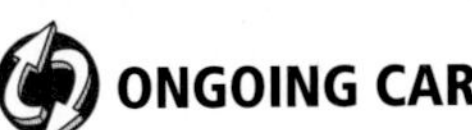

ONGOING CARE

FOLLOW-UP RECOMMENDATIONS

Follow up for recurrent episodes.

Patient Monitoring

Usually self-limiting condition.

PROGNOSIS

Favorable to good.

REFERENCES

1. Akpek EK, Uy H, Christen W, et al. Severity of episcleritis and systemic disease association. *Ophthalmology* 1999;106:729–731.
2. Okhravi N, Odufuwa B, McCluskey P, et al. Scleritis. *Surv Ophthalmol* 2005;50:351–363.
3. Jabs DA, Mudun A, Dunn JP, et al. Episcleritis and scleritis: Clinical features and treatment results. *Am J Ophthalmol*. 2000;130:469–476.

ADDITIONAL READING

- Pearlstein ES. Episcleritis. In Krachmer JH, Mannis MJ, Holland EJ (eds.), *Cornea: Fundamentals, Diagnosis, and Management*, vol 1, 1337–1342.

CODES

ICD9

- 379.00 Scleritis, unspecified
- 379.09 Other scleritis

CLINICAL PEARLS

- Mild, self-limiting disease, can be recurrent
- Diffuse or sectorial injection
- Nodular type more frequently associated with underlying systemic condition
- 2.5% phenylephrine will blanch the affected vessels in simple episcleritis
- Majority can be treated with artificial tears and cool compresses

ESOTROPIA: COMITANT

Barry N. Wasserman
David R. Lally

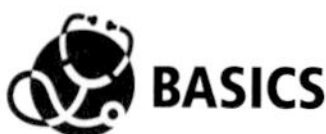

BASICS

DESCRIPTION

- Form of strabismus in which an eye deviates inward toward the nose (formerly called "internal strabismus").
  - Comitant esotropia: Angle of strabismus is similar in all gaze positions.
  - Can be intermittent or constant.
  - Types include accommodative or nonaccommodative, sensory, congenital/infantile non accommodative(see chapter), consecutive after surgery for exotropia, and cyclic
  - Rarely associated with ocular myasthenia, or thyroid eye disease.

EPIDEMIOLOGY

Incidence

1 study found incidence of 111.0 (95% confidence interval, 99.9–122.1) per 100,000 patients younger than 19 years of age. (1).

Prevalence

Approximately 2.0% of all children younger than 6 years (1).

RISK FACTORS

- Poor vision in one or both eyes (sensory esotropia).
- Premature birth.
- Cerebral palsy.
- Seizure disorders.
- Developmental delay.
- Hyperopia.

Genetics

- Likely multifactorial (environmental, polygenic).
- Accommodative esotropia: 23% have affected 1st-degree relative, 91% have any affected relative (2).
  - 1–7% of orthotropic relatives of patients with esotropia have monofixation syndrome.
  - If underlying cause of sensory esotropia then the genetics of that primary disorder may apply although the incidence of esotropia may show variable expression.

GENERAL PREVENTION

- Early correction of significant hyperopia may reduce risk of accommodative esotropia.
  - Compliance with hyperopic correction for accommodative esotropia my prevent secondary nonaccommodative esotropia from developing.
  - Correction of causes of low vision in one or both eyes.

PATHOPHYSIOLOGY

- Most cases have no known pathophysiology attributed to ocular muscles, orbit or cranial nerves.
  - Accommodative esotropia: Increased accommodative effort to overcome hyperopia yields excessive convergence.

ETIOLOGY

- Accommodative esotropia: Etiology related to high hyperopia (3).
  - Acute comitant esotropia: Possible gliomas and other tumors, Chiari type 1 malformations, hydrocephalus, thalamic disease, or seizures.
  - Sensory esotropia: Intraocular pathology including cataract and retinoblastoma.

COMMONLY ASSOCIATED CONDITIONS

- Amblyopia.
  - Refractive error (hyperopia).
  - Latent, manifest latent or manifest (sensory esotropia) nystagmus.
  - Other developmental delays or neurologic disorders, cerebral palsy.

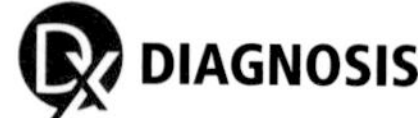

DIAGNOSIS

HISTORY

- Esotropia may start intermittently and then become constant.
- Frequently noticed by parents in pediatric cases.
  - Can present with diplopia in acute cases.
  - History of low vision in one or both eyes.
  - History of neurologic abnormalities or developmental delay.
  - History of prematurity.

PHYSICAL EXAM

- Complete eye examination including cycloplegic refraction (may need atropine for 2–3 days before visit to ensure cycloplegia complete).
  - Stereoacuity testing.
  - Strabismus evaluation including multiple gaze positions and distance and near (ratio of accommodative convergence to accommodation, AC/A ratio).

DIAGNOSTIC TESTS & INTERPRETATION

Lab

- In suspected ocular myasthenia, consider antiacetylcholine receptor antibody titers.
  - In suspected thyroid eye disease, thyroid function studies.

Imaging

- Only done in cases of suspected neurological pathology, consider in cases of acute esotropia or esotropia with other neurologic signs.
  - MRI of head and orbits.

Diagnostic Procedures/Other

Consider tensilon test if myasthenia considered.

DIFFERENTIAL DIAGNOSIS

- Pseudoesotropia: Prominent epicanthal folds that yield the appearance of esotropia when no true deviation is present, positive-angle kappa.
  - Incomitant esotropia (see chapter).
  - Myasthenia gravis.
  - Thyroid eye disease.

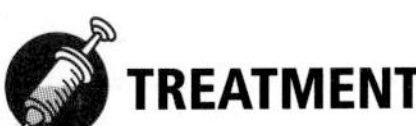

TREATMENT

MEDICATION

First Line

- Oral steroids or Mestinon specifically for myasthenia.
  - Otherwise no medications indicated.

Second Line

Phospholine iodide, an anticholinesterase miotic eye drop, has been used to facilitate accommodation without stimulating convergence.

ADDITIONAL TREATMENT

General Measures

- Glasses or contact lenses for full cycloplegic refraction in cases of accommodative esotropia <4 years old and as tolerated in older children (use of atropine at start of glasses wear may help older child tolerate full hyperopic correction if unable to relax latent hyperopia).
  - Bifocal glasses maybe necessary in cases of high AC/A ratio.

Issues for Referral

- Consider neurosurgery or neurology consultation for cases of suspected intracranial pathology or myasthenia, respectively.
  - Consider orbital specialist for cases of thyroid eye disease.

Additional Therapies

Occlusive therapy with patches or atropine 1% drops for amblyopia as indicated.

COMPLEMENTARY & ALTERNATIVE THERAPIES

Vision therapy is not indicated.

SURGERY/OTHER PROCEDURES

- Strabismus surgery performed in cases of stable nonaccommodative esotropia after other treatments (e.g., glasses for hyperopia in accommodative esotropia) fail to obtain acceptable ocular alignment.
  - Strabismus surgery can be performed on 1 eye (recession/resection) or both eyes (usually bilateral medial rectus recession).

IN-PATIENT CONSIDERATIONS

Initial Stabilization

- Only for cases of intracranial pathology.
  - Strabismus usually outpatient surgery.

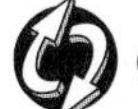

ONGOING CARE

FOLLOW-UP RECOMMENDATIONS

- Follow-up examinations based on findings at each visit.
  - For stable accommodative esotropia, follow up every 3–4 months depending on the stability of the esotropia control to check for ocular alignment and vision. Serial re-evaluation in cases of variable esotropia.

Patient Monitoring

- Patient can note diplopia frequency.
  - Parents can monitor child's alignment.

PATIENT EDUCATION

- Important to differentiate issues of vision (amblyopia) from alignment (strabismus).
  - In adults with intermittent or variable strabismus, important to know time and frequency.
  - Stress importance of glasses wear and in accommodative esotropia that it is "normal" for eye to be esotropic without glasses on.

PROGNOSIS

- Accommodative esotropia: Approximately 1/3 always need hyperopic correction (glasses or contact lenses) for straight eyes, 1/3 "grow out" of need for glasses and maintain straight eyes uncorrected, 1/3 need strabismus surgery for nonaccommodative esotropia.
  - Guarded with acute comitant esotropia—depends on etiology.
  - In cases of cerebral palsy or developmental delay esotropia may increase over time.

COMPLICATIONS

- Amblyopia.
- Surgery for esotropia can result in under- or overcorrections.
  - Strabismus surgery also associated with rare complications including infection, hemorrhage, loss of vision, slipped, or lost muscles.

REFERENCES

1. Louwagie CR, Diehl NN, Greenberg AE, Mohney BG. Is the incidence of infantile esotropia declining? A population-based study from Olmsted County, Minnesota, 1965 to 1994. *Arch Ophthalmol* 2009;127(2):200–203.
2. Birch EE, Fawcett SL, Morale SE, Weakley DR Jr, Wheaton DH. Risk factors for accommodative esotropia among hypermetropic children. *Invest Ophthalmol Vis Sci* 2005;46(2):526–529.
3. Campos EC. Why do the eyes cross? A review and discussion of the nature and origin of essential infantile esotropia, microstrabismus, accommodative esotropia, and acute comitant esotropia. *J AAPOS* 2008;12(4):326–331.

CODES

ICD9

- 378.00 Esotropia, unspecified
- 378.05 Alternating esotropia
- 378.20 Intermittent heterotropia, unspecified

CLINICAL PEARLS

- Must evaluate ocular alignment and motility in multiple gaze positions to assess comitance.
- Full cycloplegic refraction essential in accommodative esotropia.
- Always monitor for amblyopia.

E

ESOTROPIA: INCOMITANT

David R. Lally
Barry N. Wasserman

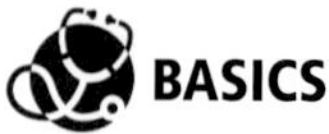

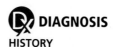

BASICS

DESCRIPTION

- Manifest convergent misalignment of the visual axes that varies quantitatively with different fields of gaze.
- Congenital or acquired

EPIDEMIOLOGY

Incidence

Varies depending on underlying cause, but overall strabismus prevalence (including comitant deviations) is 1–4%.

Prevalence

More common in adults

RISK FACTORS

- Brain injury or increased intracranial pressure
  - Thyroid eye disease
  - Myasthenia gravis
  - Family history or genetic predisposition (isolated or syndromic)
  - Orbital trauma (medial orbital wall fracture, medial fat and fibrous trauma), tumor or infiltration
  - Eye muscle surgery (excessively resected medial rectus muscle or over recessed lateral rectus muscle)
  - Craniofacial disorders

Genetics

- See chapter on craniofacial disorders
- Congenital cranial dysinnervation disorders (CCDD):
  - See chapters on Duane syndrome, Brown syndrome, Moebius syndrome
  - Also Congenital fibrosis of the extraocular muscles (but usually exotropia): CFEOM1 – autosomal dominant, K1F21 A gene (12cen); CFEOM2 – autosomal recessive, ARIX/PHOX2 A (11q13); CFEOM3 – autosomal dominant, TUBB3 (16q24.2–24.3)
  - Also horizontal gaze palsy with progressive scoliosis (HGPPS) – autosomal dominant, ROBO3 (11q23–25)

GENERAL PREVENTION

Genetic counseling

PATHOPHYSIOLOGY

Unbalanced functioning of horizontal rectus muscles whether due to structural muscle change, muscle restriction, or muscle innervation dysfunction

ETIOLOGY

- Paresis of cranial nerve VI
  - Infiltration of medial recti: Thyroid eye disease, leukemia, pseudotumor
  - Myasthenia gravis
  - Muscle entrapment/injury/restriction: Orbital trauma (medial orbital wall fracture, medial fat and fibrous trauma, or lateral orbital hemorrhage), infiltration, tumor, or eye muscle surgery
  - Congenital/genetic: CCDD, hypoplastic lateral recti, craniofacial disorders with absent/anomalous muscles

COMMONLY ASSOCIATED CONDITIONS

- Brain injury or increased intracranial pressure
  - Thyroid eye disease
  - Orbital trauma, infiltration, tumor, hemorrhage
  - Horizontal rectus muscle surgery
  - Craniofacial disorders

DIAGNOSIS

HISTORY

- Binocular, horizontal diplopia that is worse at distance and in lateral gaze
  - Orbital trauma
  - Prior infections, head trauma, ocular surgeries
  - Family history of CCDD or craniofacial disorder
  - Hyperthyroidism or myasthenia gravis

PHYSICAL EXAM

- Full ocular examination with emphasis on extraocular muscle functioning and ocular alignment in 9 positions of gaze (up, down, right, left, up right, up left, down right, and down left) as well as near
  - Measured esodeviation angle increases in lateral gaze
  - Determination of fixation pattern and visual acuity with best correction (cycloplegic refraction)
  - Cranial nerve and sensory exam
  - Forced-duction testing if necessary to distinguish lateral rectus from medial rectus dysfunction and to distinguish paresis from restriction
  - Proptosis and lid retraction may be seen with thyroid eye disease
  - Evaluate anomalous head positions, often manifest to maintain binocularity
- Congenital bilateral sixth and seventh cranial nerve palsies may indicate Moebius syndrome. Also assess for other cranial nerve palsies and defects of the neck, tongue, chest, and limbs
  - Congenital abduction deficit with an aberrant lateral rectus innervation and globe retraction ion attempted adduction may indicate Duane syndrome.

DIAGNOSTIC TESTS & INTERPRETATION

Lab

Initial lab tests

- Thyroid function tests if thyroid eye disease suspected
- Acetylcholine receptor antibody test if myasthenia gravis suspected

Follow-up & special considerations

Even if initial thyroid function or myasthenia gravis tests are normal, consider repeating at later date if clinical suspicion persists.

Imaging

- If acute-onset or neurological signs and symptoms are present, neuroimaging is necessary to rule out intracranial pathology.
- Consider orbital CT scan with suspected thyroid eye disease, or to rule out orbital mass, fracture, infiltration, or inflammatory lesions.
- Consider CT scan to evaluate for orbital fracture

Diagnostic Procedures/Other

B scan orbital ultrasound may be useful.

Pathological Findings

- CCDDs: Absent cranial nerve nuclei, absent or hypoplastic cranial nerve, fibrotic/hypoplastic extraocular muscle
  - See thyroid eye disease and myasthenia gravis chapters

DIFFERENTIAL DIAGNOSIS

- Comitant esotropia (accommodative or non-accommodative)
- Pseudo-abduction defect in infantile large angle esotropia with cross fixation
  - Esophoria
  - Negative angle kappa
  - Hyperopic anisometropia with varying deviation as fixation changes between eyes

TREATMENT

MEDICATION

- Consider systemic steroid for orbital inflammatory disease or ocular myasthenia.
- See also chapters on thyroid eye disease and myasthenia gravis.
- Medical management of increased intracranial pressure/cerebral edema.

ADDITIONAL TREATMENT

General Measures

- Amblyopia treatment as indicated
  - Fresnel press-on prisms to correct primary gaze diplopia
  - Complete remission usually occurs without intervention in sixth cranial nerve palsies if the palsy is caused by a vascular condition or increased intracranial pressure/cerebral edema.

Issues for Referral

- Neurosurgery consult if intracranial etiology is detected
  - Notify primary care physician if thyroid eye disease suspected, consider endocrinology consultation.
  - Consider neurology or neuro-ophthalmology if myasthenia gravis
  - Consider genetic counseling/geneticist where appropriate

Additional Therapies

- Smoking cessation in thyroid eye disease
- Beyond the amblyogenic age range, occlusion of one eye may be used to eliminate symptomatic diplopia

COMPLEMENTARY & ALTERNATIVE THERAPIES

None proven or indicated

SURGERY/OTHER PROCEDURES

- Surgery for a cranial nerve palsy VI or thyroid eye disease is indicated when spontaneous resolution does not occur after 6 months
  - Botox injections into the medial rectus may be useful with traumatic cranial VI paresis (1)
  - Muscle transposition is indicated with cranial VI total paralysis
  - Rectus muscle recession is the preferred surgery for thyroid eye disease
  - Orbital fracture may require liberation of entrapped tissues and fracture repair
  - Neurosurgical intervention for intracranial process if indicated

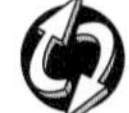

ONGOING CARE

FOLLOW-UP RECOMMENDATIONS

- For children in amblyopic age range, frequent follow-ups recommended for close monitoring of visual acuity
  - Primary care physician for glucose and blood pressure control if underlying vascular disorder suspected
  - Neurosurgery if intracranial pathology is suspected
  - Endocrinology if systemic thyroid disease is suspected
- Serial evaluations helpful in cases of variable strabismus including thyroid eye disease and ocular myasthenia
  - Stability of strabismus important before pursuing surgical intervention

Patient Monitoring

- Observation for acute neurological changes
  - Observe for amblyopia in children

PATIENT EDUCATION

- Strict glucose and blood pressure control if vascular causes of cranial nerve VI palsy are suspected
- Parents of strabismic children should be educated about the child's risk of developing amblyopia and impaired binocular depth perception
  - Diplopia management strategies

PROGNOSIS

- Dependent upon type. Some types can be improved with strabismus surgery
- In CCDDs the primary goal is improved head position and orthophoria in primary gaze
- Cranial VI palsies usually resolve spontaneously, especially if congenital or due to increased intracranial pressure
  - About one-third of palsies in older patients are associated with intracranial lesions
  - See chapters on thyroid eye disease and myasthenia gravis

COMPLICATIONS

- Amblyopia in children
  - Anomalous head posture
  - Loss of binocularity
  - Diplopia

REFERENCE

1. Rowe FJ, Noonan CP. Botulinum toxin for the treatment of strabismus. *Cochrane Database Syst Rev* 2009 ;(2):CD006499.

ADDITIONAL READING

- Volk AE, Fricke J, Strobl J, et al. Analysis of the CHN1 gene in patients with various types of congenital ocular motility disorders. *Graefes Arch Clin Exp Ophthalmol* 2010;248(9):1351–7.

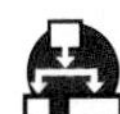

See Also (Topic, Algorithm, Electronic Media Element)

- Esotropia algorithm

CODES

ICD9

- 378.00 Esotropia, unspecified
- 378.9 Unspecified disorder of eye movements

CLINICAL PEARLS

- Esotropia varies in size with different positions of gaze
- Most common symptom is a binocular, horizontal diplopia that is worse with lateral gaze
- Differential diagnosis is restrictive versus paralytic muscle disease
- Common causes include cranial nerve VI palsy, thyroid eye disease, or medial orbital trauma
- A careful neurological exam is important to rule out an intracranial lesion
- Treat the underlying condition. Patching may be necessary in children of amblyopic age range

ESOTROPIA: INFANTILE

Donelson Manley
Jonathan Salvin

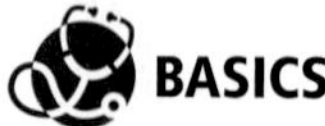

BASICS

DESCRIPTION

- A large angle (>35 prism diopters) esotropia developing within the first 6 months of life in an otherwise normal infant with no significant refractive error and no limitation of ocular movements.
  - Associated with lower incidence of amblyopia at presentation.
  - Associated with secondary findings of inferior oblique overaction, latent nystagmus, dissociated vertical deviation (DVD); often as later findings.

EPIDEMIOLOGY

Incidence

- 8% of all childhood esotropia
  - Esotropia (all) has an incidence of 111 per 100,000 under the age of 19 years

Prevalence

2% of all children under the age of 6 years

RISK FACTORS

Family history of strabismus

PATHOPHYSIOLOGY

- Studies in primates reveal that early abnormal binocular sensory input results in the creation of infantile esotropia and its related complications
  - Early restoration of normal binocular function resulted in improved alignment and decreased incidence of late findings (2)[C]

COMMONLY ASSOCIATED CONDITIONS

- Amblyopia inferior oblique overaction
  - Latent nystagmus
  - Dissociated vertical deviations
  - Cross fixation and pseudoabduction deficit

DIAGNOSIS

HISTORY

- Onset of inward crossing of the eyes seen at birth or soon thereafter (under the age of 6 months)
  - Full extraocular movements
  - Usually early cross-fixation

PHYSICAL EXAM

- Large angle of esotropia, usually over 35 prism diopters.
- Constant and comitant angle of deviation
- Refractive error usually <+2 diopters (normal for this age group).
- Ophthalmic examination is otherwise normal.
- Fixation may alternate. A lack of alternation may indicate amblyopia is present.

- Fixation with the crossed eye may suggest a lateral rectus underaction. Full abduction can be demonstrated by covering the fixating eye or Doll's eye maneuver. (3)[A]

DIAGNOSTIC TESTS & INTERPRETATION

Imaging

Neuroimaging may be indicated if esotropia associated with abnormal ductions/versions or manifest nystagmus.

DIFFERENTIAL DIAGNOSIS

- Pseudoesotropia
  - Duane syndrome Type 1 (4)[C]
  - Moebius syndrome (5)[C]
  - Congenital sixth nerve palsy
  - Orbital tumor
  - Nystagmus blockage syndrome
  - Cianca syndrome

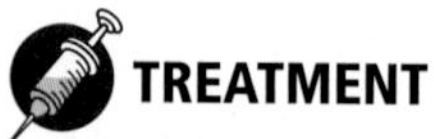

TREATMENT

ADDITIONAL TREATMENT

General Measures

- Strabismus surgery (6)[A]. Usually bimedial rectus recession, although larger deviations may be managed by additional lateral rectus recession

- Amblyopia treatment as indicated

Additional Therapies

- Treat underlying amblyopia if present, generally prior to surgery
- Treat high hyperopia to rule out accommodative component

SURGERY/OTHER PROCEDURES

- Alignment of the eyes should be achieved prior to 24 months of age to achieve binocularity. (3)[A], (7)[A]

- Some data suggests that early surgery is beneficial.
- NOTE: Spontaneous resolution without surgery may rarely occur.

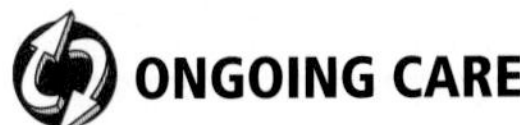

ONGOING CARE

FOLLOW-UP RECOMMENDATIONS

- Long term follow-up for recurrent strabismus, inferior oblique overaction, and DVD all of which may require later surgery
  - Second strabismus surgery needed in up to 50% of patients by the age of 10 years

Patient Monitoring

- Monitor for amblyopia and refractive errors
- Secondary accommodative component may develop and need to be treated with glasses
  - Monitor for recurrent/consecutive strabismus
  - Monitor for late complications

PATIENT EDUCATION

- Long-term monitoring for recurrent strabismus or late associated findings
  - Polycarbonate safety glasses required if dense amblyopia remains

PROGNOSIS

- Usually normal vision in both eyes
  - Poorly developed stereoacuity without early intervention

COMPLICATIONS

- Recurrent or consecutive strabismus may develop and require additional surgical treatment
- Amblyopia

REFERENCES

1. Greenberg AE, Mohney BG, Diehl NN, et al. Incidence and types of childhood esotropia. A population-based study. *Ophthalmology* 2007;114:170–174.
2. Wong AMF, Foeller P, Bradley D, et al. Early versus delayed repair of infantile strabismus in macaque monkeys: I. ocular motor effects. *J AAPOS* 2003;7:200.
3. Pediatric Eye Disease Investigator Group. The clinical spectrum of early-onset esotropia: Experience of the Congenital Esotropia Observational Study. *Am J Ophthalmol* 2002;133(1):102–108.
4. Alexandrakis G, Saunders RA. Duane retraction syndrome. *Ophthlmol Clin North Am* 2001; 14(3):407–417f
5. Miller MT, Strömland K. The Möbius sequence: A relook. *JAAPOS* 1999;3(4):199–208.
6. Ing M, Costenbader FD, Parks MM, et al. Early surgery for congenital esotropia. *Am J Ophthalmol* 1966;61(6):1419–1427.
7. Louwagie CR, Diehl N, Geenberg AE, et al. Long-term follow-up of congenital esotropia in a population-based cohort. *J AAPOS* 2009;13:8–12.

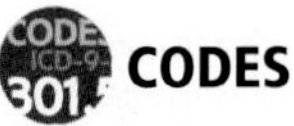

CODES

ICD9

- 378.00 Esotropia, unspecified
- 379.50 Nystagmus, unspecified
- 379.56 Other forms of nystagmus

CLINICAL PEARLS

- Infantile esotropia is an early-onset, large angle, usually alternating esotropia.
- The best outcomes are obtained with surgical intervention before the age of 24 months.
- Late associated findings including inferior oblique overaction, dissociated deviations, amblyopia, and latent nystagmus.

E

EXODEVIATIONS COMITANT

Donelson Manley
Bruce Schnall

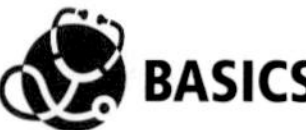

BASICS

DESCRIPTION

A horizontal divergence of the eyes that measures the same in left and right gaze as in the primary position for a given testing distance.

EPIDEMIOLOGY

Incidence

1 in 185 children by age 10 years.

Prevalence

Approximately 1% of all children <11 years old.

RISK FACTORS

Maternal cigarette smoking during pregnancy and low birth weight.

Genetics

- Multifactorial inheritance
- Autosomal-dominant inheritance has been reported

PATHOPHYSIOLOGY

- Horizontal eye muscle imbalance that results in divergent horizontal strabismus. May progress from exophoria to intermittent exotropia to constant exotropia.
  – Neurobiologic pathophysiology unknown

ETIOLOGY

Unknown

COMMONLY ASSOCIATED CONDITIONS

- May be associated with oblique muscle dysfunction, A or V patters
- Amblyopia is infrequent but may occur
- More common if refractive error is myopic

DIAGNOSIS

HISTORY

- A turning outward of the eyes, which is usually noticed in early childhood. At first it may be intermittent in the distance and then become more constant with time. It may be noticed more often during illness or fatigue
- Closing one eye outdoors in bright sunlight.
- Horizontal diplopia.
- Asthenopia with reading is common with convergence insufficiency.

PHYSICAL EXAM

Types:

- Exophoria: A tendency for the eyes to turn outward, which is controlled by fusion. This is usually not noticed. Fusion and stereopsis are good.
- Intermittent exotropia: The deviation is latent at times and manifest at others. This type of deviation may be noticed and may cause diplopia. The variability is related to a high AC/A ratio and accommodative convergence, which modify the distant exodeviation and lessen it at near. Fusion and stereopsis are good when the eyes are aligned.
- Constant exotropia: The eyes turn out constantly. Amblyopia is more common in this group. Fusion and stereopsis are lacking.
- Divergence excess: The deviation is greater at distance.
- Basic: The measurements at distance and near are the same.
- Convergence insufficiency: The near deviation is greater than distance.
- Sensory exotropia: Exotropia develops as a result of longstanding poor vision in one eye.
- Consecutive exotropia: An exotropia that occurs following treatment for esotropia. May be comitant or incomitant.

DIAGNOSTIC TESTS & INTERPRETATION

Diagnostic Procedures/Other

- Cover testing should be performed with glasses being worn, if necessary. The distant and near deviations are measured with prisms.
- An assessment of the control of an intermittent exotropia should be made. Good control-fusion is rapidly realigned after cover testing. Fair control-fusion is regained after blinking or refixation. Poor control-eye remains exotropic for an extended period of time.
- May require prolonged cover (20 minute patch test) to elicit deviation.
- Sensory exotropia is measured by Krimsky with the prism being placed over the fixing eye.
  – Fixation on a far distant target (e.g., out a window) may be required to elicit maximum deviation.

Pathological Findings

Normal extraocular muscle

DIFFERENTIAL DIAGNOSIS

- Rule out incomitant deviation (see chapter on Incomitant Exodeviation)
  – Myopia

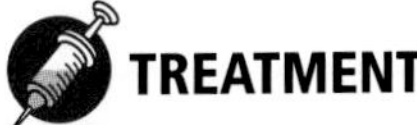

TREATMENT

ADDITIONAL TREATMENT

General Measures

- Glasses should be prescribed when indicated, especially if myopic. Some children may be offered additional minus lens power to stimulate accommodative convergence. Can add up to 3.00 diopters of minus to cycloplegic refraction
- Amblyopia if present should be treated.
- Part-time patching of preferred eye.
- Convergence training or orthoptics are most effective in treating convergence insufficiency
- Base-in prisms can help to maintain fusion and prevent diplopia. Long-term use of base-in prism is likely to result in a reduction of fusion vergence amplitudes.

Issues for Referral

- Deviations not controlled by glasses or patching or the recurrence of amblyopia despite medical treatment are indications for surgery
  - Reconstruction of a normal appearance is an indication for surgery, provided medical treatment has failed and amblyopia treated. Surgery is indicated when there is poor control of an intermittent exotropia, progression toward constant exotropia, diplopia, or asthenopia.

SURGERY/OTHER PROCEDURES

- Surgery involves recession of one or both lateral rectus muscles, which may be combined, with resection of one or both medial recti muscles. The decision on which muscles to recess or resect is based upon the size of the deviation and whether the exotropia is greater at the distance or near.
- Sensory exotropia is treated with recession of the lateral rectus and resection of the medial rectus in the deviated eye.
- Immediately following recession of both lateral recti for intermittent exotropia, a consecutive esotropia is commonly seen which should resolve within 2 weeks.

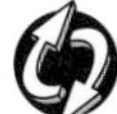

ONGOING CARE

FOLLOW-UP RECOMMENDATIONS

Patient Monitoring

- Intermittent exotropia may progress and patients may need to be monitored at 3– 6 month intervals to look for progression.
- Following strabismus surgery, patients need to be monitored for recurrence of exotropia, consecutive esotropia, and amblyopia.
  - Amblyopia monitoring as indicated based on age, depth of amblyopia (See Amblyopia chapter)

PATIENT EDUCATION

- Families should keep track of frequency of deviation
  - Importance of patching and glasses; wear as indicated

PROGNOSIS

- Untreated, up to 75% may progress over time.
- Surgical outcome is dependent upon length of follow-up. Reported success rate at 1 year is approximately 80% and 50–70% at 5 years.

COMPLICATIONS

- Surgical overcorrection of intermittent exotropia can result in diplopia and amblyopia
  - Most common reason for reoperation is residual exotropia, although consecutive esotropia may also occur

ADDITIONAL READING

- Pediatric Ophthalmology and Strabismus, Basic and Clinical Science Course, Section 6, American Academy of Ophthalmology, 2010–2011.
- Haggerty H, Richardson S, Hrisos S, et al. The Newcastle Score; a new method of grading the severity of intermittent exotropia. *Br J Ophthalmol* 2004;88(2):233–235.
- Mohney BG, Huffaker RK. Common forms of childhood exotropia. *Ophthalmology* 2003;110(11):2093–2096.
- Hunter DG, Ellis FJ. Prevalence of systemic and ocular disease in infantile exotropia: Comparison with infantile esotropia. *Ophthalmology* 1999; 106(10):1951–1956.

CODES

ICD9

- 378.10 Exotropia, unspecified
- 378.20 Intermittent heterotropia, unspecified

CLINICAL PEARLS

- Amblyopia is uncommon in intermittent exotropia.
- Serial follow-up is critical as early intervention can prevent the development of constant exotropia.
- Myopic correction may be a useful therapy prior to surgery.

EXODEVIATIONS INCOMITANT

Donelson Manley
J. Mark Engel

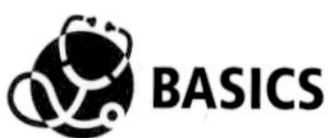

BASICS

DESCRIPTION

- Exotropia is incomitant if it measures differently in different fields of gaze. This occurs most commonly in A and V pattern exotropia where the measurements differ in upgaze and downgaze. If the exotropia is greater in upgaze than downgaze, it is termed V pattern exotropia. If the exotropia is greater in downgaze than upgaze, it is termed A pattern exotropia.
- Incomitant exotropia also occurs if the measurements differ on lateral gaze. This is commonly secondary to overaction of the oblique muscles, and can also be associated with A and V pattern exotropias.
  - Exotropia can differ in lateral gaze secondary to restriction or paralysis of the extraocular muscles.

EPIDEMIOLOGY

Incidence

The incidence of incomitant exotropia increases with cranial nerve palsies, thyroid disorders, and after previous strabismus procedures.

Prevalence

Approximately 25% of exotropia is incomitant.

RISK FACTORS

- Underlying disorders that affect the action of the medial or lateral rectus muscle
- Prior strabismus surgery

Genetics

- Heredity, in general, plays a significant role in exodeviations, and is multifactorial.
  - Underlying conditions associated with incomitant exotropia (e.g., craniosynostoses) may have a genetic basis unrelated to the strabismus.

GENERAL PREVENTION

Meticulous strabismus surgical techniques, which avoid excessive scarring, and restriction of the extraocular muscles.

PATHOPHYSIOLOGY

- It is not certain whether there are anatomical differences in patients with A or V pattern incomitant exotropia versus those with comitant exotropia.
- Downslanting palpebral features have been correlated with inferior oblique overaction, and upslanting palpebral fissures with superior oblique overaction.

ETIOLOGY

- A and V patterns may be associated with oblique overaction.
- Incomitance can also be caused by restriction or paresis of muscles, in particular, the horizontal recti

COMMONLY ASSOCIATED CONDITIONS

- Facial asymmetry
- Birth trauma
- Craniosynostoses
- Spina bifida
- Aberrant regeneration of the third cranial nerve
- Previous eye muscle surgery
- Hyperthyroidism
- Brain tumor or aneurysm
- Increased intracranial pressure
- Head trauma
- Orbital trauma, inflammation, hemorrhage, or tumor

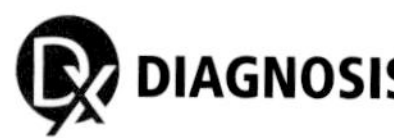

DIAGNOSIS

HISTORY

- Birth history, developmental and neurologic history should be obtained.
- A previous strabismus or other surgery, which involves or could involve the extraocular muscles, should be asked, including previous sinus surgery, orbital decompression surgery, repair of orbital floor fracture, and retinal detachment surgery.
- Possible anomalous head position (for example, a chin-down position in A pattern exotropia, or face turn in cranial VI palsy).

PHYSICAL EXAM

- Alternate cover test should be performed with and without glasses
- Measure with prisms while fixating on a distant target preferably 20 feet away in primary position, in 25 degrees of upgaze and 25–35 degrees of downgaze.
- Measurements in lateral gaze should also be made, and primary and secondary deviations should be noted if present.
- Oblique overaction should be determined by evaluating the adducting eye in full adduction when the patient is in lateral gaze. This is usually obtained by covering the abducting eye, and having the adducting eye follow a fixation target to full lateral gaze, and then uncovering the abducting eye to see if the adducting eye is higher or lower than the abducting eye.
- Change in the vertical misalignment should be noted on head tilt to the right and left, as well as all 6 positions of gaze.

DIAGNOSTIC TESTS & INTERPRETATION

Lab

In general, no special laboratory testing is necessary, unless a thyroid condition or myasthenia gravis is suspected (see those chapters).

Imaging

Initial approach

- In general, imaging is not necessary in the diagnosis and treatment of most incomitant exotropia.
- After previous complicated strabismus or retinal surgery, especially if a loss muscle is suspected, or to determine the presence of changes from thyroid disease an MRI scan be performed.
- MRI scan should also be ordered if recent onset cranial nerve palsy, head trauma, or other neurologic signs present.
- Consider CT scan if suspect orbital trauma.
- There has been a suggestion that the pulley system may be responsible for the A and V patterns in exotropia, and high resolution MRI scanning may be of theoretical use to determine the anatomical abnormality causing the incomitance.

Follow-up & special considerations

Radiologists may be unfamiliar with some of the information wanted by the strabismologist in high resolution MRI scans, and should be contacted directly before the study is performed.

Diagnostic Procedures/Other

- Forced duction and forced generation testing can be performed in the office with topical anesthesia if a paralytic or restricted muscle is suspected.
- Binocular fields are considered by some to be helpful in certain incomitant exotropias to determine the area of single binocular function.

Pathological Findings

Not applicable except as related to other disorders (e.g., see chapter on Thyroid Ophthalmolopathy)

DIFFERENTIAL DIAGNOSIS

- Infantile esotropia
- Duane syndrome
- Cranial III or VI Paralysis
- Internuclear ophthalmoplegia
- Isolated medial rectus weakness related to myasthenia gravis or multiple sclerosis.
- Consecutive exotropia following surgery for esotropia.
- Certain craniofacial syndromes can cause the appearance of an incomitant exotropia.
- Unilateral ptosis can also cause an appearance of an incomitant strabismus.
- A significant anisometropia can cause a misdiagnosis of incomitance if the primary and secondary deviations are measured without correction.

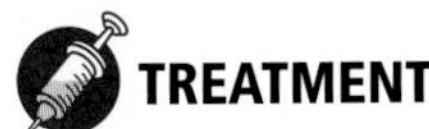

TREATMENT

MEDICATION

In general, except for certain systemic syndromes such as thyroid ophthalmopathy and myasthenia gravis, strabismus is not correctable with medications.

ADDITIONAL TREATMENT

General Measures

- Refractive errors should be corrected.
- Prisms can be helpful in some cases of diplopia or significant anomalous head position.
  - Treat secondary amblyopia.

Issues for Referral

- Endocrinology if suspect thyroid eye disease
- Neurology if suspect intracranial process
- Genetics if suspect craniofacial disorder

Additional Therapies

Should be directed at the underlying neurologic or systemic abnormality if present.

COMPLEMENTARY & ALTERNATIVE THERAPIES

In general "vision training" and orthoptic therapy have not been of proven value in most forms of strabismus, especially when incomitant.

SURGERY/OTHER PROCEDURES

- Surgical intervention is indicated if the incomitant exotropia is causing:
  - 1) Anomalous head position
  - 2) Diplopia (not correctable with prisms)
  - 3) To correct significant deformity that the strabismus is causing
  - 4) To expand binocular field and visual function of the adult or child
  - 5) Recurrent amblyopia
- The surgical correction of incomitant exotropia is usually more complicated than correcting an exotropia which is comitant, and adjustable sutures may be utilized to increase the success rate of the procedure.
- Botulinum toxin injection has also been used to correct incomitant exotropias, and can be indicated in small angle incomitant exotropias.

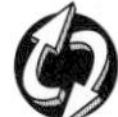

ONGOING CARE

FOLLOW-UP RECOMMENDATIONS

If the incomitance is not secondary to a cranial nerve palsy or intracranial lesion, then usually the child is followed every 6–12 months unless concerns for amblyopia or diplopia warrant more frequent follow-up.

Patient Monitoring

- Check for changes in refractive error
- Monitor amblyopia treatment (see Amblyopia chapter)

PATIENT EDUCATION

The patient should be educated to the cause and treatment options of the incomitant exotropia.

PROGNOSIS

In general, except if the incomitance of the exotropia is caused by cases of paralytic or restrictive muscle, the patient should be told that their condition is correctable, although several strabismus procedures may be necessary.

COMPLICATIONS

- Amblyopia
- May require more than one strabismus surgery
- Diplopia

ADDITIONAL READING

- Demer JL. A 12-year prospective study of extraocular muscle imaging in complex strabismus. *JAAPOS* 2003;6:337–347.
- Durtic TH, Stout AU, Drack AV, et al. Giant orbital cysts after strabismus surgery. *Am J Ophthalmol* 2006;142:698–699.
- Haggerty H, Richardson S, Hrisos S, et al. The Newcastle Score; a new method of grading the severity of intermittent exotropia. *Br J Ophthalmol* 2004;88(2):233–235.
- Hunter DG, Ellis FJ. Prevalence of systemic and ocular disease in infantile exotropia: Comparison with infantile esotropia. *Ophthalmology* 1999; 106(10):1951–1956.
- Mohney BG, Huffaker RK. Common forms of childhood exotropia. *Ophthalmology* 2003; 110(11):2093–2096.
- Pediatric Ophthalmology and Strabismus, Basic and Clinical Science Course, Section 6, American Academy of Ophthalmology, 2010–2011.
- Rosenbaum AL, Santiago AP. Clinical strabismus management. *Principles and Surgical Techniques*. WB Saunders Company: Philadelphia, 1999; 219–229.
- Stidwill D. Epidemiology of strabismus. *Ophthalmic Physiol Opt* 1997;17:536–539.

CODES

ICD9

- 378.10 Exotropia, unspecified
- 378.13 Monocular exotropia with v pattern
- 378.17 Alternating exotropia with v pattern

CLINICAL PEARLS

- Incomitant exotropia may be due to paresis or restriction of an eye muscle due to an intracranial or orbital process or due to systemic disease such as thyroid eye disease or myasthenia gravis
- Patients may present with amblyopia, diplopia, or an anomalous head position.
- Prior strabismus surgery is a not uncommon cause of incomitant exotropia.

EXPOSURE KERATOPATHY

Brad H. Feldman

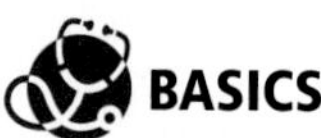

BASICS

DESCRIPTION

Corneal damage due to evaporative tear loss and disrupted tear dynamics in the setting of improper lid closure and movement.

EPIDEMIOLOGY

Incidence

Uncommon

Prevalence

Low overall, but prevalence increases with age.

GENERAL PREVENTION

Identification of at risk patients and prompt intervention to prevent serious corneal complications

PATHOPHYSIOLOGY

- The lack of normal movement of the eyelids (especially the upper lid) leads to loss of the normal protective tear film over the surface of the cornea.
- Without normal eyelid movements the tear film is disrupted for several reasons:
  - Evaporation loss of tears exposed within the palpebral fissure
  - Decreased spread of replenished tears across the cornea
  - Abnormal mixing of tear layer components (mucin, lipid, and aqueous)
  - Inadequate drainage of tears through the nasolacrimal system with loss of normal tear recycling

ETIOLOGY

- Neurogenic
  - Facial nerve palsy (e.g., Bell's palsy)
- Anatomic
  - Cicatricial or restrictive diseases of the lids
  - Prior blepharoplasty
  - Skin/mucous membrane disorders (e.g., Stevens–Johnson Syndrome)
  - Ocular proptosis (e.g., Orbital tumors, Graves' disease)
- Degenerative
  - For example, Parkinson's, Alzheimer's, dementia
- Altered mental state

ALERT

Especially common under general anesthesia or in the intensive care unit if the eyelids are not properly closed and/or lubricated

COMMONLY ASSOCIATED CONDITIONS

- Bell's palsy
- Parkinson's disease
- Lower lid ectropion
- Corneal neurotrophism

DIAGNOSIS

HISTORY

- Typically can elicit a history of one of the etiologies listed above
- May elicit a history of lid opening at night (nocturnal lagophthalmos)
- Typically subacute or chronic in presentation
- Symptoms may include the following:
  - Foreign body sensation
  - Photophobia
  - Tearing
  - Decreased visual acuity

ALERT

Be aware that patients with associated neurotrophic defects may not complain of foreign body sensation, photophobia, or tearing but may have advanced corneal damage.

PHYSICAL EXAM

- External examination may demonstrate:
  - Failure of lids to close fully on blink or voluntary closure (lagophthalmos)
  - Decreased frequency of blink
  - Widened palpebral fissure
  - Ectropion or lid position abnormalities
  - Brow ptosis (in cases of facial paralysis)
- Slit-lamp examination may demonstrate:
  - Corneal punctate epithelial erosions (most dense inferiorly but may be diffuse if severe exposure or if markedly decreased blink frequency)
  - Decreased tear break up time
  - Decreased tear production (in cases of facial paralysis)
  - Corneal ulceration, infection, thinning, scarring, or perforation if severe or prolonged

DIAGNOSTIC TESTS & INTERPRETATION

Diagnostic Procedures/Other

- Observe spontaneous blink rate and eyelid closure prior to placing anesthetic
  - Ask patient to close eyes gently and measure palpebral fissure
  - Ask patient to forcibly close eyes and measure palpebral fissure
- Check corneal sensation prior to placing anesthetic to rule out neurotrophic disease
- Stain corneal surface with fluorescein to help identify punctate erosions and measure tear break up time
- Consider measuring tear production with a Schirmer's test
- Note: In office, testing of Bell's phenomenon may be misleading as it does not often correlate well with corneal position during sleep or during involuntary lid closure.

DIFFERENTIAL DIAGNOSIS

- Dry eye syndrome
- Sjögren's syndrome
- Neurotrophic keratopathy
- Medicamentosa
- Blepharitis

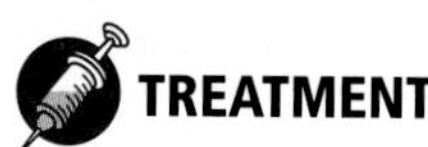

TREATMENT

MEDICATION

First Line

- Lubrication: Strategy and aggressiveness of lubrication varies with etiology (e.g., although nocturnal lagophthalmos may only require ointment at bed time, a Bell's palsy patient with a wide palpebral fissure will require frequent instillation) (1)
  - Artificial tear supplements (short-lived effect, use $\geq$4 times/day)
  - Viscous gels (longer effect)
  - Ointments (longest lasting effect)
- Eyelid taping/placement of cellophane dressing over eyelids during sleep, obtundation, or unconsciousness (e.g., general anesthesia)

Second Line
Surgical procedures to improve lid closure may be considered when lubrication and lid taping are either insufficient or intolerable, or if the condition becomes a chronic disability

ADDITIONAL TREATMENT
Issues for Referral
Lid procedures such as gold weight placement are typically performed by oculoplastics-trained ophthalmologists.

ALERT
Patients with a combination of neurotrophism and exposure are at considerable risk for sight-threatening complications and should be managed in conjunction with a corneal specialist.

Additional Therapies
- Moisture chambers/moisture goggles
- Punctal occlusion
- Contact lenses
  - Limited role for high-water content silicone hydrogel lenses in patients with decreased blink rate or mild lagophthalmos (use with caution due to risk of infection or disease exacerbation)
  - Scleral lenses (Boston Ocular Surface Prosthesis) if tolerated may help resolve keratopathy and enhance vision by providing a reservoir of aqueous and a stable refractive surface (2)

SURGERY/OTHER PROCEDURES
- Lid abnormality repair (e.g., ectropion repair or lid tightening procedure such as a lateral tarsal strip)
- Upper lid gold weight placement if due to decreased orbicularis function (90% will improve) (3)[B]
- Recession of upper eyelid retractors in cases of eyelid retraction
- Lower eyelid elevation
- Orbital decompression or removal of orbital lesion if exposure is secondary to proptosis
- Partial (typically temporal) or full tarsorrhaphy may be needed if patient has progressive or chronic keratopathy not responsive to other measures
- Botulinum toxin injection into Müller's muscles and levator to induce ptosis (may take $\geq$4 days for full effect and gives variable coverage)

ONGOING CARE

FOLLOW-UP RECOMMENDATIONS
Patients need to be followed closely if their disease is of acute onset or is acutely exacerbated as they are at risk for sight-threatening complications.

PATIENT EDUCATION
Patients should be informed that they must seek urgent care if they experience a sudden worsening of vision or an increase in pain, photophobia, or redness as this may signify a serious complication.

PROGNOSIS
Varies depending on etiology and severity

COMPLICATIONS
Corneal ulceration, infection, thinning, scarring, or perforation

REFERENCES

1. Rahman I, Sadiq SA. Ophthalmic management of facial nerve palsy: A review. *Surv Ophthalmol* 2007;52:121–144.
2. Rosenthal P, Croteau A. Fluid-ventilated, gas-permeable scleral contact lens is an effective option for managing severe ocular surface disease and many corneal disorders that would otherwise require penetrating keratoplasty. *Eye Contact Lens* 2005;31:130–134.
3. Snyder MC, Johnson PJ, Moore GF, et al. Early versus late gold weight implantation for rehabilitation of the paralyzed eyelid. *Laryngoscope* 2001;111:2109–2113.

ADDITIONAL READING

- Morris CL. Lagophthalmos Evaluation and Treatment. *EyeNet*. April 2008. Accessed at http://www.aao.org/publications/eyenet/200804/pearls.cfm
- Feldman B. Chapter 14: A patient diagnosed with Bell's palsy 2 days ago presents with lagophthalmos and moderate punctate keratopathy inferiorly on the cornea. How should I treat her? *Curbside Consultation in Cornea and External Disease*. Ed. Francis Price Jr. Thorofare: Slack Publishers, 2010. 59–63.

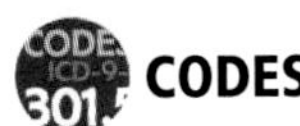

CODES

ICD9
370.34 Exposure keratoconjunctivitis

CLINICAL PEARLS

- Untreated, exposure keratopathy can lead to sight-threatening complications.
- Lubrication is the mainstay of treatment for most cases.
- More severe cases often require prompt surgical intervention.

EYELID LACERATION

Rachel K. Sobel
Jacqueline Carrasco

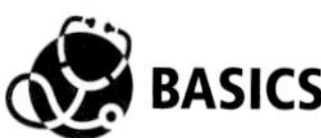

BASICS

DESCRIPTION

- Eyelid lacerations occur 3 ways: Sharp trauma (e.g., pencil), blunt trauma (e.g., fist), or diffuse trauma (e.g., motor vehicle accident). Lacerations can affect 3 regions of the eyelid.
  - Non-marginal eyelid
  - Marginal eyelid
  - Canalicular system, with or without avulsion of medial canthal tendon

EPIDEMIOLOGY

Prevalence

- 25% of eyelid trauma affects the margin (1)
- 15% of eyelid trauma involves the canaliculus (1)

RISK FACTORS

- For canalicular lacerations:
  - Average age is 24 years (2)
  - 80% are males (2)

GENERAL PREVENTION

- Work or recreational spectacles
- The glasses or goggles should say "ANSI Z87.1" This means that they meet the safety standards of the American National Standards Institute.
- See OSHA (Occupational Safety and Health Administration) and ASTM (American Society for Testing and Material) for other work and recreational eye protection standards.

PATHOPHYSIOLOGY

- Sharp trauma directly tears the eyelid skin, margin, or canaliculus. Many sharp objects have been reported to be the cause, including finger, nail, scissor, door handle, tree branch, fishing pole, and glass bottle.
- Blunt and diffuse trauma tears the skin and margin by traction. Sudden lateral displacement of the eyelid ruptures the medial canthal tendon and canalicular tissue. This can be the case with dog bites.

COMMONLY ASSOCIATED CONDITIONS

- 44% of eyelid trauma is associated with injury to the globe. (1)
- 25% of patients with canalicular lid laceration have globe injury (2).
- 65% of patients with canalicular lid laceration have associated injury including: (2)
  - Globe rupture
  - Facial fractures
  - Optic neuropathy
  - Retinal detachment
  - Head trauma

DIAGNOSIS

HISTORY

- Ophthalmology consult can be obtained once life-threatening injuries are dealt with.
- Obtain details of how and when injury occurred. Understanding the mechanism may point to further injuries such as an occult orbital foreign body.
- Prior visual status
- Tetanus status

PHYSICAL EXAM

- Full ocular examination to rule out ruptured globe or suspected orbital or ocular foreign body.
- Measure length of laceration.
- Estimate depth, that is, full thickness versus partial thickness.
- Determine if laceration involves the margin.
- Look for prolapsed orbital fat which could indicate septum violation and levator muscle injury.
- If the laceration is medial to the puncta, canalicular involvement has most likely occurred.

DIAGNOSTIC TESTS & INTERPRETATION

Imaging

Initial approach

Small lid lacerations, as with a puncture site, may indicate possible occult orbital foreign body. If history and examination are suspects, consider CT scan without contrast of orbits, thin cuts, axial and coronal, to help rule out foreign body.

Diagnostic Procedures/Other

To test whether or not the canalicular system has been injured, an ophthalmologist may perform a probing and irrigation of the canalicular system.

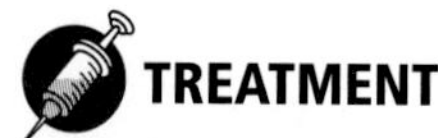

TREATMENT

MEDICATION

First Line

- Tetanus should be up to date.
- Oral antibiotics for lid lacerations are anecdotally driven. If used, a first generation cephalosporin is recommended. (3)[C]
- Lid lacerations due to animal or human bites should be treated prophylactically with antibiotics. (4)[C]

ADDITIONAL TREATMENT

Issues for Referral

- If lid margin or canalicular system is involved, refer to ophthalmic surgeon. Keep laceration moist with wet dressing if eye is not ruptured.
- Often the lacerated area may appear to have missing tissue because of skin and orbicularis muscle contraction. Only rarely is there tissue loss.
- If there is tissue loss, more complicated repair is indicated. These cases should be referred to an oculoplastic specialist.

SURGERY/OTHER PROCEDURES

- Repair can be done, depending upon the extent of laceration, in a small procedure room or in the operating room under monitored anesthesia care or general anesthesia.
- Surgery and treatment for ocular injury should precede eyelid repair.
- Repair should be done within 24–48 hours (5)
- Non-marginal repair depending upon depth may include a layered closure with 5–0 or 6–0 Vicryl and skin closure with 6–0 plain or fast gut.
- Marginal repair should be referred to an ophthalmic surgeon for closure.
- Canalicular involvement by an ophthalmic surgeon or oculoplastic specialist may utilize bi-canalicular intubation with Crawford tubes, pigtail probe, or monocanalicular stents, such as a Mini-Monoka tube.

IN-PATIENT CONSIDERATIONS

Admission Criteria

Ruptured Globe

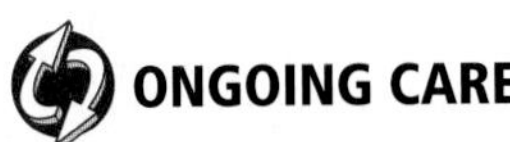

ONGOING CARE

FOLLOW-UP RECOMMENDATIONS

Small strip of antibiotic ointment should be placed over sutured wound 2–3 times daily. Depending upon the extent of wound, patient should be seen for follow-up 3–7 days following repair.

PATIENT EDUCATION

Patient should be educated about the signs of infection: Redness, swelling, and pain.

PROGNOSIS

Typically very good. Once the wound is closed, satisfactory functional and cosmetic results can be achieved.

COMPLICATIONS

- Infection
- Tearing
- Trichiasis
- Lagophthalmos and corneal exposure
- Dislodged silicone stent
- Notched eyelid margin
- Note: Patients may need further surgeries to repair symptomatic eyelid deformities

REFERENCES

1. Herzum H, Holle P, Hintschich C. Eyelid injuries: Epidemiological aspects. *Ophthalmologe* 2001;98:1079–82.
2. Naik M, Kelapure A, Rath S, et al. Management of canalicular lacerations. *Am J Ophthalmol* 2008;145:377–380.
3. Reifler D. Management of canalicular laceration. *Surv Ophthalmol* 1991;36:113–132.
4. Long J. Tann T. Adnexal Trauma. *Ophthalmol Clin North Am* 2002;15(2):179–184.
5. Nerad J. Eyelid and orbital trauma. *Techniques in Ophthalmic Plastic Surgery.* Saunders 2010; 355–368.

ADDITIONAL READING

- http://www.geteyesmart.org/eyesmart/injuries/eyewear.cfm

CODES

ICD9

- 870.1 Laceration of eyelid, full-thickness, not involving lacrimal passages
- 870.2 Laceration of eyelid involving lacrimal passages
- 870.8 Other specified open wounds of ocular adnexa

CLINICAL PEARLS

- Eyelid lacerations are often associated with globe and other facial injuries. Treat eye injuries first, than the lacerations.
- Suspect an orbital foreign body if a lid laceration is small and the history is compelling.
- Surgical treatment varies depending upon whether or not the laceration involves the margin or canaliculus. Refer to an ophthalmologist or oculoplastic specialist for marginal or canalicular lacerations.
- Prophylactic antibiotics are recommended for facial lacerations, especially animal bites.

EYELID NEOPLASMS, BENIGN

Michael P. Rabinowitz
Jacqueline R. Carrasco

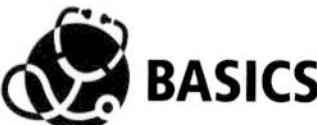

BASICS

DESCRIPTION

- The skin of the eyelids includes the epidermis, dermis, and deeper, adnexal tissue.
- The epidermis is comprised of four layers of keratinocytes, as well as Merkel cells, Langerhans cells, and melanocytes.
- The dermis is thicker than the epidermis, containing vessels, nerves, and lymphatics.
- The adnexa lies deep to the dermis and contains holocrine, apocrine, sebaceous, eccrine, and meibomian glands.
- Abnormal growth of any of these structures may fall under the rubric of benign eyelid neoplasms.
- This chapter will focus on the more common neoplasms and provide an overview therein.

EPIDEMIOLOGY

Incidence

- Of all eyelid tumors, 54–84% are benign.
- Incidence of lesions varies widely by study.
- Studies show the most common benign eyelid tumors encountered by the comprehensive ophthalmologist include chalazia and epidermal inclusion cysts.
- Capillary hemangiomas are one of the most common lid tumors in infancy; incidence is approximately 1.0–2.6% of live births.
- The following are data points from a recent review of patients whose neoplasms were surgically removed (1):
- 26% of benign lesions are squamous cell papillomas.
- 21% of benign lesions are seborrheic keratosis. Other studies note their ubiquitous nature amongst the elderly, citing that 80–100% of people older than 50 have them.
- Melanocytic nevi, hidrocystomas, and xanthoma/xanthelasma are the next most common benign eyelid tumors.
- Premalignant lesions such as actinic keratosis, Bowen disease, and keratoacanthomas are beyond the scope of this chapter and will not be further discussed.

Prevalence

- Eyelid tumors are the most common neoplasm encountered in a general ophthalmology practice.
- Overall prevalence depends on tumor type.

RISK FACTORS

- Meibomian gland inspissation and ocular rosacea may lead to chalazia and hordeolum formation.
- Female gender is a risk factor for capillary hemangiomas (3:1 female:male ratio).
- Eyelid trauma is a risk factor for epidermoid cysts.
- Eyelid surgery and infection are risk factors for inflammatory lesions and cysts.
- HPV (human papilloma virus) is a risk factor for squamous cell papillomas (particularly those in the oral mucosa).
- Sun exposure, equatorial origin, and advanced age predispose to lesions such as actinic keratosis and keratoacanthomas. Moreover, they are risk factors for progression to malignancy.
- Hypercholesterolemia and familial lipid disorders predispose to xanthelasma/xanthoma.

Genetics

It depends on lesion involved and is beyond the scope of the overview provided in this chapter.

GENERAL PREVENTION

- Limitation of ultraviolet ray and sun exposure as well as sunscreen use are perhaps the most important means of prophylaxis against the development of UV ray-associated eyelid neoplasms.
- Lid hygiene may reduce occurrences of chalazia and various cysts.
- Improved lipid metabolism may prevent and/or treat xanthoma formation.

PATHOPHYSIOLOGY

- Chalazion: Retained sebaceous secretions
- Epidermal inclusion cyst: Epidermis implanted in the dermis, usually from trauma or surgery
- Capillary hemangioma: Hamartomatous proliferation of benign vascular endothelium, likely of placental origin
- Squamous cell papilloma: Benign epithelial tumor
- Seborrheic keratosis: Originating in keratinocytes with acanthosis from basaloid cell proliferation. Somatic fibroblast growth factor receptor 3 mutations and activating transmembrane tyrosine kinase receptor mutations have been identified.
- Melanocytic nevus: Clumps of neural-crest derived melanocytes that migrate to the dermis and epidermis during development
- Xanthoma/Xanthelasma: Concentration of lipocytes

ETIOLOGY

- Chalazion: A chronic lipogranulomatous inflammatory lesion that is sterile. It may affect the meibomian glands, the glands of Zeis, or both. When superinfected, termed a hordeolum.
- Epidermal inclusion cyst: A superficial epidermal round keratin-filled lesion.
- Capillary hemangioma: A pink to faint red to violaceous macular lesion composed of vascular channels surrounded by a white halo. They typically undergo three stages: A proliferative phase, a stable period, and then involution. See the Treatment section.
- Squamous cell papilloma: Pedunculated "finger-like" projections often compared to fibroepithelial polyps found elsewhere on the body.
- Seborrheic keratosis: Usually multiple gray-brown greasy, scaly, sharply demarcated papules/plaques that may appear anywhere on the body except the palms and soles, with a predilection for the face and upper torso/back.
- Melanocytic nevi: Typically a flat lesion, ranging from smooth to verrucous, from well demarcated to slightly irregular, and from deeply pigmented to light (amelanotic).
- Apocrine hidrocystoma: Involving the glands of Moll, cysts and nodules can also involve any gland (Zeis, sweat, meibomian) of the eyelids. Pathology and histology depend on subtype.
- Xanthoma/xanthelasma: Yellow subcutaneous papules or plaques usually on the nasal upper eyelids. May also occur at lateral canthi.

COMMONLY ASSOCIATED CONDITIONS

- Ocular rosacea may be associated with chalazion and hordeolum formation.
- Visceral hemangiomas may be associated with multiple cutaneous capillary hemangiomas. Large hemangiomas may be associated with high-output cardiac failure or Kasabach–Merritt syndrome (thrombocytopenia, anemia, and low coagulant levels). Rarely, Maffucci syndrome, which has involvement of the feet and long bones, may be associated.
- Seborrheic keratoses may be associated with internal malignancies and may serve as cutaneous markers thereof.
- Dysplastic nevus syndrome, when multiple dysplastic nevi occur, is associated with increased risk of cutaneous/conjunctival/uveal melanomas.
- Corneal arcus in young age group, in the presence of xanthelasma, may signify hypercholesterolemia.
- Muir–Torre syndrome, Gorlin–Goltz syndrome, and xeroderma pigmentosum are syndromes associated with systemic malignancies/malformations but are associated with malignant skin tumors and will not be further discussed.

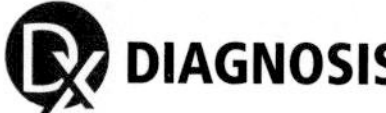

DIAGNOSIS

HISTORY

- Close attention should be paid to the duration of the lesion and to the pace of its growth, as noninflammatory benign lesions are typically slow growing or do not grow at all.
- Bleeding and necrosis are warning signs, as feeder blood vessels and tumors outgrowing their blood supply may signify malignancy.
- Previous history of skin lesions, benign or malignant, similar to or different from current pathology may provide insight into etiology of lesion or associations thereof.
- History of ocular surgery or trauma should be noted.
- History of systemic malignancies may be related.
- Previous treatment of inflammatory conditions such as allergies or blepharitis. These may predispose to eyelid cysts or chalazia. Unfortunately, chronic, unilateral blepharitis may be a misdiagnosis for a potentially malignant underlying etiology (e.g., sebaceous cell carcinoma).
- History of blistering sunburns, chronic UV exposure, and proximity to equator must be investigated.
- Previous history of radiation therapy should be taken into account.

PHYSICAL EXAM

- Thorough examination of the eyelids, including lid-flipping to examine tarsal conjunctiva, and adnexa for additional lesions, should be performed.
- Preauricular, submaxillary, cervical lymph nodes must be palpated.
- Lesions themselves must be inspected for ulcerations, necrosis, and neovascularization, all potential warning signs.
- Skin changes overlying the tumor itself are important in narrowing the differential diagnosis.
- Bleeding and discharge should be noted.
- Madarosis (loss of eyelashes), poliosis (whitening of eyelashes), and meibomian gland destruction should be noted, both locally and remote from lid lesions.

- Thorough slit-lamp and fundus examination should be performed in all patients.
- Capillary hemangiomas must be frequently monitored for facial distortion, interference with physiologic functioning (respiration, swallowing, hearing), strabismus, amblyopia, and bleeding.

DIAGNOSTIC TESTS & INTERPRETATION

Lab

- Any discharge may be sent for culture.
- Systemic laboratory tests are unnecessary unless malignancy or systemic involvement/associations are suspected.

Imaging

Imaging for benign eyelid lesions is unnecessary unless malignancy or systemic/orbital involvement is suspected.

Pathological Findings

- Chalazion: Inflammatory reaction composed primarily of epithelial, lymphocytic, and plasma cells with neutrophils and eosinophils on occasion.
- Epidermal inclusion cyst: Cavity lined by stratified squamous epithelium within the deeper dermis, filled with keratin.
- Capillary hemangioma: Nonencapsulated vascular channels of varying size in the dermis and subcutaneous tissue.
- Squamous cell papilloma: Vascular connective tissue encased by acanthotic, hyperkeratotic, and parakeratotic epithelium.
- Seborrheic keratosis: At least 6 variants, including acanthotic, reticulated, hyperkeratotic, clonal, inflamed, and melanoacanthoma subtypes. Histopathology depends on subtype.
- Melanocytic nevi: May be junctional, compound, or intradermal, with diagnosis being made by nest-like cellular arrangement.
- Xanthoma/xanthelasma: Dermal lipid-laden histiocytes with or without giant cells.

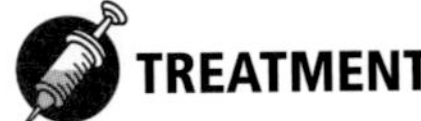

TREATMENT

Organized by Lesion Etiology

Chalazia:

First line

- Warm compresses with light massage at least q.i.d. for 10 min each time, with lid hygiene, are useful.
- Topical ophthalmic antibiotic is used for draining lesions or associated blepharitis.

Second line

- Incision and curettage are required.
- Steroid injection, dosage of which may depend on size of lesion, may be used. Triamcinolone can lead to depigmentation and skin atrophy.
- Oral doxycycline (100 mg PO b.i.d.) may be considered, particularly if associated with ocular rosacea.

Cysts:

First line

- Marsupialization, whereby the top of the lesion is amputated and contents are allowed to drain with secondary epithelialization, is required to be performed.
- Complete excision of the entire lesion in an attempt to keep capsule intact is required.

Second line

- Oftentimes complete excision follows failed marsupialization (rare).
- Nonsurgical modalities including injection of trichloroacetic acid have been shown to be useful for large or confluent apocrine hydrocystomas.

Capillary Hemangiomas:

First line

- 50% of lesions regress within 5 years, and 70% within 7 years. They often continue to fade into the early teens. Oftentimes frequent observation is warranted as a result.
- Therapy is undertaken for aggressive lesions as described above and is often individualized.
- Oral steroids at 2–4 mg/kg per day may be indicated for rapidly growing or distorting lesions.

Second line

- If the visual axis is involved, intralesional triamcinolone or betamethasone acetate may be administered (side effects include skin necrosis, adrenal suppression, growth retardation, and retinal artery occlusion).
- Interferon alpha-2a may be injected in refractory and particularly aggressive cases.
- Vascular-specific pulsed dye lasers can be effective in promoting involution of smaller lesions.
- Recently, propranolol has been administered for progressive lesions. Dose is usually 1 mg/kg per day in 3 equal doses for 1 week, doubled after 1 week, then tapered as seen fit. Typically propranolol is monitored in conjunction with child's pediatrician. See the 'Hemangioma in children' chapter.

Xanthelasma/Xanthoma:

First line

- Laser ablation or surgical excision is required.

Second line

- Oral simvastatin has recently been shown to resolve xanthelasma in association with lowered systemic lipid levels (2).

Papillomas/Seborrheic Keratosis/Nevi:

First line

- Treatment remains optional and cosmetic for all clinically benign lesions. However, lesions can grow and cause irritation and/or bleeding which necessitate excision.
- For cosmetic removal, laser ablation and cryotherapy are viable first-line options.
- Surgical excision of lesion, with wide margins entailing small portions of surrounding normal tissue, is required.

Second line

- For any suspicious lesion, biopsy must be performed.
- Incisional biopsies are common.
- Excisional biopsy with wide margins is preferable, and margins should be sent for both permanent and frozen sections.
- Mohs' micrographic surgery is an alternative intraoperative technique to ensure full resection in alternative to frozen sections.
- Map biopsy may be performed if diffuse local involvement is seen or suspected.
- Sentinel node biopsy may be indicated.

ADDITIONAL TREATMENT

General Measures

Reserved for malignant lesions: Include radiotherapy and/or chemotherapy. These are outside the scope of this chapter.

Issues for Referral

- Babies being treated for aggressive hemangiomas should be done so with consult to pediatric endocrinology, general pediatrics, and pediatric cardiology depending on treatment.
- Xanthoma/xanthelasma patients, particularly young (<50 years), may warrant referral to internists for evaluation of hyperlipidemia.

IN-PATIENT CONSIDERATIONS

Initial Stabilization

Neonates on propranolol for hemangiomas require vital sign checks every 30 min for 4 h after beginning the treatment. This should be done in collaboration with pediatric cardiology (3).

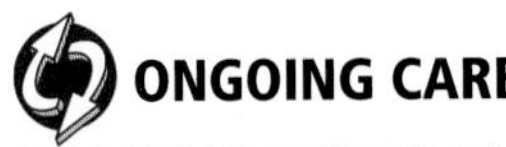

ONGOING CARE

FOLLOW-UP RECOMMENDATIONS

- All treated lesions should be followed chronically for recurrence. Care must be taken to differentiate recurrence from incomplete excision in surgical cases, as recurrences may involve different, potentially malignant pathology.
- Neonates with capillary hemangiomas should be examined twice weekly for 2 weeks after discharge, and then weekly by their internist. Ophthalmic evaluation frequency is subjective, but may be monthly to monitor aggressively for amblyopia (3).
- Care of premalignant and malignant lesions is outside the scope of this chapter.

DIET

Low cholesterol diet encouraged in patients with xanthomas/xanthelasmas

PATIENT EDUCATION

Specific to associations and risk factors as above

PROGNOSIS

Good for all benign lesions

REFERENCES

1. Deprez M, Uffer S. Clinicopathological features of eyelid skin tumors. A retrospective study of 5504 cases and review of the literature. *Am J Dermatopathol* 2009;31(3):256–262.
2. Shields CL, Mashayekhi A, Shields JA, et al. Disappearance of eyelid xanthelasma following oral simvastatin (Zocor). *Br J Ophthalmol* 2005;89: 639–640.
3. Manunza F, Syed S, Laguda B, et al. Propranolol for complicated infantile haemangiomas: A case series of 30 infants. *Br J Dermatol* 2010;162(2):466–468.

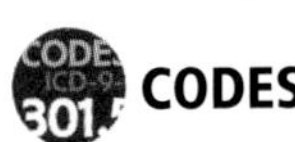

CODES

ICD9

- 216.1 Benign neoplasm of eyelid, including canthus
- 228.09 Hemangioma of other sites
- 374.51 Xanthelasma of eyelid

E

EYELID NEOPLASMS, MALIGNANT

Amanda Matthews
Jacqueline R. Carrasco

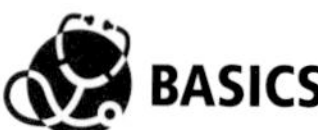

BASICS

DESCRIPTION

- The ocular adnexa contain virtually every tissue type and therefore, many types of malignant tumors can arise in this area.
- Early recognition and diagnosis of eyelid tumors are crucial to prevent local tissue destruction and distant spread.
- Metastasis can occur with many eyelid lesions and can cause significant morbidity and mortality.
- The most common malignant eyelid neoplasms include basal cell carcinoma (BCC), squamous cell carcinoma (SCC), sebaceous gland carcinoma, and malignant melanoma.
- Other extremely rare malignant tumors that can affect the eyelids are cutaneous T-cell and MALT lymphoma (see Ocular Adnexal Lymphoma chapter for further information), Merkel cell carcinoma, and Kaposi sarcoma.

EPIDEMIOLOGY

Incidence

- Varies by geographic region with degree of solar exposure.
- Approximately 5–10% of all skin cancers occur in the eyelid.
- Basal cell carcinoma: Approximately 14.35 cases per 100,000 population (80–90% of all malignant eyelid tumors).
- Squamous cell carcinoma: Between 0.09 and 2.42 cases per 100,000 population (5–10% of all malignant eyelid tumors).
- Non-basal cell and non-squamous cell tumors: Between 1.6 and 2.1 cases per 100,000 population (includes sebaceous gland carcinoma, 1–5% of all malignant eyelid tumors, malignant melanoma, 1% or less, and the very rare lymphoma, Merkel cell carcinoma and Kaposi sarcoma).

RISK FACTORS

Chronic sun exposure (the single most important risk factor), Caucasian race or fair skin color, older age, previous skin malignancy, immune dysfunction, focal dermatologic trauma (especially thermal burns), history of ionizing radiation, and exposure to trivalent inorganic arsenic.

GENERAL PREVENTION

Limit sun exposure, especially in childhood and adolescence.

PATHOPHYSIOLOGY

Chronic UV light exposure leads to defects in DNA repair that allows for malignant transformation and unchecked growth of tumor cells.

ETIOLOGY

- **Basal cell carcinoma:**
  - Neoplastic transformation of basal cells of epidermis
  - Abnormal basal cells proliferate and invade the dermis as nodules or strands
  - No premalignant lesion
  - Tumor enlargement is usually slow and rarely metastasizes
  - Potential to be locally invasive, especially with medial canthal involvement.
  - Occur most frequently on lower eyelid followed by medial canthus, upper eyelid, and lateral canthus.
  - Distant spread rarely occurs but does so by both hematogenous and lymphatic pathways.
  - Classified into 4 groups:
  - Localized (nodular, nodulo-ulcerative, and cyst): The classic, pearly BCC lesion that is indurated and firm with characteristic telangiectases over the tumor margins. It may display central ulceration. Rarely, a cystic variant is seen.
  - Diffuse (morpheaform, sclerosing): Flat, firm, white-pink to yellow subcutaneous lesion with indistinct clinical margins. Surface epidermis remains intact, that is, no ulceration. Complete surgical excision difficult and may result in large eyelid defect.
  - Superficial, multifocal: More irregular surface than nodular BCC and diffuse multicentric involvement of epidermis and dermis.
  - Fibroepitheliomatous basal cell carcinoma of Pinkus: Usually seen on the trunk.
- **Squamous cell carcinoma**:
  - Arises from prickle-squamous cell layer of epidermis
  - Spreads by extension into dermis
  - Multiple precursor lesions including actinic keratosis, Bowen's disease, and radiation dermatoses.
  - Occur most frequently on lower eyelid, followed by medial canthus, upper eyelid, and lateral canthus.
  - Variable presentation and can be mistaken for basal cell carcinoma.
  - Most commonly appear as painless nodular or plaque-like lesions.
  - Metastasis to regional lymph nodes but distant spread uncommon.
  - Perineural infiltration of SCC of the eyelids allows spread into the orbit, intracranial cavity, and periorbital structures.
- **Sebaceous gland carcinoma**:
  - Arises from the meibomian glands of the upper eyelid or the glands of Zeis.
  - Can occur many decades after radiation to the eyelids and face.
  - Often presents as small nodules and confused as recurrent chalazia or intractable blepharoconjunctivitis (known as the "masquerader").
  - There are two types of SGC based on the pattern of infiltration and include the nodular and non-nodular type.
  - The nodular type is minimally invasive and usually located on the tarsus or eyelid margin.
  - The non-nodular type is moderately-to-highly infiltrative and epithelial changes are more common.
  - There are also two types of intraepithelial spread and include pagetoid spread and replacement of the full thickness surface epithelium, resembling squamous cell carcinoma in situ.
  - Loss of eyelashes in the region of the tumor may help to differentiate SGC from more benign lesions.
  - SGC can be multicentric and has true metastatic potential.
  - Direct orbital extension into the orbit, paranasal sinuses, and intracranial cavity is possible.
  - Spread through lymphatic channels makes regional and systemic metastasis possible.
  - Local tumor recurrence after surgical excision is common and frequent surveillance is necessary.
  - Medical and oncologic referrals are important.
- **Malignant melanoma**:
  - Neoplastic proliferation of melanocytes.
  - Leading cause of death from primary skin tumors.
  - Four types including superficial spreading, nodular, lentigo maligna, and acral lentiginous melanoma.
  - Superficial spreading melanoma of the eyelid is elevated above the skin, has distinct borders, and displays a wide variety of colors including black, tan, rose, or gray.
  - Nodular melanoma has spherical nodularity and has a uniform blue–black color.
  - Lentigo maligna melanoma arises from a longstanding tan-colored macule and demonstrates surface elevation and nodule formation.
  - There are 2 methods to express depth of invasion and these are based on the anatomic level (Clark level) or the depth of invasion in millimeters (Breslow depth). The Breslow depth is the most important of the two classifications.
  - Stages I and II have no metastatic disease, stage III has regional lymph node involvement, and stage IV has distant metastasis.
  - Initial evaluation should include thorough history and physical, with special attention on the CNS, bone, and GI systems.
  - Medical and oncologic referrals are important.

COMMONLY ASSOCIATED CONDITIONS

- The basal cell nevus syndrome (Gorlin-Goltz syndrome) is autosomal dominant with high penetrance.
  - Mutation in PTCH gene on chromosome 9.
  - Multiple basal cell carcinomas, which can be seen early in childhood.
  - Associated with odontogenic cysts of the jaw, skeletal anomalies, and keratinizing pits on the palms and soles.
- Bazex syndrome is an x-linked dominant disorder.
  - Multiple basal cell carcinomas that develop on the face in childhood and adolescence.
  - Typical "ice-pick marks" on the extremities caused by atrophic dermal changes.
- The linear unilateral basal cell nevus syndrome
  - Unilateral distribution of basal cell carcinomas, multiple comedones, epidermoid cysts, and areas of striae-like atrophy.
  - Associations with scoliosis and atherosclerotic heart disease.
- Xeroderma pigmentosum is an autosomal recessive disease causing a defect in DNA repair.
  - Multiple squamous cell carcinomas, basal cell carcinomas, and melanomas develop on sun-exposed areas and arise in the first 2 decades of life.
- Albinism is an inherited disorder of melanin synthesis.
  - Lack of melanin leads to damage by solar radiation and an increased risk for all skin malignancies.
  - One-third of all basal cell carcinomas in black Africans occur in patients with albinism.

DIAGNOSIS

- Any patient presenting with an asymptomatic or irritating eyelid lesion should have a prompt biopsy performed by an experienced surgeon (1)[A].
  - Incisional biopsy when malignancy suspected, except with malignant melanoma where excisional biopsy with wide surgical margins is preferred.
  - Margins of potential sebaceous gland carcinoma and malignant melanoma are sent for permanent section.
  - Sentinel node biopsy may be necessary depending on depth of invasion by eyelid melanoma.
- Histopathologic confirmation.

HISTORY

- The following apply for all malignant eyelid tumors:
  - Duration
  - Slow versus rapid growth
  - Previous malignant skin lesion
  - History of radiation therapy
  - History of arsenic exposure
  - History of inflammatory or allergic condition

PHYSICAL EXAM

- Skin ulceration and signs of inflammation
- Distortion/disruption of normal eyelid anatomy
- Abnormal color or texture
- Persistent crusting and/or bleeding
- Focal loss of eyelashes (madarosis)
- Focal whitening of eyelashes (poliosis)
- Presence of abnormal vessels
  - Sentinel or feeder vessels
  - Telangiectatic vessels at tumor margins
- Orbital signs (proptosis, diplopia, external ophthalmoplegia) are extremely concerning for orbital invasion.

DIAGNOSTIC TESTS & INTERPRETATION

Pathological Findings

- Basal cell carcinoma: Proliferation of cells with oval nuclei and scant cytoplasm. These cells form large nests and have the characteristic "basaloid" appearance. Cells at the periphery of each nest are usually arranged in a radial, or "palisading," pattern.
- Squamous cell carcinoma: Intraepidermal squamous cell carcinoma is characterized by full-thickness atypia of the epidermis. When the atypical cells invade through the basement membrane, it becomes invasive SCC. Cells are typically polygonal with abundant cytoplasm and dyskeratotic cells with keratin pearls are present.
- Sebaceous gland carcinoma: Numerous sebaceous elements with mitotic figures. Large anaplastic cells are seen with prominent nuclei in foamy or frothy cytoplasm. This foamy appearance is a result of the presence of lipid vacuoles. Highly characteristic is spread of the tumor in the form of infiltrating lobules, nests and cords, as well as superficially.
  - Stain positive for lipid with oil red O stain.
- Malignant melanoma: The most common type, superficial spreading melanoma has a radial growth phase characterized by increased numbers of intraepithelial melanocytes that are large and atypical and arranged haphazardly at the dermoepidermal junction. These cells show upward migration (pagetoid spread). Dermal invasion confers metastatic potential.

DIFFERENTIAL DIAGNOSIS

See "Benign Eyelid Neoplasms".

TREATMENT

- Basal cell carcinoma and squamous cell carcinoma:
  - Excision with Mohs micrographic surgery (1)[A] OR
  - frozen-section or permanent-section control (1)[A]
  - These treatments yield the highest cure rate and lowest recurrence.
  - Excise entire tumor with clear margins
  - If contraindications to surgery, cryotherapy may be used in a double freeze-thaw method to eradicate the tumor cells (1,2,3)[A]
- Sebaceous gland carcinoma:
  - Mohs' micrographic surgery (1)[A]
  - Excision with frozen-section control combined with conjunctival map biopsies (1)[A]
  - Some recommend supplemental cryotherapy at the time of excision and topical chemotherapy (mitomycin C) if there is any question of residual involvement (1,6,7)[B]
  - If contraindication to surgery, electron beam radiotherapy is an alternative treatment (1,4,5)[B]
  - If orbital invasion, exenteration is the preferred treatment (1,6,8)[A]
- Malignant melanoma:
  - Recommendations for treatment are varied and often conflicting
  - Treatment often depends on Breslow thickness: <1.0 mm- excision with 1.0-cm margins (1)[A], 1.0–2.0 mm- excision with 3.0-cm margins (1)[A]
  - Stage III or IV disease: A sentinel node biopsy and lymph node mapping should be performed (1,9,10)[A]
  - Stage II-IV disease: Administration of adjuvant interferon should be considered (1,11)[B]

ADDITIONAL TREATMENT

General Measures

Suntan lotion and other protective measures against UV sunlight exposure.

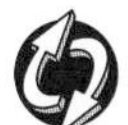

ONGOING CARE

FOLLOW-UP RECOMMENDATIONS

- Ophthalmologist follow-up
  - Initially every 1–2 weeks to ensure proper healing of surgical site
  - Reevaluation every 6–12 months thereafter, more frequent visits if an aggressive tumor type was identified such as sebaceous gland carcinoma or malignant melanoma.
- Family physician or dermatologist for thorough, full-body, skin examinations.
- Oncology follow-up is important in patients with sebaceous gland carcinoma and malignant melanoma.
- Refer to radiation oncologist if there is need for radiotherapy.

PATIENT EDUCATION

www.skincancer.org

COMPLICATIONS

- Local tissue destruction with loss of normal anatomy and function.
- Orbital, periorbital, intracranial, and systemic spread can occur with any malignant eyelid neoplasm.
- Loss of vision.
- Potentially death if there is intracranial spread or metastasis.

ADDITIONAL READING

- Bartley GB, Garrity JA, Waller RR, et al. Orbital exenteration at the Mayo Clinic: 1967–1986. *Ophthalmology* 1989;96:468–473.
- Cook BE, Bartley GB. Treatment options and future prospects for the management of eyelid malignancies. *Ophthalmology* 2001;108: 2088–2098.
- Curtis ME, Waltz K. Major review: Basal cell carcinoma of the eyelid and periocular skin. *Surv of Ophthalmology* 1993;38:169–192.
- Esmaeli B. Sentinel lymph node mapping for patients with cutaneous and conjunctival malignant melanoma [review]. *Ophthal Plast Reconstr Surg* 2000;16:170–172.
- Gennari R, Bartolomei M, Testori A. Sentinel node localization in primary melanoma: Preoperative dynamic lymphoscintigraphy, intraoperative gamma probe, and vital dye guidance. *Surgery* 2000;127: 19–25.
- Hendley RL, Rieser JC, Cavanagh HD, et al. Primary radiation therapy for meibomian gland carcinoma (case report). *Am J Ophthalmology* 1979;87: 206–209.
- Ide CH, Ridings GR, Yamashita T, Buesseler JA. Radiotherapy of a recurrent adenocarcinoma of the meibomian gland. *Arch Ophthalmology* 1968;79:540–544.
- Lens MB and Dawes M. Interferon alpha therapy in malignant melanoma: A systematic review of randomized controlled trials. *J Clin Oncol* 2002;20:1818–1825.
- Lisman RD, Jakobiec FA, Small P. Sebaceous carcinoma of the eyelids. The role of adjunctive cryotherapy in the management of conjunctival pagetoid spread. *Ophthalmology* 1989;96: 1021–1026.
- Shields JA, Demirci H, Marr BP, et al. Sebaceous carcinoma of the eyelids; Personal experience with 60 cases. *Ophthalmology* 2004;111:2151–2157.
- Tuppurainen K. Cryotherapy for eyelid and periocular basal cell carcinomas: Outcome in 166 cases over an 8 year period. *Graefes Arch Clin Exp Ophthalmology* 1995;223:205–208.

CODES

ICD9

- 172.1 Malignant melanoma of skin of eyelid, including canthus
- 173.1 Other malignant neoplasm of skin of eyelid, including canthus

FABRY'S DISEASE

Ethan H. Tittler
Hong Wei
George L. Spaeth

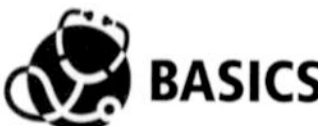

BASICS

DESCRIPTION

- Also known as Anderson–Fabry disease and α-galactosidase A deficiency, Fabry disease is a rare, X-linked recessive lysosomal storage disorder that, when left untreated, is potentially fatal. Defect in the GLA gene coding for the enzyme α-galactosidase A (α-GAL), which leads to an accumulation of glycosphingolipids, in particular globotriaosylceramide (GL-3), throughout the body. Elevated GL-3 causes cellular dysfunction, most notably in the vasculature, with resulting damage to the renal, cardiac, and vascular systems. Life expectancy shortened by 20 years in males and 15 years in females, often from renal failure, cardiomyopathy, and early stroke.
- Systemic manifestations include angiokeratomas characteristically found between the umbilicus and knees, intermittent pain crises, and hypohidrosis/anhydrosis.
- Ocular manifestations appear early and include whorl-like corneal deposits (cornea verticillata), distinctive spoke-like posterior cataracts, and vascular tortuosity of the bulbar conjunctiva and retina. Rarely affects vision.

EPIDEMIOLOGY

Incidence

Estimated 1:40,000 to 1:170,000, though newborn screening has demonstrated 1:3,100 males.

Prevalence

1:80,000 to 117,000.

RISK FACTORS

Family history, male sex, though heterozygous females can express the Fabry phenotype at various levels of severity due to random variations in X-chromosome inactivation.

Genetics

- X-linked recessive, mutation of GLA gene at Xq22.1 locus.
  - Over 150 mutations at this locus have been linked to a deficiency in the enzyme α-galactosidase A.

GENERAL PREVENTION

- Genetic counseling and prenatal chorionic villus sampling (10–12 weeks) or amniocentesis (15–18 weeks).
- Early treatment may prevent secondary complications of Fabry disease.

PATHOPHYSIOLOGY

- The glycosphingolipid metabolic pathway is responsible for breaking down glycosphingolipid components of the plasma membrane of cells. In this pathway, α-galactosidase A (α-GAL) converts globotriaosylceramide (GL-3) to lactosyl ceramide.
- Mutation of GAL gene causes α-GAL deficiency, which causes an accumulation of the upstream substrate GL-3 within lysosomes.
- High levels of GL-3 are found throughout the body and in the fluids of patients with Fabry disease, most notably in the lysosomes of endothelial, perithelial, and smooth-muscle cells of blood vessels.

ETIOLOGY

Mutation in gene coding for α-GAL causes enzyme deficiency and build-up of toxic substrate.

COMMONLY ASSOCIATED CONDITIONS

- Dermatologic
  - Clusters of angiokeratomas (non-blanching, individual, punctuate, dark red to blue-black telangiectasias) most dense between the umbilicus and knees
  - Hypo/anhydrosis
- Neurologic
  - Acroparesthesias (periodic crises of severe pain in the extremities) appear early
  - Early TIA or stroke
  - Hearing loss (CN VIII)
- Ocular
  - Cornea verticillata (whorl-like inferior corneal subepithelial deposits)—an early finding
  - Distinctive spoke-like posterior cataracts; wedge-shaped anterior cataracts
  - Vascular tortuosity and aneurismal dilation of the bulbar conjunctiva and retina
- Cardiac
  - Mitral insufficiency, left ventricular hypertrophy
  - Dysrhythmias
  - Cardiomyopathy
- Renal
  - Mild proteinuria appears in childhood/ adolescence
  - Progressive renal insufficiency leading to end-stage renal disease

DIAGNOSIS

HISTORY

- Classically, symptom onset in childhood or adolescence (acroparesthesias, angiokeratomas, ocular findings, hypohidrosis).
- Gradually progressive renal insufficiency in the 3rd to 5th decade and eventually death due to renal disease, heart failure, or cerebrovascular accident (55% of males, 45% of females).
  - Later-onset patients' initial presentation may be for renal, cardiovascular, and/or cerebrovascular symptoms.

PHYSICAL EXAM

- Ocular findings are visible early (as early as age 1)
  - Cornea verticillata (95% of males, 88% of females)
  - Spoke-like posterior cataracts (70% of males, 35% of females)
  - Vascular tortuosity and aneurismal dilation of the bulbar conjunctiva and retina (77% of males, 19% of females)
- Skin
  - Angiokeratomas between the umbilicus and knees (66% of males, 36% of females). Occasionally seen intraperiorally and periorally
  - Hypo/anhydrosis (almost constant finding)
- Cardiac
  - Arrhythmias, murmurs, chest heave, laterally displaced PMI
- Abdomen
  - Tenderness, hyperactive bowel sounds

DIAGNOSTIC TESTS & INTERPRETATION

Lab

Initial lab tests

- α-GAL enzyme activity assay of both plasma and leukocytes
- Heterozygous females may have normal enzyme activity, so molecular genetic testing may be necessary
- During childhood and adolescence, urinalysis

Imaging

Initial approach

No special imaging necessary for diagnosis.

Follow-up & special considerations

- Additional confirmation can be made by identifying mutation in α-GAL gene with molecular genetic testing.
- CBC, CMP for systemic manifestations.
- Secondary complications of Fabry disease may require imaging
  - Cardiac: ECG, chest X-ray, echo
  - Vascular: Duplex Doppler, angiogram
  - Neurologic: CT, MRI
  - Skin: electron microscopy of Fabry angiokeratomas demonstrate characteristic electron-dense, lamellar (zebra-like) inclusions within endothelial and other cell types

Diagnostic Procedures/Other

- Decreased α-GAL enzyme activity is diagnostic of Fabry disease, and confirmation can be made with molecular genetic testing.
- Any patient with a constellation of intermittent acroparesthesias, anhydrosis, angiokeratomas, left ventricular hypertrophy, corneal and/or lenticular opacities, and renal insufficiency of unknown etiology should be worked up for Fabry disease.

Pathological Findings

- Early on, urinalysis demonstrates protein, casts, red cells, and characteristic "Maltese crosses" in sediment, progressing to end-stage renal disease with electrolyte disturbances and anemia.
- Cardiac dysrhythmias including ST segment changes, T-wave inversion, and intermittent supraventricular tachycardia
- Left ventricular hypertrophy
- Multifocal cerebral small vessel involvement with thromboses, aneurisms, intracranial bleeds and areas of ischemia

DIFFERENTIAL DIAGNOSIS

- Angiokeratomas of Fabry
  - Can be confused with petechiae, pyogenic granulomas, eruptive angiomas, or angiokeratomas of Fordyce spots
  - Other metabolic syndromes that cause angiokeratomas include fucosidosis, aspartylglycosaminuria, galactosialidosis, Schindler/Kanzaki disease, mannosidosis
- Cornea verticillata
  - Long-term therapy with amiodarone, aminoquinolines, atovaquone, clofazimine, gold, ibuprofen, indomethacin, mepacrine, monobenzone, naproxen, perhexiline maleate, phenothiazines, suramin, tamoxifen, tilorone hydrochloride
  - Environmental exposure to silica dust.
  - Multiple myeloma
- Pain crises
  - Rheumatic fever, neurosis, erythromelalgia, rheumatoid arthritis, juvenile arthritis, SLE, "growing pains," Raynaud syndrome, multiple sclerosis

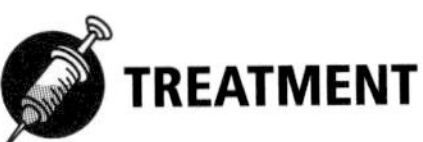

TREATMENT

MEDICATION

First Line

- Enzyme replacement therapy (ERT) as early as possible in all males and in females carriers with significant disease:
  - Agalsidase beta (Fabrazyme) 1 mg/kg body weight infused every 2 weeks as an IV infusion. The initial IV infusion rate should be no more than 0.25 mg/min (15 mg/h).
- For acroparesthesias:
  - Diphenylhydantoin
  - Carbamazepine
  - Gabapentin
- For renal disease:
  - ACE inhibitor (benazepril 40 mg per day) and ARB (losartan 100 mg PO per day)
- Antiplatelet agents (clopidogrel 75 mg PO per day) may be recommended for prophylaxis against stroke and central retinal artery occlusion.
- Lipid- (simvastatin 40 PO per day) and blood pressure (diltiazem 360 mg PO per day) lowering agents may be recommended for those with cardiac ischemia

Second Line

- Thiazide diuretic (hydrochlorothiazide 25–50 mg PO per day)
- Beta-blocker (atenolol 100 mg PO per day)
- Hydralazine

ADDITIONAL TREATMENT

General Measures

Chronic hemodialysis, if needed.

Issues for Referral

- Fabry disease is a rare, complex, and serious disease that requires consultation with and coordination amongst many specialists:
  - Pediatricians
  - Nephrologists
  - Neurologists
  - Cardiologists
  - Dermatologists
  - Ophthalmologists
  - Geneticists
  - Psychiatrists and psychologists
  - Social workers

Additional Therapies

- Mental health consultations for psychosocial impact of disease on patient
- Nutrition and exercise to decrease risk of cardiovascular disease

COMPLEMENTARY & ALTERNATIVE THERAPIES

Antioxidants and omega-3 fatty acids may have benefit by reducing vascular damage.

SURGERY/OTHER PROCEDURES

- Allograft kidney transplant can be curative of renal dysfunction (engrafted kidney has normal enzyme activity)
- For angiokeratomas:
  - Laser therapy

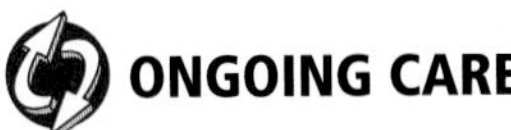

ONGOING CARE

FOLLOW-UP RECOMMENDATIONS

Annual (or more frequent) renal, cardiology, and hearing evaluations.

Patient Monitoring

- Patient should be followed by specialists in the organ systems most affected by Fabry disease.
  - Cardiology: ECG, echo, BNP
  - Neurology: Diphenylhydantoin levels (if prescribed)
  - Nephrology: CMP, urinalysis, creatinine
- Siblings and female offspring of affected patients should be tested for Fabry disease.

DIET

Low-fat, low salt diet may reduce or delay cardiovascular and renal dysfunction.

PATIENT EDUCATION

Lifelong care from various specialists will be required to maintain health beyond middle age.

PROGNOSIS

- Without treatment for end-stage renal disease, mean age of death is 41 years.
- With enzyme replacement therapy, patients can expect stabilization of their renal function, improved cardiac function, and decreases in neuropathy and gastrointestinal symptoms.

REFERENCES

1. Eng CM, Ioannou YA, Desnick RJ. Alpha-Galactosidase a deficiency: Fabry disease. *The Metabolic and Molecular Bases of Inherited Disease*. In: Scriver C, Beaudet A, Sly W, et al, eds. New York: McGraw Hill, 2001:3733–3774.
2. Pinto LLC, Vieira TA, Giugliani R, Schwartz IVD. Expression of the disease on female carriers X-linked lysosomal disorders: A brief review. *Orphanet J Rare Dis* 2010;5(1):14.
3. Samiy N. Ocular features of fabry disease: Diagnosis of a treatable life-threatening disorder. *Surv Ophthalmol* 2008;53(4):416–423.

ADDITIONAL READING

- Larralde Margarita M, Luna Paula C, "Chapter 136. Fabry Disease" (Chapter). In: Wolff K, Goldsmith LA, Katz SI, Gilchrest B, Paller AS, Leffell DJ, eds. Fitzpatrick's Dermatology in General Medicine, 7e: http://www.accessmedicine.com/content.aspx?aID = 2976828.
- Mehta A, Hughes DA, "Fabry Disease". *GeneReviews*[Internet]. In: Pagon RA, Bird TC, Dolan CR, Stephens K, eds.Seattle (WA): University of Washington, Seattle; 1993–2002 Aug 05, Feb 2008 update.

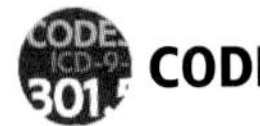

CODES

ICD9

- 272.7 Lipidoses
- 371.10 Corneal deposit, unspecified
- 743.31 Congenital capsular and subcapsular cataract

CLINICAL PEARLS

- The presentation of angiokeratomas in a "bathing suit pattern" (umbilicus to knees) with cornea verticillata (whorl-like inferior corneal deposits) is practically pathognomonic.

FAMILIAL EXUDATIVE VITREORETINOPATHY

Jared D. Peterson
Allen Chiang
Arunan Sivalingam

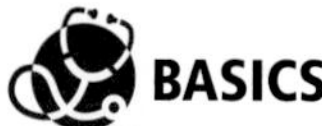

BASICS

DESCRIPTION

- Familial exudative vitreoretinopathy (FEVR) is a rare, inherited disorder in which one of several known gene mutations results in abnormal development of the retinal vasculature, characterized by a peripheral avascular zone.
- Secondary neovascularization (NV) may develop in response to retinal ischemia and may progress to fibrosis, retinal folds, macular ectopia, and ultimately, tractional retinal detachment (TRD). Cataract, neovascular glaucoma, and band keratopathy may occur in advanced stages.
- Phenotypic variability exists within families and even between eyes of the same patient; most are asymptomatic, while some suffer partial or even complete loss of vision.
- The clinical course can vary as well, from a nonprogressive or only slowly progressive course over a lifetime to a rapidly progressive course with total retinal detachment at a young age.
- Originally thought to stabilize in early adult life, FEVR is now recognized to have the potential of progressing even after years of stability.
- FEVR is usually bilateral, but may be markedly asymmetric.

EPIDEMIOLOGY

Incidence

Unknown (many are asymptomatic).

Prevalence

Unknown, yet likely underestimated given that molecular testing has suggested up to 90% of affected individuals may be asymptomatic (1).

RISK FACTORS

Family history of FEVR.

Genetics

- Autosomal dominance is the most common mode of inheritance, with autosomal recessive and X-linked recessive cases also being reported.
- Penetrance estimated to be 90–100% when using indirect ophthalmoscopy and fluorescein angiography to evaluate.
- Highly variable phenotypic expressivity ranging from asymptomatic disease to complete blindness in infancy.
- Thus far, 4 loci have been mapped, with genes from 3 of these loci identified:
  - The EVR1 locus localizes to chromosome 11q13-q23; the EVR1 gene is FZD4.
  - The EVR2 locus is the X-linked recessive locus and localizes to chromosome Xp11.4; the EVR2 gene is NDP, the same mutated gene in Norrie disease (X-linked recessive disorder characterized by congenital blindness as well as sensorineural deafness and mental deficiencies in 30% of patients).
  - The EVR3 locus localizes to chromosome 11p12-p13; the specific gene at this locus has not yet been identified.
  - The EVR4 locus localizes to a region within the original EVR1 locus, near FZD4; the EVR4 gene is LRP5.
  - A recent study suggests at least a 4th locus for autosomal dominant FEVR, indicating FEVR to be even more heterogeneous than formerly realized (2).
- Proteins encoded by the 3 known FEVR genes are part of a signaling complex in the Norrin-β-catenin pathway, which is pivotal to retinal vasogenesis.
  - Recently, Junge et al. (3) identified TSPAN12, (another component of this signaling complex) and Poulter et al. (4) showed TSPAN12 mutations lead to autosomal dominant FEVR.

GENERAL PREVENTION

None.

PATHOPHYSIOLOGY

- Gene mutations lead to defective protein products within a signaling complex that activates the Norrin-β-catenin pathway, which is vital to proper development of retinal vasculature.
- Defects in this pathway lead to incomplete retinal vascularization, leaving a peripheral avascular zone, which is thought to be the primary event in all affected patients.
- Complications secondary to the resulting peripheral retinal ischemia may ultimately result in variable degrees of vision loss.
- 20% of FEVR cases experience partial or total blindness (2).

ETIOLOGY

One of several gene mutations results in incomplete development of the retinal vasculature. Subsequently, peripheral ischemia leads to multiple complications and visual morbidity.

COMMONLY ASSOCIATED CONDITIONS

Patients with FEVR due to mutations in LRP5 have been shown to have reduced bone mass, a finding not yet reported in other forms of FEVR (1).

DIAGNOSIS

HISTORY

- A complete family history as well as history of any prematurity and/or oxygen therapy should be ascertained.
- Earlier studies suggested roughly 1/2 of affected individuals are asymptomatic. Recent molecular testing suggests this figure could be as high as 90% (1).
- Diagnosis of asymptomatic patients is typically made when family members of suspected or known cases are examined.
- Most infants present with failure to fix/follow, pendular nystagmus, heterotropia, or rarely, leukocoria from large retinal detachment (RD) or significant lipid exudation.
- Most children/adults present with a decrease in vision caused by RD, retinal folds, or macular ectopia.
- Some may present with pseudoexotropia (positive angle kappa due to ectopic macula).

PHYSICAL EXAM

- Visual acuity ranges from 20/20 to <20/200.
- Complete dilated fundus examination including scleral depression
- Avascular zone in the peripheral retina is present in all patients and may be the lone manifestation. It is usually confined to the temporal periphery, but may extend 360°
  - Visualization of avascular zone enhanced with green filter during ophthalmoscopy
- Other funduscopic findings may include the following:
  - Brushlike appearance of retinal vessels near the avascular zone
  - Extensive branching of retinal vasculature
  - Dilated vessels with temporally bent course
  - Neovascularization
  - Vitreous hemorrhage
  - Subretinal exudation
  - Fibrotic reaction manifest as vitreoretinal opacities
  - Retinal traction leading to retinal folds, macular ectopia (optic disc and retina dragged temporally), or TRD

DIAGNOSTIC TESTS & INTERPRETATION

Imaging

- Fluorescein angiography (FA) with peripheral sweeps, or ultrawide field FA
- Key angiographic features include the following (5)[B]:
- Abrupt capillary closure (avascular zone)
- Dragging of perimacular capillaries and vessels temporally toward periphery
- Dilation of perimacular capillaries with mild leakage
- Abnormal tortuous and stretched vessels
- Peripheral AV shunts with leakage

Pathological Findings

Cases to date have shown total retinal detachment with prominent fibrovascular membranes. In addition, some cases have shown intraretinal and subretinal cells/exudates, and focal retinal inflammation (6).

DIFFERENTIAL DIAGNOSIS

- The condition that most closely resembles FEVR is retinopathy of prematurity (ROP).
  - Positive family history and lack of history of prematurity help distinguish FEVR from ROP.
- Other conditions that may mimic FEVR: Persistent fetal vasculature, X-linked retinoschisis, Norrie disease, incontinentia pigmenti, Coats' disease, pars planitis, and Toxocara infection (7).

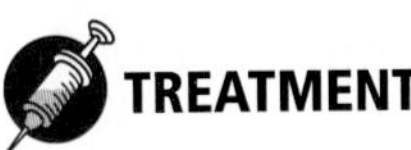

TREATMENT

ADDITIONAL TREATMENT

Additional Therapies

- Anti-VEGF therapy:
  - 1 case series (8)[C] of 4 patients with increasing exudates despite standard therapy were given a single injection of pegaptanib sodium. After 11 months, all patients had evidence of decreased exudation. However, traction continued to progress, possibly even accelerated by the anti-VEGF agent.
  - More data needed to assess role/long term complications of VEGF inhibitors in FEVR

SURGERY/OTHER PROCEDURES

- The following recommendations are based on a retrospective case series by Pendergast and Trese (9)[C]:
  - Eyes with presence of avascular zone only should be observed.
  - Eyes with early stages of neovascularization or exudate without retinal detachment should receive laser ablation or cryotherapy if there is significant exudation and retinal elevation.
  - Eyes with mild TRD not involving the fovea may respond well to scleral buckling alone, while more advanced detachments require pars plana vitrectomy as well.

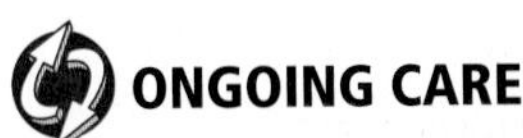

ONGOING CARE

FOLLOW-UP RECOMMENDATIONS

- Children require regular monitoring for early detection of neovascularization, exudate, and TRD.
- Asymptomatic patients whose only manifestation is the peripheral avascular region may require annual follow-up only.
- Those with neovascularization or exudate should undergo treatment and close observation.
- Those with retinal traction should be followed at intervals based on stability of clinical findings.

Patient Monitoring

See Follow-Up Recommendations section.

PATIENT EDUCATION

- Genetic counseling appropriate to the mode of inheritance should be offered.
- Family members should be educated on the chronic, progressive course and variable nature of the disease and should undergo screening examination.

PROGNOSIS

- Benson (7) reported a poor visual prognosis with onset of symptoms prior to age 3; older patients were thought to have a better prognosis due to more asymmetric involvement.
- Even those considered stable for years have the potential to progress.
- Patients with early exudation in which the abnormal vessels respond to laser or cryotherapy appear to have the best prognosis.

COMPLICATIONS

Neovascularization, hemorrhage, exudation, AV malformations, falciform folds and macular ectopia, retinal tears and TRD, blindness.

REFERENCES

1. Toomes C, Downey L. Familial exudative vitreoretinopathy, autosomal dominant. In: Pagon RA, Bird TC, Dolan CR, Stephens K, (eds). *Gene Reviews*. University of Washington: Seattle; 1993–2005, Dec 2008 update.
2. Toomes C, Downey LM, Bottomley HM, et al. Further evidence of genetic heterogeneity in familial exudative vitreoretinopathy; exclusion of EVR1, EVR3, EVR4 in a large autosomal dominant pedigree. *Br J Ophthalmol* 2005;89(2):194–197.
3. Junge HJ, Yang S, Burton JB, et al. TSPAN12 regulates retinal vascular development by promoting Norrin-but not Wnt-induced FZD4/beta-catenin signaling. *Cell* 2009;139:299–311.
4. Poulter JA, Manir A, Gilmour DF, et al. Mutations in TSPAN12 cause autosomal-dominant familial exudative vitreoretinopathy. *Am J Hum Genet* 2010;86:248–253.
5. Nijhuis FA, Deutman AF, Aan de Kerk AL. Fluorecein angiography in mild stages of dominant exudative vitreoretinopathy. *Mod Probl Ophthalmol* 1979;20:107–114.
6. Boldrey EE, Egbert P, Gass DM, et al. The histopathology of familial exudative vitreoretinopathy. *Arch Ophthalmol* 1985;103: 238–41.
7. Benson WE. Familial Exudative vitreoretinopathy. *Trans Am Ophthalmol Soc* 1195;93:473–521.
8. Quiram PA, Dresner KA, Lai MM, et al. Treatment of vascularly active familial exudative vitreoretinopathy with pegaptanib sodium (Macugen). *Retina* 2008;28(3):S8–S12.
9. Pendergast SD, Trese MT. Familial exudative vitreoretinopathy. Results of surgical management. *Ophthalmology* 1998;105:1015–1023.

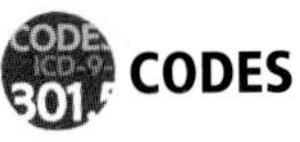

CODES

ICD9

- 362.12 Exudative retinopathy
- 362.16 Retinal neovascularization nos

CLINICAL PEARLS

- The sentinel event in FEVR is a genetic defect that results in incomplete development of retinal vasculature. Visual morbidity arises secondary to complications from retinal ischemia associated with a peripheral avascular zone.
- Genetic mutations within a signaling complex that activates the Norrin-β-catenin pathway, which regulates retinal vasogenesis, have been identified.
- FEVR has wide phenotypic variability:
  - Mild forms of disease are often asymptomatic and show only peripheral abnormalities such as an avascular zone, AV malformations, and increased vascular branching.
  - More severe forms show neovascularization, vitreous hemorrhage, subretinal exudation, and fibrosis with retinal traction, tears, detachment, and/or macular ectopia.
- Family members of FEVR patients should be screened to promote early detection.
- FEVR is a lifetime disease and may continue to progress years after considered to be "stable."

F

FETAL ALCOHOL SYNDROME

Tiffany Shiau
Esther Lee
Alex V. Levin

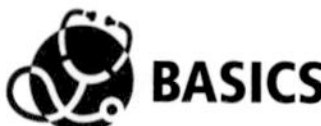

BASICS

DESCRIPTION

- Fetal Alcohol Syndrome (FAS) is the most severe end on the continuum known as Fetal Alcohol Spectrum Disorders (FASD), an umbrella term that encompasses the adverse effects to developing fetuses from alcohol exposure in utero.
- With the proposed clarifications to the Institute of Medicine's 1996 diagnostic criteria, children with FAS must fulfill 3 domains. Growth retardation (≤10th percentile for height or weight), facial anomalies that satisfy ≥2 of the 3: short palpebral fissures, thin vermilion border of upper lip and smooth philtrum, and lastly central nervous system abnormalities (structural or small head circumference).
- The presence or absence of maternal alcohol exposure divides FAS into 2 subcategories (1)[A]: FAS with confirmed maternal alcohol exposure and FAS without confirmed maternal alcohol exposure.
- Further, partial FAS characterizes those who satisfy the aforementioned facial malformations but have anomalies in only 1 of the other domains (CNS function/structure or growth).

EPIDEMIOLOGY

Incidence

With 4 billion babies born worldwide every year with in utero ethanol exposure, an estimated 1000–6000 have FAS (2)[C].

Prevalence

0.5–2.0 cases per 1000 live births (2)[C].

RISK FACTORS

- Consuming ≥1 drinks per day or binges of >5 drinks each episode (3)[C]
- Threshold not clearly defined because even 0.5 drink daily has been linked to adverse outcomes

Genetics

- High recurrence rates in siblings
- Higher rates have been detected for African Americans and Native Americans vs. non-Hispanic whites
- Different genotypes of alcohol dehydrogenase 1B (ADH1B), a gene (2)[A] which encodes the enzyme that catalyzes the breakdown of ethanol to acetaldehyde, has been found to carry unique risks for FAS.
- Most studies on ADH1B found a higher risk of alcohol-caused birth defects when the fetal genotype is homozygous for a particular at risk allele. The same genotype was also associated with a higher drinking frequency at conception. This does not explain the higher FAS occurrence in African Americans and Native Americans, the groups that have lower prevalence of the genotype.
- Another ADH1B allele seems to be a protective factor.
- Sequence variation in the cytochrome P450 E1 (CYP2E1) gene, which is involved in ethanol metabolism, has been suggested to yield a higher risk for FAS, even after adjusting for alcohol intake.

GENERAL PREVENTION

- FAS is entirely preventable (4)[A] if the pregnancy is alcohol-free. A strong predictor of alcohol use during pregnancy is consumption prior to conception.
- The U.S. Preventive Services Task Force recommended screening and behavioral counseling interventions in the primary care setting to lower alcohol abuse.

PATHOPHYSIOLOGY

- Mechanisms not well understood and most knowledge based on animal studies (5)[C]
- Craniofacial manifestations of FAS are likely due to teratogenic effects of ethanol and/or its metabolites such as acetaldehyde, before or during gastrulation and neurulation.
- Alcohol intoxication induces oxidative stress with production of free radicals and disturbance of antioxidant activities.
- Immunocytochemical assays performed with bromouridine incorporated into ethanol-exposed rats' retina and optic nerve demonstrated diminished transcription activity in the eye tissues.

ETIOLOGY

- Prenatal exposure to alcohol, a proven teratogen
- Polymorphisms in certain genes may predispose the growing fetus to FAS.

COMMONLY ASSOCIATED CONDITIONS

- Poor adaptive and communication skills, including poor understanding of social cues and registering information in social contexts (6)[A]
- Lower IQ
- Learning disabilities, seen in subjects such as language comprehension and mathematics
- Substance abuse
- Mental health problems
- Congenital heart defects and other medical conditions

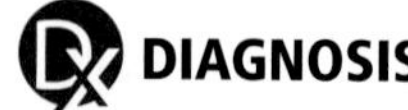

DIAGNOSIS

HISTORY

- Exposure to alcohol in utero
- NOTE: Patients often underreport consumption due to stigmatization.

PHYSICAL EXAM

- Ophthalmological findings are frequently seen in children with FAS, the most common findings are (7)[A] the following:
  - short palpebral fissures, ptosis, epicanthus, telecanthus
  - microphthalmos
  - strabismus (especially esotropia)
  - reduced acuity, unilaterally, or bilaterally
  - refractive error, most often myopia
  - anterior segment and media opacities,
  - retinal dysplasia, tortuous retinal vessels
  - optic nerve hypoplasia
  - cortical visual impairment in severe cases
- Also look for the nonophthalmologic/facial anomalies including head circumference

DIAGNOSTIC TESTS & INTERPRETATION

Lab

- No reliable biochemical markers available
- Markers proposed for identifying drinking in pregnant women include fatty acid ethyl ester levels in meconium and hair samples, gamma-glutamyl transferase (GGT), hemoglobin-associated acetaldehyde, and carbohydrate-deficit transferrin. However, none has been proven to have high sensitivity and specificity (3)[C].

Imaging

CT/MRI of brain to detect associated anomalies.

Diagnostic Procedures/Other

Electroretinogram results have been inconsistent, further research necessary before considering using ERG to diagnose FAS (7)[C].

DIFFERENTIAL DIAGNOSIS

- Many infants born with congenital syndromes and malformations have characteristics that resemble ophthalmologic features seen in children with FAS and they have coincidentally been exposed to alcohol in-utero (1)[A]
- Velocardiofacial syndrome (VCFS).
- Williams syndrome
- Blepharophimosis syndrome
- Dubowitz syndrome

TREATMENT

MEDICATION

- None for ophthalmologic abnormalities
- Stimulant medications such as methylphenidate and dextroamphetamine have some efficacy in treating children with concomitant psychiatric problems (e.g., ADHD), but larger-scale studies are needed to confirm this (6)[A].

ADDITIONAL TREATMENT

General Measures

- In children with amblyopia, patching of the better eye should be attempted
- Treat refractive errors with corrective lens

Issues for Referral

If there are characteristics inconsistent with the diagnosis, consider referral to a clinical geneticist or dysmorphologist.

Additional Therapies

- Medical services for any comorbid conditions
- For associated ocular conditions as needed (6)[A]

SURGERY/OTHER PROCEDURES

For associated strabismus or ptosis as indicated.

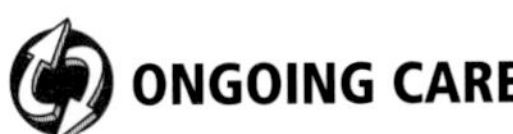

ONGOING CARE

FOLLOW-UP RECOMMENDATIONS

- As needed for amblyopia detection and treatment
- Low vision services as indicated

PATIENT EDUCATION

- Parents of should be educated on the nature of FAS, e.g., to recognize behavioral issues as a manifestation of the syndrome and learn to cope with their children's symptoms caused by FAS (6).
- http://www.faslink.org/
- http://www.nofas.org/living/resources.aspx
- Mothers who engage in alcohol abuse prenatally are likely to continue after the birth of their child. Appropriate interventions (e.g., Alcoholics Anonymous) should be recommended.

PROGNOSIS

Improvement in vision depends on early identification and intervention, in infancy or preschool age.

COMPLICATIONS

Irreversible loss in visual acuity if amblyopia from strabismus or refractive error not corrected

REFERENCES

1. Hoyme HE, May PA, Kalberg WO, et al. A practical clinical approach to diagnosis of fetal alcohol spectrum disorders: clarification of the 1996 Institue of medicine criteria. *Pediatrics* 2005; 115(1):39–47.
2. Strömland K. Visual impairment and ocular abnormalities in children with fetal alcohol syndrome. *Addict Biol* 2004;9(2):153–157; discussion 159–160.
3. Green RF, Stoler JM. Alcohol dehydrogenase 1B genotype and fetal alcohol syndrome: a HuGE minireview. *Am J Obstet Gynecol* 2007;197(1): 12–25.
4. Sokol RJ, Delaney-Black V, Nordstrom B. Fetal Alcohol Spectrum Disorder. *JAMA* 2003;290(22): 2996–2999.
5. Floyd RL, Weber MK, Denny C, O'Connor MJ. Prevention of fetal alcohol spectrum disorders. *Dev Disabil Res Rev* 2009;15(3):193–199.
6. Strömland K, Pinazo-Durán MD. Ophthalmic involvement in the fetal alcohol syndrome: clinical and animal model studies. *Alcohol Alcohol* 2002;37(1):2–8.
7. Paley B, O'Connor MJ. Intervention for individuals with fetal alcohol spectrum disorders: treatment approaches and case management. *Dev Disabil Res Rev* 2009;15(3):258–267.

ADDITIONAL READING

- http://www.cdc.gov/ncbddd/fasd/index.html

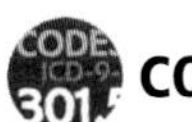

CODES

ICD9

- 374.89 Other disorders of eyelid
- 743.61 Congenital ptosis of eyelid
- 760.71 Alcohol affecting fetus or newborn via placenta or breast milk

CLINICAL PEARLS

- FAS is part of the FASD continuum and specific facial anomalies are necessary for the diagnosis, one of which is short palpebral fissures.
- FAS is entirely preventable when women refrain from consuming alcohol during their pregnancies. Physicians should screen all women of child-bearing age regarding their alcohol use as prevention is most effective when begun prior to conception.
- Many ophthalmic findings in FAS are nonspecific, therefore consider FAS a diagnosis of exclusion after other medical conditions presenting with similar features have been ruled out.
- After a thorough ophthalmic examination, necessary interventions should begin as early as possible to preserve visual acuity.
- No reliable laboratory markers are currently available to diagnose FAS.
- Treatment for FAS needs to be multidisciplinary as children frequently suffer from comorbid medical/psychiatric conditions.

FLOPPY EYELID SYNDROME

Thaddeus S. Nowinski

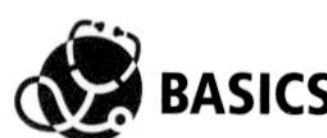

BASICS

DESCRIPTION
A loose and unstable upper eyelid associated with a chronic papillary conjunctivitis and spontaneous eversion of the eyelid during sleep (1)[C]

EPIDEMIOLOGY
Incidence
- Males > female
- Obesity (2)[C]
- Unilateral or bilateral

RISK FACTORS
- Obstructive sleep apnea—hypopnea syndrome (OSAHS)
- Recurrent mechanical rubbing

GENERAL PREVENTION
CPAP for treatment of sleep apnea may improve floppy eyelid.

PATHOPHYSIOLOGY
Upregulation of elastin-degrading enzymes (matrix metalloproteinases) secondary to reperfusion ischemia and repeated mechanical trauma on sleeping side or by repeated rubbing.

ETIOLOGY
- Unknown
- Elongation of tarsal plate allows flaccidity of upper eyelid
- Ischemia secondary to obstructive sleep apnea – hypopnea syndrome leads to optic neuropathy, papilledema, glaucoma (3)[C], (4)[C]

COMMONLY ASSOCIATED CONDITIONS
- Obstructive sleep apnea—hypopnea syndrome (OSAHS), >90%
- High body mass index
- Keratoconus on sleeping side

DIAGNOSIS

HISTORY
- Chronic mucous secretion
- Foreign body sensation—worse upon awakening
- Eversion of upper eyelid during sleep
- Sleeps on affected side of face
- Snoring
- Smoking

PHYSICAL EXAM
- Downward pointing upper eyelashes—lash ptosis
- Easily everted upper eyelid
- Soft and rubbery consistency of upper eyelid tarsal plate
- Horizontal laxity upper and possibly lower eyelids
- Chronic papillary conjunctivitis of upper eyelid
- Ptosis
- Lagophthalmos with secondary corneal punctuate keratitis

DIAGNOSTIC TESTS & INTERPRETATION
Lab
Initial lab tests

Sleep study.

Follow-up & special considerations

ALERT
- Strong association of OSAHS and systemic sequelae.
  - Cardiovascular disease
  - Stroke
  - Obesity
  - Metabolic syndrome
  - Cognitive and emotional disorders
  - Drowsiness-related accidents

DIFFERENTIAL DIAGNOSIS
- Ptosis
- Chronic blepharoconjunctivitis
- Ectropion
- Vernal conjunctivitis
- Giant papillary conjunctivitis
- Superior limbic keratoconjunctivitis

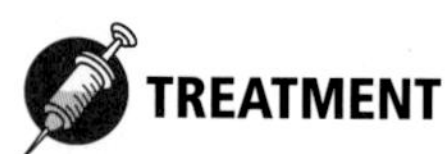

TREATMENT

MEDICATION
First Line
- Viscous ocular lubrication
  - Artificial tears, gel, ointment

Second Line
Oral doxycycline 100 mg b.i.d.

ADDITIONAL TREATMENT
General Measures
- Bedtime patching/taping shut
- Eye shield
- CPAP unit

Issues for Referral
Ophthalmologist 1–2 weeks.

Additional Therapies
- OSAHS
  - Behavioral
  - Mandibular advancement device
  - Surgery including UPPP, tonsillectomy, tracheostomy

SURGERY/OTHER PROCEDURES
- Defer surgery if possible until after OSAHS treated
- Surgical procedures
  - Full thickness eyelid resection (may also improve ptosis)
  - Horizontal eyelid/canthal tightening
- Recurrences and repeated surgeries common

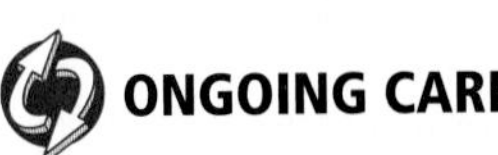

ONGOING CARE

FOLLOW-UP RECOMMENDATIONS
Ophthalmologist 1–2 weeks to monitor cornea.

PATIENT EDUCATION
Importance of treatment of obstructive sleep apnea is stressed to decrease ocular and systemic morbidity.

PROGNOSIS
Treatment of sleep apnea with CPAP unit may improve floppy eyelid syndrome and its associated ocular and systemic pathologies.

COMPLICATIONS
- Corneal abrasion, ulcer, scarring, perforation
- Optic neuropathy—nonarteritic
- Glaucoma—normal tension
- Papilledema

REFERENCES

1. Pham T, Perry J. Floppy eyelid syndrome. *Curr Opin Ophthalmol* 2007;18:430–433.
2. Cheung N, Wong TY. Obesity and eye diseases. *Surv Ophthalmol* 2007;52:180–195.
3. McNab A. The eye and sleep. *Clin Exp Ophthalmol* 2005;33:117–125.
4. Karakucuk S, Goktas S, Aksu M, et al. Ocular blood flow in patients with obstructive sleep apnea syndrome (OSAS). *Graefes Arch Clin Exp Ophthalmol* 2008;246:129–134.

ADDITIONAL READING

- Ezra DG, Beaconsfield M, Sira M, et al. Long-term outcomes of surgical approaches to the treatment of floppy eyelid syndrome. *Ophthalmology* 2010; 117:839–846.
- Ezra DG, Beaconsfield M, Sira M, Bunce C, Wormald R, Collin R. The associations of floppy eyelid syndrome: a case control study. *Ophthalmology* 2010;117:831–838.

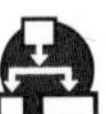

See Also (Topic, Algorithm, Electronic Media Element)
- www.asoprs.org
- Ectropion

CODES

ICD9
- 372.39 Other conjunctivitis
- 374.10 Ectropion, unspecified
- 374.89 Other disorders of eyelid

CLINICAL PEARLS
- Floppy eyelid syndrome is associated with severe cardiovascular and cerebral sequelae of obstructive sleep apnea—hypopnea syndrome (OSAHS).
- Floppy eyelid syndrome may improve with CPAP therapy.
- Floppy eyelid syndrome is associated with severe ocular sequelae including corneal, optic nerve, and glaucoma disorders.

FOREIGN BODY INTRAORBITAL

Omaya H. Youssef

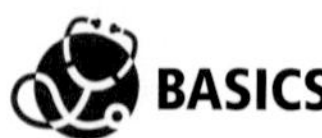

BASICS

DESCRIPTION

Intraorbital foreign bodies (IOFBs) occur as a result of a high-velocity penetrating injury or direct impalement of an object.

EPIDEMIOLOGY

The majority are male, typically of young age (less than 30 years old).

GENERAL PREVENTION

Education and protective eyewear.

PATHOPHYSIOLOGY

Traumatic insertion of a foreign body through the eyelid or conjunctiva.

ETIOLOGY

- Projectile, usually metallic, foreign bodies such as BB pellets and firearms
- Penetrating trauma from nonmetallic foreign bodies, either organic (e.g., tree branch, pencil) or inorganic (glass, plastic, or stone)

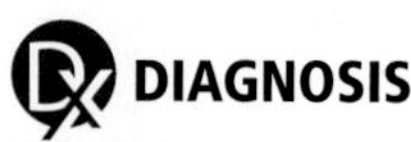

DIAGNOSIS

HISTORY

- A history of periocular trauma is usually elicited.
- A delayed presentation from the time of injury is not uncommon, especially with children or patients who sustain trauma while under the influence of various substances.
- A detailed history is essential in patients who present with orbital infections or inflammation.

PHYSICAL EXAM

- Visual acuity can range from normal to complete loss of vision, depending on associated ocular and orbital injuries.
- Afferent papillary defect may be present if optic nerve is involved.
- Extraocular muscle underaction, if extraocular muscles are affected
- Gaze-evoked amaurosis (with apical IOFBs)
- Blepharoptosis
- Proptosis
- Orbital inflammation
- Careful examination of the periocular skin and conjunctiva, especially the fornices, to identify entry wound

DIAGNOSTIC TESTS & INTERPRETATION

Lab

- Wound culture (aerobic, anaerobic, fungal)
- Foreign body culture
- CBC may reveal elevated serum white cell count secondary to chronic orbital inflammation

Imaging

- Plain film radiographs for metallic IOFBs
- CT
  - Excellent for identifying metal or glass
  - Safe in the presence of ferromagnetic metallic foreign bodies
  - Inorganic IOFBs (e.g., wood) can mimic air on CT
  - Quantitative CT with wide bone window settings can distinguish wood from low-density signals of air or fat
- MRI if CT scan is negative and non-metallic IOFB is suspected
  - MRI can be used to localize BB pellets, which are made of steel, and coated with copper or zinc
- Ultrasound (US) can be used to localize the IOFB; however it does not image the orbital apex reliably.

Follow-up & special considerations

- Orbitocranial extension should be ruled out, especially in children who have thinner orbital bones.
  - Coronal and parasagittal images should be obtained in suspected transorbital, intracranial penetration.

Diagnostic Procedures/Other

Electroretinography (ERG) to assess for photoreceptor toxicity if iron or copper containing IOFB is adjacent to sclera.

Pathological Findings

With organic IOFBs: Chronic inflammation with or without granulomatous reaction and fibrosis.

DIFFERENTIAL DIAGNOSIS

- Orbital cellulitis
- Idiopathic orbital inflammation
- Orbital neoplasm (children)

TREATMENT

MEDICATION

- Broad-spectrum antibiotic therapy with anaerobic coverage, in cases of orbital cellulitis secondary to chronically retained IOFBs (more common with organic IOFBs)
- Antitetanus prophylaxis

SURGERY/OTHER PROCEDURES

- Surgical removal depends on visual status, composition of IOFB, and location within the orbit.
- Surgical removal is indicated for the following:
  - Neurological compromise
  - Ocular motility restriction
  - All organic IOFBs
  - Inorganic IOFBs if they are located in the anterior orbit and are easily accessible
- Inorganic IOFBs that are located posteriorly may be left in place, unless they are causing orbital complications.
- Percutaneous US and fluoroscopy can be used intraoperatively to localize the IOFB.

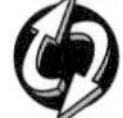

ONGOING CARE

FOLLOW-UP RECOMMENDATIONS

- Ophthalmologist
- Neurosurgeon (if intracranial involvement)

PROGNOSIS

- Vision loss is generally related to initial injury and not as a result of complications from IOFB or management.
- Retained metallic IOFBs are usually well-tolerated and have a good visual prognosis. The exception is metallic IOFBs containing copper, which can cause a chronic suppurative orbital inflammation.
- Organic IOFBs have a higher incidence of vision-threatening complications, and a higher risk of orbital and cerebral infections.

COMPLICATIONS

- Acute orbital cellulitis (usually from organic material such as wood)
- Chronic suppurative orbital inflammation (from copper foreign bodies)
- Sterile abscess
- Orbitocutaneous fistula
- Orbital wall osteomyelitis
- Cerebral infection

ADDITIONAL READING

- Finkelstein M, Legmann A, Rubin PA. Projectile metallic foreign bodies in the orbit: a retrospective study of epidemiological factors, management, and outcomes. *Ophthalmology* 1997;104:96–103.
- Fulcher TP, McNab AA, Sullivan TJ. Clinical Features and Management of Intraorbital Foreign Bodies. *Ophthalmology* 2002;109:494–500.
- Ho VH, Wilson MW, Fleming JC, et al. Retained Intraorbital Metallic Foreign Bodies. *Ophthal Plast Reconstr Surg* 2004;20:232–236.
- Nasr AM, Haik BG, Fleming JC, et al. Penetrating Orbital Injury with Organic Foreign Bodies. *Ophthalmology* 1999;106:523–532.
- Shelsta HN, Bilyk JR, Rubin PA, et al. Wooden Intraorbital Foreign Body Injuries: Clinical Characteristics and Outcomes of 23 Patients. *Ophthal Plast Reconstr Surg* 2010;26:238–244.

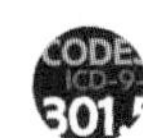

CODES

ICD9

- 360.60 Foreign body, intraocular, unspecified
- 870.4 Penetrating wound of orbit with foreign body

CLINICAL PEARLS

- Rule out intracranial involvement of IOFB prior to removal.
- All organic IOFBs should be removed.
- Inorganic IOFBs that are easily accessible in the anterior orbit should be removed, while those in the posterior orbit can be left in place unless causing orbital complications.

FOVEAL HYPOPLASIA

Michael J. Bartiss

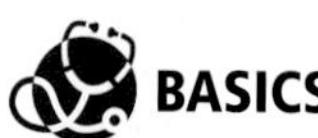

BASICS

DESCRIPTION

- Clinical condition characterized by an abnormal funduscopic appearance of the macula and decrease or absence of the foveal reflex and varying degrees of macular hypoplasia
- Macular vessels often traverse near or across the normally avascular zone of the fovea.
- Optic nerves and peripheral retina may appear normal.
- Visual acuity typically in the 20/100–20/200 range but variable depending on degree of hypoplasia

EPIDEMIOLOGY

Unknown.

RISK FACTORS

- Commonly associated with albinism and aniridia
- Family history

Genetics

- When seen in combination with aniridia or albinism the genetics of those syndromes apply. Also reported with Axenfeld–Reiger spectrum.
- Isolated autosomal dominant macular hypoplasia may be due to mutations in PAX6 (11p13).
- Autosomal recessive inheritance also reported including foveal hypoplasia with anterior segment dysgenesis (FHASD, 16q23.2–24.2).

GENERAL PREVENTION

Genetic counseling and/or prenatal testing (if mutated gene known or syndrome recognized in family).

PATHOPHYSIOLOGY

- Results from incomplete development of the fovea.
- In albinism, the absence of melanin in the retinal pigmented epithelium leads to a failure of induction of proper macular development
- In aniridia or isolated macular hypoplasia due to PAX6 mutation it is presumed that there is a failure of induction of a gene(s) downstream from PAX6, responsible for macular differentiation.

ETIOLOGY

Thought to result from incomplete embryologic development of the fovea, which typically develops in stages:

- Stage 1: Indistinct pigmented area
- Stages 2 and 3: Development of the annular reflex
- Stage 4: Appearance of the foveal pit
- Stage 5: Development of the foveal reflex

COMMONLY ASSOCIATED CONDITIONS

- Achromatopsia
- Albinism
- Aniridia
- Less common: Axenfeld–Reiger
- Nystagmus
- Reduced vision

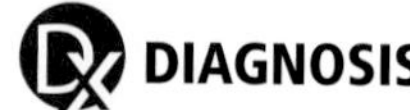

DIAGNOSIS

HISTORY

Poor vision, possible nystagmus.

PHYSICAL EXAM

- Full ocular examination including careful evaluation of the macula
- Careful examination with indirect ophthalmoscope by noting presence or absence of annular ring and foveal light reflex and anomalous patterns of macular vessels
- Assess vision, nystagmus

DIAGNOSTIC TESTS & INTERPRETATION

Lab

Initial lab tests

None needed.

Follow-up & special considerations

Consider molecular genetic testing where appropriate.

Imaging

Initial approach

- OCT can be used for grading.
  - Widespread thickening of the retina throughout the entire fovea with no difference in thickness from the surrounding macula
  - High reflectivity of the inner retina

Diagnostic Procedures/Other
Visual field, especially Goldmann, may be helpful.

Pathological Findings
- Absence of foveal differentiation and red-free zone
- Continuation of ganglion cell layer throughout macula
- Associated with reduction in the thickness of the optic nerve and in the volume of gray matter in the visual cortex
- Abnormalities in the length and mean surface area of the calcarine fissure present in visual cortex

DIFFERENTIAL DIAGNOSIS
- Epiretinal membrane
- Macular drag (e.g., retinopathy of prematurity, familial exudative retinopathy)
- High myopia
- Blonde fundus
- Congenitally anomalous retinal vascular (e.g., macrovessel, tortuosity)
- Optic atrophy with secondary macular nerve fiber loss
- Optic nerve hypoplasia
- Retinal/macular dystrophy

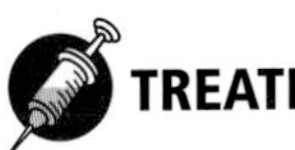

TREATMENT

MEDICATION
None.

ADDITIONAL TREATMENT

General Measures
- Amblyopia therapy as indicated
- Genetic counseling
- If photophobia consider Corning lenses

Issues for Referral
- Genetic counseling/ocular genetics
- Low vision

Additional Therapies
Maximization of vision potential with spectacles, contact lenses, and/or low-vision aids.

COMPLEMENTARY & ALTERNATIVE THERAPIES
None proven or indicated.

SURGERY/OTHER PROCEDURES
- None for foveal hypoplasia
- Strabismus and nystagmus surgery as indicated (nystagmus surgery unlikely to yield great visual acuity improvement)

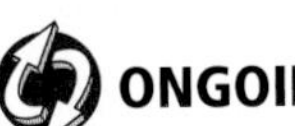

ONGOING CARE

FOLLOW-UP RECOMMENDATIONS
- As needed for amblyopia and strabismus monitoring and treatment
  - Low-vision evaluation

Patient Monitoring
- Monitor patients for associated conditions of aniridia and albinism and congenital nystagmus
- Visual development and function
- If asymmetric, amblyopia can occur.
- Strabismus.

PROGNOSIS
- Visual prognosis based on associated conditions and degree of macular hypoplasia
- Presence of anomalous blood vessels in macula (e.g., crossing midline raphe, extending close or through putative fovea) associated with worse visual prognosis

COMPLICATIONS
Low vision, nystagmus, amblyopia, strabismus.

ADDITIONAL READING

- Brodsky MC, Baker RS, Hamed LM. *"Pediatric Neuro-Ophthalmology"*, 2nd ed. Springer: New York, New York, 1996:304–307,314.
- Schroeder HW, et al. Hereditary foveal hypoplasia. *Klin Monbl Augenheikd* 2003;220(8):559–562.
- Holmstrom G, et al. Optical coherence tomography is helpful in the diagnosis of foveal hypoplasia. *Acta Ophthalmol* 2010;88(4):439–442.
- Mietz H, et al. Foveal hypoplasia in complete oculocutaneous albinism. A histopathologic study. *Retina* 1992;12(3):254–260.
- Huynh SC, et al. Macular and nerve fiber layer thickness in amblyopia: the Sydney Childhood Eye Study. *Ophthalmology* 2009;116(9):1604–1609.

CODES

ICD9
362.89 Other retinal disorders

CLINICAL PEARLS
- Look for this condition in patients with significant subnormal vision and without nystagmus.
- Look closely for this condition in patients who do not respond as expected to amblyopia therapy.

FRACTURES, ORBITAL FLOOR

Paul B. Johnson
Jacqueline R. Carrasco

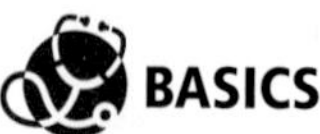

BASICS

DESCRIPTION
- Traumatic defect in the bony floor of the orbit
- Can extend from fractures of the inferior orbital rim
- Indirect (blowout) fractures of the orbital floor are not associated with fracture of the orbital rim.

EPIDEMIOLOGY
Incidence and prevalence variable

RISK FACTORS
- Male gender
- Younger age (15–30 years)
- Participation in sports
- Substance abuse

GENERAL PREVENTION
Wear eye protection when engaging in sports involving objects that move at high velocity (baseball, softball, hockey).

PATHOPHYSIOLOGY
Two theories:
- A nonpenetrating object strikes orbital entrance causing a sudden increase in intraorbital pressure. The contents of the orbit are compressed posteriorly toward the apex of the orbit. The orbital bones break at their weakest point, usually the posterior medial part of the floor in the maxillary bone.
- The striking object causes a compressive force at the inferior rim, which leads directly to buckling of the orbital floor.

ETIOLOGY
Trauma (see above)

COMMONLY ASSOCIATED CONDITIONS
- Globe rupture
- Hyphema/microhyphema
- Traumatic iritis
- Commotio retinae
- Choroidal rupture
- Traumatic optic neuropathy

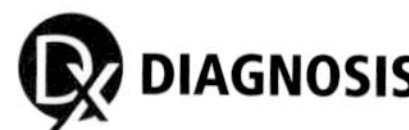

DIAGNOSIS

HISTORY
- Inquire about the timing and specific circumstances of the trauma
- Classic history involves the orbital entrance being struck by an object larger than the diameter of the orbital opening (e.g., fist, dashboard, ball)
- Nausea, vomiting, and bradycardia can indicate entrapment

PHYSICAL EXAM
- Eyelid ecchymosis
- Eyelid edema
- Diplopia with limitation on upgaze, downgaze, or both
- **Forced duction test:** Instill anesthetic eyedrops followed by lidocaine 2% gel. Grasp the insertion of the inferior rectus muscle through the conjunctiva with a toothed forceps, and attempt to rotate the globe up and down. Restriction when rotating the globe upward indicates possible entrapment.
- Enophthalmos
- Hypoglobus
- Infraorbital hypesthesia
- Emphysema of the eyelids and orbits
- Step-off deformity of orbital rim palpated

DIAGNOSTIC TESTS & INTERPRETATION

Imaging
CT scan of the orbits with coronal and axial views demonstrates a defect in the bony floor of the orbit with possible entrapment of soft tissue and/or extraocular muscle.

DIFFERENTIAL DIAGNOSIS
- Orbital hemorrhage and edema without a fracture: No fracture on CT
- Cranial nerve palsy: normal forced-duction test

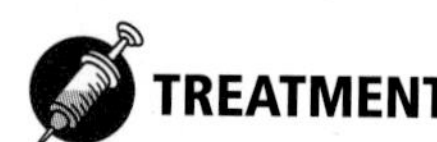

TREATMENT

MEDICATION
- Broad-spectrum oral antibiotics, especially if patient has a history of sinusitis, diabetes, or is immunocompromised: cephalexin 250–500 mg p.o. q.i.d. or erythromycin 250–500 mg p.o. q.i.d. for 7 days
- Methylprednisolone (Medrol) dose pack if patient has extensive swelling

ADDITIONAL TREATMENT

General Measures
- No nose blowing
- Nasal decongestants
- Ice packs

Issues for Referral
- If not a surgical candidate, referral should be made to a general ophthalmologist to be seen within 7–10 days of the initial trauma.
- If a surgical candidate, referral should be made to an oculoplastic surgeon within 7–10 days of the initial trauma.
- Any patient with nausea, vomiting, or bradycardia secondary to entrapped extraocular muscle should be evaluated by an oculoplastic surgeon at the time of initial exam to evaluate the need for urgent repair.

Pediatric Considerations

A pediatric patient with an entrapped extraocular muscle should be evaluated by an oculoplastic surgeon at the time of initial exam to evaluate the need for urgent repair (24–48 hours).

SURGERY/OTHER PROCEDURES

- Not all fractures need to be repaired.
- Indications for surgical repair:
  - Fracture involving at least 50% of the orbital floor, especially associated with large medial wall fractures on CT
  - Enophthalmos greater than 2 mm that is cosmetically unacceptable to the patient
  - Diplopia with limitation of upgaze and/or downgaze within 30° of primary gaze
- Should take place within 2 weeks of initial trauma
- Involves releasing entrapped tissue and placing an orbital implant to separate the orbit from the maxillary sinus

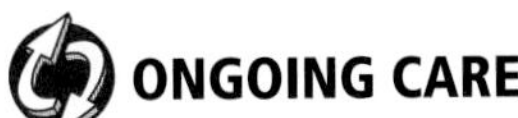

ONGOING CARE

FOLLOW-UP RECOMMENDATIONS

- Ophthalmologist
- Otolaryngologist/oral maxillofacial surgeon as needed

PATIENT EDUCATION

www.nlm.nih.gov/medlineplus/eyeinjuries.html

PROGNOSIS

Depends on the extent of associated injuries

COMPLICATIONS

- Decreased vision
- Diplopia
- Enophthalmos
- Infraorbital hypesthesia
- Orbital cellulitis

ADDITIONAL READING

- Egbert JE, May K, Kersten RC, et al. Pediatric orbital floor fracture—direct extraocular muscle involvement. *Ophthalmology* 2000;107:1875–1879.
- Harris GJ, Garcia GH, Logani SC, et al. Correlation of preoperative computed tomography and postoperative ocular motility in orbital blowout fractures. *Ophthal Plast Reconstr Surg* 2000;16:179–187.
- Hawes MJ, Dortzbach RK. Surgery on orbital floor fractures: influence of time of repair and fracture size. *Ophthalmology* 1983;90:1066–1070.
- Jordan DR, Allen LH, White J, et al. Intervention within days for some orbital floor fractures: the white-eyed blowout. *Ophthal Plast Reconstr Surg* 1998;14:379–390.
- Okulicz JF, Shah RS, Schwartz RA, et al. Oculocutaneous albinism. *European J Eur Acad Dermatol Venereol* 2003;17:251–256.
- Putterman AM, Stevens T, Urist MJ. Nonsurgical management of blowout fractures of the orbital floor. *Am J Ophthalmol* 1974;77:232–239.

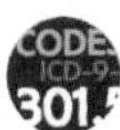

CODES

ICD9

- 802.6 Closed fracture of orbital floor (blow-out)
- 802.7 Open fracture of orbital floor (blow-out)
- 871.0 Ocular laceration without prolapse of intraocular tissue

CLINICAL PEARLS

- Pediatric orbital blowout fractures with entrapment of extraocular muscles should be considered for urgent repair.
- Optimal time for nonentrapped, orbital floor fracture repair is within 2 weeks of the initial trauma.
- Orbital CT scans with axial and coronal cuts are the key for making the diagnosis and surgical planning.
- A "white-eyed" blowout fracture can occur, especially in pediatric population, with entrapped muscle, poor motility, and very little external signs. See White Eyed Blow Out Fracture.

FRACTURES, ORBITAL MEDIAL WALL

Paul B. Johnson
Jacqueline R. Carrasco

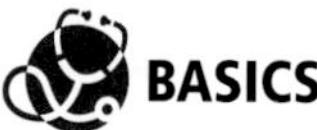

BASICS

DESCRIPTION
- Traumatic defect in the bony medial wall of the orbit
- Can extend from fractures of the maxilla, lacrimal bone, and ethmoid bones
- Indirect (blowout) fractures of the medial wall are not associated with fracture of the orbital rim

EPIDEMIOLOGY
Incidence and prevalence variable

RISK FACTORS
- Male gender
- Younger age (15–30 years)
- Participation in sports
- Substance abuse

GENERAL PREVENTION
Wear eye protection when engaging in sports involving objects that move at high velocity (baseball, softball, and hockey).

PATHOPHYSIOLOGY
- Blowout fractures of the medial wall are frequently extensions of orbital floor blowout fractures.
- Isolated medial wall blowout fractures can also occur.

ETIOLOGY
Trauma (see above)

COMMONLY ASSOCIATED CONDITIONS
- Globe rupture
- Hyphema/microhyphema
- Traumatic iritis
- Commotio retinae
- Choroidal rupture
- Traumatic optic neuropathy

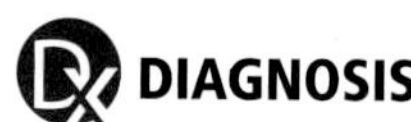

DIAGNOSIS

HISTORY
- Inquire about the timing and specific circumstances of the trauma
- Classic history involves the orbital entrance being struck by an object larger than the diameter of the orbital opening (e.g., fist, dashboard, and ball).
- Nausea, vomiting, and bradycardia can indicate entrapment (more common in children and with associated floor fractures).

PHYSICAL EXAM
- Emphysema of the eyelids and orbit
- Eyelid ecchymosis
- Eyelid edema
- Diplopia
- Globe dystopia

DIAGNOSTIC TESTS & INTERPRETATION
Imaging
Computer tomographies (CT) of the orbits with coronal and axial views demonstrate a defect in the bony medial wall of the orbit with possible entrapment of soft tissue and/or extraocular muscle.

DIFFERENTIAL DIAGNOSIS
- Orbital hemorrhage and edema without a fracture: No fracture on CT
- Cranial nerve palsy: Normal forced-duction test

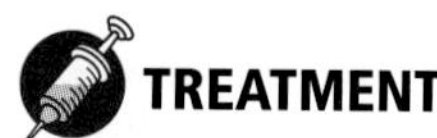

TREATMENT

MEDICATION
- Broad-spectrum oral antibiotics, especially if patient has a history of sinusitis, diabetes, or is immunocompromised: Cephalexin 250–500 mg PO q.i.d or erythromycin 250–500 mg PO q.i.d for 7 days
- Medrol dose pack if patient has extensive swelling

ADDITIONAL TREATMENT
General Measures
- No nose blowing
- Nasal decongestants
- Ice packs

Issues for Referral
- If not a surgical candidate, referral should be made to a general ophthalmologist to be seen within 7–10 days of the initial trauma.
- If a surgical candidate, referral should be made to an oculoplastic surgeon within 7–10 days of the initial trauma.
- Any patient with nausea, vomiting, or bradycardia secondary to entrapped extraocular muscle should be evaluated by an oculoplastic surgeon at the time of initial exam to evaluate the need for immediate repair.

Pediatric Considerations

A pediatric patient with an entrapped extraocular muscle should be evaluated by an oculoplastic surgeon at the time of initial exam to evaluate the need for immediate repair.

SURGERY/OTHER PROCEDURES

Indications:

- Fracture contiguous with a floor fracture involving a significant portion of the orbital floor on CT
- Enophthalmos >2 mm that is cosmetically unacceptable to the patient
- Diplopia
  - Should take place within 2 weeks of initial trauma
  - An eyelid or transconjunctival approach can allow for exploration of the orbital floor that can be continued up along the medial wall
  - The medial orbital wall can also be approached through a transcaruncular approach

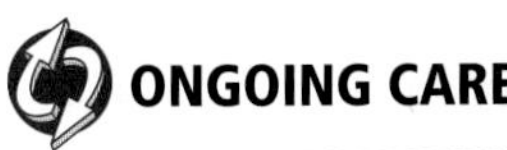

ONGOING CARE

FOLLOW-UP RECOMMENDATIONS

- Ophthalmologist
- Otolaryngologist/oral maxillofacial surgeon as needed

PATIENT EDUCATION

- www.nlm.nih.gov/medlineplus/eyeinjuries.html

PROGNOSIS

Depends on the extent of associated injuries

COMPLICATIONS

- Decreased vision
- Diplopia
- Enophthalmos
- Orbital cellulitis

ADDITIONAL READING

- Gilbard SM, Mafee MF, Lagouros PA, et al. Orbital blowout fractures: The prognostic significance of computed tomography. *Ophthalmology* 1985;92(11):1523–1528.
- Harris GJ, Garcia GH, Logani SC, et al. Correlation of preoperative computed tomography and postoperative ocular motility in orbital blowout fractures. *Ophthal Plast Reconstr Surg.* 2000;16(3):179–187.
- Jordan DR, Allen LH, White J, et al. Intervention within days for some orbital floor fractures: The white-eyed blowout. *Ophthal Plast Reconstr Surg.* 1998;14(6):379–390.
- Nolasco FP, Mathog RH. Medial orbital wall fractures: Classification and clinical profile. *Otolaryngol Head Neck Surg* 1995;112(4):49–56.

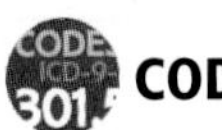

CODES

ICD9

- 802.8 Closed fracture of other facial bones
- 802.9 Open fracture of other facial bones

CLINICAL PEARLS

- Fractures of both the medial orbital wall and floor are associated with the highest rates of enophthalmos.
- Optimal time for repair is within 2 weeks of the initial trauma.
- Orbital CT scans are key for making the diagnosis and surgical planning.

F

FRACTURE, WHITE-EYED BLOWOUT

Jurij R. Bilyk

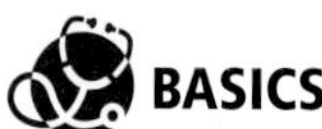

BASICS

DESCRIPTION

- Greenstick fracture of the orbital floor or medial orbital wall resulting in ischemic entrapment of an extraocular muscle.
- Typically seen in the pediatric population, although young adults in their early 20s may be affected.
- Minimal external signs of trauma (lack of swelling, ecchymosis) mask the severity of the orbital injury, ergo the term "white-eyed blowout fracture" (WEBOF).
- System: ophthalmic
- Synonyms: trapdoor orbital fracture

EPIDEMIOLOGY

- Occurs in children and young adults
- No racial predilection
- No gender predilection is reported. However, in general males are more often involved in trauma
- The orbital floor is more commonly involved than the medial orbital wall (lamina papyracea).
- The etiology is typically due to a blunt force sports-related injury, motor vehicle accident, or physical altercation.
- Incidence and prevalence are unknown

RISK FACTORS

- Pediatric age group
- Recent trauma

GENERAL PREVENTION

- Avoidance of eye trauma
- WEBOF in children is most commonly due to sports injury, but it may also occur from other mechanisms (motor vehicle accident, altercation, etc.).
- The use of eye protection in the form of polycarbonate safety glasses, goggles, or eye shields is advised in all children involved in sports.
- The use of appropriate restraining devices is advised in all children in motor vehicles.

PATHOPHYSIOLOGY

- A blowout fracture of the orbital bones is postulated to occur through two mechanisms:
  - A blow to the globe and orbit momentarily increases intraorbital pressure, causing the thin bones of the orbital floor and/or medial wall to "blowout" into the adjacent paranasal sinus.
  - A blow to the inferior orbital rim causes the orbital floor to buckle and break into the maxillary sinus.
- The bones of children have not fully calcified and in general are more pliable than those of adults.
  - When a child sustains a blow to the periocular region, the thin bone of the orbital floor or medial orbital wall cracks and momentarily opens into the adjacent sinus. The increased intraorbital pressure causes orbital fat and the adjacent extraocular muscle to herniate into the fracture.
  - In adults, the fractured bone usually remains in place within the sinus. Because of the pliability of pediatric bones, the fractured orbital bone immediately snaps back into position, much like a trapdoor on a hinged spring.
  - This results in tight incarceration of the orbital soft tissue (fat and muscle), leading to ischemic contracture (Volkmann's contracture) of the extraocular muscle.
  - The entrapped muscle limits ocular movement with resultant diplopia (double vision). On attempted ocular movement, the child experiences an oculocardiac reflex (Aschner phenomenon), a vagal response stimulated by a connection between the trigeminal and vagus nerves.
  - The oculocardiac reflex manifests as nausea, vomiting, and sometimes fainting, mimicking symptoms of concussion. This can be the cause of bradycardia and heart block.

ETIOLOGY

As described above

COMMONLY ASSOCIATED CONDITIONS

- Intraocular injury (including hyphema, vitreous hemorrhage, and choroidal rupture)
- Oculocardiac reflex, bradycardia, heart block
- Concussion and intracranial injury, including hemorrhage, are uncommon associations in the vast majority of WEBOFs.

DIAGNOSIS

HISTORY

- Blunt trauma to the periocular region.
- Diplopia.
- Pain of attempted eye movement.
- Nausea and vomiting, especially with attempted eye movements.
- Loss of consciousness is NOT a typical feature of WEBOF.

PHYSICAL EXAM

- External examination with minimal signs of injury: minimal eyelid edema or ecchymosis, subconjunctival hemorrhage
- Severe restriction in upgaze (with orbital floor fractures) or in abduction (with medial wall fractures). The child often refuses to open the eye because of discomfort.
- Cheek numbness from infraorbital nerve contusion
- Signs and symptoms can often be confused for a concussion if the eye is not examined.

DIAGNOSTIC TESTS & INTERPRETATION

Lab

Drug and alcohol screening as indicated for preoperative clearance for general anesthesia

Imaging

Initial approach

- CT of the orbits with axial and coronal images. Coronal images are crucial for diagnosis. Sagittal images are optional.
- Both bone and soft tissue windows should be examined. WEBOFs are notoriously easy to miss on imaging without a high degree of suspicion because often the trapdoor fracture snaps back into an almost normal or normal position.
- If there is a suspicion of intracranial injury, head CT should be obtained.
- A head CT is NOT equivalent to orbital CT and will not afford adequate views of the orbital bones.
- Use of age- and weight-adjusted CT radiation doses in children to minimize radiation exposure.
- Avoid plain films.
- Avoid MRI because of poor bony detail.

Follow-up & special considerations

No additional imaging is needed postoperatively unless there is a question about the effectiveness of the surgical repair or positioning of the orbital implant.

Diagnostic Procedures/Other

If bradycardia and oculocardiac reflex are severe and persistent, cardiac monitoring may be necessary in a minority of cases. If indicated, the patient should be admitted to the pediatrics service.

Pathological Findings

- Incarceration and ischemia of the inferior (or less commonly medial) rectus muscles within a trapdoor fracture
- Alternatively, the perimuscular fascia and orbital fat may be caught within the fracture.

DIFFERENTIAL DIAGNOSIS

- Intracranial injury or concussion
- Contusion injury to the extraocular muscle. In many cases of orbital fracture, soft tissue contusion and edema manifest clinically as diplopia and external ophthalmoplegia. However, such cases typically lack a significant oculocardiac reflex and patients do not complain of severe nausea and vomiting.

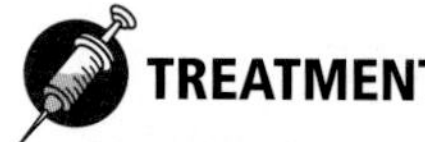

TREATMENT

MEDICATION

- WEBOF requires urgent surgical exploration (within 72 h) in essentially all cases
- Medical therapy is a secondary issue
- Some clinicians will prescribe a 1-week course of postoperative systemic antibiotic therapy as prophylaxis against infection. There is no evidence that this is effective in an otherwise healthy patient.
- Some clinicians will prescribe a 1-week course of postoperative systemic corticosteroids to decrease posttraumatic inflammation and fibrosis in the hopes of decreasing the incidence of restrictive strabismus. There is no evidence that this is effective.
- Antiemetics may be prescribed for severe nausea and vomiting but may not be effective.

ADDITIONAL TREATMENT

General Measures

- The patient is made NPO and cleared for general anesthesia.
- Because of the possibility of intraoperative paranasal sinus bleeding into the nasopharynx, laryngeal mask anesthesia should be avoided. Instead, endotracheal intubation for more complete airway protection is recommended for all orbital fracture repairs.
- The risks of surgery, including visual loss, infraorbital hypesthesia, and persistent diplopia, which could require additional surgery or prisms, are discussed in detail with the patient and parents. The option of conservative observation should be offered with caution, since this may result in severe extraocular muscle fibrosis.
- The patient and parents should be aware that in the immediate postoperative period, the diplopia may worsen. Nausea and vomiting resolve almost immediately. Diplopia and extraocular motility typically take weeks to months to improve or resolve.

Issues for Referral

Urgent referral to the appropriate orbital specialist is indicated in all patients with WEBOF to optimize timing of surgical repair and minimize the possibility of posttraumatic strabismus and diplopia.

SURGERY/OTHER PROCEDURES

- Surgical exploration with release of the entrapped tissue
- Repair of the trapdoor fracture. If adequate realignment of the fracture occurs with no evidence of soft tissue herniation, an orbital implant may not be needed.

- In most cases, an orbital wall defect is present after soft tissue release, potentially allowing for recurrent soft tissue entrapment. An orbital implant (usually an absorbable or nonabsorbable alloplastic sheet, based on surgeon preference) is placed to bridge the defect.
- Most WEBOF repair can be performed transconjunctival without a lateral canthotomy/cantholysis.

IN-PATIENT CONSIDERATIONS

Initial Stabilization

- Full ophthalmic examination to rule out intraocular and optic nerve injury
- Orbital imaging
- Cardiac monitoring as indicated

Admission Criteria

- Intractable nausea and vomiting
- Bradycardia or heart block

IV Fluids

- In many cases, patients with WEBOF have severe nausea and vomiting from the oculocardiac reflex.
- Some patients present without oral intake since the initial trauma, which may have occurred several days prior.
- Because of the possibility of dehydration, patients should be rehydrated preoperatively as indicated with the assistance of a pediatrician or anesthesiologist.

Nursing

- Following fracture repair, most patients with WEBOF experience immediate relief of their nausea and vomiting, and oral intake normalizes quickly. Antiemetics are typically not needed following successful repair.
- There is a risk of orbital hemorrhage with potential compressive optic neuropathy in any patient undergoing orbital surgery. Visual and pupillary function should be monitored over the first 12 hours postoperatively. If the nursing staff is unfamiliar with examination techniques, then the physician should assume these responsibilities.
- Any excessive swelling, pain, or bleeding should be reported to the physician immediately.
- Frequent iced or cold compresses are essential during the first 12 hours following fracture repair to decrease postoperative edema and pain. Many clinicians recommend compresses 20 minutes on and 20 minutes off while the patient is awake.
- Oral or intermuscular narcotics for pain management. This is usually unnecessary following most WEBOF repair.
- Diplopia often persists for days, weeks, or months following WEBOF repair and is not an indication of a postoperative complication.
- Antibiotic ophthalmic ointment to the conjunctival incision site

Discharge Criteria

- Resolution of nausea and vomiting. Vasovagal complaints resolve almost immediately. If they persist for more than 24 h postoperatively, then reexploration may be necessary to rule out inadequate initial release or postoperative reentrapment.
- Resolution or marked decrease in pain with eye movement
- No evidence of postoperative hemorrhage or optic neuropathy
- Diplopia will be present postoperatively in a significant proportion of patients, and it is not an indication to delay discharge.
- Most patients can be discharged home within 24 h of WEBOF repair.

ONGOING CARE

FOLLOW-UP RECOMMENDATIONS

- Depending on surgeon preference, the surgery can be performed on an outpatient or inpatient basis.
- Patients are usually seen within 1 week following repair.
- Ophthalmic ointment is typically discontinued 1–2 weeks following repair.
- Systemic antibiotics and corticosteroids, if prescribed, are usually discontinued within the first 2 weeks following repair.
- Iced or cold compresses are continued for the first 2–3 days following repair.
- The patient and his or her family are instructed to avoid any nose blowing, heavy lifting, exercise, or sports activities for 2 weeks following repair. Air travel is avoided for 1–2 weeks following repair. If essential, then the patient is instructed to use intranasal decongestants before take-off and landing to help equalize paranasal sinus pressure.
- The patient is given detailed instruction for monitoring of visual function and symptoms of orbital hemorrhage.
- An emergency telephone number is clearly included in the instruction sheet in case of visual problems or signs suggestive of orbital hemorrhage.
- The use of aspirin and related products may resume as needed 2 weeks after repair but should be avoided in the early postoperative period to reduce the potential for orbital hemorrhage.
- If diplopia persists postoperatively, the patient can occlude one eye with either a "pirate patch" or with adhesive tape over one lens of their glasses. Occlusion amblyopia is not a concern in patients older than 6 years. In children younger than 4 years, care must be taken to avoid prolonged occlusion of one eye; in this age group, alternating occlusion of each eye on a daily basis is recommended.
- A dilated fundus exam should be repeated at 6–12 weeks to assure that there are no late peripheral retinal abnormalities.

Patient Monitoring

- As already mentioned, postoperative diplopia and limited motility of the affected extraocular muscle is common after successful WEBOF repair. The patient and his or her family should be counseled about this probability preoperatively.
- No attempt at strabismus surgery should be made for at least 6 months following WEBOF repair. In most cases, if timely fracture repair was performed initially, extraocular motility will improve markedly over the ensuing weeks to months and in many cases, diplopia will resolve completely.
- After the initial postoperative follow-up visit, the patient is instructed to return 3–4 weeks later. If the diplopia has resolved, no additional therapy is indicated. If diplopia is still present, then initial strabismus pattern measurements are made utilizing prism bars and the patient is rechecked at regular intervals over the ensuing 6–9 months.

DIET

Regular, without restrictions

PROGNOSIS

- If repaired in a timely fashion, the prognosis for WEBOF is excellent, with most patients experiencing complete resolution of diplopia in useful gaze positions. Diplopia in extremes of gaze (typically upgaze) is usually left untreated.
- Clinical studies have shown that a significant delay in surgical repair (>2 weeks) results in a higher incidence of posttraumatic diplopia, which may not be amenable to further correction—thus the mantra of urgent surgical repair of WEBOF.
- Since there is a possibility of persistent diplopia from WEBOF even with timely repair, it behooves the surgeon to minimize excessive delay in surgical intervention. Most experts agree that repair within 72 h of injury is reasonable.

COMPLICATIONS

- Initial misdiagnosis as concussion or "normal" orbital CT, which may delay definitive treatment
- Persistent diplopia
- Optic neuropathy from intraoperative injury or postoperative orbital hemorrhage
- Persistent infraorbital dysesthesia (hypesthesia or neuralgia)
- Enophthalmos or hypoglobus. Unlikely given the small size of the initial fracture
- Incisional scarring
- Lid retraction or other eyelid malposition
- Implant migration or extrusion
- Postoperative infection (including sinusitis and orbital cellulitis)

F

REFERENCES

1. Bansagi ZC, Meyer DR. Internal orbital fractures in the pediatric age group. Characterization and management. *Ophthalmology* 2000;107:829–836.
2. Egbert JE, May K, Kersten RC, et al. Pediatric orbital floor fracture. Direct extraocular muscle involvement. *Ophthalmology* 2000;107:1875–1879.
3. Jordan DR, Allen LH, White J, et al. Intervention within days for some orbital floor fractures: The white-eyed blowout. *Ophthal Plast Reconstr Surg* 1998;14:379–390.
4. Lane K, Penne RB, Bilyk JR. Evaluation and management of pediatric orbital fractures in a primary care setting. *Orbit* 2007;26:183–191.
5. Parbhu KC, Galler KE, Li C, et al. Underestimation of soft tissue entrapment by computed tomography in orbital floor fractures in the pediatric population. *Ophthalmology* 2008;115:1620–1625.

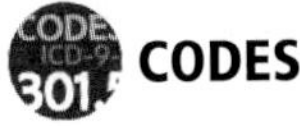

CODES

ICD9

- 368.2 Diplopia
- 802.6 Closed fracture of orbital floor (blow-out)
- 921.2 Orbital contusion

CLINICAL PEARLS

- WEBOF is often confused with concussion because of posttraumatic nausea and vomiting. Closely check and document extraocular motility in children and young adults following blunt-force trauma to the face.
- WEBOF is often difficult to diagnose on CT because of small fracture size and minimal bony displacement. Carefully check coronal bone windows for cracks in the orbital walls and coronal soft tissue windows for any distortion of the extraocular muscle contour.
- If WEBOF is suspected clinically and radiographically, do not delay referral for urgent surgical repair.

FUCHS' CORNEAL DYSTROPHY

Hall F. Chew

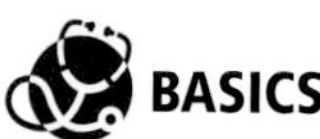

BASICS

DESCRIPTION

- Fuchs' corneal dystrophy is a progressive, bilateral, noninflammatory condition characterized by the development of focal excrescences of Descemet's membrane with resultant guttae, loss of endothelial cells, and resultant stromal edema. See Figures 1–3.
- The loss of the ion transport system and barrier function of the compromised endothelial cell layer leads to progressive stromal edema and eventual formation of epithelial bullae.
- Symptoms include glare and blurred vision worse upon awakening. This may progress to pain, photophobia and epiphora from erosions and rupture of the epithelial bullae.

EPIDEMIOLOGY

- Predominant gge: 5th and 6th decades (exception= Early-onset variant Fuchs' endothelial corneal dystrophy in first decade [rare])
- Predominant sex: Females > Males, 3.5:1

Incidence

Unknown.

Prevalence

4% of the population >40 years old.

RISK FACTORS

- Patient age
- Raised intraocular pressure
- Ocular inflammation

Genetics

- Autosomal dominant inheritance, often with incomplete penetrance and asymmetric presentation (1)
- Genetic locus:
  - Fuchs endothelial corneal dystrophy (FECD) 13pTel-13q12.13, 15q, 18q21.2-q21.32
  - Early-onset variant FECD 1p34.3-p32
- Gene:
  - Early-onset variant FECD collagen type VIII, Alpha 2-*COL8A2*

PATHOPHYSIOLOGY

- Primary dysfunction of the endothelial cell layer causes abnormal production of Descemet's membrane.
- Descemet's membrane becomes 2–3 times thicker with guttae excrescences of excess collagen visible with PAS and H&E staining.
- Reduction in the number of endothelial cells, followed by variations in size (polymegathism) and shape (polymorphism) are characteristic.
- The compromised endothelial cell layer leads to progressive stromal edema and eventually formation of epithelial bullae and corneal erosions.
- In end stage disease subepithelial fibrosis, anterior basement membrane changes, ± superficial neovascularization of the cornea can occur

ETIOLOGY

- Endothelial cell loss increases with age
- Average endothelial cell density = 6000 cells/mm^2 in infants and 2400 cells/mm^2 in adults
- Significant reduction of endothelial cells after intraocular surgery—especially cataract surgery. Fuchs' patients already have compromised endothelial cells.
- Loss of the endothelial layer's barrier function and Na^+/K^+-ATPase pump function leads to increased permeability of the endothelial layer producing stromal and epithelial edema.

COMMONLY ASSOCIATED CONDITIONS

- Cataracts
- Recurrent erosions from bullae
- Open-angle glaucoma
- Angle-closure glaucoma
- Keratoconus (rare)

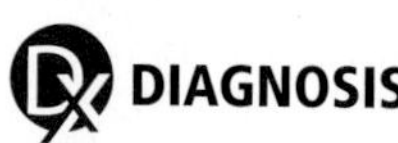

DIAGNOSIS

HISTORY

- Any previous cataract surgery
- Any previous ocular surgery
- Glare, blurred vision worse upon awakening
- Pain, photophobia, and epiphora from erosions and bullae
- Past history of glaucoma or uveitis

PHYSICAL EXAM

- Full ophthalmic examination including measurement of intraocular pressure and dilated fundus examination
- B-scan ultrasound to rule out posterior segment pathology if unable to visualize secondary to corneal or lenticular changes
- Slit-lamp examination shows:
  - In early stages—central corneal guttae on direct illumination and retroillumination
  - Later stages—guttae spread peripherally, with a beaten metal endothelial appearance secondary to increased pigmentation of the guttae, thickening of Descemet's membrane
  - Corneal edema is initially in the posterior stroma and also posterior to Bowman's membrane seen best with sclerotic scatter.
  - Worsening edema leads to folds in Descemet's membrane, microcystic epithelial edema that coalesces and forms bullae.
  - Peripheral superficial corneal neovascularization occurs in end stage Fuchs' as well as bullae formation.

DIAGNOSTIC TESTS & INTERPRETATION

Lab

Initial lab tests

- Slit-lamp examination (as mentioned in previous section)
- Ultrasound pachymetry to measure central corneal thickness
- Specular microscopy to measure endothelial cell counts, guttae, and levels of endothelial cell polymegathism and polymorphism

Follow-up & special considerations

- Slit-lamp examination
- Ultrasound pachymetry
- Specular microscopy
- Significant clinical findings require treatment using hypertonic saline topical drop and/or ointment, or surgery
- Evaluation of cataract if present

Diagnostic Procedures/Other

Confocal microscopy can identify and diagnose endothelial cell findings in patients with severe corneal edema that precludes slit-lamp examination.

Pathological Findings

- Diffusely thickened Descemet's membrane
- Anvil-shaped excrescences of basement membrane (guttae) within Descemet's membrane
- Paucity of endothelial cells
- Varying degrees of subepithelial fibrosis and anterior basement membrane changes
- Bullous keratopathy ± neovascularization of the epithelium may be present

DIFFERENTIAL DIAGNOSIS

- Pseudophakic/aphakic corneal edema
- Posterior polymorphous dystrophy
- Congenital hereditary endothelial dystrophy
- Macular dystrophy
- Interstitial keratitis
- Central herpetic disciform keratitis
- Chandler's syndrome (iridocorneal endothelial syndrome)
- Corneal pseudoguttae from the following:
  - Trauma
  - Intraocular inflammation
  - Infection
  - Toxins

TREATMENT

MEDICATION

First Line

- Topical hypertonic saline (5%) drops (1 drop q.i.d.) and ointment (q.h.s. or if preferable q.i.d. instead of drops). No contraindications.

Second Line

- If pressure is elevated, add antiglaucoma medications (see Glaucoma section).

ADDITIONAL TREATMENT

General Measures

- Initial treatment is reduction of corneal edema and pain relief.
- If epithelial bullae rupture, can manage with a therapeutic bandage contact lens. Risk for corneal ulcer is increased.
- Use a hair dryer on the eyes to dehydrate the cornea.
- Surgical intervention is required for visual rehabilitation when there is significant reduction of vision that fails all medical therapy.

Issues for Referral

- Worsening vision
- Corneal ulcer

SURGERY/OTHER PROCEDURES

- Full-thickness penetrating keratoplasty (PKP) is required for compliant patients with advanced Fuchs' dystrophy who have central anterior scarring, anterior basement membrane changes, or subepithelial fibrosis.
- In patients without central anterior stromal scarring or subepithelial fibrosis, an endothelial keratoplasty (EK) may be required, either
  - Descemet's stripping endothelial keratoplasty (DSEK/DSAEK)
  - Descemet's membrane endothelial keratoplasty (DMEK)—relatively new procedure
- Compared with PKP, EK is preferred as recovery time is less, less induced astigmatism, less chance for wound dehiscence.
- Patients with Fuchs' dystrophy and visually significant cataract may benefit from cataract surgery alone, or combined cataract surgery with keratoplasty (PKP or EK as in guidelines earlier.).
  - The current guidelines recommend a combined cataract surgery with keratoplasty be considered when the endothelial cell count is $<1000/mm^2$ or central corneal thickness is >650 mm, although other clinical factors should be considered by the surgeon (2).

ONGOING CARE

FOLLOW-UP RECOMMENDATIONS

- Depends on severity of disease
- Typically follow-up every 3–12 months
- In cases with ruptured bullae and epithelial defects, follow-up as in corneal abrasions

Patient Monitoring

- Continued follow-up with complete ophthalmic examination and slit-lamp examination
- Ultrasound pachymetry and specular microscopy as required

PATIENT EDUCATION

- This is usually a slowly progressive condition
- Primarily autosomal dominant
- Hypertonic saline treatment can halt progression in most cases
- Hypertonic saline topical drops cause stinging and patients should be reassured that this is normal to maximize compliance
- Hypertonic saline topical ointment does not cause stinging, but causes blur. It is ideally used at bedtime or in eyes that already have significantly reduced vision
- If vision is worse in the morning it is usually attributed to Fuchs' dystrophy as corneal edema increases while sleeping
- Patients with Fuchs' dystrophy undergoing cataract surgery should be warned that there is a higher probability of postoperative corneal edema that may require corneal transplantation (keratoplasty)
- Keratoplasty by itself will accelerate cataract formation so if the patient is still phakic, cataract extraction with keratoplasty is usually performed (depending on surgeon's discretion)

PROGNOSIS

- Fuchs' dystrophy is a progressive disease that worsens over time; however, the course is variable.
- After any intraocular surgery, endothelial cell loss occurs.
- Prognosis after PKP is good with most patients (>80%) with clear corneal transplants from 2 to 5 years after surgery, but long-term prognosis is not as good.
- DSEK and DMEK are relatively new procedures. Results for DSEK at 12 months are excellent (98% >20/40) (3–4).

COMPLICATIONS

- Painful bullous keratopathy
- Corneal ulceration with infectious keratitis
- Post keratoplasty:
  - Rejection
  - Graft failure
  - Glaucoma
  - Astigmatism
  - Anisometropia
  - Corneal ulcer
  - Wound dehiscence
  - Uveitis
  - Epithelial downgrowth
  - Retinal detachment
  - Endophthalmitis

REFERENCES

1. Weiss JS, Moller HU, Lisch W, et al. The IC3D classification of the corneal dystrophies. *Cornea* 2008;27Suppl.2:S26–S28.
2. Eghrari AO, Daoud YJ, Gottsch JD. Cataract surgery in Fuchs' corneal dystrophy. *Curr Opin Ophthalmol* 2010;21:15–19.
3. Lee WB, Jacobs DS, Musch DC, et al. Descemet's stripping endothelial keratoplasty: Safety and outcomes: A report by the American Academy of Ophthalmology. *Ophthalmology* 2009;116: 1818–1830.
4. Terry MA, Shamie N, Chen ES, et al. Endothelial keratoplasty for Fuchs' dystrophy with cataract: Complications and clinical results with the new triple procedure. *Ophthalmology* 2009;116: 631–639.

ADDITIONAL READING

- Melles GR, Ong TS, Ververs B, et al. Descemet membrane endothelial keratoplasty (DMEK). *Cornea* 2006;25:987–990.
- Sundin OH, Jun AS, Broman KW, et al. Linkage of late-onset Fuchs corneal dystrophy to a novel locus at 13pTel-13q12.13. *Invest Ophthalmol Vis Sci* 2006;47:140–145.
- Weisenthal RW, Streeten BW. Posterior Membrane Dystrophies, In: Krachmer JH, Mannis MJ, Holland EJ, (eds). *Cornea*, 2nd ed, 2005;938:948.

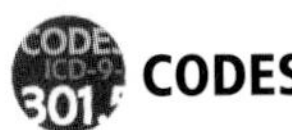

CODES

ICD9

371.57 Endothelial corneal dystrophy

CLINICAL PEARLS

- There is a hyperopic shift (+0.71 to +1.50 D) following DSEK. If planning a staged procedure with cataract surgery first and a possible DSEK surgery in the future, the intraocular lens power for cataract surgery should be made more myopic in case a DSEK is required.

FUCH'S HETEROCHROMIC IRIDOCYCLITIS

Anita P. Schadlu
Ramin Schadlu

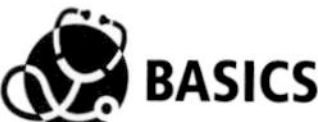

BASICS

DESCRIPTION

- Typically FHI is a unilateral chronic, recurrent anterior uveitis that can be asymptomatic or cause mild blurring and decreased vision. Recent articles have suggested a greater bilateral incidence than previously reported.
  - The causative role of rubella virus in FHI has been established (3).
  - There is a high association of glaucoma and cataract with FHI.

Pediatric Considerations

The number of cases of Fuchs heterochromic iridocyclitis (FHI) has decreased among those born after introduction of the rubella vaccination program in 1969 in the US. Parents of children diagnosed with FHI should be questioned regarding vaccination history (1)[A].

Pregnancy Considerations

Pregnant patients with clinical findings consistent with FHI should be tested for rubella immunity due to the risk of congenital rubella syndrome, which is especially serious when the virus is contracted during early pregnancy (2)[B].

EPIDEMIOLOGY

Incidence

- FHI accounted for less than 6% of all cases of anterior uveitis in a tertiary care setting (1).
  - The incidence of FHI decreased dramatically in patients born after 1968 due to the introduction of the rubella vaccine in 1969 (1).

Prevalence

The prevalence is <1%, but is likely underreported due to the lack of symptoms, and minimal signs in the majority of patients.

RISK FACTORS

- Risk factors include no personal or maternal history of rubella vaccination, or coming from a country without a rubella vaccination program.
  - Due to the minimally symptomatic uveitis, patients who do not receive regular examinations may present with vision loss secondary to cataract and/or advanced glaucoma.

Genetics

No genetic associations for FHI have been found.

GENERAL PREVENTION

Universal rubella vaccination is recommended.

PATHOPHYSIOLOGY

- Most cases are associated with chronic rubella virus infection.
  - The ocular inflammation associated with FHI is a local immune response driven by the rubella virus antigen. A CD8-positive T cell immune response mediates the inflammation (3).

ETIOLOGY

- Elevated levels of rubella antibodies (measured via a modified Goldmann–Witmer Index) were identified in the aqueous humor of 52 of 52 patients with FHI (3).
- The rubella virus (a single-stranded RNA virus) genome was identified in 5 of 28 specimens tested. Persistent virus genome is preferentially detected in younger patients (3).

COMMONLY ASSOCIATED CONDITIONS

- Cataracts are present in approximately $^3/_4$ of patients with FHI.
- Glaucoma is associated with FHI in 15% of patients (4).

DIAGNOSIS

HISTORY

- Patients are typically young and often asymptomatic.
  - Complaints may include progressive iris heterochromia, unilateral mild visual disturbance, mild ocular discomfort, and occasionally floaters.
  - Eye pain and redness are rare.

PHYSICAL EXAM

- Heterochromia is common (70% of patients) (4).
  - An affected dark eye will appear lighter due to iris atrophy. If the eyes are blue, the affected eye may appear darker due to visualization of the underlying iris pigment epithelium.
  - Heterochromia will not be evident in bilateral cases of FHI (6% of cases) (3).
- The affected eye typically is white and quiet on external exam.
- The characteristic diffuse, stellate nongranulomatous keratic precipitates are ubiquitous, although may not be evident on presentation.
- Cataracts develop in approximately $^3/_4$ of eyes with FHI (4).
- Glaucoma occurs in approximately 15% of eyes and may require surgical intervention (4).
- Abnormal bridging vessels in the anterior chamber angle may be seen on gonioscopy.
- Vitreous opacities may be present, and can cause visual symptoms. Chorioretinal scars may also be seen (2)
  - Posterior segment involvement is otherwise uncommon in FHI, although cystoid macular edema may be seen.
- Peripheral anterior synechiae and posterior synechiae are not typical for FHI.

DIAGNOSTIC TESTS & INTERPRETATION

Lab

Initial lab tests

- Clinical signs may be sufficient to make the diagnosis of FHI. However, often the signs are not present at the same time. A laboratory supported diagnosis may be made by detection of intraocular rubella antibody (100% specificity). Absence of rubella antibody in the aqueous humor makes the diagnosis of FHI unlikely.
  - Increased rubella antibody index (AI) (modified Goldmann–Witmer Index) is not specific when <40. However in conjunction with clinical findings, an increased AI has a very high positive predictive value.
- Oligoclonal IgG has 87% sensitivity for FHI and can be used for screening of unspecified ocular inflammation (3)[A].

Follow-up & special considerations

FHI is a chronic disease. Patients must be followed at regular intervals to monitor intraocular pressure and cataract formation.

Imaging

External photos and slit lamp photos may be obtained to monitor heterochromia, iris atrophy, and cataracts.

Pathological Findings

Infiltrating plasma cells and lymphocytes seen in pathological specimens support viral-induced inflammation as the etiology for FHI.

DIFFERENTIAL DIAGNOSIS

- Other causes of unilateral anterior uveitis.
  - Herpes Simplex Virus
  - Herpes Zoster Virus
  - Toxoplasmosis
  - Posner–Schlossman syndrome (glaucomatocyclitic crisis)
- Other causes of iris heterochromia.
  - Horner's syndrome
  - Malignant melanoma of the iris

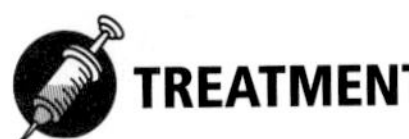

TREATMENT

MEDICATION

- Topical steroid treatment may be withheld if the inflammation is mild. The effect of steroid eyedrops in controlling FHI-related inflammation is minimal, and may hasten cataract formation and cause secondary glaucoma. However, patients should be monitored closely for worsening inflammation.
- Secondary glaucoma should be treated aggressively with topical drops and surgery, if indicated.

ADDITIONAL TREATMENT

Issues for Referral

Patients in whom the intraocular pressure is not controlled with topical drops, or who have progressive visual field loss, should be referred to a glaucoma specialist.

SURGERY/OTHER PROCEDURES

- Cataract surgery and glaucoma surgery may be complicated by intraoperative or postoperative hyphema due to the abnormal vessels bridging the anterior chamber angle (Amsler's sign).
  - Perioperative topical and/or oral steroid treatment should be used to minimize surgery-induced inflammation.
  - Posterior capsule opacification, glaucoma, and vitreous opacity may limit visual outcomes following cataract surgery (4).
- Pars plana vitrectomy may be indicated to clear visually-significant vitreous opacities.

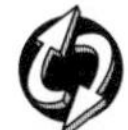

ONGOING CARE

FOLLOW-UP RECOMMENDATIONS

Patients need regularly scheduled follow-up visits depending on the presence of glaucoma and cataracts. Since FHI is often asymptomatic, patients may not notice recurrences.

PATIENT EDUCATION

Patients should be educated on the need for regular follow-up and the importance of compliance with glaucoma medications.

PROGNOSIS

Visual prognosis can be good, as long as glaucoma and any posterior segment complications are controlled.

REFERENCES

1. Birnbaum AD, Tessler HH, Schultz KL, et al. Epidemiologic relationship between fuchs heterochromic iridocyclitis and the United States rubella vaccination program. *Am J Ophthalmol* 2007;144:424–428.
2. Rothova A. The riddle of fuchs heterochromic uveitis. *Am J Ophthalmol* 2007;144:447–448.
3. Quentin CD, Reiber H. Fuchs heterochromic iridocyclitis: Rubella virus antibodies and genome in aqueous humor. *Am J Ophthalmol* 2004;138: 46–54.
4. Velilla S, Dios E, Herreras JM, Calonge M. Fuchs' heterochromic iridocyclitis: A review of 26 cases. *Ocul Immunol Inflamm* 2001;9:169–175.

ADDITIONAL READING

- de Visser L, Braakenburg A, Rothova A, de Boer JH. Rubella virus-associated uveitis: Clinical manifestations and visual prognosis. *Am J Ophthalmol* 2008;146:292–7.
- Van Gelder RN. Idiopathic no more: Clues to the pathogenesis of fuchs heterochromic iridocyclitis and glaucomatocyclitic crisis. *Am J Ophthalmol* 2008;145:769–71.

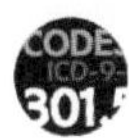

CODES

ICD9

- 364.10 Chronic iridocyclitis, unspecified
- 364.21 Fuchs' heterochromic cyclitis
- 365.62 Glaucoma associated with ocular inflammations

CLINICAL PEARLS

- Fuchs heterochromic iridocyclitis is most commonly a unilateral, episodic anterior uveitis that can be asymptomatic. It is often complicated by secondary glaucoma and cataract formation.
- Rubella virus has been implicated as the causative antigen in FHI.

GIANT CELL ARTERITIS

Helen Danesh-Meyer

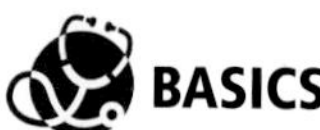

BASICS

DESCRIPTION

- Giant cell arteritis (GCA) is also known as temporal arteritis or granulomatous arteritis.
- It is a systemic inflammatory vasculitis that affects medium-sized to large arteries.
- Arterial wall inflammation leads to luminal occlusion and tissue ischemia, which cause the clinical manifestations of this vasculitis.
- Vision loss is a frequent complication of GCA, and once it occurs it tends to be both permanent and profound.
- Bilateral involvement is not uncommon.
- Causes of visual loss include arteritic anterior ischemic optic neuropathy (AAION), central retinal artery occlusion, posterior ischemic optic neuropathy, ocular ischemic syndrome, cilioretinal artery occlusion, and branch retinal artery occlusion.

EPIDEMIOLOGY

Incidence

- GCA predominantly affects Caucasians over 50 years of age, with women affected at least twice as often as men.
- Overall incidence is 15 to 25 per 100,000/year in individuals over the age of 50 years; however, incidence increases with age: from 2.3 per 100,000/year among patients in their 6th decade of life, to 44.7 per 100,000/year among patients in their ninth decade and older.
- GCA is more frequent among people of Scandinavian and Northern European descent, irrespective of their place of residence.
- There is some evidence to suggest an inherited component.

Genetics

- Some studies have found an association with HLA-DR4 haplotype and 60% of patients express the B1*0401 or B1*0404/8 variant of the HLA-DR4 haplotype.
- The intercellular adhesion molecule 1 (ICAM-1) genes may also predispose to GCA. ICAM-1 is strongly expressed in the inflammatory infiltrate of the temporal artery in GCA and G/R 241 polymorphisms in the ICAM-1 gene are associated with GCA susceptibility.

GENERAL PREVENTION

Prevention of visual loss depends on early diagnosis with adequate and timely intervention.

PATHOPHYSIOLOGY

- Both the adaptive and innate immune systems have been implicated.
- The acute-phase response mediated by the innate immune system is responsible for the systemic inflammatory component of GCA.
- Interleukin-6 being is critical by stimulating the production of acute-phase proteins.
- Circulating monocytes are a major source of interleukin-6; however, the mechanism and site of monocyte activation in GCA are unknown.
- Inappropriate activation of the adaptive immune system by dendritic cells is thought to cause the vascular lesions seen in GCA.
- Both T-cells and macrophages are attracted to the vessel wall via the vasa vasorum.
- In the adventitial layer, selective clonal expansion of CD4+ T cells leads to the release of cytokines such as interferon gamma (IFN-γ), which recruit macrophages into the vessel wall to form a prominent granulomatous reaction.
- Intimal hyperplasia, tissue ischemia and luminal occlusion also occur.

ETIOLOGY

The exact etiology of GCA is unknown, a variety of infectious agents have been suggested as potential immune triggers for the disease, including herpes virus, parainfluenza virus, cytomegalovirus, parvovirus B19, chlamydia, and mycoplasma.

COMMONLY ASSOCIATED CONDITIONS

- Giant-cell arteritis and polymyalgia rheumatica frequently occur together in the same patient.
- Polymyalgia rheumatica is a systemic inflammatory disease that manifests as myalgias of the neck, shoulder, and pelvic girdle.

DIAGNOSIS

HISTORY

- Patients should be specifically interrogated for the following symptoms:
- Constitutional: Poor appetite, weight loss, fatigue, night sweats, general malaise, fever or unknown origin.
- Symptoms associated with polymyalgia rheumatic: stiff and painful shoulder, girdle muscles.
- Symptoms associated with arteritis of carotid arteries and their branches: **Headaches** that are new and severe. **Scalp tenderness**, or direct temporal artery tenderness. **Jaw claudication** (highly specific for GCA). Less frequent are tongue claudication, facial pain.
- Visual symptoms: Transient visual loss, diplopia, sudden visual loss, graying of vision, eye pain.
- Ocular involvement without the presence of other GCA symptoms, or occult GCA, occurs between 5 and 38%.

PHYSICAL EXAM

- AAION: Chalky white optic disc edema (unlike nonarteritic anterior ischemic optic neuropathy [NAION], which shows a hyperemic swollen optic nerve), at times associated retinal edema. This produces abnormalities in optic nerve function: relative afferent papillary defect, dyschromatopsia, decrease visual acuity, visual field defect.
  - Central retinal artery—Note the lack of an embolic plaque in artery. Also, there is no sparing of the cilioretinal artery.
  - Diplopia due to 4th, 6th, or 3rd cranial nerve ischemia.
  - Changes in temporal arteries: Loss of pulse, tender to palpation.

DIAGNOSTIC TESTS & INTERPRETATION

Lab

- There is no single clinical symptom, sign or laboratory test specific for GCA.
- **Westergren erythrocyte sedimentation rate (WESR):** Approximately 80% of patients with GCA will have elevated ESR. But ESR is a nonspecific indicator of inflammation and can also be increased in malignancy, infection, connective tissue disorders, trauma, anemia, and hypercholesterolemia.
- "Normal" ESR is present in up to 17% of diagnosed cases, and thus cannot be used to exclude GCA.
- WESR increases with age. Upper limit is and has been defined as the age divided by two for men, and the age plus 10 divided by 2 for women.
- **C-reactive protein (CRP)** is an acute-phase protein. An elevated CRP has a specificity of up to 97.5% in patients with GCA, and may be elevated in the presence of a normal ESR. CRP is considered to be more sensitive than an elevated ESR.
- **ESR and CRP together** have higher sensitivity than either individually.
- **Other tests:** Elevated platelet count, normochromic normocytic anemia, fibrinogen, interleukin-6 (IL-6) and a2- and β-globulins have been found in GCA.

Imaging

- **Fluorescein angiography** may show prolonged choroidal and central retinal arterial filling times, and choroidal nonperfusion or filling defects suggestive of AAION.
- **Ultrasonography** of affected arteries is a may demonstrated changes in the arterial or be used to track the arterial course prior to biopsy.

Diagnostic Procedures/Other

- **Temporal artery biopsy (TAB)** is the gold standard for the diagnosis of GCA and should be performed on all patients in whom the diagnosis of GCA is suspected.
- Histological confirmation is recommended since long-term corticosteroid treatment is not without complications.
- TAB should never delay the instigation of treatment.
- TAB should be performed within one week of initiating systemic corticosteroids; however, histological evidence remains up to 6 weeks following treatment.
- Minimum length of 20 mm should be obtained to avoid skip lesions.
- If the TAB result is negative and the suspicion of GCA is high, a contralateral TAB should be performed.

Pathological Findings
- GCA is characterized by granulomatous inflammation affecting all layers of medium-sized and large arteries that have an internal elastic lamina.
- The inflammatory infiltrate is composed of activated CD4+ T cells, macrophages, and giant cells.
- Giant cells are not necessary for a diagnosis of GCA.
- Luminal stenosis or occlusion may be visualized due to intimal hyperplasia and subsequent mural thickening secondary to myofibroblast migration and proliferation.
- "Skip lesions" or segments of uninvolved regions adjacent to areas of inflammation are common.

DIFFERENTIAL DIAGNOSIS
NAION.

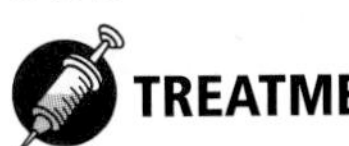

TREATMENT

The goal of treatment is to prevent ongoing ischemic damage. If the visual loss is the major symptom, the aim is to halt the progression of visual loss in the affected eye and prevent involvement of the contralateral eye.

MEDICATION
First Line
- **Systemic corticosteroids** are the mainstay of treatment. Intravenous methylprednisolone 1 g/d, usually for a minimum of 3 days, is recommended if there is visual loss.
- High-dose oral prednisone 1 mg/kg for GCA without visual symptoms.

Improvement of systemic symptoms usually occurs within 24–72 hours after initiation of therapy, but normalization of ESR may take several weeks.

Second Line
Methotrexate has been shown to have some benefit as a steroid-sparing agent.

ADDITIONAL TREATMENT
General Measures
Elderly patients being treated with high-dose prednisone should be admitted to hospital.

Issues for Referral
- A referral to a general physician should be made for prevention and management of potential complications of long-term high-dose corticosteroid treatment.
- These include diabetes, loss of bone density, GI disturbance, mood alteration, difficulty sleeping.

Additional Therapies
- Bone maintenance treatments: Calcium, vitamin D, bisphosphonates. This needs to be managed in consultation with general physician.
- GI disturbance: Patients are often treated with proton pump inhibitors (omeprazole) to prevent GI disturbance.
- Sleep difficulties: Patients may need additional medication to assist with sleeping.

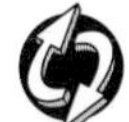

ONGOING CARE

FOLLOW-UP RECOMMENDATIONS
Systemic Steroid Dosage
- Most patients will remain on oral prednisone 1 mg/kg for a minimum of 4 weeks after which steroids should be tapered on the basis of symptoms and serial monitoring of inflammatory markers.
- The rate of steroid taper is about 10 mg per month initially (or 10% of the total daily dose every 1–2 weeks), then decreased to 5 mg per month, and even as low as 1 mg per month, once a dose of 10 or 15 mg per day is reached.
- Most patients will require treatment for a minimum of 1 to 2 years.
- Patients will need continued treatment with bone sparing agents, proton pump inhibitors and management of diabetes, and other possible complications of corticosteroid use.

Patient Monitoring
In most GCA patients with ESR/CRP elevation, it can be used accurately to monitor disease activity along with patients' symptoms.

PATIENT EDUCATION
- Patients should be educated about the side effects of corticosteroid use.
- Relapses are associated with a recurrence of symptoms or a rise in ESR/CRP. They are most common in the first 18 months, with a median time of around 7 months. Patients should be educated to contact their doctor if they have any recurrence of their GCA symptoms.

PROGNOSIS
- The prognosis for visual recovery is poor.
- Progressive visual loss may occur despite the early institution of high-dose corticosteroid treatment.
- Visual deterioration occurs in about 27% of eyes despite high-dose intravenous methylprednisolone.
- The greatest risk of visual deterioration is in the first 6 days.
- Treatment with intravenous corticosteroids is effective in reducing the likelihood of fellow eye involvement. Without treatment the risk of fellow eye involvement is 54 to 95%

COMPLICATIONS
- Causes of mortality associated with GCA include cardiovascular, neurological, and gastrointestinal events. Vasculitis of the coronary arteries may result in myocardial infarction or congestive heart failure. Ischemic brain damage is the second most common cause of GCA-related death after cardiac disease.
- Necrotizing segments of bowel are uncommon, but can also be fatal.

REFERENCES

1. Danesh-Meyer HV, Savino PJ. *Curr Opin Ophthalmol* 2007;18(6):443–449.
2. Niederkohr RD, Levin LA. Management of the patient with suspected temporal arteritis. A decision-analytic approach. *Ophthalmology* 2005;112:744–756.
3. Piggott K, Biousse V, Newman NJ, Goronzy JJ, Weyand CM. Vascular damage in giant cell arteritis. *Autoimmunity* 2009;42(7):596–604.
4. Weyand CM, Goronzy JJ. Medium and large-vessel vasculitis. *N Engl J Med* 2003;349:160–169.

ADDITIONAL READING

- Danesh-Meyer H, Savino PJ, Gamble GD. Poor prognosis of visual outcome after visual loss from giant cell arteritis. *Ophthalmology* 2005;112: 1098–1103.
- Foroozan R, Deramo VA, Buono LM, et al. Recovery of visual function in patients with biopsy-proven giant cell arteritis. *Ophthalmology* 2003;110: 539–542.
- Danesh-Meyer HV. Giant cell arteritis: A medical emergency. *New Zealand Medical Journal* 2008;23:10–13.

CODES

ICD9
- 362.31 Central retinal artery occlusion
- 377.41 Ischemic optic neuropathy
- 446.5 Giant cell arteritis

CLINICAL PEARLS

- The most common reason that GCA leads to blindness is failure of early diagnosis. The key to diagnosis is having a high index of suspicion in patients older than 50 years of age. The visual symptoms include transient visual blurring, diplopia, and acute visual loss in one or both eyes.
- Most common cause of blindness from GCA is arteritic anterior ischemic optic neuropathy that presents with sudden loss of vision and pallid disc edema.
- Once the clinician suspects GCA, the patient should be started immediately on high-dose corticosteroid treatment while the investigative process is underway.
- Temporal artery biopsy (TAB) is considered the reference standard for the diagnosis of GCA.

GOLDENHAR SYNDROME

Anam Qureshi
Jonathan H. Salvin

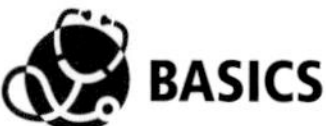

BASICS

DESCRIPTION
- Goldenhar syndrome is part of the oculoauriculovertebral spectrum (OAVS).
- Characterized by epibulbar choristomas, preauricular appendages, vertebral anomalies, and hemifacial microsomia (1)[C].

EPIDEMIOLOGY

Incidence
- 1 in 3500 to 5600 births (2)[C]
- Male predominance (3:2)

Prevalence
Unknown.

RISK FACTORS
None definitively identified.

Genetics
- Most cases are sporadic.
- Autosomal dominant (often bilateral auricular involvement) and autosomal recessive have been reported (3)[C].
- Chromosomal aberrations have been reported including chromosome 5p terminal deletion and del22q11.2 (4)[C].
- At least 4 specific loci and 1 identified gene, *SALL1* gene (16q12.1).

PATHOPHYSIOLOGY
Congenital disorder; see Etiology section.

ETIOLOGY
- Impaired migration of neural crest cells resulting in anomalies of 1st and 2nd branchial arches (5)[C].
- Ocular manifestations second to anomalous formation of first branchial arch, maxillary division (2)[C].

COMMONLY ASSOCIATED CONDITIONS
- Hemifacial microsomia (1)[C].
- Cardiovascular, nervous, musculoskeletal, and urogenital abnormalities.
- Nasal abnormalities.
- Hearing loss/deafness.
- Torticollis due to vertebral anomalies.

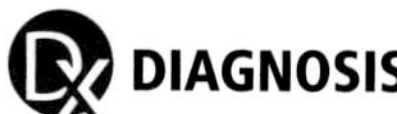

DIAGNOSIS

HISTORY
Family history.

PHYSICAL EXAM
- Full ocular examination
  - Limbal, ipsilateral, inferotemporal epibulbar dermoid (most frequent ocular sign); may have protruding cilia and induced astigmatism (2)[C].
  - Lipodermoid typically found temporally (2)[C].
  - Assess for ocular motility disorders, especially Duane syndrome (1)[C].
  - Examine for other signs: Upper eyelid coloboma with possible adhesion to the globe, blepharoptosis/shortening of palpebral fissure (uncommon), lacrimal drainage system anomalies (1)[C].
  - Evaluate for corneal anesthesia, decreased tear production, neuroparalytic corneal ulcers (uncommon) (6)[C].
  - Assessment of visual function as induced astigmatism can frequently cause amblyopia (2)[C].
  - Facial examination for preauricular appendages, hemifacial asymmetry, and microtia (1)[C].
  - Microphthalmia with or without hypoplasia of optic nerve and macula (uncommon) (5)[C].
  - Caruncle may be absent or ectopic.
- Full systemic exam for other associated findings.

DIAGNOSTIC TESTS & INTERPRETATION

Lab
- None, if no other systemic findings.
- Appropriate laboratory testing if genitourinary involvement.

Imaging
Initial approach
- Neurologic and facial imaging as indicated.
- Cervical spine imaging.

Follow-up & special considerations
Monitor for amblyopia.

Diagnostic Procedures/Other
- Audiology evaluation
- Genetics consultation
- Renal ultrasound as indicated

Pathological Findings
Epibulbar dermoids consist of collagenous connective tissue covered by conjunctival or corneal epithelium with possible epidermal appendages.

DIFFERENTIAL DIAGNOSIS
- Treacher–Collins syndrome
- Pierre Robin syndrome
- Cervico-oculo-acusticus syndrome
- Town–Brocks syndrome
- Oculoectodermal syndrome

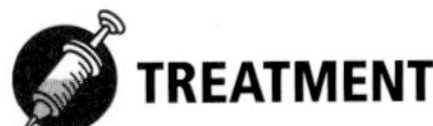

TREATMENT

MEDICATION

None for the primary disorder but may need for secondary complications.

ADDITIONAL TREATMENT

General Measures

Amblyopia treatment as indicated.

Issues for Referral

- Craniofacial/plastic surgery evaluation for cosmetic repair.
- Otolaryngology evaluation for external ear and audiology testing.
- Genetics for diagnosis, testing, and counseling.

SURGERY/OTHER PROCEDURES

- Surgical excision of limbal dermoid indicated for cosmetic reconstruction, presence of symptoms (redness, foreign body sensation), induced astigmatism causing amblyopia, secondary corneal complications (1)[C].
- Excision of lipodermoid with caution due to extraocular muscle involvement.
- Eyelid repair
- Craniofacial/plastic surgery for facial malformations

IN-PATIENT CONSIDERATIONS

Initial Stabilization

In-patient care only required for nonocular associations.

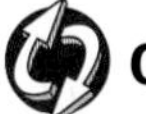

ONGOING CARE

FOLLOW-UP RECOMMENDATIONS

- As needed for secondary complications.
- Monitor for amblyopia, full refractive correction and symptoms requiring excision of limbal dermoid.

PATIENT EDUCATION

- Genetic counseling
- Appropriate educational services for hearing impairment
- Goldenhar Syndrome Support Network Society, http://barbmiles.tripod.com/
- Goldenhar Family Support Group (UK), http://www.goldenhar.org.uk/
- AboutFace, http://www.aboutfaceinternational.org/

PROGNOSIS

Ocular prognosis is good if amblyopia treated.

COMPLICATIONS

- Corneal dellen, exposure or ulcer
- Amblyopia

REFERENCES

1. Mansour AM, Wang F, Henkind P, Goldberg R, Shprintzen R. Ocular findings in the facioauriculovertebral sequence (Goldenhar-Gorlin Syndrome). *Am J Opthalmol* 1985;100(4):555–559.
2. Caca I, Unlu K, Ari S. Two cases of goldenhar syndrome. *J Pediatr Opthalmol Strabismus* 2006;43:107–109.
3. Vendramini-Pittoli S, Kokitsu-Nakata NM. Oculoauriculovertebral spectrum: report of nine familial cases with evidence of autosomal dominant inheritance and review of the literature. *Clin Dysmorphol* 2009;18(2):67–77.
4. Ala-Mello S, Siggberg L, Knuutila S, Von Koskull H, Taskinen M, Peippo M. Further evidence for a relationship between the 5p15 chromosome region and the oculoauriculovertebral anomaly. *Am J Med Genet* 2008;146A:2490–2494.
5. Margolis S, Aleksic S, Charles N, McCarthy J, Greco A, Budzilovich G. Retinal and optic nerve findings in Goldenhar-Gorlin Syndrome. *Ophthalmology* 1984;91(11):1327–1333.
6. Baum JL, Feingold M. Ocular aspects of Goldenhar's syndrome. *Am J Ophthalmol* 1973;75(2):250–257.

CODES

ICD9

- 224.3 Benign neoplasm of conjunctiva
- 367.20 Astigmatism, unspecified
- 756.0 Congenital anomalies of skull and face bones

CLINICAL PEARLS

- Carefully evaluate patients with epibulbar dermoids for Goldenhar syndrome.
- Refer for full systemic workup with a focus on cardiac, renal, vertebral, and central nervous system abnormalities.
- Evaluate and treat astigmatism early as a potential cause of amblyopia.
- Evaluate for hearing loss.

GRANULOMATOUS UVEITIS

Chirag Patel
Jeffrey L. Olson
Naresh Mandava
Scott C.N. Oliver

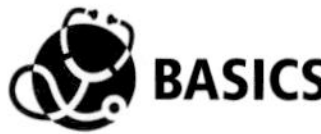

BASICS

DESCRIPTION

- Nonspecific term describing intraocular granulomatous inflammation.
- Symptoms may include painful red eye, photophobia and decreased vision.
- Classically presents with large keratic precipitates (KPs) on the corneal endothelium (mutton-fat KPs).
- Inflammation can involve only the anterior eye (iritis), vitreous (intermediate uveitis), retina and/or choroid (posterior uveitis), or the entire eye (panuveitis).
- More commonly associated with systemic disease or underlying ocular syndrome than nongranulomatous uveitis.
- Can be unilateral or bilateral
- Can be acute or chronic
- May occur at any age

RISK FACTORS

- Geographic location (e.g., endemic areas for Lyme disease)
- Exposure to animals (e.g., cats for toxoplasmosis)
- Ethnicity (e.g., sarcoidosis more prevalent in African Americans and Scandinavians)
- Prior injury to fellow eye for sympathetic ophthalmia
- Disruption of lens capsule (traumatic or surgical) for lens associated uveitis

Genetics

Associated diseases may have genetic markers (e.g., HLA-DR1 and HLA-DR4 for VKH).

PATHOPHYSIOLOGY

- Exact pathophysiology unknown
- May result from an autoimmune reaction
- May depend on the host's immune response to a systemic infectious process

ETIOLOGY

- Idiopathic in 50% of cases
- May be associated with a number of systemic conditions or infectious processes

COMMONLY ASSOCIATED CONDITIONS

- Sarcoidosis
- Syphilis
- Herpes zoster virus
- Herpes simplex virus
- Cytomegalovirus
- Lens associated uveitis
- Lyme disease
- Toxoplasmosis
- Vogt–Koyanagi–Harada (VKH) disease
- Sympathetic ophthalmia
- Tuberculosis (TB)
- Leprosy
- Wegener granulomatosis
- Coccidioidomycosis
- Brucellosis

DIAGNOSIS

HISTORY

- Review all medical conditions, surgeries, and ocular history.
- Obtain a complete and detailed review of systems (joint pain, rashes, shortness of breath, swollen lymph nodes, recent headaches, hearing difficulties, hair loss, pigmentary skin changes, history of ocular trauma, recent insect bites, sexually transmitted diseases, tuberculosis exposure, pet or animal exposure, and recent travel).

PHYSICAL EXAM

- Vision: May be unchanged or decreased depending on amount of inflammation.
- Intraocular pressure (IOP): Usually decreased because inflammation of the ciliary body causes decreased production of aqueous humor. Increased IOP may suggest a viral etiology or secondary glaucoma from chronic disease.
- External findings: Enlarged lacrimal glands, enlarged parotid glands, and cranial nerve seven palsy may suggest sarcoidosis.
- Conjunctiva: Generalized redness of the bulbar conjunctiva may be present. The eye may have a perilimbal injection termed ciliary flush. Perilimbal vitiligo (Sugiura sign) is a sign of VKH disease, occurring within a month of disease onset.
- Cornea: KPs are found on the endothelium and are clusters of white blood cells (WBCs) usually located in the lower half of the cornea. Classic mutton-fat KPs are large and greasy in appearance.
- Anterior chamber: Cells and flare are usually present.
- Cells floating in the anterior chamber are found with anterior segment inflammation. They can be graded under high-magnification slit lamp examination in a 1 × 1 mm field of light, as described by The SUN Working Group Grading Scheme (1)[A].
  - 0 < 1
  - 0.5 = 1–5 cells
  - 1+ = 6–15 cells
  - 2+ = 16–25 cells
  - 3+ = 26–50 cells
  - 4+ = More than 50 cells
- Flare is the result of extra protein in the aqueous. It can be graded using the SUN Working Group Grading Scheme:
  - 0 = None
  - 1+ = Faint
  - 2+ = Moderate (iris and lens details clear)
  - 3+ = Marked (iris and lens details hazy)
  - 4+ = Intense (fibrin or plastic aqueous)
- Iris: Peripheral anterior synechiae and posterior synechiae may be present. Inflammatory nodules on the iris represent accumulations of inflammatory cells. They can be present in the pupillary border, the iris surface or the anterior chamber angle.
- Lens: Lenticular precipitates may be visible on the anterior lens capsule. Posterior subcapsular cataracts may be present if the patient has had repeated episodes of iritis or ongoing chronic inflammation.
- Vitreous: Inflammatory cells in the vitreous imply involvement of the posterior segment. Aggregation of cells in the vitreous are called snowballs.
- Posterior segment: Optic nerve edema, sheathing of venules or arterioles, focal retinal and choroidal lesions, and exudative retinal detachment may be present.

DIAGNOSTIC TESTS & INTERPRETATION

Lab

- The patient's medical history, review of systems and physical examination should guide the laboratory evaluation.
- All patients who present with granulomatous uveitis should receive a diagnostic evaluation even if it is their first episode.
- As a minimum, CBC with differential and fluorescent treponemal antibody absorption (FTA-ABS) or other specific antitreponemal syphilis serology should be ordered.
- The following tests should be considered based in the history:
  - Purified protein derivative (PPD) test or gold quantiferon testing for TB.
  - ACE and lysozyme can be obtained if sarcoidosis is suspected.
  - Lyme serology
  - Toxoplasmosis IgG and IgM by ELISA
  - Antineutrophil cytoplasmic autoantibodies (ANCA): c-ANCA is found in 80–95% of active cases of Wegener granulomatosis.
  - PCR may be obtained for HSV 1, HSV 2, VZV, CMV, and toxoplasma.

Imaging

Initial approach

- If media opacity blocks the view of the posterior segment, B-scan ultrasonography may identify exudative detachment, subretinal granulomas, and optic nerve edema.
- Fluorescein angiography may identify vasculitis, papillitis, and choroiditis.
- Indocyanine green angiography may demonstrate defects of the choroid with greater detail than fluorescein angiography.
- Chest radiography may identify hilar adenopathy associated with sarcoidosis and tuberculosis.

Follow-up & special considerations

If chest radiography is equivocal, a chest CT or gallium scan can be considered if sarcoidosis is strongly suspected.

Diagnostic Procedures/Other

Lacrimal gland or conjunctival nodule biopsy is highly specific for sarcoidosis if positive.

Pathological Findings

Histopathology classically shows epithelioid and giant cells.

DIFFERENTIAL DIAGNOSIS
- Endophthalmitis
- Intraocular lymphoma
- Chronic retinal detachment
- Phacoanaphylactic glaucoma

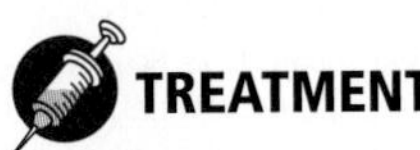

TREATMENT

MEDICATION
First Line
- Topical corticosteroids (e.g., prednisolone acetate), should be used aggressively initially and tapered with response to treatment.
- Cycloplegic agents (e.g., cyclopentolate or homatropine) should be used to treat pain and photophobia and to prevent iris synechiae.
- Patients with a known etiology for their inflammation (e.g., tuberculosis or toxoplasmosis) should be treated for the underlying cause in addition to steroids and cycloplegic agents.

Second Line
- After excluding infectious etiologies, oral, or periocular steroid may be required if inflammation does not adequately respond to topical steroids.
- Mid- to long-term oral steroids use should be accompanied by supplementary calcium and vitamin D to reduce the risk of osteoporosis.
- Prophylaxis against peptic ulcers should be considered using H2 blockers or proton pump inhibitors when systemic steroids are administered.
- Immunomodulatory and immunosuppressive agents may be considered in patients unresponsive to steroids or in patients needing long-term immunosuppressive (>3 mths) treatment (2)[A].
- Intravitreal steroid (e.g., triamcinolone acetonide 4 mg in 0.1 cm^3) may be administered for severe cases. Risk of cataract and ocular hypertension must be discussed. Infectious etiologies must be ruled out prior to administration of intraocular steroid.

ADDITIONAL TREATMENT
General Measures
Patients may develop increased intraocular pressure which should be treated with topical IOP lowering drops.

Issues for Referral
- All patients who need long-term treatment with oral steroids should be followed by a primary care provider to monitor blood sugars, blood pressure, and bone densitometry.
- All patients who require immunomodulatory or immunosuppressive agents may be referred to a rheumatologist for initiation and management of therapy.
- If an underlying etiology for inflammation is identified, an appropriate consultation should be made to treat the systemic condition (e.g., pulmonology for sarcoidosis, infectious disease for TB).
- Elevated intraocular pressure may necessitate a referral to glaucoma specialist.
- Development of cystoid macular edema (CME) may necessitate a referral to a vitreoretinal specialist.
- Uncontrolled or persistent inflammation requires referral to a uveitis specialist.

SURGERY/OTHER PROCEDURES
- Patients with chronic or recurrent episodes of uveitis may be candidates for a fluocinolone (Retisert) implant (3)[B].
- Treatment with steroids may cause a cataract resulting in the need for cataract extraction and intraocular lens implantation.
- Ocular hypertension unresponsive to topical medications may require a trabeculectomy or valve implantation.
- Pars plana vitrectomy may reduce the severity of posterior uveitis in some cases.

IN-PATIENT CONSIDERATIONS
Admission Criteria
- Usually not required if inflammation only affects the eye.
- Rarely may be indicated for treatment of systemic infections such as neurosyphilis, or for administration of IV medication, such as ganciclovir or acyclovir for viral retinitis.

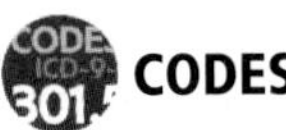

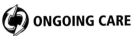

ONGOING CARE

FOLLOW-UP RECOMMENDATIONS
Patients should be followed closely, and steroids should be tapered slowly as inflammation resolves.

Patient Monitoring
Once inflammation has resolved patients should be seen at regular intervals to monitor for recurrences.

PATIENT EDUCATION
- Patients should be educated about signs and symptoms of flare ups of inflammation so they can return for prompt treatment.
- The often chronic or recurrent nature of granulomatous uveitis should be explained to the patient.
- The possibility of irreversible vision loss and even loss of the globe in the setting of untreated disease should be explained to the patient.

PROGNOSIS
- Many patients will have recurrent episodes of inflammation.
- Visual prognosis is good in the absence of cataract, glaucoma or CME.

COMPLICATIONS
- Cataract
- Glaucoma
- Cystoid macular edema
- Exudative retinal detachment
- RPE atrophy
- Band keratopathy

REFERENCES

1. Jabs DA, Nussenblatt RB, Rosenbaum JT. Standardization of uveitis nomenclature for reporting clinical data: Results of the First International Workshop; Standardization of Uveitis Nomenclature (SUN) Working Group. *Am J Ophthalmol* 2005;140:509–516.
2. Jabs DA, Rosenbaum JT, Foster CS, et al. Guidelines for the use of immunosuppressive drugs in patients with ocular inflammatory disorders: Recommendations of an expert panel. *Am J Ophthalmol* 2000;130(4):492–513.
3. Jaffe GJ, Martin D, Callanan D, et al. Fluocinolone acetonide implant (Retisert) for noninfectious posterior uveitis: Thirty-four-week results of a multicenter randomized clinical study. *Ophthalmology* 2006;113(6):1020–1027.

ADDITIONAL READING

- Nusenblatt RB, Whitcup SM. *Uveitis: Fundamentals and Clinical Practice*, 4th ed. Philadelphia, PA: Mosby, 2010.

CODES

ICD9
- 360.12 Panuveitis
- 363.21 Pars planitis
- 364.10 Chronic iridocyclitis, unspecified

CLINICAL PEARLS
- Patients with granulomatous uveitis should undergo a workup for systemic infectious and inflammatory etiologies.
- Aggressive anti-inflammatory therapy should be applied to suppress inflammation.
- Vision threatening complications may occur from uncontrolled uveitis.

GUILLAIN–BARRÉ SYNDROME AND FISHER SYNDROME VARIANT

Mark L. Moster

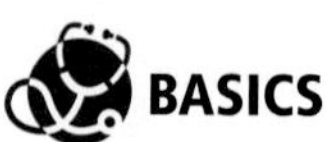

BASICS

DESCRIPTION

- A syndrome of acute inflammatory demyelination of peripheral (including cranial) nerves.
- Spectrum includes typical Guillain–Barré syndrome (GBS, also known as acute inflammatory demyelinating polyneuropathy; AIDP), Fisher syndrome (FS), and Bickerstaff Brainstem Encephalitis (BBE) and some other variants
- Often postinfectious

ALERT

Ascending paralysis in GBS may be rapid and lead to respiratory failure. Close monitoring is imperative.

EPIDEMIOLOGY

Incidence

- GBS: 0.6–4/100,000
- FS accounts for 1–7% in western countries but up to 25% in Japan.
- Men > women
- Caucasian > African
- Most often 3rd to 7th decade with bimodal peak for FS in 4th and 6th decade.

RISK FACTORS

- Infection:
  - Campylobacter jejuni
  - Hemophilus influenza
  - Viral—CMV, EBV
- Surgery
- Immunization

PATHOPHYSIOLOGY

- Immune inflammatory demyelination of peripheral nerve.
  - Perivascular inflammatory infiltrates
  - Axonal involvement may occur
- Wallerian degeneration

ETIOLOGY

Exposure to antigen with generation of autoimmune response.

COMMONLY ASSOCIATED CONDITIONS

Antecedent infection in 2/3 of patients.

DIAGNOSIS

HISTORY

- Acute weakness
- Most often beginning in distal lower extremities and ascending over hours to days
- Variable numbness
- Often ascends to involve cranial nerves with facial droop, ptosis, diplopia
- FS presentation—diplopia and gait disturbance

PHYSICAL EXAM

- Weakness, usually ascending
- Weakness in bulbar distribution may lead to apnea.
- Loss of deep tendon reflexes
- Ptosis and ophthalmoparesis may occur with all GBS subtypes but are the hallmark of FS.
- Classic triad of FS variant
  - Ptosis and ophthalmoparesis
  - Ataxia
  - Areflexia
- Ophthalmoparesis may have both peripheral and central nervous system features including: combinations of 3rd, 4th, 6th nerve paresis, symmetric patterns that do not fit one nerve or muscle, internuclear ophthalmoplegia, vertical gaze palsy, nystagmus, and other supranuclear patterns. GBS (especially FS) is the most common cause of complete bilateral ophthalmoparesis.
- BBE includes ophthalmoparesis, ataxia, impaired consciousness and ***hyper*** reflexia
- Many patients have mydriasis with poor pupillary light reaction. Light near dissociation may occur.

DIAGNOSTIC TESTS & INTERPRETATION

Lab

- Lumbar Puncture—"albumino-cytologic dissociation" —elevated protein with few WBCs. May take a few days until protein elevates.
- Electromyography—peripheral neuropathy with demyelinating and sometimes axonal features.
- AntiGQ1b antibody—especially elevated in FS (>85%). Clinically correlates with ophthalmoplegia and ataxia.

Imaging

- Consider MRI for differential diagnosis of brainstem infarction, Wernicke encephalopathy, brainstem encephalitis.
- Rarely see brainstem signal changes in GBS.
- May see enhancement of cranial nerves.

Pathological Findings

Perivenular inflammatory infiltrate and demyelination of peripheral nerves.

DIFFERENTIAL DIAGNOSIS

- Brainstem encephalitis, infarction, mass, or hemorrhage
- Myasthenia gravis
- Demyelinating disease
- Wernicke's encephalopathy
- Botulism
- Cavernous sinus lesion

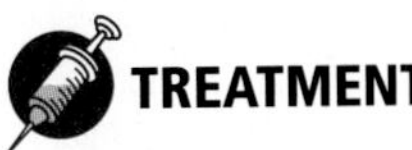

TREATMENT

MEDICATION

- For GBS
- Plasmapheresis (1)[A]
- Intravenous immunoglobulin (2)[A]
- No controlled trial of treatment in FS

ADDITIONAL TREATMENT

General Measures

- ICU monitoring
- Respiratory support
- Monitoring for autonomic dysfunction

Additional Therapies

- Physical therapy for weakness
- Monocular occlusion or prism for acute or nonresolving diplopia
- Care for corneal exposure with facial paresis

SURGERY/OTHER PROCEDURES

With suboptimal recovery of ptosis or ophthalmoparesis-strabismus, or lid surgery.

IN-PATIENT CONSIDERATIONS

Initial Stabilization

With typical GBS and ascending paralysis frequent monitoring of respiratory status and cardiac rhythm.

Admission Criteria

All GBS patients except relatively stable FS patients.

ALERT

- With GBS—ICU monitoring for potential respiratory failure or autonomic dysfunction (arrhythmia).
- Early intubation with progressive respiratory failure.

Discharge Criteria

Plateau in progression of weakness or improvement.

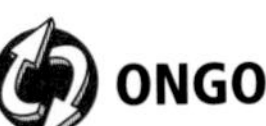

ONGOING CARE

FOLLOW-UP RECOMMENDATIONS

Continued follow up until recovery is complete or plateaued.

PROGNOSIS

- Good for significant recovery within 3 months of onset with FS. Recovery often begins within 2 weeks.
- Good for significant recovery with GBS.
- A subgroup of GBS patients will have recurrent episodes or continued progression into chronic inflammatory demyelinating polyneuropathy (CIDP).

REFERENCES

1. Guillain–Barré Study Group. Plasmapheresis and acute Guillain-Barré syndrome. *Neurology* 1985;35:1096–1104.
2. Plasma Exchange/Sandoglobulin Guillain-Barré Syndrome Trial Group. Randomized trial of plasma exchange, intravenous immunoglobulin, and combined treatments in Guillain-Barré syndrome. *Lancet* 1997;349:225–230.

ADDITIONAL READING

- Snyder LA, Rismondo V, Miller NR. The fisher variant of Guillain-Barre syndrome (Fisher Syndrome). *J Neuro-Ophthalmol* 2009;29:313–324.
- Vucic S, Kiernan MC, Cornblath DR. Guillain-Barre syndrome: An update. *J Clin Neurosci* 2009;16: 733–741.

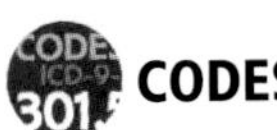

CODES

ICD9

- 323.81 Other causes of encephalitis and encephalomyelitis
- 357.0 Acute infective polyneuritis
- 374.30 Ptosis of eyelid, unspecified

G

GYRATE ATROPHY

Avni Vyas

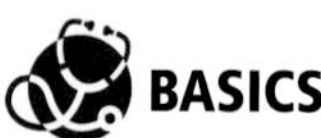

BASICS

DESCRIPTION

Gyrate atrophy is an autosomal recessive chorioretinal dystrophy that initially presents with nyctalopia and decreased peripheral vision during the first decade of life with progressive constriction of the visual field and eventual loss of central vision.

EPIDEMIOLOGY

Incidence

- Rare disease
- Most commonly reported in Finland with an incidence of approximately 1 in 50,000.
- Generally, presents in the first decade of life

RISK FACTORS

Has been diagnosed in several countries with the largest number of patients reported in Finland (1)[A].

Genetics

- Autosomal recessive inheritance
- Linked to chromosome 10q26, with more than 60 reported mutations

PATHOPHYSIOLOGY

- Patients have a deficiency of ornithine aminotransferase (OAT), which leads to a 10- to 20-fold increase in plasma ornithine levels.
- It is proposed that high ornithine levels may be toxic to the retinal pigment epithelium (RPE).

ETIOLOGY

Enzyme deficiency of OAT.

COMMONLY ASSOCIATED CONDITIONS

- EEG abnormalities and hair abnormalities have been reported in patients with gyrate atrophy.
- Skeletal muscle changes have been reported on CT and MRI.
- White matter lesions and atrophy have been noted on brain MRIs.

DIAGNOSIS

HISTORY

- In the first decade of life, patients typically present with nyctalopia, decreased peripheral vision, myopia, and astigmatism.
- In the second decade of life, patients develop posterior subcapsular cataracts.
- Patients develop progressive constriction of their visual fields with advancing age.
- Patients report a gradual decline in vision with loss of central visual acuity by the fifth decade.

PHYSICAL EXAM

- All patients with gyrate atrophy are myopic, generally with refractive errors−4.00 to −20.00D. Many patients have astigmatism as well.
- By adolescence, posterior subcapsular cataracts are evident.
- Dilated fundus exam initially shows multiple round well-circumscribed areas of chorioretinal atrophy in the periphery and midperiphery of both eyes, generally in a symmetric pattern.
- These areas coalesce with age and move towards the posterior pole, eventually involving the entire fundus.
- Typically, there is a scalloped border between the remaining normal retina and the atrophic retina.

DIAGNOSTIC TESTS & INTERPRETATION

Lab

Plasma ornithine levels should be checked and are generally 10 to 20 times higher than the general population.

Imaging

- Fluorescein angiography typically shows hyperfluorescence of the atrophic areas with possible leakage at the margins between normal and atrophic tissue.
  - Optical coherence tomography may demonstrate cystoid macular edema or an epiretinal membrane.

Diagnostic Procedures/Other

Early electroretinographic (ERG) testing shows reduced scotopic and photopic responses. By adulthood, ERG responses are nondetectable.

DIFFERENTIAL DIAGNOSIS

Advanced choroideremia—This is an X-linked recessive disorder with atrophy of the RPE and choriocapillaris.

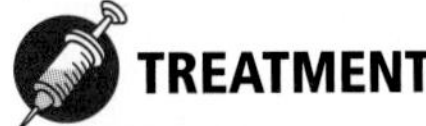

TREATMENT

MEDICATION

First Line

- Studies have suggested that long-term compliance with a low-protein, low-arginine diet can slow the progression of chorioretinal degeneration (2)[A]. However, even with good compliance, there is still a progressive decline in retinal function. One study of sibling pairs showed that younger siblings with earlier commencement of arginine-restriction had slower progression compared with older siblings with later commencement of dietary modification (3)[A].
- Supplementation with vitamin B6 (pyridoxine) has also been suggested, with additional dietary protein restriction based on ornithine levels. However, the majority of patients with gyrate atrophy are not pyridoxine responders. The dose of pyridoxine supplementation is not well established.

Second Line

Consider cataract extraction when the posterior subcapsular cataracts become visually significant. Patients should be educated that the postoperative visual potential is limited by their retinal disease.

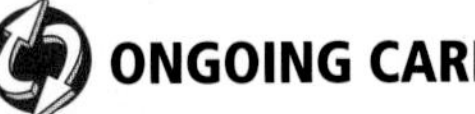

ONGOING CARE

FOLLOW-UP RECOMMENDATIONS

- Gyrate atrophy is a chronic progressive disorder with progressive loss of visual acuity and peripheral vision.
- Patients should be followed routinely for cataract and retinal evaluation.

DIET

See Treatment section.

PATIENT EDUCATION

Consider genetic counseling.

PROGNOSIS

Long-term visual prognosis is poor.

REFERENCES

1. Potter MJ, Berson EL. Diagnosis and treatment of gyrate atrophy. *Int Ophthalmol Clin* 1993;33: 229–236.
2. Kaiser-Kupfer ML, Caruso RC, Valle D, Reed GF. Use of an arginine-restricted diet to slow progressionof visual loss in patients with gyrate atrophy. *Arch Ophthalmol* 2004;122:982–984.
3. Kaiser-Kupfer ML, Caruso RC, Valle D. Gyrate atrophy of the choroid and retina. *Arch Ophthalmol* 2002;120:146–153.
4. Takki KK, Milton RC. The natural history of gyrate atrophy of the choroid and retina. *Ophthalmology* 1981;88:292–301.

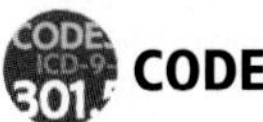

CODES

ICD9

- 363.54 Central choroidal atrophy, total
- 363.57 Other diffuse or generalized dystrophy of choroid, total
- 368.60 Night blindness, unspecified

CLINICAL PEARLS

- Early intervention with a low-protein, low-arginine diet may help slow progression of the disease.

G

HALLUCINATIONS, VISUAL

Tulay Kansu

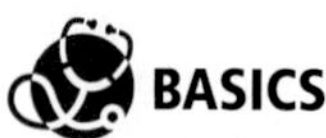

BASICS

DESCRIPTION

- Visual hallucinations are visual sensory perceptions without external stimulation associated with ophthalmologic, neurologic, metabolic, toxic, and psychiatric diseases.
- Charles Bonnet syndrome (CBS) is vivid, detailed, but nonthreatening hallucinations in visually deprived but cognitively unimpaired patients (1).

EPIDEMIOLOGY

Incidence

The incidence of the Charles Bonnet syndrome varies among different population groups. Common in patients with dementia or confusional states secondary to metabolic insults.

Prevalence

The prevalence of visual hallucinations in a range of ophthalmological populations, is around 10%, varying between 0.4% and 63%, significantly associated with an age over 64 years and a visual acuity in the best eye of 0.3 or less (2,3).

RISK FACTORS

Dementia, psychiatric disorders, drugs, alcohol, social isolation, visual loss, female sex, and old age.

PATHOPHYSIOLOGY

- Visual loss due to certain conditions produces a state of sensory deprivation that releases the visual cortex from regulation by external stimuli, resulting in visual hallucinations (cortical release phenomenon-deafferentation).
- Ictal hallucinations are caused by spontaneous or iatrogenic stimulation of the occipital or temporal cortex.
- Hallucinogenic agents have effects on serotonergic and limbic system structures.
- Migraine aura is caused by cortical spreading depression, which is a wave of electro-physiological hyperactivity followed by a wave of inhibition, usually in the visual cortex.

ETIOLOGY

- Ophthalmologic diseases (Visual loss due to enucleation, cataract, glaucoma, optic nerve, or retinal disease)
- Neurologic disorders (Epilepsy, migraine, narcolepsy, brainstem disorders, hemispheric lesions, Alzheimer, Parkinson, and Lewy body disease)
- Toxic and metabolic conditions (encephalopathies, drugs, alcohol, and withdrawal syndromes)
- Psychosis

COMMONLY ASSOCIATED CONDITIONS

- Hallucinogenic agents
- Visual deprivation
- Psychosis
- Delirium, delirium tremens
- Dementia (Alzheimer disease, vascular dementia, Dementia with Lewy bodies (DLB), Creutzfeldt–Jakob disease)

DIAGNOSIS

HISTORY

- Detailed description of seeing things
- Any clues to the cause anywhere in the body
- Neurologic or ophthalmologic symptoms
- Smoking, alcohol, illicit drugs
- Most patients are reluctant to admit hallucinations due to fear of being labeled with a psychiatric disease. Therefore, directed questioning of susceptible patients is essential.

PHYSICAL EXAM

- Visual acuity
- Visual fields
- Full neurologic examination

DIAGNOSTIC TESTS & INTERPRETATION

Lab

- Drug levels if patient is on medications
- Electroencephalography (EEG) for seizure disorders and encephalopathy

Imaging

MRI if brainstem or hemispheric lesion is suspected.

DIFFERENTIAL DIAGNOSIS

- Delusions are abnormal beliefs that are endorsed by patients as real.
- Confabulations are fabricated facts or events and occur primarily in patients with memory disturbances.
- Visual illusions are abnormal visual perceptions of a viewed object (metamorphopsia, cerebral diplopia, polyopia, and palinopsia).
- Hallucinations are the visual sensation that does not correspond to a real object.
  - Simple (flashes, sparkles, haloes, lights, shapes, patterns, phosphenes)
  - Complex (flowers, animals, people)
- Release hallucinations represent images formed from memory traces which would ordinarily be blocked by incoming sensory data.
- Charles Bonnet syndrome (CBS) is characterized by complex formed and recurrent visual hallucinations in psychologically normal people, and is often associated with eye pathology.
- Ictal hallucinations are brief, stereotyped visual experiences. Ictal hallucinations tend to be unformed when associated with occipital lesions and formed when associated with temporal lobe lesions.
- Peduncular hallucinosis is colorful, vivid images associated with midbrain, pontine, and thalamic lesions due to damage to the ascending reticular activating system.
- Migraine aura is a disturbance of vision consisting unformed black and white flashes, multicolored lights, dazzling zigzag lines (scintillating scotoma); and fortifications (teichopsia).
- "Alice in Wonderland" syndrome is a rare form of migraine aura. The most distinctive symptom is metamorphopsia, a distortion of body image and perspective.
- Hypnagogic hallucinations are dreamlike hallucinations associated with narcolepsy that occur as a person is falling to sleep.
- Schizophrenia sufferers experience auditory, visual, tactile, olfactory, and taste hallucinations. Auditory hallucinations are more common.
- Hallucinations are primarily visual in delirium which can be caused by drugs or metabolic diseases.

Pediatric Considerations

- Children may have hallucinations associated with substance abuse, psychosis, night terrors, decongestant medications, and seizures. Vivid recall of visual images with hallucinatory character can occur in some children.
- "Alice in Wonderland" syndrome can occur at any age, but is more commonly experienced by children.

Geriatric Considerations

- Elderly people, especially who are suffering with dementia might see people, animals, complicated scenes, and other bizarre scenarios.
- Hallucinations associated with:
  - 25% of Parkinson's disease
  - 25% of Alzheimer disease
  - 57% of patients with a variety of causes of visual loss (Charles Bonnet Syndrome)
  - Hallucinations and agitation are especially troublesome in dementia with Lewy bodies (DLB). Clinical characteristics include progressive dementia, persistent visual hallucinations, extrapyramidal syndrome, and severe sensitivity to neuroleptics.

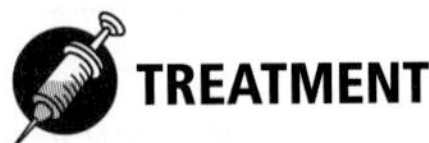

TREATMENT

Current evidence of treatment comes from case reports. No controlled clinical trials have been reported. The treatment is dependent on the underlying cause.

MEDICATION

First Line

- Antipsychotics
  - Drug selection should be individualized to the patient's previous history of antipsychotic use, current medical conditions, potential drug interactions, and side effects of the medication.
- In dementia with Lewy bodies, if symptoms are mild, no medical treatment may be necessary.
  - Therapeutic strategies include prescription of L-dopa and cholinesterase inhibitors such as rivastigmine, and avoidance of anticholinergic medications and neuroleptics.
  - Atypical neuroleptics are recommended such as clozapine, quetiapine, or aripiprazole when cholinesterase inhibitors are ineffective (4)
  - Caution is also required when prescribing memantine to patients with possible DLB.
- Antiepileptics in seizure disorders

Second Line

Selective serotonin reuptake inhibitors and tricyclic antidepressants (3).

ADDITIONAL TREATMENT

General Measures

Visual improvement and reassurance are the mainstays of treatment.

Issues for Referral

Ophthalmology, Psychiatry, Neurology consultations for related problems

SURGERY/OTHER PROCEDURES

Not indicated except tumors causing ictal hallucinations

IN-PATIENT CONSIDERATIONS

Initial Stabilization

Make sure that the metabolic status is normalized.

Admission Criteria

Metabolic disorders, delirium, agitation.

IV Fluids

Given as supplement and to correct the metabolic status.

Nursing

Careful monitoring for agitation and self-destruction.

Discharge Criteria

When the metabolic status is normalized

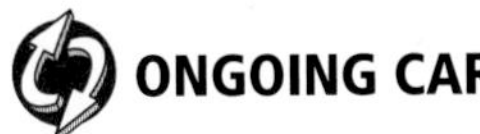

ONGOING CARE

FOLLOW-UP RECOMMENDATIONS

Reassurance and regulation of medications

Patient Monitoring

Metabolic side effects should be closely monitored in this population.

DIET

No specific diet, thiamine in alcohol withdrawal

PATIENT EDUCATION

Reassurance

PROGNOSIS

- Depends on the cause and complications
- Most patients are relieved by reassurance and medications but resolution of symptoms over time does not always occur.

COMPLICATIONS

Hallucinations may be persistent despite the treatment

REFERENCES

1. Ffytche DH. Visual hallucinatory syndromes: Past, present, and future. *Dialogues Clin Neurosci* 2007;9:173–189.
2. Ffytche DH. Visual hallucinations in eye disease. *Curr Opin Neurol* 2009;22:28–35.
3. Schadlu AP, Schadlu R, Shepherd JB 3rd. Charles Bonnet syndrome: A review. *Curr Opin Ophthalmol* 2009;20:219–222.
4. Gold G. Dementia with Lewy bodies: Clinical diagnosis and therapeutic approach. *Front Neurol Neurosci* 2009;24:107–113.

ADDITIONAL READING

- Cummings JL, Miller BL. Visual hallucinations. Clinical occurrence and use in differential diagnosis. *West J Med* 1987;146:46–51.
- Khan JC, Shahid H, Thurlby DA, et al. Charles Bonnet syndrome in age-related macular degeneration: The nature and frequency of images in subjects with end-stage disease. *Ophthalmic Epidemiol* 2008;15:202–208.
- Teeple RC, Caplan JP, Stern TA. Visual hallucinations: Differential diagnosis and treatment. *Prim Care Companion J Clin Psychiatry* 2009;11:26–32.

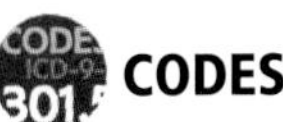

CODES

ICD9

368.16 Psychophysical visual disturbances

CLINICAL PEARLS

- Visual hallucinations can be caused by release phenomena, seizures, migraine, cognitive deficits, retinal disease, alcohol, drugs, hallucinogens, or metabolic disturbances.
- Charles Bonnet syndrome is vivid, detailed but nonthreatening hallucinations in visually deprived patients. Patients are not cognitively impaired.
- Occipital seizures cause simple unformed hallucinations. Temporal lobe seizures may lead to complex imagery or formed hallucinations. Electroencephalography can be diagnostic.
- Avoid neuroleptics such as haloperidol in a dementia patient with Lewy body disease.

HARD EXUDATES

Vikram J. Setlur

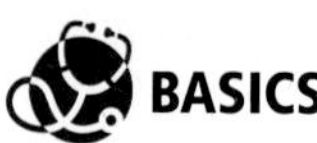

BASICS

DESCRIPTION

- Hard exudates in theundus represent leakage of lipid and protein from incompetent vessels in the retina, choroid, or optic disc.
  - Hard exudates are usually present in the outer plexiform layer of the retina but can dissect into the subretinal space as well as into other retinal layers.

EPIDEMIOLOGY

Incidence

Difficult to quantify

RISK FACTORS

Underlying vascular diseases such as diabetes, hypertension, and dyslipidemia

GENERAL PREVENTION

Control of blood glucose, blood pressure, and blood lipid levels can reduce the risk of common causes of hard exudates, such as diabetic retinopathy, hypertensive retinopathy, retinal arterial macroaneurysm, and retinal vascular occlusion.

PATHOPHYSIOLOGY

Increased vascular permeability allows leakage of protein and lipid into the retina.

ETIOLOGY

- Numerous retinal vascular diseases can cause hard exudates, including:
  - Diabetic retinopathy
  - Hypertensive retinopathy
  - Retinal vascular occlusion
  - Retinal arterial macroaneurysm
  - Radiation retinopathy
  - Coats' disease
  - Capillary hemangioma of the retina (i.e., von Hippel lesion)
  - Neuroretinitis
  - Choroidal neovascularization (e.g., age-related macular degeneration)

COMMONLY ASSOCIATED CONDITIONS

Macular edema is often present with hard exudates.

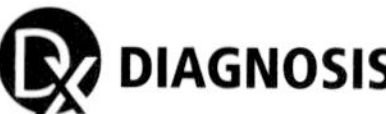

DIAGNOSIS

HISTORY

- Decreased vision if hard exudates are present in the macula
- Underlying medical diseases

PHYSICAL EXAM

- Fundus examination reveals discrete, yellow–white deposits most frequently in the posterior pole.
- Can be globular, linear, circinate surrounding a leaking vessel, or large and confluent. A macular star can be seen with neuroretinitis or hypertensive retinopathy.

DIAGNOSTIC TESTS & INTERPRETATION

DIFFERENTIAL DIAGNOSIS

- Cotton-wool spots
- Myelinated nerve fiber layer
- Retinitis
- Drusen
- Chorioretinal atrophy
- Hollenhorst plaque
- Crystalline retinopathy (see the Talc retinopathy chapter)

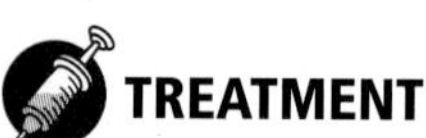

TREATMENT

MEDICATION

First Line

Treatment of the underlying disorder is required.

Second Line

For diabetic retinopathy and diabetic macular edema, a common cause of hard exudates, treatment of the underlying macular edema with laser photocoagulation and/or injection of intraoular steroid or anti-VEGF medication can lead to resolution of the hard exudates (1,2)[C].

SURGERY/OTHER PROCEDURES

Submacular surgery has been used to remove massive diabetic submacular hard exudates.

ONGOING CARE

COMPLICATIONS

- Macular edema is often associated with hard exudates.
- Patients with neuroretinitis may have an afferent pupillary defect, but this often resolves with time.

REFERENCES

1. Larsson J, Kifley A, Zhu M, et al. Rapid reduction of hard exudates in eyes with diabetic retinopathy after intravitreal triamcinolone: Data from a randomized, placebo-controlled, clinical trial. *Acta Ophthalmol* 2009;87:275–280.
2. Ciardella AP, Klancnik J, Schiff W, et al. Intravitreal triamcinolone for the treatment of refractory diabetic macular oedema with hard exudates: An optical coherence tomography study. *Br J Ophthalmol* 2004;88:1131–1136.

ADDITIONAL READING

- Naito T, Matsushit S, Sato H, et al. Results of submacular surgery to remove diabetic submacular hard exudates. *J Med Invest* 2008;55:211–215.

CODES

ICD9

- 250.50 Diabetes mellitus with ophthalmic manifestations, type ii or unspecified type, not stated as uncontrolled
- 362.01 Background diabetic retinopathy
- 362.82 Retinal exudates and deposits

CLINICAL PEARLS

- Discrete, yellow–white deposits of lipid and protein in the fundus from leaking vessels in the retina, choroid, or optic disc.
- First-line treatment is aimed at the underlying disorder, not the hard exudates themselves.
- Macular edema is frequent association, and may need treatment independent of underlying systemic diseases (if present).

HEMANGIOMA IN CHILDREN

Mary O'Hara

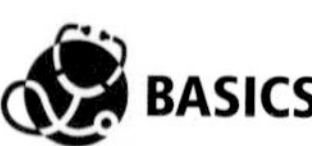

BASICS

DESCRIPTION
Rapidly growing benign blood vessel tumor of the periorbital tissues

EPIDEMIOLOGY
1–2.6% of neonates (1)[C]

RISK FACTORS
- Female sex (1)[C]
- Caucasian race (1)[C]
- Prematurity (1)[C]
- Chorionic villus sampling (2)[C]
- Family history

Genetics
- Most are sporadic without hereditary component
  - Familial form is a highly penetrant autosomal dominant trait with variable expression, linkage to chromosome 5q31–33 (2)[C]

GENERAL PREVENTION
Genetic counseling for familial form

PATHOPHYSIOLOGY
Increased local expression of vascular endothelial growth factor (VEGF) during proliferative stage. During involutional phase, VEGF expression decreases (2)[C].

ETIOLOGY
Hamartomatous growth of blood vessels.

COMMONLY ASSOCIATED CONDITIONS
- PHACES: Posterior fossa malformations, hemangiomas (usually large facial), arterial anomalies, coarctation of the aorta and other cardiac defects, eye abnormalities (especially optic nerve malformation), sternal clefting and supraumbilical raphe
- Kasabach-Merritt syndrome: Consumptive coagulopathy with thrombocytopenia, associated with very large capillary hemangiomas
- Diffuse neonatal hemangiomatosis
- Maffucci syndrome: Endochondromas, bony deformities, and diffuse hemangiomas
- Klippel-Trenaunay syndrome: Rare triad of capillary or cavernous hemangioma, venous malformations, and soft tissue or bony hypertrophy

DIAGNOSIS

HISTORY
- Rapid growth and proliferation of a vascular lesion in the first 6 months of life
  - Presentation is variable, may be red macule or no lesion noted
- Spontaneous involution begins during second year of life and may continue for almost 10 years.

PHYSICAL EXAM
- Full ocular examination with special attention to refraction (can induce myopia or astigmatism)
- Measure size of lesion/photograph if possible
- Systemic examination for other anomalies
- Vascular nature of lesion gives it a reddish color if superficial and bluish–purple color if subcutaneous
- Lesion is compressible and blanches to touch
- Mass may swell and become more violaceous when baby cries or when placed in Trendelenburg position.
- Attention to obstruction of visual axis, preference of fixation, and chin lift (indicating likely binocular fusion).
- Assess for proptosis, optic nerve compression, or fullness of temporal fossa.

DIAGNOSTIC TESTS & INTERPRETATION

Lab

Initial lab tests
- None if no systemic involvement
- CBC with platelet count for large lesions or if other signs of small vessel bleeding (e.g., petechia)

Follow-up & special considerations
- Counsel parents that wheezing may indicate airway hemangioma and to seek immediate medical care
- Bleeding or petechia indicate consumptive coagulopathy (Kasabach-Merritt syndrome)

Imaging

Initial approach
- Ultrasound of the lesion demonstrates compressibility, internal reflectivity, and indiscrete borders
  - Computed tomography (CT) less favored because of radiation to the infant, but can determine if there is any associated bony erosion.
  - Magnetic resonance imaging (MRI) demonstrates indiscrete margins and vascularity when comparing T1- and T2-weighted images.
  - Orbital and brain imaging if proptosis, full temporal fossa, indication of optic nerve compression (e.g., afferent pupillary defect).

Follow-up & special considerations
Close follow-up of the ophthalmic examination during the proliferative phase as astigmatism, anisometropia, and ptosis can cause profound amblyopia.

Diagnostic Procedures/Other
- Doppler of lesion demonstrates vascularity
  - Biopsy may be necessary if cannot rule out rhabdomyosarcoma

Pathological Findings
Proliferative phase marked by rapid proliferation of capillaries lined by endothelial cells with high mitotic rates and accompanying fibroblasts, pericytes, and mast cells. During involution there is drop-off of mitosis with apoptosis of endothelial cells.

DIFFERENTIAL DIAGNOSIS
- Rhabdomyosarcoma (usually superior temporal or nasal)
- Lymphangioma
- Cavernous hemangioma
- Nevus flammeus (does not gain volume)
- Port wine mark (does not gain volume until much later in childhood)
- Arteriovenous malformation
- Neuroblastoma
- Encephalocele (usually superior nasal)
- Lacrimal sac mucocele (inferior nasal)

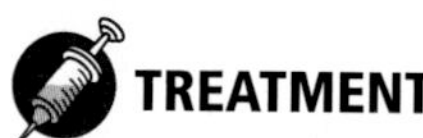

TREATMENT

MEDICATION
Only indicated when visual axis obstructed and amblyopia unresponsive to penalization or occlusion of the contralateral eye.

First Line
- Beta-blocker therapy is rapidly becoming first-line treatment modality (3)[C]
  - Systemic treatment with 1–2 mg/kg/d of propranolol divided b.i.d has produced dramatic involution of lesions. There is no universally accepted protocol for initiation of therapy. A history of bronchospasm, cardiac disease, or CNS vascular anomaly may be a contraindication to therapy.
- Topical treatment with timolol eyedrops or gel has produced results similar to systemic treatment in isolated cases but has not been rigorously studied (4)[C].

Second Line

- Corticosteroid therapy has been the most commonly used treatment modality until recently (1)[C]
  - Oral therapy has a 30–90% response rate. Particularly useful in treating deep orbital lesions. Complications include pituitary/adrenal suppression, immunological suppression, and Cushing syndrome. Dose 1–2 mg/kg/d. Some have used as much as 4 mg/kg/d
  - Intralesional steroid therapy has a 60–80% response rate. Potential complications: Central retinal artery occlusion, eyelid necrosis, eyelid depigmentation, and subcutaneous fat atrophy. Adrenal suppression also reported.
  - Topical steroid therapy may be helpful. Skin changes have been reported and adrenal suppression can be seen with high-dose, extended treatment.
- Interferon alfa can be effective but rarely used because of high rate of toxicity in children. Efficacy may be increased if used with steroids.
  - Spastic diplegia, seizures, coma
  - Liver toxicity
  - Hematologic abnormalities

ADDITIONAL TREATMENT

General Measures

- Observation if no obstruction of visual axis or significant astigmatism
- Treatment of amblyopia with atropine penalization or occlusion of the contralateral eye along with spectacle if indicated

Issues for Referral

- Prompt ENT referral for airway hemangiomas
- Genetic counseling if familial form or associated conditions
- Hematology consultation if Kasabach-Merritt syndrome
- Neurosurgical consultation if orbital/brain involvement

Additional Therapies

- Laser therapy may occasionally benefit superficial lesions. Several different types of laser have been used
  - Carbon dioxide (CO_2)
  - Argon
  - Neodymium:Yttrium-aluminum-garnet (Nd:YAG)
  - Pulsed dye lasers

COMPLEMENTARY & ALTERNATIVE THERAPIES

None proven or indicated

SURGERY/OTHER PROCEDURES

- Embolectomy usually not indicated for orbital and adnexal lesions.
- Complete or partial excision of sight-threatening lesions resistant to other treatment modalities may be necessary on rare occasions.
- Surgical excisions/facial plastic procedures may be done after involution.

IN-PATIENT CONSIDERATIONS

Initial Stabilization

If airway concerns, this is primary consideration.

Admission Criteria

Some have recommended inpatient initiation of systemic beta-blocker treatment with appropriate monitoring.

ONGOING CARE

FOLLOW-UP RECOMMENDATIONS

- Rebound recurrence of the lesion has been seen on cessation of all forms of steroid and beta blocker therapy.
- Close follow-up during proliferative phase as amblyopia is common
  - Spectacles for significant astigmatism
  - Penalization/occlusion therapy as needed
  - Medically treat if not responsive to conservative therapy
- Subsequent follow-up for appearance issues
  - Defer surgery until involution complete, if possible

Patient Monitoring

- Vision/refraction
- Psychosocial interactions

PATIENT EDUCATION

Family support network: National Organization of Vascular Anomalies (NOVA): http://www.novanews.org

PROGNOSIS

- Approximately 40% of lesions spontaneously involute by 4 years old and 70% by 7 years old.
- Astigmatic refractive errors are seen in 20–46% of patients with eyelid or orbital capillary hemangiomas (5)[C].
- One-third of patients with anisometropia had visual acuity of 20/60 or worse in the affected eye (5)[C].

COMPLICATIONS

- Lid deformity
- Scarring, hypopigmentation, or atrophy of skin
- Facial asymmetry
- Psychosocial issues related to appearance

REFERENCES

1. Ceisler EJ, Santos L, Blei F. Periocular hemangiomas: What every physician should know. *Pediatr Dermatol* 2004;21:1–9.
2. Phung TL, Hochman M, Mihm MC. Current knowledge of the pathogenesis of infantile hemangiomas. *Arch Facial Plast Surg* 2005;7: 319–321.
3. Zimmerman AP, Wiegand S, Werner JA, et al. Propranolol therapy for infantile haemangiomas: Review of the literature. *Int J Pediatr Otorhinolaryngol* 2010;74:338–342.
4. Guo S, Ni N. Topical treatment for capillary hemangioma of the eyelid using beta-blocker solution. *Arch Ophthalmol* 2010;128:255–256.
5. Schwartz SR, Kodsi SR, Blei F, et al. Treatment of capillary hemangiomas causing refractive and occlusional amblyopia. *J AAPOS* 2007;11: 577–583.

ADDITIONAL READING

- http://emedicine.medscape.com/article/1218805-overview

CODES

ICD9

228.01 Hemangioma of skin and subcutaneous tissue

CLINICAL PEARLS

- Follow closely for amblyopia in the proliferative phase of the lesion.
- Wheezing warrants evaluation for airway hemangioma.
- Most lesions do not warrant treatment and spontaneously resolve over the first decade of life.

H

HERPES SIMPLEX

Peter R. Laibson

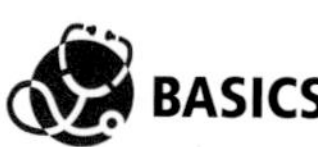

BASICS

DESCRIPTION

- Herpes simplex virus type 1 causes ocular infection following introduction of the virus in childhood as a subclinical or mild systemic infection. The HSV becomes latent in ganglion around the eye (trigeminal). The virus or viral genome may remain latent for decades before reactivating to cause various forms of herpetic keratitis.
- Conjunctival inflammation precedes corneal vesicles, Superficial Punctate Keratitis (SPK), and then branching epithelial ulcer, a classic dendritic ulcer which may enlarge to a geographic form.
- Deeper corneal forms of herpes simplex virus keratitis (HSVK) may follow days/weeks later. Disciform keratitis is an immune form of HSV involving corneal endothelium leading to edema. With persistence, corneal scarring, thinning, and rarely, perforation.

EPIDEMIOLOGY

Incidence

- HSV type 1 is the leading cause of blindness from an infectious corneal disease. By age 5 years, over 60% show antibody evidence systemic HSV.
- About 1% of HSV infected patients develop ocular HSV.

Prevalence

- There are about 20,000 new primary cases of HSVK seen yearly. Most are dendritic keratitis.
- About 30,000 recurrent HSVK cases are seen annually.

RISK FACTORS

Fever, URI, ocular trauma, menses, high stress, CL use, all have been considered risk factors, but not proven.

Genetics

Probably exist but not defined.

GENERAL PREVENTION

Oral antivirals are useful to prevent recurrent HSVK. Most helpful with previous hx of multiple recurrences of HSVK.

PATHOPHYSIOLOGY

Systemic viremia of HSV early in life seeds ganglia around the eye. Later reactivation of latent virus causes infection.

COMMONLY ASSOCIATED CONDITIONS

Fever blisters around the mouth, nose, and eye often accompany ocular HSV.

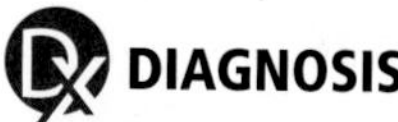

DIAGNOSIS

HISTORY

Ocular inflammation and eye irritation (pain) often precede HSVK. Blurred VA when the infection is in the visual axis.

PHYSICAL EXAM

Slit-lamp examination is critical to diagnose ocular HSV. Vital dyes such as fluorescein, lissamine green, or Bengal rose are very helpful.

DIAGNOSTIC TESTS & INTERPRETATION

Lab

Most often lab tests such as culture are not necessary as slit-lamp diagnosis of dendritic keratitis is very specific. With more complicated, deeper forms of HSVK, culture, PCR, or immune tests are used.

Imaging

None.

Pathological Findings

Pathological studies are rarely performed.

DIFFERENTIAL DIAGNOSIS

Can be confused with herpes zoster keratitis, Epstein Barr, acanthamoeba, fungal keratitis, and other persistent unusual deeper corneal infections.

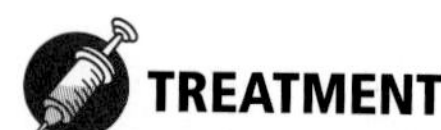

TREATMENT

MEDICATION

First Line

Dendritic keratitis responds well to trifluridine drops topically and third generation topical gels such as ganciclovir. Oral antivirals, acyclovir and valacyclovir are useful. Steroids should be avoided for ocular surface HSVK, but are used with antivirals for stromal HSVK, disciform, necrotizing and uveitis.

SURGERY/OTHER PROCEDURES

Penetrating keratoplasty for severe stromal scarring, thinning, or perforation is helpful.

ONGOING CARE

FOLLOW-UP RECOMMENDATIONS

Patient Monitoring

With HSV dendritic keratitis follow-up, slit-lamp exams as necessary until resolution, with stromal disease, very long term follow-up is critical. Herpes is forever.

PATIENT EDUCATION

Discussion of long-term therapy. Not to self-medicate with recurrences, but to expedite office examination.

PROGNOSIS

Good for initial and early recurrent dendritic keratitis with topical Rx. Or oral Rx. Guarded for stromal HSV.

COMPLICATIONS

Significant morbidity and visual loss with stromal HSV.

Pediatric Considerations

Infants and children can develop HSVK after loss of maternal antibodies. Steroids should never be used for a red eye in this group unless a slit-lamp examination is done.

ADDITIONAL READING

- Young RC, Hodge DO, Liesegang TJ, et al. Incidence, recurrence, and outcomes of herpes simplex virus eye disease in Olmsted County, Minnesota, 1976–2007: The effect of oral antiviral prophylaxis. *Arch Ophthalmol* 2010;128(9):1178–1183.
- Knickelbein JE, Hendricks RL, Charukamnoetkanok P. Management of hsv stromal keratitis: An evidence-based review. *Surv Ophthal* 2009; 54(2):226–234.

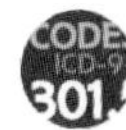

CODES

ICD9

- 054.42 Dendritic keratitis
- 054.43 Herpes simplex disciform keratitis

CLINICAL PEARLS

- Always suspect possible ocular HSV in patients. With acute red eye and do slit-lamp examination with vital dye to avoid treating HSV with topical steroids especially in children.

HERPES ZOSTER OPHTHALMICUS

Neelofar Ghaznawi
Kristin M. Hammersmith

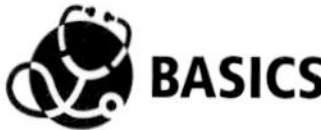

BASICS

DESCRIPTION

- Acute, painful, vesicular eruption distributed along the ophthalmic branch of the trigeminal nerve (1).
- Ocular inflammation without characteristic rash: Zoster sine herpete (2).

EPIDEMIOLOGY

Incidence

- 200,000 new cases per year in the US.
- 1% life time risk (3).

RISK FACTORS

- Increasing age.
- Immune compromise (i.e., HIV, cancer, immunosuppression) (4).

GENERAL PREVENTION

- CDC recommendation (2008)—routine vaccination of all individuals 60 years or older with Varicella Zoster Vaccination (Zostavax®), including those with prior history of herpes zoster or chronic medical conditions.
- The vaccine is not licensed for the treatment of acute HZ or post herpetic neuralgia (PHN), or for the prevention of HZ in patients aged younger than 60 years (5).

PATHOPHYSIOLOGY

- Reactivation of latent virus from trigeminal ganglia with viremia and spread of virus from sensory axons to skin.
- Age-related decline in varicella-zoster virus specific cell mediated immunity increases susceptibility to viremia (5).

DIAGNOSIS

HISTORY

- Painful vesicular eruption in a single dermatome.
- Fever, malaise, headache, and pain in the affected dermatome.
- Affective disorder: Anorexia, lassitude, mood changes, antisocial behavior, depression, and insomnia (6).

PHYSICAL EXAM

- Rash involving the V1 dermatome evolving from an erythematous lesion with macules, papules and vesicles with pustules and crusts developing subsequently.
- Slit-lamp examination.
  - Early:
    - Eyelid: Hyperemia, edema, ptosis.
    - Conjunctiva: Hyperemia, petechial hemorrhages, vesicles, pseudodendrites, papillae, follicles, pseudomembranes.
    - Sclera/episclera: Limbal vasculitis, sclerokeratitis, posterior scleritis.
    - Cornea:
    - Epithelium: Pseudodendrites, punctate epithelial keratitis.
    - Stroma: Nummular stromal keratitis, disciform keratitis (7).
    - Iris/uvea: Segmental iris edema, granulomatous keratouveitis with keratic precipitates (8), secondary glaucoma (9).
    - Retina/optic nerve: Retinal perivasculitis, ischemic optic neuritis, necrotizing retinopathy.
  - Late (1 month after rash):
    - Eyelid: Cicatricial entropion/ectropion, trichiasis.
    - Conjunctiva: Hyperemia, pseudomembranes.
    - Sclera/episclera: Limbal vasculitis, sclerokeratitis, posterior scleritis.
    - Cornea:
    - Epithelium: Delayed pseudodendrites (mucous plaque keratitis), punctate epithelial keratitis, neurotrophic ulceration, band keratopathy (10).
    - Stroma: Nummular stromal keratitis, disciform keratitis, lipid deposition, anterior and posterior stromal scarring, chronic edema (7).
    - Iris/Uvea: Segmental iris atrophy, granulomatous keratouveitis with KP, secondary glaucoma.
    - Retina: Acute retinal necrosis (ARN), progressive outer retinal necrosis (PORN).
- Neuroophthalmic examination.
  - Extraocular muscles: Transient EOM palsy and diplopia (11).
  - Cranial nerves: CN III, IV, or VI can be involved indicating vasculitis within the orbital apex (orbital apex syndrome) or brainstem dysfunction (12).
  - Acute pain: Characterized as lancinating, burning, aching, and/or itching.
  - Post-herpetic neuralgia (PHN)—pain lasting more than 1 month after disease onset. Characterized as constant or intermittent aching or burning, sudden lancinating pain, allodynia (pain from nonpainful stimuli), and/or a constant or intermittent itch (13).

DIAGNOSTIC TESTS & INTERPRETATION

Lab

No laboratory work up is necessary unless there is a high index of suspicion for HIV.

Imaging

Initial approach

Slit-lamp examination including intraocular pressure assessment, corneal sensation, and dilated funduscopic examination.

Follow-up & special considerations

- Starting oral antiviral therapy shortens the duration of acute pain, virus shedding, rash, acute, and late-onset anterior segment complications, and the incidence and severity of PHN (12).
- Depending on severity of ocular inflammation, patient should be re-evaluated within 5–7 days and frequency of follow-up visits should be dictated by severity of slit-lamp findings.

ALERT

Treatment with valacyclovir in severe immunocompromise has been associated with thrombocytopenic purpura/hemolytic uremic syndrome and is therefore not FDA approved for use in this subset of patients.

Diagnostic Procedures/Other

- PCR can be used to document the presence of VZV DNA in aqueous samples in patients with evidence of uveitis but without clinical eruption (14).
- Evolution of IgG antibody titers between acute and convalescent phase specimens demonstrating a 4-fold increase can confirm evidence of HZO in the absence of skin involvement (15).

DIFFERENTIAL DIAGNOSIS

Orbital cellulitis, poison ivy, herpes simplex keratitis.

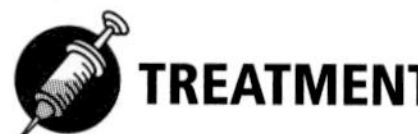

TREATMENT

MEDICATION

First Line

- Oral antiviral therapy starting with 72 hours of rash onset. Duration of therapy—10 days.
  - Acyclovir 800 mg PO, 5 times daily†
  - Valacyclovir 1000 mg PO, 3 times daily†*
  - Famciclovir 500 mg PO, 3 times daily†*

†Acute renal failure: May occur in elderly patients (with or without reduced renal function) Use with caution in elderly patients and reduce dosage in patients with renal impairment (16).

*Note: Use of valacyclovir and famciclovir has been associated with decreased occurrence of PHN.

Second Line

There are no FDA-approved alternative therapies.

ADDITIONAL TREATMENT

Additional Therapies

- Acute HZO:
  - Rash: Topical antibiotic ointment for areas of pustule and crust formation.
  - Pain: Prednisone 60 mg/day for the first 7 days, 30 mg/day on days 8 to 14, and 15 mg/day on days 15 to 21 for moderate to severe pain (17).
  - Anterior segment complications:
  - Dry eye syndrome (DES): Frequent lubrication with topical artificial tear formulations.
  - Stromal scarring: Cautious use of low potency topical steroid to control inflammation.
  - Iritis: Topical steroids (7).
- Chronic HZO:
  - PHN: Tricyclic antidepressants, opioids, anticonvulsants, and topical analgesics have proven benefit. Refer to neurologist/pain specialist for further management (13).
  - Anterior segment complications:
  - DES: lubrication, punctal occlusion, autologous serum.
  - Neurotrophic ulceration: autologous serum, conjunctival flap, amniotic membrane transplant, tarsorrhaphy.
  - Keratouveitis/Interstitial keratitis: Topical steroid therapy (7).
  - Pseudodendritiform keratitis (mucous plaque keratitis): Lubrication and off label use of topical antiviral ointment (acyclovir, vidarabine, or ganciclovir) has demonstrated potential benefit (10).
  - ARN/PORN: Intravitreal and intravenous antiviral therapy. Seek retina consult immediately.

SURGERY/OTHER PROCEDURES

- Tarsorrhaphy: Neurotrophic ulceration not responsive to lubrication.
- Corneal glue: Perforations 1 mm or less in diameter.
- Amniotic membrane transplant/Gunderson flap: Neurotrophic ulceration and thinning.
- Penetrating keratoplasty (PK): Visually significant scarring or ulceration not responsive to tarsorrhaphy alone (7).

ALERT

Tarsorrhaphy should be strongly considered in patients undergoing PK.

IN-PATIENT CONSIDERATIONS

Admission Criteria

- Pediatric patients requiring intravenous antiviral therapy
- Elderly patients unable to self-administer oral medications or those with zoster in multiple dermatomes
- Patients with severe immune compromise at risk for disseminated disease

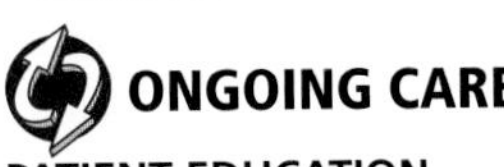

ONGOING CARE

PATIENT EDUCATION

Immunization with varicella zoster vaccine is recommended after resolution of disease.

PROGNOSIS

New lesion formation in the primary dermatome frequently stops in 3–7 days in the healthy individual and the affected dermatome often heals within 2 weeks, but may not resolve for 4 to 6 weeks (1).

COMPLICATIONS

- Chronic disease occurs in 30% of patients over 60 and approaches 70% in patients older than 80 years (18)
- Ophthalmic complications include the following:
  - Stromal scarring
  - Cataract
  - Corneal perforation
  - Glaucoma
  - Neurotrophic ulceration
  - Secondary infectious keratitis
  - Necrotizing retinitis
  - Optic neuritis
- Systemic complications
  - PHN
  - Stroke (19)

REFERENCES

1. Liesegang TJ. Herpes zoster ophthalmicus: Natural history, risk factors, clinical presentation and morbidity. *Ophthalmology* 2008;115:S3–S12.
2. Lewis GW. Zoster sine herpete. *Br Med J* 2958;2: 418–421.
3. Ragozzino MW. Population based study of herpes zoster and its sequelae. *Medicine* 1982;61: 310–316.
4. Cohen PR, Grossman ME. Clinical features of HIV-associated disseminated HZV infection—A review of literature. *Clin Exp Dermatol* 1989;14: 273–276.
5. Harpaz R, Ortega-Sanchez IR, Seward JF. Advisory Committee of Immunization Practices (ACIP) Centers for Disease Control and Prevention. Prevention if herpes zoster: recommendations of the Advisory Committee of Immunization Practices (ACIP). [published correction appears in *MMWR Recomm Rep*. 2008;57(28):779; *MMWR Recomm Rep* 2008;57(RR-5):1–30; http://www.cdc.gov/mmwr/preview/mmwrhtml/rr5705a1.htm. Accessed July 10, 2010.
6. Burke BL. Immune response to varicella-zoster in the aged. *Arch Intern Med* 1982;142:291–293
7. Liesegang TJ. Corneal complications from herpes zoster ophthalmicus. *Ophthalmol* 1985;92: 316–324.
8. Yamada K. Cutaneous eruption with or without ocular complications in patients with herpes zoster involving the trigeminal nerve. *Graefes Arch Clin Exp Ophthalmol* 1990;228:1–4.
9. Cobo M. Observations on the natural history of herpes zoster ophthalmicus. *Curr Eye Res* 1987;6:195–199.
10. Pavan-Langston D. Delayed herpes zoster pseudodendrites. PCR detection of viral DNA and a role for antiviral therapy. *Arch Ophthalmol* 1995;13:1381–1385.
11. Marsh RJ. Extraocular motor palsies in ophthalmic zoster: a review. *Br J Ophthalmol* 1977;61: 677–682.
12. Kattah JC, Kennerdel JS. Orbital apex syndrome secondary to herpes zoster ophthalmicus. *Am J Ophthalmol* 1978;85:378–382.
13. Pavan-Langston D. Herpes zoster: Antivirals and pain management. *Ophthalmol* 2008;115: S13–S20.
14. Starrou P. Detection of varicella zoster virus DNA in ocular samples from patients with uvietis but no cutaneous eruption. *Eye* 1994;8:684–687.
15. Gilden DH. Varicella zoster virus reactivation without rash. *J Infect Dis* 1992;166:S30–S34.
16. http://dailymed.nlm.nih.gov/dailymed/archives/fdaDrugInfo.cfm?archiveid=13284. Accessed 7/26/10.
17. Gnann JW Jr, et al. Acyclovir with and without prednisone for the treatment of herpes zoster. A randomized, placebo-controlled trial. The National Institute of Allergy and Infectious Diseases Collaborative Antiviral Study Group. *Ann Intern Med* 1996;125:376–383.
18. Harding SP. Management of ophthalmic zoster. *J Med Virol* 1993;S 97–101.
19. Lin HC. Herpes zoster ophthalmicus and the risk of stroke: A population-based follow-up study. *Neurology* 2010;74:792–797.

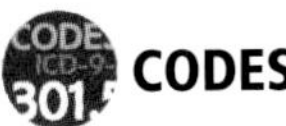

CODES

ICD9

- 053.21 Herpes zoster keratoconjunctivitis
- 053.22 Herpes zoster iridocyclitis
- 053.29 Herpes zoster with other ophthalmic complications

CLINICAL PEARLS

- Recognition and prompt treatment of HZO is necessary to reduce the incidence of complications.
- HZO can have a chronic and complicated course and therefore requires frequent follow-up.
- Herpes zoster vaccination should be recommended to all individuals meeting immunization criteria.

HIV/AIDS-RELATED RETINOPATHIES

Brad Ballard
Mark L. Nelson

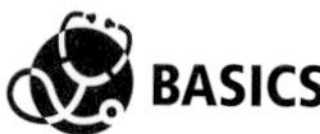

BASICS

DESCRIPTION

- HIV retinopathy and CMV retinitis are by far the most common ocular manifestations of HIV.
- Cytomegalovirus (CMV) retinitis is the most important AIDS-associated illness to affect the eyes. It is a full thickness retinal infection that can lead to necrosis and to retinal tears and detachments.
- Other ocular manifestations of HIV infection include HIV retinopathy, various opportunistic infections including toxoplasmosis, syphilis, pneumocystis carinii, cryptococcus, and herpes-family virus infections, especially CMV retinitis and progressive outer retinal necrosis. Kaposi Sarcoma, intraocular lymphoma, and conjunctival squamous cell carcinoma also occur.

Pediatric Considerations

Congenital CMV infection can cause significant neurological and developmental abnormalities.

Pregnancy Considerations

Mothers with CMV primary infections can pass the virus on to fetus transplacentally causing congenital CMV infection.

EPIDEMIOLOGY

Incidence

In the pre-HAART era, CMV retinitis had a cumulative lifetime incidence of 25–40%. The incidence has decreased considerably in recent years.

Prevalence

- HIV retinopathy occurs in 50–60% of patients infected with HIV.
- Historically, CMV retinitis occurred in up to 40% of patients with HIV and is an AIDS-defining illness; however, it is much less common in the HAART era.

RISK FACTORS

The main risk factor for development of CMV retinitis is a low CD4 count, typically below 50.

GENERAL PREVENTION

HAART therapy has shown great benefit for reduction in CMV retinitis, as it often maintains a CD4 count above 50.

PATHOPHYSIOLOGY

- CMV reaches the retina hematogenously. It then infects the retinal vascular endothelium.
- On histopathology, infected cells show pathognomonic cytomegalic inclusions with large eosinophilic intracellular bodies.
- Electron microscopy can show CMV particles within infected cells.
- Histopathology shows full thickness retinal necrosis, coagulative vasculitis, and choroiditis.

ETIOLOGY

- Cytomegalovirus (CMV) is a member of the herpes virus family.
- There is a high prevalence of CMV antibodies in the general population and most people are thought to have been infected at one time or another.
- In healthy people, CMV infection may manifest as a mild mono-like illness, or may be asymptomatic.

COMMONLY ASSOCIATED CONDITIONS

- Although CMV retinitis occurs most commonly in patients with AIDS, it can also occur in severely immunocompromised individuals, such as those receiving chemotherapy.
- Before HAART, a diagnosis of CMV retinitis was associated with a median survival time of 6 months.

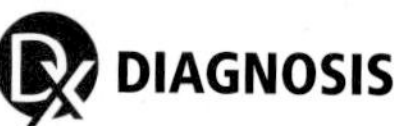

DIAGNOSIS

HISTORY

- Patients may present with decreased visual acuity, flashing lights (photopsias), or blind spots (scotomata).
- One study found that 54% were asymptomatic.

PHYSICAL EXAM

- Physical exam shows yellow–white areas of retinal necrosis with some retinal hemorrhages that often start in the periphery and follow the vasculature centripetally.
- There may also be hard exudates, and mottling of the retinal pigment epithelium.
- Each lesion is most active at the borders.
- As most patients are severely immunocompromised, there is usually minimal vitreitis.
- Very early CMV may resemble cotton wool spots, but with lesions larger than 750 μm, CMV must be considered.
- Funduscopy may show a granular pattern, a fulminant/hemorrhagic appearance, or "frosted branch" angiitis.

DIAGNOSTIC TESTS & INTERPRETATION

Lab

- CD4 count and viral load are important lab tests to follow. It is not necessary to draw CMV blood serology as CMV has a high prevalence in the population.
- Aqueous sampling with PCR analysis can be used to identify CMV DNA.

Imaging

- Serial fundus photographs are helpful to document progression of disease.
- Fluorescein angiography is not usually helpful in diagnosis.

DIFFERENTIAL DIAGNOSIS

The differential diagnosis includes cotton wool spots from other causes, herpetic retinitis syndrome such as ARN and PORN, and toxoplasmosis.

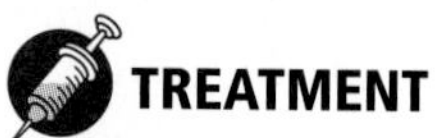

TREATMENT

MEDICATION

First Line

- In all FDA approved treatments of CMV retinitis, there is an initial period of high-dose antiviral induction followed by continuous maintenance. Initially, oral valganciclovir (the oral pro-drug of ganciclovir) 900 mg b.i.d for 21 days of induction followed by 900 mg q day for maintenance therapy can be used. The major side effect of valganciclovir/ganciclovir is bone marrow suppression.
  – However, in eyes with macula threatening disease, IV ganciclovir should still be considered.
- IV ganciclovir can be administered 5 mg/kg IV b.i.d for 2 weeks followed by 5 mg/kg IV for maintenance therapy. The major toxicity of ganciclovir is myelosuppression. Granulocyte-macrophage colony stimulating factor should be used concomitantly to avoid myelosuppression.
- Oral ganciclovir can be used as maintenance therapy, but recurrence is more frequent than with valganciclovir or IV ganciclovir, and the fellow eye is at greater risk of developing CMV retinitis.

- IV foscarnet at 90 mg/kg b.i.d for 2 weeks followed by 90–120 mg/kg daily for maintenance is another option. The principle toxicity of foscarnet is renal dysfunction, electrolyte abnormalities, and possibly seizures.
- Institution of HAART therapy is critical. It has raised the survival time from 0.65 years to >1 year, it has reduced the odds of CMV progression, and the number of new CMV cases has declined.
- Maintenance therapy may be discontinued in patients with CD4 >100 cells/μL who show no signs of progression AND who are on HAART.

Second Line

- Intravitreal administration of ganciclovir 200 μg–2 mg weekly and foscarnet 2.4 mg weekly. Induction with intravitreal injections is twice a week for 2–3 weeks. Intravitreal injection to one eye obviously does not protect the other eye from developing CMV retinitis.
- A ganciclovir intravitreal implant (Vitrasert) may be considered in patients who do not tolerate systemic treatment, but it does not provide systemic protection against CMV nor does it protect the other eye from CMV. It typically lasts 2 years if CMV resistance to ganciclovir does not develop.
- The risks of intravitreal injections include cataract, vitreous hemorrhage, retinal detachment, and infectious endophthalmitis.
- IV cidofovir at 5 mg/kg weekly for 2 weeks, then 5 mg/kg every other week for maintenance. Cidofovir may cause hypotony and anterior uveitis.

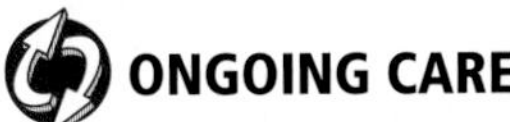

ONGOING CARE

FOLLOW-UP RECOMMENDATIONS

Patients should be followed closely, especially if they have discontinued therapy as CMV retinitis has a high recurrence rate in patients with a CD4 count <100.

PROGNOSIS

- The prognosis was almost uniformly fatal prior to the advent of HAART.
- Now it carries a much better prognosis, but even with HAART, and anti-CMV therapy, mortality is still increased after CMV retinitis develops.

COMPLICATIONS

- Immune Recovery Uveitis (IRU) is a potential complication of recovery from low CD4 counts. Patients who had CMV retinitis, who then have reconstitution of their immune system, may develop anterior or intermediate uveitis, cystoid macular edema, and epiretinal membranes. Patients complain of vision loss, pain, photophobia, and floaters.
- Other complications of IRU include posterior subcapsular cataracts, proliferative vitreoretinopathy, and optic nerve neovascularization.
- CMV retinitis can cause retinal detachments. Regular monitoring is needed.

ADDITIONAL READING

- Martin DF, Sierra-Madero J, Walmsley S, et al; Valganciclovir Study Group. A controlled trial of valganciclovir as induction therapy for cytomegalovirus retinitis. *N Engl J Med*. 2002;346(15):1119–1126. Erratum in: *N Engl J Med* 2002;347(11):862.
- Goldberg DE, Smithen LM, Angelilli A, et al. HIV-associated retinopathy in the HAART Era. *Retina* 2005;25(5):633–649.
- Thorne JE, Jabs DA, Kempen JH, et al; Studies of Ocular Complications of AIDS Research Group. Incidence of and risk factors for visual acuity loss among patients with AIDS and cytomegalovirus retinitis in the era of highly active antiretroviral therapy. *Ophthalmology* 2006 Aug;113 (8):1432–1440.
- Holland GN. AIDS and Ophthalmology: The first quarter century. *Am J Ophthalmol* 2008;145(3): 397–408.
- Musch DC, Martin DF, Gordon JF, et al. Treatment of cytomegalovirus retinitis with a sustained-release ganciclovir implant. The Ganciclovir Implant Study Group. *N Engl J Med*. 1997;337(2):83–90.

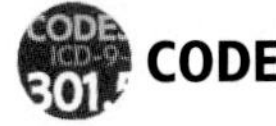

CODES

ICD9

- 078.5 Cytomegaloviral disease
- 363.20 Chorioretinitis, unspecified

CLINICAL PEARLS

- After HIV retinopathy, CMV retinitis is the most common ocular manifestation of AIDS. It is an AIDS defining illness.
- Patients may be asymptomatic or may have vision loss, floaters, flashes, or blind spots. Retinal findings of vascular angiitis, yellow–white retinitis with a granular appearance, and hemorrhage can be seen.
- Treatment is usually started with oral valganciclovir and HAART treatment is necessary to achieve any lasting remission.
- Prognosis is improved since HAART, but is still poor.

HOMOCYSTINURIA

Douglas M. Wisner

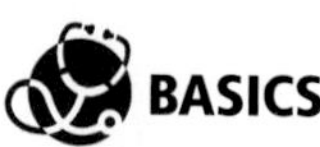

BASICS

DESCRIPTION

- Homocystinuria compromises a group of inborn errors of methionine metabolism that result in elevated levels of homocysteine in the urine (homocystinuria) and blood (homocysteinemia).
- Cystathione β-synthetase deficiency (classic homocystinuria) is the most common cause and is discussed here.
- Other defects leading to elevated levels of plasma and urine homocysteine include defects in methylcobalamin formation and methylenetetrahydrofolate reductase deficiency.
- Signs and symptoms of classic homocystinuria are systemic, primarily involving the ocular, nervous, cutaneous, skeletal, and hematologic systems.
- Ocular involvement is marked by progressive myopia (nearsightedness) and ectopia lentis (dislocation of the native lens).

EPIDEMIOLOGY

Incidence

- Varies by region; the highest incidence in the world, a ratio of about 1:3000 live births, is found in Qatar. Other nations with high incidence include Norway (1:6400), Germany (1:17,800), and Ireland (1:65,000).
- General incidence is estimated to be 1:200,000 to 1:300,000 live births.

RISK FACTORS

Genetics

- Classic homocystinuria is autosomal recessive.
- The gene for cystathionine β-synthetase is located on chromosome 21q22.3.
- Patients typically harbor 2 different mutations in the gene for cystathionine β-synthetase (i.e., compound heterozygotes).
- Varying disease manifestations are felt to be related to the particular mutations inherited.

GENERAL PREVENTION

- Newborn screening
  - Not available in all states
  - Tests for methionine levels
    - High false-negative rates secondary to normal neonatal levels during the first few days of life
- Genetic counseling

PATHOPHYSIOLOGY

- Progressive lenticular myopia and eventual ectopia lentis
- Acute glaucoma secondary to pupillary block
- Thromboembolism secondary to increased vascular endothelial adhesiveness and platelet activation

ETIOLOGY

- Incompetence and disruption of the zonular fibers
- Ischemia to brain and vital organs

COMMONLY ASSOCIATED CONDITIONS

- Developmental delay (common)
- Thromboembolic disease (common)

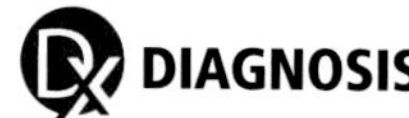

DIAGNOSIS

HISTORY

- Birth history
  - Neonatal screening performed?
- Development
  - Speech delay
  - Mental retardation
  - Behavioral/psychiatric disturbances
- Family history
  - Consanguinity
  - Thromboembolic death at an early age
- Ocular history
  - Poor vision
  - Profound nearsightedness (reading material held very close to face)
  - Eye pain

PHYSICAL EXAM

- General
  - Poor speech/interaction for age
  - Marfanoid habitus
  - Scoliosis
  - Pectus excavatum or carinatum
  - Genu valgum
  - Pes cavus
  - High arched palate
  - Dental crowding
  - Malar flush
  - Generalized osteoporosis
- Ocular
  - Thick glasses/progressive and severe myopia
  - Increased intraocular pressure
  - Red eye
  - Ectopia lentis with disrupted zonular fibers
    - Usually after age 2
  - Cataract
  - Retinal detachment
  - Optic atrophy
  - Staphyloma

DIAGNOSTIC TESTS & INTERPRETATION

Lab

- Classic homocystinuria is a clinical diagnosis affirmed by laboratory and genetic testing.
- Laboratory testing reveals elevated levels of plasma methionine and plasma homocysteine.
- Urinary levels of homocysteine are elevated. This should be a freshly voided specimen as the compound is unstable.
- Pyridoxine (B_6) challenge differentiates B_6 responders from nonresponders and dictates treatment.
  - 100 mg pyridoxine PO $\times$ 1.
  - Plasma amino acids measured in 24 hours.
  - A reduction of 30% or more in plasma homocystine and/or plasma methionine concentration suggests B_6 responsiveness.
    - If no significant change occurs, 200 mg pyridoxine PO $\times$ 1, then reassess as above.
    - If still no change has occurred, 500 mg of pyridoxine is given in a child or adult.
  - If plasma homocystine and methionine concentrations are not significantly decreased after the last dose of pyridoxine, it is concluded that the individual is B_6-nonresponsive.
    - Note: Infants should not receive more than 300 mg of pyridoxine. This can lead to ventilator-dependent respiratory failure.

Imaging

- MRI with stroke protocol if any suggestion of focal CNS lesion on examination.
- DEXA scan for osteoporosis monitoring.

Diagnostic Procedures/Other

- Prenatal diagnosis possible with amniocentesis.
- Molecular genetic testing is available to isolate the genetic mutations.
- Liver biopsy can be used to assay for cystathionine β-synthetase.

Pathological Findings

- Disrupted zonular fibers (as opposed to Marfan syndrome where fibers tend to be stretched).
- Ectopia lentis in homocystinuria can occur in any direction (contrary to classical teaching).

DIFFERENTIAL DIAGNOSIS
- Trauma
- Isolated ocular disease
  - Buphthalmos
  - Aniridia
  - Ectopia lentis et pupillae
  - Familial ectopia lentis
  - Persistent hyperplasia of the primary vitreous/persistent fetal vasculature
  - Coloboma
- Infectious
  - Syphilis
- Metabolic/syndromic
  - Marfan syndrome
  - Weill–Marchesani syndrome
  - Sulfite oxidase deficiency
  - Xanthine oxidase deficiency
  - Molybdenum cofactor deficiency
  - Hyperlysinemia
  - Methylenetetrahydrofolate reductase deficiency

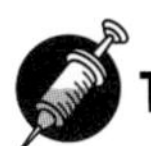

TREATMENT

MEDICATION
- B_6/pyridoxine
  - 200–1000 mg/24 hr B_6
  - 1–5 mg/24 hr pyridoxine
    - Drives methionine metabolism forward
    - Patients with some residual enzyme activity (40% of affected) will respond.
- B_{12} supplementation
- Betaine (1)[C]
  - 200–250 mg/kg/day
  - Remethylates homocysteine to methionine

ADDITIONAL TREATMENT

General Measures
- Address refractive error with glasses or contact lens.
- Treat amblyopia, which can result from anisometropia.
- Hydration to prevent thromboembolism.

SURGERY/OTHER PROCEDURES
- Patients are at extremely high risk of intraoperative stroke and thrombosis.
- Urgent lens extraction for acute glaucoma caused by ectopia lentis
- Elective lens extraction for extreme myopia or to prevent acute glaucoma
  - Accomplished via pars plana lensectomy with successful long-term outcome (2)[C].
- Thrombolysis for acute stroke

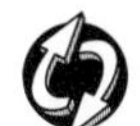

ONGOING CARE

FOLLOW-UP RECOMMENDATIONS
- Pediatric ophthalmologist
- Contact lens specialist (if aphakic)
- Pediatric metabolic disease specialist
- Hematology evaluation

Patient Monitoring
- Special intraoperative antithrombotic measures are indicated if patients require a surgical procedure (3)[C].
- See "Follow-up" section.

DIET
Methionine-restricted diet.

PATIENT EDUCATION
- Genetics Home Reference: Homocystinuria (http://ghr.nlm.nih.gov/condition=homocystinuria)

PROGNOSIS
- Usually limited lifespan (thromboembolism) and intelligence.
- If B_6 therapy instituted at an early age in a responsive patient, developmental delay and ectopia lentis can be prevented (4)[C].

COMPLICATIONS
- Visual loss
- Death (thromboembolism)
- Fractures (osteoporosis)

REFERENCES

1. Lawson-Yuen A, Levy HL. The use of betaine in the treatment of elevated homocysteine. *Mol Genet Metab* 2006;88(3):201–207.
2. Wu-Chen W, Letson R, Summers C. Functional and structural outcomes following lensectomy for ectopia lentis. *J Am Assoc Pediatric Ophthal Strabismus* 2005;9(4):353–357.
3. Lowe S, Johnson D, Tobias J. Anesthetic implications of the child with homocystinuria. *J Clin Anesth* 1994;6(2):142–144.
4. Burke JP, O'Keefe M, Bowell R, Naughten ER. Ocular complications in homocystinuria–early and late treated. *Br J Ophthalmol* 1989;73:427–431.

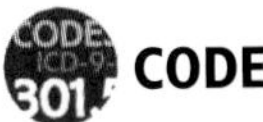

CODES

ICD9
- 270.4 Disturbances of sulphur-bearing amino-acid metabolism
- 367.1 Myopia
- 743.37 Congenital ectopic lens

CLINICAL PEARLS
- Newborn screening currently has high false-negative rates.
- Early treatment can reduce long-term complications.
- Patients are at extremely high risk of intraoperative stroke and thrombosis.
- Parents of patients with classic homocystinuria are at increased risk for thromboembolism as heterozygotes.

HORNER SYNDROME

Deepak P. Grover
Ann P. Murchison
Jurij R. Bilyk

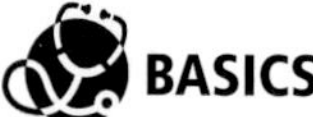

BASICS

DESCRIPTION

- Horner syndrome (HS) refers to the clinical triad of ptosis, miosis, and at times anhydrosis, which results from an interruption in the oculosympathetic pathway.
- May have iris heterochromia if congenital.
- Transient conjunctival hyperemia
- Congenital or acquired.

EPIDEMIOLOGY

Incidence

- Pediatric HS: 1.42 per 100,000 patients.
- Acquired adult HS: Unknown.

Prevalence

- Congenital HS: 1 in 6,250 births.
- Acquired adult HS: Unknown.

RISK FACTORS

- Head and neck trauma
- Brainstem or cervical spine pathology
- Neck or lung apex pathology, including benign tumors, malignancy, and inflammation

Genetics

A rare genetic form is likely an autosomal dominant trait. The vast majority of HS is sporadic and acquired from a localized abnormality.

GENERAL PREVENTION

None

PATHOPHYSIOLOGY

- First-order central sympathetic fibers descend from the hypothalamus through the midbrain and pons, and terminate in the intermediolateral cell column of the spinal cord (ciliospinal center of Budge) at the level of C8-T2.
- Second-order preganglionic sympathetic fibers exit the spinal cord at the level of T1, enter the cervical sympathetic chain near the pulmonary apex and the subclavian artery, then travel up the sympathetic chain and synapse in the superior cervical ganglion at the level of the bifurcation of the common carotid artery (C3–C4).
- Third-order postganglionic fibers exit the superior cervical ganglion, ascend along the internal carotid artery and enter the orbit through the optic canal and cavernous sinus/superior orbital fissure. Intraorbitally, the fibers travel with sensory nerves and arteries to innervate the iris dilator and Müller muscle.

ETIOLOGY

- First-order neuron lesions: Intracranial or cervical spine pathology.
- Second-order neuron lesions: Lung apex and neck to level of carotid bifurcation.
- Third-order neuron lesions: Carotid bifurcation to cavernous sinus.
- N.B.: Although migraine and cluster headaches may rarely present as HS, carotid dissection must be ruled out in any patient presenting with pain (including headache).
- N.B.: Cavernous sinus lesions rarely present as an *isolated* HS. Typically cranial neuropathy (e.g., abducens nerve palsy) is also present.
- N.B.: Orbital lesions *never* cause an isolated HS.

COMMONLY ASSOCIATED CONDITIONS

See Table 1 in "Online Resources".

DIAGNOSIS

HISTORY

- By far, the most frequent complaint is new onset, unilateral ptosis.
- Patients rarely complain of visual problems secondary to miosis.
- Transient redness of the affected eye.
- Forehead anhydrosis is an infrequent complaint.
- Duration of symptoms is important to elicit.
- The most important symptom to obtain from the patient is the presence of any head, periorbital, or neck pain (sometimes described by the patient as a dull ache).
- Additional history may be obtained on directed questions
- Associated neurologic symptoms:
  - Hemisensory loss
  - Dysarthria
  - Dysphagia
  - Ataxia
  - Vertigo
  - Nystagmus
- Recent or distant head, neck, or chest trauma, including surgery.
- Any history of respiratory disease, including smoking.
- Any history of cancer.

PHYSICAL EXAM

- 1–3 mm of upper eyelid ptosis secondary to Müller muscle paresis
- Reverse ptosis (slight elevation) of the lower lid secondary to denervation of the inferior tarsal muscle. This finding is not always present, but is highly specific.
- Miosis
- Anisocoria that increases in the dark. Dilation lag is usually present (the affected pupil dilates slowly in a dark room).
- Anhydrosis is variable and difficult to test.
- Conjunctival hyperemia may be noted in the first 2 weeks of onset, but is usually a transient phenomenon.
- Iris heterochromia (hypopigmented iris) can be seen in congenital HS or in acquired pediatric HS (within a few months of birth).

DIAGNOSTIC TESTS & INTERPRETATION

Lab

Initial lab tests

- Initial lab studies are not necessary in the diagnosis of the HS.
- Lab tests may be considered depending on localization and suspected etiology:
  - ACE and PPD placement if chest imaging is abnormal.
  - Urine test (vanillylmandelic acid [VMA], homovanillic acid [HVA]) to rule out neuroblastoma in pediatric HS.

Follow-up & special considerations

Inspect old photographs for evidence of HS.

Imaging

Initial approach

- Correct imaging is critical in the management of HS.
- In many cases of HS, the history will provide important clues as to the etiology of the HS.
- Any acute HS (<4 weeks) presenting with head/neck pain or discomfort requires urgent imaging to rule carotid artery dissection.
- As a rule, the work-up of HS necessitates imaging from the level of the cavernous sinus (skull base) to the lung apex. Note that imaging of the brain above the skull base, as is usually done in routine brain CT and MRI, is unnecessary and inadequate.
- A combination of conventional imaging and angiography of the head and neck is recommended (MRI/MRA or CT/CTA).
- Extracranial Doppler ultrasonography is unreliable for diagnosing carotid artery dissection of the skull base.
- Chest CT or MRI to rule out apical lung mass.
- MRI of the thorax and abdomen to rule out neuroblastoma in children.
- Conventional arteriography is usually unnecessary (unless stenting of the carotid artery dissection is recommended in rare cases) and is contraindicated as a first imaging modality.

Follow-up & special considerations

- Multiple pharmacologic tests (cocaine, hydroxyamphetamine, phenylephrine, apraclonidine) are available for the diagnosis of HS. Note that many cannot be performed on the same day. The clinician should therefore carefully choose the test best suited for the patient. (See Table 2 in "Online Resources")
- In general, cocaine and apraclonidine are the most useful and most frequently used agents.
  - Should not be used in infants younger than 6 months without cardiopulmonary monitoring. Apraclonidine may cause lethargy, bradycardia, and respiratory depression in infants.
- Hydroxyamphetamine and dilute phenylephrine testing are impractical and usually unnecessary.

DIFFERENTIAL DIAGNOSIS

- Involutional ptosis with physiologic anisocoria. Both conditions are common and may coexist. In physiologic anisocoria, the amount of anisocoria will not change in bright and dim lighting, distinguishing it from that seen in HS.
- Cranial nerve III palsy. An incomplete CN-III paresis may present with ptosis. If anisocoria is present, the affected pupil is larger than the normal side.
- Holmes-Adie tonic pupil. The affected pupil is larger.
- Use of ipsilateral miotic (e.g., pilocarpine) or contralateral mydriatic agent
- Iris sphincter muscle damage (usually causes mild mydriasis). The most common cause is cataract surgery.

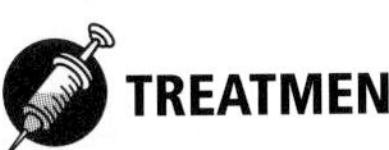

TREATMENT

MEDICATION

- Dependent upon the specific etiology.
- Carotid artery dissection.
  - Antiplatelet or anticoagulant agents.
- Neuroblastoma
- Antineoplastic agents if secondary to neoplasia.
- Anti-inflammatory or anti-metabolite agents if inflammatory (e.g., sarcoidosis).

Geriatric Considerations

Cautionary use of topical cocaine and hydroxyamphetamine in elderly and in patients who may undergo urine testing in their occupation.

Pediatric Considerations

Cautionary use of topical cocaine, hydroxyamphetamine, or apraclonidine in infants or children.

Pregnancy Considerations

- Cocaine, hydroxyamphetamine, and apraclonidine are Class C agents.
- Cocaine and apraclonidine testing is contraindicated if breastfeeding due to high risk of significant adverse effects to infant/breast milk production.
- Caution is advised for topical hydroxyamphetamine during lactation.

ADDITIONAL TREATMENT

Issues for Referral

- Neurologic consultation for CVA, mass, meningitis, or medical management for carotid artery dissection
- Interventional radiology, vascular surgery, and/or neurosurgical consultation for carotid artery dissection or aneurysm for possible angioplasty and carotid artery stenting
- Oncology or infectious disease consultation for neoplastic or infectious etiology
- Pediatric oncology consultation for neuroblastoma
- Pulmonology consultation for management of sarcoidosis or lung mass.
- Oculoplastic consultation for ptosis repair

SURGERY/OTHER PROCEDURES

- Dependent upon specific etiology.
- Miosis is asymptomatic and does not require medical or surgical intervention.
- Eyelid repair
  - Conjunctivomullerectomy for ptosis repair

IN-PATIENT CONSIDERATIONS

Dependent upon etiology.

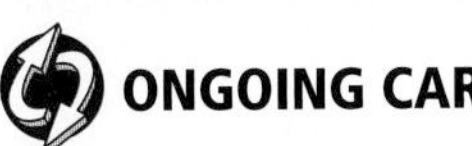

ONGOING CARE

FOLLOW-UP RECOMMENDATIONS

Dependent upon etiology

DIET

Nutrition for children with neuroblastoma is important during therapy for adequate caloric intake for growth and development.

ADDITIONAL READING

- Almog Y, Gepstein R, Kesler A. Diagnostic value of imaging in Horner syndrome in adults. *J Neuroophthalmol* 2010;30(1):7–11.
- Chen PL, Chen JT, Lu DW, et al. Comparing efficacies of 0.5% apraclonidine with 4% cocaine in the diagnosis of Horner syndrome in pediatric patients. *J Ocul Pharmacol Ther* 2006;22(3):182–187.
- Smith SJ, Diehl N, Leavitt JA, et al. Incidence of pediatric Horner syndrome and the risk of neuroblastoma: A population-based study. *Arch Ophthalmol* 2010;128(3):324–329.
- Arnold M, Baumgartner RW, Stapf C, et al. Ultrasound diagnosis of spontaneous carotid dissection with isolated Horner syndrome. *Stroke* 2008;39(1):82–86.
- Mughal M, Longmuir R. Current pharmacologic testing for Horner syndrome. *Curr Neurol Neurosci Rep* 2009;9(5):384–389.
- Kadkhodayan Y, Jeck DT, Moran CJ, et al. Angioplasty and stenting in carotid dissection with or without associated pseudoaneurysm. *AJNR Am J Neuroradiol* 2005;26(9):2328–2335.
- Trobe JD. The evaluation of Horner syndrome. *J Neuroophthalmol* 2010;30(1):1–2.
- Koc F, Kavuncu S, Kansu T, et al. The sensitivity and specificity of 0.5% apraclonidine in the diagnosis of oculosympathetic paresis. *Br J Ophthalmol* 2005; 89:1442–1444.
- Biousse V, D'Anglejan-Chatillon J, Touboul PJ, et al. Time course of symptoms in extracranial carotid artery dissections. A series of 80 patients. *Stroke* 1995;26:235–239.
- Glatt HJ, Putterman AM, Fett DR. Müller's muscle-conjunctival resection procedure in the treatment of ptosis in Horner's syndrome. *Ophthalmic Surg* 1990;21(2):93–96.

CODES

ICD9

- 337.09 Other idiopathic peripheral autonomic neuropathy
- 374.31 Ptosis of eyelid, paralytic
- 379.42 Miosis (persistent), not due to miotics

CLINICAL PEARLS

- HS in the presence of ipsilateral head, facial, or neck pain or discomfort requires urgent and correctly ordered imaging to rule out a carotid artery or vertebral artery dissection: CT/CTA or MRI/MRA of the head and neck.
- Imaging of the lung apex should be performed if other imaging is normal, but is not urgent.
- The anisocoria of HS is greater in dim light.
- "Reverse ptosis" of the lower lid is a helpful finding in the diagnosis of HS.
- Horner syndrome may be the first manifestation of neuroblastoma in the pediatric age group.
- Cocaine and apraclonidine are the most useful agents for pharmacologic testing of HS.
- Cocaine and apraclonidine should be used with caution in children younger than 6 months.

HYPERTENSIVE RETINOPATHY

Julie M. Rosenthal
Sunir Garg

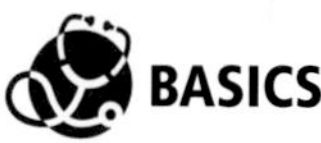

BASICS

DESCRIPTION

Systemic hypertension leads to characteristic changes in the retina, choroid, and optic nerve. It can be divided into acute and chronic findings

Pregnancy Considerations

In women of child-bearing age with uncontrolled hypertension, check pregnancy status as these patients may have eclampsia/pre-eclampsia.

EPIDEMIOLOGY

Incidence

- 6.0% of patients in Beaver Dam Eye Study developed hypertensive retinopathy (1).
  - Arterial narrowing was seen in 9.9% of patients.
  - AV nicking was observed in 6.5% of patients (1).

Prevalence

- Occurs in 2–15% of people older than 40 years of age.
- Greater in African American than Caucasian population.
- No reliable association with age or gender (2).

RISK FACTORS

- Elevated systolic and diastolic blood pressure.
- Diabetes.

Genetics

There are likely multiple genetic factors that play a role in the development of hypertension.

GENERAL PREVENTION

- Maintenance of normotensive blood pressure.
- Antihypertensive medication.
- Regular blood pressure monitoring.

PATHOPHYSIOLOGY

- As blood pressure rises, retinal blood vessels undergo vasoconstriction.
- Over time, the blood vessel walls thicken.
- The blood–retinal barrier becomes compromised, leading to exudation and ischemia.

ETIOLOGY

- Essential hypertension
- Hypertension secondary to eclampsia, renal artery stenosis, and other systemic conditions

COMMONLY ASSOCIATED CONDITIONS

- Diabetes
- Hyperlipidemia
- Atherosclerosis
- Retinal artery macroaneurysm
- Branch vein or artery occlusion
- Stroke
- Cognitive decline
- Possible increased risk of coronary artery disease
- Age-related macular degeneration—possible link
- Glaucoma—possible link

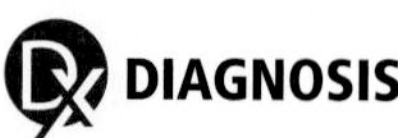

DIAGNOSIS

HISTORY

- May or may not have diagnosis of hypertension/ elevated blood pressure.
- Many will have no history of eye disease.

PHYSICAL EXAM

- Findings from acute, accelerated or malignant, hypertension
  - Fibrinoid necrosis of choroid/retinal pigment epithelium causes a deep, yellow - gray whitening in the acute phase
  - Later these areas become hyperpigmented and are called Elschnig spots. Hyperpigmented flecks that are arranged in a linear fashion (following areas of choroidal infarction) are called Siegrist streaks.
  - Optic disc edema—this can result from ischemia to the optic nerve to intracranial hypertension. must be present for diagnosis of malignant hypertension.
  - Retinal hemorrhages, which may be ranging from mild intraretinal hemorrhages to severe subinternal limiting mimbane or subretinal hemorrhage
  - Cotton wool spots
  - Serous retinal detachment (4).
- Findings from chronic hypertension.
  - Arteriolar narrowing—decreased artery to vein ratio (normal is 2:3).
  - Copper wiring—light reflex widens and the vessel takes on the appearance of copper wire.
  - Silver wiring occurs when the vessel becomes so narrow that blood flow through the artery is not visible on ophthalmoscopy.
  - Arterior–venous nicking occurs when the artery compresses the vein in their common adventitial sheath (Gunn sign).
  - Vein may be deflected as it crosses the arteriole (Salus sign).
  - Microaneurysms

DIAGNOSTIC TESTS & INTERPRETATION

Lab

Initial lab tests

Blood pressure measurement.

Follow-up & special considerations

In patients with diabetes, controlling blood pressure decreases the risk of progression of retinopathy (3).

Imaging

Initial approach

- None needed unless secondary cause of blood pressure elevation is suspected.
- Fluorescein angiography may demonstrate microaneurysms, retinal telangiectasias, retinal/choroidal ischemia, and diffuse capillary and/or optic nerve leakage.

Follow-up & special considerations

- Close monitoring of both systolic and diastolic blood pressure is essential.
- Many acute changes may resolve with treatment of blood pressure.

Pathological Findings

- The Scheie classification of hypertensive retinopathy is the following:
  - Grade 0: Normal fundus
  - Grade 1: Mild arteriolar narrowing
  - Grade 2: Obvious arteriolar narrowing with focal vessel irregularity
  - Grade 3: Grade 2 with exudates or hemorrhages
  - Grade 4: Grade 3 with optic disc edema

DIFFERENTIAL DIAGNOSIS
- Diabetic retinopathy
- Radiation retinopathy
- Juxtafoveal telangiectasis
- Retinal artery occlusions
- Vasculitis (lupus, lyme disease, sarcoidosis)
- Giant cell arteritis

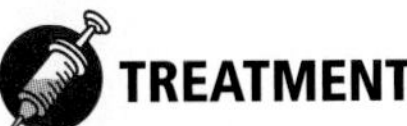

TREATMENT

MEDICATION

First Line
Oral antihypertensive medications.

Second Line
Intravenous antihypertensive medication.

ADDITIONAL TREATMENT

General Measures
Treatment should be initiated with direction from the primary care physician.

Issues for Referral
- All patients with suspected hypertensive retinopathy should be referred to their primary doctor for further workup and treatment.
- Patients with signs of malignant/acute hypertension may require emergency inpatient stabilization.

IN-PATIENT CONSIDERATIONS

Initial Stabilization
Blood pressure lowering medications (see earlier).

Admission Criteria
Hypertensive emergency/malignant hypertension (diastolic blood pressure >120, with end-organ damage, which includes optic disc edema.

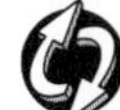

ONGOING CARE

FOLLOW-UP RECOMMENDATIONS
- Blood pressure should be closely monitored by the primary care doctor.
- Patients should undergo regular dilated fundus examination to rule out the above complications.

DIET
For salt-responsive patients, diets low in salt may aid in blood pressure lowering.

PATIENT EDUCATION
Inform patients of the need to maintain a normotensive blood pressure and to regularly take their blood pressure medications to reduce their risk of visual complications.

PROGNOSIS
Patients who maintain their blood pressures at a normotensive level, with drugs, diet or otherwise, usually maintain excellent vision.

COMPLICATIONS
- Retinal vein occlusion
- Retinal artery macroaneurysm (women > men)
- Retinal arterial occlusion
- Optic nerve ischemia/neuropathy

REFERENCES

1. Klein R, Klein BEK, Moss SE. The relation of systemic hypertension to changes in the retinal vasculature. *Trans Am Ophthalmol Soc* 1997;95:329–348.
2. Wong TY, Mitchell P. Hypertensive retinopathy. *N Engl J Med* 2004;351(22):2310–2317.
3. The UK Prospective Diabetes Study Group. Tight blood pressure control and risk of macrovascular and microvascular complications in type 2 diabetes: UKPDS 38. *Br Med J (Clin Res Ed)* 1998;317: 703–713.
4. Dellacroce JT, Vitale AT. Hypertension and the eye. *Curr Opin Ophthalmol* 2008;19(6):493–498.

ADDITIONAL READING

- Chobanian AV, Bakris GL, Black HR, et al. Seventh report of the joint national committee on prevention, detection, evaluation, and treatment of high blood pressure. *Hypertension* 2003;42:1206–1252.

CODES

ICD9
362.11 Hypertensive retinopathy

CLINICAL PEARLS
- Hypertensive retinopathy is a common finding in those with elevated blood pressure. It can be divided into chronic and acute changes.
- In young women with otherwise unexplained hypertensive retinopathy, consider pre-eclampsia as a cause and obtain an urine pregnancy screen.

H

HYPHEMA

Michael A. DellaVecchia

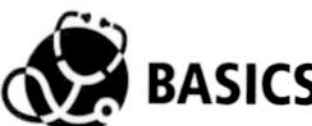

BASICS

DESCRIPTION
Blood in the anterior chamber (segment).

GENERAL PREVENTION
Safety eyewear protection

PATHOPHYSIOLOGY
Bleeding from the structures of the anterior segment of the eye; for example, an iris tear, iridodialysis, or cyclodialysis secondary to trauma and rarely from vascular abnormalities or bleeding diaphyses.

ETIOLOGY
Usually associated with trauma; including intraocular manual and laser surgery.

COMMONLY ASSOCIATED CONDITIONS
- Hematodyscrasias and coagulopathies (pathologic and pharmaceutic)
- Intraocular neoplasm and infections

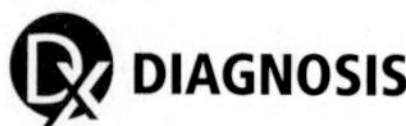

DIAGNOSIS

HISTORY
- When nonsurgical trauma is suspected, a definitive history of the mechanism should be acquired. This should include the description of the object, its momentum and direction, and the exact location of impact. For example: A fist of a large assailant with a side strike to the brow versus a forceful explosion with sharp shrapnel hitting the globe directly while not wearing spectacles
- Inquire about predisposing factors, such as anticoagulants or conditions that may cause a bleeding diathesis

PHYSICAL EXAM
- Rule out ruptured globe/ intraocular foreign body (IOFB)
- Take baseline examination: Va, IOP, Slit Lamp Exam (SLE), Dilated Fundus Exam (DFE)
- Clotted, layered, or suspended blood in the anterior chamber which is best visualized by slit-lamp examination

DIAGNOSTIC TESTS & INTERPRETATION

Lab
- Initial examination and testing is intended to assess the degree of visual compromise, possible additional ocular injury, and establish a baseline to monitor resolution or progression of the hyphema.
- Visual acuity (VA)
- Intraocular pressure (IOP)
- Measurement of clot, layer, or degree of suspended blood to monitor resolution or rebleeds
- Blood studies as indicated

Imaging

Initial approach

If a rupture globe or IOFB is suspected, direct visualization and/or imaging to include ultrasound (careful if there is possibly an open globe) and CT. MRI is contraindicated in cases of possible metallic IOFB's. Vegetable matter, such as wood, may be difficult to image.

Follow-up & special considerations

Direct at monitoring resolution of hyphema and avoidance of complications such as pressure rise, rebleeds, and corneal staining.

Diagnostic Procedures/Other
- B scan imaging if visualization is poor
- UBM if more detailed imaging of the anatomical angle is needed

Pathological Findings
Clotted, layered, or suspended blood in the anterior chamber, which is best visualized by slit-lamp examination.

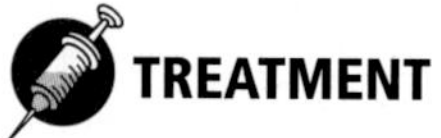

TREATMENT

ADDITIONAL TREATMENT

General Measures
Treatment is directed to
- Stabilize the patient
- Stop bleeding
- Stop strenuous physical activity
- Shield eye from further trauma with clear eye shield or safety spectacles. Do not block vision with patches and so on because the patient must be able to assess changes in his/her vision
- Promote healing
- Have the patient remain upright with bed rest at 30 degree angle to have the blood settle and clot. This will help the patient's visual acuity and promote aqueous fluid drainage. In a pediatric or poorly compliant patient, bed rest may be advisable.
- Decrease inflammation
- A penetrating topical steroid (e.g., prednisolone acetate 1%) 4–8 ×/day. If there is an associated corneal abrasion, use with caution or begin after epithelialization occurs.
- Avoid complications
- Synechiae – keep the eye dilated. This also helps to immobilize the iris, which may be a location of bleeding. Long acting dilation with Atropine 1%, Homatropine 2%, or scopolamine 0.25 % are generally used b.i.d.

- Pressure rise
- This may be delayed and transient as the RBC's are filtering through the trabecular meshwork. Initiation of treatment should be based on the extent and duration of the pressure rise as well as the patient profile for optic nerve risk factors.
- Appropriate patients should be screened for sickle cell disease/trait (Sickledex test) or other hemoglobinopathies (hemoglobin electrophoresis) because of possible complications from some pharmacologic agents, such as brinzolamide (Azopt) & dorzolamide (Trusopt) topically and systemic diuretics.
- Beta blockers are generally used as an initial agent.
- Alpha antagonists are used with caution because of systemic side effects.
- Oral diuretics if topical methods of antiocular hypertensive therapy are in effective. Avoid agents that may promote sickling in patients at risk.
- Avoid prostaglandin analogs, due to their promotion of intraocular inflammation effects.
- Anterior chamber paracentesis is controversial in hyphema. It requires an extremely cooperative patient. Anterior chamber structures are poorly visible, the procedure may result in a secondary rebleed, and the effects are temporary.
- Aminocaproic acid is seldom used and is usually reserved for hospitalized pediatric patients who have had rebleed episodes.
- Corneal blood staining. A late but gravid complication whereby hemoglobin and iron from lysed RBC's enters the corneal stroma. Generally a result of a longstanding large hyphema in a hypertensive eye. Patients at risk for this complication should be evaluated for an anterior chamber wash out.

Additional Therapies

- Shield the eye at all times with protective spectacles or eye shield – including when at rest.
- Limit physical activity for 1 week after resolution of the hyphema.
- Keep the head elevated to promote RBC settlement; including 30 degree bed rest
- Antiemetics for nausea and vomiting and stool softeners to prevent Valsalva.
- Avoid aspirin products or NSAIDs as an analgesic because of bleeding tendencies.

SURGERY/OTHER PROCEDURES

If surgical washout of the anterior chamber (AC) is indicted, the patient should be prepared according to intraocular surgery protocols. Irrigation and aspiration of the AC is cautiously performed to evacuate hematologic contents without disrupting ocular structures or tearing clots and causing a rebleed.

IN-PATIENT CONSIDERATIONS

Initial Stabilization

- Rule out ruptured globe/IOFB
- Take baseline examination: Va, IOP, SLE, DFE
- Stabilize IOP if necessary

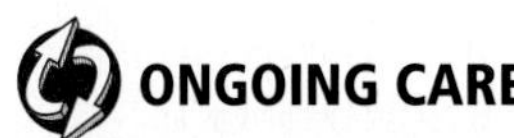

ONGOING CARE

FOLLOW-UP RECOMMENDATIONS

Patient Monitoring

The patient should be observed until there is resolution of the hyphema, cessation of therapy, and the pupils return to normal size and function. Gonioscopy should be performed. Follow-up should be at 6 months initially, then annually for evaluation of angle recession glaucoma.

ADDITIONAL READING

- Ehlers JP, Shah CP. (eds). The Wills Eye Manual, 5th (ed). Lippincott Williams & Wilkins, Philadelphia, 2008:19–23.

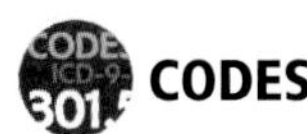

CODES

ICD9

364.41 Hyphema of iris and ciliary body

HYPOTONY

Marlene R. Moster
Parul Ichhpujani

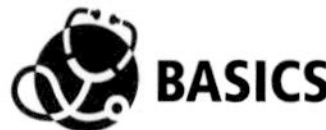

BASICS

DESCRIPTION
- "Statistical" hypotony can be defined as an intraocular pressure (IOP) less than 6.5 mm Hg, which corresponds to more than 3 standard deviations below the mean.
- "Clinically significant" hypotony represents the condition where the IOP is low enough to result in visual loss.

EPIDEMIOLOGY
Incidence
- **Transient hypotony:** Common following glaucoma surgery, surgeries involving a pars plana approach, or following trauma. The rate of hypotony following uncomplicated cataract surgery is extremely low. The incidence of hypotony following trabeculectomy increases with the use of antifibrotic agents such as Mitomycin-C.
- **Chronic hypotony:** Hypotony leading to phthisis is rare and occurs only in eyes with severe damage.

RISK FACTORS
- Young, male, myopes (low scleral rigidity).
- Uveitis.

GENERAL PREVENTION
- Hypotony following glaucoma surgery can be prevented in several ways.
  - Exposure time and the concentration of antimetabolites can be reduced, if used.
  - Using releasable sutures or placing extra sutures in the trabeculectomy flap may prevent overfiltration.
  - For tube shunts, choosing a valved device or modifying the shunt with a ligature suture can slow drainage.
  - Leave the anterior chamber inflated with viscoelastic at the end of the case.
  - Aggressive use of anti-inflammatory agents can help prevent the cycle of iridocyclitis and hypotony.

PATHOPHYSIOLOGY
- Hypotony occurs when aqueous humor production does not keep pace with outflow.
- **Impaired outflow:** Outflow may be greater than usual, as seen with wound leak, overfiltering bleb, or cyclodialysis cleft.
- **Impaired production:** Conditions that alter ciliary body function, such as iridocyclitis, tractional detachment, or hypoperfusion.
- **Role of inflammation:** It causes increased permeability of the blood–aqueous barrier.
- **Altered equation of conventional and uveoscleral outflow:** Flow through the conventional route ceases when IOP declines below the episcleral venous pressure, usually 9 mm Hg. Therefore, uveoscleral outflow predominates at low IOPs.
- Choroidal fluid is believed to accumulate as a result of enhanced uveoscleral outflow and decreased aqueous humor production, a cycle that is often perpetuated once choroidal effusions develop. A ring of anterior choroidal fluid can cause forward rotation of the ciliary body, impairing aqueous humor production.

ETIOLOGY
- Unilateral hypotony is seen with the following:
  - Wound leak
  - Overfiltering or inadvertent bleb
  - Cyclodialysis cleft
  - Inflammation—Iridocyclitis or trauma
  - Retinal detachment
  - Ocular ischemia
  - Scleral perforation with needle or suture, or scleral rupture following trauma
  - Chemical cyclodestruction from antimetabolites
  - Photocoagulation or cryoablation of the ciliary body
  - Pharmacologic aqueous humor suppression
- Bilateral hypotony is seen with the following:
  - Systemic hypertonicity or acidosis—dehydration, uremia, uncontrolled diabetes, or use of hyperosmotic agents
  - Myotonic dystrophy

COMMONLY ASSOCIATED CONDITIONS
Direct trauma with undiagnosed eye wall perforation.

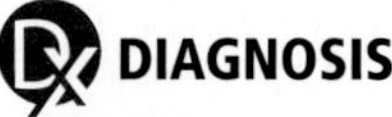

DIAGNOSIS

HISTORY
- Recent trauma or surgery, especially primary glaucoma surgery with antimetabolites
- Blurred vision
- Eye pain (usually a deep ache), especially with choroidal detachment (hemorrhagic choroidal detachment can cause extreme pain)
- History of eye inflammation or systemic illnesses predisposing to uveitis
- Signs and symptoms associated with retinal detachment

PHYSICAL EXAM
- Seidel positive wound leak
- Large bleb following trabeculectomy or tube shunt
- Shallowing of the anterior chamber
- Corneal edema and decompensation
- Synechiae formation
- Corneal astigmatism
- Inflammatory cells and flare in the anterior chamber
- Accelerated cataract formation
- Cyclodialysis cleft
- Ciliochoroidal detachment—serous or hemorrhagic
- Hypotony maculopathy
- Retinal folds
- Vascular engorgement and tortuosity
- Optic disc swelling
- Retinal detachment

DIAGNOSTIC TESTS & INTERPRETATION
Lab
Initial lab tests
- Hypotony is usually diagnosed based on only the history and the physical examination.
- In patients with undiagnosed but suspected uveitis, evaluate for systemic inflammatory disease, especially if the condition is recurrent
- In patients with bilateral hypotony, test for glucose, BUN, and creatinine

Imaging
Initial approach
- **B-scan ultrasonography:** Useful when the fundus is not easily visualized. It can help in determining the size and the extent of ciliochoroidal detachment, choroidal hemorrhage, and retinal detachment.
- **Ultrasonic biomicroscopy or anterior optical coherence tomography (ASOCT):** These can help to further evaluate the anterior chamber depth, the position of the ciliary body, and the presence of anterior ciliary detachment or cyclodialysis cleft.
- **OCT:** OCT scan of the posterior pole can help to better demonstrate subtle macular fluid or folds.

Follow-up & special considerations
- OCT to see resolution of macular fluid and folds of the choroid
- Close and frequent follow-up for uveitic patients and diabetics

Diagnostic Procedures/Other
Fluorescein angiography is helpful in demonstrating the chorioretinal folds, which in relatively mild degrees may be overlooked.

Pathological Findings
- Corneal changes
- Accelerated cataract formation
- Choroidal fluid
- Choroidal folds
- Maculopathy with disturbance of the retinal pigment epithelium (RPE)
- Cystoid macular edema
- Optic disc edema

DIFFERENTIAL DIAGNOSIS
- Idiopathic chorioretinal folds
- Choroidal detachment
- Postoperative endophthalmitis
- Scleral inflammation
- Uveitic glaucoma
- Hyphema
- Corneoscleral laceration
- Postoperative retinal detachment
- Rhegmatogenous retinal detachment
- Tractional retinal detachment
- Uveitis

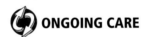

TREATMENT

MEDICATION

First Line

- Hypotony is best managed by correcting the underlying problem. The anterior chamber may be reformed with viscoelastic as a temporizing measure.
- Steroids may improve aqueous humor production by decreasing ciliary body inflammation.
- Atropine and other cycloplegics deepen the anterior chamber to lessen iris–corneal touch.

Second Line

- Drainage of the choroidal detachment.
- Tighten the sclera flap with additional sutures or revise the trabeculectomy.
- Tie off the tube shunt with a permanent or dissolving suture.
- Large bandage contact lens for seidel positive leak in the bleb or at the limbus
- Patching after atropine
- Systemic medications for treatment of iridocyclitis
- Repair cyclodialysis cleft if present.

ADDITIONAL TREATMENT

General Measures

- The patient should avoid lifting, bending, and strenuous activity. Sudden movement or straining could cause a vessel, which already is stretched in the suprachoroidal space, to bleed and create a suprachoroidal hemorrhage.
- The patient should avoid any direct pressure on the eye that could cause further decompression.
- An eye shield at bedtime is advisable.

Issues for Referral

- Unresolved macula folds
- Persistent wound leak
- Cyclodialysis repair
- Kissing choroidals
- Flat chamber with touch of the iris to the edge of the pupil or involving the pupil with corneal folds and decompensation

Additional Therapies

- Nonsteroidal medications topically and orally to decrease inflammation and avoid papillary membrane formation
- Immediate reformation of the anterior chamber with viscoelastic if the chamber is flat and involving the pupil or if there is corneal decompensation

COMPLEMENTARY & ALTERNATIVE THERAPIES

- Encourage oral hydration.
- Laxatives and avoid Valsalva to decrease the chance of a suprachoroidal hemorrhage when the eye is hypotonus.

SURGERY/OTHER PROCEDURES

- Treatment of wound leaks:
- Small wound leaks with a well-formed anterior chamber: Conservative management with patching or a large diameter bandage contact lens
- Focal leak: Cyanoacrylate glue application with a contact lens placed over the glue
- Large wound leaks causing clinically significant hypotony: Surgical revision using a round bodied needle to prevent leaks from suture tracts
- Cyclodialysis cleft: Treatment options include argon laser photocoagulation, cryotherapy, and ciliary body suturing.
- Conjunctival flaps can work well for diffusely incompetent blebs due to tissue thinning and avascularity.
- For chronic hypotony, surgical wound revision with resuturing of the flap, and/or conjunctival advancement or autograft is the procedure of choice.
- Treatment of uveitis:
- Anti-inflammatory agents are the mainstay of treatment. Intravitreal steroid injections can be tried in prephthisical eyes.
- Surgical removal of a cyclitic membrane may release tractional detachment of the ciliary body.
- Vitrectomy and placement of silicone oil may be useful in refractory cases.

IN-PATIENT CONSIDERATIONS

This condition can be monitored and treated as an outpatient.

ONGOING CARE

FOLLOW-UP RECOMMENDATIONS

Close observation of visual acuity. The patient should report subjective improvement as the hypotony resolves.

Patient Monitoring

Every few days if the chamber is shallow or flat, or if there is a wound leak. When a bandage lens is in place, the treatment involves coverage with a topical fluoroquinolone q.i.d.

DIET

Patients at risk for hypotony should maintain good hydration.

PATIENT EDUCATION

- Educate patients about the cause and the implications of this condition. Better understanding may help the patient to be more compliant with treatment and follow-up care.
- Patients should also be warned that improvement in visual acuity often lags behind the resolution of hypotony.

PROGNOSIS

Prognosis varies with the cause and the extent of hypotony.

COMPLICATIONS

- Corneal decompensation, synechiae, cataract formation, and chronic retinal edema or folds may occur.
- If suprachoroidal hemorrhage develops, the results may be catastrophic for the eye; however close observation and drainage after 10 days when the blood is liquefied will often yield an excellent result.
- Prolonged hypotony may lead to pre-phthisis or phthisis bulbi.

REFERENCES

1. Fine HF, Biscette O, Chang S, Schiff WM. Ocular hypotony: A review. *Compr Ophthalmol Update* 2007;8(1):29–37.
2. Costa VP, Wilson RP, Moster MR, Schmidt CM, Grandham S. Hypotony maculopathy following the use of topical mitomycin C in glaucoma filtration surgery. *Ophthalmic Surg* 1993;24:389–394.
3. Fannin LA, Schiffman JC, Budenz DL. Risk factors for hypotony maculopathy. *Ophthalmology* 2003;110:1185–1191.

ADDITIONAL READING

- Leen MM, Mills RP. *Ophthalmic surgery: Principles and practice*. 3rd ed. Philadelphia, PA: Saunders, 2003, 379.

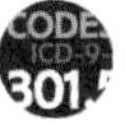

CODES

ICD9

- 360.30 Hypotony of eye, unspecified
- 360.31 Primary hypotony of eye
- 360.33 Hypotony associated with other ocular disorders

CLINICAL PEARLS

- Modifications of the surgical technique, such as tighter scleral flap suturing and postoperative gradual increase in outflow with laser suture lysis or releasable sutures, should be used to avoid overfiltration and the occurrence of hypotony maculopathy.

H

IDIOPATHIC JUXTAFOVEAL RETINAL TELANGIECTASIA

Adam T. Gerstenblith
Marc Spirn

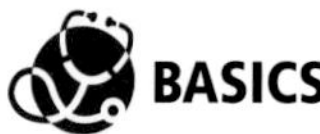

BASICS

DESCRIPTION

- Idiopathic juxtafoveal retinal telangiectasia (IJRT) is characterized by the presence of small perifoveal or parafoveal telangiectatic retinal vessels in the absence of an identifiable systemic or ocular disease.
  - Typically occurs temporal to the fovea
  - May be scattered throughout the macula
- Classified on the basis of biomicroscopic and fluorescein angiographic appearance into 3 groups (1,2,3) and 2 sub-groups (A and B)

EPIDEMIOLOGY

Incidence

Rare

Prevalence

Unknown

RISK FACTORS

No clear risk factors identified

PATHOPHYSIOLOGY

- Multifactorial visual loss
  - Macular edema from vascular leakage
  - Retinal ischemia from capillary occlusion
  - Secondary choroidal neovascularization (CNV)

ETIOLOGY

- Not well understood
  - May be a result of retinal Muller cell dysfunction

COMMONLY ASSOCIATED CONDITIONS

- Most often an isolated condition
- An association exists with abnormal glucose metabolism (2).

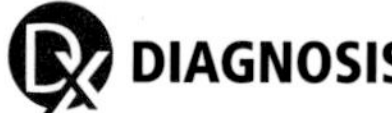

DIAGNOSIS

HISTORY

Unilateral or bilateral disruption of central vision

PHYSICAL EXAM

- Slit-lamp examination:
  - Peri- or parafoveal dilated, tortuous, and irregular capillaries seen most often in the temporal macula
  - "Right-angle" veins may be seen draining the telangiectatic areas.
  - Small refractile deposits on the surface of the retina
  - Retinal pigment epithelial hyperplasia may develop in long-standing disease.

DIAGNOSTIC TESTS & INTERPRETATION

Imaging

- Intravenous fluorescein angiography (IVFA) demonstrates the abnormal retinal vessels and may also show:
  - Areas of leakage or capillary occlusion
  - Presence of CNV
- OCT shows:
  - Areas of hyporeflectivity representing cystic intraretinal spaces
  - Intraretinal and subretinal fluid as well as outer retinal atrophy, particularly in IJRT group 2A

Pathological Findings

Endothelial cell and pericyte degeneration with retinal capillary narrowing

DIFFERENTIAL DIAGNOSIS

- Various vascular disorders may mimic IJRT including:
  - Diabetic retinopathy
  - Retinal vein occlusion
  - Radiation retinopathy
  - Carotid-occlusive disease
  - Sickle cell retinopathy
  - Coats' disease

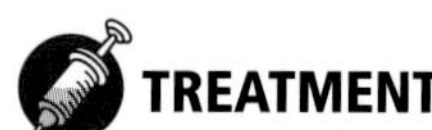

TREATMENT

SURGERY/OTHER PROCEDURES

- Laser photocoagulation may improve the macular edema (3)[C].
  - This treatment is limited in IJRT due to the proximity of the lesions to the fovea.
- For treatment of CNV:
  - Anti-VEGF agents (ranibizumab and bevacizumab) and photodynamic therapy (PDT) may be beneficial, although large studies are lacking (4,5)[C].

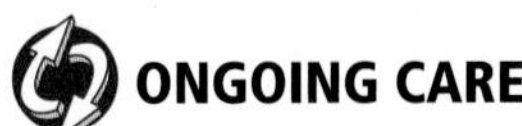

ONGOING CARE

FOLLOW-UP RECOMMENDATIONS

- Yearly dilated fundus examinations at the minimum
  - Should complications such as macular edema or CNV develop, the patient should be referred to a retinal specialist for further evaluation and management with IVFA and/or OCT.

Patient Monitoring

Patients should be counseled to return to the ophthalmologist if any changes in vision occur.

PROGNOSIS

- Vision is normal or only mildly affected in the absence of macular edema, macular ischemia, or CNV.
  - The extent of vision loss is directly correlated with the development and severity of the above-mentioned complications.

COMPLICATIONS

- Macular edema
- Macular ischemia
- Choroidal neovascularization

REFERENCES

1. Gass JDM, Oyakawa RT. Idiopathic juxtafoveal retinal telangiectasis. *Arch Ophthalmol* 1982;100: 769–780.
2. Milay RH, Klein ML, Handelman IL, et al Abnormal glucose metabolism and parafoveal telangiectasia. *Am J Ophthalmol* 1986;102:363.
3. Chopdar A. Retinal telangiectasis in adults: Fluorescein angiographic findings and treatment by argon laser. *Br J Ophthalmol* 1978;62:243–250.
4. Konstantinidis L, Mantel I, Zografos L, et al. Intravitreal ranibizumab as primary treatment for neovascular membrane associated with idiopathic juxtafoveal retinal telangiectasia. *Graefes Arch Clin Exp Ophthalmol* 2009;247(11):1567–1569.
5. Kovach JL, Rosenfeld PJL. Bevacizumab (avastin) therapy for idiopathic macular telangiectasia type II. *Retina* 2009;29:27–32.

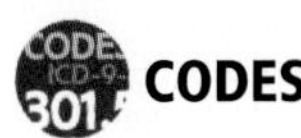

CODES

ICD9

362.15 Retinal telangiectasia

CLINICAL PEARLS

- Idiopathic condition characterized by abnormal telangiectatic capillaries most often located in the temporal macula
- Unilateral or bilateral presentation
- Complications include macular edema, macular ischemia, and choroidal neovascularization

IDIOPATHIC ORBITAL INFLAMMATORY SYNDROME (ORBITAL PSEUDOTUMOR)

Katherine A. Lane
Jurij R. Bilyk

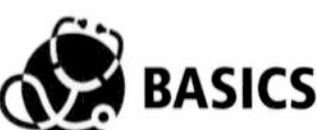

BASICS

DESCRIPTION

- Idiopathic orbital inflammatory syndrome (IOIS) is a nonspecific inflammation of orbital tissue with no identifiable local or systemic cause.
- IOIS is a diagnosis of exclusion, made only after other entities have been ruled out.
- IOIS can involve any orbital tissue individually or in combination; often subcategorized based on anatomic location of inflammation:
  – Myositis
  – Dacryoadenitis
  – Posterior scleritis
  – Inflammation of the orbital fat
  – Inflammation of the orbital apex

EPIDEMIOLOGY

Incidence

- Unknown
- Accounts for ~5% of orbital disorders
- Peak incidence between 40 and 60 years of age, but may occur at any age

Prevalence

Unknown

RISK FACTORS

- No clear risk factors
- On occasion, patients with IOIS also have or develop other autoimmune diseases. This may simply be an epiphenomenon.
- IOIS never progresses to lymphoma.

Genetics

No known hereditary pattern

GENERAL PREVENTION

None known

PATHOPHYSIOLOGY

- The signs and symptoms of IOIS most likely represent the clinical manifestations of a variety of autoimmune and cell-mediated processes for which the trigger(s) has yet to be determined.
- There is no evidence that IOIS is part of the spectrum of lymphoproliferative diseases (see Ocular Adnexal Lymphoma chapter).

ETIOLOGY

See pathophysiology

COMMONLY ASSOCIATED CONDITIONS

- Idiopathic
- Possible associations have been reported with Crohn's disease, systemic lupus erythematosus, rheumatoid arthritis, diabetes, and ankylosing spondylitis. This may be an epiphenomenon.

DIAGNOSIS

HISTORY

- The 'classic' presentation includes the abrupt onset of one or more of the following signs and symptoms:
  – Periorbital pain. Absence of pain is an atypical feature of IOIS.
  – Diplopia
  – Visual changes
- There may be a history of autoimmune disease.
- Complete review of systems, including the presence of constitutional symptoms (particularly in children), history of malignancy, respiratory symptoms, autoimmune disease, or immunosuppression

PHYSICAL EXAM

- Complete ophthalmic and orbital exam. Some or all of the following may be seen:
  – Boggy eyelid edema
  – Erythema, which is usually more pink than red
  – Conjunctival chemosis and/or injection
  – Proptosis
  – External ophthalmoplegia
  – Choroidal detachment and optic disc swelling may be seen in cases of posterior scleritis.
- Children may present with bilateral findings, either simultaneously or sequentially.

DIAGNOSTIC TESTS & INTERPRETATION

Lab

Initial lab tests

- Baseline serologic work-up may include:
  – CBC with differential, ACE, cANCA, ANA, SPEP, and serum lactate dehydrogenase

Follow-up & special considerations

- Follow-up with primary care doctor (± rheumatologist) if lab studies reveal positive findings.

Imaging

- All cases of clinically suspected IOIS require orbital imaging. The diagnosis of IOIS should never be made on clinical grounds alone.
- CT
  – Focal or diffuse mass, poorly demarcated, which enhances with contrast
  – Bone erosion is highly atypical for IOIS.
- MRI
  – T1: low signal intensity
  – T2: increased signal intensity
  – Gadolinium: + homogenous enhancement
- Echography
  – Not widely used, but may be very useful for suspected posterior scleritis: scleral thickening with a squared-off optic nerve entry (T-sign) may be seen.

Diagnostic Procedures/Other

- Orbital biopsy may not be required for diagnosis:
  – Should be attempted in patients who present in an atypical fashion, in patients who do not respond to corticosteroid treatment, and in patients with recurrent episodes of inflammation
  – A low threshold for biopsy is also indicated in patients with a known history of local or distant malignancy.
  – Some experts will also perform biopsy on all patients presenting with lacrimal gland inflammation, because this area is easily accessible and, on occasion, a malignancy can present with secondary inflammation.

Pathological Findings

Nonspecific paucicellular infiltrate of lymphocytes, plasma cells, and histiocytes, and varying degrees of fibrosis

DIFFERENTIAL DIAGNOSIS

- Acute bacterial cellulitis: This is especially important to rule out in children before beginning corticosteroid therapy.
- Sarcoidosis
- Wegener granulomatosis
- Lymphoproliferative disease, including lymphoma
- Tolosa–Hunt syndrome
- Benign neoplasm
- Malignancy: primary or metastatic
- Thyroid eye disease

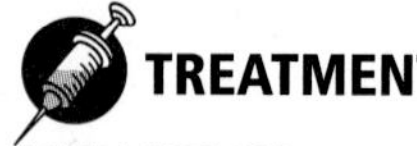

TREATMENT

MEDICATION

First Line

- Oral corticosteroids:
  – Starting dosage of 1.0–1.5 mg/kg/day
  – A prompt and complete response is expected, and may be considered part of the diagnostic algorithm.
  – Symptom rebound during steroid taper may occur and may respond to a slower taper.
  – Inflammation not sensitive to the effects of steroids or an inability to taper off steroids is considered 'atypical', and alternative diagnoses should be sought.
  – Note that a course of corticosteroids may mask the true diagnosis if biopsy is needed at a later date. This is particularly true for inflammatory (e.g., sarcoidosis) or lymphoproliferative lesions.

Second Line

- Parenteral corticosteroids
  – Often reserved for cases of IOIS-related optic neuropathy
- Non-steroidal anti-inflammatory medications:
  – Typically used as bridging therapy at the tail end of the corticosteroid taper in patients who re-flare at lower corticosteroid doses
  – Some experts advocate the use of NSAIDs as first-line therapy.

- Local intralesional corticosteroid injections (off-label use of triamcinolone acetonide)
  - May be used in cases of local inflammatory masses or dacryoadenitis.
  - Use is controversial because of potential side effects and risks of injection.

ADDITIONAL TREATMENT

General Measures

- Observation:
  - Inflammation often resolves slowly without treatment.

Issues for Referral

- Referral for orbital biopsy should be considered in cases that present in an atypical fashion, in patients with a history of malignancy, or in those treated empirically with corticosteroids if:
  - Minimal or sub-total response to adequate corticosteroid treatment
  - Relapse of symptoms

Additional Therapies

- Orbital radiotherapy
  - May be used in steroid-resistant cases or those unable to tolerate corticosteroids
  - Biopsy should be obtained prior to radiotherapy if the tissue is accessible without excessive morbidity.
- Immuno-modulating agents may be used in steroid-resistant cases, but it is preferable to obtain tissue biopsy first. All therapies listed below are off-label uses of the specific agent:
  - Antimetabolites (e.g., methotrexate, azathioprine)
  - Alkylating agents (e.g., cyclophosphamide, chlorambucil)
  - T-cell inhibitors (e.g., cyclosporine, tacrolimus)
  - Biologic agents (e.g., infliximab, enteracept)

SURGERY/OTHER PROCEDURES

- Tissue biopsy for confirmation should be performed in all atypical cases.
- The threshold for biopsy is lower in patients with a history of malignancy.
- Some experts will biopsy all cases of inflammatory dacryoadenitis.
- Complete excision is typically not needed and is, usually, technically not feasible without significant local morbidity.

IN-PATIENT CONSIDERATIONS

Admission Criteria

- Comorbidities (e.g., brittle diabetes) which preclude the use of corticosteroids on an outpatient basis
- Postoperative observation following deep orbital biopsy

IV Fluids

As needed for inpatient corticosteroid therapy.

Nursing

As needed for inpatient corticosteroid therapy or postoperative care

Discharge Criteria

Response to therapy and stability of comorbidities

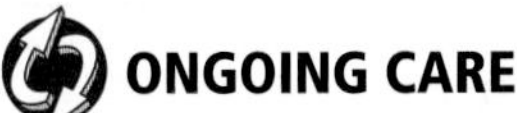

ONGOING CARE

FOLLOW-UP RECOMMENDATIONS

Long-term follow-up is recommended after the resolution of a patient's acute symptoms, as an episode of 'idiopathic' orbital inflammation may be a harbinger of systemic disease.

Patient Monitoring

- As required during the treatment period:
  - Monitoring patient's response to treatment and treatment-related side effects, including blood sugar elevation
- Bi-annual or annual follow-up after resolution to monitor for signs of recurrence

PATIENT EDUCATION

- IOIS is a diagnosis often made based on clinical grounds, without pathologic confirmation.
  - Patients must understand that they need to be followed prospectively for the development of an alternate diagnosis.

PROGNOSIS

- Most patients respond well and completely to treatment.
  - Patients with severe disease or multiple recurrences may, in rare cases, develop orbital scarring, permanent diplopia, or loss of vision.

COMPLICATIONS

- Treatment-related (see Treatment section)
- Permanent orbital scarring
- Complications related to tissue biopsy (e.g., visual loss, diplopia, hypesthesia, ptosis, infection)

ADDITIONAL READING

- Harris G. Idiopathic orbital inflammation: A pathogenetic construct and treatment strategy. *Ophthal Plast Reconst Surg* 2006;22:79–86.
- Yuen SJ, Rubin PA. Idiopathic orbital inflammation: Distributions, clinical features and treatment outcome. *Arch Ophthalmol* 2003;121:491–499.
- Rose GE. A personal view: Probability in medicine, levels of (un)certainty, and the diagnosis of orbital disease (with particular reference to orbital "pseudotumor"). *Arch Ophthalmol* 2007;125:1171–1172.
- Lane KA, Bilyk JR. Current concepts in the diagnosis and management of idiopathic orbital inflammation. In: Guthoff R, Katowtiz JA, eds. *Essentials in ophthalmology: oculoplastics and orbit: Aesthetic and functional oculofacial plastic problem-solving in the 21st century.* Berlin: Spring-Verlag, 2010:47–63.

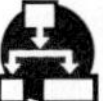

See Also (Topic, Algorithm, Electronic Media Element)

- Idiopathic Orbital Inflammatory Syndrome, Typical and Atypical (online algorithm)

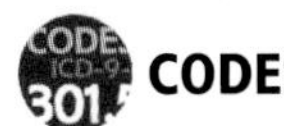

CODES

ICD9

- 375.00 Dacryoadenitis, unspecified
- 376.00 Orbital inflammation, unspecified
- 376.11 Inflammatory orbital pseudotumor

CLINICAL PEARLS

- IOIS is a diagnosis of exclusion. The clinician should always maintain a degree of uneasiness with this diagnosis and follow the patient over the long term.
- Typical features of IOIS include sudden, painful onset; varying degrees of external signs of inflammation; orbital soft tissue infiltration with lack of bone erosion on imaging; and rapid, dramatic response to appropriate systemic corticosteroid therapy (Table 1).
- All other presentations should be considered atypical and lower the threshold for tissue biopsy (Table 2).
- A history of cancer lowers the threshold for tissue biopsy.
- Some experts advocate biopsy of all cases of suspected inflammatory dacryoadenitis.
- Systemic corticosteroid therapy may mask pathologic processes on subsequent tissue biopsy.

INTERMEDIATE UVEITIS AND PARS PLANITIS

Fatima K. Ahmad

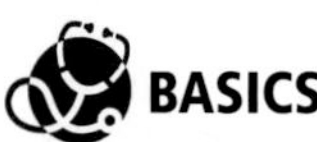

BASICS

DESCRIPTION

- Intermediate uveitis (IU) is inflammation primarily, of the anterior vitreous, ciliary body, and peripheral retina.
- Pars planitis is a subset of IU for which there is no associated infection or systemic disease.

EPIDEMIOLOGY

- IU comprises ~15% of all cases of uveitis
- No gender predisposition
- Bilateral in 70–90% of cases, but can be asymmetric
- Pars planitis accounts for 85–90% of intermediate uveitis
  - It has a bimodal distribution; the younger age group is 5–15 years, and older age group is 20–40 years

RISK FACTORS

Genetics

Pars planitis has been shown to be associated with HLA-DR15 and HLA-DR51

PATHOPHYSIOLOGY

- The pathophysiology of IU/pars planitis is not well understood
  - It is probably an autoimmune reaction against an ocular antigen
- Peripheral retinal veins are the primary foci for inflammation

COMMONLY ASSOCIATED CONDITIONS

- Sarcoidosis
- Multiple sclerosis
- Infectious conditions
  - Syphilis
  - Tuberculosis
  - Lyme's disease
  - Toxocariasis
  - HTLV-1
  - Bartonella
- Pars planitis has no associated systemic condition

DIAGNOSIS

HISTORY

- Patients present with floaters and decreased vision
- Usually a white, quiet eye, but patients can experience redness and photophobia (more commonly in children).

PHYSICAL EXAM

- Anterior vitreous cellular reaction
- Snowballs, which are aggregates of vitreous cells
- Snowbanks, which are inflammatory pars plana exudates, typically found inferiorly
  - Tends to indicate more severe disease
- Vascular tortuosity and peripheral retinal phlebitis

Pediatric Considerations

In children, IU tends to cause greater anterior chamber inflammation

DIAGNOSTIC TESTS & INTERPRETATION

Lab

- Complete blood count (CBC) with differential count
- Erythrocyte sedimentation rate (ESR)
- Purified protein derivative (PPD) skin test
- Angiotensin-converting enzyme (ACE) level, which can be elevated in sarcoidosis
- Consider serologic testing for Lyme's, syphilis, and Bartonella

Imaging

- Chest X-ray to assess for sarcoidosis and tuberculosis
  - If chest X-ray is negative, consider gallium scan or computed tomography (CT) to rule out sarcoidosis if clinical suspicion is high

Diagnostic Procedures/Other

- Fluorescein angiography is helpful in determining presence of cystoid macular edema (CME), retinal phlebitis, and neovascularization.
- Ultrasound biomicroscopy (UBM) can demonstrate pars plana exudates and vitreitis in cases with small pupil
- Diagnostic vitrectomy may be needed in cases where there is suspicion of intraocular lymphoma, endophthalmitis, or in cases refractory to medical therapy

Pathological Findings

- Histologic findings show lymphocytic infiltration of retinal veins
- Pars plana exudates consist of fibroglial tissue with inflammatory cells

DIFFERENTIAL DIAGNOSIS

- Primary central nervous system lymphoma
- Endophthalmitis
- Other uveitic conditions, including Vogt–Koyanagi–Harada disease and Fuch's heterochromic cyclitis

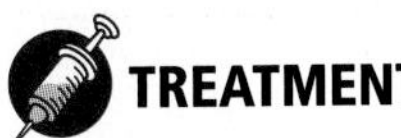

TREATMENT

MEDICATION

First Line

- Treat underlying cause of disease if infectious etiology is present
- For other cases, corticosteroids are indicated if patient is symptomatic or has vision loss.
  - Periocular corticosteroids are first line
  - Oral corticosteroids is indicated if local therapy is ineffective, or if there is bilateral severe disease
  - Intravitreal injection for refractory cases

Second Line

- Immunomodulatory therapy if corticosteroids fail or side effects cannot be tolerated
  - Methotrexate
  - Cyclosporine
  - Azathioprine
  - Mycophenolate mofetil
  - Tacrolimus

SURGERY/OTHER PROCEDURES

- If drug therapy fails, cryotherapy and laser photocoagulation can be performed to peripheral retina for ablation of pars plana exudates and neovascularization
- Pars plana vitrectomy (PPV) for chronic inflammation or structural complications such as retinal detachment
  - PPV is helpful in reducing CME

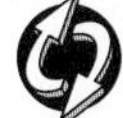

ONGOING CARE

FOLLOW-UP RECOMMENDATIONS

- Ophthalmology
- Rheumatology or infectious disease specialist, depending on etiology

PROGNOSIS

- IU generally has a chronic course with exacerbations and remissions, although a small subset of patients have self-limiting disease
  - Of all subsets of uveitis, IU tends to have the longest duration, most cases last for 5–15 years but can be longer
- Visual outcome is related to severity of disease and presence of CME
  - Pars plana exudate indicates poorer prognosis
- Pars planitis has an overall favorable visual prognosis

COMPLICATIONS

- Chronic inflammation from IU can lead to CME.
- Cataracts result from both chronic inflammation and corticosteroid therapy
  - Perioperative use of corticosteroids is needed to control inflammation.
- Glaucoma, both angle closure and open angle
- Band keratopathy
- Peripheral retinal neovascularization
- Vitreous hemorrhage
- Retinal detachment

ADDITIONAL READING

- Bloch-Michel E, Nussenblatt RB. International Uveitis Study Group recommendations for the evaluation of intraocular inflammatory disease. *Am J Ophthalmol* 1987;103:234–235.
- Jabs DA, Nusenblatt RB, Rosenbaum JT. Standardization of Uveitis nomenclature (SUN) working group. Standardization of uveitis nomenclature for reporting clinical data. Results of the First International Workshop. *Am J Ophthalmol* 2005;140:509–516.

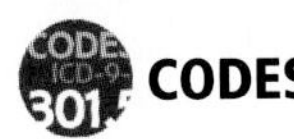

CODES

ICD9

- 363.21 Pars planitis
- 364.3 Unspecified iridocyclitis

I

INTERNUCLEAR OPHTHALMOPLEGIA

Sarkis M. Nazarian

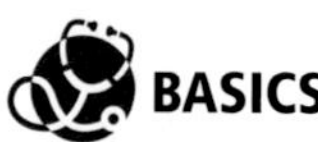

BASICS

DESCRIPTION

- Internuclear ophthalmoplegia (INO) is an ocular motility disturbance manifest by intact abduction of ipsilateral eye but impaired adduction of contralateral eye during ipsilateral horizontal gaze attempts. It is always named after the impaired adducting eye (i.e., a right INO is only observed with gaze to left). It is due to interruption of the pathway [medial longitudinal fasciculus (MLF)] from the ipsilateral abducens nucleus to the contralateral oculomotor nucleus. The abducting eye usually develops coarse end-gaze horizontal nystagmus. Convergence is generally preserved.
  - Partial INO, manifest by slowed saccadic velocity in the adducting eye, is much more common than full INO.
  - If the lesion encompasses both MLFs and the eyes are exotropic in primary position, the condition is termed wall-eyed bilateral INO (WEBINO). Convergence is usually lost with WEBINO.
  - If the lesion encompasses both the MLF and the ipsilateral abducens nucleus/PPRF complex, ipsilateral gaze palsy and contralateral INO occurs; the only normal movement is abduction of contralateral eye. This syndrome is called one-and-a-half syndrome (3 of the 4 horizontal half-movements, 2 in each eye, are affected).

EPIDEMIOLOGY

Incidence

No data available on incidence

Prevalence

INO prevalence in multiple sclerosis (MS) patients is common; 30% of fifty patients in a VA clinic were found to have INO. (1) (C). Exact prevalence is unknown.

RISK FACTORS

Strokes have been associated with 38%, MS with 34%, and unusual causes with 28% of INO cases in a retrospective study in Los Angeles (2)[C]

Genetics

No genetic pattern

GENERAL PREVENTION

Prevention consists of medical control of underlying condition (e.g., stroke risk, MS).

PATHOPHYSIOLOGY

Demyelinating or vascular occlusion affecting the MLF in its course between the abducens and contralateral oculomotor nucleus

ETIOLOGY

- The most common etiology of INO is MS, which often results in bilateral INOs. Asymmetric involvement is the rule.
  - In the elderly, small pontine or midbrain strokes often lead to unilateral INO.
  - Medications such as anticonvulsants, opioids, etc.

COMMONLY ASSOCIATED CONDITIONS

- Multiple sclerosis
- Optic neuritis
- Small-vessel (lacunar) strokes
- Brainstem hemorrhage
- Brainstem tumors
- Trauma
- Overdose of sedative medications

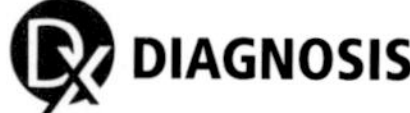

DIAGNOSIS

HISTORY

- Most patients with partial INO are asymptomatic, although they may complain of transient horizontal diplopia during rapid eye movements.
  - As skew deviation may accompany INO, patients may also complain of vertical or oblique diplopia.

PHYSICAL EXAM

- Attempt to gaze in contralateral direction of INO results in normal abduction, but impaired adduction. This latter can range from inability to move eye past midline to slower velocity of the adduction saccade. The abducting eye often has coarse horizontal nystagmus.
- In one-and-a-half syndrome, contralateral gaze is impaired; attempts at ipsilateral gaze result in abduction of ipsilateral eye only.
- In WEBINO, INO is seen with attempts to look in either horizontal direction. Exotropia is usually present, and convergence is usually impaired.
- The presence of ptosis, fatiguable weakness, or other extraocular muscle weakness points to a different etiology. The most common confounder of INO is pseudo-INO, which is usually associated with myasthenia gravis.

DIAGNOSTIC TESTS & INTERPRETATION

Lab

No specific testing is available

Imaging

Initial approach

MRI of the brain is the preferred imaging method. CT scan of the brain does not have sufficient resolution to identify the lesion. The usual finding is a small white matter lesion, best seen on FLAIR imaging. For acute demyelinating lesions in patients with MS, the lesion may enhance with gadolinium contrast. Acute lacunar strokes may show up on diffusion-weighted MR imaging. Often the brainstem is normal on imaging.

Follow-up & special considerations

Repeat imaging for stable or improving INO is not necessary. Infrared oculography can be used to confirm the presence of INO, although the diagnosis is usually made by clinical examination alone.

Diagnostic Procedures/Other

INO commonly occurs as a consequence of a small lacunar infarct or an inflammatory demyelinating lesion. Diagnostic procedures are aimed at finding the causes of stroke or to document the presence of MS or other demyelinating CNS disease.

DIFFERENTIAL DIAGNOSIS

Pseudo-INO due to myasthenia can occur.

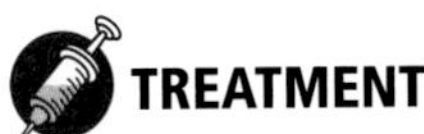

TREATMENT

ADDITIONAL TREATMENT

General Measures

Not applicable

Issues for Referral

Selected patients may need to be referred to a neurologist specializing in MS or stroke management.

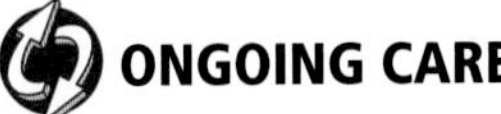

ONGOING CARE

FOLLOW-UP RECOMMENDATIONS

Patients should be re-examined in 3–6 months.

DIET

If the cause of the INO is determined to be due to a lacunar stroke, a diet resulting in lowering of vascular disease risk is indicated.

PATIENT EDUCATION

Appropriate to the etiology, usually MS or stroke

PROGNOSIS

INO prognosis is dependent on the etiology; those due to MS, trauma, tumors, strokes, or hemorrhages tend to persist, whereas those due to infections (e.g., brainstem encephalitis) or drug overdoses improve or resolve with treatment.

REFERENCES

1. Downey AL, Stahl JS, Asiri RB, Derwenskus J, Adams NL, Ruff RL, Leigh RJ. *Ann N Y Acad Sci* 2002;956:438–440.
2. Keane JR. Internuclear ophthalmoplegia: Unusual causes in 114 of 410 patients. *Arch Neurol* 2005;62:714–717.

ADDITIONAL READING

- Prasad S, Galetta SL. Eye movement abnormalities in multiple sclerosis. *Neurologic Clinics* 2010;28: 641–655.
- Zee DS. Internuclear ophthalmoplegia: Pathophysiology and diagnosis. *Baillieres Clin Neurol* 1992;1:455–470.
- Baloh RW, Yee RD, Honrubia V. Internuclear ophthalmoplegia. 1. Saccades and dissociated nystagmus. *Arch Neurol* 1978;35:484–489.
- Cogan DG. Internuclear ophthalmoplegia, typical and atypical. *Arch Ophthalmol* 1970;84:583–589.
- National Multiple Sclerosis Society of America http://www.nmss.org.
- Multiple Sclerosis International Federation http://www.ifmss.org.uk.
- The Multiple Sclerosis Society of Great Britain and Northern Ireland http://www.mssociety.org.uk.
- MS Research Trust http://www.msresearchtrust.org.uk.
- MedSupport FSF International http://www.medsupport.org.
- Consortium of Multiple Sclerosis Centers http://www.mscare.org.
- Computer Literate Advocates for Multiple Sclerosis http://www.clams.org.
- National Institute of Neurological Disorders and Stroke http://www.ninds.nih.gov/health_and_medical/disorders/multiple_sclerosis.htm.
- http://www.mult-sclerosis.org/internuclearophthalmoplegia.html.
- Jooly's Joint http://www.mswebpals.org.

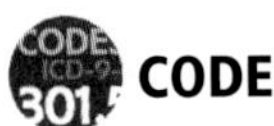

CODES

ICD9

378.86 Internuclear ophthalmoplegia

CLINICAL PEARLS

- INO is the most reliable localizing sign in the CNS, pinpointing the ipsilateral pons or midbrain as the site of pathology.
- Bilateral INO usually means MS; unilateral INO usually means stroke.
- Pseudo-INO, which is clinically indistinguishable from INO, may occur in myasthenia gravis.

I

INTERSTITIAL KERATITIS (IK)

Nicole R. Fram
Eliza Hoskins
Doug S. Holsclaw

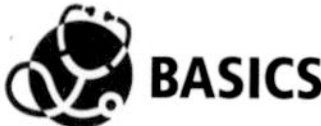

BASICS

DESCRIPTION

- Interstitial keratitis (IK) or immune stromal keratitis (ISK) is nonsuppurative (nonmelting) inflammation and cellular infiltration of the corneal stroma
- Often accompanied by corneal vascularization
- Minimal primary involvement of the epithelium (non-ulcerative) or endothelium in the active stage of inflammation
- However, corneal thinning can occur as a result of chronic inflammation.
  - Active disease is characterized by pain, tearing, and photophobia
  - Typically associated with systemic disease
  - Often diagnosed as a late sequelae of disease characterized by ghost vessels and corneal scarring

ETIOLOGY

- Congenital syphilis has been described as the most common cause of IK worldwide (1).
  - Worldwide 90% of IK
  - Congenital (87%) versus acquired (3%)
  - F>M is 2:1 for congenital and acquired syphilis
- However, herpetic eye disease and idiopathic causes appear to be the most common causes of active IK in North America (2).
- Herpetic eye disease and syphilis comprise >50% of cases of IK in the US.
- IK is responsible for 2–5% of penetrating keratoplasties(3, 4).

RISK FACTORS

- Bacterial, viral, or parasitic infections (see Differential Diagnosis)
- Systemic diseases (see Differential Diagnosis)

PATHOPHYSIOLOGY

- Lymphocytic infiltration and neovascularizaion (typically) of the corneal stroma. Late findings of ghost vessel and corneal scarring.
- Type IV hypersensitivity response to infectious organisms or antigens in the corneal stroma

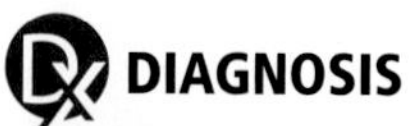

DIAGNOSIS

HISTORY

- Targeted history: onset, duration, location, quality of symptoms, associated systemic conditions (hearing loss), contact lens wear, sexually transmitted diseases, trauma, travel history, and tick or insect bites
- Unilateral or bilateral
- Active inflammation is characterized by pain, tearing, and photophobia.

Past Medical History and Medications

- **Review of systems (ROS):**
  - **Constitutional:** fever, night sweats, chills [tuberculosis (TB)]
  - **Skin/mucocutaneous:** oral ulcers (herpes simplex virus (HSV), vesicular lesions (herpetic disease), erythema migrans (Lyme's disease), stigmata of Hansen's (leprosy)
  - **Dental/ENT:** incisor and molar deformation (congenital syphilis), saddle nose (syphilis), hearing loss, tinnitus, vertigo (Cogan's syndrome), parotiditis [Epstein Barr Virus (EBV), mumps]
  - **Respiratory:** Shortness of breath (sarocoidosis), productive cough (TB)
  - **Cardiovascular:** AV block (Lyme's disease)
  - **Musculoskeletal:** Migratory joint pain (Lyme's disease); saber shins (syphilis)
  - **Genitourinary:** Genital ulcers (syphilis)
  - **Neurological:** Cranial nerve palsies (CN V, VII, and VIII) (herpetic disease, Lyme's disease, Cogan's syndrome, leprosy)

PHYSICAL EXAM

- Visual acuity, intraocular pressure (IOP)
- Pupillary function, confrontational visual fields, and ocular motility/alignment
- **External exam:** Rashes (Lyme's disease, syphilis, herpetic disease, leprosy)
- **Eyelids:** Vesicles (herpetic), lid chancre (syphilis)
- **Conjunctiva/sclera:** Conjunctival injection, scleritis, conjunctival granuloma (sarcoidosis, TB, leprosy)
- **Cornea:** Stromal white blood cell infiltrate, epithelium typically intact, corneal scarring (diffuse, sectoral, central, circumferential, or multifocal), decreased corneal sensation (herpetic disease, EBV, leprosy), stromal vascularization**,** lipid exudation/keratopathy, ghost vessels**,** corneal scarring, and corneal thinning (late)
- **Iris:** Iris atrophy (herpetic disease, syphilis), iris pearls (leprosy), posterior synechiae
- **Anterior chamber:** Iritis, fine keratic precipitates (KP)
- **Posterior Segment:** Salt and pepper fundus (syphilis), vasculitis ± choroiditis (sarcoidosis, herpetic disease, TB, syphilis)

DIAGNOSTIC TESTS & INTERPRETATION

- Slit lamp examination
- Confocal microscopy may be useful in cases where fungal or acanthamoeba infection is suspected.

Lab

- VDRL or RPR (syphilis)
- FTA-ABS or MHA-TP (syphilis)
- Lyme's Ab (ELISA IgG and IgM)
- Lyme's Western Blot
- HSV-1, HSV-2 (herpetic disease)
- Purified protein derivative (PPD) or quantiferon, chest X-ray [CXR (TB)]
- Cogan's syndrome: Leukocytosis and mild eosinophilia
- EBV (positive heterophil antibody test)

DIFFERENTIAL DIAGNOSIS

- Bacterial
  - Syphilis
  - Tuberculosis
  - Lyme's disease
  - Leprosy
  - Brucellosis
  - *Chlamydia trachomatis*
- Viral
  - Herpes simplex virus (HSV)
  - Varicella zoster virus (VZV)
  - Epstein–Barr Virus (EBV)
  - Mumps
  - Rubella
- Parasitic
  - Leishmaniasis
  - Onchocerciasis
  - Trypansomiasis
  - Acanthamoeba
  - Microsporidiosis
- Systemic disease
  - Cogan's syndrome
  - Sarcoidosis
  - Lymphoma
  - Idiopathic

DESCRIPTION OF ETIOLOGIES[1]

Syphilitic Interstitial Keratitis

- Triad of Hutchinson [IK, deafness (CN VIII), Hutchinson's incisors (dental deformation]
- **Congenital Syphilitic IK**
  - *Treponema pallidum*
  - Crosses placenta in primary, secondary, or early latent phase
  - Clinical disease is rarely present at birth
  - Age of onset: 5–20 years; Peak incidence 9–11 years; rare after age 30
  - 80% bilateral; unilateral disease at presentation, diffuse stromal disease, deep stromal vessels with overlying "salmon patch" edema, associated iritis in active disease
  - Second eye involved after days to years (~1 year)
  - Corneal involvement in 40% of congenital IK
  - Late phase characterized by ghost vessels ± corneal scarring, guttae-like excrescences on Descemet's membrane
- **Acquired Syphilitic IK**
  - Very uncommon and less severe
  - 10 years after primary infection
  - Probable corneal invasion of spirochetes
  - Bulbar conjunctival, limbal, or lid chancre
  - Unilateral in >60%
  - Often remains sectoral with vascularization
  - Regresses rapidly with anti-syphilitic therapy

TUBERCULOSIS

- *Mycobacterium Tuberculosis*
- Infection enters body via inhalation
- Granulomatous inflammation; 2% of IK cases
- Typically, unilateral, sectoral, and peripheral; frequently involves inferior cornea
- Stromal vascularization (minimal)
- Dense sectoral scar ± thinning
- Associated conditions: uveitis, choroiditis, retinal vasculitis, conjunctivitis, and scleritis
- Host response to antigen rather than active disease and natural course is weeks to months.

LYME'S DISEASE
- *Borrelia burgdorferi*
- Spirochete; *Ixodes scapularis* from tick
- Bilateral, focal, and avascular
- Poorly defined nebulous lesions seen in all stromal levels; iritis and fine KP may be present
- May progress to vascularization and scarring
- IK is a late manifestation and is immune- mediated
- Associated disease: Erythema migrans rash, constitutional symptoms, migratory joint and muscle pain, cranial nerve palsies, and optic neuritis

HERPETIC INTERSTITIAL KERATITIS
- **Herpes Simplex Virus**
  - Unilateral, diffuse or sectoral
  - Frequently begins as disciform keratitis
  - Followed by deep corneal infiltrates associated with iritis
  - Deep and superficial vessels
  - Reduced corneal sensation
  - HSV serologies useful only for exclusion
- **Hepes Zoster Virus (Varicella Zoster Virus)**
  - Develops 2–3 weeks after acute epithelial keratitis or dermatitis (shingles)
  - Unilateral, anterior stromal infiltrates, disciform keratitis, Wessely ring (immune ring infiltrate)
  - Sequelae: lipid deposition, scarring, deep neovascularization
  - Immune-mediated
  - Reduced corneal sensation
  - May be seen in inactive stage

COGAN'S SYNDROME
First described by Cogan in 1945 as nonsyphilitic IK with vestibuloauditory symptoms
- **Typical Cogan's**
  - IK and vestibuloauditory symptoms (vertigo, tinnitus, and hearing loss)
- **Atypical Cogan's:**
  - Vestibuloauditory disease (as above)
- **Ocular inflammatory disease other than IK**
  - Posterior uveitis, subconjunctival hemorrhage, scleritis, episcleritis, retinal hemorrhage, disk edema, conjunctivitis, and orbital inflammation
- **Systemic associations**
  - 10% systemic large vessel vasculitis:
  - Polyarteritis, aortic insufficiency, coronary stenosis, and brain infarcts
  - Underlying rheumatologic disease in up to 50% of patients with atypical Cogan's
  - Polyarteritis nodosum, Wegener's granulomatosis, rheumatoid arthritis, Crohn's disease, and relapsing polychondritis
- Usually bilateral, sudden-onset severe pain, tearing, and photophobia
- **Early:** peripheral subepithelial keratitis with faint nummular lesions; begins peripherally and superficially
- **Late:** involves deep stroma; ± uveitis; variable mild late vascularization
- Vestibuloauditory symptoms develop within 1 month (before or after IK)
- Autoimmune hypersensitivity reaction to antigen present in corneal stroma and inner ear; can be preceded by upper respiratory infection (URI)
- Can progress to deafness in 3 months if untreated.

Other
Epstein–Barr Virus (EBV)
- Bilateral nummular keratitis
- Vascularization variable (usually avascular)
- Parotiditis
- Mononucleosis confirmed by positive heterophil antibody test

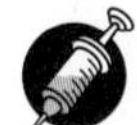

TREATMENT

SYPHILIS
- Topical corticosteroids and cycloplegics
- Primary, secondary, and early latent stages:
  - 2.4 million units PCN G IM × 1
- Late congenital:
  - 2.4 million units PCN G i.v. or i.v. for 10 days
- Lumbar puncture to r/o neurosyphilis:
  - 24 million units PCN G i.v. for 10–14 days

TUBERCULOSIS (TB)
- Topical corticosteroid and cycloplegics
- Treat underlying TB: usually multidrug Rx
  - Isoniazid
  - Rifampin
  - Pyrazinamide
  - Streptomycin or ethambutol

LYME'S DISEASE
- Topical corticosteroid and cycloplegics
- Systemic antibiotics if no prior treatment:
  - i.v. penicillin
  - Ceftriaxone
  - Cefotaxime
  - Tetracycline/doxycycline

HERPETIC DISEASE
- Topical corticosteroid ± trifluridine 1% and cycloplegics[3]
- Oral antiviral agents:
  - Acyclovir (ACV)
  - Valcyclovir
  - Famciclovir
- Although oral antivirals did not reduce established stromal inflammation, in the treatment group of topical steroid and trifluridine, the addition of oral antiviral was superior to placebo in causing visual improvement at 6 months follow-up (5).
- Prophylactic treatment of HSV stromal keratitis patients with oral acycolvir resulted in a statistically significant reduction of ocular (14% treated vs. 28% placebo) and orofacial recurrences during a 12-month treatment and 6-month follow-up period. Consider antiviral prophylaxis ACV 400 mg b.i.d if >1 episode (6).

COGAN'S DISEASE
- Topical corticosteroids and cycloplegics
- Prednisone 2 mg/kg for first week; slow taper
- Systemic immunosuppression for underlying systemic disease or disease unresponsive to corticosteroids alone.
- Check MRI inner ear, audiogram, and echocardiogram if diagnosis is suspected and start high-dose steroids.

SURGERY/OTHER PROCEDURES
- Penetrating keratoplasty (PKP)
- Deep anterior lamellar keratoplasty (DALK) (7)
- High-risk of graft rejection with active corneal neovascularization
- Consider antiviral prophylaxis in herpetic disease and PKP (8).

ONGOING CARE

FOLLOW-UP RECOMMENDATIONS

Patient Monitoring
- Follow patients weekly until inflammation is controlled.
- Goal is to have patients on least amount of topical corticosteroid to control inflammation and permanent corneal scarring
- Infectious Disease consult when indicated

REFERENCES

1. Knox MC, Holsclaw DS. Interstitial keratitis. *Int Ophthalmol Clin*. 1998;38:183–195. [A]
2. Schwartz GS, Harrison AR, Holland EJ. Etiology of immune stromal (interstitial) keratitis. *Cornea* 1998 May;17:271–281. [A]
3. Liu E, Slomovic AR. Indications for penetrating keratoplasty in Canada, 1986–1995.*Cornea* 1997;16:414–419. [A]
4. Dorrepaal SJ, Cao KY, Slomovic AR. Indications for penetrating keratoplasty in a tertiary care referral centre In Canada, 1996–2004. *Can J Ophthalmol* 2007;42:244–250. [A]
5. Wilhelmus KR, Gee L, Hauck WW, et al: Herpetic eye disease study. A controlled trial of topical corticosteroids for herpes simplex stromal keratitis. *Ophthalmology* 1994;101:1883–1895; discussion 95–96.
6. Herpetic Eye Disease Study Group: Oral Acyclovir for herpes simplex virus:effect on prevention of epithelial keratitis and stromal keratitis. *Arch Ophthalmol* 2000;118:1030–1036.
7. Sarnicola V, Toro P. Deep anterior lamellar keratoplasty in herpes simplex corneal opacities. *Cornea* 2010;29:60–64.
8. Tambasco FP, Cohen EJ, Nguyen LH, et al. Oral acyclovir after penetrating keratoplasty for herpes simplex keratitis.*Arch Ophthalmol* 1999;117: 445–449.

CODES

ICD9
- 053.21 Herpes zoster keratoconjunctivitis
- 090.3 Syphilitic interstitial keratitis
- 370.50 Interstitial keratitis, unspecified

CLINICAL PEARLS
- **Unilateral:** Acquired syphilis, TB, mumps, herpetic disease, and Cogan's syndrome
- **Bilateral:** Congenital syphilis, leprosy, EBV, Lyme's disease, Cogan's syndrome, and onchocerciasis

INTRAOPERATIVE FLOPPY IRIS SYNDROME (IFIS)

Brad H. Feldman
Mark H. Blecher

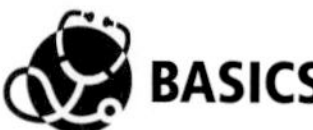

BASICS

DESCRIPTION

- An iris abnormality that may manifest preoperatively with poor pupil dilation and may manifest intraoperatively with some or all of the following findings:
  - Billowing of the iris stroma during normal irrigation
  - Iris prolapse to corneal incisions
  - Poor maintenance of dilation with progressive miosis (pupil constriction)
  - Ineffectiveness of pupillary stretching to maintain pupil expansion

EPIDEMIOLOGY

Occurs in males > females

Prevalence

In the US, occurs in ~2–3% of cataract surgeries

RISK FACTORS

- Most frequent and severe in patients exposed to selective α_1-antagonists
  Associated α_1-antagonists:
  - 1A selective
    - Tamsulosin (Flomax): up to 90% of patients taking this drug may have IFIS
    - Alfuzosin (Uroxatral): up to 15% of patients taking this drug have IFIS
    - Silodosin (Rapaflo): unknown%
  - Nonselective: lower risk
    - Terazosin (Hytrin)
    - Doxazosin (Cardura)
    - Naftopidil (Flivas)
    Use of other medicines/supplements: lowest risk
  - 5-alpha reductase inhibitors
    - Finasteride
    - Dutasteride (Avodart)
  - Saw palmetto
  - Antipsychotic drugs

GENERAL PREVENTION

Avoidance of associated medications

PATHOPHYSIOLOGY

- Alpha 1A iris smooth muscle adrenoreceptor may be blocked by associated antagonists.
- Blockage may lead to loss of dilator muscle tone.
- Decreased dilator tone may lead to poor dilation and intraoperative floppiness.

ETIOLOGY

IFIS may occur even with short-term exposure to associated medications (≥2 days reported) or use in the distant past

COMMONLY ASSOCIATED CONDITIONS

Any condition treated with associated medications

- Benign prostatic hypertrophy
- Prostate cancer
- Urinary retention (men/women)
- Hypertension
- Hair loss
- Psychiatric disturbances

Geriatric Considerations

The incidence of benign prostatic hyperplasia (BPH) is ~50% in men >50 years and 90% in men >85 years of age.

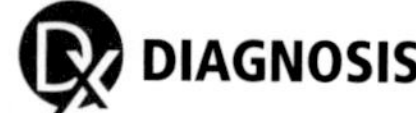

DIAGNOSIS

HISTORY

Important to screen all patients for current or past use of all associated agents

PHYSICAL EXAM

Poor or slow dilation preoperatively may suggest IFIS

DIFFERENTIAL DIAGNOSIS

- Poor preoperative dilation
  - Prior injury, inflammation, infection, or topical miotic use
- Iris prolapse
  - Short or inadequately constructed wounds
  - High intracameral pressure

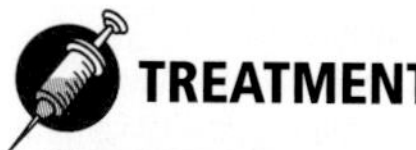

TREATMENT

MEDICATION

- Stopping associated agent preoperatively
  - May improve dilation but will not typically decrease IFIS severity
  - Most surgeons do not stop these agents
- Preoperative atropine
  - Improves dilation but does not reliably decrease IFIS severity
- Intracameral α_1-agonist injections (preservative-free only)
  - Epinephrine 1:1000 mixed 1:3 or 1:4 with balanced salt solution to buffer
  - Phenylephrine (not available in the US)

ADDITIONAL TREATMENT

General Measures

- Highly cohesive ophthalmic viscoelastic devices (OVD)
  - Sodium hyaluronate 2.3% (Healon5) may facilitate pupil expansion and prevent iris movement
- Other specialized viscoelastics
  - Hyaluronic acid 1.6% and chondroitin sulfate 4.0% (DisCoVisc) may remain in the eye longer with higher flow rates

SURGERY/OTHER PROCEDURES

- Longer, more stable, wound tunnels may decrease iris prolapse
- Pupil expansion
  - Pupillary rings: Malyugin (Microsurgical technology), Graether silicone ring (Eagle Vision), 5S Pupil Ring (Morcher GmbH), Perfect Pupil (Milvella Ltd.)
  - Iris retractors/hooks: Disposable 6–0 nylon (Alcon) or reusable 4–0 polypropylene (Katena Products, FCI, Oasis Medical)

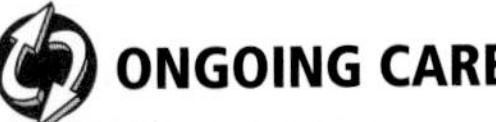

ONGOING CARE

PATIENT EDUCATION

- Patients should be informed of risks of associated medicines.
- Prescribing physicians should consider referring patients to an ophthalmologist for consultation before starting these medicines.
- Patients must inform their ophthalmologists if they are currently or have ever taken these medicines.

COMPLICATIONS

- IFIS is associated with a higher rate of posterior capsule rupture, vitreous loss, and iris damage.
- The rate of complication is highest when the ophthalmologist is unaware of patient use of associated medicines.

ADDITIONAL READING

- Chang DF, Braga-Mele R, Mamalis N, et al. ASCRS white paper: Clinical review of floppy-iris syndrome. *J Cataract Refract Surg* 2008;34:2153–2161.
- Chang DF, Campbell JR. Intraoperative floppy-iris syndrome associated with tamsulosin. *J Cataract Refract Surg* 2005;31:664–673.
- Chang DF, Osher RH, Wang L, et al. Prospective multicenter evaluation of cataract surgery in patients taking tamsulosin (Flomax). *Ophthalmology* 2007;114:957–964.

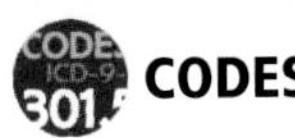

CODES

ICD9

364.81 Floppy iris syndrome

CLINICAL PEARLS

- IFIS is associated with α_1-antagonist use.
- Outcomes are best if IFIS risk is identified preoperatively.
- Several strategies can be used to successfully manage IFIS intraoperatively.
- Patients and physicians should be educated about IFIS risks.

I

IRIDOCORNEAL ENDOTHELIAL (ICE) SYNDROME

Michael J. Pro

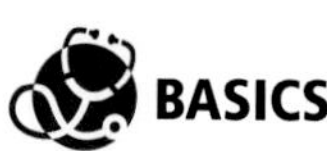

BASICS

DESCRIPTION

An acquired and usually unilateral condition affecting young and middle-aged women. The condition causes various degrees of iris abnormalities, corneal edema, and glaucoma in affected individuals. The etiology is unknown, but is thought to be due to a viral infection. It affects all races. The hallmark of the condition is an abnormal corneal endothelium, which advances onto the anterior chamber angle and iris.

Pediatric Considerations

It rarely affects children. A case of an 11-year-old girl with ICE syndrome and glaucoma was reported (1).

Geriatric Considerations

Older patients may have limitation in vision in the affected eye due to corneal disease and/or glaucomatous optic nerve damage.

Pregnancy Considerations

Glaucoma medications may need to be adjusted during pregnancy and nursing.

EPIDEMIOLOGY

ICE syndrome is a very rare condition with no known genetic risk factors.

GENERAL PREVENTION

There is no known preventive measure ICE syndrome.

ETIOLOGY

Thought to be due to a viral infection. In one study 5 out of 9 corneal specimens were positive for herpes simplex virus (HSV) DNA in the corneal endothelium. The specimens were negative for herpes zoster virus or Epstein–Barr virus DNA (2).

COMMONLY ASSOCIATED CONDITIONS

- There are 3 variants that have slightly different presentations and courses. All 3 variants are associated with corneal disease and glaucoma.
- Essential or progressive iris atrophy is notable for corectopia (distorted pupil) or pseudopolycoria (a "second" pupil). Marked iris atrophy is a hallmark of this variant. Severe anterior segment abnormalities may include extensive peripheral anterior synechiae (PAS). PAS formation is progressive, leading to angle closure and frequently elevated intraocular pressure (IOP). Secondary angle-closure glaucoma is present in at least 50% of individuals.
- Iris nevus syndrome (Cogan Reese) is notable for the presence of a large nevus covering a large part of the iris or multiple iris nodules. Specimens from eyes enucleated for presumed malignancy demonstrated iris tissue in these nevi.
- Chandler's syndrome is notable for a corneal endothelium with a characteristic "hammered silver" appearance. Chandler's syndrome variant has a lower incidence of glaucoma and a higher incidence of corneal edema due to dysfunction of normal endothelial function.

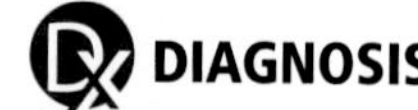

DIAGNOSIS

HISTORY

Signs and symptoms:

- Almost always has a unilateral presentation
- Decreased vision due to corneal edema, which is frequently worse in the morning upon awakening
- Pain is usually due to corneal edema, but may be from elevated IOP later on in the course of the disease.
- Iris abnormalities noticed by patient or family and friends
- Decreased visual function due to glaucoma is present in advanced disease.

PHYSICAL EXAM

Slit lamp exam can demonstrate corneal edema and abnormal corneal endothelial appearance. Areas of abnormal corneal endothelium may be seen in the fellow eye. Iris atrophy and pupillary irregularity or decentration are hallmarks of progressive iris atrophy. Gonioscopy can reveal complete angle closure, especially in essential iris atrophy.

DIAGNOSTIC TESTS & INTERPRETATION

- Visual acuity may be reduced in the affected eye and may fluctuate with varying degrees of corneal edema.
- Visual field may be abnormal if there is co-existing glaucomatous optic neuropathy.

Imaging

- Optic nerve imaging can be helpful in establishing diagnosis of glaucoma or assisting in detection of glaucoma progression. Imaging devices include optic nerve photography, optical coherence tomography (OCT), confocal scanning laser ophthalmoscopy (Heidelberg Retina Tomograph – HRT), and scanning laser polarimetry (GDx).
- Corneal disease is mostly followed clinically, but specular microscopy can demonstrate characteristic endothelial cell abnormality with variability in cell size and shape as well as loss of the normal clear hexagonal margins.
- Pachymetry can be useful to quantify corneal thickening.

DIFFERENTIAL DIAGNOSIS

- Fuch's dystrophy may have a similar corneal appearance, but with no anterior chamber abnormalities.
- PPMD—may appear similar, but is familial and bilateral
- Axenfeld Riegers is congenital and bilateral and may have systemic findings, such as dental abnormalities.
- Iris melanomas can appear similar to pure Cogan–Reese syndrome.

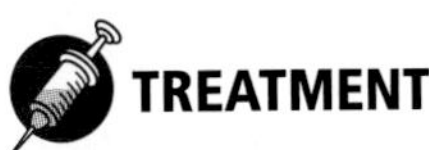

TREATMENT

ADDITIONAL TREATMENT

General Measures

- Corneal edema can be treated with hypertonic saline drops or ointment (sodium chloride solution or ointment 5%).
- Elevated IOP and glaucoma can be treated with anti-glaucoma drops.
- Laser trabeculoplasty is not usually beneficial in this type of chronic angle-closure glaucoma.
- Laser peripheral iridotomy does not halt the progression of progressive angle closure that is a hallmark of this condition.

SURGERY/OTHER PROCEDURES

- Cataract surgery can be complicated by poor papillary dilation and the presence of an ICE membrane over the anterior capsule.
- Corneal transplants are performed for chronically edematous and hazy corneas. Newer partial-thickness corneal transplant procedures may reduce the incidence of rejection. Descemet Stripping Automated Endothelial Keratoplasty (DSAEK) involves Descemet's and endothelial membrane transplant.
- Iris reconstruction surgery for improved cosmetic appearance or to ameliorate glare can be undertaken alone or at the time of cataract surgery. The iris tissue is often friable and difficult to suture. Artificial iris implantation can be useful (3).
- Glaucoma in ICE syndrome may be more severe and refractory to surgical management. Trabeculectomy may fail more frequently, and this is thought to be partially due to growth of abnormal corneal endothelium over the internal scleral ostium. Trabeculectomy in patients with Chandler's syndrome may be more successful than in the other variants.
- Trabeculectomy may be more successful if performed with an anti-metabolite such as mitomycin C
- Glaucoma drainage implants (tube shunts) may be more successful than trabeculectomy as they may be less likely to be blocked with an endothelial membrane (4).

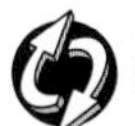

ONGOING CARE

FOLLOW-UP RECOMMENDATIONS

Patient Monitoring

- Affected individuals should be followed up periodically for routine eye care. Mild cases without glaucoma may be seen yearly.
- Monitoring for development of glaucoma includes evaluation of optic nerve appearance with either direct or indirect ophthalmoscopy. Visual field testing and optic nerve imaging may also be appropriate.
- Individuals with glaucoma or corneal disease may need more frequent monitoring
- Corneal decompensation and glaucoma may require sub-specialty referral.

PROGNOSIS

- Visual prognosis is mostly related to severity of glaucoma but may be affected by success in restoration of corneal clarity.
- Complications from cataract surgery can also affect visual prognosis.
- Visual prognosis is generally more poor for individuals who reject multiple corneal transplants.
- Irregular refractive errors after corneal surgery may require use of specialty contact lenses.

REFERENCES

1. Salim S, Shields MB, Walton D. Iridocorneal endothelial syndrome in a child. *J Pediatr Ophthalmol Strabismus* 2006;43:308–310.
2. Alvarado JA, Underwood JL, Green WR, et al. Detection of herpes simplex viral DNA in the iridocorneal endothelial syndrome. *Arch Ophthalmol* 1994;112:1601–1609.
3. Khng C, Snyder ME. Iris reconstruction with a multipiece endocapsular prosthesis in iridocorneal endothelial syndrome. *J Cataract Refract Surg* 2005;31:2051–2054.
4. Doe EA, Budenz DL, Gedde SJ, Imami NR. Long-term surgical outcomes of patients with glaucoma secondary to the iridocorneal endothelial syndrome. *Ophthalmology* 2001;108:1789–1795.

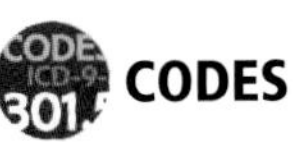

CODES

ICD9

- 365.43 Glaucoma associated with other anterior segment anomalies
- 371.20 Corneal edema, unspecified

IRIS ATROPHY

Anita P. Schadlu
Ramin Schadlu

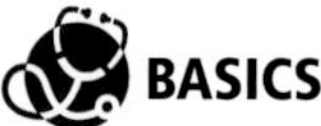

BASICS

DESCRIPTION

- Iris atrophy can be caused by a myriad of ocular disorders.
  - The etiology can be determined by careful history taking and physical examination.

Pediatric Considerations

Iris atrophy in the pediatric population may indicate syndromes such as ocular albinism or Axenfeld–Rieger syndrome.

Pregnancy Considerations

Iris atrophy with uveitis in a pregnant patient may suggest a diagnosis of herpes simplex, herpes zoster, or Fuchs' heterochromic iridocyclitis (linked to rubella virus). All of these infectious etiologies should be addressed.

EPIDEMIOLOGY

Incidence

The incidence varies depending upon the etiology and the population in question. Iridocorneal endothelial (ICE) syndrome is quite rare, whereas herpes zoster iritis occurs in ~43% of patients with herpes zoster ophthalmicus, a fairly common condition (1).

Prevalence

The prevalence varies depending upon the etiology of the iris atrophy. In patients with Fuchs' heterochromic iridocyclitis, the prevalence of iris atrophy approaches 90% (2).

RISK FACTORS

History of common causes of iris atrophy such as chronic or recurrent uveitis and certain types of glaucoma

Genetics

- Axenfeld–Rieger syndrome is autosomal dominant. The responsible gene has been isolated to chromosome 4q25.
- Ocular albinism follows all of the inheritance patterns, including X-linked recessive pattern.

PATHOPHYSIOLOGY

- In cases of chronic inflammation, iris atrophy manifests as loss of detail and density of the anterior iris as the iris stroma breaks down.
- In Axenfeld–Rieger syndrome, iris atrophy results from abnormal embryologic development of the iris and anterior chamber angle.
- In ocular albinism, the number of melanosomes in the iris pigment epithelium is decreased, resulting in transillumination defects.

ETIOLOGY

- Herpes simplex uveitis
- Herpes zoster uveitis
- Fuchs' heterochromic iridocyclitis
- Pigment dispersion syndrome and secondary glaucoma
- Pseudophakic pigment dispersion from iris chafing
- Traumatic or iatrogenic
- ICE syndrome
  - Essential iris atrophy subtype
  - Minimal iris atrophy may also be seen in Chandler's syndrome and Cogan–Reese syndrome subtypes.
- Axenfeld–Rieger syndrome
- Ocular albinism
- Ischemic iridopathy
  - Diabetic
  - Ocular ischemic syndrome
  - Systemic cryoglobulinemia

COMMONLY ASSOCIATED CONDITIONS

- Chronic uveitis
- Glaucoma
- Cataract

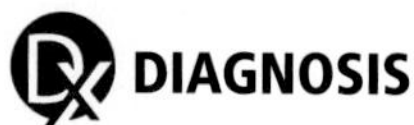

DIAGNOSIS

HISTORY

Patients may be any age. They should be questioned for a history of recurrent red eye, pain, glaucoma, and visual loss.

PHYSICAL EXAM

- The patient's visual acuity and intraocular pressure should be accurately determined.
  - Increased intraocular pressure can be seen in:
    - Herpes simplex uveitis, herpes zoster uveitis, Fuchs' heterochromic uveitis, any form of chronic uveitis, ICE syndrome, Axenfeld–Rieger syndrome, and pigment dispersion glaucoma
- Laterality of the iris atrophy is important in making the diagnosis of the underlying disease.
- Fuchs' heterochromic iridocyclitis and herpetic uveitis are typically unilateral, but can be bilateral. ICE syndrome is unilateral, whereas Axenfeld—Rieger syndrome is bilateral.
- Iris atrophy can be subtle. It is best detected by performing transillumination in the slit-lamp exam.
- Different patterns of iris atrophy may suggest the underlying disorder
  - Iris atrophy at the pupillary margin and/or persistent pupillary dilation suggests herpes simplex uveitis (3).
  - Sectoral iris atrophy suggests herpes zoster uveitis or herpes simplex uveitis (4).
  - Diffuse atrophy suggests Fuchs' heterochromic iridocyclitis.
  - Radial iris atrophy suggests pigment dispersion syndrome (which can cause secondary glaucoma). This pattern results from the lens zonules eroding the iris pigment epithelium.
  - Iris corectopia, ectropion uveae, and/or iris hole formation can be seen in ICE and Axenfeld–Rieger syndromes.
- The corneal exam can also aid in diagnosis.
  - Corneal edema can be seen in ICE syndrome.
  - Keratic precipitates on the corneal endothelium suggest prior or current anterior uveitis. Diffuse keratic precipitates are seen in herpetic uveitis and Fuchs' heterochromic uveitis.
- Gonioscopy should be performed.
  - Peripheral anterior synechiae suggest prior uveitis or ICE syndrome.
  - Heavily pigmented trabecular meshwork suggests pigment dispersion syndrome.
- The presence of a cataract can suggest chronic uveitis.
- The posterior segment examination is important in the workup of iris atrophy.
  - The optic nerve should be evaluated for glaucomatous cupping.
  - The retina should be examined for signs of ocular albinism as well as ischemic processes.

DIAGNOSTIC TESTS & INTERPRETATION

Lab

Initial lab tests

- Laboratory testing is not often indicated, but can be directed by the suspected underlying diagnosis.
  - PCR can be performed on aqueous samples to detect herpes simplex, varicella zoster, or rubella virus.

Follow-up & special considerations

Patients with iris atrophy from any etiology should be monitored for glaucoma, cataract formation, and visual loss.

Imaging
- Slit-lamp photographs with and without transillumination may be obtained to document the degree of iris atrophy.
- In cases where iris-chafe from an intraocular lens implant or dislocated crystalline lens is suspected, anterior-segment high-resolution biomicroscopy can be performed to identify the lens location.

DIFFERENTIAL DIAGNOSIS
- Herpes simplex uveitis
- Herpes zoster uveitis
- Fuchs' heterochromic iridocyclitis
- Pigment dispersion syndrome and secondary glaucoma
- Pseudophakic pigment dispersion
- Iatrogenic
- Trauma
- ICE syndrome
- Axenfeld–Rieger syndrome
- Ocular albinism
- Ischemic iridopathy
  - Diabetic
  - Ocular ischemic syndrome
  - Systemic cryoglobulinemia

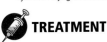

TREATMENT

MEDICATION
- The underlying condition should be treated, if indicated, with topical steroids or oral antivirals.
- Glaucoma should be treated with topical drops and surgery if indicated.

ADDITIONAL TREATMENT
Issues for Referral
- Patients in whom the IOP is not controlled with topical drops, or who have progressive visual field loss, should be referred to a glaucoma specialist.
- Patients with suspected Axenfeld–Rieger syndrome or ocular albinism should be evaluated by a pediatrician and a geneticist.

SURGERY/OTHER PROCEDURES
Cataract surgery and glaucoma surgery may be indicated in the management of patients with iris atrophy due to various causes.

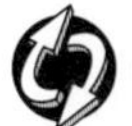

ONGOING CARE

FOLLOW-UP RECOMMENDATIONS
Patients need regularly scheduled follow-up visits depending on the presence of glaucoma and cataracts.

PATIENT EDUCATION
- Patients should be educated on the need for regular follow up and the importance of compliance with glaucoma medications.
- Patients with genetic causes of iris atrophy should receive genetic counseling.

PROGNOSIS
Visual prognosis varies depending on the etiology of the iris atrophy.

REFERENCES

1. Thean JH, Hall AJ, Stawell RJ. Uveitis in herpes zoster ophthalmicus. *Clin Experiment Ophthalmol* 2001;29:406–410.
2. Tugal-Tutkun I, Güney-Tefekli E, Kamaci-Duman F, et al. A cross-sectional and longitudinal study of Fuchs uveitis syndrome in Turkish patients. *Am J Ophthalmol* 2009;148:510–515.
3. Goldstein DA, Mis AA, Oh FS, et al. Persistent pupillary dilation in herpes simplex uveitis. *Can J Ophthalmol* 2009;44:314–316.
4. Van der Lelij A, Ooijaman FM, Kijlstra A, et al. Anterior uveitis with sectoral iris atrophy in the absence of keratitis: A distinct clinical entity among herpetic eye diseases. *Ophthalmology* 2000;107:1164–1170.

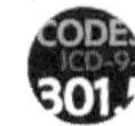

CODES

ICD9
- 270.2 Other disturbances of aromatic amino-acid metabolism
- 364.3 Unspecified iridocyclitis
- 364.59 Other iris atrophy

CLINICAL PEARLS
- Iris atrophy is an important finding that can alert the clinician to the presence of underlying vision-threatening disease.
- The detection of iris atrophy requires careful slit-lamp examination with transillumination.

IRIS MELANOMA

Carlos Bianciotto
Carol L. Shields

ALERT
Any pigmented iris lesion should be carefully checked for tumor seeding, secondary glaucoma, and intrinsic vessels, features that are found with iris melanoma.

Pediatric Considerations

A study of 40 young patients with uveal melanoma (age <20 years) by Shields and associates indicated that iris melanoma in this patient age group is more common (12%) than in adults (4%; ref. 1)[A].

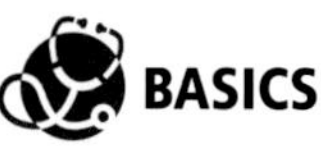

BASICS

DESCRIPTION

- Iris melanoma represents a malignant melanocytic neoplasm arising from the iris stroma. Iris melanoma is uncommon, representing only 4% of all uveal melanomas. In a series of 169 consecutive patients with iris melanoma, elevated intraocular pressure (IOP) was found in 30% of cases. The main mechanism for the elevated pressure was mechanical obstruction of aqueous outflow from solid tumor or seeding (2)[A].
- Iris melanoma has potential to metastasize to liver, lungs, or skin.
- Iris melanoma can assume different clinical presentations such as circumscribed, diffuse, tapioca, or trabecular meshwork configuration. Size, shape, and degree of pigmentation can vary from case to case. Similar to iris nevus, iris melanoma can cause corectopia and ectropion of the pupillary margin. More than 80% of iris melanomas are located in the inferior half of the iris.
  - Circumscribed iris melanoma is the most common type and presents as a well-defined mass in the iris stroma.
  - Diffuse iris melanoma is less common and tends to produce acquired hyperchromic heterochromia with secondary glaucoma due to infiltration of the trabecular meshwork by tumor cells. It can affect the entire iris or only patches of its surface.
  - Tapioca melanoma is a rare variant that presents characteristic translucent, fine nodules on the surface of the tumor resembling tapioca pudding.
  - Trabecular meshwork melanoma affects the angle without the presence of a distinct mass, and it is usually associated with secondary ipsilateral glaucoma, which can cause a delay in diagnosis due to its resemblance to pigmentary glaucoma.
  - Other less common presentations include spontaneous hyphema or iridocyclitis.
  - Seeding of tumor cells on the iris surface or on the anterior chamber angle is a characteristic finding in many cases of iris melanoma. It is usually visualized as clumps of fine pigmented cells on slit-lamp exam or gonioscopy.

EPIDEMIOLOGY

Incidence

Iris melanoma represents <5% of all uveal melanomas. (Uveal melanoma has an estimated incidence of 6 cases per million per year in the US).

RISK FACTORS

- White race
- Inferior iris location (>80% of iris melanomas are located below the horizontal meridian of the iris)
- In an article by Territo and associates, the features that were associated with enlargement of the lesion included medial location of the mass on the iris and presence of pigment dispersion onto the adjacent iris and anterior chamber angle structures (3)[A]. Another article by Kliman and coworkers found a strong association between light iris color (blue, gray, or green) and the presence of iris melanocytic lesions (4)[A].

Genetics

- Iris melanomas can demonstrate monosomy, partial monosomy, or disomy of chromosome 3, 6, or 8 on genetic testing performed with microarray through fine needle aspiration biopsy (FNAB).
- These genetic features have been proven to be related to high risk (monosomy) or low risk (disomy) for systemic metastasis.

GENERAL PREVENTION

- Decrease sun exposure
- Periodic follow-up of suspicious iris lesions with ophthalmologist

PATHOPHYSIOLOGY

Malignant transformation of melanocytic iris stromal cells

ETIOLOGY

Unknown

COMMONLY ASSOCIATED CONDITIONS

- Unilateral secondary glaucoma
- Ocular melanocytosis

DIAGNOSIS

HISTORY

- Slow-growing pigmented or non-pigmented iris lesion (iris melanoma) noticed by the patient or the ophthalmologist on a routine eye visit
- Can be associated with pain or decreased vision in cases of iris melanoma with secondary glaucoma

PHYSICAL EXAM

- Secondary glaucoma with iris nevi is rare; therefore, elevated IOP should raise suspicion of malignancy. In a series of 169 patients with iris melanoma described by Shields and associates, the mean age at the time of diagnosis was 43 years, all patients were white, the mean tumor base was 6 mm, mean tumor thickness was 2 mm, the mean number of clock hours of tumor involvement in the iris as well as tumor seeding on the iris and on the anterior chamber angle was 4, and extraocular extension was present in 10 eyes (6%; ref. 5)[A].
- Other common features of iris melanoma are intrinsic and feeder vessels.

DIAGNOSTIC TESTS & INTERPRETATION

Lab

Initial lab tests

- Imaging tests include ultrasonographic biomicroscopy (UBM), anterior segment optical coherence tomography (AS-OCT), and anterior segment photography.
- Liver function tests, liver MRI, chest X-Ray, and complete physical exam

Imaging

Initial approach

- Slit-lamp examination and anterior segment photography
- IOP measurement
- Perform gonioscopy to assess angle involvement by tumor or seeds
- Perform transillumination to rule out ciliary body involvement
- UBM to measure thickness and to rule out associated ciliary body involvement or the presence of a cystic lesion
- AS-OCT can also be useful for imaging small, nonpigmented iris lesions, although it is limited by posterior shadowing in more pigmented, larger lesions

Follow-up & special considerations

- Follow-up every 6 months after treatment of iris melanoma to evaluate tumor regression and rule out recurrence
- Slit-lamp examination, anterior segment photography, UBM, gonioscopy, IOP measurement, and transillumination should be repeated at every visit.
- Systemic work up should be performed every 6 months lifelong to rule out the presence of systemic metastasis.
- Physical exam and liver function tests twice a year and liver MRI and chest X-Ray once a year, lifelong.

Diagnostic Procedures/Other

FNAB for cytology or cytogenetic analysis is a useful tool in the diagnosis of borderline iris lesions. The specimen should be interpreted by an experienced ophthalmic cytopathologist.

Pathological Findings

- Jakobiec and associates described the histopathologic features of 189 cases of excised iris melanomas and found that only 13% of them presented spindle B and epithelioid cells (6)[A].
- Some borderline cases of iris nevus are difficult to differentiate from low-grade iris melanoma, even for experienced pathologists.

DIFFERENTIAL DIAGNOSIS

- Iris nevus
- Iris melanocytoma
- Foreign body in the anterior chamber
- Irido-corneal endothelial (ICE) syndrome
- Iris lymphoma
- Iris pigment epithelium (IPE) cysts
- Adenoma (epithelioma) of the IPE
- Iris metastasis
- Iris granuloma
- Iris juvenile xanthogranuloma (JXG)

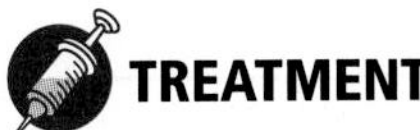

TREATMENT

MEDICATION

First Line

Currently, there are no effective medications for the treatment of iris melanoma.

Second Line

After surgical treatment, either with plaque brachytherapy or excision, atropine 1% once a day and Maxitrol (ointment) 3 times a day for a period of 6 weeks are prescribed to decrease inflammation, pain, and to avoid the formation of posterior synechiae.

- Bevacizumab (Avastin) 0.05 mg intravitreal or intracameral injection can be used in association with plaque radiotherapy or surgical excision, because iris melanoma was demonstrated to have vascular endothelial growth factor (VEGF) receptors according to reports from the ophthalmic literature.

ADDITIONAL TREATMENT

Issues for Referral

Glaucoma-filtering procedures such as trabeculectomy should be avoided because of the risk for spread of tumor cells outside the eye through the opening. A preferred method for lowering the IOP in these cases is through the use of glaucoma medications or laser cyclophotocoagulation.

SURGERY/OTHER PROCEDURES

- Lesions with unequivocal documented growth require treatment.
- Excisional biopsy (iridectomy, iridocyclectomy, or iridogoniocyclectomy for cases with concomitant ciliary body involvement) should be considered in circumscribed tumors, in the absence of seeds or elevated IOP.
- Plaque radiotherapy can be used to treat selected cases of unresectable iris melanoma or when the tumor is located in the patient's only eye with useful vision. It can be used for larger tumors, those with a diffuse configuration, and in cases with tumor seeding in the anterior chamber or angle. Plaque is an alternative for eyes with iris melanoma in cases that would have been enucleated in the past (7)[A].
- Enucleation should be considered for diffuse tumors affecting more than half of the iris surface and trabecular meshwork, in cases with secondary glaucoma not responsive to IOP-lowering medications, diffuse tumor seeding into the anterior chamber and/or painful eye. Visual status of the contralateral eye should be assessed before proceeding with enucleation.

IN-PATIENT CONSIDERATIONS

Iris melanoma is managed on an outpatient basis.

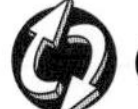

ONGOING CARE

FOLLOW-UP RECOMMENDATIONS

Biannual eye evaluations including slit-lamp exam, gonioscopy, anterior segment photography, UBM, transillumination, and IOP measurement

Patient Monitoring

- In a report by Shields and associates, radiation-related complications after plaque brachytherapy for iris melanoma at 5-year follow-up included corneal epitheliopathy (9%), cataract (70%), and neovascular glaucoma (8%). After treatment, the incidence of elevated IOP at 5 years was 33%. Tumor recurrence was found in 8%, and enucleation was necessary in 13% at 5 years (7)[A].
- Systemic work up should include physical exam and liver function tests twice a year and MRI of the liver and chest X-ray once a year to rule out the presence of metastasis.

DIET

No dietary restrictions

PATIENT EDUCATION

Avoid excessive sun exposure

PROGNOSIS

In a recent retrospective study of 8033 cases of uveal melanoma, there were 285 iris melanoma cases. The authors found a rates of metastasis of 0.5%, 4%, and 7% at 3, 5, and 10 years, making this tumor less likely to metastasize than choroidal melanoma (8)[A].

- Metastases from iris melanoma are more common in older patients, patients with secondary glaucoma, extraocular extension, and angle involvement (risk factors; ref. 5)[A].

COMPLICATIONS

- Cataract formation after surgical treatment with either surgical resection or plaque radiotherapy
- Secondary glaucoma (more common in patients with seeding and angle involvement)

REFERENCES

1. Shields CL, Shields JA, Milite J, et al. Uveal melanoma in teenagers and children. A report of 40 cases. *Ophthalmology* 1991;98:1662–1666.
2. Shields CL.Materin M, Shields JA, et al. Factors associated with elevated intraocular pressure in eyes with iris melanoma. *Br J Ophthalmol* 2001;85:666–669.
3. Territo C, Shields CL, Shields JA, et al. Natural course of melanocytic tumors of the iris. *Ophthalmology*1988;95:1251–1255.
4. Kliman GH, Augsburger JJ, Shields JA. Association between iris color and iris melanocytic lesions. *Am J Ophthalmol* 1985;100:547–548.
5. Shields CL, Shields JA, Materin M, et al. Iris melanoma: risk factors for metastasis in 169 consecutive patients. *Ophthalmology* 2001;108: 172–178.
6. Jakobiec FA, Silbert G. Are most iris "melanomas' really nevi? A clinicopathologic study of 189 lesions. *Arch Ophthalmol* 1981;99:2117–2132.
7. Shields CL, Naseripour M, Shields JA, et al. Custom designed plaque radiotherapy for non resectable iris melanoma in 38 patients: tumor control and ocular complications. *Am J Ophthalmol* 2003;135: 648–656.
8. Shields CL, Furuta M, Thangappan, et al. Metastasis of uveal melanoma millimeter-by-millimeter in 8033 consecutive eyes. *Arch Ophthalmol* 2009;127:989–998.

ADDITIONAL READING

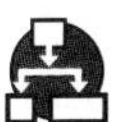

See Also (Topic, Algorithm, Electronic Media Element)

- www.fighteyecancer.com
- www.malignantmelanomainfo.com
- www.retinoblastomainfo.com
- www.eyecancerinfo.com
- www.eyecancerbook.com
- www.etrf.org

CODES

ICD9

190.0 Malignant neoplasm of eyeball, except conjunctiva, cornea, retina, and choroid

CLINICAL PEARLS

The management of iris melanoma with elevated IOP is challenging and requires enucleation in approximately 60% of cases. Filtering glaucoma procedures should be avoided in these patients due to the risk of extraocular extension.

IRIS NEVUS

Carlos Bianciotto
Carol L. Shields

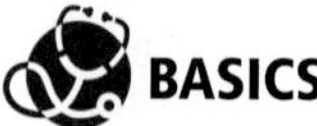

BASICS

DESCRIPTION

- Melanocytic tumors of the iris stroma include a wide spectrum of lesions, ranging from benign iris nevus to malignant iris melanoma.
- They can display a varied clinical presentation in terms of size, shape, and degree of pigmentation.
- Iris nevi are differentiated from freckles in that they efface the normal iris stromal architecture. Iris freckles can be found in >50% of the population and have no malignant potential.
- Iris nevi usually become clinically apparent during puberty or young adulthood.
- A special variant of iris nevus is melanocytoma, which is more darkly pigmented and can undergo necrosis and pigment dispersion, with subsequent secondary glaucoma through obstruction of the trabecular outflow—a condition referred to as "melanocytomalytic glaucoma". It can also present with an associated ciliary body component. Similar to other iris nevi, it can rarely undergo malignant transformation.
- Iris nevi can rarely grow into a melanoma, with a 5% rate of transformation of suspicious borderline iris nevi into melanoma within 5 years of diagnosis.

ALERT
A pigmented iris tumor that shows progressive enlargement could represent a melanoma.

Geriatric Considerations

Iris nevi are usually discovered in childhood and remain stable into adulthood.

Pediatric Considerations

Iris nevi are typically discovered in childhood, often in the preteen years, as a pigmented lesion of the iris.

EPIDEMIOLOGY

Prevalence

- Iris freckles can be found in ~60% of the population.
- Iris nevi occur in ~5% of the population.

RISK FACTORS

- White race
- Inferior iris location (>80% of iris nevi and melanomas are located below the horizontal meridian of the iris)
- A report by Kliman and associates found a strong correlation between light iris color (blue, gray, or green) and the presence of iris melanocytic lesions.

GENERAL PREVENTION

- Decrease sun exposure
  - Periodic follow-up of suspicious iris lesions with ophthalmologist

ETIOLOGY

Unknown

COMMONLY ASSOCIATED CONDITIONS

Ocular melanocytosis in the case of sector iris nevi

DIAGNOSIS

HISTORY

Stable iris lesion noticed by the patient or the ophthalmologist on a routine eye visit

PHYSICAL EXAM

- Iris nevus can assume multiple clinical presentations and can appear as small or large, circumscribed or diffuse, flat or dome shaped, and pigmented or non-pigmented lesions. Iris nevi can produce secondary changes such as corectopia, ectropion, secondary iris pigment epithelial cyst, or cataract. Further, iris nevi can stimulate the development of intrinsic and feeder vascularity.
- Secondary glaucoma with iris nevi is rare; therefore, elevated IOP should raise suspicion of malignancy.
- Another type of iris nevus is the sector iris nevus, in which the lesion extends from the pupillary margin to the angle and can affect 1 or multiple clock-hour positions. This is considered by some authors to be a localized form of ocular melanocytosis.
- Tapioca nevus presents with a multinodular surface that resembles tapioca pudding, similar to some iris melanoma cases.
- Diffuse iris nevus, also called Cogan–Reese syndrome, is part of the iridocorneal endothelial (ICE) syndrome and is not a true nevus.

DIAGNOSTIC TESTS & INTERPRETATION

Lab

Initial lab tests

Ultrasound biomicroscopy (UBM), anterior segment optical coherence tomography (AS-OCT), gonioscopy, and transillumination.

Imaging

Initial approach

- Slit-lamp examination and anterior segment photography
- Measurement of IOP
- Perform gonioscopy to assess angle involvement by tumor or seeds
- Perform transillumination to rule out ciliary body involvement
- UBM to measure thickness and to rule out associated ciliary body involvement or the presence of a cystic lesion
- AS-OCT can also be useful for imaging small, non-pigmented iris lesions, although it is limited by posterior shadowing in more pigmented, larger lesions

Follow-up & special considerations

- Follow-up every 6 months for iris nevi to document stability.
- Slit-lamp examination, anterior segment photography, UBM, gonioscopy, IOP measurement, and transillumination should be repeated at every visit.
- Follow up every 62 months to document stability of the lesion by an ophthalmologist.

Diagnostic Procedures/Other

Fine needle aspiration biopsy (FNAB) for cytologic analysis plays a key role in the diagnosis of suspicious iris lesions. The specimen should be interpreted by an experienced cytopathologist.

Pathological Findings
Iris nevi are usually composed of low-grade spindle cells. Some borderline cases of iris nevus are difficult to differentiate from low-grade iris melanoma, even for experienced pathologists.

DIFFERENTIAL DIAGNOSIS
- Iris melanoma
- Iris melanocytoma
- Ocular melanocytosis
- Foreign bodies in the anterior chamber
- ICE syndrome
- Iris lymphoma
- Iris pigment epithelium (IPE) cysts
- Adenoma (epithelioma) of the IPE
- Iris metastasis
- Iris granuloma
- Iris juvenile xanthogranuloma (JXG)

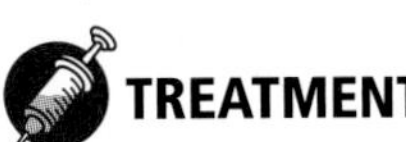

TREATMENT

MEDICATION
None

ADDITIONAL TREATMENT
General Measures
- Iris nevi only require observation every 6 months by an ophthalmologist, and baseline photographs and other pertinent tests, such as UBM, anterior segment OCT, gonioscopy, and transillumination, should be performed.
- If documented growth is evidenced, then the iris lesion should be treated like an iris melanoma.

Issues for Referral
Documentation of growth or secondary IOP elevation in an eye with a melanocytic iris lesion

Additional Therapies
Topical glaucoma medications should be used in patients with secondary IOP elevation, and cycloplegics and topical steroids should be used in patients with associated hyphema.

SURGERY/OTHER PROCEDURES
Only lesions that show documented growth require treatment.

IN-PATIENT CONSIDERATIONS
Outpatient management only

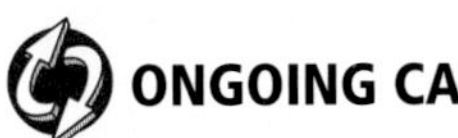

ONGOING CARE

FOLLOW-UP RECOMMENDATIONS
Biannual eye evaluations including slit-lamp exam, gonioscopy, anterior segment photography, UBM, transillumination, and IOP measurement

Patient Monitoring
Every 6–12 months by ophthalmologist

DIET
No dietary restrictions necessary

PATIENT EDUCATION
Avoid excessive sun exposure

PROGNOSIS
Good; the rate of malignant transformation of iris nevi is very low (<5% at 5 years of follow-up), based on a study by Territo and associates.

COMPLICATIONS
- Secondary cataract formation
- Secondary glaucoma (more common in patients with seeding and angle involvement)

ADDITIONAL READING

- Territo C, Shields CL, Shields JA, et al. Natural course of melanocytic tumors of the iris. *Ophthalmology* 1988;95:1251–1255.
- Kliman GH, Augsburger JJ, Shields JA. Association between iris color and iris melanocytic lesions. *Am J Ophthalmol* 1985;100:547–548.
- Fineman M, Shields JA, Eagle RC, et al. Melanocytomalytic glaucoma in eyes with necrotic iris melanocytoma. *Ophthalmology* 1998;105: 492–496.
- Shields JA, Sanborn GE, Augsburger JJ. The differential diagnosis of malignant melanoma of the iris: A clinical study of 200 cases. *Ophthalmology* 1983;90:716–720.
- Shields CL, Shields JA, Shields MB. Prevalence and mechanisms of secondary intraocular pressure elevation in eyes with intraocular tumors. *Ophthalmology* 1987;94:839–846.

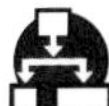

See Also (Topic, Algorithm, Electronic Media Element)

- www.fighteyecancer.com
- www.malignantmelanomainfo.com
- www.retinoblastomainfo.com
- www.eyecancerinfo.com
- www.eyecancerbook.com
- www.etrf.org

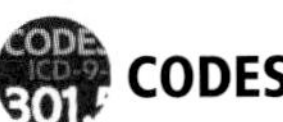

CODES

ICD9
224.0 Benign neoplasm of eyeball, except conjunctiva, cornea, retina, and choroid

CLINICAL PEARLS

- Only ~5% of untreated suspicious melanocytic iris lesions show growth over the first 5 years after diagnosis.

IRITIS-UVEITIS IN CHILDREN

Sharon S. Lehman

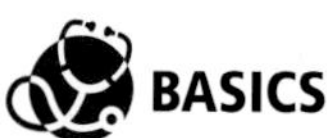

BASICS

DESCRIPTION
- Uveitis: intraocular inflammation
  - Anterior: involving iris and ciliary body (e.g., iritis, iridocyclitis)
  - Intermediate: involving pars plana (i.e., pars planitis)
  - Posterior: involving retina (i.e., retinitis) and choroid (i.e., choroiditis), and, possibly, the optic nerve (papillitis or optic neuritis) and vitreous (vitreitis)
  - Panuveitis: 2 or more of the above

EPIDEMIOLOGY
Incidence
4.3–6.9 per 100,000

Prevalence
- 30 cases per 100,000 (1)[A]
- Uveitis is much less common in children than in adults

RISK FACTORS
- Genetic predisposition (HLA-B27)
  - Juvenile idiopathic arthritis (JIA) is the most common cause other than idiopathic causes and trauma
  - Pauciarticular disease
  - Age <7 years at presentation
  - ANA positive, RF negative
  - Female gender
- Other autoimmune diseases
- Pre- or postnatal infection (e.g., toxoplasmosis, toxocariasis, tuberculosis)
- See Etiology

Genetics
- HLA-B27
  - Associated with anterior uveitis, ankylosing spondylitis, Reiter syndrome, inflammatory bowel disease, and psoriatic arthritis
- Genetic predisposition may be coupled with environmental trigger to produce disease

GENERAL PREVENTION
- Appropriate monitoring of systemic disease and periodic ophthalmologic examination of those at risk
- Avoidance of infection

PATHOPHYSIOLOGY
- Dependent upon etiology
- JIA: Pathophysiology unknown

ETIOLOGY
- Anterior
  - Juvenile idiopathic arthritis (JIA)
    - Most common cause of noninfectious anterior uveitis
    - Oligoarticular: greatest risk of uveitis
    - Systemic: least risk of uveitis
    - Eye involvement may precede joint activity
    - No correlation between eye and joint disease
    - Onset and activity is asymptomatic with white, quiet eye
    - ~50% may require long-term treatment
    - Enthesis-related (HLA-B27): ankylosing spondylitis, Reiter syndrome, inflammatory bowel disease, psoriatic arthritis
  - Idiopathic
  - Trauma
  - Behçet's disease
  - Sarcoidosis
  - Kawasaki disease
  - Tubulointerstitial nephritis and uveitis (TINU)
  - Masquerade syndromes:
    - Retinoblastoma
    - Lymphoma or leukemia
    - Trauma and/or intraocular foreign body
    - Juvenile xanthogranuloma (JXG)
    - Coat's disease
  - Infectious
    - Herpes simplex or varicella zoster virus
    - Syphilis, tuberculosis, Lyme's disease
    - Parasitic infection (e.g., toxoplasmosis)
- Intermediate
  - Idiopathic
  - Sarcoidosis
  - Inflammatory bowel disease
  - Multiple sclerosis
  - Lyme's disease
  - Uncommon in JIA
- Posterior
  - Infectious
    - Toxoplasmosis: most common
    - Less frequent: toxocariasis, tuberculosis, syphilis, Lyme's disease, cat scratch disease, parasitic, fungal, bacterial, and viral including HSV, varicella, and cytomegalovirus
  - Noninfectious
    - Masquerade syndrome
    - Sarcoidosis
    - Sympathetic ophthalmia
    - Vogt–Koyanagi–Harada disease
- Panuveitis
  - Infection
  - Systemic disease
  - Masquerade syndrome

COMMONLY ASSOCIATED CONDITIONS
Cataract, glaucoma, band keratopathy, posterior synechiae, chorioretinal scar, exudative retinal detachment, hypotony, and visual loss

DIAGNOSIS

HISTORY
- May be key to determining diagnosis
- Ocular symptoms (NOTE: absence of symptoms does not rule out uveitis, especially in JIA)
- Medical illnesses
- Review of systems, family history, sexual history, and travel history

PHYSICAL EXAM
- General physical exam
- Complete ophthalmologic examination
  - Visual acuity testing
  - Intraocular pressure
  - Conjunctiva
    - Ciliary flush, nodules, episcleritis, and scleritis
  - Cornea
    - Edema from inflammation or glaucoma
    - Keratitic precipitates: collections of inflammatory cells deposited on endothelium; small-nongranulomatous; larger with greasy appearance—granulomatous (Mutton Fat)
    - Band keratopathy
    - Dendrite or geographic ulcer with HSV
    - Interstitial keratitis
  - Anterior chamber
    - Cells measured +1 to +4 or cells/slit-lamp field
    - Flare: leakage of protein
    - Hypopyon: white blood cells settled in lower anterior chamber
    - Pseudohypopyon: tumor cells
  - Iris
    - Posterior synechiae: adhesion between iris and lens capsule
    - Peripheral anterior synechiae: adhesion between iris and peripheral cornea
    - neovascularization
  - Lens: cataract
    - Gonioscopy
  - Vitreous cells, blood, or membranes
  - Retina
    - Cystoid macular edema, cotton wool spots, hemorrhage, vascular sheathing, neovascularization, or detachment
  - Choroid
    - Dalen–Fuchs nodules: yellowish lesions with hyperpigmentation seen with sarcoid and sympathetic ophthalmia
  - Pars plana
    - Snowbanking: white masses
    - Neovascularization
  - Optic nerve: swelling, atrophy, neovascularization, and infiltration

DIAGNOSTIC TESTS & INTERPRETATION

Directed work up based on history and physical findings

Lab

- Blood work if no clear cause
  - ACE, ANA, calcium, CBC with differential, ESR, Lyme titer (if geographic risk), RF, VDRL/FTA-ABS
- Urinalysis

Imaging

- CXR
- Ocular ultrasound if no view

Diagnostic Procedures/Other

- Hand and SI joint radiographs
- CT/MRI brain and sinuses
- High-frequency ultrasonographic biomicroscopy
- Lumbar puncture
- ANCA, HLAB27, other antibodies or titers, T-cell counts, or HIV
- Stool for ova and parasites
- Skin testing: allergy, anergy, and PPD
- Additional ophthalmic testing
  - ERG, VEP
  - Fluorescein angiography
  - OCT
  - Visual field testing
- Biopsy: conjunctiva, lacrimal gland, aqueous, vitreous, or retina

Pathological Findings

Dependent upon etiologic agent

DIFFERENTIAL DIAGNOSIS

- Retinoblastoma
- Leukemia or lymphoma
- Trauma
- Intraocular foreign body
- Retinitis pigmentosa
- Coat's disease
- Juvenile xanthogranuloma

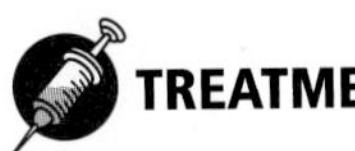

TREATMENT

MEDICATION

First Line

- Topical steroid: 1 drop in affected eye ranging from q.i.d to every 15 min, based on initial severity and taper based on clinical picture
- Cycloplegic agent to prevent synechiae and for pain control

Second Line

- Periocular injection of steroid
- Systemic therapy should be prescribed and managed by physician familiar with therapies and monitoring for complications (e.g., rheumatologist).
- Least toxic systemic therapy should be instituted when topical therapy is insufficient.
- Systemic steroid (e.g., oral, intravenous)
- Nonsteroidal anti-inflammatory drugs: topical or systemic have a minor role
- Nonsteroidal immunosuppressives
  - Antimetabolites
    - Methotrexate (for JIA first line, if failing topical steroids)
    - Mycophenolate mofetil
  - Anti-tumor necrosis factor antibody medications (second line for JIA)
    - Infliximab, etanercept, adalimumab
  - B-cell-directed therapy: Rituximab
  - Immunosuppressives: Cyclosporine, tacrolimus, or azathioprine
  - Alkylating agents: Cyclophosphamide, chlorambucil, etc.

ADDITIONAL TREATMENT

General Measures

Based on underlying disease and disability when present

Issues for Referral

- Rheumatology evaluation in all patients without obvious etiology
- Infectious disease, oncology, and other specialties as indicated

Additional Therapies

- Low-vision services
- Counseling for adjustment to vision loss and living with chronic disease

COMPLEMENTARY & ALTERNATIVE THERAPIES

None known to be helpful

SURGERY/OTHER PROCEDURES

- Chelation for band keratopathy
- Cataract surgery
- Glaucoma surgery
- Retinal laser, detachment repair
- Drug-delivery implant

IN-PATIENT CONSIDERATIONS

Admission Criteria

Only required if systemic disease warrants or treatment with short-term intravenous pulse steroids

ONGOING CARE

FOLLOW-UP RECOMMENDATIONS

- Frequent eye examination to address ocular complications of disease
- Control systemic disease
- Monitor systemic treatment

Patient Monitoring

- Appropriate testing based on therapy
- Medication doses based on weight periodically need to be adjusted as child grows.

DIET

No typical dietary restrictions

PATIENT EDUCATION

- www.aapos.org/faq_list/iritis
- www.uveitis.org/
- www.mdjunction.com/arthritis-juvenile-rheumatoid
- www.pgcfa.org

PROGNOSIS

- Early and aggressive therapy can often prevent or delay vision loss.
- Visual disability can significantly impact quality of life (2)[A].

COMPLICATIONS

- Band keratopathy
- Cataract
- Posterior synechiae
- Glaucoma
- Cystoid macular edema (CME)
- Hypotony
- Disc edema
- Vitreous hemorrhage
- Vitreoretinal membrane
- Phthisis
- Permanent vision loss
  - May occur in up to 1/3 of uveitis patients
  - Posterior uveitis, CME, and hypotony associated with significant vision loss (3)[A]

REFERENCES

1. Nagpal A, Leigh JF, Acharya NR. Epidemiology of uveitis in children. *Int Ophthalmol Clin* 2008 Summer;48:1–7.
2. Angeles-Han ST, Griffin KW, Lehman JT, et al. The importance of visual function in the quality of life of children with uveitis. *J AAPOS* 2010;14:163–168.
3. Smith JA, Mackensen F, Sen N. Epidemiology and course of disease in childhood uveitis. *Ophthalmol* 2009;116:1544–1551.

ADDITIONAL READING

- http://aappolicy.aappublications.org/cgi/content/full/pediatrics;117/5/1843.

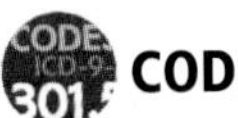

CODES

ICD9

- 364.00 Acute and subacute iridocyclitis, unspecified
- 364.3 Unspecified iridocyclitis
- 714.30 Chronic or unspecified polyarticular juvenile rheumatoid arthritis

CLINICAL PEARLS

- Aggressive elimination of inflammation should be the goal of treatment.
- Multidisciplinary approach is necessary for successful treatment.
- Always rule out leukemia and masquerade syndromes.

ISOLATED OCULOMOTOR NERVE (CRANIAL NERVE III) PALSY

Edsel B. Ing

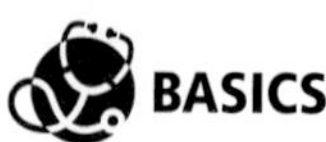

BASICS

DESCRIPTION

The 3rd cranial nerve innervates the levator palpebrae superioris, superior rectus, medial rectus, inferior oblique, and inferior rectus. The pupillary fibers follow the inferior oblique muscle. Pupil involvement in CN III palsy is an efferent defect (unrelated to a relative afferent pupillary defect).

ALERT

In patients with non-traumatic cranial nerve III palsy and ipsilateral pupillary dilation (efferent defect), posterior communicating artery aneurysm must be excluded.

Pediatric Considerations

Children <8 years of age should be closely monitored for amblyopia. Congenital 3rd nerve palsies may be caused by birth trauma. Compared with adults, it is rare for aneurysms to cause CN III palsy in children. Ophthalmoplegic migraine is a diagnosis of exclusion, with onset in childhood. Ophthalmoplegic migraine is uncommon and the ophthalmoplegia develops days after the onset of head pain.

Pregnancy Considerations

It is not common to have 3rd nerve palsy in pregnancy. Exclude pituitary apoplexy, gestational diabetes, or hypertension.

PATHOPHYSIOLOGY

The pupillary fibers of the oculomotor nerve are located superficially along the medial aspect of the nerve, close to the posterior communicating artery. The pupillary fibers travel in the outer layers of the nerve and are closer to the vasa nervorum nutrient blood supply. As such, the pupillary fibers are less likely to be affected by microvascular ischemia; however, they can be compressed by a posterior communicating artery aneurysm.

ETIOLOGY

- Microvascular (e.g., diabetes, hypertension)
- Aneurysm
- Trauma
- Tumor/infiltration (e.g., lymphoma, carcinoma)
- Inflammation (e.g., sarcoidosis)
- Vasculitis
- Infection (e.g., meningitis)

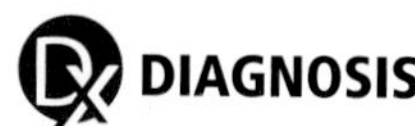

DIAGNOSIS

HISTORY

The patient may have binocular diplopia with diagonal separation. If the ptosis is severe enough to occlude the visual axis, the patient will not complain of diplopia.

PHYSICAL EXAM

- With a complete 3rd nerve palsy, there is a ptosis, and the eye is positioned downward and outward.
  - A truly pupil-sparing 3rd nerve palsy shows normal pupillary function but complete loss of eyelid and eye movement subserved by the oculomotor nerve.
  - Aberrant regeneration may occur if the disrupted 3rd cranial nerve fibers reroute themselves along anomalous pathways. Most commonly, the ptotic lid will elevate on adduction or infraduction if there is lid-gaze synkinesis. The pupil may constrict with adduction with pupil-gaze synkinesis.
  - Aberrant regeneration is primary if there is no preceding acute 3rd nerve palsy, and it is seen with cavernous sinus lesions such as meningioma or aneurysm. Aberrant regeneration is secondary if it follows recovery from a 3rd nerve palsy (e.g., post-trauma or compression).

DIAGNOSTIC TESTS & INTERPRETATION

Lab

Blood sugar, glycosylated hemoglobin if is diabetes suspected. Serum lipids can be drawn. Westergren erythrocyte sedimentation rate and C-reactive protein if giant cell arteritis is suspected

Imaging

Initial approach

CT angiogram or MR angiogram, if the pupil is involved

Follow-up & special considerations

In patients that were not initially imaged, but have persistent non-improving deficit at 4 months, consider MRI.

Diagnostic Procedures/Other

Lumbar puncture may be considered if neuroimaging and blood tests are not diagnostic.

DIFFERENTIAL DIAGNOSIS

- Myasthenia can mimic pupil-sparing 3rd nerve palsy. An "isolated medial rectus palsy" is unlikely to represent a partial 3rd nerve palsy, but is more likely to be an internuclear ophthalmoplegia or, perhaps, myasthenia. Giant cell arteritis can cause extraocular muscle ischemia or 3rd nerve palsy appearance. Closely check for intorsion to ensure that CN IV is intact, and check CN V1 and V2 sensation to exclude a cavernous sinus lesion.
- If there is isolated efferent pupillary dysfunction with intact lid function and eye movement in an alert patient, Adie's pupil should be suspected.

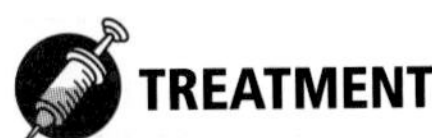

TREATMENT

MEDICATION

If giant cell arteritis is suspected, give intravenous steroids or minimum 60 mg p.o. prednisone.

ADDITIONAL TREATMENT

General Measures

Optimize the patient's blood pressure, blood sugar, and cholesterol. If the adult patient has bothersome diplopia, the palsied eye can be patched. Prism glasses can be attempted but usually are of limited benefit because there is marked incomitance. Children <8 years of age should be monitored closely to determine the need for amblyopia treatment.

Issues for Referral

Pupil involving 3rd nerve palsy requires referral to neurosurgery or neurology. Diabetes, hypertension, collagen vascular disease, or temporal arteritis suspects should be referred to primary care doctor or medicine service.

IN-PATIENT CONSIDERATIONS

Admission Criteria

Pupil involving CN III palsies requiring neuroimaging (e.g., CT angiogram or MR angiogram) should be assessed by neurosurgery or neurology

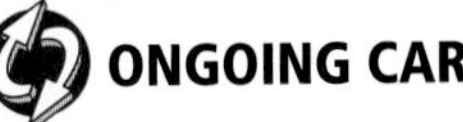

ONGOING CARE

FOLLOW-UP RECOMMENDATIONS

In patients with new-onset CN III palsy and pupil-sparing, follow the pupil daily for 5–7 days to ensure the pupil does not become involved.

PROGNOSIS

Patients with ischemic 3rd nerve palsies may have significant recovery of function. If patients with CN III palsy have not recovered after 12 months, strabismus surgery or ptosis repair can be considered. The surgical rehabilitation of partial 3rd nerve palsy is better than that for complete 3rd nerve palsy. With complete 3rd nerve palsy, fixation of the globe to the medial canthal tendon and frontalis sling for ptosis may provide cosmetic improvement; however, the patient may have chronic diplopia. In patients with severe ptosis and poor Bells' phenomenon, corneal exposure may be a relative contraindication to frontalis sling ptosis repair.

COMPLICATIONS

Aneurysmal 3rd nerve palsy is a potentially life-threatening condition. Unrecognized giant cell arteritis may lead to bilateral blindness.

REFERENCES

1. Lanning B. Kline. *Neuro-ophthalmology review manual*, 6th ed. Slack Incorporated: Thorofare, NJ, 2008.
2. Lanning B. Kline. *Neuro-ophthalmology. Section 5. Basic and Clinical Science Course*. American Academy of Ophthalmology: San Francisco, CA, 2009.
3. Burde RM, Savino PJ, Trobe JD. *Clinical decisions in neuro-ophthalmology*, 3rd ed. Mosby: St. Louis, MO, 2002.

CODES

ICD9

- 378.51 Third or oculomotor nerve palsy, partial
- 378.52 Third or oculomotor nerve palsy, total

CLINICAL PEARLS

- With new-onset 3rd nerve palsy, pupil involvement in the absence of trauma suggests cerebral aneurysm.
- Patients with apparent pupil-sparing 3rd nerve palsy should be followed for a week to ensure there is no pupillary involvement.
- "Medial rectus palsies" are usually not partial 3rd nerve palsies. Internuclear ophthalmoplegia (e.g., demyelination/stroke) or myasthenia should be suspected.
- Significant head trauma is usually required before a 3rd nerve palsy will occur.
- Pain does NOT distinguish between compression and microvascular infarction.
- Aberrant regeneration does NOT occur after ischemic 3rd nerve palsy.

I

ISOLATED TROCHLEAR NERVE (CRANIAL NERVE IV) PALSY

Edsel Ing

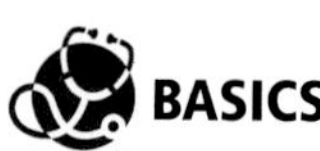

BASICS

DESCRIPTION

4th nerve palsy is caused by weakness or paralysis of the superior oblique muscle, and may result in diplopia.

EPIDEMIOLOGY

Prevalence

4th nerve palsy occurs frequently after closed head trauma due to its unique anatomic dorsal midbrain decussation.

ETIOLOGY

- Trauma and microvascular ischemia are the most common causes of acquired 4th nerve palsy. Congenital 4th nerve palsies are also common. Review of childhood photos showing head tilt to the side opposite the palsy can help determine the chronicity of the lesion.
- Tumor (e.g., pinealoma, tentorial meningioma), aneurysm, meningitis, and giant cell arteritis are uncommon causes of trochlear nerve palsy.

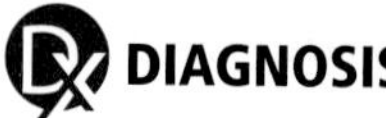

DIAGNOSIS

HISTORY

- Patients with 4th nerve palsy usually complain of binocular diplopia with vertical or diagonal separation that worsens on downgaze. They may complain that objects appear tilted in the affected eye.
- Patients often indicate that, when they tilt their head to the side opposite the palsy, they have less or no diplopia.

PHYSICAL EXAM

- On the palsied side, there may be deficient inferior movement of the eye, when the patient looks downward and inward. The antagonist inferior oblique muscle may appear to overact (over-elevation in adduction) on affected side.
- The vertical separation between the 2 eyes often increases when the head is tilted to side of the 4th nerve palsy, explaining why patients usually tilt their head to the side opposite the palsy.
- Alternate-cover tests in different positions of gaze, (3-step test) may help confirm the diagnosis of 4th nerve palsy.
- Patients with congenital 4th nerve palsy often have a high vertical fusional amplitude (>3 prism diopters).
- Patients with 4th nerve palsy should not have ptosis, but may volitionally close 1 eye to avert diplopia.

DIAGNOSTIC TESTS & INTERPRETATION

Lab

In adults, work-up for diabetes, hypertension and hypercholesterolemia should be considered.

Imaging

If a suspected 4th nerve palsy does not improve after a few months, neuroimaging should be performed.

DIFFERENTIAL DIAGNOSIS

- Bilateral 4th nerve palsies can occur, especially after trauma. Myasthenia gravis, Graves ophthalmopathy, and skew deviation may mimic a 4th nerve palsy. Patients with ocular myasthenia often have variable ptosis and variability in their eye misalignment with diurnal variation. Patients with Graves ophthalmopathy may show lid retraction, proptosis, conjunctival chemosis, and often have abnormal TSH. It is difficult for a non-specialist to differentiate 4th nerve palsy from skew deviation. Patients with skew deviation may have stroke history or brainstem findings, show incyclotorsion on Maddox rod testing, and often have less vertical strabismus in the supine, compared to upright, position.
- Rarely giant cell arteritis may mimic or cause 4th nerve palsy
  - Patients with superior oblique myokymia (due to neurovascular compression of the 4th cranial nerve root exit zone, multiple sclerosis, or posterior fossa tumor) may complain of episodic tilting.

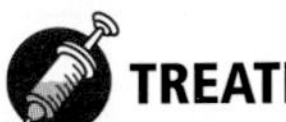

TREATMENT

ADDITIONAL TREATMENT

General Measures

Patients may find it helpful to tilt their head away from the side of the palsied nerve. Prism glasses are often helpful if there is vertical or diagonal diplopia. If the patient has intolerable torsional diplopia, patching or translucent tape over a glasses lens can be of help.

Issues for Referral

Any non-resolving 4th nerve palsy should be referred for ophthalmic assessment.

SURGERY/OTHER PROCEDURES

If new-onset diplopia does not improve after a year, and prism glasses do not help the patient, strabismus surgery can be considered.

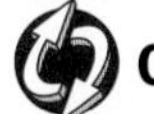

ONGOING CARE

PROGNOSIS

Many patients with microvascular or traumatic 4th nerve palsy have some improvement 3–9 months after presentation.

REFERENCES

1. Lanning B. Kline. *Neuro-ophthalmology review manual*, 6th ed. Slack Incorporated: Thorofare, NJ, 2008.
2. Lanning B. Kline. *Neuro-ophthalmology. Section 5. Basic and Clinical Science Course*. American Academy of Ophthalmology: San Francisco, CA, 2009.
3. Burde RM, Savino PJ, Trobe JD. *Clinical decisions in neuro-ophthalmology*, 3rd ed. Mosby: St. Louis, MO, 2002.

CODES

ICD9

- 368.2 Diplopia
- 378.53 Fourth nerve palsy

CLINICAL PEARLS

- With 4th nerve palsy, there is a characteristic head tilt to the side opposite to the palsy. Review of old photos (e.g., photo I.D.) may help determine chronicity of 4th nerve palsy.
- 4th nerve palsy can occur even after relatively minor head trauma.

JUVENILE IDIOPATHIC ARTHRITIS-RELATED UVEITIS

Darrell E. Baskin

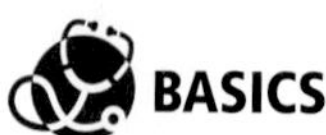

BASICS

DESCRIPTION

- Juvenile idiopathic arthritis (JIA)-related uveitis is a group of idiopathic arthritides with an onset before 16 years of age that persists longer than 6 weeks.
- There are 7 subtypes of JIA
  - Systemic arthritis: Arthritis in one or more joints accompanied or preceded by fever and accompanied by one of the following: Evanescent, erythematous rash, generalized lymph node enlargement, hepatomegaly and/or splenomegaly, or serositis
  - Oligoarthritis: Arthritis in 1–4 joints in the first 6 months of disease. Oligoarthritis is further subcategorized as persistent oligoarthritis (affecting not more than 4 joints throughout the disease course) or extended oligoarthritis (affecting a total of more than 4 joints after the initial 6 months)
  - Polyarthritis (RF negative): Arthritis in 5 or more joints in the initial 6 months and a negative test for rheumatoid factor (RF)
  - Polyarthritis (RF positive): Arthritis in 5 or more joints in the initial 6 months and a positive test for RF on 2 occasions at least 3 months apart during the first 6 months of disease
  - Psoriatic arthritis (PsA): Arthritis and psoriasis or arthritis and at least 2 of the following: Dactylitis, nail-pitting or onycholysis, or psoriasis in a first-degree relative
  - Enthesitis-related arthritis (ERA): Arthritis and/or enthesitis (tenderness at the insertion of a tendon, ligament, fascia, or capsule to bone) with at least 2 of the following: Presence or history of sacroiliac joint tenderness, HLA-B27 antigen, onset of arthritis in male over 6 years of age, acute (symptomatic) anterior uveitis, or history of ankylosing spondylitis, ERA, sacroiliitis with inflammatory bowel disease, Reiter syndrome or acute anterior uveitis in a first-degree relative
  - Undifferentiated arthritis: Arthritis that fulfills criteria in no category or in 2 or more of the above categories

EPIDEMIOLOGY

Incidence

The exact incidence of JIA is unknown. The reported incidence varies from 0.008–0.226 per 1,000 children per year.

Prevalence

- The exact prevalence of JIA is unknown. The reported prevalence varies from 0.07–4.01 per 1,000 children.
- The prevalence of uveitis within known JIA populations varies from 4–38% worldwide. Analysis of pulled data suggests a cumulative prevalence of uveitis of 8.3% of JIA patients.

RISK FACTORS

Risk factors for developing JIA uveitis include ANA positivity, early age at onset of arthritis (<6 years), and female sex.

Genetics

- HLA-DRB1 has been linked with an increased susceptibility to develop JIA.
- HLA-DRB1*13 has been associated with the development of JIA uveitis.

PATHOPHYSIOLOGY

- Abnormal immune responses have been documented in JIA patients, but the precise etiology remains unknown.
- Serologic abnormalities such as antineutrophil antibody (ANA), RF, and anticyclic citrullinated peptide (anti-CCP) have implicated self-targeting antibodies, but the exact target remains unknown.

ETIOLOGY

Etiology is unknown.

COMMONLY ASSOCIATED CONDITIONS

See 7 subtypes in "Description".

DIAGNOSIS

HISTORY

- Many patients with JIA uveitis do not have any ocular symptoms, which is the reason for regular ophthalmic screening examinations according to disease subtype.
- One should inquire about decreased vision, history of pink eye, and photophobia.

PHYSICAL EXAM

- Patients may be categorized according to type of uveitis as standardized by the SUN group (see "Additional Reading").
  - Acute anterior uveitis: Anterior uveitis that is sudden in onset and has <3 months duration
  - Recurrent anterior uveitis: Anterior uveitis of less than 3 months duration but with recurrent episodes that occur >3 months apart without medication
  - Chronic anterior uveitis: Anterior uveitis that lasts longer than 3 months
  - Anterior uveitis with vitreitis: Anterior uveitis with vitreitis and this does not include snowbanking or spillover cells in the vitreous
- Ophthalmic features of JIA uveitis may include:
  - Bilateral anterior uveitis with a chronic course; in most cases, both eyes are involved within a few months of each other.
  - It is usually a nongranulomatous uveitis; however, recent studies suggest that granulomatous inflammation may be more common than previously thought, particularly in African–Americans and ANA-positive children.
  - One should look for uveitic complications, such as posterior synechiae, cataract, band keratopathy, glaucoma, hypotony, and cystoid macular edema (CME).
  - Chronic anterior uveitis is the most common, followed by acute anterior uveitis, recurrent anterior uveitis, and finally, anterior uveitis with vitreitis.

DIAGNOSTIC TESTS & INTERPRETATION

Lab

- There are no confirmatory tests since JIA is a diagnosis of exclusion. One may consider the following tests if the diagnosis has not already been made:
- Erythrocyte sedimentation rate, C-reactive protein, platelet count, ANA, RF, and anti-CCP. One may consider laboratory tests for Lyme disease and sarcoidosis as well.

Imaging

One may consider optical coherence tomography if CME is suspected.

DIFFERENTIAL DIAGNOSIS

- Sarcoidosis is the disease that most closely mimics JIA uveitis.
- Other diseases to consider include: Lyme disease, trauma, Kawasaki disease, and herpetic keratouveitis.

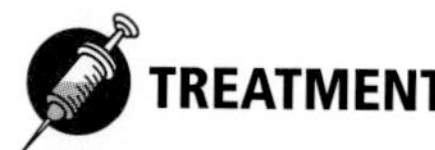

TREATMENT

MEDICATION

First Line

- Topical corticosteroids are first line therapy to treat anterior uveitis (treat cells, not flare). The dose is titrated according to the cellular reaction, the presence of posterior synechiae, and band keratopathy. The goal is to use the least amount of steroid that will maintain quiescence. If the steroid drop must be used more than 4 times per day, then a second line drug should be used.
- Short-acting mydriatics and cycloplegics should be used. Short acting allows the pupil to move and not develop synechiae either in a dilated or non-dilated state. Be careful not to induce amblyopia by constant cycloplegia.

Second Line

- Periocular injections of steroids may be necessary. But they carry a higher risk of glaucoma and cataract formation.
- Oral corticosteroids should not be used for prolonged periods of time given the adverse impact on growth and bony development.
- Naproxen may have some benefit as a steroid-sparing agent; it is the most frequent nonsteroidal anti-inflammatory drug prescribed for patients with JIA.
- Methotrexate (MTX) is the most commonly used agent when adjunctive therapy is needed. It usually takes 4–8 weeks for an effect to be seen. Liver enzymes and CBC should be monitored every 4–6 weeks.
- Cyclosporine and azathioprine have also been used with success.
- The biologics are also being increasingly utilized. Although etanercept works well for joint disease, in a randomized, controlled trial, it was no better than placebo for JIA uveitis. However, infliximab and adalimumab appear to be effective for treating JIA uveitis.

ADDITIONAL TREATMENT

General Measures

If uveitic complications develop, surgery may be warranted to address these. See "Surgery/Other Procedures."

SURGERY/OTHER PROCEDURES

- Cataract formation is the most common vision-threatening complication of JIA uveitis. Up to 60% of children with JIA uveitis develop cataract due to chronic inflammation and/or corticosteroid use.
  - In the past, pars plana lensectomy, anterior vitrectomy and removal of the capsule were performed. This required lifelong dependence on aphakic spectacles or contact lenses.
  - Recently, success has been achieved with phacoemulsification, posterior capsulorrhexis, anterior vitrectomy, and intraocular lens placement (often accompanied by an injection of triamcinolone acetonide into the anterior chamber).
- Glaucoma may be managed by topical therapy; but if drops do not control the intraocular pressure, then trabeculectomy and antimetabolite use or glaucoma drainage device placement may be necessitated.
- Band keratopathy may require chelation therapy, but recurrences are common.

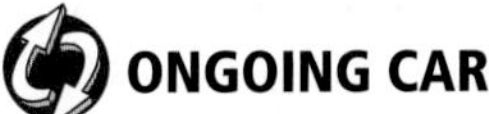

ONGOING CARE

FOLLOW-UP RECOMMENDATIONS

- Pediatric ophthalmologist
- Pediatric rheumatologist
- Consider uveitis specialist

Patient Monitoring

Screening for eye disease once JIA is diagnosed is mandatory. Referral to ophthalmologist should be performed promptly. Current guidelines for screening are summarized in Table.

PATIENT EDUCATION

Parents should be taught that the ocular inflammation in JIA is often asymptomatic and therefore, regular screening appointments are necessary. They should also be taught that any pink eye should not be dismissed as viral until evaluated by an ophthalmologist.

PROGNOSIS

In some of the more recent studies, over 90% of eyes with JIA uveitis, at final visit, had a visual acuity of 20/40 or better; and over 97% of patients (using better-seeing eye) had 20/40 or better vision.

COMPLICATIONS

See "Surgery/Other Procedures"

ADDITIONAL READING

- Jabs DA, Nussenblatt RB, Rosenbaum JT; Standardization of Uveitis Nomenclature (SUN) Working Group. Standardization of uveitis nomenclature for reporting clinical data. Results of the First International Workshop. *Am J Ophthalmol*. 2005;140:509–516.
- Kesen MR, Setlur V, Goldstein DA. Juvenile idiopathic arthritis-related uveitis. *Int Ophthalmol Clin*. 2008; 48(3):21–38.
- Sabri K. Saurenmann RK, Silverman ED, et al. Course, complications, and outcome of juvenile arthritis-related uveitis. *J AAPOS*. 2008; 12:539–545.
- American Academy of Pediatrics Section on Rheumatology and Section on Ophthalmology: Guidelines for ophthalmologic examinations in children with juvenile rheumatoid arthritis. *Pediatrics*. 1993;92(2):295–296.

Table 1 Frequency of Ophthalmologic Visits for Children With Juvenile Rheumatoid Arthritis (JRA) and Without Known Iridocyclitis*

	Age of Onset	
JRA Subtype at Onset	**<7y**†	**≥7**‡
Pauciarticular		
+ ANA	H§	M
− ANA	M	M
Polyarticular		
+ ANA	H§	M
− ANA	M	M
Systemic	L	L

*High Fttk (H) indicates ophthalmologic examinations every 3–4 months. Medium risk (M) indicates ophthalmologic examinations every 6 months. Low risk (L) indicates ophthalmologic examinations every 12 months. ANA indicates antinuclear antibody lest.

†All patients are considered at low risk 7 years after the unset of their arthritis and should have yearly ophthalmologic examinations Indefinitely

‡All patients are considered at low risk 4 yrs after the onset of their arthritis and should have yearly ophthalmologic examinations Indefinitely.

§AL high-risk patients are considered at medium risk 4 year after the onset of their arthritis.

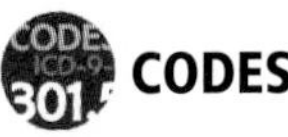

CODES

ICD9

- 364.00 Acute and subacute iridocyclitis, unspecified
- 364.3 Unspecified iridocyclitis
- 714.30 Chronic or unspecified polyarticular juvenile rheumatoid arthritis

J

JUVENILE XANTHOGRANULOMA (NEVOXANTHOENDOTHELIOMA)

Kristina Pao

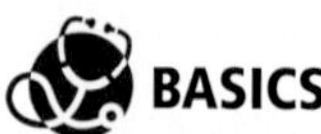

BASICS

DESCRIPTION

- Juvenile xanthogranuloma (JXG) is a nonneoplastic form of non-Langerhans cell group (class II) of histiocytic proliferative disorders typically seen in infants and children.
  - Usually a self-limited dermatologic disorder consisting of skin lesions on the head, neck, and trunk.
  - Extracutaneous JXG occurs in 4–5%.
  - May involve the eye, lung, GI tract, bone, and muscles.
- Ocular JXG occurs in about 10% of all JXG.
  - May involve the iris, eyelid, cornea, conjunctiva, ciliary body, choroid, episclera, posterior segment, or orbit.

EPIDEMIOLOGY

Incidence

- Frequency is unknown.
  - Incidence may be higher than reported as lesions may spontaneously regress by 5 years of age.
- More common in Caucasians.
- Single cutaneous lesion occurs in 83–90% of patients with JXG.
  - Median age of presentation with solitary skin lesion is 2 years old.
  - Median age of presentation with multiple skin lesions is 5 months old.
  - Increased predominance in males if multiple skin lesions present.
  - 10% of cases occur at birth.
  - 85% of cases occur by 1 year of age.
- Ocular involvement before age 2 occurs in 92%.
  - Most often unilateral.
  - 50% of patients with ocular involvement have skin lesions.

PATHOPHYSIOLOGY

Believed to result from a granulomatous reaction of histiocytes in response to a nonspecific physical or possibly infectious stimulus.

COMMONLY ASSOCIATED CONDITIONS

- Neurofibromatosis-1
  - Inherited disorder in which neurofibromas form in the skin, CNS, and bones.
  - Café au lait macules + JXG is associated with epilepsy in 20%.
- Niemann–Pick disease
  - A lysosomal storage disease due to acid sphingomyelinase deficiency characterized by cherry red spot, macular halo, optic atrophy
  - Systemic manifestations affect the lungs and bone marrow without mental retardation.
- Urticaria pigmentosa
  - Common form of cutaneous mastocytosis in which minor skin irritation results in massive mast cell release and urticaria
- Juvenile myelomonocytic leukemia
  - Chronic myeloproliferative disorder affecting children age 1–4 years old

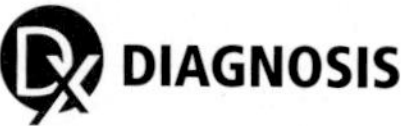

DIAGNOSIS

- Cutaneous features of JXG include the following:
  - Firm tan-orange papillomacular lesion(s) on the head, neck, trunk, or extremities
  - Café au lait spots (20%)
- Ophthalmic features of oculocutaneous and ocular JXG include various degrees of the following:
  - Spontaneous hyphema.
  - Corneal blood staining.
  - Unilateral glaucoma.
  - Vascular yellow-brow iris lesion.
  - Heterochromia iridis.
  - Conjunctival mass.
  - Unilateral uveitis.
  - Proptosis.
  - Cataract.
  - Vascular occlusion.
  - Retinal detachment.
  - Amblyopia.

HISTORY

- Most patients with JXG are asymptomatic.
- Acute pain and photophobia due to secondary glaucoma

PHYSICAL EXAM

- Exam head, neck, trunk, and extremities for cutaneous lesions
- Complete ophthalmic examination for ocular manifestations

DIAGNOSTIC TESTS & INTERPRETATION

Diagnostic Procedures/Other

- Skin biopsy
- Iris biopsy
  - Fine-needle biopsy
  - Iridectomy
  - Iridocyclectomy

Pathological Findings

In ocular JXG, histology reveals Touton giant cells in a background of plasma cells, lymphocytes, and histiocytes. Touton giant cells are present in 85% of cases and appear as a wreath of foamy lipid surrounding a ring of nuclei. Histology may also reveal foam cells and foreign body giant cells. Histiocytes stain with antibodies against factor XIIIa, HAM 56, KP1 (CD 68), HF35, Ki-M1P, vimentin, CD 163, fascin, and CD 14. Histiocytes do not stain with CD 1a or S-100.

DIFFERENTIAL DIAGNOSIS

- Leukemic involvement of the iris
- Iris nevus
- Iris melanoma
- Langerhans cells histiocytosis
- Rhabdomyosarcoma
- Fibrous dysplasia
- Dermoid
- Xanthoma
- Hemangioma
- Neurofibroma
- Molluscum contagiosum

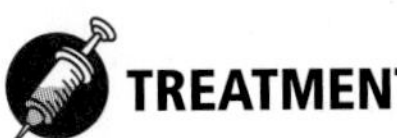

TREATMENT

ADDITIONAL TREATMENT

General Measures

- Systemic corticosteroids
- Rarely immunomodulatory therapy
- Rarely radiation therapy
- Treat spontaneous hyphema with topical cycloplegia and corticosteroids as well as hyphema precautions (wear eye shield, keep head upright, no strenuous lifting, minimize anticoagulants)
- Topical corticosteroids and pharmacologic agents to reduce intraocular pressure should secondary glaucoma develop
- Treat amblyopia, which can result from strabismus or anisometropia due to corneal blood staining, cataract formation, or secondary glaucoma

SURGERY/OTHER PROCEDURES

- Local resection
- Cataract extraction

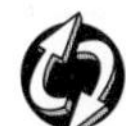

ONGOING CARE

FOLLOW-UP RECOMMENDATIONS

- Ophthalmologist
- Primary care doctor or dermatologist for periodic skin examinations

PATIENT EDUCATION

- The Histiocytosis Association of America (http://www.histio.org/).

PROGNOSIS

- Normal lifespan, development, intelligence, fertility
- Most cutaneous lesions spontaneous regress

COMPLICATIONS

- Secondary glaucoma
- Profound vision loss

ADDITIONAL READING

- Shields JA, Shields CL. Clinical spectrum of histiocytic tumors of the orbit. *Trans Pa Acad Ophthalmol Otolaryngol* 1990;42:931–937.
- Wertz FD, Zimmerman LE, McKeown CA, et al. Juvenile xanthogranuloma of the optic nerve, disc, retina, and choroid. *Ophthalmology* 1982;89:1131–1135.
- Zimmerman LE. Ocular lesions of juvenile xanthogranuloma. *Am J Ophthalmol* 1965;60:1011–1035.

CODES

ICD9

272.7 Lipidoses

CLINICAL PEARLS

- Suspect JXG in spontaneous hyphema, unilateral glaucoma, or exophthalmos in an infant
- Monitor for secondary glaucoma
- Look for café au lait macules given association with epilepsy

KAWASAKI DISEASE

Denise A. Hug

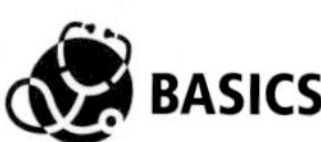

BASICS

DESCRIPTION

- Multisystem acute vasculitis usually involving the small to mid-size arteries during infancy and early childhood.
- Fever for at least 5 days duration plus 4 of the 5 major criteria
  - bilateral conjunctival injection
  - erythema of the lips or oropharynx
  - nonpurulent cervical lymphadenopathy
  - erythema and edema of palms and soles with desquamation
  - polymorphous truncal rash (1)

EPIDEMIOLOGY

Incidence

- Variable depending on race
  - Asian American and Pacific Island: 32.5 per 100,000 children younger than 5 years old.
  - African American: 16.9 per 100,000 children younger than 5 years old.
  - Hispanic American: 11.1 per 100,000 children younger than 5 years old.
  - Caucasian American: 9.1 per 100,000 children younger than 5 years old (2).

Prevalence

- Approximately 4200 hospitalizations associated with Kawasaki disease per year.
  - 1.5:1 boy to girl ratio.
  - 76% of children are <5 years old.
  - More common in winter and early spring.
  - Peak mortality occurs 15–45 days after onset of fever (3).

RISK FACTORS

- Genetic susceptibility
- Delayed diagnosis
- Prolonged fever is risk for development of aneurysmal coronary artery disease.

Genetics

Genetic susceptibility: Polymorphism of ITPKC gene (19q13.2) (2)

GENERAL PREVENTION

Sequelae of disease are avoided with early diagnosis and treatment.

PATHOPHYSIOLOGY

- Acute vasculitis of all blood vessels with the mid-size arteries being most predominantly affected.
  - Early phase: Neutrophil infiltration with edema and a rapid transition to mononuclear cells (primarily CD8 T-cells, IgA plasma cells, monocytes, and macrophages).
  - Second phase: Production of matrix metalloproteinase, which destructs the internal elastic lamina and media.
  - Final phase: Replacement of the vessel intima and media with fibrous connective tissue (2).

ETIOLOGY

Thought to be triggered by unidentified infection in genetically susceptible children.

COMMONLY ASSOCIATED CONDITIONS

- Coronary artery aneurysm with secondary thrombosis/ischemia
- Arthritis/arthralgia
- Diarrhea, vomiting, abdominal pain
- Myocarditis
- Anterior uveitis (usually mild)
- Less common conditions
  - Superficial punctuate keratitis
  - Choroiditis
  - Papilledema

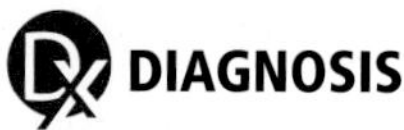

DIAGNOSIS

HISTORY

- Fever of at least 5 days duration plus 4 of the 5 major criteria.
  - History of recently affected family member may be present.

PHYSICAL EXAM

- Fever (often 104°F or higher)
- Bilateral bulbar conjunctival injection
- Erythema of oropharyngeal mucosa with strawberry tongue
- Dry, cracked lips without ulceration
- Erythema, desquamation, edema of hands and feet (may also affect gluteal cleft). Periungual desquamation of the fingers and toes begins 1–3 weeks after onset.
- Truncal rash
- Nonsuppurative cervical lymphadenopathy
- Other findings may include extreme irritability, aseptic meningitis, diarrhea, mild hepatitis, hydrops of gallbladder, pyuria, otitis media, and arthritis.

DIAGNOSTIC TESTS & INTERPRETATION

Lab

Initial lab tests

- No diagnostic laboratory test but certain findings are often present:
  - Anemia (normocytic, normochromic)
  - Leukocyte count normal to elevated with neutrophil shift
  - Platelet count initially normal
  - Elevated ESR and CRP
  - Elevated hepatic transaminases
  - Pyuria (1)[B]

Follow-up & special considerations

Rapid elevation of platelets in second week of illness.

Imaging

Initial approach

- Echocardiogram during acute phase of illness.
  - Coronary artery aneurysm/ectasia may be present in as many as 25% of children with Kawasaki disease (3)[C].

Follow-up & special considerations

- If coronary artery aneurysm is present repeat echocardiogram is needed until resolved.
- For uncomplicated cases, follow-up echocardiogram should be performed at 2 and 8 weeks after onset
- Cardiac stress testing is recommended for children with Kawasaki disease and coronary artery abnormality.
  - Angiography is needed if evidence of cardiac ischemia is present.

DIFFERENTIAL DIAGNOSIS

- Scarlet fever
- Toxic shock syndrome
- Measles
- Adenovirus infection
- Drug hypersensitivity (Steven–Johnson syndrome)
- Epidermolysis bullosa
- Conjunctivitis
- Collagen vascular disease (e.g., lupus)

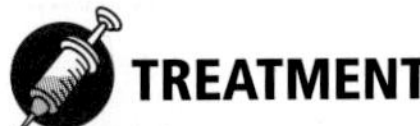

TREATMENT

MEDICATION

First Line

- Single infusion of IVIG at 2 g/kg given within 10 days of onset (2,3) [A].
  - Aspirin at 80–100 mg/kg/d given in 4 divided doses (2,3) [C].
  - Topical steroids for iritis usually not necessary.

Second Line

- IV prednisolone may play a role in decreasing duration of disease but no standard dose is recommended (3)[C].
- Pentoxifylline has been used as adjunct therapy in small clinical trials but its role is uncertain (3)[C].

ADDITIONAL TREATMENT

General Measures

- Low-dose aspirin (3–5 mg/kg/d) is continued until 6–8 weeks after onset of illness if no coronary changes are present (3)[C].
  - Patients not responsive to standard treatment may benefit from repeat IVIG, steroids, or infliximab (3)[C].

Issues for Referral

- Infectious disease and rheumatology consultation may be useful in establishing diagnosis.
  - Pediatric cardiologist should be involved in the patient's care.

Additional Therapies

- Antiplatelet agents (clopidogrel, dipyridamole) may be considered.
- Anticoagulant therapy (warfarin, heparin) may be used in patients at risk of thrombus formation.
- Treatment of acute coronary occlusion secondary to thrombus is controversial but streptokinase, urokinase, and tissue plasminogen activator has been reported (3)[C].
- Activity restriction guided by anticoagulation therapy and cardiac stress testing.

SURGERY/OTHER PROCEDURES

- Cardiac catheterization with stent placement has been useful in specific clinical conditions.
- Coronary bypass graft may be used in children with recurrent myocardial infarct.
  - Rarely, cardiac transplant is justified.

IN-PATIENT CONSIDERATIONS

Admission Criteria

Children with at least 4 days of fever with suspected Kawasaki should be admitted for further testing and treatment.

IV Fluids

Use as needed particularly if abdominal symptoms.

Discharge Criteria

- Afebrile for 48 hours after initiating treatment.
  - Appropriate testing complete.
  - Longer hospitalization may be required if significant coronary disease is present.

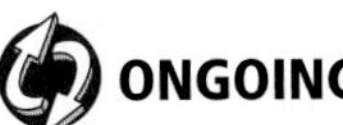

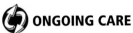

ONGOING CARE

FOLLOW-UP RECOMMENDATIONS

- Ophthalmologic follow-up is needed only in presence of anterior uveitis or more severe ocular manifestations.
- Systemic follow-up is directed by coronary artery involvement (3)[C].
  - Cardiovascular risk assessment recommended at 5 year intervals for children with no coronary artery changes.
  - Cardiovascular risk assessment recommended at 3 year intervals for children with transient coronary artery ectasia.
  - Annual cardiology follow-up with echocardiogram and electrocardiogram in addition to stress testing every 2 years recommended in children with an isolated small/medium coronary aneurysm.
  - Biannual cardiology follow-up with echocardiogram, electrocardiogram and stress testing is recommended for children with large coronary artery aneurysms or coronary artery obstruction.

PATIENT EDUCATION

- Kawasaki Support Group http://www.patient.co.uk/support/Kawasaki-Support-Group.htm
- Kawasaki Disease Foundation http://www.kdfoundation.org/
- Activity restrictions must be discussed in patients taking anticoagulants as well as in patients with severe coronary artery disease.
  - Signs and symptoms of ischemic heart disease need be discussed with patient and family.

PROGNOSIS

Early diagnosis and treatment with IVIG and aspirin reduce coronary artery disease to 2–4% (2)[C].

COMPLICATIONS

- Coronary ischemia and arterial thrombosis resulting in myocardial infarction.
- Sudden death

REFERENCES

1. Perrin L, Letierce A, Guitton C, et al. Comparative study of completer versus incomplete Kawasaki disease in 59 pediatric patients. *Joint Bone Spine* 2009;76:481–485.
2. Gedalia A, Cuchacovich R. Systemic vasculitis in childhood. *Curr Rheumatol Rep* 2009;11:402–409.
3. Newburger JW, Takahashi M, Gerber MA, et al. Diagnosis, treatment, and long-term management of Kawasaki disease: A statement for health professionals from the Committee on Rheumatic Fever, Endocarditis and Kawasaki Disease, Council on Cardiovascular Disease in the Young, American Heart Association. *Pediatirics* 2004;114: 1708–1733.

ADDITIONAL READING

- Yellen ES, Gauvreau K, Takahashi M, et al. Performance of 2004 American Heart Association recommendations of treatment of kawasaki disease. *Pediatrics* 2010;125:e234–e241.

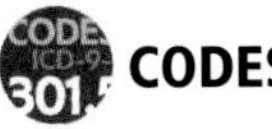

CODES

ICD9

- 364.3 Unspecified iridocyclitis
- 372.71 Hyperemia of conjunctiva
- 446.1 Acute febrile mucocutaneous lymph node syndrome (mcls)

CLINICAL PEARLS

- Cardiac evaluation is essential when Kawasaki disease is suspected or confirmed. Children with incomplete Kawasaki disease seem to have a risk of coronary artery aneurysm at least as great as that of children who fulfill the classic criteria.
- Early diagnosis and treatment is key to decreasing morbidity and mortality.
- Iritis rarely needs topical intervention and is usually self-limiting and benign.
- More severe ophthalmic involvement is uncommon.

KERATOCONUS

Brad H. Feldman

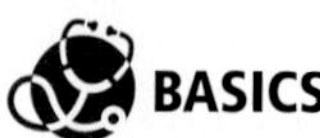

BASICS

DESCRIPTION

A disorder of corneal instability, thinning, steepening, and protrusion that develops in the absence of neovascular inflammation. The name derives from the conical shape of the cornea in advanced disease. Clinical disease is characterized by the following:

- Progressive astigmatism ± myopia.
- Loss of best spectacle-corrected visual acuity.
- Decreased tolerance of contact lens wear.
- Central corneal scar formation and opacification.

EPIDEMIOLOGY

Incidence

Highest in puberty and early adulthood.

Prevalence

50–230 per 100,000 (1).

RISK FACTORS

- Eye rubbing
  - A significant risk factor in susceptible individuals
- Nocturnal pressure on the cornea
  - A suspected risk factor in susceptible individuals
- 1st degree relative with keratoconus
  - 3–4% prevalence within families of affected individuals

Genetics

- No clear inheritance pattern (2).
  - Some support for incomplete autosomal dominant pattern.
  - Less than full concordance in monozygotic twins.

GENERAL PREVENTION

Avoidance of corneal rubbing is recommended.

PATHOPHYSIOLOGY

- Progressive instability and irregularity in anterior and posterior corneal contours lead to irregular astigmatism.
- Breaks in Bowman's layer result in fibrosis and corneal scarring.
- Breaks in Descemet's layer lead to acute corneal edema (hydrops).

ETIOLOGY

Not yet fully elucidated.

COMMONLY ASSOCIATED CONDITIONS

- Floppy lid syndrome/lid laxity (odds ratio >19) (3).
- Sleep apnea.
- Atopy.
- Allergic conjunctivitis.
- Congenital disorders of low vision, including the following:
  - Leber's congenital amaurosis, retinopathy of prematurity, and aniridia
- Congenital disorders of developmental delay (and eye rubbing), including the following:
  - Down's syndrome.
- Connective tissue disorders, including the following:
  - Ehlers–Danlos Marfan's and Osteogenesis imperfecta.
- Corneal dystrophies, including the following:
  - Fuchs' endothelial, posterior polymorphous, granular, and lattice

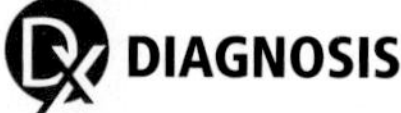

DIAGNOSIS

HISTORY

- Progressive asymmetric vision and contrast sensitivity loss, glare, distortion, or monocular diplopia
- Progressive asymmetric astigmatism (noticed commonly as distorted vision)
- May manifest clinically as unilateral (but >95% show bilateral topographic changes).
- Eye rubbing/pressure on eye during the day or during sleep (4)
  - Many patients directly and forcibly rub the globe (in a pattern often distinct from allergic rubbing)
  - May describe a discomfort relieved by rub
  - Preferred sleeping side often correlates with more affected eye.
- Difficulty or intolerance of contact lenses
  - May describe progression from astigmatism correcting soft-to-rigid lenses.

PHYSICAL EXAM

- Fluctuating refraction with increasing astigmatism and, usually, myopia over time
- Irregular retinoscopic reflex (scissoring)
- Irregular shadowing of red reflex
- External examination abnormalities may include the following:
  - V-shaped indentation of lower lid with depression (Munson's sign)
  - Conical prominence and/or displacement of apex on lateral view
  - Upper lid laxity ± upper lid lash misdirection
- Slit lamp abnormalities may include the following:
  - Iron deposition in basal epithelium around base of cone (Fleischer ring)
  - Corneal scarring (mild haze to severe opacification typically at apex)
  - Irregular corneal thickness and curvature seen with slit beam
  - Prominent corneal nerves
  - Posterior stromal striae (Vogt striae) which are typically central and vertical—these may fade with external pressure
  - Corneal edema, bullae, and posterior scars in cases of Descemet's membrane rupture (Hydrops)
- Manual keratometry: Irregular rings ± steep readings

DIAGNOSTIC TESTS & INTERPRETATION

Imaging

- Placido-based keratoscopy or topography may demonstrate some or all of the following (5):
  - High keratometric values, inferior steepening (elevated I–S values), high astigmatism, skewed radial axes.
- Scanning-slit beam with placido-disc topography (Orbscan IIz, Bausch & Lomb) or rotating Scheimpflug imaging (Pentacam, Oculus) may demonstrate above abnormalities plus
  - Anterior and posterior corneal elevation abnormalities.
  - Abnormal corneal thickness profiles with decentered thinnest points.
- Optical coherence tomography (Visante, Carl Zeiss) may demonstrate abnormal corneal thickness profiles with decentered thinnest points.
- Wavefront aberrometry may demonstrate increased higher order aberrations (especially vertical coma).
- High-frequency ultrasound (Artemis, ArcScan, Inc.) may demonstrate abnormal corneal epithelial thickness profile.

Pathological Findings

- All corneal layers may be affected in the disease process, including the following:
  - Central epithelial thinning with changes in epithelial cell morphology
  - Degenerated basal epithelial cells with accumulation of ferritin particles between cells
  - Breaks in epithelial layer
  - Fragmentation of and breaks in Bowman's layer
  - Alteration of normal stromal collagen architecture
  - Endothelial cell pleomorphism and polymegathism
- Note that pathologic findings may vary

DIFFERENTIAL DIAGNOSIS
- Physiologic astigmatism
- Postrefractive surgery ectasia
- Pellucid marginal degeneration
- Keratoglobus
- Traumatic corneal scar
- Contact lens warpage

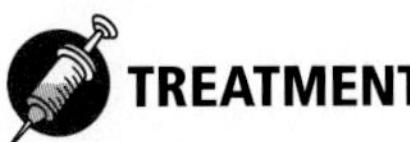

TREATMENT

MEDICATION
- For acute hydrops:
  - Cycloplegia $\pm$ patching or bandage contact lens for comfort
  - Hypertonic solution/ointment (5% sodium chloride) b.i.d. to q.i.d.

ADDITIONAL TREATMENT
General Measures
- Important to stop rubbing eyes
- Avoid pressure on eyes during sleep
- Spectacle correction if possible
- Contact lens fitting
  - Possible if there is not significant scarring or edema.
  - Soft lenses for low levels of regular astigmatism
  - Rigid gas-permeable (RGP) lenses are most often successful.
  - If unable to fit in an RGP, try piggybacking with soft lens or use a hybrid or scleral lens

Issues for Referral
- Contact lens fitting is often difficult and is best performed by an experienced fitter.
- Patients intolerant of contact lens wear should seek consultation with a cornea specialist to consider surgical options.
- Consider polysomnography to test for undiagnosed sleep apnea.

SURGERY/OTHER PROCEDURES
- Intrastromal ring segments (Intacs, Addition Technology)
  - May improve vision and contact lens tolerance
- Corneal stromal crosslinking is an investigational therapy that may help decrease progression of vision loss
- Corneal transplantation is the gold standard
  - Full-thickness penetrating keratoplasty
  - Trephinated versus noncylindrical variations (manual or Femtosecond-assisted)
  - Deep anterior lamellar keratoplasty

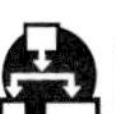

ONGOING CARE

FOLLOW-UP RECOMMENDATIONS
- At minimum every 12 months, more frequently if progressing rapidly.
- Every 1–4 weeks during a hydrops episode until it resolves (vision may improve due to corneal flattening after hydrops, if edema persists over months, surgery may be indicated).

PROGNOSIS
- Disease severity and rates of progression are widely variable, but even milder forms of disease may lead to significant decreases in vision-related quality of life.
- Significant visual loss over 5–7 year period more likely if better baseline acuity, steeper keratometric values, or fundus abnormalities (6).

COMPLICATIONS
Corneal perforation is rare.

REFERENCES

1. Krachmer JH, Feder RS, Belin MW. Keratoconus and related noninflammatory corneal thinning disorders. *Surv Ophthalmol* 1984;28:293–322.
2. Wang Y, Rabinowitz YS, Rotter JI, et al. Genetic epidemiologic study of keratoconus: Evidence for major gene determination. *Am J Med Genet* 2000;93:403–409.
3. Ezra DG.Beaconsfield M, Sira M, et al. The Associations of Floppy Eyelid Syndrome: A case control study. *Ophthalmology* 2010;4:831–838.
4. Carlson AN. Keratoconus. *Ophthalmology* 2009;116:2036–2037.
5. Rabinowitz YS. Videokeratographic indices to aid in screening for keratoconus. *J Refractive Surg* 1995;11:371–379.
6. Davis LJ, Schechtman KB, Wilson BS, et al. Longitudinal changes in visual acuity in keratoconus. *Invest Ophthalmol Vis Sci* 2006;47:489–500.

ADDITIONAL READING

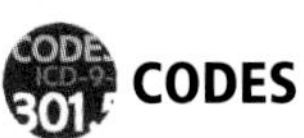

See Also (Topic, Algorithm, Electronic Media Element)

- Elevated keratometric values on the sagittal curvature mapping.
- Decreased corneal thickness with a decentered thinnest point on corneal thickness mapping.
- Significant anterior corneal elevation over a best-fit sphere on elevation (front) mapping.
- Significant posterior corneal elevation over a best-fit sphere on elevation (back) mapping.

CODES

ICD9
- 371.00 Corneal opacity, unspecified
- 371.60 Keratoconus, unspecified

K

LACRIMAL GLAND TUMORS

Michael P. Rabinowitz
Jacqueline R. Carrasco

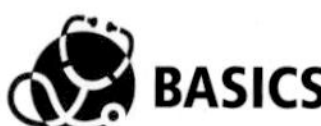

BASICS

DESCRIPTION

- Lacrimal gland tumors include a wide variety of masses that may be epithelial or nonepithelial, benign or malignant, and primary or metastatic.
- Historically, ~50% of lacrimal gland lesions were epithelial, and 50% benign. It seems that these numbers were subject to referral bias to tertiary care institutions. Rarer, interesting, and/or malignant lesions may be more likely to be reported. Further, reviews of these subjects reveal that some cases reported individually were also included in series.
- Current guidelines show the following (1):
  - 10% of orbital lesions are in the lacrimal gland.
  - 20% are epithelial, and 80% are nonepithelial.
  - Of nonepithelial cases, idiopathic orbital inflammation seems most common, followed by non-Hodgkin's B-cell lymphoma.
  - Of epithelial cases, 55% are benign while 45% are malignant.
  - Of benign epithelial tumors, dacryops (ductal cyst of the palpebral lobe) seems most common (37%).
  - Of malignant epithelial tumors, adenoid cystic carcinoma is most common (~60%).
  - Thus, this chapter focuses on inflammatory, benign epithelial, and adenoid cystic etiologies with greatest detail.

EPIDEMIOLOGY

Varies widely based on tumor etiology

- Adenoid cystic carcinoma: Mean age at presentation is 40 years, with recognized cases historically presenting in the first two decades as well. Can occur in any age.
- Dacryops: Common (6%), usually in young or middle-aged patients, and rarely symptomatic (only around 21% in reported series require excision).
- Orbital lymphoma/reactive lymphoproliferative processes: Equal incidence of males and females, with age range including all ages, mean age 55 years.
- Idiopathic orbital inflammation (IOI): Wide age range, from teens to 70s in many series, with a mean age of 45 years and an even gender distribution.
- Sarcoidosis: Can occur in any age, but most common between 20 and 40 years, and rare after 50 years.
  - Within the orbit, the lacrimal gland is most commonly involved (up to 61%).
  - In North America, highest incidence amongst African Americans: 35.5 cases per 100,000
  - In the world, highest incidence amongst Northern Europeans: up to 60 cases per 100,000

RISK FACTORS

- Malignant epithelial lesions: Incomplete resection of prior lesion, whether benign or malignant
- Lymphoma: Sjögren's syndrome predisposes to orbital adnexal lymphoma.
- Idiopathic inflammation: Viral and environmental factors are proposed triggers.
- Sarcoidosis: Environmental triggers such as pesticides and pollutants have been postulated but are largely theoretical.

Genetics

- Lymphoma: Largely depends on the type of lymphoma. T(11;18)(q21;q21) may represent an important developmental event in marginal zone lymphomas, resulting in a gene fusion on chromosome 11 and the development of the MALT1 gene on chromosome 18.
- Idiopathic inflammation: Unknown.
- Sarcoidosis: Two genome-wide scans may be biased by population selection:
  - White Germans – chromosomes 3p and 6p
  - African Americans – chromosomes 5p and 5q.

GENERAL PREVENTION

Depends on the etiology of orbital tumor, but largely unknown in most cases.

PATHOPHYSIOLOGY

Varies widely based on tumor etiology. See the "Pathological findings" section for histologic detail of tumor entity.

ETIOLOGY

- Epithelial lesions (in order of decreasing incidence in patients warranting referral to an ophthalmic oncology service):
  - Dacryops, adenoid cystic carcinoma, pleomorphic adenoma, pleomorphic adenocarcinoma, prolapsed lacrimal gland, mucoepidermoid carcinoma
- Nonepithelial lesions (in order of decreasing incidence in patients warranting referral to an ophthalmic oncology service):
  - Dacryoadenitis (pseudotumor), non-Hodgkin's lymphoma, benign reactive lymphoid hyperplasia, atypical lymphoid hyperplasia, plasmacytoma, lymphoepithelial hyperplasia
- Sarcoidosis: See previous epidemiology
- Leukemia, metastases, dermoids, lipomas, Wegener's granulomatosis, and plasmacytomas
- Infectious: tuberculosis, syphilis, and mumps
- A recent review of patients with lacrimal gland enlargement referred to the Wills Eye Institute Oculoplastics and Orbital Surgery service shows that 43% of lacrimal gland lesions were nongranulomatous inflammation, 20% were sarcoidosis, 10% were reactive lymphoid hyperplasia, 6% were lymphoma, and 5% were atypical lymphoid hyperplasia.

COMMONLY ASSOCIATED CONDITIONS

- Salmon patch: Pink subconjunctival lesion may represent extension of orbital lymphoma.
- Sjögren's syndrome: May precede lacrimal gland lymphoma or be associated with sarcoidosis infiltration of the lacrimal gland, parotid, and conjunctiva
- Lofgren's syndrome: Arthritis, erythema nodosum, and bilateral hilar adenopathy with sarcoidosis
- Arthritis: Rheumatoid or juvenile rheumatoid with sarcoidosis
- Heerfordt syndrome: Parotid enlargement, anterior uveitis, and cranial nerve palsies with sarcoidosis.
- Blau's syndrome (familial juvenile systemic granulomatosis): Children may present with granulomatous arthritis, skin and eye pathology with sarcoidosis.

DIAGNOSIS

HISTORY

- Careful history must be taken regarding previous malignancies, lacrimal gland biopsies, or surgeries.
- Epithelial and nonepithelial malignancies: Inferior and nasal globe displacement with proptosis. Lesions are typically painless, although pain may be seen with bony erosion or perineural involvement (typical of adenoid cystic carcinoma). Ptosis, motility disturbances, and diplopia may occur with lacrimal gland malignancies.
- Benign epithelial tumors: Typically a long history of painless proptosis ± globe displacement. "S-shaped" proptosis seen in orbital lobe involvement.
- IOI: Explosive onset of pain and swelling predominantly in the outer one-third of the upper eyelid. Tearing, injection, diplopia, and decreased vision. If previous episodes exist, rapid response to corticosteroids is the norm.
- Infectious: May appear similar to IOI, which exists along a spectrum of inflammation with scleritis, but with purulent discharge in bacterial cases or frequent bilateral involvement with preauricular nodal involvement with viral etiologies. Fevers, chills, sweats, and other systemic symptoms should be screened for but are nonspecific.
- Sarcoidosis: Systemic symptoms such as fevers, chills, sweats, and weight loss. Adnexal involvement marked by pain, proptosis, and lacrimal gland enlargement. Sarcoidosis most commonly affects the lungs, eyes, and skin, so history may be tailored toward a targeted review of systems accordingly.

PHYSICAL EXAM

- Physical exam should be a thorough ophthalmologic evaluation with consideration of all aforementioned potential etiologies.
- Visual acuity, intraocular pressure, visual fields, and extraocular motility should be evaluated in all patients.
- All cranial nerves should be evaluated, and the presence or absence of ptosis should be documented.
- Optic nerve involvement and infiltration should be evaluated with visual fields, color plates, and pupillary examination.
- Anterior slit lamp exam includes evaluation of conjunctival nodules, conjunctivitis, episcleritis, scleritis, dry eyes, corneal edema, keratic precipitates (may be granulomatous, particularly in a triangular distribution on the inferior corneal endothelium), anterior chamber cell and flare, peripheral anterior synechiae, and posterior synechiae given differential diagnosis including sarcoidosis and blood dyscrasias.
- Posterior slit lamp and indirect exam should evaluate for peripheral retinal neovascularization, periphlebitis and peripheral retinal vein sheathing, intermediate uveitis, and optic nerve edema.
- Full physical exam should evaluate for tachypnea, arthritis, lymphadenopathy, hepatosplenomegaly, erythema nodosum (most commonly found over shins), and skin rashes.
  - Imaging and further evaluation as below.

DIAGNOSTIC TESTS & INTERPRETATION

Lab

- Angiotensin converting enzyme (ACE): Elevated in 60–90% of patients with active sarcoidosis. Rates higher in those with active signs and symptoms
- CBC with differential and serum protein electrophoresis if malignancies suspected. Blood smear to further pursue etiology.
- PPD with anergy panel to evaluate tuberculosis, and to rule it out if steroid therapy anticipated.
- Antineutrophil cytoplasmic antibody (cANCA), ANA, RPR, FTA-Abs to evaluate for autoimmune and infectious causes as history and exam warrant.

Imaging

Initial approach

- Orbital CT with axial and coronal views. Look at the lacrimal gland fossa (superotemporal orbit) for the presence of any bony erosion.
- MRI if suspicion of intracranial extension
- Chest X-ray to evaluate for sarcoidosis, tuberculosis, primary malignancy, or metastases
- Chest CT if initial imaging nondiagnostic

Follow-up & special considerations

- Systemic evaluation and full medical examination should be performed by an internist as etiology or suspected etiology demands.
- Hematology/oncology evaluation when malignancy, both epithelial and nonepithelial, is diagnosed or suspected.
- Systemic or neurologic involvement should involve internal medicine, pulmonology, rheumatology, and/or neurologic referral as primary etiology calls for. Further evaluation and treatment, as below, is often performed in conjunction with healthcare practitioners in those fields.

Diagnostic Procedures/Other

- Note: Do not biopsy lesions suspected to be dermoids! Ruptured dermoids may cause dramatic inflammatory reactions.
- Note: Do not biopsy or incompletely excise benign mixed tumors! Incomplete excision may result in orbital seeding and recurrence with our without malignant transformation.
- Lacrimal gland biopsy is considered if lesions are accessible, diagnosis is uncertain, and malignancy is suspected. The orbital lobe of the lacrimal gland is the preferred site of biopsy, in order to preserve lacrimal ductules in the palpebral lobe.
- Typical granulomas need evaluation with special stains (methenamine-silver to rule out tuberculosis and fungal infections, and acid-fast to look for mycobacteria). In sarcoidosis, lacrimal gland biopsy has a 60% yield.
- Conjunctiva may be biopsied in sarcoidosis suspects: Yield of blind conjunctival biopsy is 66% in sarcoidosis patients, and 80% in those with conjunctival involvement.
- Skin lesions may be biopsied in sarcoidosis: The edges of lesions should be sampled. Erythema nodosum does not contain pathologic changes.
- Whole-body gallium scan, when combined with positive ACE, is up to 73% sensitive and 100% specific for sarcoidosis.
- Bronchoscopy with pulmonary biopsy may be performed with consideration from a pulmonologist and/or cardiothoracic surgeon in cases with pulmonary involvement by the primary etiology. Other distant organ system involvement, either metastatic or primary, warrants diagnostic evaluation by the appropriate subspecialist.

Pathological Findings

- Adenoid cystic carcinoma: Solid cords of bland-appearing malignant epithelial cells with well-defined borders of five subtypes, including basaloid, cribriform, sclerosing, tubular, and comedocarcinoma
- Benign epithelial neoplasms: Myoepithelial cells are present in adjacent tissue, as opposed to adenoid cystic carcinoma, which has clearly defined borders.
- Sarcoidosis: Noncaseating granulomas, or congregations of epithelioid cells and macrophages, with negative special stains as above
- IOI: Cellular infiltrate consisting of mature lymphocytes, plasma cells, neutrophils, eosinophils, macrophages, and occasionally histiocytes with stromal and vascular changes, fibrosis, and tissue edema

DIFFERENTIAL DIAGNOSIS

- See etiologies.
- Prolapsed retro-orbital fat in the anterior, superotemporal quadrant may simulate lacrimal gland enlargement.
- Perilacrimal gland tumors not involving the gland itself may simulate lacrimal gland masses.

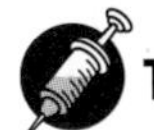

TREATMENT

- Adenoid cystic carcinoma and other epithelial malignancies: Orbital exenteration is usually indicated, particularly in adenoid cystic carcinoma. Neoadjuvant intracarotid chemotherapy or systemic chemotherapy may improve prognosis, and postexenteration orbital irradiation (55–60 Gy) has been recommended, although long-term follow-up data are not available.
- Dacryops/benign epithelial tumors: Complete excision
- Lymphoid tumors: Initial biopsy with local radiation and corticosteroids in indolent cases if confined to the orbit; chemotherapy with subsequent irradiation for systemic involvement
- Sarcoidosis: Systemic immunosuppression with corticosteroids initially followed by steroid-sparing agents; however, high-dose NSAIDs standard of care in the UK. Systemic immunomodulators if steroids fail or are poorly tolerated. Surgical debulking or radiation therapy.
  - Majority of sarcoidosis regresses spontaneously, but observation not recommended.
- IOI: Oral prednisone 80–100 mg daily with GI prophylaxis usually induces prompt response. Low-dose radiation may be used in nonresponders. Treatment refractory cases are atypical may warrant evaluation for other causes of lacrimal gland inflammation.

ADDITIONAL TREATMENT

Issues for Referral

- Neurology and neuro-ophthalmic consultation to evaluate for central neurologic involvement.
- Systemic or other organ involvement warrants referral for evaluation and management as stated previously.

IN-PATIENT CONSIDERATIONS

- As above, IOI not responding promptly to corticosteroids should prompt evaluation, including biopsy, for other etiologies of lacrimal gland inflammation/enlargement.
- Lacrimal gland malignancies warrant internal medicine/oncology subspecialist evaluation for metastatic work-up.

Admission Criteria

Compressive, inflammatory, or vascular optic neuropathies may warrant intravenous corticosteroids, orbital decompression, or other intervention necessitating admission and urgent management.

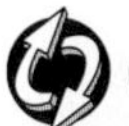

ONGOING CARE

FOLLOW-UP RECOMMENDATIONS

- Epithelial and nonepithelial malignancies must be followed as per recommendations by the hematology/oncology subspecialist for appropriate management.
- Inflammatory conditions: Follow-up intervals depend on severity of inflammation, and patients are usually followed every 1–7 days. Steroid doses, whether topical or oral, are adjusted according to response to treatment, and are tapered as clinical progress allows.

Patient Monitoring

- IOP and cataract development should be followed in patients treated with steroids.
- Patients treated with oral steroids should be seen by their primary care physicians every 3–6 weeks for general exams and blood work to evaluate blood pressures and blood sugars, for example.

PROGNOSIS

- Varies greatly based on the etiology of lacrimal gland mass
- Within epithelial lesions, adenoid cystic carcinoma carries worse prognosis than other lesions.
- Benign lesions completely excised usually do not recur.
- IOI and sarcoidosis often promptly respond to steroids, but may recur.

REFERENCE

1. Shields JA, et al. Primary epithelial malignancies of the lacrimal gland: The 2003 Ramon L. Font Lecture. *Ophthal Plast Reconstr Surg* 2004; 20(1):10–21.

ADDITIONAL READING

- Ehlers JP, Shah CP. *The wills eye manual*, 5th ed. Lippincott Williams & Wilkins, 2008.
- Shields JA, Shields CL, Scartozzi R. Survey of 1264 patients with orbital tumors and simulating lesions: The 2002 Montgomery Lecture, part 1. *Ophthalmology* 2004;111(5):997–1008.

CODES

ICD9

- 190.2 Malignant neoplasm of lacrimal gland
- 198.4 Secondary malignant neoplasm of other parts of nervous system
- 224.2 Benign neoplasm of lacrimal gland

LAGOPHTHALMOS & LID RETRACTION

Vladimir Yakopson
Jacqueline Carrasco

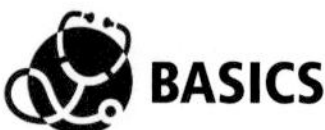

BASICS

DESCRIPTION

- Lagophthalmos = incomplete lid closure
- Lid retraction = presence of scleral shown above the superior or below the inferior limbus, with eyes in primary gaze, brows relaxed, and head in normal posture

EPIDEMIOLOGY

Incidence

- Depends on etiology
- Lid retraction is the most common sign of thyroid eye disease (TED).

RISK FACTORS

Depend on etiology

Genetics

N/A, depends on etiology

GENERAL PREVENTION

Prevention of postoperative lid retraction and lagophthalmos involves judicious removal of skin in blepharoplasty, reformation of the lateral canthal tendon if a canthotomy and cantholysis has been performed, possible placement of traction sutures to prevent contracture, severing of fascial attachments of inferior rectus (IR) during recession surgery.

PATHOPHYSIOLOGY

- Lagophthalmos:
  - Reduced ability of lids to cover the entire globe may be due to several possibilities:
    - Globe is proptotic, e.g., TED, retrobulbar mass or hemorrhage; normal variant in patients with shallow orbits
    - Scarring of anterior lamella (skin and orbicularis), e.g., post op, post herpes zoster, post trauma
    - Loss of anterior lamella, e.g., post tumor excision, post aggressive blepharoplasty
    - Posterior lamella (conjunctiva and tarsus) scarring limiting lid excursion, e.g., ocular cicatricial pemphigoid (OCP), chemical burn, trachoma
    - Neurogenic: Facial nerve (CNVII) palsy or weakness. Orbicularis oculi muscle is responsible for eyelid closure and is innervated by CNVII.
- Lid retraction:
  - Sclera is visible above or below the limbus due to eyelid malposition.
  - Differential as above; however, the abnormality (lid retraction) is present at rest, in primary gaze.
- Lower eyelid retraction may co-occur with severe ectropion.

ETIOLOGY

Depends on the following conditions:

- Autoimmune (e.g., TED, OCP)
- Inflammatory (e.g., post op, trachoma, leprosy)
- Neurogenic (e.g., CNVII palsy)
- Mechanical (e.g., shallow orbits, lower lid tumor, anterior lamella scarring)
- Involutional/senile (e.g., ectropion)

COMMONLY ASSOCIATED CONDITIONS

- TED
- Facial palsy
- Ectropion
- Postsurgical state

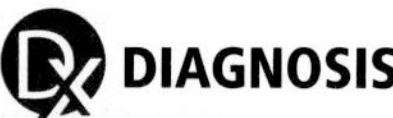

DIAGNOSIS

- Lid retraction – sclera is visible above and/or below the limbus in primary (straight ahead) gaze with brows relaxed.
- Lagophthalmos – incomplete lid closure; patient is asked to close eyes normally (not squeezing maximally) and checked for the presence of a gap between eyelids.

HISTORY

Inquire about

- timing of onset
- tearing, irritation, foreign body sensation, pain
- periorbital ache
- pain with eye movement
- diplopia
- change in vision
- history of prior eyelid or facial surgery or trauma
- history of herpes zoster or simplex infection on face/neck
- history of chronic ophthalmic medication use (possible cause of pseudo-OCP)
- history of chemical burn to eyes/lids/facial skin

PHYSICAL EXAM

- Lid position
- Lid closure
- Examine tarsal conjunctiva for evidence of scarring
- Check for the presence of symblepharon formation
- Visual acuity
- Pupillary reaction (check for rAPD)
- Ocular motility
- Ocular alignment
- Presence of other external signs (e.g., facial scarring, facial nerve palsy/weakness)
- Hertel Exophthalmometry (measures proptosis)
- Anterior segment exam, with careful attention to corneal surface, presence of superficial punctate keratopathy (SPK), corneal erosions or scarring, areas of iris atrophy, presence of active uveitis
- Funduscopy (presence of choroidal folds, optic nerve swelling may indicate the presence of a retrobulbar mass)

DIAGNOSTIC TESTS & INTERPRETATION

Lab

- TSH, T3, free T4, thyroid stimulating immunoglobulin
- Conjunctival biopsy in cases of suspected OCP

Imaging

- CT/MRI of orbits as indicated, e.g., to evaluate for the presence of extraocular muscle enlargement (TED) or mass
- MRI/MRA of brain/brainstem as indicated during work-up of CNVII palsy

Diagnostic Procedures/Other

- Visual field testing (may have various defects in cases of optic neuropathy due to orbital mass or TED)
- External photography (document current lid position, may compare to old family photos to assess for change vs. normal variant as in shallow orbits)
- Color plate deficiencies (decreased color perception may be an indicator of optic neuropathy)

Pathological Findings

Depend on underlying etiology

- TED: Focal and diffuse mononuclear cell infiltrates within EOMs and orbital fat in active disease, fibrotic changes in inactive disease
- OCP: Deposition of IgG, IgA, C3, C4 in conjunctival membrane

DIFFERENTIAL DIAGNOSIS

- Depends on etiology (see the Etiology section):
  - DDx of proptosis (TED, tumor, shallow orbits, etc.)
  - DDx of anterior and posterior lamella scarring
  - DDx of CNVII palsy
- Lower lids may appear falsely retracted in patients with chronic neck flexion forcing chronic chin down head posture and resulting in chronic upgaze.

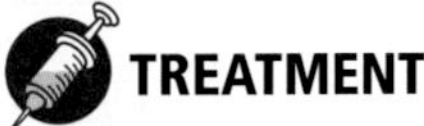

TREATMENT

ADDITIONAL TREATMENT

General Measures

- If asymptomatic and the cornea is well lubricated, the patient may be observed.
- Both lid retraction and lagophthalmos may result in corneal exposure with symptoms and signs of ocular irritation (pain, foreign body sensation, gritty/sandy sensation, redness, excessive tearing, photophobia, etc.).
- Treatment is directed at alleviating the above symptoms.
- Initial measures include frequent lubrication with artificial tears, use of artificial tear gels or ointments at bedtime to protect the corneal surface.
- Eyelids may be taped closed at night.
- Avoiding excessively dry environments is recommended (e.g., if fans are used in the bedroom, they should be pointed away from the patient; use of humidifiers is considered, etc.).
- Concurrent conditions such as blepharitis or ocular allergies are treated appropriately.
- Underlying conditions (e.g., TED, OCP) treated as appropriate.

SURGERY/OTHER PROCEDURES

- If no relief with supportive treatments, surgery may be indicated.
- In cases of CNVII involvement need for surgery is determined by prognosis for CNVII recovery. If no recovery is expected, the upper eyelid retraction, lagophthalmos, and paralytic ectropion should be surgically addressed.
- Eyelid surgery:
  - Approach depends on the underlying condition (e.g., in postoperative lower lid retraction due to aggressive blepharoplasty a skin graft may be required whereas in the case of paralytic ectropion secondary to CNVII palsy the lower lid may need to be horizontally shortened and tightened).
  - Goal is to restore eyelid closure, coverage during blink, reduce symptoms of exposure.
  - Secondary goal is to improve cosmesis, restoring a more normal appearance.
  - Temporary or permanent tarsorrhaphies (parts of the upper and lower lid are sutured together) may be placed.
  - In cases of anterior lamella deficit, a skin graft may be required.
  - Upper eyelids:
    - Transcutaneous or transconjunctival approaches may be utilized. Upper eyelid retractors (Muller's muscle and/or levator palpebrae) are cut (recessed).
    - Gold or platinum weight placement into the upper eyelid is used to improve lid closure.
    - Eye springs may be used.
  - Lower eyelids:
    - Lower lid retractors may be recessed.
    - Spacer graft (AlloDerm, buccal mucosa, banked sclera, etc.) may be used to replace posterior lamella and to elevate the lower lid.
    - Lower lids may be tightened (lateral canthoplasty).
    - Mini-tendon grafting may be performed.

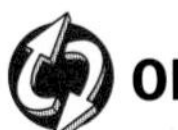

ONGOING CARE

FOLLOW-UP RECOMMENDATIONS

- Primary care provider and/or endocrinologist involved if thyroid disease is suspected.
- Ophthalmologist with subspecialty involvement of an oculoplastic surgeon can manage eye complications and surgery.
- Others may include neurology, ENT, or neurosurgery in cases of CNVII palsy.

Patient Monitoring

Frequency depends on severity of corneal disease: Daily or possible inpatient admission in cases of corneal ulcers to yearly if mild or stable.

PATIENT EDUCATION

Patients are informed about the status of their cornea and/or underlying condition and advised as to the recommended treatment and prognosis.

PROGNOSIS

Depends on underlying etiology and extent of corneal exposure. Ranges from severe visual loss and possible loss of the eye in cases of severe nonhealing or perforated corneal ulcers to mild or asymptomatic cases which require supportive care and monitoring only.

COMPLICATIONS

- Visual loss
- Disfigurement

ADDITIONAL READING

- Abenavoli FM, De Gregorio A, Corelli R. Upper eye lid loading with autologous cartilage in paralytic lagophthalmos. *Plast Reconstr Surg* 2006;117(7): 2511–2512.
- Garg RK. Unusually thickened ulnar nerve and lagophthalmos in leprosy. *Am J Trop Med Hyg* 2010;82(5):758.
- Golio D, De Martelaere S, Anderson J, Esmaeli B. Outcomes of periocular reconstruction for facial nerve paralysis in cancer patients. *Plast Reconstr Surg* 2007;119(4):1233–1237.
- Hassan AS, Frueh BR, Elner VM. Müllerectomy for upper eyelid retraction and lagophthalmos due to facial nerve palsy. *Arch Ophthalmol* 2005;123(9): 1221–1225.
- Liao SL, Shih MJ, Lin LL. A procedure to minimize lower lid retraction during large inferior rectus recession in graves ophthalmopathy. *Am J Ophthalmol* 2006;141(2):340–345.

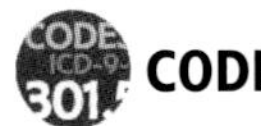

CODES

ICD9

- 374.20 Lagophthalmos, unspecified
- 374.22 Mechanical lagophthalmos
- 374.41 Lid retraction or lag

CLINICAL PEARLS

- Lid retraction is most common sign of TED.
- Severe corneal exposure can lead to visual loss.
- Simple measures such as use of over-the-counter artificial tears and gels may be the extent of required treatment.
- Head posture should be assessed as it can affect gaze position and apparent lid position.

LATTICE CORNEAL DYSTROPHY

Brandon D. Ayres

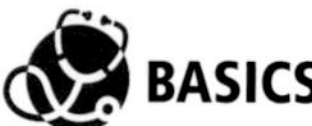

BASICS

DESCRIPTION

- Two major categories of lattice corneal dystrophy are described by the International Committee for Classification of Corneal Dystrophies (IC3D) (1).
- A dystrophy is a process that is noninflammatory and bilateral.
- Lattice corneal dystrophy type I (LCD I) is typically an autosomal dominant corneal dystrophy that leads to frequent recurrent corneal erosions and can progress to severe visual impairment.
- The onset of symptoms is in the first decade of life, with visual impairment often by the fourth decade.
- With this dystrophy protein (amyloid) deposits in the corneal stroma creating refractile branching lines the resemble lattice work. In LCD I, the branching lines do not reach the corneal limbus.
- Synonyms of LCD I include classic LCD and Biber-Haab-Dimmer dystrophy.
- Lattice corneal dystrophy type II (LCD II) has similar corneal changes but the lattice lines start peripherally and move centrally.
- Onset of symptoms is typically in third to fourth decade of life
- Often LCD II is associated with systemic amyloidosis and can be associated with central and peripheral neuropathy, carpal tunnel syndrome, autonomic disturbances, and cardiac arrhythmia
- Synonyms of LCD II include Meretoja syndrome, Amyloidosis V, Familial amyloidotic polyneuropathy IV, Familial amyloidosis, Finnish.
- Autosomal recessive variants of LCD are known, but are very rare. Most patients with have Japanese ancestry.

EPIDEMIOLOGY

LCD is the most common of the stromal corneal dystrophies but is still relatively rare.

RISK FACTORS

- Family history of LCD. Spontaneous mutation in the TGFβI gene can lead to the dystrophy in the absence of a family history.
- Family history of systemic amyloidosis is a risk factor for LCD II. Spontaneous mutation in the Gelsolin (9q34) is responsible for sporadic cases.

Genetics

- LCD I is linked to the transforming growth factor-β-induced (TGFβI) gene on chromosome 5q31 as are many other corneal stromal dystrophies. This gene was once called the BIGH3 gene.
- LCD II is linked to the gelsolin gene 9q34.

GENERAL PREVENTION

Genetic screening

PATHOPHYSIOLOGY

- Accumulation of amyloid protein in the corneal stroma leads to branching refractile lines. When these deposits of amyloid are close to the surface of the corneal erosions of corneal epithelium can occur. Corneal epithelial erosions lead to pain, light sensitivity, and in some cases reduced vision.
- Multiple recurrences of epithelial erosions will lead to scar formation on the corneal leading to a decline in best corrected vision.

ETIOLOGY

Genetic mutation in either the TGFβI or Gelsolin gene. Multiple mutations have been documented in the FAS1 domain of the TGFβI gene, all leading to the phenotype of LCD.

COMMONLY ASSOCIATED CONDITIONS

- LCD I has no commonly associated conditions.
- LCD II is part of a systemic amyloidosis and can be associated with any or all of the following:
  - Cranial neuropathy leading to facial drooping and corneal anesthesia
  - Peripheral neuropathy
  - Autonomic dysfunctions such as postural orthostatic tachycardia syndrome, vasovagal syncope, and neurally mediated hypotension

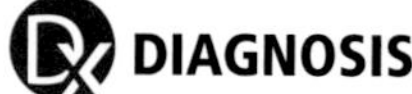

DIAGNOSIS

HISTORY

- Younger patients will complain of spontaneous foreign body sensation.
- Tearing and photophobia will occur in one or both eyes.
- Erosions in the visual axis will reduce vision.
- Older patients will additionally experience a reduction in best corrected vision.

PHYSICAL EXAM

- In early disease the slit lamp exam of the cornea may show subepithelial faint opacities usually close to the apex of the cornea.
- With time the opacities form branching lattice lines that migrate peripherally and deeper into the cornea.
- Repeated corneal epithelial erosions will eventually cause scar formation in the anterior cornea.
- Corneal sensation is often reduced which made reduce healing time.
- In LCD II, the lattice lines may start at the periphery and move centrally over time, and they are more likely to include the periphery.
- Recurrent erosions are less likely in LCD II, but neurotrophic epithelial defects are often a problem.

DIAGNOSTIC TESTS & INTERPRETATION

Diagnostic Procedures/Other

Diagnosis is based on physical exam.

Pathological Findings

- Pathology will show deposits in the cornea of amyloid protein.
- Amyloid protein will stain with congo red stain.
- Amyloid protein will also show apple green birefringence with polarized light.

DIFFERENTIAL DIAGNOSIS

- Recurrent corneal erosion
- Amyloid corneal degeneration
- Granular dystrophy
- Macular dystrophy

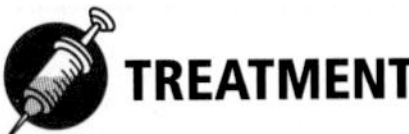

TREATMENT

MEDICATION

First Line

- Treatment of the recurrent erosions with:
  - Topical antibiotics, usually a fluoroquinolone
  - Hypertonic saline drops/ointment
  - Frequent lubricating drops
  - Cyclopedias to reduce photophobia

Second Line

- Epithelial debridement can accelerate the healing of an epithelial erosion.
- Bandage contact lenses are helpful in reducing the pain of an erosion and may speed healing. Antibiotic prophylaxis is a must in these cases with close follow-up.

ADDITIONAL TREATMENT

General Measures

- Routine health care is a must.
- Communication with primary care provider is essential especially in cases of LCD II.
- Reassurance of the patient that while no cure is available, excellent treatments are available.

Issues for Referral

- Referral to a corneal/external disease specialist may be indicated once erosions become problematic or best-corrected vision becomes reduced.
- Frequency of follow-up will depend on severity of symptoms and corneal changes.

SURGERY/OTHER PROCEDURES

- Reduced best-corrected vision from LCD is usually due to progressive scar formation and irregularity in the cornea.
- In early stages, erosions and mild scars can be treated with superficial keratectomy and diamond burr debridement.
- More significant superficial scars can be treated with phototherapeutic keratectomy (PTK) (2).
- Deeper scars require treatment by full or partial thickness corneal transplantation.
- Watch for slower epithelial healing in patients with LCD (3).
- LCD will eventually return in the transplanted cornea.

IN-PATIENT CONSIDERATIONS

Initial Stabilization

Inpatient admission for LCD is very unusual unless it is for systemic complications of familial amyloidosis.

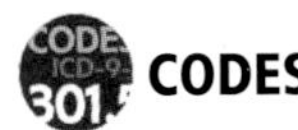

ONGOING CARE

FOLLOW-UP RECOMMENDATIONS

- Regular follow-up with a comprehensive ophthalmologist or cornea specialist is recommended.
- Frequency of follow-up will depend on severity of corneal changes.
- If patients have had a corneal transplant, regular follow-up is needed to ensure transplant success and watch for recurrence of dystrophy.

Patient Monitoring

Any patient who is on topical steroids long time after corneal transplant must be monitored for steroid-related complications such as cataract progression and elevation in eye pressure.

PATIENT EDUCATION

- Patient education is essential.
- www.cornealdystrophyfoundation.org

PROGNOSIS

- Patients with LCD I are very likely to need corneal surgery by the fourth decade. With proper follow-up and management the prognosis for good vision is excellent.
- Longevity of life is normal in these patients.
- Patients with LCD II are less likely to need corneal surgery, but much more likely to suffer from health problems related to systemic amyloidosis.

COMPLICATIONS

- Infectious keratitis can be seen with corneal epithelial erosions and from chronic steroid use.
- Recurrence of lattice dystrophy in the transplanted corneal is common.
- Steroid-induced glaucoma is observed in transplant patients.
- Corneal transplant rejection.

REFERENCES

1. Weiss JS, et al. The IC3D classification of the corneal dystrophies. *Cornea* 2008;27:S1–S42.
2. Ayres BD, Rapuaon CJ. Excimer laser phototherapeutic keratectomy. *Ocular Surface* 2006;4(4):196–206.
3. Foerster CG, Langenbucher A, Cursliefen C, et al. Delayed epithelial healing after keratoplasty for lattice corneal dystrophy. *Cornea* 2007;26: 1182–1183.

CODES

ICD9

371.54 Lattice corneal dystrophy

L

LATTICE DEGENERATION

Brett J. Rosenblatt

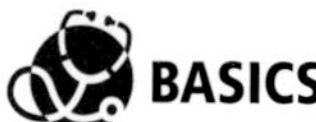

BASICS

DESCRIPTION

Lattice degeneration is a common vitreoretinal degeneration associated with retinal thinning, and subsequent retinal tears or detachments.

EPIDEMIOLOGY

Prevalence

- Found in 6–10% of the population
- More common in myopic eyes
- Found in 20% of eyes with retinal detachments (1)[C]

RISK FACTORS

- Myopia
- Family history
- Systemic disorders such as Stickler's and Wagner's syndromes

GENERAL PREVENTION

None

PATHOPHYSIOLOGY

Inner retinal atrophy with overlying pockets of liquefied vitreous with adherence of formed vitreous to the borders of the areas of lattice degeneration

ETIOLOGY

Unknown, but there is likely a genetic predisposition.

COMMONLY ASSOCIATED CONDITIONS

- Axial myopia
- Atrophic holes
- Chorioretinal atrophy
- Stickler's or Wagner's syndrome

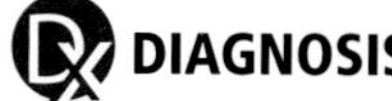

DIAGNOSIS

HISTORY

- Symptoms of vitreous or retinal detachment, such as flashes or floaters
- History of retinal tears or detachments in the fellow eye
- Family history of retinal tears or detachment
- History of myopia (patients may have had laser vision correction or cataract surgery, and should be specifically asked)

PHYSICAL EXAM

- Careful inspection of vitreous for signs of dispersed pigment (indicating tear or detachment)
- Presence of posterior vitreous scleral detachment
- Peripheral retinal exam including depression ophthalmoscopy reveals varied appearance of lattice degeneration:
  - Usually there are linear, pigmented lesions, anterior to the equator that parallel the ora serrata.
  - Variable retinal thinning
  - Sclerotic vessels or white atrophic spots
  - Atrophic retinal holes or branching white lines may be present within the patches of lattice degeneration.

DIFFERENTIAL DIAGNOSIS

- Cobblestone degeneration
- Peripheral retinoschisis
- Microcystic degeneration
- Chorioretinal scar
- Previous laser treatment
- Chronic retinal detachment
- Hereditary vitreoretinal degenerations such as Stickler's syndrome
  - Stickler's syndrome is characterized by mid-face hypoplasia and small chin; bifid uvula or cleft palate; cataract; lattice degeneration; and a high risk of retinal detachment. It is caused by mutations in COL2A1 or in COL11A1 (2,3)[C]

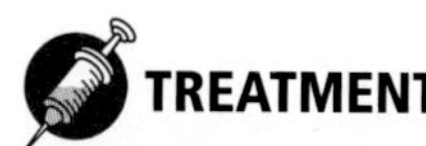

TREATMENT

ADDITIONAL TREATMENT

General Measures

- If no symptoms or tears, then treatment is not indicated even if atrophic holes are present (4,5)[C].
- Consider treating the asymptomatic eye if the fellow eye has had retinal tears or detachment.
- If symptomatic (flashes and/or floaters), consider offering laser demarcation.
- Treat retinal tears with laser or cryoretinopexy.
- Retinal detachments should be treated in a standard fashion.

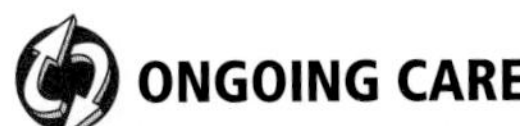

ONGOING CARE

FOLLOW-UP RECOMMENDATIONS

- Recommended follow-up depends on the extent of lattice, symptoms, and presence of tears or retinal detachments.
- Patients with high myopia and patients with a history of retinal detachment in the fellow eye should be watched closely.

PATIENT EDUCATION

Symptoms of retinal tears should be explained. If new flashes, floaters, or scotoma develop, prompt evaluation is critical.

PROGNOSIS

- For patients with lattice degeneration, the risk of retinal detachment is only 1% over a 10-year period.
- Prognosis is excellent unless retinal detachment develops.
- Delay in treatment of retinal detachment can lead to permanent vision loss.

REFERENCES

1. Benson WE, Morse PH. The prognosis of retinal detachment due to lattice degeneration. *Ann Ophthalmol* 1978;10:1197–1200. [C]
2. Edwards AO. Clinical features of the congenital vitreoretinopathies. *Eye* 2008;22:1233–1242. [C]
3. Ang A, Poulson AV, Goodburn SF, et al. Retinal detachment and prophylaxis in type 1 Stickler syndrome. *Ophthalmology* 2008;115:164–168. [C]
4. Byer NE. Long-term natural history of lattice degeneration of the retina. *Ophthalmology* 1989;96:1396–1402. [C]
5. Wilkinson CP. Evidence-based analysis of prophylactic treatment of asymptomatic retinal breaks and lattice degeneration. *Ophthalmology* 2000;107(1):12–15; discussion 15–18. [C]

CODES

ICD9

- 362.63 Lattice degeneration of retina
- 367.1 Myopia

CLINICAL PEARLS

- Lattice is commonly found in asymptomatic patients.
- Risk of detachment is small.
- Prompt treatment of retinal tears or detachments is necessary to prevent loss of vision.
- Patients with Stickler's syndrome should have prophylactic laser retinopexy.

L

LEBER HEREDITARY OPTIC NEUROPATHY

Kenneth C. Kubis
Susan Whitmer
Margaret MacClary

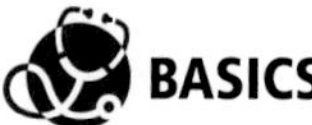

BASICS

DESCRIPTION

- Leber hereditary optic neuropathy (LHON) is usually a unilateral acute or subacute painless profound visual loss (20/200 or worse), followed in weeks to months by loss of vision in the fellow eye (50% of cases in 2–3 months).
- It usually starts as a central scotoma that becomes larger and obscures vision.
- It is caused by optic nerve dysfunction resulting from maternally inherited mitochondrial DNA (mtDNA) mutations.
- Predominantly in males, mean onset is 18–35 years of age (80–90%), but the age of onset can be early or late in life.

EPIDEMIOLOGY

Incidence

Estimated to be 1:30,000 to 1:50,000 in European populations

Prevalence

1:8,500 in the USA

RISK FACTORS

- Maternal carrier with known mtDNA mutation
- Excessive smoking and alcohol consumption have been linked to higher rates of visual loss in susceptible individuals.

Genetics

- Maternally inherited mtDNA mutation
- "Primary mutations" (single mutation sufficient to cause disease) are G3460A, G11778A, and T14484C accounting for 95% of LHON cases.
- G11778A accounts for 50%.
- >18 mutations have been reported.
- Many sporadic and singleton cases have been reported.
- Risk of visual loss from all mutations is 46% for men and 11% for women.
- ~15% of LHON patients demonstrate heteroplasmy (mutant and normal mtDNA will coexist); this may explain the disease threshold with more mutant alleles leading to higher rates of disease and transmission in susceptible individuals.
- Although the rates of homoplasmy or heteroplasmy are measured, they may not directly correlate to levels at the optic nerve.

GENERAL PREVENTION

- Avoid excessive use of tobacco and alcohol if there is a known maternal family member with the disease or carrier state.
- Avoid cyanide-containing products, medications with mitochondrial toxicity, and environmental toxins especially in the acute phase of the disease.

PATHOPHYSIOLOGY

- Each mtDNA mutation affects a subunit of NADH dehydrogenase in the oxidative phosphorylation pathway, which supplies energy to cells.
  - It is thought that these mutations cause LHON because of the increased energy requirement of the optic nerve.
  - The leading theory is that disease results when some individually determined minimal energy requirement threshold is breeched.

ETIOLOGY

First described in 1871 by Theodor Leber, Professor of Ophthalmology at the University of Gottingen

COMMONLY ASSOCIATED CONDITIONS

- Visual dysfunction is usually the only manifestation of the disease. However, cardiac conduction abnormalities and other conditions can rarely manifest.
  - Preexcitation syndromes, Wolf–Parkinson–White, Lown–Ganong–Levine, and prolonged QT interval (rare)
  - Palpitations, syncope, and sudden death have also been reported (rare)
  - Additional neurologic abnormalities have also been reported (rare)
  - Deafness, dystonia, hyperreflexia, cerebellar ataxia, tremor, movement disorders, muscle wasting, gaze evoked nystagmus

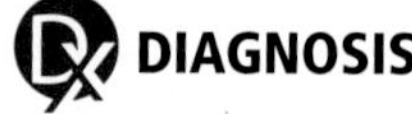

DIAGNOSIS

HISTORY

- At onset most patients complain of painless central vision loss in one eye.
- Patients may complain of the sensation of a blur that obscures vision, or loss of color perception.
- Patients may have associated headache, eye discomfort, flashes of light, color disturbance, limb paresthesias, or dizziness.
- Pedigree analysis may reveal maternal male relatives with profound visual loss.

PHYSICAL EXAM

- Color vision often affected earlier than visual acuity
- Central visual field defects
- Decreased visual acuity usually <20/200
- The classic signs on exam are circumpapillary telangiectatic microangiopathy, nerve fiber layer swelling around the disc, and absence of leakage from the disc on fluorescein angiography; however, these signs may not be seen.
- The classic LHON findings may assist in diagnosis, but their presence is not required for diagnosis.

DIAGNOSTIC TESTS & INTERPRETATION

Lab

Initial lab tests

Genetic testing for mtDNA mutations (see the "Genetics" section)

Follow-up & special considerations

- EKGs can reveal cardiac conduction abnormalities present in some forms of LHON.
- CSF analysis is normal; however, a Leber-plus disease has been described in patients with a multiple sclerosis-like syndrome.
- Formal color testing with D-15 panel and Farnsworth Munsell 100 Hue tests can show optic nerve dysfunction before visual loss.
- Pattern reversal visual evoked potentials (VEPs) may be absent or show prolonged latencies and decreased amplitudes.

Imaging

Initial approach

- Fluorescein angiography can confirm LHON funduscopic features and lack of disc leakage.
- Orbital ultrasound, CT, and MRI can show distended optic nerve sheaths.

Follow-up & special considerations

- Patients with LHON and carriers may show impaired mitochondrial metabolism within limb muscle and occipital lobes on Phosphorus-31 MRI.
- Abnormal lactate production with exercise may be seen in both LHON patients and carriers.

Diagnostic Procedures/Other

Genetic testing

Pathological Findings

Muscle biopsies fail to show morphologic changes of mitochondria and are therefore thought to have limited value.

DIFFERENTIAL DIAGNOSIS

- Other inherited optic neuropathies: Dominant optic neuropathy, Wolfram syndrome
- Acquired optic neuropathies: Tobacco–alcohol amblyopia
- Multiple sclerosis
- Leber's-Plus

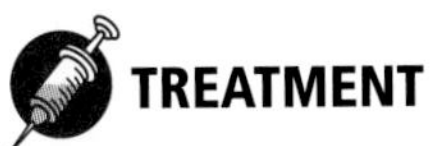

TREATMENT

MEDICATION

First Line

As of 2010 there is no evidence supporting any intervention in the management of mitochondrial disorders.

Second Line

Studies are ongoing in gene therapy.

ADDITIONAL TREATMENT

General Measures

Four main categories

- Vitamins and cofactors (Coenzyme Q10(CoQ10)) (doses up to 3000 mg daily, typically <400 mg daily), folic acid, vitamin B12, thiamine, riboflavin (100 mg daily), L-carnitine (3 g daily), and creatine (3 g b.i.d.)
- Electron acceptors (vitamin C (4 g daily), menadiol (40 mg daily))
- Free radical scavengers (CoQ10, idebenone (75 mg/kg daily), alpha-lipoic acid (600 mg daily), and vitamin E (400 IU daily))
- Inhibitors of toxic metabolites (dichloroacetate DCA)

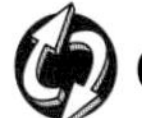

Issues for Referral

Patients suspected of having LHON should be followed by a neuro-ophthalmologist.

SURGERY/OTHER PROCEDURES

- Optic nerve sheath decompression showed no improvement.
- Older literature suggested that craniotomy with lysis of chiasmal arachnoid adhesions resulted in visual improvement.
  - This study has not been repeated and the distance from the site of involvement, at the retinal ganglion cells, makes it difficult to support in light of known spontaneous recovery.

ONGOING CARE

FOLLOW-UP RECOMMENDATIONS

Patient Monitoring

Frequent follow-up for visual acuity can indicate regression of the disease.

DIET

- A balanced diet rich in antioxidants, for example, vitamins A, C, and E, selenium, and zinc, is recommended.
- Patients have been treated with antioxidant dietary supplements.

PATIENT EDUCATION

- Low vision assistance can help patients use vision that remains intact, usually peripheral.
- Genetic counseling is crucial once the diagnosis has been made. This affords understanding of disease transmission. It is critical for female carriers to be identified and educated.

PROGNOSIS

- Rates of spontaneous recovery vary by mutation.
- Patients with 14484 have 37–71% chance of some recovery.
- 11778 typically shows the worst prognosis, spontaneous recovery 4%.
- Other favorable prognostic factors are age of onset <20 (better <10) and larger optic disc vertical diameter on OCT.

REFERENCES

1. Geromel V, Darin N, Chretien D, et al. Coenzyme Q(10) and idebenone in the therapy of respiratory chain diseases: Rationale and comparative benefits. *Mol Genet Metab* 2002;77:21.
2. Newman NJ. Hereditary optic neuropathy, is there a treatment? *Neuro-Ophthalmology: Annual Meeting Syllabus* 2010.
3. Newman NJ. Hereditary optic neuropathies, In: Miller NR, Newman NJ, Biousse V, Kerrisioon JB (eds). *Walsh & Hoyt's Clinical Neuro-Ophthalmology*, 6th ed. Baltimore: Williams & Wilkins, 2005:465–501.
4. Newman NJ. Leber hereditary optic neuropathy: Bad habits, bad vision? *Brain* 2009:132:2306–2308
5. Newman NJ, Lott MT, Wallace DC. The clinical characteristics of pedigrees of Leber's hereditary optic neuropathy with the 11778 mutation. *Am J Ophthalmol* 1991;111:750–762.
6. Nikoskelainen EK, Huopnen K, Juvonen V, et al. Ophthalmoscopic findings in Leber hereditary optic neuropathy, with special reference to mtDNA mutations. *Ophthalmology* 1996;103:504–514.
7. Newman NJ: "Chapter 11: Hereditary optic neuropathies". *Walsh and Hoyt's Clinical-Neurology*. 6th ed. Miller NR, Newman NJ, Biousse V, Kerrison JB. Philadelphia: Lippincott Williams & Wilkins, 2005.

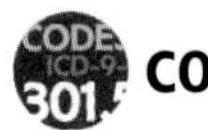

CODES

ICD9

- 368.41 Scotoma involving central area
- 377.9 Unspecified disorder of optic nerve and visual pathways
- 377.16 Hereditary optic atrophy

LENS-INDUCED UVEITIS

Vikram J. Setlur
Sunir Garg

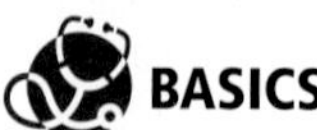

BASICS

DESCRIPTION

- Lens-induced uveitis results from an autoimmune reaction to crystalline lens protein released from surgical or accidental trauma (phacoantigenic endophthalmitis) or leaked from a hypermature cataract (phacolytic glaucoma). Phacoantigenic endophthalmitis was formerly known as phacoanaphylactic endophthalmitis (1)[C], (2)[C].
- Uveitis-glaucoma-hyphema (UGH) syndrome is a complication of intraocular lens (IOL) implantation.

EPIDEMIOLOGY

Rare cause of uveitis, exact incidence and prevalence unknown.

RISK FACTORS

- Lens-induced uveitis occurs with cataract extraction surgery, ocular trauma with disruption of the anterior lens capsule, or a hypermature cataract.
- UGH syndrome is more commonly seen with iris-fixated, anterior chamber IOLs, and sulcus placed posterior chamber IOLs.

PATHOPHYSIOLOGY

- Immune reaction to lens protein in the anterior chamber causes lens-induced uveitis. Inflammation can result from surgery or trauma that disrupts the anterior lens capsule. This inflammation can be granulomatous and severe (phacoantigenic endophthalmitis).
- Leakage of hypermature lens protein through an intact capsule can stimulate a nongranulomatous anterior uveitis with elevated intraocular pressure (phacolytic glaucoma).
- UGH syndrome is caused by contact between the uveal tissue and the IOL haptic or optic.

ETIOLOGY

- In lens-induced uveitis, lens proteins are exposed through trauma (either surgical or accidental) or leakage from a hypermature cataract through an intact lens capsule.
- Iris chafe in UGH syndrome is caused by iris-clipped IOLs, inappropriately sized IOLs, malpositioned IOLs, or rigid closed-loop haptics. It may also occur with poorly manufactured IOL edges and decentered posterior chamber IOLs.

DIAGNOSIS

HISTORY

- Recent history of surgery or eye trauma for lens-induced uveitis
- UGH syndrome more often seen with history of IOL implantation one or more years prior to presentation
- Symptoms include pain, redness, photophobia, and blurred vision.

PHYSICAL EXAM

- Lens-induced uveitis may cause an anterior uveitis than can be mild or severe and granulomatous or nongranulomatous. Posterior synechiae and elevated intraocular pressure are common. Cells may be present in anterior vitreous. Integrity of anterior lens capsule should be assessed.
- The uveitis in UGH syndrome is nongranulomatous and may be accompanied by transillumination defects in the iris, pigment dispersion, hyphema, and elevated intraocular pressure.

DIAGNOSTIC TESTS & INTERPRETATION

Imaging

Ultrasound biomicroscopy (UBM) of the anterior segment may demonstrate IOL contact with uvea for UGH syndrome (3)[C].

Diagnostic Procedures/Other

- Diagnosis in lens-induced uveitis can be confirmed by cytologic analysis of cells obtained via anterior chamber paracentesis (4)[C].
  - Infectious endophthalmitis can be ruled out by analysis of vitreous or aqueous cultures.

Pathological Findings

Lens protein can be observed with anterior chamber paracentesis.

DIFFERENTIAL DIAGNOSIS

- Infectious endophthalmitis, especially following surgery
- Other causes of acute anterior uveitis (e.g. HSV, VZV, idiopathic, sarcoidosis, HLA-B27, and others)

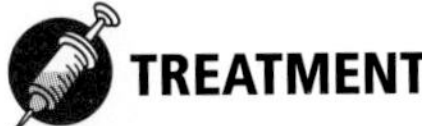

TREATMENT

MEDICATION

First Line

- Topical corticosteroids, with systemic corticosteroids if needed
- Topical antiglaucoma medications for elevated intraocular pressure

SURGERY/OTHER PROCEDURES

- UGH syndrome patients may require IOL explantation for persistent inflammation, glaucomatous nerve damage, or recurrent hyphemas (6)[C].
- Prompt removal of all lens remnants can be curative for lens-induced uveitis:
  - Optimal treatment involves controlling intraocular inflammation and pressure prior to surgery.

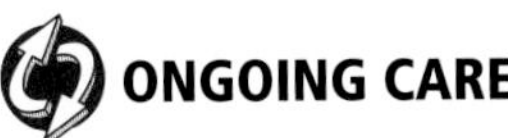

ONGOING CARE

FOLLOW-UP RECOMMENDATIONS

Close follow-up to ensure that intraocular inflammation and pressure are controlled

COMPLICATIONS

Phthisis, glaucomatous visual field loss, central retinal artery occlusion (secondary to elevated intraocular pressure)

REFERENCES

1. Apple DJ, Mamalis M, Steinmetz RL, et al. Phacoanaphylactic endophthalmitis associated with extracapsular cataract extraction and posterior chamber intraocular lens. *Arch Ophthalmol* 1984;102:1528–1532.
2. Marak GE Jr. Phacoanaphylactic endophthalmitis. *Surv Ophthalmol* 1992;36(5):325–329.
3. Piette S, Canlas OA, Tran HV, et al. Ultrasound biomicroscopy in uveitis-glaucoma-hyphema syndrome. *Am J Ophthalmol* 2002;133(6): 839–841.
4. Kalogeropoulos CD, Malamou-Mitsi VD, Asproudis I, et al. The contribution of aqueous humor cytology in the differential diagnosis of anterior uvea inflammations. *Ocul Immunol Inflamm* 2004;12(3): 215–225.
5. Abrahams IW. Diagnosis and surgical management of phacoanaphylactic uveitis following extracapsular cataract extraction with intraocular lens implantation. *J Am Intraocul Implant Soc* 1985;11(5):444–447.
6. McMahon MS, Weiss JS, Riedel KG, Albert DM. Clinically unsuspected phacoanaphylaxis after extracapsular cataract extraction with intraocular lens implantation. *Br J Ophthalmol* 1985;69(11): 836–840.

CODES

ICD9

- 360.19 Other endophthalmitis
- 364.23 Lens-induced iridocyclitis
- 365.51 Phacolytic glaucoma

CLINICAL PEARLS

- Lens-induced uveitis can result from trauma, surgery, or a hypermature cataract that leaks lens protein.
- Management of lens-induced uveitis includes corticosteroids, antiglaucoma medications, and prompt surgical removal of the lens and lens remnants.
- UGH syndrome results from IOL contact with uveal tissue.

L

LEPROSY

Sriranjani P. Padmanabhan
Jennifer Cohn
Vatinee Y. Bunya

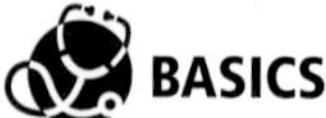

BASICS

DESCRIPTION

- Chronic granulomatous disease caused by *Mycobacterium leprae*
- Also called Hansen's disease
- Primarily affects peripheral nerves, upper respiratory tract mucosa, and skin
- Secondarily affects eyes, nose, ears, muscle, bone, and testes
- Considered one of the 13 neglected tropical diseases
- WHO classification: Paucibacillary (PB) or multibacillary (MB)
  - PB form is also known as tuberculoid leprosy (TT) or borderline tuberculoid (BT) in the Ridley–Jopling classification system. It does not show intraocular manifestations.
  - MB form is also known as lepromatous leprosy (LL), borderline lepromatous (BL), or borderline (BB).
- Ocular leprosy tends to be slow and progressive, can be blinding.
- Eye thought to be a source of re-infection in previously treated generalized disease
- Blindness is especially debilitating as patients may also have compromised mobility and sense of touch.

EPIDEMIOLOGY

Incidence

- WHO estimated ~400,000 new cases in 2004.
- Worldwide incidence currently has a declining trend.

Prevalence

- ~400,000 to 20 million cases have been estimated worldwide.
- 2–3 million suffer permanent disability from leprosy.
- ~5–7% of infected individuals suffer from leprosy related blindness.
- Regions of highest prevalence include India, sub-Saharan Africa, Latin America, and Caribbean.
- Prevalence has dramatically decreased since the 1980s due to advent of multidrug therapy.

RISK FACTORS

- Poverty/squalor
- Impaired cell-mediated immunity
- Residence in endemic areas
- Close contact with infected persons, particularly those with MB disease
- Males affected more than females
- Host genetic susceptibility (see the "Genetics" section below)

Genetics

- Genes involved in innate immune response thought to increase host susceptibility to *M. leprae* and subsequent immune activation: HLA-DRB1, HLA-DRDQ, TNFSF15, RIPK2, NOD2, PARK2, LRRK2.

GENERAL PREVENTION

- Single-dose rifampin in close contacts of patients with newly diagnosed disease provides 57% reduction in subsequent 2-year incidence.
- BCG vaccination or dapsone prophylaxis is marginally effective and not recommended.

PATHOPHYSIOLOGY

- Granulomatous infiltration of peripheral nerves
- Predilection for "cooler" areas; hence ocular leprosy limited to anterior segment
- Infiltration of lids and globe related to tracking along CN VII, corneal nerves, ciliary (uveal) nerves

ETIOLOGY

- Infection with *M. leprae*
- Transmission thought to occur via respiratory route

COMMONLY ASSOCIATED CONDITIONS

- HIV/AIDS
- Intestinal helminth infections

DIAGNOSIS

HISTORY

- Recent close contact with an infected patient
- HIV status/impaired cell-mediated immunity
- Origin from or travel to endemic areas
- Photophobia, epiphora, decreased vision
- May not have pain due to corneal hypoesthesia

PHYSICAL EXAM

- Cornea: Leprous pannus superiorly, prominent corneal nerves (early ocular finding), hypoesthesia, exposure, corneal pearls (chalky white stromal avascular deposits), interstitial keratitis
- Conjunctiva: conjunctivitis, leproma (superficial granulomatous nodule)
- Lens: Cataract, PSC (often treatment induced)
- Uvea: iridocyclitis (can occur even after treatment), iris pearls (miliary leproma)
- External: CN VII palsy, lagophthalmos, cicatricial entropion/ectropion, brow and lash madarosis (loss of hair, late finding), dacryocystitis/fibrosis with resulting dry eye
- Rarely affects *posterior segment*; retinal pearls and/or uveal effusions have been reported
- Systemic: Thickening of facial skin ("leonine facies"), thickened peripheral nerves, decreased sensation to touch and temperature, variable skin lesions including erythema nodosum, hypopigmented or erythematous macules, papules or nodules, Lucio phenomenon (ulcerated erythematous lesions)

DIAGNOSTIC TESTS & INTERPRETATION

- Routine lab tests used primarily to rule out other disease or evaluate drug-related toxicities and/or contraindications:
  - PPD and chest x-ray to rule out TB prior to systemic steroids
  - *T. pallidum* agglutination/RPR for syphilis
  - LFTs depending on treatment regimen

Diagnostic Procedures/Other

- Must establish a tissue diagnosis:
  - Can accomplish via conjunctival or corneal scrapings, AC tap, or skin smears or biopsy

Pathological Findings

- Modified Fite's stain to visualize acid-fast lepra bacilli
- Caseous granulomas causing axonal degeneration is pathognomonic.

DIFFERENTIAL DIAGNOSIS

- Onchocerciasis
- Trachoma
- Syphilis
- Neurofibromatosis
- Leishmaniasis
- Sarcoidosis
- Autoimmune granulomatous uveitides

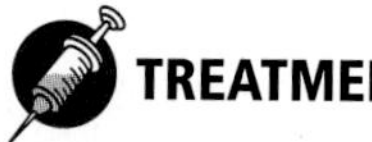

TREATMENT

MEDICATION

First Line

Systemic therapy

- Provided free of charge by WHO to all leprosy patients worldwide
- WHO recommendations for multidrug therapy:
  - PB form: 6-month duration of therapy
    - Adults: rifampicin 600 mg once monthly, dapsone 100 mg daily
    - Pediatric: rifampicin 450 mg once monthly, dapsone 50 mg daily
  - MB form: 12-month duration of therapy
    - Adults: rifampicin 600 mg once monthly, clofazimine 300 mg once monthly, dapsone 100 mg once monthly; then clofazimine 50 mg daily and dapsone 100 mg daily
    - Pediatric: rifampicin 450 mg once monthly, clofazimine 150 mg once monthly, dapsone 50 mg once monthly; then clofazimine 50 mg daily and dapsone 50 mg daily

Pediatric Considerations
Multidrug therapy recommended for children older than 10 years of age. Weight-based dose adjustment necessary for younger children.

Pregnancy Considerations
Leprosy is exacerbated in pregnancy. There are no current contraindications to the above multidrug therapy regimens in pregnancy.

Second Line
Ophthalmic therapy
- Must be concurrent with multidrug therapy
- Many sources suggest escalation and prolongation of multidrug therapy with ocular disease; however, no official guidelines exist
- Artificial tears and other topical lubricants for corneal and lid pathology
- Topical and/or systemic steroids for keratitis and iridocyclitis
- Topical fluoroquinolones if necessary for corneal ulceration or dacryocystitis (ofloxacin shown to be effective against *M. leprae*)
- Often requires definitive surgical therapy for globe protection and visual rehabilitation (see the "Surgery/Other Procedures" section)

ADDITIONAL TREATMENT
Issues for Referral
- Management of multidrug therapy and systemic disease with infectious disease specialist or leprologist, and dermatologist
- Referral of close contacts to infectious disease specialist for prophylaxis (see the "Prevention" section)
- Consider referral for psychological/social support given long history of social stigma

SURGERY/OTHER PROCEDURES
- *Conjunctiva:* Pterygium excision, if applicable, may considerably reduce bacillary load
- *Cornea*: Penetrating keratoplasty for corneal scarring
- *Uvea/glaucoma:* Sector iridectomy for iris bombe, consider enucleation in blind, painful, glaucomatous eye
- *Trichiasis*: Epilation or electrolysis
- *Lagophthalmos:* Should be corrected if >5 mm, decreased corneal sensation, monocular, or for cosmesis. Tarsal shortening procedures, tarsorrhaphy, or frontalis muscle transfer.
- *Entropion/ectropion*: Should be corrected by clinically appropriate procedure

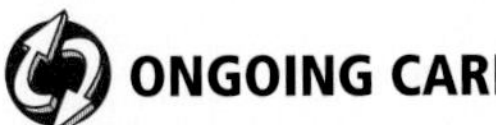

ONGOING CARE

FOLLOW-UP RECOMMENDATIONS
Regular follow-up with ophthalmologist given possibility of recurrent uveitis despite multidrug therapy

PATIENT EDUCATION
International Federation of Anti-Leprosy Associations (ILEP) (http://www.ilep.org.uk/)

PROGNOSIS
- May have recurrent uveitis despite multidrug therapy
- Poor visual morbidity if MB form is untreated for prolonged period of time
- May be confounded by poverty

COMPLICATIONS
- Decreased vision
- Blindness
- Disfiguration
- Death
- Social stigma

ADDITIONAL READING

- Citirik M, et al. Lepromatous iridiocylcitis. *Ocul Immunol Inflamm* 2005;13:95–99.
- Hotz PJ, et al. Control of neglected tropical diseases. *N Engl J Med* 2007;357:1018–1027.
- Johnson GJ. Update on ocular leprosy. *Community Eye Health* 2001;14(38):25–26.
- Moet FJ, et al. for the COLEP Study Group: Effectiveness of single dose rifampicin in preventing leprosy in close contacts of patients with newly diagnosed leprosy: Cluster randomised controlled trial. *BMJ* 2008;336(7647):761–764.
- Mondal K, Biswas S. Review of ocular leprosy. *J Indian Med Assoc* 2006;104(7):401–403, 407.
- WHO Multi-Drug Therapy: Elimination of Leprosy. http://www.who.int/lep/mdt/en/ (accessed March 15, 2010).
- Zhang FR, et al. Genomewide association study of leprosy. *N Engl J Med* 2009;361(27):2609–2618.

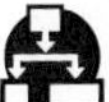

See Also (Topic, Algorithm, Electronic Media Element)

- WHO – Leprosy Elimination (http://www.who.int/lep/en/)

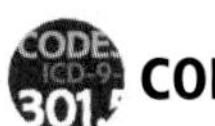

CODES

ICD9
- 030.0 Lepromatous leprosy (type l)
- 030.9 Leprosy, unspecified
- 364.3 Unspecified iridocyclitis

CLINICAL PEARLS

- Iris and corneal pearls are pathognomonic for ocular leprosy.
- Bilateral iridocyclitis is the primary cause of blindness in leprosy.

L

LEUKEMIA/BLOOD DYSCRASIAS

Paul S. Baker

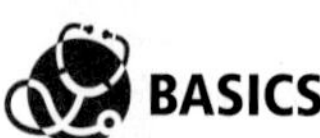

BASICS

DESCRIPTION

Intraocular leukemia is an uncommon ophthalmic disorder, which is due to an accumulation of circulating leukemic cells in the choroid, iris, ciliary body, neural retina, optic nerve, vitreous, and anterior chamber. Leukemia also causes a hemorrhagic retinopathy.

Geriatric Considerations

- Acute myelogenous leukemia is the predominant leukemia type in adults. Compared to children, survival rate is significantly lower.
- Chronic leukemias are generally found in older individuals and often appear in an indolent manner.

Pediatric Considerations

Acute lymphocytic leukemia is the predominant leukemia type in children and has a 50% cure rate.

EPIDEMIOLOGY

Incidence

- The cumulative lifetime incidence of intraocular leukemia in the United States is about 1 case per 2000–2500 persons.
- Peak incidence of intraocular lesions mirrors that of leukemia in general.

Prevalence

- 1 out of every 6 patients with leukemia develops ophthalmic symptoms that lead to referral to an ophthalmologist.
- Ocular findings are more common in acute leukemia compared to chronic leukemia.
- In a small prospective series, 62% of 120 newly diagnosed acute leukemia patients had some level of retinopathy (1)[A].
- In another series of 288 newly diagnosed acute leukemia patients, 35% had ocular findings but only 10% had symptoms (2)[A].
  - Ocular findings are more common in adults than in children.
- 10% of all detected intraocular lesions in leukemic patients are infiltrative.

RISK FACTORS

- Previous cancer treatment (certain chemotherapy and radiation therapy)
- Genetic diseases (i.e., Down syndrome)
- Blood disorders (i.e., myelodysplastic syndromes)
- High levels of radiation
- Certain chemicals (i.e., benzene)
- Smoking
- Family history of leukemia

ETIOLOGY

History of leukemia, which is a cancer of the blood or bone marrow characterized by an abnormal proliferation of blood cells, usually leukocytes

DIAGNOSIS

HISTORY

- Decreased vision or asymptomatic
- Signs and symptoms of leukemia:
  - Coagulopathy (decreased platelets)
  - Frequent infection (dysfunctional leukocytes and a compromised immune system)
  - Dyspnea and pallor (anemia)
  - Constitutional symptoms, such as fevers, chills, persistent fatigue, and weight loss
  - Enlarged lymph nodes

PHYSICAL EXAM

- Leukemic infiltrates:
  - Can involve many intraocular structures – choroidal most common, but retinal changes are most recognizable
  - Most characteristic clinical intraocular lesions
  - Unifocal or multifocal, and one or both eyes
  - Typical lesions are fuzzy, flat, white retinal patch often associated with retinal hemorrhages and overlying vitreous cells.
  - Other infiltrative lesions include vitreous cells, retinal vessel sheathing, optic disc infiltration, retinal pigment epithelial detachment, exudative retinal detachment, localized or diffuse choroidal infiltration, neoplastic pseudohypopyon, and iris infiltration.
- Leukemic retinopathy:
  - Hemorrhages are the most common finding, frequently multifocal and bilateral. May be sub-, intra-, or preretinal with potential breakthrough into vitreous cavity. Cotton wool spots are also seen.
  - Significantly more common than true malignant infiltrates
  - Usually secondary to associated anemia and thrombocytopenia
  - Larger intraretinal hemorrhages may have prominent white centers, known as Roth spots, some of which may represent small leukemic infiltrates.
  - Peripheral retinal capillary nonperfusion and microaneurysm formation has been observed in patients with chronic myelogenous leukemia, which rarely leads to neovascularization.
- Hyperviscosity syndrome:
  - Pathologic mechanism related to increased blood viscosity
  - Results from high white cell count (leukemia), red blood cell count (polycythemia vera), monoclonal gammopathy (i.e., Waldenstroms, multiple myeloma)
  - Venous stasis retinopathy can include vascular tortuosity, microaneurysm formation (posterior and peripheral), retinal hemorrhages, peripheral nonperfusion, neovascularization, intra- and subretinal fluid, mild central retinal vein occlusion appearance,
  - Suspected with bilateral changes
- Opportunistic infections:
  - CMV retinitis is the most common infectious retinitis
  - Progressive outer retinal necrosis
  - Ocular toxoplasmosis
  - Fungal infection

DIAGNOSTIC TESTS & INTERPRETATION

Lab

- Evaluation for suspected leukemic intraocular infiltrate includes a complete hematologic workup in conjunction with an internist.
  - Complete blood count
  - Bone marrow aspiration or biopsy
  - Systemic staging evaluation
  - Lumbar puncture for cerebrospinal fluid evaluation
  - Serum protein electrophoresis for hyperviscosity syndrome

Imaging

- Magnetic resonance imaging of the orbits and brain if optic nerve infiltration
- Serous macular detachments with hyperviscosity can show a characteristic silent fluorescein angiogram with minimal leakage (3)[B].

Diagnostic Procedures/Other

- Fine-needle aspiration biopsy or diagnostic pars-plana vitrectomy if diagnosis in doubt:
  - Patients with leukemia are often immunosuppressed from their disease and/or chemotherapy treatment, making it difficult to clinically distinguish between leukemic infiltrates and other infectious lesions by opportunistic organisms.

Pathological Findings

- In an autopsy series, choroidal infiltration is most common.
- At the time of death, 28–80% of patients have ocular involvement on autopsy (4)[B].
- Leukemic infiltration observed in the uvea, optic disc, retina, vitreous, lumen of choroidal and retinal blood vessels.

DIFFERENTIAL DIAGNOSIS

- Infectious infiltrate:
  - Candida
  - Syphilis
  - Lyme
  - Nocardia
  - Cryptococcus
- Noninfectious infiltrate:
  - Sarcoid granuloma
  - Pars planitis
- Primary intraocular lymphoma

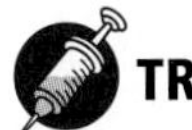

TREATMENT

MEDICATION

First Line

- Systemic chemotherapy is administered to control underlying problem.
- Intraocular manifestations of leukemia usually are not treated directly.

Second Line

When leukemic infiltrates fail to respond to systemic chemotherapy, ocular radiation is often recommended.

ADDITIONAL TREATMENT

General Measures

- Supportive measures (i.e., blood transfusions) are recommended for patients with severe anemia or thrombocytopenia.
- High-dose chemotherapy may increase susceptibility for radiation retinopathy at otherwise safe radiation doses.

Issues for Referral

Treatment of blood dyscrasia, such as leukemia, is always performed by an experienced hematologist/oncologist.

Additional Therapies

- Hyperviscosity syndrome often improves with treatment of underlying disorder
  - In acute setting, leukapheresis (for leukemia) or plasmapheresis (for Waldenström's and multiple myeloma) can be successfully utilized.

SURGERY/OTHER PROCEDURES

Panretinal photocoagulation is used in the setting of peripheral nonperfusion and retinal neovascularization.

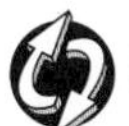

ONGOING CARE

FOLLOW-UP RECOMMENDATIONS

- Full evaluation, staging and treatment by an oncologist/hematologist
- Given the large percentage of leukemia patients with retinopathy, routine ocular examination is recommended for all patients with newly diagnosed acute leukemia.
- More frequent ophthalmic follow-up is recommended in the setting of significant leukemic infiltrates, retinopathy, or hyperviscosity syndrome.

PROGNOSIS

- Leukemic retinopathy has prognostic significance based on multiple studies.
  - In 63 patients with childhood leukemia, 5-year survival was lower in those with leukemic retinopathy on presentation than in those without ophthalmic involvement (21% vs 46%) (5)[B].
- If anemia and thrombocytopenia are addressed, hemorrhagic retinopathy can improve.
- Leukemic infiltrates are viewed as a poor prognostic sign.

REFERENCES

1. Schachat AP, Markowitz JA, Guyer DR, et al. Ophthalmic manifestations of leukemia. *Arch Ophthalmol* 1989;107:697–700.
2. Reddy SC, Jackson N, Menon BS. Ocular involvement in leukemia – a study of 288 cases. *Ophthalmologica* 2003;217:441–445
3. Ho AC, Benson WE, Wong J. Unusual immunogammopathy maculopathy. *Ophthalmology* 2000;107:1099–1103.
4. Kincaid MC, Green WR. Ocular and orbital involvement in leukemia. *Surv Ophthalmol* 1983;27:211–232.
5. Ohkoshi K, Tsiaras WG. Prognostic importance of ophthalmic manifestations in childhood leukaemia. *Br J Ophthalmol* 1992;76:651–655.

CODES

ICD9

- 208.90 Unspecified leukemia, without mention of having achieved remission
- 362.42 Serous detachment of retinal pigment epithelium
- 362.81 Retinal hemorrhage

L

LOW VISION

Scott A. Edmonds
Susan E. Edmonds
Ryan P. Edmonds

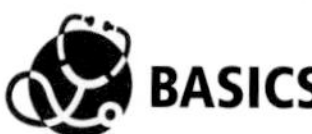

BASICS

DESCRIPTION

Condition where there is a permanent loss in vision due to any disease or disorder where some usable vision remains but desired life function is limited. Some common causes are macular degeneration, diabetic retinopathy, optic neuropathy, and disorders of the visual pathways.

Geriatric Considerations

- Extra time is required to evaluate this population.
- Concentration on near tasks is required.
- Clinical picture can be affected by dementia and cognitive disorders.

Pediatric Considerations

- Accommodation can compensate for magnification.
- Presbyopia occurs very early due to the need for close working distances.
- Telescopes and distance magnification often required.

EPIDEMIOLOGY

Incidence

1/28 for Americans over 40

Prevalence

- 3.3 million adults in the USA
- 0.65–2.75/1000 children
- Difficult to determine due to different definitions for low vision and impairment

RISK FACTORS

- Follows cardiovascular risk factors
- Genetic
- Diet
- Exercise
- Smoking
- UV light exposure

Genetics

- Follows ocular genetic patterns for many causes
- Retinitis pigmentosa
- Stargardt's
- Optic atrophy
- Macular degeneration

GENERAL PREVENTION

- Maintain ocular health
- Protect eyes from UV light
- Maintain cardiovascular health
- Control systemic disease
- Diabetes

PATHOPHYSIOLOGY

- Varies with underlying cause
- Media disorders
- Retinal disorders
- Neurological disorders

ETIOLOGY

Ocular disorders that result in permanent vision loss

COMMONLY ASSOCIATED CONDITIONS

- Diabetes
- Vascular disorders
- Macular degeneration
- Glaucoma
- Optic neuropathy

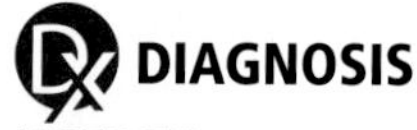

DIAGNOSIS

HISTORY

- Medical
- Ocular
- Functional
- Reading
- Driving
- Educational needs
- Personal independence

PHYSICAL EXAM

- Visual acuity
- Distance
- Near
- Slit lamp exam:
  - Media integrity
- K reading or topography
- Fundus examination:
  - Photographic
- Refraction:
  - Encourage eccentric viewing
  - Trail frame
  - Large steps ±0.50, ±1.00, ±2.00
  - Diagnostic tests & hand held cross cylinder testing
  - Bracket to end point
- Magnification testing:
  - Inverse of distance acuity formula 20/200 . . . 200/20 = +10.00 Add
  - Test at focal length of Add
  - Increase Plus until target near acuity is achieved (0.8 M)
- Reading function testing:
  - Sloan Cards, MN Read, or equivalent
- Telescope testing:
  - 2.2× wide angle telescope over best refraction in trial frame
  - Increase magnification until desired distance acuity is achieved

DIAGNOSTIC TESTS & INTERPRETATION

Diagnostic Procedures/Other

- Refractive, magnification testing, and reading tests:
  - Provide an excellent overview of the patient's function:
    - Are the patient's specific goals realistic?
    - Can rehabilitation bridge the gap?
- Rehabilitation will require repetitive reading tasks at home:
  - Follow-up visits are required to monitor progress and introduce other low vision aids to meet patient goals.
  - Visual fluctuations or changes in the disease will require reevaluation.

TREATMENT

ADDITIONAL TREATMENT

Rehabilitation

- First line:
  - Establish eye movement patterns consistent with reading or the accurate identification of details:
    - Large print
    - Regular print
- Second line:
  - Magnification devices to achieve specific goals
  - Near spotting tasks like shopping, menus, setting stove, thermostat, and dials
  - Hand held magnifiers
  - Reading books, magazines, mail
  - Spectacles mounted microscopes (high adds)
  - Personal management
  - Closed circuit TV or electronic magnifiers
  - Distance tasks
  - Telescopic lenses

General Measures

- Occupational therapy
- Home evaluation

Issues for Referral

- Depression or mental health issues
- Psychology/psychiatry

Additional Therapies

- Close follow-up with specialty ophthalmology to manage underlying ocular disease
- Close follow-up with other medical specialties to manage underlying systemic disease (diabetes)

SURGERY/OTHER PROCEDURES

If low vision management cannot achieve required life goals, aggressive surgical options must be considered.

ONGOING CARE

FOLLOW-UP RECOMMENDATIONS

- Patients need aggressive follow-up during rehabilitation and introduction of new low vision aids:
  - 2–4 weeks, 3 months, 6 months

Patient Monitoring

Annual

DIET

Diet or supplements consistent with management of underlying ocular problem, i.e., Macular Degeneration – AREDS recommendations

PATIENT EDUCATION

- Educate the patient on the underlying ocular disease
- Educate the patient on goals and progress of low vision rehabilitation
- Educate the patient on required lifestyle changes (i.e., driving)
- Educate the patient on other resources that may be available to assist him or her:
  - Support groups
  - Para-transit
  - Large print
- Review new low vision aids and strategies on annual follow-up

PROGNOSIS

- Based on underlying ocular disease
- Based on underlying systemic disease

COMPLICATIONS

- Mental health issues
- Progression of related disease

ADDITIONAL READING

- Edmonds SA, Edmonds SE. New evidence that vision rehabilitation is a key component in the management of patients with macular degeneration. *Curr Opin Ophthalmol* 2006;17(3):278–280.
- Faye EE. *Clinical low vision*, 2nd ed. Boston: Little Brown and Company, 1984.
- Freeman P, Jose R. *The art and practice of low vision*. Boston: Butterworth Heinemann, 1997.
- Rosenthal B, Thompson B. Awareness of age-related macular degeneration in adults: The results of a large-scale international survey. *Optometry* 2003;74(1):16–24.
- Scheiman M, Scheiman M, Whittaker SG. *Low vision rehabilitation: A practical guide for occupational therapists*. Thorofare, NJ: Slack Inc., 2006.

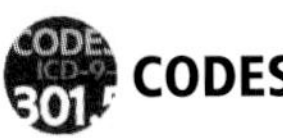

CODES

ICD9

369.9 Unspecified visual loss

CLINICAL PEARLS

- Positive attitude throughout evaluation and treatment is required to manage low vision problems
- Manage refractive problems first
- Consider contact lenses
- Consider prism
- Extensive counseling and patient education
- Follow patients closely, consider changes in management plan, and work closely with referring eye doctors and other specialists
- Refer for ancillary services
- Occupational therapy
- Mental health
- Orientation and mobility training
- Support groups

LOWE SYNDROME

Ahmara V. Gibbons
Alex V. Levin

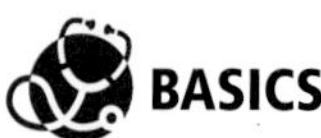

BASICS

DESCRIPTION

- Lowe syndrome is a multisystem disorder characterized by anomalies affecting the eye, nervous system, and kidney (1)[B].
- It is also known as oculo-cerebral-renal syndrome of Lowe.

EPIDEMIOLOGY

Incidence

There have been ~190 known living cases in the United States as of 2000 (1)[B].

Prevalence

1 in 10 affected males in 1,000,000 inhabitants of the United States (1)[B]

RISK FACTORS

X-linked recessive: Female carriers with each pregnancy have a 25% risk of having an affected son, 25% risk of having a carrier daughter, 25% risk of having an unaffected son, and 25% risk of having a noncarrier daughter (2,3)[C,B].

Genetics

- Caused by mutations in OCRL1 gene (Xq24–26); 30% of affected males due to de novo mutations
- Germline and somatic mosaicism in 4.5% of patients
- Rare female affectation due to chromosomal aberration or adverse lyonization (2,3)[C,B]

GENERAL PREVENTION

Genetic counseling

PATHOPHYSIOLOGY

- Cataract: Altered migration of lens embryonic epithelium causes dense cataracts that are present at birth and usually involve the posterior lens.
- Glaucoma due to goniodysgenesis:
  - Other manifestations due to accumulation of phosphatidylinositol biphosphate (PiP2) cause a disequilibrium in phosphoinositides.
  - Convoluted cytoskeleton remodeling and dysfunctional membrane trafficking cause dysregulation of endocytosis, defective maintenance of tight and adherens junctions, and protein trafficking abnormalities (2)[C].

ETIOLOGY

The OCRL1 gene is an inositol polyphosphate 5 phosphatase (a phosphatidylinositol).

COMMONLY ASSOCIATED CONDITIONS

- Ocular manifestations: Infantile cataract, infantile glaucoma conjunctival cheloids (25% of patients) (4)[C], late-onset retinal dystrophy
- Neurologic manifestations: Hypotonia, absence of deep tendon reflexes, compromised suck reflex, developmental delay behavior disturbances (87%), seizures (50%) (1,5) [B]
- Renal manifestations: Fanconi syndrome (proteinuria, proximal renal tubular acidosis, renal phosphate wasting, hypercalciuria, aminoaciduria, and hypokalemia) with secondary failure to thrive and eventual chronic renal failure (5)
- Renal wasting is associated with the presentation of renal rickets, osteomalacia, and pathological fractures.
- Hypercalciuria is associated with nephrocalcinosis and nephrolithiasis.
- Hyperkaliemia is associated with secondary hyperaldosteronism.
- Cryptorchidism (1)[B]
- Characteristic facies

DIAGNOSIS

HISTORY

- Family history
- Visual deficit due to cataract
- Signs and symptoms of infantile glaucoma (buphthalmus, photophobia, epiphora, corneal clouding)
- Failure to thrive
- Developmental delay, seizures
- Symptoms/signs of renal disease or chronic renal failure (1)[B]

PHYSICAL EXAM

- Facial dysmorphisms are often present and consist of vertically elongated and prominent forehead, fair complexion.
  - Plot height, weight, and head circumference on growth curves. Full ocular examination with attention to evidence of cataract, glaucoma (may require sedation or anesthesia for exam), or corneal/conjunctival keloids is required.
  - Neurologic assessment for hypotonia with absent deep tendon reflex and poor suck reflexes needs to be done.
  - Examine mother for radiating dot lenticular opacities which signify the carrier state. Mother may also have signs of the disease including mild difficulties with mentation, retinal dystrophy, or other signs (1,4) [B,C].

DIAGNOSTIC TESTS & INTERPRETATION

Lab

Initial lab tests

- Renal function studies and urinalysis
- Urine amino acids
- OCRL mutation analysis

Follow-up & special considerations

- Renal function must be monitored over time as worsening will likely occur.

Imaging

Initial approach

- Brain MRI may show mild ventriculomegaly and multiple periventricular cystic lesions (6)[B].
  - MRI findings stabilize with time and currently has no clinically significant meaning (6)[B].

Diagnostic Procedures/Other

- B-scan ultrasound if no fundus view
- Photography of optic nerves recommended to allow for monitoring of sequential change due to glaucoma

Pathological Findings

- Cataracts are small and discoid containing posterior lenticonus.
  - Fetal nucleus may show retention of the lens nuclei with lens capsular excrescences.
- Patients show embryonic anterior chamber angle with anterior displacement of rudimentary ciliary processes.
  - Histology may show segmental hypoplasia of the iris dilator muscle.
- Retina shows Lange's folds with peripheral retinal cystoid changes.
- Some cases may show hyalinized retinal vessels and mild gliosis.
- The anterior lens of carrier females has many small, irregular, punctate spots, clustered in zones or wedges.
- Carrier females may also present with round, conical, white plaque in the central portion just inside the back capsule (or shell) of the lens (7)[B].

DIFFERENTIAL DIAGNOSIS

- Congenital rubella
- Peroxisomal disorders
- Mitochondriopathies
- Numerous syndromes combine developmental delay and cataract but the renal and glaucoma features will help to narrow differential diagnosis.

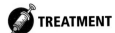

TREATMENT

MEDICATION

- Antiseizure medication as needed
- Psychoactive medication for behavior issues:
  - Renal management often includes sodium or potassium citrate and sodium bicarbonate. Renal rickets is treated with phosphate supplementation and vitamin D. Treatment should be targeted toward maintaining serum calcium and parathyroid hormone within the normal range.
  - Glaucoma management may involve medical control unless infantile presentation and gonioscopy indicate surgery (see the Infantile Glaucoma chapter)

ADDITIONAL TREATMENT

General Measures

- Aphakic/pseudophakic rehabilitation
- Low vision intervention as indicated
- At risk for amblyopia – treat as indicated

Issues for Referral

- Consult medical genetics
- Genetic counseling (3)[B]
- Nephrology
- Neurology:
  - Developmental pediatricians, occupational therapists, physical therapists, speech therapists
  - Psychology/psychiatry for behavioral issues or general surgery if cryptochidism

SURGERY/OTHER PROCEDURES

- Glaucoma surgery as indicated (see the Infantile Glaucoma chapter) (1)[B]. Usually initial surgery is goniotomy or trabeculotomy.
- Cataract surgery as indicated
- Renal transplantation may be needed.

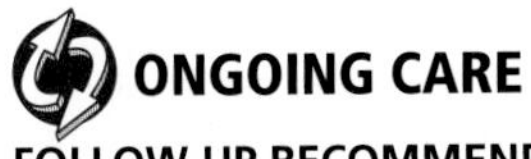

ONGOING CARE

FOLLOW-UP RECOMMENDATIONS

- Periodic examination for glaucoma and cataract assessment
- Renal monitoring
- Patients should follow up with a neurologist for appropriate treatment of seizures (1)[B]
- Developmental support

DIET

As indicated for renal issues

PATIENT EDUCATION

Lowe's Syndrome Association: 972-733-1338 (http://www.lowesyndrome.org/)

PROGNOSIS

- Death usually occurs between the end of second decade and the beginning of fourth decade.
- In first years of life, death occurs as a consequence of renal disease, hypotonia, or susceptibility to infectious disease.
  - Respiratory or gastrointestinal infections are common.
- Most frequent causes of death are respiratory disease, epileptic seizures, and sudden death while sleeping.
- Longest reported survival is 54 years old (1)[B].
- Visual prognosis limited by ultimate retinal dystrophy
- Early response to cataract and glaucoma intervention can be positive.

COMPLICATIONS

- Amblyopia
- Glaucoma
- Cataract
- Retinal dystrophy
- Seizure disorders
- Renal insufficiency
- Developmental delay
- Respiratory issues

REFERENCES

1. Loi M. Lowe syndrome. *Orphanet J Rare Dis* 2006;1:16.
2. Monnier N, et al. OCRL1 mutation analysis in French Lowe syndrome patients: Implications for molecular diagnosis strategy and genetic counseling. *Hum Mutat* 2000;16(2):157–165.
3. Cau M, et al. A locus for familial skewed X chromosome inactivation maps to chromosome Xq25 in a family with a female manifesting Lowe syndrome. *J Hum Genet* 2006;51(11):1030–1036.
4. Tripathi RC, Cibis GW, Tripathi BJ, Pathogenesis of cataracts in patients with Lowe's syndrome. *Ophthalmology* 1986;93(8):1046–1051.
5. Scriver CR. *The metabolic & molecular bases of inherited disease*, 8th ed. New York: McGraw-Hill, 2001;4v:6338.
6. Demmer LA, Wippold FJ, 2nd, Dowton SB. Periventricular white matter cystic lesions in Lowe (oculocerebrorenal) syndrome. A new MR finding. *Pediatr Radiol* 1992;22(1):76–77.
7. Tripathi RC, Cibis GW, Tripathi BJ. Lowe's syndrome. *Trans Ophthalmol Soc UK* 1980; 100(Pt 1):132–139.

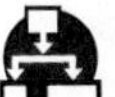

See Also (Topic, Algorithm, Electronic Media Element)

- See also Algorithm.
- For more on the treatment of Infantile Glaucoma read the comprehensive glaucoma section.

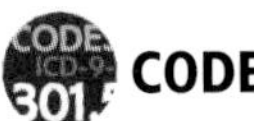

CODES

ICD9

- 270.8 Other specified disorders of amino-acid metabolism
- 365.14 Glaucoma of childhood
- 366.00 Nonsenile cataract, unspecified

CLINICAL PEARLS

- Lowe syndrome or the oculo-cerebro-renal syndrome of Lowe is a multisystem disorder characterized by anomalies that affect the eye, nervous system, and kidney.
- Lowe syndrome is a rare X-linked recessive disease marked by mutations in OCRL1 (Xq26.1).
- Neonates present with bilateral cataracts and severe hypotonia.
- Infants (>6 weeks or months) present with proximal Falconi-type renal tubulopathy, glaucoma, and cheloids.
- Molecular and enzymatic testing is available for prenatal detection and confirmation of the diagnosis.
- Treatment options are multidisciplinary and should include cataract extraction, glaucoma control, physical and speech therapy, correction of tubular acidosis, and complications and chronic renal failure.

LYME DISEASE

Donelson Manley

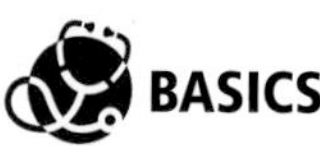

BASICS

DESCRIPTION

- Lyme disease is a worldwide inflammatory, immune-mediated, multisystem disease that begins with a pathognomonic skin rash. Later, neurologic, cardiac, rheumatologic, dermatologic, and ophthalmologic manifestations may occur.
- It is named after the village of Lyme, Connecticut, where a group of children were studied who had an unusual rash associated with rheumatoid arthritis. As they developed the illness during the warmer months a tick transmission was suspected.
- It commonly begins in the spring, summer, and fall owing to the timing of the tick's blood meals. Less common in winter.

EPIDEMIOLOGY

- The Centers for Disease Control and Prevention (CDC) began surveillance for Lyme disease in 1982. In 1991, Lyme was classified as a nationally reportable disease.
- It is the most common tick-borne disease in the temperate northern hemisphere, in the USA and Europe.
- It is one of the fastest growing infectious diseases in the USA.
- It has been reported in 49 of the 50 states, but the majority of cases are confined to five geographical areas (New England, Mid-Atlantic, East-North Central, South Atlantic, and West North-Central). It has also been reported in China, Europe, Japan, and parts of the former Soviet Union.

Incidence

- In the 10 states where Lyme disease is most common, the average was 31.6 cases for every 100,000 persons for the year 2005.
- In 2006, 19,931 new cases were reported in the USA.

Prevalence

Of cases reported to the US CDC, the ratio of Lyme disease infection is 7.9 cases for every 100,000 persons.

RISK FACTORS

It is present in an area where one could be bitten by a tick.

GENERAL PREVENTION

- Avoidance of tick bites is the most important way to prevent Lyme disease.
- Avoide the woods, high brush, and grasses where ticks are present.
- Wear protective clothing when out of doors; long pants, long sleeves, and light colored clothing make it easier to spot ticks.
- Apply tick repellant (DEET) to clothing.
- Remove clothing before entering the house.
- Take a shower and examine skin for ticks soon after returning from wooded areas or areas with high grass or brush. Complete inspection of the skin and scalp in children is recommended.
- Remove attached ticks as soon as possible.
- Use care when handling outdoor pets inside homes.
- Reduce deer population in suburban and rural areas.
- Reduce the number of primary hosts on which the deer tick depends, such as rodents.
- A vaccine was developed for its cure, but was voluntarily withdrawn from the market in 2002 by the manufacturer due to poor sales.

PATHOPHYSIOLOGY

- Because the bacteria's flagellae are located inside the periplasm between the inner and outer cell membranes, the cell is able to travel through bodily fluids and tissues.
- It is believed that the bacteria use a variety of mechanisms to evade the host immune response. The bacteria produce specific outer surface proteins in order to successfully invade and inhabit certain organisms. The bacterial outer surface proteins are able to bind host factor H, a regulator in the complement activating pathway. By binding this regulator, the bacteria may be able to protect themselves from complement killing.
- Once the bacteria have entered the host, it becomes very invasive and can spread quickly throughout the entire system.
- The exact mechanisms for its pathology are still trying to be understood.
- The outer membrane of *Borrelia burgdorferi* is composed of various unique outer surface proteins. These can be varied in response to immune attack.
- Another way *B. burgdorferi* evades the immune system is to establish a chronic infection. The exact mechanisms for its pathology are not completely understood.

ETIOLOGY

- *B. burgdorferi* is the infectious agent. It is Gram-negative spirochete in the genus *Borrelia* and is named for Willy Burgdorfer who isolated it from the intestine of the Ixodes tick in 1982.
- Its life cycle is complex and requires ticks, rodents, and deer at various times. The white-footed mouse is the primary reservoir for the bacteria.
- The bacteria are maintained in a natural cycle of infection by ticks. The ticks acquire and transmit the bacteria by feeding on the mouse, which acts as a reservoir. Ixodes ticks harbor the bacteria in their stomachs.
- After attaching themselves to deer, the ticks transfer the bacteria during a blood meal. The ticks fall off onto vegetation and are transferred inadvertently to humans as they travel in tick-infected areas and are bitten.
- Once the bacteria enter the host it becomes very invasive and can spread very quickly throughout the entire system.
- The disease is not transmitted from one human to another.

DIAGNOSIS

- Ocular symptoms: Blurred vision, eye pain, injection of conjunctiva, diplopia, floaters, progressive visual loss, paresthesias
- Ocular manifestations: Third, fourth, or sixth cranial nerve palsies with diplopia, conjunctival injection, follicular conjunctivitis, keratitis, exposure keratopathy (facial nerve palsy) with hypesthesia, idiopathic orbital inflammation, episcleritis, scleritis, granulomatous anterior uveitis, pars planitis, vitreitis, afferent pupillary defect, optic and retrobulbar neuritis, ischemic optic neuropathy, retinal arteriole occlusion, optic nerve edema, retinitis
- Ocular complaints usually occur during stages I and II (see the 'Physical Exam' section below).

HISTORY

- Travel to an endemic area
- Tick bite

PHYSICAL EXAM

- Complete systemic, neurologic, and ophthalmologic examinations

Stage 1:

- The diagnosis of Lyme disease is based on clinical features in a person who has traveled to or lives in an endemic area during the spring, summer, or fall.
- After the tick bite, the first symptom is a skin rash called erythema migrans, which is usually a flat, reddish rash that spreads from the site of the bite.
- The rash is usually >2 inches wide and can grow larger.
- It often develops a central clear area known as a "bull's eye." The rash doesn't itch or hurt.
- Some individuals do not recall the rash.
- Ophthalmological manifestations include conjunctivitis and periorbital edema.
- Other symptoms at this stage can include fever, chills, nausea, muscle and joint aches, fatigue, headache, severe stiff neck, and swollen lymph nodes.

Stage 2:

- Early infection (1–4 months) occurs when the spirochete has disseminated to many organs including the skin, heart, joints, and nervous system. Fatigue may be present.
- The original skin lesion may fade and then recur and become chronic and may appear in other areas of the body.
- Ophthalmological manifestations include blepharospasm, iritis/uveitis, panophthalmitis, choroiditis, optic disc edema, macular edema, pseudotumor cerebri, optic neuropathy, nonarteritic ischemic optic neuropathy, temporal arteritis, optic atrophy, Horner's syndrome, and Argyll Robertson pupil.

- Cardiac effects include palpitations, arrhythmias, and A-V blocks.
- Neurologic changes include meningitis, meningoencephalitis, cranial neuritis, and radiculoneuritis. Severe headaches, nausea, vomiting, and photophobia may occur.

Stage 3:

- Clinical manifestations may continue for years.
- Ophthalmological manifestations include stromal keratitis, episcleritis, orbital myositis, and cortical blindness.
- Skin changes called acrodermatitis chronica atrophicans may be present as a red swollen skin area that causes the underlying skin to atrophy.
- Arthritis may occur and be present in the majority of patients and may simulate rheumatoid arthritis.

DIAGNOSTIC TESTS & INTERPRETATION

Diagnostic Procedures/Other

- Two-step diagnosis with a screening assay and confirmatory Western blot for *B. burgdorferi*.
- Serum RPR and FTA-ABS. High positive FTA-ABS titer may produce a low false-positive antibody titer against *B. burgdorferi*.
- Consider lumbar puncture when meningitis is suspected or neurologic signs or symptoms are present.

DIFFERENTIAL DIAGNOSIS

The differential diagnosis of retinitis and optic nerve edema includes cat-scratch disease, syphilis, acute retinal necrosis, and toxoplasmosis.

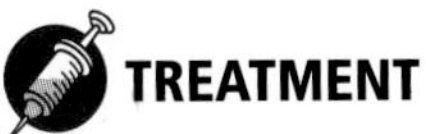

TREATMENT

ADDITIONAL TREATMENT

General Measures

B. burgdorferi bacteria are very slow growing, with a doubling time of 12–18 h. Since most antibiotics kill bacteria only when they are dividing, this longer doubling time necessitates the use of relatively longer treatment courses for Lyme disease.

Ocular:

- Topical corticosteroids for anterior segment inflammation

Early Lyme disease (including Lyme-related uveitis, keratitis, or seventh nerve palsy):

- Doxycycline 100 mg PO b.i.d for 10–21 days
- In children, pregnant women, and those who cannot take doxycycline, substitute amoxicillin 500 mg PO t.i.d., cefuroxime axetil 500 mg PO b.i.d., clarithromycin 500 mg PO b.i.d., or azithromycin 500 mg PO daily.

Patients with neuro-ophthalmic signs of recurrent or resistant infection:

- Ceftriaxone 2 g intravenously daily for 2–3 weeks
- Alternatively, penicillin G, 20 million units intravenously daily for 2–3 weeks

SURGERY/OTHER PROCEDURES

Tick removal: Removal with forceps is preferred. The tick should not be crushed or squeezed; this may cause regurgitation of blood from the tick into the skin thereby increasing the likelihood of *Borrelia* transmission. After the tick has been removed the site should be cleansed.

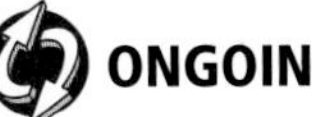

ONGOING CARE

FOLLOW-UP RECOMMENDATIONS

Every 1–3 days until improvement is demonstrated, and then weekly until resolved

PATIENT EDUCATION

- Wear protective light colored clothing so as to make it easier to spot ticks.
- Carefully inspect skin for ticks.
- Remove ticks rapidly.
- Remove clothing when entering the house.
- Shower after entering the house.

PROGNOSIS

- Most patients respond well to antibiotics.
- Prognosis depends upon promptness of diagnosis and treatment.

COMPLICATIONS

Ophthalmic complications include visual loss from a variety of mechanisms.

ADDITIONAL READING

- Aaberg TM. The expanding ophthalmologic spectrum of Lyme disease. *Am J Ophthalmol* 1981:77–80.
- Ehlers J, Shah C. (Eds). *The Wills eye manual*. 5th edn. Wolters Kluwer/Lippincott, Williams and Wilkins, 2007:371–372.
- Nau R, Christen HJ, Eiffert H. Lyme disease – current state of knowledge. *Deutsches Ärzteblatt Int* 2009;106(5):72–82.
- Winterkorn JMS. Lyme disease: Neurologic and ophthalmologic manifestations. *Surv Ophthalmol* 1990;35(3):191–204.
- Winward KE, Smith JL, Culbertson WW, et al. Ocular Lyme borreliosis. *Am J Ophthalmol* 1989;108: 651–657.

CODES

ICD9

- 088.81 Lyme disease
- 370.50 Interstitial keratitis, unspecified
- 372.39 Other conjunctivitis

CLINICAL PEARLS

- Lyme disease has many ophthalmic manifestations, including uveitis, optic neuropathy, and arteritis.
- Lyme disease has many systemic manifestations, including meningoencephalitis and cardiac arrhythmias.
- Lyme disease can be prevented by avoiding tick bites.
- Timely diagnosis and initiation of treatment improve prognosis of Lyme disease.

MACULAR CORNEAL DYSTROPHY

Hall F. Chew

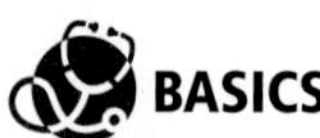

BASICS

DESCRIPTION

- Macular corneal dystrophy (Groenouw corneal dystrophy Type II, Fehr spotted dystrophy) is an autosomal recessive, progressive, bilateral, noninflammatory condition characterized by multiple opacifications with intervening haze within the corneal stroma.
- Patients present with corneal clouding by ages 3–9 years.
- Opacities are focal, gray-white, ill-defined, and extend to the peripheral cornea. They can present throughout the entire thickness of the stroma and, in advanced cases, extend to Descemet's membrane and the endothelium producing guttae excrescences and corneal edema. The opacities are typically superficial centrally and more posterior peripherally.
- Compared to other corneal stromal dystrophies (granular and lattice), macular corneal dystrophy is:
  - the least common
  - has reduced vision at an earlier age
  - has thinner central corneal thickness in the early stages of the disease
  - has no clear areas between opacities
  - extends to the peripheral cornea
  - requires corneal transplantation at an earlier age
  - has the lowest frequency for corneal transplant replacement; however, recurrence of the opacities from macular dystrophy can still occur in the transplant (1).
- Symptoms include: progressive vision loss (usually severe by second to third decade), glare, photophobia, recurrent erosions.

EPIDEMIOLOGY

Incidence/Prevalence

Uncommon, no reports in literature

RISK FACTORS

Consanguinity (2)

Genetics

- Autosomal Recessive
- Genetic locus: 16q22
- Gene: Carbohydrate sulfotransferase 6 gene—*CHST6* (3,4)

PATHOPHYSIOLOGY

- The opacities are glycosaminoglycans (GAGs or mucopolysaccharides) that accumulate intracellularly and extracellularly in the corneal stroma, Descemet's membrane, and endothelium.
- In macular corneal dystrophy, GAGs accumulate in the endoplasmic reticulum of cells, whereas in systemic mucopolysaccharidoses, GAGs accumulate in lysosomal vacuoles.
- GAGs stain with Alcian blue, Hale colloidal iron, metachromatic dyes, and Periodic Acid-Schiff (PAS).
- Electron microscopy shows that the GAGs stain positively in keratocytes and endothelial cells. They also stain positively in the extracellular matrix fibrillogranular material.

ETIOLOGY

- Autosomal recessive, progressive, bilateral, noninflammatory condition characterized by multiple opacifications with intervening haze within the corneal stroma.
- The opacities are glycosaminoglycans (GAGs or mucopolysaccharides) with corneal clouding by ages 3–9 years.

DIAGNOSIS

HISTORY

- Macular corneal dystrophy is an autosomal recessive, progressive, bilateral, noninflammatory condition characterized by multiple opacifications with intervening haze within the corneal stroma.
- Presents with corneal clouding by ages 3–9 years
- Symptoms include: Progressive vision loss (usually severe by the second to third decade), glare, photophobia, recurrent erosions.
- Possible history for consanguinity in parents

PHYSICAL EXAM

- Full ophthalmic examination including measurement of intraocular pressure and dilated fundus examination
- B-Scan ultrasound to rule out posterior segment pathology if unable to visualize secondary to corneal opacification
- Ultrasound pachymetry to measure central corneal thickness
- Specular microscopy to measure endothelial cell counts if possible
- Slit-lamp examination shows:
  - Focal, gray-white opacities that are ill-defined and extend to the peripheral cornea
  - Opacities can present throughout the entire thickness of the stroma and, in advanced cases, extend to Descemet's membrane and the endothelium, producing guttae excrescences and corneal edema.
  - The opacities are typically superficial centrally and more posterior peripherally.
  - There are no clear areas between opacities.
  - Opacities extend to the peripheral cornea.

DIAGNOSTIC TESTS & INTERPRETATION

Lab

Initial lab tests

ELISA may be used to measure sulfated keratan sulfate.

Follow-up & special considerations

- Slit-lamp examination
- Ultrasound pachymetry
- Specular microscopy

Pathological Findings

- The opacities are glycosaminoglycans (GAGs, mucopolysaccharides) that accumulate intra- and extracellularly in the corneal stroma, Descemet's membrane, and endothelium.
- In macular corneal dystrophy, GAGs accumulate in the endoplasmic reticulum of cells, whereas in systemic mucopolysaccharidoses, GAGs accumulate in lysosomal vacuoles.
- GAGs stain with Alcian blue, Hale colloidal iron, metachromatic dyes, and PAS.
- Electron microscopy shows that the GAGs stain positively in keratocytes and endothelial cells. They also stain positively in the extracellular matrix fibrillogranular material.
- Immunoreactivity of an antibody specific for sulfate epitopes on antigenic keratan sulfate (AgKS) delineates the three variants of macular corneal dystrophy. Clinical presentation is similar between the three types (2)
  - Type 1
    - AgKS nonreactive to cornea and serum
  - Type 1 A
    - AgKS reactive to keratocytes
    - AgKS nonreactive to extracellular matrix and serum
  - Type 2
    - AgKS reactive to cornea and serum

DIFFERENTIAL DIAGNOSIS

- Granular corneal dystrophy
- Schnyder's crystalline corneal dystrophy (SCCD)
- Avellino corneal dystrophy
- Lattice corneal dystrophy

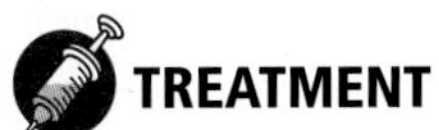

TREATMENT

MEDICATION

- Artificial tears for recurrent erosions. No contraindications.
- Topical hypertonic saline (5%) drops (1 drop q.i.d) and ointment (q.h.s). No contraindications.

ADDITIONAL TREATMENT

General Measures

- Tinted contact lenses to reduce photophobia
- Pressure patch of eye to allow healing of epithelial defect
- Therapeutic contact lenses for recurrent corneal erosions with topical antibiotic coverage (1 drop q.i.d.)
- Risks of corneal infection possible with patching and contact lens use. Patient requires frequent follow-up until healed.

Issues for Referral

- Worsening vision
- Nonhealing epithelial defects

SURGERY/OTHER PROCEDURES

- Phototherapeutic keratectomy (PTK):
  - Early onset disease with anterior stromal opacities
  - Treatment of recurrent erosions (5)
- Keratoplasty (corneal transplantation) for more posterior stromal opacities leading to significant visual loss
  - Lamellar keratoplasty (LK)
  - Deep anterior lamellar keratoplasty (DALK)
    - In cases without opacities in Descemet's membrane or endothelium
    - DALK has a reduced risk of endothelial rejection of the corneal transplant
  - Full-thickness penetrating keratoplasty (PKP)

IN-PATIENT CONSIDERATIONS

Discharge Criteria

- Risks of corneal infection possible with patching and contact lens use
- Patients with recurrent erosions should be followed closely until the epithelial defect has healed.

ONGOING CARE

FOLLOW-UP RECOMMENDATIONS

Periodic follow-up to monitor status of opacities and vision

Patient Monitoring

- Timing of outpatient follow-up is dependent on severity of disease.
  - Patients who are stable can be followed every 6–12 months.
  - Patients with recurrent erosions should be followed every 1–7 days, until healed.
  - Patients with pressure patch should be seen every 24–48 hours.

PATIENT EDUCATION

- Patients should be advised to seek medical attention immediately if there are any symptoms of pain, acute visual loss, redness, purulent discharge, or severe photophobia.
- As the disease is progressive, patients may be advised a surgical procedure (PTK or corneal transplantation) if there is significant visual loss.

PROGNOSIS

Patients have progressive vision loss (usually severe by second to third decade), glare, photophobia, and recurrent erosions.

COMPLICATIONS

- Progressive vision loss with glare, photophobia, and recurrent erosions
- Despite successful treatment with PTK and/or corneal transplantation, recurrences can still occur.

REFERENCES

1. Marcon AS, Cohen EJ, Rapuano CJ, Laibson PR. Recurrence of corneal stromal dystrophies after penetrating keratoplasty. *Cornea* 2003;22:19–21.
2. Pandrowala H, Bansal A, Vemuganti GK, Rao GN. Frequency, distribution, and outcome of keratoplasty for corneal dystrophies at a tertiary eye care center in South India. *Cornea* 2004;23: 541–546.
3. Weiss JS, Moller HU, Lisch W, et al. The IC3D classification of the corneal dystrophies. *Cornea* 2008;27(Suppl 2):S19–S20.
4. Klintworth GK, Smith CF, Bowling BL. CHST6 mutations in North American subjects with macular corneal dystrophy: A comprehensive molecular genetic review. *Mol Vis* 2006;12:159–176.
5. Szentmáry N, Seitz B, Langenbucher A, et al. Histologic and ultrastructural changes in corneas with granular and macular dystrophy after excimer laser phototherapeutic keratectomy. *Cornea* 2006;25:257–263.

ADDITIONAL READING

- De Sousa LB, Mannis MJ. The stromal dystrophies. In: Krachmer JH, Mannis MJ, Holland EJ (eds). *Cornea*. 2nd ed. Philadelphia, PA: Elsevier Mosby, 2005;907–927.

CODES

ICD9

371.55 Macular corneal dystrophy

CLINICAL PEARLS

- Never prescribe topical anesthetics for patients with pain secondary to recurrent erosions.
- Never patch contact lens wearers.
- Patients treated with a patch or therapeutic contact lens for recurrent erosions must be followed closely due to increased risk for infection.
- Compared to other corneal stromal dystrophies (granular and lattice), macular requires corneal transplantation at an earlier age, but has the lowest frequency for corneal transplant replacement due to recurrence. However, recurrence of the opacities from macular dystrophy can still occur in the transplant.

M

MACULAR HOLE

Nicholas G. Anderson

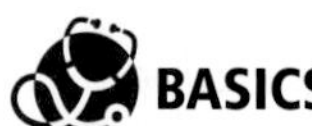

BASICS

DESCRIPTION
Partial or full-thickness retinal defect in the central macula.

EPIDEMIOLOGY

Incidence
- 7.8–8.7 cases/100,000 persons/year
- Peak incidence in seventh decade of life

Prevalence
- 0.02–0.8%
- Women affected more than men
- Typically affects patients over age 55 years

RISK FACTORS
Recent trauma

PATHOPHYSIOLOGY
Vitreoretinal traction contributes to macular hole formation.

ETIOLOGY
- Most macular holes are idiopathic
- Trauma may also cause a macular hole

DIAGNOSIS

HISTORY
- Patients notice blurry central vision, metamorphopsia, or a central scotoma in one eye.
- Acute or subacute onset
  - Symptoms often first noted when fellow eye is incidentally covered.
- History of trauma may be elicited.

PHYSICAL EXAM
- Visual acuity ranges from 20/25 to 20/400 depending on the size and stage of hole.
  - Average acuity is 20/200 for a full-thickness macular hole.
- Diagnosis primarily based on biomicroscopic examination
  - Hand-held indirect lens or fundus contact lens
  - Typically dark, round defect noted in central fovea
  - Small neurosensory detachment may be present as a fluid "cuff" surrounding the hole.
  - Yellow–white dots may be present at the level of retinal pigment epithelium.
  - Pseudo-operculum may be visible overlying hole
- Biomicroscopic (Gass) classification (1)[C]
  - Stage 1: Impending hole
    - Central yellow spot (Stage 1-A) or yellow ring (Stage 1-B) with loss of foveolar depression
  - Stage 2: Small (<400 micron) full-thickness defect visible in the fovea
  - Stage 3: Large (>400 micron) full-thickness defect
  - Stage 4: Full-thickness defect with posterior vitreous detachment present
- Watzke-Allen test utilized to differentiate full-thickness from lamellar hole and other lesions
  - Macular lens and slit lamp utilized to focus thin beam through central macula. Patients with macular hole will note a break or "compression" in the slit beam.

DIAGNOSTIC TESTS & INTERPRETATION

Lab
Laboratory testing not indicated

Imaging
- Optical coherence tomography (OCT)
  - Shows full thickness defect involving the macula.
  - May show vitreoretinal adhesion
  - A pseudo-operculum may be visible

Diagnostic Procedures/Other
- Laser aiming beam test
  - 50-micron laser aiming beam focused in center of lesion. Patients with full-thickness macular hole will be unable to see the spot, whereas patients with other lesions typically are able to see the spot.

Pathological Findings
Surgical specimens are typically not obtained.

DIFFERENTIAL DIAGNOSIS
- Epiretinal membrane with pseudohole
- Cystoid macular edema
- Macular cyst
- Lamellar macular hole
- Pigment epithelial detachment
- Central serous retinopathy
- Vitreomacular traction

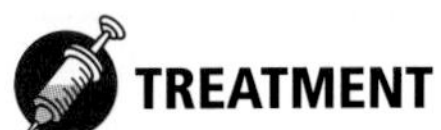

TREATMENT

MEDICATION

No medications indicated

ADDITIONAL TREATMENT

Issues for Referral

Referral to vitreoretinal surgeon indicated.

COMPLEMENTARY & ALTERNATIVE THERAPIES

None indicated.

SURGERY/OTHER PROCEDURES

- Surgery is the only successful treatment option.
- Pars plana vitrectomy with gas tamponade (2)[C]
  - Internal limiting membrane peeling in many cases (3)[B]
- Non-emergent or urgent, but surgery typically performed within 1–2 months of diagnosis
- Extensive postoperative face-down positioning, lasting several days to weeks, is usually required.
- Subsequent cataract extraction may be required in phakic patients.

IN-PATIENT CONSIDERATIONS

Initial Stabilization

Outpatient management indicated.

ONGOING CARE

FOLLOW-UP RECOMMENDATIONS

- Referral to a vitreoretinal surgeon is indicated.
- Routine postoperative examinations on postoperative day 1, 1 week, 2–3 weeks, and 6–12 weeks after surgery.

PATIENT EDUCATION

- Fellow eye develops a macular hole in 5–20%
  - Educate patient to monitor symptoms in fellow eye
- Educate patient on signs and symptoms of retinal tear and detachment postoperatively and need for urgent evaluation if symptoms develop.

PROGNOSIS

- Hole closure rates >90% with surgery (3)[B], (4)[C]
- Postoperative visual acuity variable but can be good with successful hole closure

COMPLICATIONS

- Surgical complications
  - Cataract (common)
  - Retinal tear or detachment (uncommon)
- Macular hole associated retinal detachment (rare)

REFERENCES

1. Gass JD. Reappraisal of biomicroscopic classification of stages of development of a macular hole. *Am J Ophthalmol* 1995;119:752–759.
2. Kelly NE, Wendel RT. Vitreous surgery for idiopathic macular holes. Results of a pilot study. *Arch Ophthalmol* 1991;109:654–659.
3. Christensen UC, Kroyer K, Sander B, et al. Value of internal limiting membrane peeling in surgery for idiopathic macular hole stage 2 and 3: A randomised clinical trial. *Br J Ophthalmol* 2009;93:1005–1015.
4. Kumagai K, Furukawa M, Ogino N, et al. Long-term outcomes of internal limiting membrane peeling with and without indocyanine green in macular hole surgery. *Retina* 2006;26:613–617.

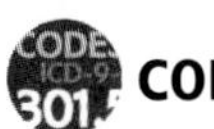

CODES

ICD9

362.54 Macular cyst, hole, or pseudohole of retina

CLINICAL PEARLS

- Macular pseudohole can often be differentiated from macular hole by a negative Watzke-Allen sign and relatively good visual acuity.
- Patients with suspected macular hole should be referred to a vitreoretinal surgeon for evaluation and consideration of surgery.
- Visual prognosis variable but often good with timely surgery.

MALIGNANT GLAUCOMA

Anand V. Mantravadi

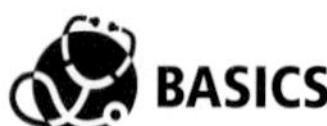

BASICS

DESCRIPTION

- An uncommon form of secondary glaucoma occurring post intraocular surgery characterized by a flat or shallow anterior chamber, absence of pupillary block, and elevated intraocular pressure. Expansion in vitreous volume due to sequestration of aqueous in the posterior segment with resultant anterior shift in the lens iris diaphragm.
- "Malignant glaucoma" – named by Von Graefe in 1869 – refers to the likelihood that this progressive condition will not improve spontaneously.
  - Synonyms: Aqueous misdirection syndrome, ciliary block glaucoma, and ciliovitreal block.

EPIDEMIOLOGY

Incidence

- 2–4% in eyes undergoing glaucoma filtration surgery for angle closure glaucoma (1)
- Can occur at any time following surgery
- No established racial, sexual predilection

RISK FACTORS

- Small eyes with small anterior hyaloid surface
- Filtering surgery in eye with history of angle closure such as shallow chamber and peripheral anterior synechia
- History of malignant glaucoma in fellow eye

Genetics

Unknown for malignant glaucoma – but smaller eyes with angle closure have predisposition to development of malignant glaucoma, and eye size has a genetic basis with many genes associated with angle closure (2).

GENERAL PREVENTION

Involves preoperative identification of high risk eyes – small eyes with a history of angle closure or that of malignant glaucoma.

PATHOPHYSIOLOGY

- Under homeostatic conditions, aqueous volume flows predominantly anteriorly exiting through trabecular and uveoscleral outflow pathways and, to a lesser degree, aqueous circulates posteriorly into and around the vitreous body.
- Under pathologic conditions, a shift to greater aqueous flow posteriorly occurs incited by sudden anterior chamber decompression (i.e., anterior chamber entry, overfiltration). When combined with a fundamentally decreased rate of aqueous exchange from the ciliary processes both across the anterior hyaloid and through the vitreous gel, the result is vitreous volume expansion through aqueous sequestration, and an anterior shift of the lens–iris diaphragm axis. The anterior chamber space is consequentially shallowed or flattened, further obstructing aqueous outflow through angle closure resulting in elevated IOP.

ETIOLOGY

- The exact initiating event is not known but appears strongly related to an abnormal interaction between the ciliary processes, the lens, and the anterior vitreous face, seemingly induced by postoperative anterior chamber decompression leading to an anterior shift in the lens–iris diaphragm and diversion of aqueous into the vitreous cavity (3).
- Smaller/hyperopic eyes – with tendency toward angle closure glaucoma, have correspondingly smaller anterior hyaloid surface area, and less space between the ciliary processes and the anterior hyaloid. Consequentially, if a shift in the lens–iris diaphragm occurs abruptly, contact between the ciliary processes and anterior hyaloid occurs. Aqueous is then disproportionately circulated posteriorly with resultant vitreous volume expansion and further flattening of the anterior chamber with elevation in intraocular pressure.

COMMONLY ASSOCIATED CONDITIONS

- Chronic angle closure
- Hyperopia
- Nanophthalmos

DIAGNOSIS

HISTORY

Malignant glaucoma can present any time after any intraocular surgery in phakic, pseudophakic, or aphakic eyes, but most typically arises in eyes with a history of angle closure undergoing glaucoma filtration surgery. It has been reported rarely after laser iridotomy and miotic administration.

PHYSICAL EXAM

- Shallow anterior chamber: Uniform decrease in anterior chamber depth centrally and peripherally.
- Absence of pupillary block: Reflected by presence of patent iridotomy/iridectomy.
- Elevated intraocular pressure (IOP)
  - IOP may not be present, or only modestly elevated in the early stages of ciliary block in the presence of a filtering procedure.
- Absence of simulating conditions causing posterior volume expansion: Choroidal effusion, hemorrhage: As visualized with indirect ophthalmoscopy.

DIAGNOSTIC TESTS & INTERPRETATION

Lab

- Slit-lamp exam may reveal elevated bleb initially with gradual flattening and disappearance upon further posterior misdirection and sequestration of aqueous.
- Gonioscopy may reveal closed angle or obscured angle structures, and possibly visualization through the iridotomy of ciliary processes pushed forward.

Imaging

- Ultrasound biomicroscopy (UBM) can demonstrate irido-corneal contact, decreased anterior chamber depth, forward displacement of the lens–iris diaphragm, and ciliary processes.
- B-mode ultrasound can confirm absence of posterior space-occupying mechanism such as choroidal hemorrhage or effusion if visualization is poor with indirect ophthalmoscopy.

Diagnostic Procedures/Other

- Anterior-segment optical coherence tomography (AS-OCT): Can noninvasively demonstrate anterior chamber angle structures and quantitatively assess the anterior chamber angle
- Laser iridotomy: Must be performed if not already present to diagnostically exclude pupillary block, and therapeutically relieve block if present
- Fluorescein injection through peripheral vein, with visualization of fluorescein-tinged aqueous fluid flowing posteriorly shortly thereafter can confirm diagnosis

Pathological Findings

- Smaller eyes have thicker sclera with a reduced ability to remove suprachoroidal fluid.
- Malignant glaucoma has been proposed to involve a pathologic behavior of the vitreous gel with poor vitreous conductivity of fluid (4).

DIFFERENTIAL DIAGNOSIS

- **Pupillary block**
  - Will typically demonstrate elevated IOP, preserved central anterior chamber depth, closed angle, and iris bombé of variable degrees. If patency of iridotomy is doubted, then another should be performed to exclude pupillary block.
- **Choroidal effusion**
  - Serous: Gray–light brown choroidal elevation directly visualized or observed with B-scan ultrasound. Typically associated with low IOP, and shallow anterior chamber. Must consider overfiltration or wound leak if following filtration surgery.
  - Hemorrhagic: Dark-brown or red effusion directly visualized or observed with B-scan ultrasound. Typically associated with uniform anterior chamber shallowing or flattening, increased IOP, and frequently preceded by pain.
- **Overfiltration**
- Shallow anterior chamber associated with low IOP. If low IOP is accompanied by high/diffuse bleb morphology: Likely overfiltration. If low IOP is accompanied by low/flat bleb: Must exclude bleb leak.
- **Lens related angle closure:** With anterior shift of lens–iris diaphragm and resultant angle closure.
  - Phacomorphic glaucoma: Anterior shift due to intumescent lens
  - Lens dislocation: Anterior shift due to zonular laxity as in pseudoexfoliation or other predisposing condition (i.e., Marfan's, trauma, etc.)
- **Infusion misdirection syndrome**
  - Intraoperative condition due to misdirection of irrigating fluid posteriorly, potentially through iridotomy or zonular dehiscence – expanding vitreous volume and resultant anterior shift of iris/posterior capsule.

TREATMENT

MEDICATION

- Cycloplegia/mydriasis: Widens ciliary body diameter through contraction of dilator muscle of iris increasing diffusional area for aqueous; pulls lens posteriorly by tightening zonules through unopposed action of longitudinal muscle with circular muscle paralysis.
- IOP management
  - Aqueous suppression: Beta-blockers, carbonic anhydrase inhibitors, and alpha-agonist
  - Osmotic agents (Mannitol, Isosorbide): Decrease vitreous volume by increasing osmotic gradient between blood and ocular fluids causing fluid to be drawn intravascular

Geriatric Considerations

Osmotics are relatively contraindicated in patients with renal or cardiovascular compromise. Signs of atropine toxicity should be monitored in elderly patients.

Pediatric Considerations

Alpha agonists have potentially serious adverse effects in children and are contraindicated in children <2 years old.

Pregnancy Considerations

Aqueous suppressants and osmotic agents are classified as class C in pregnancy – with fetal risk revealed in animal studies, but not established or studied in humans.

ADDITIONAL TREATMENT

General Measures

- Miotics contraindicated
- If attack broken medically (chamber deepening, normalization of IOP), can taper off hyperosmotics, and aqueous suppressants with long-term use of cycloplegia/mydriasis due to risks of reoccurrence

Issues for Referral

- Patients not adequately responding to medical therapy require surgical intervention.
- Response may develop days after initiating medical therapy.

SURGERY/OTHER PROCEDURES

- **Nd: YAG laser** disruption of anterior hyaloid face: Can be attempted in typically aphakic or pseudophakic patients not responding to medical therapy (5)[C]. Response can be observed as progressive deepening of anterior chamber over hours–days. If view is precluded by posterior capsule opacification, capsulotomy should be undertaken prior to vitreous face disruption.
- **Surgical vitrectomy** with opening/disruption of anterior hyaloid face, removal of sufficient vitreous to disrupt pockets of aqueous, with ultimate goal to create unicameral eye – with a direct communication between the anterior and posterior chamber (6)[C].

IN-PATIENT CONSIDERATIONS

Initial Stabilization

Medical consultation and consideration for admission is necessary if medical comorbidities such as cardiac, respiratory, renal conditions are present.

Admission Criteria

Hospital admission may be required for monitoring during parenteral osmotic administration, and/or pain control, or urgent surgical intervention if warranted.

IV Fluids

- Osmotics agents
- Intravenous carbonic anhydrase inhibitor can be administered for aqueous suppression.

Nursing

Adherence to parenteral medication administration guidelines, and topical medication schedule administration with appropriate monitoring during therapy.

Discharge Criteria

Controlled pain, stabilization/improvement in condition.

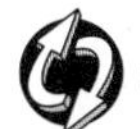

ONGOING CARE

FOLLOW-UP RECOMMENDATIONS

Degree and duration of flat anterior chamber, level of IOP, and degree of patient comfort are all carefully monitored with urgency and frequency of follow-up based on response to intervention and progress.

Patient Monitoring

- Long term surveillance for reoccurrence is required with careful monitoring upon cessation of cycloplegia.
- If any intraocular surgery is required in fellow eye, precautionary measures taken to avoid sudden anterior chamber decompression or overfiltration, and consideration should be given for pre/postoperative cycloplegia/mydriasis.

PATIENT EDUCATION

- Risks of malignant glaucoma with surgery in fellow eye, and risks of reoccurrence in operated eye should be discussed with patient.
- Adherence to prescribed medical therapy, particularly long term cycloplegia should be emphasized.

PROGNOSIS

- Approximately 50% of cases will respond medically within 5 days.
- Surgical success rates are higher in pseudophakic eyes as compared to phakic eyes (6)[C].

COMPLICATIONS

- Reoccurrence/persistence
- Corneal decompensation
- Cataract progression
- Glaucomatous progression
- Vitreous traction with retinal tear/detachment

REFERENCES

1. Luntz MH, Rosenblatt M. Malignant glaucoma. *Surv Ophthalmol* 1987;32:73–93.
2. He M, Wang D, Zheng Y, et al. Heritability of anterior chamber depth as an intermediate phenotype of angle-closure in Chinese: The Guangzhou Twin Eye Study. *Invest Ophthalmol Vis Sci* 2008;49:81–86.
3. Ruben S, Tsai J, Hitchings R. Malignant glaucoma and its management. *Br J of Ophthalmol* 1997;81:163–167.
4. Quigley H. Angle closure glaucoma – simpler answers to complex mechanisms: LXVI Edward Jackson Memorial Lecture. *Am J Ophthalmol* 2009;148:657–669.
5. Epstein D, Steiert RF, Puliafito CA. Nd:YAG laser therapy to the anterior hyaloid in aphakic malignant (ciliovitreal block) glaucoma. *Am J Ophthalmol* 1984;98:137–143.
6. Byrnes BA, Leen MM, Wong TP, Benson WE. Vitrectomy for ciliary block (malignant) glaucoma. *Ophthalmology* 1995;102:1308–1311.

ADDITIONAL READING

- Simmons RJ, Thomas JV. Malignant glaucoma. In: Ritch R, Shields MB, Krupin T (eds). *The glaucomas*. St Louis: CV Mosby, 1989:1251–1263.
- Spaeth, GL, Wilson R. Aqueous misdirection (Malignant or Ciliary Block Glaucoma). In: Eid TM, Spaeth GL (eds). *The Glaucomas*. Philadelphia: LWW, 2000:140–145.

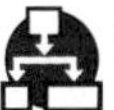

See Also (Topic, Algorithm, Electronic Media Element)

- Acknowledgment (Tasman W, Jaeger EA. The Wills Eye Hospital Atlas of Clinical Ophthalmology, Philadelphia: Lippincott Williams and Wilkins, 2001.)

CODES

ICD9

365.83 Aqueous misdirection

CLINICAL PEARLS

- Rare postoperative condition with uniform shallowing of anterior chamber, rise in IOP likely due to abnormal anatomical relationship between lens, zonules, anterior hyaloid face, and ciliary body.
- Medical and surgical management targeted towards control of IOP, chamber depth, and reestablish normal balance of aqueous circulation.
- Fellow eye is at high risk of developing malignant glaucoma if surgery is performed.

MARFAN'S SYNDROME

Caesar Luo

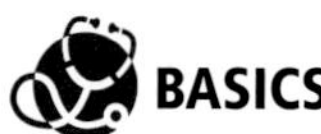

BASICS

DESCRIPTION
Autosomal dominant connective tissue disorder of the fibrillin gene that affects the cardiovascular, musculoskeletal, and ophthalmic systems.

EPIDEMIOLOGY
Prevalence
- 4–6 in 10,000 individuals
- Affects both genders equally
- 25% sporadic mutation

RISK FACTORS
- Family history
- 50% risk in each pregnancy

Genetics
- Autosomal dominant 65–75% of cases
- Defect of **fibrillin**, on 15q21 (FBNI)
- Tissue growth factor-β receptor 2 on 3p24.2–25
- High penetrance with variable manifestations

PATHOPHYSIOLOGY
- Fibrillin is essential component of microfibril assembly in extracellular matrix
- Structural function in tissues
- Fibrillin found in ciliary zonule, lens capsule, endothelium of Schlemm's canal, sclera, choroid, Bruch's membrane, lamina cribrosa, and corneal epithelium
- May explain ectopia lentis, axial myopia, glaucoma, corneal ectasia, and retinal complications
- Most common cause of nontraumatic ectopia lentis (1)[B]

ETIOLOGY
Defect in fibrillin or TFGβR2 or spontaneous mutation.

COMMONLY ASSOCIATED CONDITIONS
- Cardiac manifestations (80%)
  - Aortic root dilatation, dissecting aneurysm, mitral valve prolapse
- Musculoskeletal manifestations
  - Tall stature, scoliosis or kyphoscoliosis, chest deformities (pectus excavatum), generalized joint hypermobility
- Pulmonary manifestations
  - Spontaneous pneumothorax, apical blebs
- Neurosurgical manifestations
  - Dural ectasia

DIAGNOSIS

HISTORY
- Family history
- Focused history on cardiac, musculoskeletal, pulmonary, integumentary symptoms

PHYSICAL EXAM
- Ghent diagnostic criteria (1996)
  - Major criteria in 1 organ system and minor criteria of another with positive family history or positive genetic testing
  - With no family history, major criteria in 2 organ systems with minor in third required (2)[C]
- Ocular examination
  - Corneal ectasia, often flat cornea
  - Ectopia lentis classically superotemporal, however, all meridians have been reported. Seen in 50–80% of patients.
  - Poorly dilating pupils due to hypoplastic iris or ciliary muscle
  - Earlier onset nuclear sclerosis (10–20 years earlier)
  - Central/posterior vitreous liquefaction
  - Axial myopia
  - Retinal detachment common (8–25.6%), often in younger age (mean 22 years). Common in conjunction with ectopia lentis secondary to traction of unstable lens. Also common after lens extraction, although improved detachment rate with pars plana lensectomy versus anterior approach.

DIAGNOSTIC TESTS & INTERPRETATION
Lab
- Although mutation in FBN1 is known, molecular testing is neither sensitive nor specific (3)[C]
- Clinical and radiologic diagnosis according to Ghent criteria

Imaging
- Echocardiography
- MRI or CT
- B-scan if poorly dilated pupils with suspected retinal detachment

DIFFERENTIAL DIAGNOSIS
- Ectopia Lentis
- Trauma
- Buphthalmos
- Aniridia
- Ectopia lentis et pupillae
- Familial ectopia lentis
- Syphilis
- Weill-Marchesani syndrome
- Sulfite oxidase deficiency
- Xanthine oxidase deficiency
- Molybdenum cofactor deficiency
- Hyperlysinemia
- Methylenetetrahydrofolate reductase deficiency

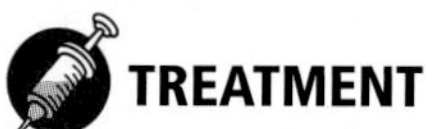

TREATMENT

MEDICATION
First Line
- β-blockers (3)[C]
- Has been shown to decrease event rates, but no effect on mortality

Second Line
- ACE inhibitors or ARB
- Currently experimental

ADDITIONAL TREATMENT
Issues for Referral
Cardiology, Pulmonary, Neurosurgery, Dermatology, and Ophthalmology/Retinal Surgery.

SURGERY/OTHER PROCEDURES

- Cataract-Pars plana lensectomy with vitrectomy preferred
- Retinal detachment
  - May need pupil stretching techniques
  - Scleral buckle-consider with minimal lens displacement with well-dilated pupil
  - Pars plana vitrectomy-consider with severe lens displacement. Additional encircling band may decrease risk of redetachment
  - Must examine fellow eye, as risk of bilateral detachment is high
  - Reported success rates for retinal reattachment is 71–89% (2)[C].

Pregnancy Considerations

Maternal risk

- Increased risk of aortic dissection, with higher risk of maternal and fetal mortality
- Progressive aortic dilatation
- Most common complications in second and third trimester
- Overall complication rate in pregnancy is low, and relatively safe in women with aortic root diameter <4.0 cm
- Consider prophylactic surgery if aortic dilatation exceeds 4.7 cm (<4.0 cm carries 10% risk of dissection).
- Consider prophylactic β-blocker with overall favorable side effect profile on the fetus.
- Vaginal delivery safe in patients with minimal aortic dilatation (<4.0 cm), but consider C-section in higher risk mothers (>4.0 cm) as hemodynamic instability during labor/delivery increases risk of dissection. Cardiac surgery can follow, or concurrent with C-section.

Fetal risk

- Variable penetrance-mildly affected mother may have severely affected fetus.
- Development of aortic dissection carries substantial risk.
- Higher rate of obstetric complications (40%) (4)[B]

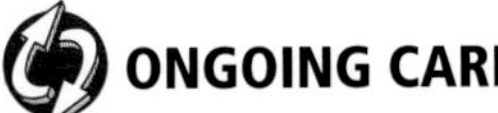

ONGOING CARE

FOLLOW-UP RECOMMENDATIONS

- Regular monitoring of valvular function and aortic diameter with echocardiography
- Elective repair of moderately regurgitant mitral valve or moderately dilated aortic root
- Low dynamic activity with avoidance of bodily collisions during exercise
- Regular ophthalmic exams

Patient Monitoring

Echocardiography

PATIENT EDUCATION

- Exercise
- Pregnancy
- Genetic counseling
- Retinal detachment warning symptoms (flashing lights, floaters, curtain over vision)

PROGNOSIS

- With modern cardiothoracic surgical techniques, average life expectancy 70 years (3)[C]
- Visual prognosis varied and is dependent on degree of involvement in regards to amblyopia, ectopia lentis, retinal detachment

COMPLICATIONS

Visual loss

REFERENCES

1. Remulla JF, Tolentino FI. Retinal detachment in Marfan's syndrome. *Int Ophth Cl* 2001;41(4): 235–240.
2. De Paepe A, Devereux RB, Dietz HC, et al. Revised diagnostic criteria for the Marfan syndrome. *Am J Med Genet* 1996;62:417–426.
3. Keane MG, Pyeritz RE. Medical management of Marfan syndrome. *Circulation* 2008;117: 2802–2813.
4. Goland S, Barrakat M, Khatri N, et al. Pregnancy in Marfan syndrome. *Card in Rev* 2009;17:253–262.

ADDITIONAL READING

- Judge DP, Dietz HC. Marfan's syndrome. *Lancet* 2005;366:1965–1976.

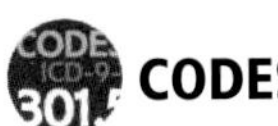

CODES

ICD9

- 367.1 Myopia
- 743.37 Congenital ectopic lens
- 759.82 Marfan syndrome

CLINICAL PEARLS

- Lens subluxation with Marfan's is classically superotemporal, versus inferior displacement in homocystinuria.
- Mutation in fibrillin gene
- 25% sporadic mutation rate
- Retinal detachment is common.

M

MEESMANN'S CORNEAL DYSTROPHY

Arvind Saini
Anthony Aldave

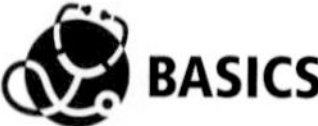

BASICS

DESCRIPTION

- Meesmann's corneal dystrophy (MCD) is an epithelial dystrophy
- Occurs early in life
- Also called Juvenile epithelial dystrophy
  - Autosomal dominant inheritance
  - Characterized by epithelial microcysts
  - Cysts contain degenerated cell products

EPIDEMIOLOGY

Incidence

- There are no incidence values.
  - Rare; patients are often misdiagnosed

Prevalence

- There are no prevalence values
- Patients are often misdiagnosed
- First described in Germany
- Has now been described worldwide

RISK FACTORS

Family History (affected parent).

Genetics

- Autosomal dominant inheritance, incomplete penetrance
- Mutation in KRT3 (1) (chromosome 12q13) and KRT12 (chromosome 17q12) (2) genes
- Genes code cornea specific proteins K3, K12

PATHOPHYSIOLOGY

- K3 and K12 proteins form meshwork filaments found in the epithelial cell cytoplasm.
- The meshwork maintains epithelial integrity, provides resistance to mechanical stress (3).
- Pain results from cyst rupture.
- Cysts appear early in life, increase with age.
- Blurry vision evolves from increased cyst formation and corneal surface irregularity.
- Scarring may develop after repeat erosions.

ETIOLOGY

Genetic inheritance

COMMONLY ASSOCIATED CONDITIONS

Other corneal dystrophies may coexist (4).

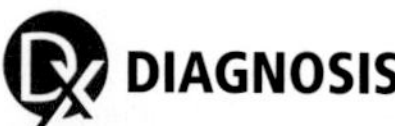

DIAGNOSIS

HISTORY

- Usually asymptomatic or have mild symptoms
- May have episodes of photophobia, tearing, blepharospasm, foreign body sensation, and mild pain from erosions due to cyst rupture
- Significant visual loss is uncommon

Pediatric Considerations

Can be a cause of corneal erosions in children.

PHYSICAL EXAM

Multiple tiny, intraepithelial, microcystic, bubble-like lesions and dot-like opacities (5)

- Usually bilateral and symmetric
- Can be unilateral
- Surrounding epithelium is usually clear
- Usually cysts are most prevalent in the interpalpebral zone or involve the entire epithelium, extending to the corneal limbus.
- Cysts may involve only the periphery, usually with spared central cornea.
- Punctate epithelial erosions, mild injection
- Central scarring, subepithelial serpiginous lines and opacities in advanced cases

DIAGNOSTIC TESTS & INTERPRETATION

Lab

Blood or saliva can be collected and sent for screening of KRT3 and KRT12 to differentiate from conditions with similar phenotypes.

Imaging

- Indirect slit-lamp illumination from the iris reveals a dust-like pattern.
- Slit-lamp retroillumination bubble-like cysts

Diagnostic Procedures/Other

- Histology and electron microscopy are useful with tissue samples from corneal biopsy or lamellar/penetrating keratoplasty.
- Confocal microscopy for in vivo study (3)

Pathological Findings
- Intraepithelial cysts, 10–70 μm in diameter
- Cysts are filled with PAS-positive granules, (5) and fibrogranular material termed "peculiar substance."
- Epithelial basement membrane is irregular, showing thickening and multilaminarity.
- Some cases have thinning of the cornea.
- Advanced disease shows disorganized epithelium with loss of cell polarity.

DIFFERENTIAL DIAGNOSIS
- Epithelial basement membrane dystrophy
- Bleb-like variant of EBMD
- Lisch corneal dystrophy
- Limbal stem cell deficiency
- Epidermolysis bullosa

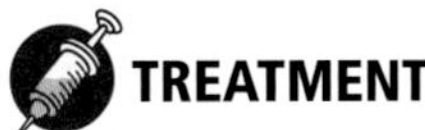

TREATMENT

MEDICATION

First Line
- Most do not require treatment
- If symptomatic, frequent lubrication with artificial tears or ointments for discomfort

Second Line
Bandage soft contact lenses.

ALERT
Patients and ophthalmologists must be aware of the increased risk for infectious keratitis.

SURGERY/OTHER PROCEDURES
- Phototherapeutic keratectomy
- Epithelial debridement
- Manual superficial keratectomy
- Penetrating keratoplasty in advanced disease
- Mitomycin C may be used after keratectomy (6), but extreme care is required with mitomycin use.

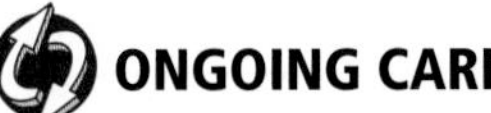

ONGOING CARE

FOLLOW-UP RECOMMENDATIONS
Routine annual examination unless other conditions exist, or if the patient is symptomatic

Patient Monitoring
If patients have frequent erosions, care should be taken to limit erosions.

PROGNOSIS
Good; most patients are asymptomatic or have mild discomfort and vision disturbances.

COMPLICATIONS
There is a risk for corneal infection and scarring with repeat erosions.

REFERENCES

1. Irvine AD, Corden LD, Swensson O, et al. Mutations in cornea-specific keratin K3 or K12 genes cause Meesmann's corneal dystrophy. *Nature Genet* 1997;16:184–187.
2. Irvine AD, Coleman CM, Moore JE, et al. A novel mutation in KRT12 associated with Meesmann's epithelial corneal dystrophy. *Br J Ophthalmol* 2002;86:729–732.
3. Patel DV, Grupcheva CN, McGhee CN. Imaging the microstructural abnormalities of Meesmann corneal dystrophy by in vivo confocal microscopy. *Cornea* 2005;24:669–673.
4. Cremona F, Ghosheh FR, Laibson PR, et al. Meesmann corneal dystrophy associated with epithelial basement membrane and posterior polymorphous cornea dystrophies. *Cornea* 2008;27:374–377.
5. Fine BS, Yanoff M, Pitts E, et al. Meesmann's epithelial dystrophy of the cornea. *Am J Ophthalmol* 1977;83:633–642.
6. Yeung JYT, Hodge QG. Recurrent Meesmann's corneal dystrophy: Treatment with keratectomy and mitomycin C. *Can J Ophthalmol* 2009;44:103–104.

ADDITIONAL READING

- Krachmer JH, Mannis MJ, Holland EJ. (eds). Cornea. *Cornea and External Disease: Clinical Diagnosis and Management: II*. Mosby: St. Louis, 1997.

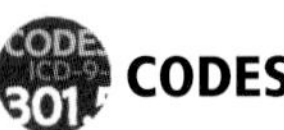

CODES

ICD9
371.51 Juvenile epithelial corneal dystrophy

CLINICAL PEARLS
- Meesmann's corneal dystrophy is often an asymptomatic condition and may be an incidental finding on examination.
- There is a strong family pattern of inheritance.
- Management should be directed at symptoms and not signs of the disease on exam.

M

METASTATIC TUMORS TO THE EYE AND ADNEXA

Aparna Ramasubramanian
Carol L. Shields

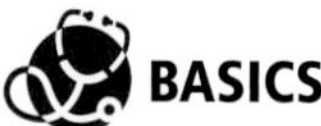

BASICS

DESCRIPTION

- Intraocular metastasis – most common tumor of the eye
- Most common site of involvement is choroid (63%)
- Other sites – iris, ciliary body (6%), vitreous, retina, optic disc, eyelid, and orbit (32%)
- 25% of patients have no known history of cancer. Primary site remains unknown in 10%
- Most common primary site - breasts in women and lungs in men

EPIDEMIOLOGY

Prevalence

- Increasing incidence paralleling improving cancer survival rates
- True incidence unknown in view of poor detection because of advanced cancer stage and asymptomatic nature of disease
- Postmortem incidence ≈10%
- Estimated prevalence of uveal metastasis – 2.3–9.2% of all patients with systemic cancer
- Estimated prevalence of orbital metastasis – 2–4.7% of all patients with systemic cancer

RISK FACTORS

- Risk factor for uveal metastasis – presence of metastatic disease in 2 or more organs
- 70–90% of patients have metastatic lesion elsewhere at time of ocular diagnosis
- Median time from diagnosis of primary cancer to ocular metastasis – 12–55 months, depending on the primary cancer site

PATHOPHYSIOLOGY

Choroid has a rich vascular supply and is recognized as the tissue with the highest metastatic efficiency index (measure of metastatic deposits in relation to blood flow).

COMMONLY ASSOCIATED CONDITIONS

- Primary cancer sites that promote ocular metastasis (pooled from multiple studies)
  - Breast cancer– 40–47%
  - Lung cancer– 14–30%
  - GI cancer– 4%
  - Prostate cancer– 1–4%
  - Melanoma – 5%
  - Kidney cancer– 2–4%

DIAGNOSIS

HISTORY

- Most cases are asymptomatic
- Blurred vision is the most common presentation
- Other features
  - **Uveal metastasis** – pain, scotoma, redness, and photophobia
  - **Orbital metastasis** – diplopia, proptosis, pain, ptosis, and visible mass

PHYSICAL EXAM

- **Choroidal metastasis**
  - Bilaterality in 20–50%
  - Multifocal lesions ≈30%
  - Commonly affects posterior choroid, especially macula
  - Usually cream colored lesions
  - Orange color in metastasis from bronchial carcinoid, renal cell carcinoma, and thyroid cancer.
  - Gray–brown color in melanoma metastasis
  - Extensive subretinal fluid in active lesions
  - "Leopard skin appearance" – due to clumps of brown pigment
- **Iris metastasis**
  - Yellow to white single or multiple nodules
  - Other likely features - iridocyclitis, hyphema, and glaucoma
- **Ciliary body metastasis**
  - Solitary sessile or dome shaped
  - Other features – cataract, iridocyclitis, and hyphema
- **Retinal metastasis**
  - Resemble occlusive vasculitis
  - Vitreous seeding may be present
- **Vitreous metastasis**
  - Tumor infiltration of vitreous resembling lymphoma
- **Optic nerve metastasis**
  - Occurs as juxtapapillary spread from choroidal metastasis or isolated optic nerve involvement
  - Unilateral optic nerve elevation
  - Significant visual loss observed
- **Orbit metastasis**
  - Mass effect causing proptosis, globe displacement, pain, chemosis, and eyelid swelling
  - Soft tissue infiltration – ptosis, restricted extraocular movement
  - Enophthalmos in scirrhous carcinoma (commonly breast and stomach metastasis)
  - Carcinoid – frequently, orbital metastasis is the first sign.
    - Primary small intestinal carcinoids typically metastasizes to orbit and bronchial carcinoid metastasizes to choroid
  - Pediatric population – metastasis are rare but the most likely primary sites are– neuroblastoma, Wilms tumor, Ewing's sarcoma, rhabdomyosarcoma
- **Eyelid metastasis**
  - Varied presentation – solitary or multiple nodules or diffuse lid infiltration

DIAGNOSTIC TESTS & INTERPRETATION

Initial approach

- Diagnosis primarily clinical
- CNS imaging of paramount importance because of coexistent brain metastasis

Imaging

- **Uveal metastasis**
  - Fluorescein angiography – early hypofluorescence and late leakage
  - Ultrasound –
    - A-scan - moderate to high internal reflectivity
    - B-scan – Acoustic solidity
    - Rarely mushroom shaped configuration noted
    - Ultrasound biomicroscopy useful for ciliary body metastasis
- **Orbital metastasis**
  - CT and MRI primary diagnostic tests – MRI provides better soft tissue resolution. CT appropriate for imaging bony lesions (e.g., Prostatic metastasis)

Diagnostic Procedures/Other

- Definitive diagnosis – fine needle aspiration biopsy or open biopsy
- Immunohistochemistry beneficial in select cases to diagnose primary cell type

Pathological Findings

- Orbital tissue metastasis rate – bone–fat-muscle ratio – 2:2:1
- Diagnosis of ocular metastasis consistent with Stage IV cancer
- Work up with oncologist required for restaging tumor and investigating for other sites of metastasis

DIFFERENTIAL DIAGNOSIS

- **Choroidal metastasis**
  - Melanoma/nevus
  - Hemangioma
  - Osteoma
  - Lymphoma
  - Inflammatory diseases
- **Iris metastasis**
  - Amelanotic melanoma/nevus
  - Granulomas
- **Orbit/Eyelid metastasis**
  - Benign and malignant orbital/eyelid tumors

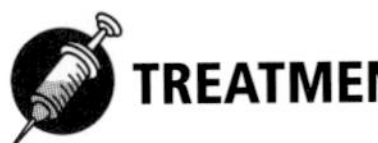

TREATMENT

Uveal Metastasis

- **External beam radiotherapy** (Grade B treatment recommendation)
  - Dose – 20–50 Gy
  - Response – 63–83%
  - Visual improvement – 27–89%
  - Complications – ocular surface changes, cataract, and radiation retinopathy
- **Systemic chemotherapy/Hormonal therapy**
  - Success based on type of primary tumor
  - Useful in breast/lung cancer
- **Plaque radiotherapy**
  - High dose targeted radiation dosage
  - Useful for solitary choroidal metastasis
  - Beneficial for recurrent tumor following external beam radiation
- **Proton beam therapy**
  - Shorter duration of therapy
  - More precise tissue targeting due to minimal scatter
- **Local therapy**
  - Transpupillary thermotherapy, laser photocoagulation, photodynamic therapy
  - Can be used as adjuvant treatment to radiation
  - Isolated reports of successful treatment with intravitreal bevacizumab – role unknown
- **Enucleation**
  - Indicated for blind painful eye due to glaucomatous damage

Orbit Metastasis

- Treatment considerations dependent on systemic features and life expectancy.
- External beam radiotherapy – primary treatment modality
  - Advantages – decrease tumor size, reduce proptosis, preserve vision
  - Dose – 20–40 Gy over 2–4 weeks
  - Complications – Cataract, Radiation retinopathy
  - Concurrent intracranial irradiation required for brain metastases
- Systemic chemotherapy – reserved for chemosensitive tumors like small cell lung cancer
- Hormonal therapy – Breast/prostate metastasis
- Orbital surgery – debulking reserved to reduce ocular pain, proptosis, and diplopia
- Exenteration – for disfiguring orbital mass

EyelID Metastasis

- Dependent on tumor size, location, extent, and systemic features.
- Excisional biopsy - Small solitary lesion
- External beam radiotherapy – for multiple/recurrent lesions
- Systemic chemotherapy/immunotherapy – for extensive systemic metastasis
- Palliative care – for terminal metastasis
- Topical Imiquimod – for cutaneous melanoma metastasis

ADDITIONAL TREATMENT

General Measures

Treatment of primary tumor and other metastatic foci

Additional Therapies

- Palliative care
- Pain management

COMPLEMENTARY & ALTERNATIVE THERAPIES

- In 3–5% of patients the primary site remains unknown after workup
- Following evaluation of all sites of metastasis, therapeutic chemotherapy trial can be attempted
- 85% of these patients die within 1 year

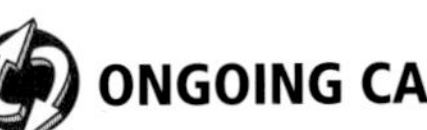

ONGOING CARE

FOLLOW-UP RECOMMENDATIONS

- Multidisciplinary coordinated care required
- Close monitoring for detection of systemic metastatic foci
- Close ophthalmic follow-up for detection of new metastasis, especially in the fellow eye

PATIENT EDUCATION

- Counsel regarding warning eye signs in patients with advanced cancers
- After diagnosis of ocular metastasis – careful monitoring is required to detect new metastasis in both eyes

PROGNOSIS

- Median life expectancy – 6–9 months
- Prognosis dependent on type of tumor and extent of metastasis
- Favorable prognosis – Breast cancer and carcinoid metastasis

ADDITIONAL READING

- Ahmad SM, Esmaeli B. Metastatic tumors of the orbit and ocular adnexa. *Curr Opin Ophthalmol* 2007;18:405–413.
- Bianciotto C, Demirci H, Shields CL, et al. Metastatic tumors to the eyelid: Report of 20 cases and review of the literature. *Arch Ophthalmol* 2009;127: 999–1005.
- Kanthan GL, Jayamohan J, Yip D, et al. Management of metastatic carcinoma of the uveal tract: An evidence-based analysis. *Clin Experiment Ophthalmol* 2007;35:553–565.
- Shields JA, Shields CL, Kiratli H, et al. Metastatic tumors to the iris in 40 patients. *Am J Ophthalmol* 1995;119:422–430.
- Shields CL, Shields JA, Gross NE, et al. Survey of 520 eyes with uveal metastases. *Ophthalmology* 1997;104:1265–1276.
- Shields JA, Shields CL. Metastatic tumors to the uvea, retina, and optic disc. In: Shields JA, Shields CL, eds. *Eyelid, Conjunctival, and Orbital Tumors. A Textbook and Atlas*, 2nd ed. Philadelphia, PA: Lippincott, Williams & Wilkins, 2007;727–745, 168–173.
- Shields JA, Shields CL. Metastatic tumors to the uvea, retina, and optic disc. In: Shields JA, Shields CL, eds. *Intraocular Tumors. A Textbook and Atlas*, 2nd ed. Philadelphia, PA: Lippincott, Williams & Wilkins, 2007;198–227.
- Shields CL, Shields JA. Metastatic cancer to the eye and adnexa. In Tasman WS, Jaeger E, eds, *Duane's Clinical Ophthalmology* Vol. 5, Chapter 34, Philadelphia, PA: Lippincott Williams & Wilkins, 2010.

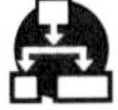

See Also (Topic, Algorithm, Electronic Media Element)

- www.fighteyecancer.com
- www.malignantmelanomainfo.com
- www.retinoblastomainfo.com
- www.eyecancerinfo.com
- www.eyecancerbook.com
- www.etrf.org

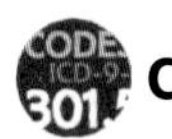

CODES

ICD9

- 198.4 Secondary malignant neoplasm of other parts of nervous system
- 198.2 Secondary malignant neoplasm of skin

CLINICAL PEARLS

- Increasing incidence of ocular metastasis
- High index of suspicion required for diagnosis
- Early diagnosis and appropriate therapy improves prognosis and visual morbidity.
- Ocular metastasis is the first presentation of malignancy in around 30%.
- Choroid is the most common site of metastasis.
- External beam radiotherapy is the treatment of choice in most patients.

M

MEWDS (MULTIPLE EVANESCENT WHITE DOT SYNDROME)

Mimi Liu

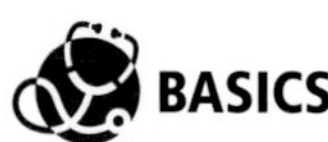

BASICS

DESCRIPTION
- Multiple evanescent white dot syndrome (MEWDS) is an idiopathic inflammatory disease of the choroid that causes mild to moderate acute vision loss (1).
- It is usually self-limited, with recovery to normal vision within several weeks without recurrence.
- It is usually unilateral.

EPIDEMIOLOGY
Incidence
- Affect younger individuals, usually in the second to fifth decades of life
- 90% of patients are female

RISK FACTORS
50% of cases are associated with a viral prodrome.

Genetics
Possible association with HLA-B51 (2).

PATHOPHYSIOLOGY
Unclear.

ETIOLOGY
- Unknown
- It is presumed to be caused by a virus.
- Genetic predisposition combined with an environmental trigger may cause the disease.

COMMONLY ASSOCIATED CONDITIONS
Acute idiopathic blind spot enlargement syndrome (AIBES)-some feel that MEWDS and AIBES (as well as a number of other "white dot" syndromes are a spectrum of the same disease) (3).

DIAGNOSIS

HISTORY
- Sudden onset of decreased central vision in one eye
- Occasionally it may be bilateral, and may occur asynchronously
- May have central scotoma or photopsias
- May have a history of a recent viral illness

PHYSICAL EXAM
- Patients often have mild myopia
- There may be a mild afferent papillary defect
- Patients may have a mild vitreitis
- Optic disc edema
- There are ill defined small white lesions in the posterior pole at the level of the RPE/outer retina
- "Orange" foveal granularity

DIAGNOSTIC TESTS & INTERPRETATION
Lab
None usually necessary as MEWDS is a clinical diagnosis.

Imaging
Initial approach
- Fluorescein angiogram shows early hyperfluorescence with late staining in a cluster or wreath-like pattern around the macula.
- OCT shows subtle disruptions of photoreceptor inner and outer segment junction (4).

Follow-up & special considerations
- ICG is usually not needed for diagnosis.
- ICG angiography usually demonstrates more numerous hypofluorescent spots than seen on fluorescein angiography.

Diagnostic Procedures/Other
An electroretinogram (ERG) may be abnormal.

DIFFERENTIAL DIAGNOSIS
- Acute idiopathic blind spot enlargement
- Acute multifocal posterior pigment epitheliopathy (AMPPE)
- Acute macular neuroretinopathy
- Multifocal choroiditis
- Birdshot retinochoroidopathy
- Primary intraocular lymphoma may rarely appear similar to MEWDS, especially in patients >50 years old (5).

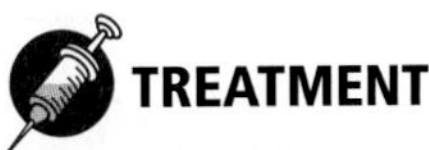

TREATMENT

MEDICATION

- Observation
- Symptoms usually resolve in 1–2 months.

ADDITIONAL TREATMENT

Issues for Referral

Consider referral to a vitreoretinal specialist.

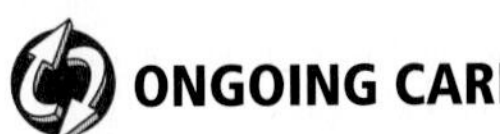

ONGOING CARE

FOLLOW-UP RECOMMENDATIONS

Monthly until symptoms resolve, then as needed.

PROGNOSIS

- Visual prognosis is good with almost all patients recovering vision >20/40.
- Recurrence is rare.

COMPLICATIONS

Choroidal neovascularization is extremely rare.

REFERENCES

1. Jampol LM, Sieving PA, Pugh D, et al. Multiple evanescent white dot syndrome. I. Clinical findings. *Arch Ophthalmol* 1984;102:671–674.
2. Borruat FX, Herbort CP, Spertini F, et al. HLA typing in patients with multiple evanescent white dot syndrome (MEWDS). *Ocular Immunol Inflamm* 1998;6:39–41.
3. Gass JD. Are acute zonal occult outer retinopathy and the white spot syndromes (AZOOR complex) specific autoimmune diseases? *Am J Ophthalmol* 2003;135:380–381.
4. Shah GK, Kleiner RC, Augsburger JJ, et al. Primary intraocular lymphoma seen with transient white fundus lesions simulating the multiple evanescent white dot syndrome. *Arch Ophthalmol* 2001;119: 617–620.
5. Nguyen MH, Witkin AJ, Reichel E, et al. Microstructural abnormalities in MEWDS demonstrated by ultrahigh resolution optical coherence tomography. *Retina* 2007;27:414–418.

ADDITIONAL READING

- Jampol LM, Wiredu A. MEWDS, MFC, PIC, AMN, AIBSE, and AZOOR: One disease or many? *Retina* 1995;15(5):373–378.
- Quillen DA, Davis JB, Gottlieb JL, et al. The white dot syndromes. *Am J Ophthalmol* 2004;137(3): 538–535.

CODES

ICD9

- 363.07 Focal retinitis and retinochoroiditis of other posterior pole
- 363.15 Disseminated retinitis and retinochoroiditis, pigment epitheliopathy
- 363.20 Chorioretinitis, unspecified

CLINICAL PEARLS

- MEWDS typically presents with unilateral acute loss of vision in healthy young women.
- Clinical examination shows outer retinal ill-defined small white lesions in the posterior pole and foveal granularity.
- MEWDS is usually self-limited with resolution of symptoms in 1–2 months.

MICROPHTHALMIA

Alex V. Levin

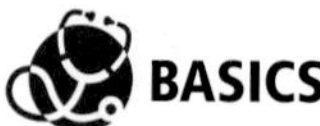

BASICS

DESCRIPTION

- Small eye, unilateral or bilateral, including axial length and corneal diameter
- With or without intraocular anomalies or systemic disease

EPIDEMIOLOGY

1–2 per 10,000 newborns (1)[C]

RISK FACTORS

- Ocular coloboma (1)[C]
- Congenital cataract
- Intrauterine infection (especially rubella)
- Wide range of chromosomal aberrations, syndromes, and congenital disorders
- Possibly some teratogens including ionizing radiation, alcohol, and isotretinoin

Genetics

- Known genes for isolated ocular involvement include CHX0, SHH, OTX2, MAF, PAX6, CRYAA, GDF6, SIX6, CMIC, RX, CRYBA4, and FOXE3. Other loci known but gene not cloned.
- Known genes with syndrome associations include CHD7 (CHARGE syndrome), DPD (developmental delay), HESX1 (septo-optic dysplasia), SOX2 (multiple anomalies), BMP4 (multiple anomalies), STRA6 (multiple anomalies, Matthew Wood syndrome), HCCS (microphthalmia with linear skin defects syndrome), ANOP1 (Lenz microphthalmia), BCOR (oculofacialcardiodental). Multiple other genes and loci known.
- Isolated and syndromic forms may be autosomal dominant or autosomal recessive. Syndromic may also be X-linked dominant or X-linked recessive.
- Sporadic cases may or may not be heritable.
- Familial cases may have variable expression. Incomplete penetrance is rare.
- Unilateral cases may be genetic (2)[B].

GENERAL PREVENTION

- Genetic counseling and/or prenatal testing (if mutated gene known or syndrome recognized in family)
- Avoidance of *in utero* exposures if known risk for infection or teratogen
- Can be detected by prenatal ultrasound at 12–13 weeks (3)[C], (4)[C]

PATHOPHYSIOLOGY

Incomplete ocular development during embryogenesis as a result of a variety of faulty processes of ocular growth, most often involving mutations in developmental genes acting as transcription factors for other downstream genes.

ETIOLOGY

- Mutated or otherwise abnormal gene(s), especially when bilateral
- Infection or teratogen exposure *in utero*
- Coloboma or rarely primary aphakia
- Idiopathic

COMMONLY ASSOCIATED CONDITIONS

- Ocular coloboma
- Congenital cataract, especially if nuclear or persistent fetal vasculature (PFV, formerly known as PHPV), or other forms of anterior segment dysgenesis (5)[C]
- Optic nerve abnormalities (e.g., hypoplasia)
- Retinal dysplasia (5)[C]
- No consistent systemic associations except perhaps developmental delay when chromosomal aberration or other systemic syndromic findings
- Anterior chamber depth usually normal (shallow in nanophthalmia)

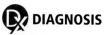

DIAGNOSIS

HISTORY

- Family history of microphthalmia or related congenital ocular disease
- Known exposure to infection or teratogen *in utero*
- Other known associated anomalies or developmental delay

PHYSICAL EXAM

- Full ocular examination including inferior nasal peripheral retinal examination for coloboma
- Systemic examination for other anomalies
- Nystagmus and strabismus may be present
- Refraction may range from high hyperopia to high myopia
- Assessment of visual function
- Clinical assessment of size of palpebral fissure and periocular tissue/bone size
- Assessment of anterior chamber depth

DIAGNOSTIC TESTS & INTERPRETATION

Lab

Initial lab tests

- None if no systemic involvement
- Karyotype if other congenital anomalies
- Specific genetic analysis based on diagnosis (e.g., FISH for microdeletion 22q11 if considering CHARGE syndrome, specific gene mutation analysis as directed by diagnosis)

Follow-up & special considerations

- Genetic consultation if systemic abnormalities or developmental delay and if family history or recognized genetic diagnosis
- Examine parents for ocular signs and peripheral asymptomatic coloboma if child has coloboma.

Imaging

Initial approach

- B-scan to assess retina and optic nerve if no view. Will also rule out primary aphakia.
- B-scan or UBM may be used to assess scleral thickness.
- A scan for axial length
- Consider neuroimaging if bilateral optic nerve involvement
- Consider CT scan if evidence of small orbit (especially if severe)

Follow-up & special considerations

- If other findings, suggesting glaucoma risk (e.g., elevated risk in aphakia) requires ongoing monitoring every 6 months for glaucoma. Sedation/anesthesia as needed.
- If coloboma, examine every 6 months to screen for retinal detachment.

Diagnostic Procedures/Other

Genetic counseling and molecular genetic testing as appropriate and available.

Pathological Findings

Incomplete ocular development possibly including retina, optic nerve, iris, and choroid.

DIFFERENTIAL DIAGNOSIS

- Anophthalmia (no evidence of a globe on imaging or on postmortem dissection of orbit)
  - Nanophthalmia
  - Microcornea without microphthalmia (1)[C]
  - Phthisis (e.g., following infection or trauma)

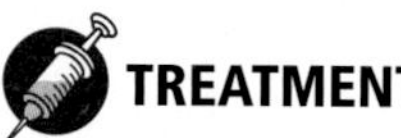

TREATMENT

MEDICATION

- None for the primary disorder but may need treatment for secondary concerns such as glaucoma
- Consider atropine (0.5% if <1 year old) if anterior chamber shallow as prophylaxis for angle closure and other complications or if glaucoma present and anterior chamber shallow/flat
- Avoid pilocarpine if anterior chamber shallow (nanophthalmia)

ADDITIONAL TREATMENT

General Measures

Amblyopia therapy as indicated

Issues for Referral

- Genetic consultation if systemic signs or family history
- Low vision evaluation and support as indicated
- Retinal surgery for detachment due to coloboma. Surgery is not beneficial in cases of congenital retinal non-attachment/retinal dysplasia and usually not helpful in congenital retinal detachment

Additional Therapies

- If nonfunctional eye and small palpebral fissure/orbital opening, consider scleral shell to encourage periocular tissue growth. Severe cases may benefit from intraorbital balloon placement by craniofacial surgeon (6)[C].
- If nonfunctional eye and microphthalmia mild, consider plus lens in spectacle for enhancing appearance of eye (enlarging) to outside observer.

COMPLEMENTARY & ALTERNATIVE THERAPIES

None proven or indicated.

SURGERY/OTHER PROCEDURES

Cataract, glaucoma, retina, and strabismus as needed.

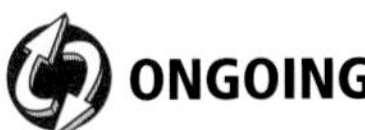

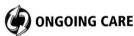

ONGOING CARE

FOLLOW-UP RECOMMENDATIONS

- As needed for amblyopia monitoring and treatment
- As needed for secondary complications (cataract, glaucoma, retinal detachment, and strabismus). Every 6 months if glaucoma risk or coloboma
- Low vision
- Follow orbital and periocular tissue growth especially in the first 5 years of life

Patient Monitoring

- School performance and development
- Patient concerns about appearance

PATIENT EDUCATION

- Genetic counseling
- Low vision intervention
- International Children's Anophthalmia and Microphthalmia Network http://www.anophthalmia.org/

PROGNOSIS

- Variable acuity – depends in part on, presence of other ocular or non ocular abnormalities. Very poor prognosis if associated with primary aphakia, retinal dysplasia, congenital retinal detachment/non attachment.
- Risk for retinal detachment if coloboma may be in excess of 2%
- Risk for glaucoma depends on associated ocular anomalies

COMPLICATIONS

- Retinal detachment if coloboma
- Glaucoma if aphakia, persistent fetal vasculature (PFV), and anterior segment dysgenesis

REFERENCES

1. Warburg M. Classification of microphthalmos and coloboma. *J med Genet* 1993;30:664–669.
2. Fleckenstein M, Maumenee IH. Unilateral isolated microphthalmia inherited as an autosomal recessive trait. *Ophthalmic Genet* 2005;26:163–168.
3. Wong HS, Parker S, Tait J, Pringle KC. Antenatal diagnosis of anophthalmia by three-dimensional ultrasound: A novel application of the reverse face view. *Ultrasound Obstet Gynecol* 2008;32: 103–105.
4. Chitayat D, Sroka H, Keating S, et al. The PDAC syndrome (pulmonary hypoplasia/agenesis, diaphragmatic hernia/eventration, Anophthalmia/microphthalmia, and cardiac defect) (Spear syndrome, Matthew-Wood syndrome): Report of eight cases including a living child and further evidence for autosomal recessive inheritance. *Am J Med Genet* 2007;143A: 1268–1281.
5. Weiss AH, Kousseff BG, Ross EA, Longbottom J. Complex microphthalmos. *Arch Ophthalmol* 1989;107:1619–1624.
6. Gossman MD, Mohay J, Roberts DM. Expansion of the human microphthalmic orbit. *Ophthalmology* 1999;106:2005–2009.

ADDITIONAL READING

http://www.einstein.edu/yourhealth/genetic/article15837.html.

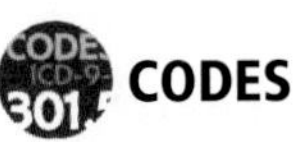

CODES

ICD9

- 743.10 Microphthalmos, unspecified
- 743.30 Congenital cataract, unspecified
- 743.49 Other congenital anomalies of anterior segment

CLINICAL PEARLS

- Visual prognosis without clear obstruction to visual pathway (e.g., cataract) uncertain, so try amblyopia therapy and glasses where indicated.
- Small diameter gas permeable contact lenses are an option for high refractive error.
- Consider possibility of associated systemic findings.
- Ensure adequate orbital and periocular tissue growth.
- Examine parents if coloboma present.
- Consider genetic consult and counseling.
- Rule out nanophthalmia (increased scleral thickness, axial length <14 mm, shallow anterior chamber, peripheral choroidal effusion)
- A microphthalmic eye in infancy and toddler years that develops glaucoma may enlarge inappropriately and have relative buphthalmia even if the size is still less than normal for age.
- If doing glaucoma tube implantation on microphthalmic eye <18–20 mm long, consider pediatric tube size to avoid contact between posterior plate and optic nerve.

M

MIGRAINE & CLUSTER HEADACHE

Scott Uretsky

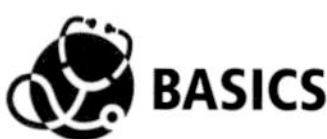

BASICS

DESCRIPTION

- Migraine headache (HA): A chronic, recurrent episodic, stereotypical HA syndrome not caused by intracranial or systemic disease (but neural-based)
  - ± associated migraine features; ± aura
  - International Headache Society (IHS): Diagnostic criteria and migraine subtypes: Migraine without aura →
    - A. At least 5 attacks fulfilling B–D
    - B. HA lasting for 4–72 hours
    - C. HA with at least 2 of the following: Unilateral location, pulsing quality, moderate to severe intensity, aggravation by or avoidance of routine activity
    - D. HA accompanied by at least 1 of following: Nausea and/or vomiting, photophobia, or phonophobia
    - E. Not attributed to another disorder
- Cluster HA: Episodic, short-lived attacks, clustered temporally, followed by pain-free interval.
  - IHS criteria:
    - A. 5 attacks fulfilling B–D
    - B. Severe, unilateral, orbital, supraorbital, or temporal pain lasting 15–80 minutes
    - C. At least 1 ipsilateral feature: Conjunctival injection/lacrimation, nasal congestion/rhinorrhea, eyelid edema, forehead/facial sweating, ptosis, miosis, restlessness or agitation
    - D. Frequency: every other day to 8 attacks/day
    - E. Not attributed to another disorder
  - Characteristic circadian & circannual features
- Initial determinations: 1) Primary (no underlying intracranial or systemic disease) versus secondary HA 2) New onset versus chronic
  - Requires emergent evaluation (e.g., neuroimaging ± lumbar puncture (LP)):
    - Acute onset, maximal at onset or focal signs; Progressive symptoms and signs; systemic symptoms (e.g., fever)
  - Other worrisome features: Onset fourth to fifth decade, accelerating pattern, history of malignancy or HIV, significant change in HA pattern, exacerbation with position change, exertion, sexual activity, or Valsalva

EPIDEMIOLOGY

Incidence

Migraine: ♀:♂ 3:1; cumulative lifetime: ♀ 43%, ♂ 18%. cluster: ♂:♀ 8:1

Prevalence

Migraine 12–15%; cluster ~69/100,000

RISK FACTORS

Family history: ↑ Risk by 50% versus controls

Genetics

Familial hemiplegic migraine 1, 19p13

GENERAL PREVENTION

Identification and avoidance of migraine triggers

PATHOPHYSIOLOGY

Central activation of pain sensitive cranial structures; serotonergic neurotransmission dysfunction; central pain sensitization

ETIOLOGY

Hereditary; pattern and mode of inheritance unclear; multiple genes contribute

COMMONLY ASSOCIATED CONDITIONS

Depression, panic disorder, epilepsy, asthma, non-HA pain

DIAGNOSIS

HISTORY

- See IHS criteria
- Assess: Inciting event, new onset/de novo versus chronic/recurrent, quality, duration, location, and time course
  - Characteristic frequency and symptom pattern?
  - Exacerbating or alleviating factors? Triggers?
  - Position, posture, or Valsalva related?
  - Age >50 years: Temporal arteritis ROS?
  - Time-intensity relationship:
    - Subarachnoid hemorrhage (SAH): Maximal intensity at onset, that is, "thunder-clap"
    - Cluster: Peaks over 3–5 minutes, maximal for 1–2 hours, tapers off.
    - Migraine: Escalates over hour(s), lasts hours to days.
  - Migraine features? Aura, nausea, vomiting, photophobia, and phonophobia
  - Cluster: Excruciating, acute, unilateral periorbital pain; crescendo within 5 minutes; ipsilateral autonomic features
    - Pathognomonic: Provoked by ETOH in ~70%
- Assess additional symptoms: Transient visual obscurations, vertigo, meningismus, amenorrhea, galactorrhea, fever, purulent nasal discharge, myalgias, scalp tenderness, jaw claudication, and cognitive dysfunction.
  - History of focal neurological symptoms?
- Past medical, psychiatric, and medication history: Neoplasm, aneurysm, or HIV history?

PHYSICAL EXAM

Complete neurological exam including funduscopy: Normal except for transient aura signs.

DIAGNOSTIC TESTS & INTERPRETATION

Lab

Initial lab tests

Exclusion of secondary causes: Metabolic panel, CBC/Platelets, ESR and CRP for age >50 years

Follow-up & special considerations

ANA, Anti-DS DNA Ab, Arterial blood gas, sleep study to r/o sleep apnea, anti TSH-receptor Ab, → tailor to individual patient

Imaging

Initial approach

- New onset HA of non-urgent nature: MRI
- Acute, severe HA, or focal signs: Urgent non-contrast CT

Follow-up & special considerations

- MRV for venous sinus thrombosis and work-up of idiopathic intracranial hypertension (IIH)
- CTA or MRI/A with axial T1 fat suppression: Optimal for ruling out dissection

Diagnostic Procedures/Other

ALERT

- LP ***must*** be obtained for suspected SAH if CT negative (prior to MRI)
- Visual aura: Include visual field to exclude homonymous defects indicating parenchymal disease
- Clinical impact scales: MIDAS, HIT, MIBS, MSQ, MPQ-5

DIFFERENTIAL DIAGNOSIS

- Differentiate from other primary HA: Tension-type, cluster, and "sinus HA" (often self-diagnosed).
- Secondary causes of HA are numerous (brief list):
  - In ER: Migraine is diagnosis of exclusion for first or "worst" HA
  - Vascular: Intracranial hemorrhage, ischemia, arterial dissection, sinus thrombosis, aneurysm, and malformations
  - Neoplasm, benign masses, and lymphoproliferative disease
  - Other: Meningitis, IIH, Chiari, malignant HTN, cranial neuralgias, infectious sinusitis, Tolosa-Hunt, acute glaucoma, hypercapnia, sleep apnea, and depression

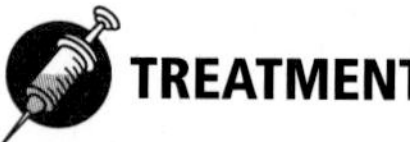

TREATMENT

MEDICATION

First Line

- Abortive/acute therapy: Used at first/premonitory migraine symptom
  - Analgesics: For mild to moderate HA
    - Acetaminophen, aspirin (ASA 900–1000 mg), ibuprofen (400–800 mg) ± antiemetic (1)[A]
    - Naproxen (500–1000 mg), Ketorolac (also IV 15–60 mg)
  - Triptans: 5-$HT_{1B/1D}$ agonists; vasoconstrictors
    - Triptan choice: Tailor to route of administration, side effect profile, tolerability, rapidity of onset of HA and drug action, recurrence history and drug half life
    - Most effective when used at earliest onset
    - Avoid in prolonged aura, hemiplegic or basilar syndromes

ALERT

SSRI + Triptan = risk of serotonin syndrome.

- Contraindications: Ischemic heart disease, angina, poorly controlled HTN
- Antiemetics: Use for GI symptoms; combine with analgesic or vasoconstrictor
  - Metoclopramide, prochlorperazine
- Ergot alkaloids: Vasoconstrictors
  - Dihydroergotamine (DHE): IV, best tolerated
  - Premedication: Prochlorperazine 5–10 mg IV + diphenhydramine 25–50 mg IV/PO
  - Test dose 0.25–0.5 mg IV
  - Useful in ER and inpatient setting; Inpatient: 0.5 mg IV q6h or 1 mg IV q8h × 8–12 doses; d/c one dose beyond aborting HA
  - Note contraindications.

Pediatric Considerations

ER therapy: Prochlorperazine IV + analgesic.

Pregnancy Considerations

Non-pharmacologic interventions; acetaminophen ± antiemetic; triptan safety unclear

- Prophylactic (daily) therapy: For frequent, prolonged, or disabling/severe attacks, poor response/contraindications to acute therapies
  - Goal: Reduce frequency/severity of attacks, use of acute therapies and disability
  - Titration to clinical response; side effects limit escalation
  - Drug class tailored to individual comorbidities & tolerability:
    - β-blockers: for example, propranolol
    - Calcium channel blockers: for example, verapamil, flunarizine
    - Anti-depressants: for example, TCA: amitriptyline, SNRI: Venlafaxine
    - Anti-epileptics (AED): For example, valproate, topiramate, and gabapentin

Pediatric Considerations

β-blocker, flunarizine

Pregnancy Considerations

Mg2+, propranolol; Avoid: NSAID in third trimester, corticosteroids in first trimester.

- Cluster HA
  - Drugs to prevent cluster attacks at onset:
    - Lithium: 600–900 mg daily; effective in chronic form
    - Verapamil: Start 80 mg t.i.d. → 120 mg t.i.d.
    - Prednisone: 60 mg daily × 7 days; rapid taper
    - Ergotamine: Useful for nocturnal attacks: 1 mg suppository q.h.s.
  - During attacks:
    - 100% oxygen inhalation by non-rebreather mask; 10 mL/min × >15 minutes
    - Intranasal lidocaine; DHE: IV or intranasal
    - Sumatriptan 6 mg subcutaneously

ALERT

Concomitant use (within 24 hours) of an ergot or MAOI and a triptan contraindicated.

Second Line

- Valproate IV (Depacon): 1 gram in 50 cc of normal saline, IV push over 5 minutes; for inpatient management may use q8–12 hours
- Limited use: Corticosteroids, combination analgesics, and opiates
- Prophylactic therapies: AED: carbamazepine, lamotrigine; SSRI: lacks conclusive trial data; MAOI: limited by diet and drug interactions
- Botulinum toxin

ADDITIONAL TREATMENT

General Measures

- Stratified pharmacotherapy: Regimen based on attack characteristics, frequency, severity, disability impact and associated features
- Manage: Obesity, anxiety, depression

Issues for Referral

Chronic/transformed migraine, frequent HA or disability, medication overuse HA, complex syndromes, and prophylaxis.

Additional Therapies

Cognitive and biobehavioral training, Mg2+, riboflavin, coenzyme Q10, and melatonin

COMPLEMENTARY & ALTERNATIVE THERAPIES

Acupuncture (2); hyperbaric oxygen therapy (3); Supplements: Feverfew, Butterbur root

SURGERY/OTHER PROCEDURES

Occipital nerve stimulation

IN-PATIENT CONSIDERATIONS

Initial Stabilization

See Treatments

Admission Criteria

Intractable HA or Status migrainosus; medication weans

IV Fluids

IV normal saline until oral hydration adequate

Nursing

Routine

Discharge Criteria

HA resolution

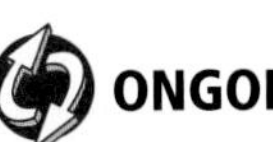

ONGOING CARE

FOLLOW-UP RECOMMENDATIONS

Determined by HA response to treatment: Primary care or Neurology

Patient Monitoring

- Recent ER visits or regimen adjustment warrants sooner follow-up: For example, 1–2 weeks.
- Poorly controlled HA may require frequent visits: For example, 2–4 weeks.

DIET

Educate: Food triggers, caffeine, balanced diet, and avoid skipping meals.

PATIENT EDUCATION

"Managing their illness": Triggers, use of medications, and overuse, side effects profiles, outcome expectations, and lifestyle

PROGNOSIS

Not clearly defined & multifactorial

COMPLICATIONS

Transformation to chronic daily HA, chronic migraine, medication overuse HA

REFERENCES

1. Kirthi V, Derry S, Moore RA, et al. Aspirin with or without an antiemetic for acute migraine headaches in adults. *Cochrane Database Syst Rev* 2010;(4):CD008041.
2. Linde K, Allais G, Brinkhaus B, et al. Acupuncture for migraine prophylaxis. *Cochrane Database Syst Rev* 2009;(1):CD001218.
3. Bennett MH, French C, Schnabel A, et al. Normobaric & hyperbaric oxygen therapy for migraine and cluster headache. *Cochrane Database Syst Rev* 2008;(3):CD005219.

ADDITIONAL READING

- Buse DC, Rupnow MFT, Lipton RB. Assessing & managing all aspects of migraine: Migraine attacks, Migraine-Related functional impairment, Common Comorbidities & Quality of Life. *Mayo Clin Proc* 2009;84:422–435.
- Goadsby PJ, Sprenger T. Current practice & future directions in the prevention & acute management of migraine. *Lancet neurology* 2010;9:285–298.
- Lewis D, Ashwal A, Hershey D, et al. Practice parameter: Pharmacological treatment of migraine in children & adolescents: Report of the AAN Quality Standards Subcommittee & the practice committee of the Child Neurology Society. *Neurology* 2004;63:2215–2224.
- Rapoport AM. Acute & prophylactic treatments for migraine: Present & future. *Neurolog Sci* 2008;29: S110–S122.

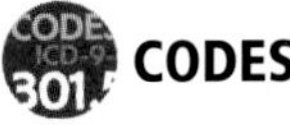

CODES

ICD9

- 339.00 Cluster headache syndrome, unspecified
- 346.90 Migraine, unspecified, without mention of intractable migraine without mention of status migrainosus

CLINICAL PEARLS

- Acute, severe HA, escalating or maximal at onset or focal signs, requires urgent non-contrast CT ± lumbar puncture
- Therapy determined by migraine characteristics and medicine profiles
- Patient education improves outcomes

MOEBIUS SYNDROME

Denise A. Hug

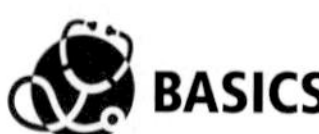

BASICS

DESCRIPTION

- Unilateral or bilateral facial weakness with impairment of ocular abduction
  - Other cranial nerves may be involved
  - Limb anomalies may be present

EPIDEMIOLOGY

Incidence

0.0002–0.002% of live births (1)

Prevalence

- Estimated 2,000 living cases worldwide (2)
- Estimated 800 living in the US (2)

RISK FACTORS

- Family history of Moebius or possibly other overlapping congenital cranial dysinnervation disorders (CCDD)
- Multiple teratogens have been suggested (1)
  - Gestational hyperthermia
  - Electric shock
  - Chorionic villus sampling
  - Abuse of benzodiazepines
  - Alcohol
  - Cocaine
  - Thalidomide
  - Misoprostol

Genetics

- Autosomal dominant, autosomal recessive and X-linked recessive have been reported.
- Variable expression and penetrance
  - MBS1 (13q12.2–q13) involved in two unrelated families (1)
  - MBS2 (3q21–q22) and MBS3 (10q21.3–q22.1) await confirmation (1)
  - Multiple chromosomal aberrations known to have Moebius as a feature

GENERAL PREVENTION

- Avoidance of *in utero* exposure to known teratogens.
- Genetic counseling

PATHOPHYSIOLOGY

- Not completely understood but felt to be secondary to rhombencephalic maldevelopment involving predominantly motor nuclei and axons traversing long tracts (3)
  - Complex disruption of development thought to occur between 21–34 days of embryogenesis (4)

ETIOLOGY

- Genetic/inherited
  - Exposure to teratogens

COMMONLY ASSOCIATED CONDITIONS

- Crenulations on sides of tongue/hypoplasia (75%): Involvement of cranial nerve XII
- Craniofacial malformations: Epicanthal folds, flat nasal bridge, micrognathia, high arched palate, external ear defects, teeth defects, and hypertelorism (90%)
- Malformations of extremities (85%)
- Feeding problems (86%)
- Duane syndrome (34%)
- Poland syndrome (11%)
  - Rare associations: Congenital heart defects, dextrocardia, arthrogryposis multiplex, urinary tract anomalies, anosmia, and hypogonadotropic hypogonadism (3)

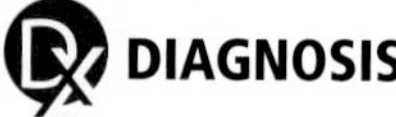

DIAGNOSIS

HISTORY

- Family history
- Known exposure to teratogen *in utero*
- Other known associated anomalies

PHYSICAL EXAM

- Complete ocular examination
  - Evaluate ocular motility and alignment (usually orthophoric in primary position)
  - Evaluate weakness of orbicularis oculi (involvement of cranial VII)
  - Evaluation of ocular surface
  - Assessment of visual function
  - Evaluate external structures for craniofacial findings
  - Complete systemic evaluation for associated anomalies

DIAGNOSTIC TESTS & INTERPRETATION

Lab

Initial lab tests

- None required
- Consider karyotype/microarray if no teratogen is identified. Gene testing not yet available specifically for Moebius, although testing of other genes known to be causative of CCDD may have a role.

Follow-up & special considerations

Consider evaluation for mitochondrial disorder including Kearn Sayres with chronic progressive ophthalmoplegia (acquired), if history of congenital involvement unclear.

Imaging

- No imaging is necessary
  - MRI of head may be performed to evaluate cranial nerves and nuclei

DIFFERENTIAL DIAGNOSIS

- Isolated cranial nerve 6 palsy
- Esotropia with pseudo-abduction deficit (especially with congenital/infantile esotropia)
- Other oromandibular limb hypogenesis syndromes: Hypoglossia-hypodactylia syndrome, Hanhart syndrome, glossopalatine ankylosis syndrome
- Chronic progressive external ophthalmoplegia and other mitochondrial disorders
- Thyroid eye disease
- Intranuclear ophthalmoplegia

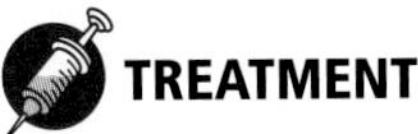

TREATMENT

MEDICATION

- Ocular lubricants as needed for ocular surface drying
- Artificial tear ointment at bedtime or taping lids close may be helpful in cases of lagophthalmos

ADDITIONAL TREATMENT

General Measures

Amblyopia therapy as needed

Issues for Referral

- These patients have multiple system involvement and often need multidisciplinary approach
  - Nutritionists, occupational therapist for feeding issues
  - Orthopedist, physical and occupational therapist for limb anomalies
  - Speech pathologist for language delay
  - ENT for tracheostomy if unable to manage their secretion
  - Dentist for teeth anomalies
  - Neuropsychologist is often helpful
  - Genetic counseling

Additional Therapies

Bandage contact lenses may be useful in the treatment of extreme corneal involvement from exposure.

COMPLEMENTARY & ALTERNATIVE THERAPIES

None proven

SURGERY/OTHER PROCEDURES

- Surgery for esotropia may be performed as needed
  - Temporary tarsorrhaphy for extreme exposure may be beneficial

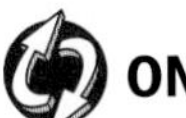

ONGOING CARE

FOLLOW-UP RECOMMENDATIONS

- Frequent follow-up required if ocular surface drying is present.
- As needed for amblyopia monitoring and treatment

Patient Monitoring

- Visual function and school performance
- Overall health and development of child
- Attention to concerns about self image

DIET

Adjust as needed in view of possible swallowing issues.

PATIENT EDUCATION

- Genetic counseling
- Family support network: Moebius Syndrome Foundation (www.moebiussyndrome.com)

PROGNOSIS

- Moebius is a nonprogressive congenital condition
  - With good supportive care, normal life expectancy

COMPLICATIONS

- Corneal ulceration and/or perforation
- Amblyopia

REFERENCES

1. Briegel W. Neuropsychiatric findings of Mobius sequence – a review. *Clin Genet* 2006;70:91–97.
2. Broussard AB, Borazjani JG. The faces of Moebius syndrome: Recognition and anticipatory guidance. *Am J Matern Child Nurs* 2008;5:272–278.
3. Verzijl HT, van der Zwaag B, Cruysberg JR, Padberg GW. Moebius syndrome redefined: A syndrome of rhombencephalic maldevelopment. *Neurology* 2003;61:327–333.
4. Miller MT, Owens P, Chen F. Mobius and Mobius-like syndromes. *J Pediatr Ophthalmol Strabismus* 1989;26:176–189.

ADDITIONAL READING

http://www.ncbi.nlm.nih.gov/omim/157900#157900_Reference41.

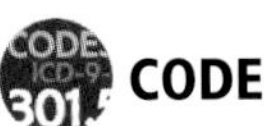

CODES

ICD9

- 346.20 Variants of migraine, not elsewhere classified, without mention of intractable migraine without mention of status migrainosus
- 378.72 Progressive external ophthalmoplegia

CLINICAL PEARLS

- Children with Moebius syndrome need multidisciplinary approach.
- Watch for corneal desiccation/exposure.

M

MORNING GLORY SYNDROME

Eugene Milder
Sunir Garg

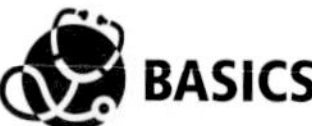

BASICS

DESCRIPTION

- Morning glory syndrome, or morning glory disc anomaly (MGDA), is a rare, congenital, funnel-like excavation of the optic disc and posterior fundus. There are several systemic conditions associated with MGDA and patients found to have this optic disc anomaly should be checked for these conditions (1)[C].
- Its name derives from the optic nerve appearance which has been likened to that of the morning glory flower.

EPIDEMIOLOGY

Incidence

(Estimated) 1/1,000,000 live births

PATHOPHYSIOLOGY

MGDA is thought to arise from incomplete development of the optic nerve during gestation. A remnant of normal glial tissue remains as a tuft at the center of the nerve (a classic finding in MGDA). Some speculate that there is a component of mesodermal dysgenesis; myocontractile elements have been found on histopathology and actual contractile movements have been observed clinically.

COMMONLY ASSOCIATED CONDITIONS

- Retinal detachment (RD)
  - There is controversy about the etiology of RD in MGDA, which occurs in about one-third of patients. Some postulate that there is a slit-like full-thickness peripapillary retinal break, while others, using optical coherence tomography (OCT), have documented schisis-like breaks leading to RD. Still others have suggested that there is an abnormal connection between the subarachnoid space at the distal end of the anomalous optic nerve and the subretinal space, leading to a serous detachment filled with cerebrospinal fluid (2)[C].
- Retinal arteriovenous malformations (rare)
- Carotid artery abnormalities
  - Stenosis or aplasia of the carotid arteries can occur, leading to cerebrovascular accidents and seizures. There are variable amounts of stenosis and there have been documented cases of spontaneous resolution of carotid stenosis.
  - Moyamoya is thought to be an inherited disease associated with cerebral artery stenosis, and has been seen in patients with MGDA. Patients with moyamoya develop exuberant collateralization in the cerebral circulation and are prone to thrombosis and hemorrhage. Moyamoya malformations have also been seen in Down syndrome, neurofibromatosis, and sickle cell disease.
- Midline cranial defects (3,4,5)[C].
  - Pituitary abnormalities, both anatomic and functional
  - Basal encephalocele
  - Absent septum pellucidum
- Renal disease (rarely)
  - Thought to be part of the spectrum of papillorenal syndromes
- Neurofibromatosis, type 2
  - Scattered reports of this association

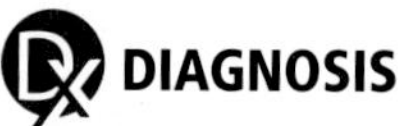

DIAGNOSIS

HISTORY

- Poor vision, can present with:
  - Strabismus
  - Leukocoria
  - Failed school vision screening
  - Acute vision change (suggests RD)
- Evidence of pituitary dysfunction
  - Growth retardation
  - Hypothyroidism
- Evidence of cerebral circulation abnormalities
  - Strokes, seizures

PHYSICAL EXAM

- Eye exam
  - Poor visual acuity. This can be highly variable, from normal vision to no light perception.
  - Refraction: Myopia is common
  - Strabismus
  - Afferent pupillary defect
  - Color vision defects
  - (Rarely) cataract
  - Morning glory disc findings (Image 1): Funnel-like excavation of the optic nerve and sclera, a large optic disc with a surrounding annular ring of pigmented uveal tissue, radial pattern of narrowed retinal vessels emanate from the far edges of the optic disc, a central white tuft of glial tissue. Rarely bilateral.
  - Retinal detachment: Can range from a shallow, localized detachment of the macula to a bullous total retinal detachment. There are rare reports of spontaneous resolution.
- Full physical exam
  - Height/weight charts for children
  - Full neurologic assessment

DIAGNOSTIC TESTS & INTERPRETATION

Lab

- Pituitary panel including TSH and GH levels
- Kidney function testing including a basic metabolic panel and urinalysis.

Imaging

Initial approach

- Cerebral imaging
  - Consider MRI/MRA in children to limit radiation exposure. CT/CTA acceptable in adults.
  - Imaging should focus on the carotid circulation, the circle of Willis, and midline structures including the pituitary.
- Fundus photography

Follow-up & special considerations
Children should be followed closely. Reversible causes of vision loss, including myopia and cataract, as well as amblyopia should be addressed. However, patching should be pursued cautiously due to the limited visual potential of eyes with MGDA.

Diagnostic Procedures/Other
Fluorescein angiography and OCT are usually needed. OCT of the peripapillary area is sometimes used in cases of RD to attempt to locate a retinal break.

Pathological Findings
Staphylomatous excavation of the optic disc and surrounding sclera. Variable amounts of myocontractile elements, glial tissue, and persistent fetal vasculature have been identified.

DIFFERENTIAL DIAGNOSIS
- Posterior staphyloma/coloboma
- Microphthalmia with cyst

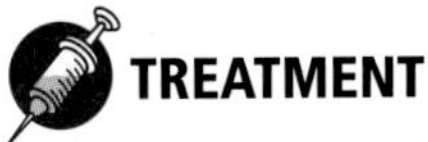

TREATMENT

MEDICATION
- Hormone therapy per endocrinology recommendations
- Anti-thrombotics per neurology recommendations if cerebral vascular anomalies exist

ADDITIONAL TREATMENT
Issues for Referral
- Pediatric ophthalmology referral is indicated in most cases to assure accurate diagnosis, refraction, strabismus assessment, and to maximize visual potential
- Retina referral is indicated for cases of RD
- Neurology referral is indicated for full neurologic evaluation, stroke, and seizure assessment and treatment.
- Endocrinology referral is indicated for cases with pituitary abnormalities
- Neurosurgical and interventional radiology referral is indicated for cases with cerebral vascular abnormalities

Additional Therapies
Monocular precautions with polycarbonate spectacles is recommended

SURGERY/OTHER PROCEDURES
Retinal detachment is usually addressed with pars plana vitrectomy and long-acting gas tamponade.

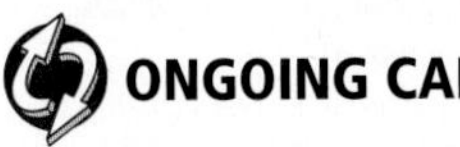

ONGOING CARE

FOLLOW-UP RECOMMENDATIONS
Yearly eye exams are advisable in children found to have MGDA.

Patient Monitoring
- Parents should monitor children for changes in vision or behavior.
- Other systemic monitoring as recommended by pediatrics

PATIENT EDUCATION
Patients and parents should be educated about the symptoms of retinal detachment. A shallow macular detachment associated with MGDA can present with subtle central metamorphopsia and micropsia.

PROGNOSIS
Visual prognosis in MGDA is often very poor. In the absence of RD, patients who present with good vision are not likely to deteriorate. Episodes of optic neuritis and progressive optic atrophy have been documented but are rare.

REFERENCES

1. Kindler P. Morning glory syndrome: Unusual congenital optic disc anomaly. *Am J Ophthalmol* 1970;69:376–384. (C)
2. Haik BG, Greenstein SH, Smith ME, Abramson DH, Ellsworth RM. Retinal detachment in the morning glory anomaly. *Ophthalmology* 1984;91: 1638–1647. (C)
3. Bakri SJ, Siker D, Masaryk T, et al. Ocular malformations, moyamoya disease, and midline cranial defects: A distinct syndrome. *Am J Ophthalmol* 1999;127:356–357.
4. Komiyama M, Yasui T, Sakamoto H, et al. Basal meningoencephalocele, anomaly of optic disc and panhypopituitarism in association with moyamoya disease. *Pediatr Neurosurg* 2000;33:100–104.
5. Krishnan C, Roy A, Traboulsi E. Morning glory disk anomaly, choroidal coloboma, and congenital constrictive malformations of the internal carotid arteries (moyamoya disease). *Ophthalmic Genet* 2000;21:21–24.

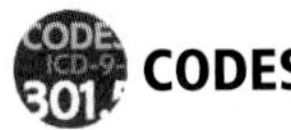

CODES

ICD9
- 361.9 Unspecified retinal detachment
- 743.57 Specified congenital anomalies of optic disc

CLINICAL PEARLS
- The 3 features that best distinguish MGDA from a typical staphyloma are: The annular ring of pigmented tissue, the central tuft of glial tissue, and the radial pattern of attenuated vessels.
- It is estimated that one-third of eyes with MGDA will develop a retinal detachment.
- The most important associated conditions of MGDA are cerebral defects including carotid vascular stenosis and midline defects such as basal encepholcele and pituitary abnormalities.

M

MULTIFOCAL CHOROIDITIS/PUNCTATE INNER CHOROIDITIS

Bradley T. Smith

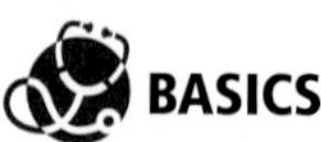

BASICS

DESCRIPTION

Multifocal choroiditis (MFC) and panuveitis consist of vitreitis, anterior uveitis, and active choroidal lesions. (1) Punctate inner choroiditis (PIC) is similar, but the lesions are confined to the posterior pole.

ETIOLOGY

- The exact cause remains unknown. Both MFC and PIC, as well as a third entity known as diffuse subretinal fibrosis (DSF) may be syndromic variations on a common disease spectrum.
- Exogenous viral pathogens that simulate antigens found within the eye may induce an autoimmune response resulting in inflammation within the eye.

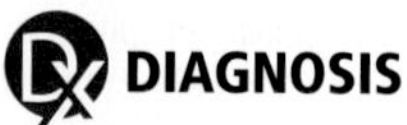

DIAGNOSIS

HISTORY

- Patients with MFC are usually otherwise healthy. Some may experience systemic symptoms of viral illness just prior to the ocular manifestation. Women tend to be affected more than men, mostly in the third decade of life. PIC usually occurs in myopic eyes.
- Common complaints include decreased or blurred vision, peripheral field loss, and floaters that have an insidious onset. The disease may be noticed only in one eye, but both eyes are usually affected.
- PIC patients often have photopsias and scotomas.

PHYSICAL EXAM

Vitreitis is present in almost all cases. Anterior segment inflammation may also be found in about half of cases. Yellow–white subretinal lesions, often with pigmented borders, are the key finding and are seen throughout the fundus. Their size may vary between 50–300 microns in diameter and represent focal areas of inflammation within the choroid. Patients with PIC have similar lesions that are localized to the posterior pole. These patients may not have an associated vitreitis on presentation. Broad zones of coalesced lesions resulting in subretinal fibrosis typify DSF.

DIAGNOSTIC TESTS & INTERPRETATION

Lab

- May be necessary (as guided by history and exam) to rule out other treatable causes of posterior uveitis. (i.e., sarcoidosis, toxoplasmosis, syphilis, lyme disease, and tuberculosis)
- Complete blood counts as well as liver function and kidney function are needed when immune modulators are used for disease control.

Imaging

Initial approach

- Fundus photography using color and red-free techniques is useful for documenting and following the course of the disease.
- Intravenous fluorescein angiography (IVFA) is helpful in these patients for several reasons. IVFA may reveal lesions that may not yet be visible clinically. Also, it is helpful in defining whether or not a particular lesion is active. Active lesions characteristically block fluorescein within the choroid, but as the study progresses these foci of inflammation will usually show hyperfluorescence due to staining. Older, inactive lesions typically show only a window defect (hyperfluorescence). In some cases lesions may show hypofluorescence due to complete loss of the choriocapillaris. IVFA also may demonstrate leakage from cystoid macular edema and abnormal hyperfluorescence from choroidal neovascular membranes that may complicate this disease.
- Optical coherence tomography (OCT) is useful for diagnosing the presence of cystoid macular edema, subretinal fluid, and choroidal neovascular membranes. Newer generation spectral-domain OCT may help in determining whether vision loss is from atrophy of photoreceptors or from a potentially treatable process such as cystoid macular edema or choroidal neovascular membrane. Serial OCT may be used to follow the course of disease and/or response to treatment.
- Visual field testing is sometimes useful for monitoring peripheral loss. These scotomas do not necessarily correspond to active choroiditis. Some patients also have an enlarged blind spot as demonstrated by formal visual field testing.

Follow-up & special considerations

- During the acute phase of inflammation, a patient may need to be seen at 1–4 week intervals depending on the severity of the disease.
- Patients should be followed to monitor for the development of choroidal neovascularization, which can occur under the macula or near the optic nerve (peripapillary). This can occur even after the acute phase of the disease is over. Self-monitoring with an Amsler grid may help the patient detect new scotomas, distortion, or blurriness that may herald the onset of new disease activity or the development of choroidal neovascularization.
- Self-monitoring with an Amsler grid may aid a patient in developing new disease activity or the development of choroidal neovascularization.

DIFFERENTIAL DIAGNOSIS

- Syphilis
- Tuberculosis
- Presumed ocular histoplasmosis
- Toxoplasmosis
- Central serous chorioretinopathy
- Age-related macular degeneration
- Trauma

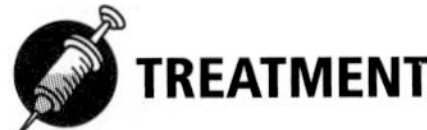

TREATMENT

MEDICATION

First Line

Topical steroid alone is generally inadequate for posterior uveitis. In general, these patients require systemic, and/or periocular steroid therapy (1). Intravitreal steroids may also be considered. Infectious causes of uveitis must be ruled out before instituting any immune- suppressing treatment.

Second Line

Systemic immune modulating drugs may be considered when long-term therapy is required and/or a patient is not a good candidate for systemic steroid therapy (i.e., uncontrolled hypertension, diabetes, elderly, etc.) (2). Caution is required when dealing with these agents due to adverse effects ranging from organ damage to fetal insult. In general, their use should be avoided during pregnancy.

ADDITIONAL TREATMENT

Issues for Referral

Posterior uveitis has many different causes and the potential for vision loss is high. In general, these cases should be promptly referred to someone who has considerable experience in the diagnosis and treatment of uveitis.

Additional Therapies

- Choroidal neovascular membranes may be treated with thermal laser, photodynamic therapy, anti-vascular endothelial growth factor agents, and/or intravitreal steroids.
- Cystoid macular edema may be treated with intravitreal steroids, periocular steroids, and/or anti-vascular endothelial growth factor.

SURGERY/OTHER PROCEDURES

- Surgical extraction of cataracts may be considered when the inflammation has been adequately controlled and remains in remission.
- Slow-release steroidal implants may be considered in some cases.
- Vitrectomy for therapeutic clearance of vitreous opacities and for diagnostic purposes may be considered when the diagnosis is unclear.

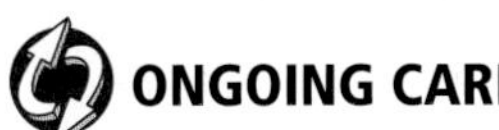

ONGOING CARE

PROGNOSIS

MFC, PIC, and DSF can often last months to years with frequent relapses resulting in a poor visual prognosis.

COMPLICATIONS

Patients with MFC/PIC are at risk for developing cystoid macular edema. Choroidal neovascularization can occur even after there is no active inflammation. Diffuse scarring as seen with DSF may occur resulting in poor visual potential. Cataracts and glaucoma can result from the disease process and as a side effect from steroid therapy. Lifetime periodic follow up is necessary to monitor for these complications.

REFERENCES

1. Dreyer RF, Gass JDM. Multifocal choroiditis and panuveitis: A syndrome that mimics ocular histoplasmosis. *Arch Ophthalmol* 1984;102: 1776–1784.
2. Michel SS, Ekong A, Baltatzis S, Foster CS. Multifocalchoroiditis and panuveitis: Immunomodulatory therapy. *Ophthalmology* 2002;109:378–383.

ADDITIONAL READING

- Quillen DA, Davis JB, Gottlieb JL, et al. The white dot syndromes. *Am J Ophthalmol* 2004;137:538–550

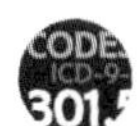

CODES

ICD9

- 360.12 Panuveitis
- 363.00 Focal chorioretinitis, unspecified
- 363.8 Other disorders of choroid

CLINICAL PEARLS

- MFC/PIC is a chronic relapsing disorder causing inflammation in the eye.
- Steroids are first line therapy.
- Long-term follow up is necessary to monitor for complications such as choroidal neovascularization.

M

MYASTHENIA GRAVIS

William A. Cantore

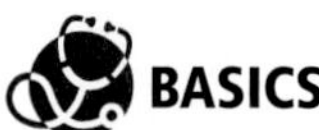

BASICS

DESCRIPTION

- Myasthenia gravis (MG) is the most common disorder of the neuromuscular junction. MG causes painless, variable, fatigable muscle weakness. Weakness can involve ocular, bulbar, limb, and respiratory muscles. Extraocular muscles are most commonly affected and patients often present with ptosis and/or diplopia.
- MG is the best characterized autoimmune disease.
- 2 clinical forms of MG:
  - Ocular MG (15%): Weakness is limited to the eyelids and extraocular muscles
  - Generalized MG (85%): Variable involvement of bulbar, limb, and respiratory muscles as well
- 2 serological forms of MG:
  - Seropositive: Patients have detectable antibodies to the acetylcholine receptor (AChR) or to the muscle-specific receptor tyrosine kinase (MuSK).
  - Seronegative: Patients do not have detectable antibody levels
    - 50% of patients with ocular myasthenia are seropositive.
    - 90% of patients with generalized myasthenia are seropositive
- The thymus is abnormal in most patients with MG.

EPIDEMIOLOGY

- Occurs at any age
- Bimodal distribution:
  - Early peak (40%) in the second and third decades.
    - Female:Male ratio is 2:1.
  - Late peak (60%) in the sixth to eighth decades.
    - Female:Male ratio is 1:2

Incidence

30 new cases per million (1)

Prevalence

- 15 per 100,000 in the US
- Approximately 60,000 patients with MG in the US
- Prevalence of MG has increased over the past 50 years

RISK FACTORS

- Familial MG
- Factors that worsen MG symptoms include stress, heat, infection, thyroid disease, pregnancy, menstruation, fever, and drugs.
  - Consider annual vaccination against influenza for MG patients.

Genetics

- No known Mendelian inheritance of MG
- Family members of patients with MG are 1,000 times more likely to develop the disease than is the general population.
- Transient neonatal MG seen in 10–20% of infants born to myasthenic mothers.
  - Transplacental passage of anti-AChR antibodies
  - Resolution in weeks to months

GENERAL PREVENTION

- Drugs may unmask or exacerbate MG
  - Aminoglycoside antibiotics and penicillamine
  - Statin treatment may be associated with a myasthenic syndrome or exacerbation of myasthenia symptoms.

PATHOPHYSIOLOGY

- Circulating anti-AChR antibodies (80%)
  - Antibodies bind to the AChR of junctional folds, cause complement-mediated destruction of the folds; results in "simplification" of postsynaptic region.
- Circulating anti-MuSK antibodies (10%)
  - MuSK-positive patients more likely to have early bulbar and respiratory symptoms
  - Women more commonly affected
- Seronegative patients clinically similar to patients with AChR antibodies

ETIOLOGY

- Thymus plays important role in early-onset MG associated with anti-AChR antibodies.
  - Gland enlarged with lymphocytic infiltrates, germinal centers, and myoid cells which express AChRs

COMMONLY ASSOCIATED CONDITIONS

- Thymus abnormal in most patients with MG:
  - Lymphoid follicular hyperplasia in 70%
  - Thymoma present in to 10–15% of patients with MG
    - Most thymic tumors in patients with MG are benign
    - The peak incidence occurs in the fourth to sixth decades, with no sex predilection
- Autoimmune thyroid disease (8% of MG patients)

DIAGNOSIS

HISTORY

- Patients with MG complain of muscle weakness
  - In most patients, ptosis or diplopia is the initial symptom.
  - Difficulty chewing, swallowing, or talking.
    - Patients may complain of choking or coughing after eating, escape of liquids through the nose when swallowing
    - Voice may become nasal or hoarse
  - Limb weakness
  - Respiratory dysfunction is rarely the presenting symptom of MG
- Weakness usually fluctuates, worsening at the end of the day or with prolonged use of the muscles
- Sensory complaints not typical of MG

PHYSICAL EXAM

- Ptosis
  - Unilateral or bilateral
  - Often fatigable
    - Can be demonstrated by observing progressive ptosis during sustained upgaze
  - Patients often compensate for ptosis by using their frontalis muscle
  - Cold applied to the eyelid may improve ptosis ("ice-pack test")
  - With rapid shift from downgaze to upgaze, may see excessive lid elevation, followed by drooping (Cogan's lid twitch sign)
- Ocular motility limitations
  - Asymmetric weakness of several muscles in both eyes typical
  - Medial rectus muscle often involved ("pseudo INO")
  - Pupil is not involved
- Weak orbicularis oculi
  - Examiner can easily pry open forcibly closed eyelids
  - When the patient tries to keep the eyes closed, slight involuntary opening may occur ("peek sign")
- Examiner may be able to manually open the jaw against resistance.

DIAGNOSTIC TESTS & INTERPRETATION

Lab

- Anti-AChR antibodies
  - Binding (sufficient in most cases), blocking, and modulating antibodies can be assayed.
  - 80–85% of all patients with MG seropositive
    - Generalized MG: 85% (2)[C]
    - Ocular MG: 50%
    - MG and thymoma: Almost 100%
- Anti-MuSK antibodies
  - Present in up to 50% of generalized MG patients seronegative for anti-AChR antibodies; absent in ocular MG
- Thyroid function tests
- Thyroid antibody test

Imaging

- CT or MRI of anterior mediastinum
  - Thymoma

Diagnostic Procedures/Other

- Ice test frequently performed in office with improvement of ptosis 2+ mm highly suggestive for MG.
- Edrophonium chloride (Tensilon) test
  - Acetylcholinesterase inhibitor
  - Allows ACh to interact longer with postsynaptic membrane, resulting in greater end-plate depolarization
  - Examiner looks for transient improvement in muscle strength (e.g., resolution of ptosis)
    - Initial dose 2 mg IV, can be followed by another 2 mg every 1 minute up to maximum of 10 mg
    - Sensitivity 80–90%
  - Atropine must be available during the edrophonium test.
  - Patients should avoid taking oral anticholinesterase inhibitors for 24 hours prior to the test.
  - With availability of serologic tests, edrophonium test is rarely performed.

- Neurophysiological tests
  - Routine EMG is not helpful in ocular MG
  - Repetitive nerve stimulation (RNS) has a sensitivity of about 55%.
  - Single-fiber EMG is more sensitive (90–95%), but less specific than RNS.

Pathological Findings

- Muscle electron microscopy
  - "Simplification" of postsynaptic region
- Immunofluorescence
  - IgG antibodies and complement on receptor membranes

DIFFERENTIAL DIAGNOSIS

- Conditions that mimic ocular MG:
  - Chronic progressive external ophthalmoplegia
  - Myotonic dystrophy
  - Cranial neuropathies
  - Guillain Barré Syndrome (Fisher variant)
  - Thyroid ophthalmopathy
- Conditions that mimic generalized MG:
  - Amyotrophic lateral sclerosis (ALS)
  - Lambert-Eaton myasthenic syndrome
  - Botulism

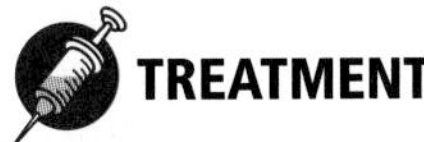

TREATMENT

MEDICATION

First Line

- Controlled clinical trials for any treatment of MG are rare.
- Acetylcholinesterase inhibitors
  - No placebo-controlled randomized studies
  - May provide symptomatic relief
  - Short half-lives necessitate frequent dosing
  - Side effects include diarrhea, sweating, salivation, and tearing
  - Rarely effective for ocular MG
  - Pyridostigmine bromide (Mestinon)
    - Available as 60 mg tablet, 180 mg sustained-release tablet, and 60 mg/5 mL syrup
    - Initial dose in adults is 30 mg t.i.d.
    - Increase dose in 30 mg increments as needed, to maximum 120 mg q3–4 h
  - Neostigmine methylsulfate (Prostigmin)
    - Available in 0.25, 0.5, and 1 mg/mL concentrations
    - Initial dose 0.5 mg subcutaneously or IM q3h
- Corticosteroids
  - Limited evidence from randomized controlled trials (3)[A]
  - Marked improvement in over 75% of MG patients
  - Ptosis and ophthalmoparesis usually respond only to immunosuppression
  - Early use of steroids in ocular MG may prevent generalization (4)[C]
  - Prednisone
    - Initial dose 60–80 mg/d PO
    - Taper very slowly
    - Switch to alternate day regimen within 2 weeks
    - May also start at 20 mg/d and gradually increase dose

Second Line

- Azathioprine: 100–200 mg/d PO
  - Most commonly used second line immunomodulator
  - Side effects include hepatotoxicity, cytopenia, and lymphoproliferative disease.
  - Regular monitoring of complete blood count, liver function tests, and renal function tests
- Mycophenolate mofetil: 1 g PO or IV b.i.d.
  - Selectively inhibits proliferation of activated B and T lymphocytes

ADDITIONAL TREATMENT

General Measures

- Assistive devices
  - Ptosis "crutches" and lid adhesives are usually not well tolerated
  - An eye patch or lens occluder eliminates diplopia
  - Prism is helpful only if the ocular misalignment is stable

Issues for Referral

Because of the likelihood of generalization and complexity of management, patients with MG should be followed by a neurologist.

SURGERY/OTHER PROCEDURES

- Thymoma
  - Surgery with or without radiotherapy
  - Value of thymectomy in patients without thymoma unclear
    - No randomized trials to date
    - In general, thymectomy is offered to younger (under age 60) anti-AChR antibody-positive patients with generalized MG.
- Neuromuscular blocking agents should be avoided by anesthesiologists.

IN-PATIENT CONSIDERATIONS

Admission Criteria

- Plasmapheresis
- IVIG
- Pulmonary infections
- Myasthenic or cholinergic crises

ALERT

Any patient with MG and difficulty breathing or swallowing is a medical emergency.

ONGOING CARE

PROGNOSIS

- The course of MG is highly variable, but usually progressive
- Ocular myasthenia "generalizes" in 50–90%, almost always within first 2 years
- Maximum weakness usually occurs within the first year
- After 15–20 years, untreated weakness becomes fixed
- Remission very rarely permanent
- 40% of patients have severe MG
  - 50% of these will require mechanical ventilation during the course of their illness
- Mortality rate less than 5%

COMPLICATIONS

- Myasthenic crisis
  - Neurological emergency
  - Intensive care unit admission
    - Ventilatory support
    - IVIG or plasma exchange to remove circulating autoantibodies

REFERENCES

1. McGrogan A, Sneddon S, de Vries CS. The incidence of myasthenia gravis: A systematic literature review. *Neuroepidemiology* 2010;34(3):171–183.
2. Meriggioli MN. Myasthenia gravis with anti-acetylcholine receptor antibodies. *Front Neurol Neurosci* 2009;26:94–108.
3. Schneider-Gold C, Gajdos P, Toyka KV, Hohlfeld RR. Corticosteroids for myasthenia gravis. *Cochrane Database Syst Rev* 2005(2):CD002828.
4. Kupersmith MJ. Ocular myasthenia gravis: Treatment successes and failures in patients with long-term follow-up. *J Neurol* 2009;256(8): 1314–1320.

CODES

ICD9

- 358.00 Myasthenia gravis without (acute) exacerbation
- 368.2 Diplopia
- 374.30 Ptosis of eyelid, unspecified

CLINICAL PEARLS

- Consider the diagnosis of MG in any patient who presents with diplopia, regardless of the pattern of ocular misalignment. MG can mimic any ocular motor abnormality, including an internuclear ophthalmoplegia.
- When suspicious of MG, ask the patient about hair (trouble combing), chairs (trouble arising), and stairs (trouble climbing).
- The differential diagnosis of variable diplopia includes MG and thyroid ophthalmopathy. Patients with MG are most symptomatic late in the day; patients with thyroid ophthalmopathy are most symptomatic early in the day (due to increased orbital congestion after being supine).

M

MYELINATED NERVE FIBERS

Michael J. Bartiss

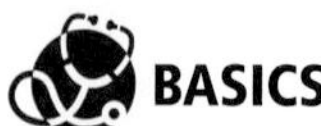

BASICS

DESCRIPTION

Myelinated (Medullated) Nerve Fibers

- White striated patches at the upper and lower poles of the optic disc of varying severity
- Frayed and feathered edges follow path of normal retinal fibers
- Retinal vessels that pass through the superficial layers of the nerve fibers are obscured
- Patches or slits of normal appearing retina may occasionally be visible within the area of myelination
- Myelinated fibers are discontinuous with the optic nerve head in approximately 20% of cases
- Can rarely be acquired after infancy and even in adulthood (trauma appears to be common denominator in these cases)

EPIDEMIOLOGY

Occurs in approximately 1% of the general population

RISK FACTORS

Genetics

- Has been reported with an autosomal dominant inheritance pattern in familial cases (uncommon)
- Has been reported with Gorlin syndrome: Multiple basal cell nevi, with possible associated medulloblastoma
- Traboulsi described an autosomal dominant vitreoretinopathy characterized by extensive bilateral myelinization of the retinal nerve fiber layer, congenitally poor vision, severe vitreous degeneration, high myopia, retinal dystrophy with night blindness with reduction of electroretinographic responses and limb deformities.

PATHOPHYSIOLOGY

- Possible mechanisms include:
  - Defect in lamina cribrosa
  - Fewer axons relative to size of scleral canal, thus allowing room for myelination to proceed into the retina
  - Late development of the lamina cribrosa may allow oligodendrocytes to migrate into the eye

ETIOLOGY

- Oligodendrocytes (responsible for myelination within the central nervous system) typically begin at the lateral geniculate nucleus at approximately 5 months gestation and terminate at the lamina cribrosa at approximately 40 weeks gestation
- Clinical appearance occurs when fibers in the retina acquire a myelin sheath

COMMONLY ASSOCIATED CONDITIONS

- Amblyopia with or without high myopia in involved eye
- Oxycephaly with abnormal length of the optic nerve (uncommon)
- Tilted disc syndrome
- Anterior segment dysgenesis
- Possibly neurofibromatosis type2 (debated)

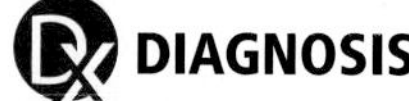

DIAGNOSIS

HISTORY

- Possible history of trauma
- History of lesser vision in one eye with or without strabismus

PHYSICAL EXAM

- Full ocular examination including careful evaluation of the optic discs and evaluation for concomitant potentially treatable amblyopia and high myopia
- Evaluate skin for evidence of Gorlin syndrome (uncommon)

DIAGNOSTIC TESTS & INTERPRETATION

Imaging

- Usually none
- Neuroimaging should be considered in any patient with suspected Gorlin syndrome to rule out associated medulloblastoma

Diagnostic Procedures/Other

OCT may be helpful

DIFFERENTIAL DIAGNOSIS

- Tilted disc syndrome with myelinated nerve fibers
- Cotton wool spots/exudate

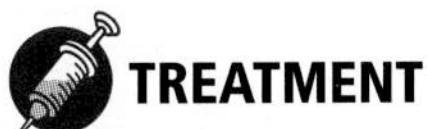

TREATMENT

MEDICATION

No medical treatment for the primary disorder

ADDITIONAL TREATMENT

General Measures

Appropriate refractive error correction as soon as appropriate with concomitant amblyopia treatment if indicated

Issues for Referral

- Dermatology, if concerned about Gorlin syndrome (uncommon)
- Genetic counseling if indicated

COMPLEMENTARY & ALTERNATIVE THERAPIES

None proven or indicated

SURGERY/OTHER PROCEDURES

Surgery for strabismus if indicated

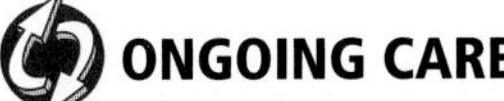

ONGOING CARE

FOLLOW-UP RECOMMENDATIONS

- Regular follow-ups to monitor for changes in refractive error
- As needed for amblyopia monitoring and treatment

PATIENT EDUCATION

Amblyopia management

PROGNOSIS

- Amblyopia associated with high myopia previously thought to be unamenable to amblyopia treatment. Evidence now indicates that some patients will respond to amblyopia therapy.
- Myelinated nerve fibers reported to disappear as a result of tabetic optic atrophy, pituitary tumor, glaucoma, central retinal artery occlusion, and optic neuritis.

COMPLICATIONS

- Amblyopia
- Strabismus
- Refractive error

ADDITIONAL READING

- Nucci. Paulo in Ophthalmic Genetics 1990;11(2): 143–145.
- Brodsky MC, Baker RS, Hamed LM. *"Pediatric Neuro-Ophthalmology."* Springer; New York: New York, 1996.
- Pollack S. The morning glory disc anomaly; contractile movement, classification, and embryogenesis. *Doc Ophthalmol* 1987;65:439–460.
- Brown G, Tasman W. *"Congenital Anomalies of the Optic Disc."* New York: New York Grune & Stratton, 1983.
- Traboulsi EI, et al. A new syndrome of myelinated nerve fibers, vitreoretinopathy and skeletal malformations. *Arch Ophthalmol* 1993;111: 1543–1545.
- Miller NR. *"Walsh and Hoyt's Clinical Neuro-ophthalmology Baltimore.* Maryland: Williams and Wilkins, 1982.

CODES

ICD9

- 367.1 Myopia
- 379.21 Vitreous degeneration
- 743.57 Specified congenital anomalies of optic disc

CLINICAL PEARLS

- Work to maximize visual potential, especially in bilateral cases.
- Protective eyewear if best corrected visual acuity is subnormal in one eye

MYOPIC DEGENERATION

Robert Bergren

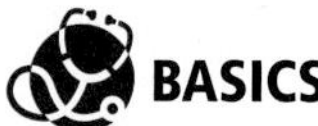

BASICS

DESCRIPTION

Myopic degeneration is a complication of severe or progressive myopia causing mild to severe central vision loss and is one of the leading causes of visual debilitation in the world. Loss of macular function occurs secondary to macular hemorrhage, retinal pigment epithelium (RPE) atrophy, or choroidal neovascularization.

- Myopia may be divided into simple, congenital, and degenerative.
- Simple and congenital myopia are not progressive and do not develop the typical degenerative changes.

EPIDEMIOLOGY

Incidence

- The incidence of myopia varies with age but it generally occurs in the grade school years. At a young age, progressive myopia can be indistinguishable from simple or congenital myopia.
- Those with degenerative myopia often have rapidly increasing myopia and axial length through adolescence. This increase can then continue until the age of 50 years.
- The macular degenerative changes often develop in the productive years of young adulthood and continue to progress indefinitely.

Prevalence

- The prevalence of myopia in developed countries is reported to be between 11–36%. The frequency of degenerative myopia has been reported to range from 27–33% of the myopic population that corresponds to rates of 1.7–2.1% in the general population.
- The prevalence of myopia shows a marked change with age, with the peak at 20 years.

RISK FACTORS

Genetics

Simple myopia has often been described as a dominant condition but the degenerative form is thought to be autosomal recessive. However, both forms are multifactorial.

PATHOPHYSIOLOGY

- The sclera is thinned at the posterior pole with sclera ectasia and posterior staphyloma.
- The choriocapillaris is thin and there is a loss of melanocytes from the choroid.
- The RPE cells are flatter and larger before they undergo degeneration.
- Bruch's membrane undergoes thinning, splitting, and rupturing.

ETIOLOGY

The cause of the degenerative process is not clearly understood but it may be the result of a biomechanical abnormality with progressive stretching of the sclera, leading to thinning of all layers in the posterior pole.

COMMONLY ASSOCIATED CONDITIONS

Retinopathy of prematurity and premature birth without ROP is associated with high myopia.

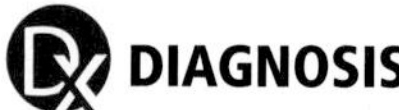

DIAGNOSIS

- Ophthalmic features of degenerative myopia include:
  - Scleral thinning, ectasia, and posterior staphyloma
  - Tilted oval disc with long vertical axis and temporal atrophy or myopic crescent
  - Thinning of the pigment epithelium and choroid allowing visibility of the larger choroidal vessels giving a "tessellated fundus" appearance.
  - Areas of pigment epithelial and choroidal atrophy with sharp margins sometime lined by pigment. These can progress and coalesce into larger irregular lesions with time
  - Lacquer Cracks (ruptured Bruch's elastic lamina) appear as irregular liner or stellate breaks in the pigment epithelium
  - Macular hemorrhage can occur with a lacquer crack in the absence of a choroidal neovascular membrane. They can be associated with trauma
- Choroidal neovascularization.
  - Hemorrhage with pigment epithelial elevation, subretinal fluid or edema
  - When occurring as a dark spot in the posterior pole, it is sometimes referred to as a Foerster-Fuch's spot.
  - May occur in up to 40% of highly myopic patients. Those with patchy atrophy and lacquer cracks are at high risk.

HISTORY
Highly myopic patients with sudden vision changes and new metamorphopsia need to be evaluated for choroidal neovascularization.

DIAGNOSTIC TESTS & INTERPRETATION
Diagnostic Procedures/Other
- Flourescein angiography
- Optical coherence testing (OCT)

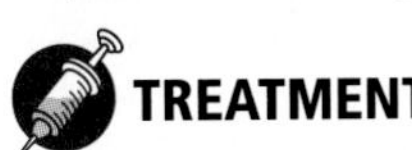

TREATMENT

- Address refractive error with glasses or contact lens
- Low vision support
- Choroidal neovascularization (CNV)
  - Laser treatment for extrafoveal CNV but not juxtafoveal CNV due to possible long term expansion of the laser scar
  - Anti-vascular endothelial growth factor (Anti-VEGF) therapy for subfoveal or juxtafoveal CNV

SURGERY/OTHER PROCEDURES
Scleral buckle or vitrectomy for retinal detachment

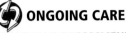

ONGOING CARE

FOLLOW-UP RECOMMENDATIONS
- Ophthalmologist for continued careful evaluation of both macular changes and possible peripheral retinal changes
- Low vision support and continued monitoring of refractive error. Declining vision can be due to both progressive macular changes and progression of the myopia.

PATIENT EDUCATION
Patients who are at high risk for choroidal neovascularization should be instructed to monitor detailed vision in each eye separately on a regular basis and consider using an Amsler grid.

PROGNOSIS
There is a guarded prognosis for those with progressive staphyloma. Risk of vision loss from macular atrophy or choroidal neovascularization increases with age.

COMPLICATIONS
- Visual loss from macular changes
- Retinal detachment

ADDITIONAL READING

- Rabb MF, Garoon I, LaFranco FP. Myopic macular degeneration. *Int Ophthalmol Clin* 1981;21:51–69.
- Hayashi K, Ohno-Matsui K, Shimada N, et al. Long-term pattern of progression of myopic maculopathy: A natural history study. *Ophthalmology* 2010; 117(8): 1595–1611.
- Chang LK, Spaide RF, Brue C, et al. Bevacizumab treatment for subfoveal choroidal neovascularization from causes other than age-related macular degeneration. *Arch Ophthalmol* 2008;126(7): 941–945.

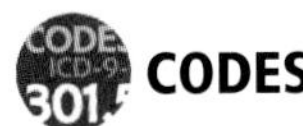

CODES

ICD9
360.21 Progressive high (degenerative) myopia

MYOTONIC DYSTROPHY

Hyung Cho
Christian Wertenbaker

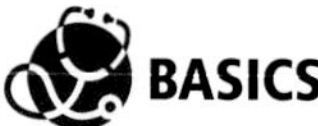

BASICS

DESCRIPTION

- Myotonic dystrophy is an inherited disorder of the muscles and other body systems.
- Type 1: DM1 (Steinert's disease)
  - Represents 98% of all cases
  - Severe congenital form with marked developmental disability
- Type 2: DM2 (Proximal myotonic myopathy)
  - Milder version of DM1 with more restricted manifestations

EPIDEMIOLOGY

- Most common muscular dystrophy affecting adults
- DM1: Age of onset is childhood to 40 years
- DM2: Age of onset is 20–60 years
- Men and women equally affected

Prevalence

- ~1 case per 8,000 population
- Varies widely in different geographic areas

RISK FACTORS

Genetics

- Myotonic dystrophy is inherited in an autosomal dominant pattern
- Exhibits anticipation, getting progressively worse with each generation
  - More severe when the disorder is passed on from the mother
- One of several known nucleotide repeat disorders
  - DM1: DPMK gene-expanded repeat of CTG on chromosome 19
  - DM2: ZNF9 gene-expanded quadruplet repeat of CCTG on chromosome 3

GENERAL PREVENTION

- Genetic counseling
- Prenatal and preimplantation diagnosis possible

PATHOPHYSIOLOGY

- CUG or CCUG repeats in the mutant RNA interact with RNA binding proteins and disrupt RNA splicing, affecting many genes
  - Skeletal muscle chloride channel: Responsible for myotonia
  - Insulin receptor
  - Cardiac troponin T

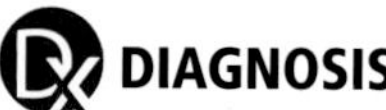

DIAGNOSIS

Ophthalmic features of myotonic dystrophy include varying degrees of:

- Cataract: Most common ocular abnormality
  - "Christmas tree cataract": Multicolored iridescent crystalline lens opacities
  - Later, stellate posterior cortical cataract
- Orbicularis weakness
- Delayed opening of eyes after forceful closure (myotonia of orbicularis)
- Ptosis: Involvement of levator muscle
- Slow saccades
- Progressive external ophthalmoplegia (diplopia rare)
- Low intraocular pressure
- Pigmentary retinopathy similar to that of Kearns Sayre syndrome

HISTORY

- Myotonia: Slow relaxation of muscles after contraction, often the first detectable finding
- Dysphagia
- Muscle weakness (and pain in DM2)
- Hypoventilation, disturbed sleep, and excessive daytime sleepiness
- Gastrointestinal symptoms: Dysphagia, constipation, abdominal pain
- Incontinence
- Infertility
- Cardiac history: Palpitations, blackouts, syncope
- Cognitive impairment/personality disturbance
- Complications of pregnancy and delivery

PHYSICAL EXAM

- Myotonia (handshake sign)
- Frontal balding
- Hollowing of the masseter and temporalis muscles
- Facial weakness
- Slackened mouth
- "Long face"
- Frontal bossing
- "Hatchet face"
- Wasting of neck and limb muscles
- Monotonous nasal voice
- Cardiac abnormalities: Bradyarrhythmias, tachyarrhythmias
- Endocrine disturbance: Insulin resistance, testicular atrophy
- Gastrointestinal disorders

DIAGNOSTIC TESTS & INTERPRETATION

Lab

- Blood work may show insulin resistance and mild to moderate elevations in serum creatine kinase
- Serum immunoglobulin studies may show IgG and IgM hypogammaglobulinemia

Imaging

- Brain MRI
  - Scattered or diffuse bilateral symmetrical white matter hyperintense lesions, with variable frontal or temporal-insular predominance

Diagnostic Procedures/Other

- Molecular analysis for the nucleotide expansions in the DMPK and ZNF9 gene is the gold standard
- Electromyography (EMG) may detect presence of myotonia
- Slit-lamp examination may show typical cataract formation
- Electrocardiography (ECG) may show atrioventricular and intraventricular conduction disturbances with prolongation of the PR interval and QRS complex
- Muscle biopsy (see path)
- Forced vital capacity (FVC) measurements to detect weakness of respiratory muscles
- Swallowing assessment to assess for dysphagia

Pathological Findings

- Centrally-located nuclei run down the centers of muscle fibers
- The myofilaments and sarcoplasmic reticulum are disrupted, and accumulations of impaired mitochondria may be found

DIFFERENTIAL DIAGNOSIS

- Other muscular dystrophies
- Other myotonic syndromes
- Mild tetanus
- Polymyositis
- Stiff person syndrome

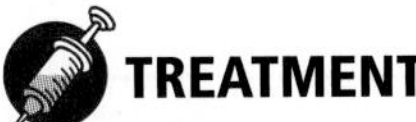

TREATMENT

ADDITIONAL TREATMENT

General Measures

- Symptomatic support
- Muscle weakness: Exercise training
- Ankle-foot-orthotics for foot drop
- Excessive daytime sleepiness: Modafinil, BiPAP
- Conduction abnormalities: Pacemaker placement
- Myotonia rarely requires treatment

SURGERY/OTHER PROCEDURES

- Cataract extraction for cataracts
- Ptosis repair for sight limiting ptosis: Caution not to precipitate exposure keratopathy

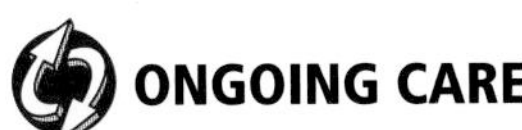

ONGOING CARE

FOLLOW-UP RECOMMENDATIONS

- Ophthalmologist
- Neurologist
- Cardiologist
- Pulmonologist
- Physical therapist
- Endocrinologist
- Rheumatologist
- Genetic counseling

PATIENT EDUCATION

- The myotonic dystrophy foundation (www.myotonic.org)
- MDA USA homepage (http://www.mda.org)
- International Myotonic Dystrophy Organization (http://www.myotonicdystrophy.com)

PROGNOSIS

- DM1: Life expectancy appears to be reduced
- DM2: Life expectancy appears to be normal

COMPLICATIONS

- High risk of cardiovascular and respiratory complications during general anesthesia

ADDITIONAL READING

- Arsenault ME, Prévost C, Lescault A, Laberge C, et al. Clinical characteristics of myotonic dystrophy type 1 patients with small CTG expansions. *Neurology* 2006;66(8):1248–1250.
- Cho DH, Tapscott SJ. Myotonic dystrophy: Emerging mechanisms for DM1 and DM2. *Biochim Biophys Acta* 2007;1772(2):195–204.
- Day JW, Ricker K, Jacobsen FJ, et al. Myotonic dystrophy type 2: Molecular, diagnostic and clinical spectrum. *Neurology* 2003;60(4):657–664.
- Machuca-Tzili L, Brook D, Hilton-Jones D. Clinical and molecular aspects of the myotonic dystrophies: A review. *Muscle Nerve* 2005;32:1–18.

CODES

ICD9

- 359.21 Myotonic muscular dystrophy
- 366.9 Unspecified cataract
- 374.30 Ptosis of eyelid, unspecified

CLINICAL PEARLS

- Myotonic dystrophy is the most common inherited neuromuscular disease in adults.
- It is a multisystem disorder characterized by skeletal muscle weakness and myotonia, cardiac conduction abnormalities, cataracts, testicular failure, hypogammaglobulinemia, and insulin resistance.
- Due to its wide range and variability of presentations, the diagnosis can often be initially missed, but it can usually be confirmed by careful attention to all the clinical features and/or by detailed family history.
- Treatment is symptomatic and there is no disease-modifying therapy available.

NANOPHTHALMOS

M. Reza Razeghinejad
L. Jay Katz

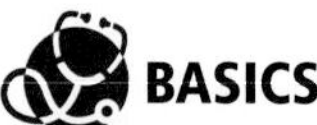

BASICS

DESCRIPTION

- Nanophthalmos (simple microphthalmos) is a rare developmental disorder characterized by a small eye with short axial length (14.5–20 mm), shallow anterior chamber, high hypermetropia (+7.25-+20.50 diopter), thick sclera, a normal or thick lens, high lens-to-eye volume ratio, and crowded optic disc (pseudopapilledema).
- Rarely, some patients have emmetropia or myopia secondary to increased refractive power of the cornea and lens.

EPIDEMIOLOGY

Prevalence

- An uncommon condition
- Equal prevalence in men and women

RISK FACTORS

Nanophthalmos is a congenital malformation without risk factor for acquisition.

Genetics

- Most cases are not inherited and are not heritable.
- Both patterns of autosomal dominant (more common) and recessive isolated nanophthalmos have been reported.
- Mutations of MFRP (membrane frizzled-related protein) that regulates axial length in autosomal recessive nanophthalmos and NNO1 on chromosome 11, an autosomal dominant locus.

PATHOPHYSIOLOGY

- It may result from an arrest in ocular development after closure of the embryonic fissure.
- A smaller than normal optic vesicle growing from the forebrain may be the cause of the reduced size of the eye, and scleral thickening could be explained by the development of a normal amount of scleral cells surrounding a smaller optic vesicle, resulting in a proportionately denser population of cells.

COMMONLY ASSOCIATED CONDITIONS

- Ocular: Hypermetropia, retinal folds and yellow macular pigmentation, macular hypoplasia, pigmentary retinal degeneration, retinitis pigmentosa, pigmentary retinal dystrophy, acquired retinoschisis, retinitis pigmentosa, and optic nerve head drusen
- Systemic: Cryptorchidism, Hallermann-Streiff syndrome

DIAGNOSIS

HISTORY

- Glasses with thick convex lenses since childhood
- Amblyopia in those who did not receive appropriate treatment in childhood
- Family history of glaucoma

PHYSICAL EXAM

- Slit lamp exam: Corneal diameter usually <12 mm, lens and iris bulging forward into a shallow anterior chamber.
- Refraction: Hyperopia
- Gonioscopy: Occludable angle
- Funduscopy: Crowded optic discs (pseudopapilledema), pigmentary retinal changes.
- Tonometry: Elevated intraocular pressure (IOP), wide pulse amplitude of mires

DIAGNOSTIC TESTS & INTERPRETATION

Lab

Initial lab tests

Ocular sonography: Axial length <20 mm, shallow anterior chamber depth, thickened sclerochoroidal wall (>1.5 mm), possible optic nerve head drusen.

Follow-up & special considerations

- In childhood, correction of refractive error to prevent amblyopia is mandatory.
- Adults without glaucoma need follow-up examination every 6 months for early glaucoma detection.
- Avoid any intraocular surgery unless absolutely necessary.
- Patients are at risk of spontaneous uveal effusion.
- High risk of malignant glaucoma and uveal effusion intra- and postoperatively.

Imaging

- Full ophthalmic examination with particular attention to possibility of angle-closure glaucoma
  - Review of systems to identify other possible syndrome findings
- A scan ocular sonography to determine the ocular axial length
  - B-scan ocular sonography to evaluate for choroidal thickening and choroidal effusion

Diagnostic Procedures/Other

Orbital MRI is done to evaluate choroidal thickening or detachment and choroidal effusion. Usually not required.

Pathological Findings

Thickened sclera with an abnormal arrangement of collagen, reduced levels of glycosaminoglycan, and elevated levels of fibronectin.

DIFFERENTIAL DIAGNOSIS

- Anterior segment microphthalmos
- Microphthalmos

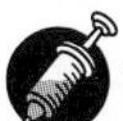

TREATMENT

- Narrow angle with a normal IOP: Follow-up every 3–6 months and consider early laser iridotomy.
- Closed angle with a normal IOP: Laser iridotomy
- Closed angle after laser iridotomy with normal or high IOP: Do ocular sonography.
  - Choroidal effusion: Treat the effusion.
  - No choroidal effusion: Peripheral iridoplasty
- High IOP without response to laser iridotomy or iridoplasty and no choroidal effusion: Start medical therapy like a case of open angle glaucoma.
  - Miotics can worsen angle obstruction by producing a relative papillary block and by relaxing lens zonules
- High IOP accompanied with peripheral anterior synechia without response to laser therapy and maximum medical therapy: Trabeculectomy, possible lens extraction in those who do not have peripheral anterior synechia.
- Modification of the trabeculectomy to avoid postoperative hypotony and perform prophylactic posterior sclerotomies in both lower quadrants. The sclerotomies should be left unsutured to allow continued drainage of suprachoroidal fluid.
- Uveal effusion, choroidal detachment, or serous retinal detachment: Systemic steroid or surgical vortex vein decompression

ADDITIONAL TREATMENT

General Measures

- Any patient with nanophthalmos by the fourth decade should have ocular sonography for detecting possible choroidal separation or effusion and gonioscopic evaluation for angle closure.
- Performing any kind of surgery including laser iridotomy may be associated with uveal effusion and exudative retinal detachment.

Issues for Referral

- Angle-closure glaucoma.
- Cataract. Holladay 2 and Hoffer Q formulas are appropriate for IOL power calculation.
- Choroidal or retinal pathologies.

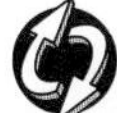

ONGOING CARE

FOLLOW-UP RECOMMENDATIONS

- All patients should be followed regularly for early glaucoma detection, especially after their fourth decade.
- Nanophthalmos associated with any ocular or systemic problems should be followed for those conditions.

PROGNOSIS

Those who develop uncontrolled glaucoma and need surgery have poor visual prognosis secondary to common posterior segment intra- and postoperative complications.

COMPLICATIONS

- Glaucoma.
- Spontaneous and intra- or postoperative uveal effusion or exudative retinal detachment.

ADDITIONAL READING

- Tay T, Smith JE, Berman Y, et al. Nanophthalmos in a Melanesian population. *Clin Experiment Ophthalmol* 2007;35(4):348–354.
- Yuzbasioglu E, Artunay O, Agachan A, et al. Phacoemulsification in patients with nanophthalmos. *Can J Ophthalmol* 2009;44(5): 534–539.
- MacKay CJ, Shek MS, Carr RE, et al. Retinal degeneration with nanophthalmos, cystic macular degeneration, and angle closure glaucoma. A new recessive syndrome. *Arch Ophthalmol* 1987;105(3): 366–371.
- Singh OS, Simmons RJ, Brockhurst RJ, et al. Nanophthalmos: A perspective on identification and therapy. *Ophthalmology* 1982;89(9):1006–1012.

CODES

ICD9

- 743.10 Microphthalmos, unspecified
- 743.11 Simple microphthalmos

CLINICAL PEARLS

- Nanophthalmos is a congenital ocular finding and may be associated with cryptorchidism and Hallermann-Streiff syndrome.
- High possibility of posterior segment complications with any surgical intervention
- The patients usually develop angle-closure glaucoma after the fourth decade.

N

NASOLACRIMAL DUCT OBSTRUCTION

Behin Barahimi
Jacqueline R. Carrasco

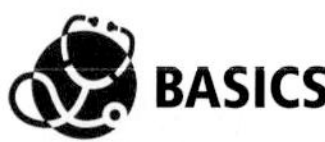

BASICS

DESCRIPTION

- The nasolacrimal duct is a bilateral structure that carries tears from the lacrimal sac into the nasal cavity at the level of the inferior turbinate. Obstruction along the course of the duct can lead to epiphora or dacryocystitis (1)[C].
- The cause of acquired nasolacrimal duct obstruction (NLDO) in adults can be divided into primary and secondary. Congenital NLDO will be discussed separately.

EPIDEMIOLOGY

Incidence

- The incidence from one retrospective study was estimated to be 20.2 per 100,000. There are no population-based studies in the literature evaluating NLDO (3)[C].
- The male to female ratio of NLDO is 1:3 (3)[C] Some have postulated that the higher incidence amongst women is due to a nasolacrimal duct with a smaller diameter (4)[C].

Prevalence

Unknown

RISK FACTORS

- Use of topical eye medications (usually seen in patients in glaucoma drops)
- Previous facial trauma
- Previous sinus or nasal surgery
- Recurrent dacryocystitis
- Recurrent conjunctivitis
- History of systemic chemotherapeutic agents such as 5-fluorouracil or Taxotere

GENERAL PREVENTION

- Wear protective eyewear with polycarbonate lenses, especially during high-risk activities such as sports to prevent trauma.
- Discuss punctal occlusion when patients are on chronic eye medications for glaucoma to minimize exposure to the nasolacrimal duct.
- In majority of cases, NLDO is unavoidable.

PATHOPHYSIOLOGY

- Primary-acquired NLDO is associated with a fibro-inflammatory process of unknown etiology (1)[C].
- Secondary-acquired NLDO can be divided up into the following categories: infectious, inflammatory, neoplastic, traumatic, and mechanical.
  - Infectious: bacteria, viruses, fungi, and parasites have all been reported as causes.
  - Inflammatory: endogenous causes such as sarcoidosis or exogenous causes such as radiation or topical eye drops.
  - Neoplastic: Primary or metastatic lesions, both of which are rare. The most common primary lesions are squamous cell papilloma and squamous cell carcinoma. Less common tumors consist of transitional cell carcinoma, adenocarcinoma, fibrous histiocytoma, lymphoid lesions, and melanoma.
  - Trauma: Iatrogenic from lacrimal probing or sinus surgery, and non-iatrogenic usually causing canalicular laceration
  - Mechanical: Foreign bodies, dacryoliths, or casts can physically block the duct (1)[C].

ETIOLOGY

See Pathophysiology.

COMMONLY ASSOCIATED CONDITIONS

- Sarcoidosis
- Wegener's granulomatosis
- Ocular cicatricial pemphigoid
- Scleroderma
- Herpetic keratitis/conjunctivitis
- History of chemotherapy
- History of radiation
- Glaucoma

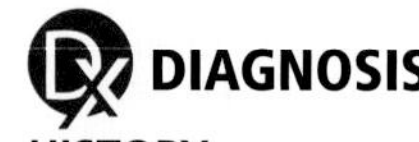

DIAGNOSIS

HISTORY

Patients often complain of constant tearing that is usually unilateral. They may also report blurry vision, difficulty reading and driving because of epiphora. One study found that over 65% of patients were embarrassed by their tearing problem (2)[B].

PHYSICAL EXAM

- Examine position of eyelids, lashes, and puncta as alternate causes for tearing.
- Thorough exam of the eyelid, conjunctiva, cornea, and anterior chamber is needed to rule out other causes of epiphora listed in the differential diagnosis.
- Increased tear lake, >2 mm is suggestive of NLDO (1)[C].
- Palpate the lacrimal sac. Reflux of purulent material is indicative of NLDO. Palpation of a firm mass above the medial canthal tendon is concerning for a neoplasm.
- Examine the nasal cavity as neoplastic, inflammatory, and structural disorders of the nasal passage that can cause NLDO.

DIAGNOSTIC TESTS & INTERPRETATION

Lab

- Lab testing is not diagnostic in NLDO
- If purulent discharge is elicited from lacrimal sac massage, collect it for Gram stain, culture, and sensitivity testing.

Imaging

- If neoplastic etiology is of concern, then CT or MRI is warranted.
- Optional work up, rarely necessary
- Dacryoscintigraphy with technetium-99 m: Assess functionality of lacrimal system.
- Dacryocystography: Visualize anatomy of lacrimal system.

Diagnostic Procedures/Other
- Irrigation and Probing
- Jones I: Functional test
- Jones II test: Anatomic test
- Schirmer test: Measure basal and stimulated tears

Pathological Findings
In the majority of cases, surgical specimens will show evidence of chronic inflammation. However, in cases where there is an underlying systemic cause such as sarcoidosis, Wegener's granulomatosis, neoplasm, and so forth, the pathology can be diagnostic. For example, in sarcoidosis, granulomas will be seen on pathology.

DIFFERENTIAL DIAGNOSIS
- Dry eye syndrome
- Blepharitis
- Conjunctivitis
- Trichiasis
- Corneal foreign body
- Entropion
- Ectropion
- Corneal abrasion
- Angle closure glaucoma
- Lacrimal sac tumor

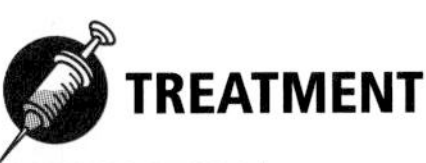

TREATMENT

MEDICATION
First Line
Definitive treatment is surgery; however, the presence of stagnant tears from NLDO can cause an infectious dacryocystitis. Treatment with oral antibiotics is necessary to prevent development of pre-septal or even orbital cellulitis. Cultures help guide antibiotic choice. Be suspicious for *Actinomyces* infections and the need to remove canalicular stones (1)[C].

ADDITIONAL TREATMENT
Issues for Referral
If the epiphora caused by NLDO is affecting the patient's quality of life, or if there is concern for an infection, refer to ophthalmology.

SURGERY/OTHER PROCEDURES
- Dacryocystorhinostomy (DCR) bypasses the usual site of obstruction in the distal nasolacrimal duct and creates a new opening at the level of the middle turbinate. A silicone tube is placed ensuring that the new ostium remains patent. The procedure can be done with an external or endoscopic approach. Each procedure has its disadvantages but both are acceptable treatments with comparable success rates (5)[C].
- Balloon dacryoplasty: This procedure has lower success rate, but may be helpful with partial nasolacrimal duct obstruction. It is often successful for congenital NLDO.
- Probing: This has not been found to be beneficial for acquired NLDO, but is often successful for congenital NLDO.

IN-PATIENT CONSIDERATIONS
Admission Criteria
Secondary orbital cellulitis is rare but would require admission if it should develop. Otherwise, NLDO is treated on an outpatient basis.

ONGOING CARE

FOLLOW-UP RECOMMENDATIONS
After DCR, the silicone tube should be left in place for at least 1 month and in some cases, up to 6 months.

Patient Monitoring
- After DCR surgery, a 1-week follow-up exam is done to ensure that the silicone tube is in the appropriate position.
- If the tube begins to extrude, it can gently be reposited. Contact your physician for any concerns.

DIET
There are no dietary recommendations for NLDO.

PATIENT EDUCATION
- Educate patients on the function of the nasolacrimal duct and the anatomy of the lacrimal system, so that they have a better understanding of the signs and symptoms caused by NLDO.
- Inform patients that they will have epiphora after DCR surgery because of the silicone tube. Once the tube is removed, the tearing will decrease.

PROGNOSIS
Good, as the success rate of DCR ranges between 75–95% (3)[C], (5)[C].

COMPLICATIONS
- Epiphora
- Bloody tears
- Purulent discharge
- Dacryocystitis
- Pre-septal cellulitis
- Orbital cellulitis
- Rare: CSF leak or meningitis

REFERENCES

1. Mills DM, Meyer DR. Acquired nasolacrimal duct obstruction. *Otolaryngol Clin N Am* 2006;39: 979–999.
2. Cheung LM, Francis IC, Stapleton F, et al. Symptom assessment in patients with functional and primary acquired nasolacrimal duct obstruction before and after successful dacryocystorhinostomy surgery: A prospective study. *Br J Ophthalmology* 2007;91: 1671–1674.
3. Woog JJ. The incidence of symptomatic acquired lacrimal outflow obstruction among the residents of Olmstead County, Minnesota, 1976–2000. *Trans Am Ophthalmol Soc* 2007;105:649–666.
4. McCormick A, Sloan B. The diameter of the nasolacrimal canal measured by computed tomography: Gender and racial difference. *Clin Exp Ophthalmol* 2009;37:357–361.
5. Patel BC. Management of acquired nasolacrimal duct obstruction: External and endonasal dacryocystorhinostomy. Is there a third way? *Br J Ophthalmol* 2009;93(11):1416–1419

ADDITIONAL READING

- Nesi F, Levine M, Lisman R. *Smith's Ophthalmic Plastic and Reconstructive Surgery*. 2nd ed. 1998:661–669.

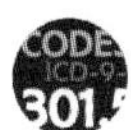

CODES

ICD9
- 375.22 Epiphora due to insufficient drainage
- 375.30 Dacryocystitis, unspecified
- 375.56 Stenosis of nasolacrimal duct, acquired

CLINICAL PEARLS

- In addition to visual symptoms, acquired NLDO can have serious, adverse emotional and social effects on patients.
- Surgical procedures available for NLDO have good success rates and can improve the daily living of patients.
- Patients who complain of persistent epiphora, that is decreasing their quality of life should be referred for ophthalmology evaluation.

NASOLACRIMAL DUCT OBSTRUCTION IN CHILDREN

Behin Barahimi

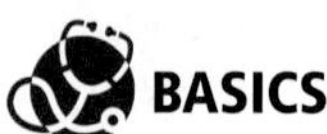

BASICS

DESCRIPTION

- The most common congenital abnormality of the lacrimal drainage system
- The nasolacrimal duct is a bilateral structure that carries tears from the lacrimal sac into the nasal cavity with an opening, the inferior meatus, under the inferior turbinate.
- Congenital nasolacrimal duct obstruction (NLDO) reportedly affects 6–20% of neonates. In 90% of the cases, symptoms spontaneously resolve by 12 months (1)[C].

EPIDEMIOLOGY

Incidence

6–20% of neonates are born with symptoms on NLDO, with the majority having spontaneous resolution (1)[C].

Prevalence

Most common lacrimal system anomaly in childhood.

RISK FACTORS

Patients with some craniofacial malformations, Down syndrome, and a wide variety of other syndromes with craniofacial or oculonasal malformations (e.g., Cornelia de Lange, Johanson-Blizzard) are at increased risk for NLDO as well as other nasolacrimal system anomalies.

Genetics

- There is no known specific causative genetic abnormality but the incidence is higher within families.
  - When associated with underlying genetic systemic syndromes, the inheritance pattern of that syndrome applies although variable expression of the nasolacrimal duct anomaly may often be seen.

PATHOPHYSIOLOGY

The nasolacrimal duct canalizes by the eighth month of gestation from the mesoderm centrally and from the surface ectoderm distally. A thin mucosal membrane at the distal end (Valve of Hasner) causes congenital NLDO.

ETIOLOGY

Unknown

COMMONLY ASSOCIATED CONDITIONS

- Down syndrome
- Craniofacial abnormalities
- Preauricular sinus
- Other systemic syndromes characterized by oculofacial involvement
- Majority of cases have no associated systemic disease

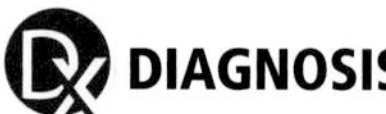

DIAGNOSIS

HISTORY

- Parents usually report history of epiphora that may or may not be accompanied by a mucopurulent discharge
- Epiphora may not occur until later in infancy
  - Discharge usually mucoid, clinging to lower lashes, not associated with conjunctival injection
  - Discharge worse upon wakening from sleep. Eyelashes often stuck together
  - May be worse with upper respiratory tract infection or outdoors on windy days

PHYSICAL EXAM

- Eyelashes may appear matted or wet.
- Digital pressure on the lacrimal sac can cause reflux of purulent material by puncta.
- Chronic skin changes of lower lid
- Increased tear lake may be visible on the side that has NLDO. If there is bilateral NLDO, this will be difficult to defect.
- Careful examination of the eyelid, conjunctiva, and cornea should be performed to rule out other causes of epiphora (see Differential Diagnosis).
  - Little or no conjunctival injection

DIAGNOSTIC TESTS & INTERPRETATION

Lab

Initial lab tests

None

Follow-up & special considerations

Should erythema and swelling with or without a mass develop in the area of the medial canthus or the inferior medial aspect of the lower lid, suspect dacryocystitis/infected lacrimal sac mucocele and treat urgently with referral to ophthalmology.

Imaging

- In the majority of cases, no imaging is needed.
- Consider CT scan if craniofacial abnormality or trauma (2)[C].

Diagnostic Procedures/Other

Dye Disappearances Test: A drop of fluorescein is placed in the eye and visualized with a cobalt blue light. If pooling persists in the eye after 5 minutes, or significantly longer than the uninvolved eye, the test is positive for an obstruction. When fluorescein is found in the nasal cavity, most commonly by inserting a cotton swab through the nares, then the system is patent.

DIFFERENTIAL DIAGNOSIS

- Dacryocele (lacrimal sac mucocele)
- Congenital entropion/ectropion
- Epiblepharon
- Trichiasis
- Congenital/infantile glaucoma
- Infectious conjunctivitis or keratitis
- Uveitis
- Foreign body
- Other lacrimal system (e.g., anomaly: Punctal/canalicular stenosis/agenesis, lacrimal fistula)

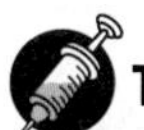

TREATMENT

MEDICATION

First Line

- Massage of lacrimal sac should be the first line of therapy. It is theorized that this will increase the hydrostatic pressure in the lacrimal system allowing the membranous obstruction to rupture (2)[C].
  - Caretaker should place forefinger on medial canthal ligament and push posteriorly (towards occiput) to compress underlying lacrimal sac, 3–4 times daily. Often done with feedings.

Second Line

Antibiotics therapy should only be used if there are signs of secondary infection (e.g., conjunctivitis) (2)[C].

ADDITIONAL TREATMENT

Issues for Referral

- A large percentage of babies are born with NLDO and resolve within the first year of life. If by age 12 months tearing persists, then referral to an ophthalmologist is warranted. Severe NLDO with copious discharge may be referred earlier, especially if there is no improvement with massage.
- Concern for dacryocystitis or pre-septal cellulitis should be referred urgently to ophthalmology.

SURGERY/OTHER PROCEDURES

- If symptoms persist past the first year of life, and massage for at least 3 months has failed, surgery may be considered and is highly successful in most cases. Earlier surgery may be considered in severe cases. The use of awake in office (as opposed to general anesthesia) is controversial. Early surgery is also indicated following secondary dacryocystitis/cellulitis.
- Probing: Probing is traditionally seen as first-line treatment (1)[C]. Approximately 78% success rate (3)[B].
- Balloon catheter dilation: Variation of standard probing. More costly. 82% success rate reported in the literature (4)[B]. May not be statistically significant.
- Nasolacrimal duct intubation: A monocanalicular or bicanalicular tube can be left in place for several months at the time of probing. One disadvantage is that the tube does need to be removed and some children may not tolerate this in the office requiring sedation. In a prospective study the success rate of intubation was 91% (5)[B]. Most often this is reserved for older children and children who have failed standard probing once or twice.
- Dacryocystorhinostomy: This is usually a last resort for patients who have had multiple failed procedures.

IN-PATIENT CONSIDERATIONS

Admission Criteria

Admission only necessary if signs of dacryocystitis, pre-septal or orbital cellulitis develop and intravenous antibiotics are needed.

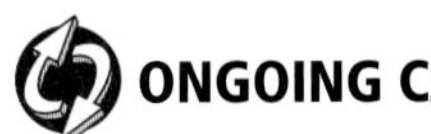

ONGOING CARE

FOLLOW-UP RECOMMENDATIONS

No follow-up required after NLDO is resolved.

Patient Monitoring

- Minimum massage time is 3 months
- Monitor for signs of cellulitis/dacryocystitis until NLDO resolved

DIET

No dietary recommendations

PATIENT EDUCATION

- Educate parents that this is a common problem that resolves spontaneously in the majority of cases with the assistance of massage. In situations where surgery is needed, outcomes are excellent.
- Patients with craniofacial abnormalities may have lower success rates even with surgery.

PROGNOSIS

Excellent

COMPLICATIONS

- Mild transient nose bleeding after surgery
- Corneal abrasion after surgery
- False passage created with probing
- Extrusion of tube
- Dacryocystitis/cellulitis
- Complications of probing are extremely uncommon

REFERENCES

1. Puvanachandra N, Trikha A, MacEwen CJ, et al. A national survey of the management of congenital nasolacrimal duct obstruction in the United Kingdom. *J Pediatr Ophthalmol Strabismus* 2010;47(2):76–80.
2. Takahashi Y, Kakizaki H, Chan WO, et al. Management of congential nasolacrimal duct obstruction. *Acta Ophthalmol* 2010;88(5): 506–513.
3. Pediatric Eye Disease Investigator Group. Primary treatment of nasolacrimal duct obstruction with probing in children less than four years old. *Ophthalmology* 2008;115(3):577–584.
4. Pediatric Eye Disease Investigator Group. Primary treatment of nasolacrimal duct obstruction with balloon catheter dilation in children less than four years old. *J AAPOS* 2008;12(5):451–445.
5. Pediatric Eye Disease Investigator Group. Primary treatment of nasolacrimal duct obstruction with nasolacrimal duct intubation in children less than four years old. *J AAPOS* 2008;12(5):445–450.

ADDITIONAL READING

- Nelson LB, Calhous JH, Menduke H. Medical management of congenital nasolacrimal duct obstruction. *Ophthalmology* 1985;92(9): 1187–1190.

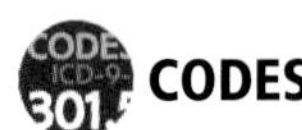

CODES

ICD9

- 375.22 Epiphora due to insufficient drainage
- 375.55 Obstruction of nasolacrimal duct, neonatal
- 743.65 Specified congenital anomalies of lacrimal passages

CLINICAL PEARLS

- The majority of patients with congenital NLDO will have spontaneous resolution by the age of 12 months using massage alone. If signs or symptoms of cellulitis/dacryocystitis occur, urgent referral to an ophthalmologist is indicated.
- Although CNLDO is common, other conditions that need immediate attention such as congenital glaucoma can have similar presentation. Therefore, a full eye examination is important.

NEONATAL CONJUNCTIVITIS

Sharon S. Lehman

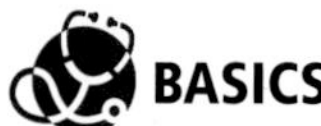

BASICS

DESCRIPTION
Conjunctivitis occurring in the first 4 weeks of life

EPIDEMIOLOGY
Incidence
- US:
  - Gonococcal: 0.3/1,000 births
  - Chlamydial: 8.2/1,000 births
- Developing countries: 15–60% of live births

Gonorrhea is a major cause of childhood blindness in some countries.

RISK FACTORS
- Maternal systemic infection
- Premature or prolonged rupture of placental membranes
- Low birth weight
- Nasal cannula, mask, or ventilator use
- Ophthalmologic examination and speculum use
- Use of silver nitrate or gentamicin for prophylaxis
- Failure to use prophylaxis
- Folk treatments including urine instilled into the eyes

Genetics
No known contribution

GENERAL PREVENTION
- Proper prenatal care
- Universal precautions and maintenance of sterility
- Ocular prophylaxis immediately after birth: Preferably 0.5% erythromycin ointment (1)[A]
  - Povidone-iodine solution is effective, safe, and cost effective but not yet approved in the US or Canada (2)[A], (3)[A].
  - Respiratory organisms through respiratory supportive care (especially intubation or mask)
  - Discourage folk treatments of conjunctivitis

PATHOPHYSIOLOGY
- Inoculation by maternal or iatrogenic routes
- Deficient infant immune defense mechanisms
- Chemical irritation: Silver nitrate and gentamicin ointment

ETIOLOGY
- Infectious: Gram-negative enteric bacteria, *Staphylococcus aureus* (including methicillin-resistant strains), *Neisseria gonorrhea*, *Streptococcus pneumoniae*, *Chlamydia trachomatis*, and herpes simplex virus
- Noninfectious: Silver nitrate toxicity, topical gentamicin toxicity

COMMONLY ASSOCIATED CONDITIONS
- Maternal infection (known or unknown)
- Premature or prolonged rupture of placental membranes
- Gonorrhea: Corneal perforation
- Herpes: Skin lesions, encephalitis, and viral sepsis
- Gentamicin toxicity: Lid skin erosions

DIAGNOSIS

HISTORY
- Maternal/birth
  - Quality of prenatal care
  - Systemic infection and history of sexually transmitted disease
  - Paternal or maternal genital discharge
  - Premature or prolonged rupture of placental membranes
- Infant
  - Low birth weight
  - Systemic disease and immunodeficiency
  - Prophylaxis not given
  - Use of silver nitrate or gentamicin prophylaxis
  - Ocular examination, use of nonsterile speculum/instruments
  - Requiring respiratory support

PHYSICAL EXAM
- Systemic physical examination
- Complete ocular exam including dilated retinal examination to rule out intraocular involvement if infectious etiology
  - Eyelids: Edema and erythema, lid skin erosions in gentamicin toxicity
  - Conjunctiva: Chemosis and injection (Note: Absence of conjunctival injection suggests nasolacrimal duct obstruction as cause of discharge)
  - Discharge: Bacterial infection and silver nitrate/gentamicin toxicity: Mucopurulent, viral infection may be clear discharge
  - Cornea
    - HSV: Dendrite, stromal infiltrate, or geographic erosion of corneal epithelium
    - Gonorrhea: Ulcer, possible perforation

DIAGNOSTIC TESTS & INTERPRETATION
Lab
Initial lab tests
- Urgent Gram stain to identify gonorrhea
- Culture for bacteria, chlamydia, and viruses
- Coordinate with lab for special stains (Giemsa for chlamydia), culture media (chocolate agar for gonorrhea), and rapid tests (for chlamydia)

Follow-up & special considerations
- If sexually transmitted disease is identified, mother and her sexual partners should be referred for testing and, as needed, for treatment.
- If sexually transmitted disease is identified, test child for other organisms: HIV and syphilis.

Imaging
- CT/MRI of brain if herpes simplex virus is identified or child is systemically unwell
- CT/MRI if concern about secondary periorbital or orbital cellulitis

Diagnostic Procedures/Other
Lumbar puncture if child is systemically unwell or concern about herpes simplex encephalitis

Pathological Findings
- Biopsy not typically performed
- Gonorrhea: Gram stain shows intracellular gram-negative diplococci
- Chlamydia: Intracellular inclusions in conjunctival epithelial scraping

DIFFERENTIAL DIAGNOSIS
- Nasolacrimal duct obstruction
- Neonatal blepharitis/blepharoconjunctivitis
- Diffuse retinoblastoma
- Neonatal leukemia with ocular involvement
- Uveitis due to prenatal infection
- Epiphora due to congenital/infantile glaucoma

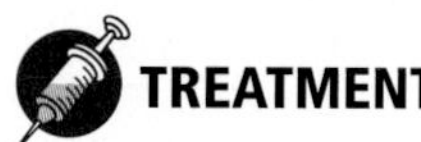

TREATMENT

MEDICATION
- Chlamydia trachomatis
  - Systemic therapy necessary to prevent respiratory infection (pneumonitis)
  - Erythromycin estolate 40–50 mg/kg per day in 4 divided doses for 14–21 days; maximum dose: 2 g/day
  - Topical therapy optional, erythromycin ointment b.i.d.
- Neisseria gonorrhea
  - Single dose of ceftriaxone (25–50 mg/kg, not to exceed 125 mg) IV or IM in healthy infant with uncomplicated conjunctivitis
  - Cefotaxime (100 mg/kg) IV or IM, also acceptable in uncomplicated cases
  - Topical therapy: Topical antibiotic, optional
  - Note: Penicillin alone is not a satisfactory treatment.

- Herpes simplex virus
  - Acyclovir 60 mg/kg per day in 3 divided doses IV for 14–21 days and possibly longer, as determined by the pediatrician.
  - Topical trifluridine 1% may be used every 1–2 hours (not to exceed 9 times per day) for 1–2 week and tapered.
  - Topical steroids should be avoided.
- Other bacterial
  - Therapy based on Gram stain and culture results
  - Consider coverage for MRSA (4)[C].
- Chemical
  - Discontinue offending agent.
  - Treat for inflammatory response and/or secondary infection.
  - Usually self-limited

ADDITIONAL TREATMENT

General Measures

Saline irrigation every 2 hours to clear mucopurulent discharge

Issues for Referral

- Cornea consult if perforation or impending perforation
  - Cornea consult if nonresolving corneal lesion due to herpes

Additional Therapies

As indicated by medical condition and etiologic agent.

COMPLEMENTARY & ALTERNATIVE THERAPIES

- Not indicated
- Do not use breast milk or urine in eyes.

SURGERY/OTHER PROCEDURES

Not typically necessary (except for trichiasis and scarring as long term result of chronic chlamydia trachomatis).

IN-PATIENT CONSIDERATIONS

Initial Stabilization

Pediatric consultation if child systemically unwell or other concerns.

Admission Criteria

- Systemically unwell
- Urgent hospital admission suggested for all purulent suspected bacterial conjunctivitis until etiology clear and for neonatal herpes simplex conjunctivitis.

IV Fluids

As needed.

Nursing

Appropriate isolation/precautions

Discharge Criteria

When parenteral antibiotics are completed, the child is systemically well, and the parents are able to continue care as needed.

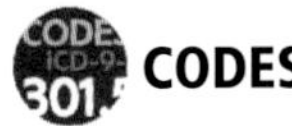

ONGOING CARE

FOLLOW-UP RECOMMENDATIONS

As needed for amblyopia therapy, if corneal scar is present.

Patient Monitoring

Visual acuity as needed for amblyopia therapy, if corneal scar is present.

DIET

No special dietary recommendations.

PATIENT EDUCATION

If sexually transmitted disease, mother and her sexual partners should be referred for diagnosis, treatment, and counseling.

PROGNOSIS

- Uncomplicated–excellent
- Complicated with corneal scar–variable depending upon severity and compliance with amblyopia therapy
- Gonorrhea corneal perforation–poor prognosis

COMPLICATIONS

Permanent vision loss from amblyopia due to corneal scar

REFERENCES

1. American Academy of Pediatrics. Prevention of ophthalmia neonatorum. In: Pickering LK, Baker CJ, Kimberlin DW, Long SS (eds). *Red Book 2009 Report of the Committee on Infectious Diseases*. 28th ed. Elk Grove Village, IL: AAP, 2009:827–829.
2. Richter R, Below H, Kadow I, et al. Effect of topical 1.25% povidine-iodine eyedrops used for prophylaxis of ophthalmia neonatorum on renal iodine excretion and thyroid-stimulating hormone level. *J Pediatr* 2006;148:401–403.
3. Keenan JD, Eckert S, Rutar T. Cost Analysis of povidine-iodine for ophthalmia neonatorum prophylaxis. *Arch Ophthalmol* 2010;128(1): 136–137.
4. Sahu DN, Thomson S, Salam A, et al. Neonatal methicillin resistant Staphylococcus aureus conjunctivitis. *Br J Ophthalmol* 2006;90(6): 794–795.

ADDITIONAL READING

whqlibdoc.who.int/bulletin/2001/issue3/79(3)262–266.pdf

CODES

ICD9

- 098.40 Gonococcal conjunctivitis (neonatorum)
- 771.6 Neonatal conjunctivitis and dacryocystitis

CLINICAL PEARLS

- Always consider gonorrhea in the evaluation of purulent neonatal conjunctivitis and evaluate urgently.
- Always consider possibility of methicillin-resistant *Staphylococcus aureus* (MRSA) in the evaluation of purulent neonatal conjunctivitis. If no discharge and no red eye, consider nasolacrimal duct obstruction or congenital/infantile glaucoma.
- Do not rely on Gram stain results alone but in case of gram-negative intracellular diplococci, treat urgently as gonorrhea.
- Avoid use of topical silver nitrate or gentamicin for prophylaxis.
- If sexually transmitted disease, refer mother and her sexual partners for testing, treatment, and counseling.
- If herpes simplex is suspected, consider possible encephalitis and viral sepsis.

N

NEOVASCULAR GLAUCOMA

Elyse R. Trastman-Caruso

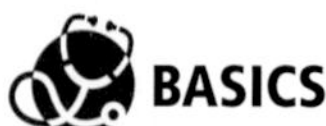

BASICS

DESCRIPTION

- Glaucoma caused by neovascularization of the angle and pupillary margin with contraction of myofibroblasts. This leads to peripheral anterior synechiae and eventual angle closure glaucoma.
- In the early stages, the abnormal blood vessels can regress after panretinal laser (PRP) or Bevacizumab treatment.
- In later stages, when fibrovascular ingrowth and contraction of the drainage angle occur, medical therapy becomes less effective for intraocular pressure control.
- Synonym(s): Hemorrhagic glaucoma, congestive glaucoma, rubeotic glaucoma, and thrombotic glaucoma.

EPIDEMIOLOGY

Incidence

- Rare
- Increased in diabetic patients after lens removal and vitrectomy or any breach in the posterior capsule.

Prevalence

- More prevalent in elderly patients
- Prevalence of neovascular glaucoma (NVG) in diabetes is overall 2%, but 21% of those with proliferative diabetic retinopathy.
- 23–33% of patients with ischemic central retinal vein occlusion (CRVO) develop NVG with the prevalence of CRVO ranging from 0.1–0.7%.

RISK FACTORS

- Any process that involves retinal ischemia (see Etiology section).
- The most frequent risk factors are the presence of a CRVO or proliferative diabetic retinopathy.

PATHOPHYSIOLOGY

- Retinal hypoxia causes production of factors promoting angiogenesis including vascular endothelial growth factor (VEGF).
- New blood vessels form in the anterior and posterior segment following chronic retinal ischemia.

ETIOLOGY

- Central retinal vein occlusion (CRVO)
- Proliferative diabetic retinopathy
- Carotid artery occlusive disease
- Central retinal artery occlusion (CRAO)
- Branch retinal vein occlusion
- Intraocular tumor
- Chronic retinal detachment
- Uveitis-glaucoma-hyphema syndrome
- Chronic or severe ocular inflammation
- Radiation retinopathy
- Coats disease
- Sickle cell retinopathy
- Eales disease
- Retinopathy of prematurity
- Carotid-cavernous fistula
- Takayasu disease
- Giant cell arteritis
- Anterior segment ischemia (previous strabismus surgery)
- Trauma

COMMONLY ASSOCIATED CONDITIONS

- Diabetes
- High blood pressure
- Atherosclerotic disease

DIAGNOSIS

HISTORY

- Red, painful eye
- Pressure sensation
- Photophobia
- Decreased vision

PHYSICAL EXAM

- New blood vessels at the pupillary margin
- Gonioscopy- new blood vessels in angle or hyphema
- Indirect ophthalmoscopy- look for the underlying cause:
  - CRVO- venous engorgement, retinal hemorrhages, disc swelling, cotton wool spots, and macular edema
  - Long-standing ischemia – optociliary shunt vessels
  - Choroidal Tumors
  - Retinoblastoma (in kids)
  - CRAO-cherry red spot
  - Proliferative diabetic retinopathy
  - Ocular ischemic syndrome- midperipheral hemorrhages, central retinal artery collapses with mild digital pressure on the globe

DIAGNOSTIC TESTS & INTERPRETATION

Lab

Depends on etiology:

- Fasting glucose, Hemoglobin A1c
- Blood pressure, cholesterol
- ESR (anyone >50 yrs old with CRAO or suspected autoimmune/inflammatory disease)
- Hyperviscosity workup- young patients with CRVO

Imaging

Initial approach

- Fluorescein angiography- to further delineate the underlying cause and the amount of neovascularization and retinal ischemia (*to assess ischemic versus nonischemic CRVO)
- B-scan, if no view of posterior fundus to eliminate tumors as the etiology of rubeosis
- ERG- can be used to assess retinal ischemia when there is no view of the fundus due to lens opacity
- Carotid ultrasound/echocardiogram- in CRAO and ocular ischemic syndrome

Follow-up & special considerations

- Gonioscopy/examination every month for the first 4 months after CRVO, since rubeosis classically appears 3 months after ischemic CRVO in 50% of eyes and 80% appears in the first 6 months
- Monthly follow-up needed for nonischemic CRVO since 15% of nonischemic CRVO converts to ischemic CRVO within 8 months and 33% convert in 3 years.

DIFFERENTIAL DIAGNOSIS

- Uveitic glaucoma
- Fuchs heterochromic iridocyclitis

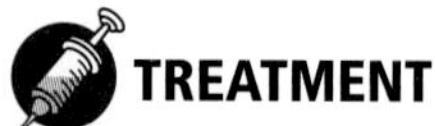

TREATMENT

MEDICATION

- Anti-VEGF (anti-vascular endothelial growth factor) intravitreal injections with PRP (1)[B], (2)[B]
  - Avastin (Bevacizumab)
  - Macugen (Pegaptanib sodium)
  - Lucentis (Ranibizumab)
  (either 1 mg/0.05 mL, 1.25 mg/0.05 mL, or 2.5 mg/0.05 mL)
- Aqueous suppressant eye drops: Beta blockers, topical and oral carbonic anhydrase inhibitors (Diamox), Brimonidine
- Contraindicated- Pilocarpine
- Steroid drops for the inflammatory response
- Atropine (cycloplegics)-decrease ocular congestion and prevent ciliary muscle spasm

ADDITIONAL TREATMENT

General Measures

- Limiting carbohydrates in diabetics
- Limiting salt intake in hypertensive patients

Issues for Referral

Retinal specialist- for PRP and Avastin

SURGERY/OTHER PROCEDURES

- Panretinal photocoagulation (PRP)-can be done with slit lamp laser, indirect laser, or endolaser at the time of vitrectomy (1)[A] 1500–2000 burns with 500 micron spot size.
  Argon, Krypton, or Diode laser (Krypton and Diode better with media opacities or blood)
  Central Retinal Vein Occlusion Study (3)[A]-PRP if ischemic CRVO caused 2 clock hours of iris neovascularization or any angle neovascularization.
- Trabeculectomy with Mitomycin C-possible, if eye is quiet 1 month after PRP/medical therapy; 61% qualified success rate with concurrent Avastin intravitreal injection (2)[B]

- Tube shunt with patch graft
  - Ahmed (S2 or FP): Especially if history of multiple surgeries; success rates vary in the literature but Netland et al. had a 73.1% success rate at 1 year that decreased to 20.6% at 5 years (4)[B].
  - Baerveldt tube shunts vary in success as well, with Sidoti et al. showing a 56% success rate at 18 months (5)[B].
- CPC (cyclophotocoagulation) (Diode or Nd:YAG transscleral laser): If poor visual potential or poor surgical candidate
- Endocyclophotocoagulation- similar to CPC but done through an intraocular approach
- Radiation or enucleation for tumor-associated rubeosis

IN-PATIENT CONSIDERATIONS

Initial Stabilization

- Diabetes or blood pressure control prior to surgery
- Treatment of hypercoagulable states if present

Admission Criteria

Inpatient admission required only in those patients who have uncontrolled systemic medical conditions.

Nursing

IV insertion and EKG monitoring perioperatively and when IV mannitol is used to decrease vitreous volume.

Discharge Criteria

Once systemic medical conditions are controlled

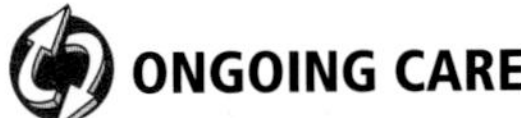

ONGOING CARE

FOLLOW-UP RECOMMENDATIONS

- Frequent follow-up is scheduled depending on the patient's response to medical glaucoma therapy.
- If guarded filtration surgery or tube shunt is indicated, then standard postoperative care is followed depending on the patient's clinical response and amount of filtration.

DIET

- Blood pressure, blood glucose, and cholesterol control
- Anticoagulation and antiplatelet agents in those at risk for stroke

PATIENT EDUCATION

- The importance of preventive medicine and routine follow-up with the patient's internist
- The need for at least routine yearly ophthalmologic examinations in patients >50 years and in all diabetics to improve prognosis with early diagnosis and treatment.

PROGNOSIS

Guarded prognosis: Success depends on prevention and treatment of neovascular glaucoma early in its course and the ability to control the underlying disease process.

COMPLICATIONS

- Chronic pain
- Complete loss of vision
- Choroidal effusions
- Suprachoroidal hemorrhage
- Phthisis
- Loss of eye

REFERENCES

1. Sivak-Callcott JA, O'Day DM, et al. Evidence-based recommendations for the diagnosis and treatment of neovascular glaucoma. *Ophthalmology* 2001; 108(10):1767–1776.
2. Fakhraie G, Katz LJ, Prasad A, et al. Surgical outcomes of intravitreal bevacizumab and guarded filtration surgery in neovascular glaucoma. *J Glaucoma* 2010;19(3):212–218.
3. The Central Vein Occlusion Study Group. A randomized clinical trial of early panretinal photocoagulation for ischemic central vein occlusion. The Central Vein Occlusion Study Group N report. *Ophthalmology* 1995;102(10): 1434–1444.
4. Netland PA. The Ahmed glaucoma valve in neovascular glaucoma (An AOS Thesis). *Trans Am Ophthalmol Soc* 2009;107:325–342.
5. Sidoti PA, Dunphy TR, Baerveldt G, et al. Experience with the Baerveldt glaucoma implant in treating neovascular glaucoma. *Ophthalmology* 1995;102(7):1107–1118.

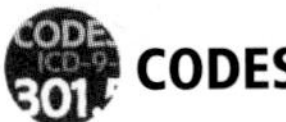

CODES

ICD9

- 362.02 Proliferative diabetic retinopathy
- 362.35 Central retinal vein occlusion
- 365.63 Glaucoma associated with vascular disorders of eye

CLINICAL PEARLS

- Gonioscopy is key! Diagnose early by performing gonioscopy and identify early signs of neovascularization.
- Continuity of care and communication between the glaucoma and retinal specialists and the patient's primary care physician is important to maximize the patient's general health and visual potential.
- Anti-VEGF intravitreal injections and PRP are the mainstays of treatment of neovascularization.
- If the intraocular pressure fails to be controlled with aqueous suppressants, guarded filtration procedures or tube shunts can be performed with a decreasing success rate over a 5 year period.
- More, larger studies need to be done regarding the long-term success rate of guarded filtration procedures and tube shunts in the era of anti-VEGF medications.

NEUROFIBROMATOSIS

Deepak P. Grover

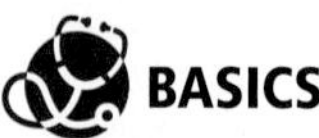

BASICS

DESCRIPTION

- Neurofibromatosis (NF) consists of 2 neurocutaneous genetic disorders that can involve the bones, the nervous system, soft tissue, and the skin. It is the most common hereditary disorder belonging to the group of hamartoses.
  - NF1, also known as von Recklinghausen's NF, is the most common subtype.
  - NF2 is also referred to as central NF.

EPIDEMIOLOGY

Incidence

- NF1: 1 case per 3,500 population
- NF2: 1 case per 37,000 population

RISK FACTORS

Genetics

- Neurofibromatosis is an autosomal dominant disorder with complete penetrance and high variability in its expression. Roughly half tend to be familial and the other half sporadic. It is independent of sex or race.
  - NF1 – The *NF1* gene has been mapped to chromosome 17q11.2. The gene encodes the protein neurofibromin.
  - NF2 – The *NF2* gene has been mapped to chromosome 22q11. The gene encodes the protein merlin.

GENERAL PREVENTION

Genetic counseling

PATHOPHYSIOLOGY

The gene products of the respective *NF* genes, neurofibromin for NF1 and merlin for NF2, act as tumor suppressors. A decrease in function of these proteins predisposes one to develop a variety of tumors involving the central and peripheral nervous systems.

ETIOLOGY

Many different mutations in the neurofibromatosis genes have been described respectively for both the *NF1* or *NF2* genes.

COMMONLY ASSOCIATED CONDITIONS

- Moyamoya disease
  - A progressive occlusive disease of the cerebral vasculature with particular involvement of the Circle of Willis
  - Linkage studies have linked one of the genes for familial Moyamoya disease to chromosome 17q25, which is in close proximity to the *NF1* gene.
  - Children often present with signs and symptoms of cerebral ischemic events, whereas, adults may present with signs and symptoms of subarachnoid or intracerebral hemorrhage.

DIAGNOSIS

HISTORY

- **Neurofibromatosis Type 1 (NF1)**
  - Parents may notice their children to have cutaneous discoloration or pathologic fractures.
  - Patients may complain of pain caused by neurofibromas or develop hypertensive headaches caused by a pheochromocytoma.
- **Neurofibromatosis Type 2 (NF2)**
  - Patients may present with gradual hearing loss, tinnitus, or vestibular dysfunction secondary to vestibular schwannomas.
  - A visual decline secondary to optic nerve sheath meningioma, posterior subcapsular cataract, combined hamartoma of the retina and RPE, or epiretinal membrane may often be a presenting complaint.

PHYSICAL EXAM

- **Neurofibromatosis Type 1 (2 of 7 criteria needed)**
  - 6 or more café-au-lait spots or hyperpigmented macules $\geq$5 mm in diameter in children younger than 10 years and to 15 mm in adults
  - Axillary or inguinal freckles
  - 2 or more typical neurofibromas or 1 plexiform neurofibroma involving the upper eyelid
  - Optic nerve glioma (seen in 15–20% of patients)
  - 2 or more Lisch nodules (iris hamartomas)
  - Sphenoid dysplasia or pseudarthrosis of long-bones
  - First-degree relative (parent or sibling) with NF1
- **Other manifestations of NF1**
  - Neurological manifestations
    - Seizure disorder
    - Pilocytic astrocytoma, meningioma, intramedullary glioma, and ependymoma
    - Vascular ectasias
    - Aneurysms
    - Chiari type 1 malformations
    - Malignant peripheral nerve sheath tumors
    - Dumbbell-shaped tumors of spinal cord
  - Ophthalmic manifestations
    - Proptosis, strabismus
  - Bone manifestations
    - Scoliosis, osteoporosis
  - Other disorders
    - Essential hypertension
    - Pheochromocytomas
    - Renal artery stenosis
    - Precocious puberty
    - Gastrointestinal stromal tumors
    - Learning disabilities or mild/moderate mental retardation
    - Vitamin D deficiency
- **Neurofibromatosis Type 2 (1 of 2 criteria needed)**
  - Bilateral cranial nerve eighth masses visualized on MRI
  - First-degree relative (parent or sibling) with NF2 and either:
    - A unilateral eighth nerve mass or,
    - 2 of the following: Neurofibroma, schwannoma, glioma, meningioma, or juvenile posterior subcapsular cataract
- **Other manifestations of NF2:**
  - Neurological manifestations
    - Nonvestibular schwannomas usually involving cranial nerves 3 and 5
    - Dumbbell-shaped spinal cord schwannoma
    - Spinal cord ependymoma, astrocytoma, and meningioma
    - Cranial nerve palsies from compression by expanding vestibular schwannoma or nonvestibular cranial nerve schwannoma
  - Ophthalmic manifestations
    - Optic nerve sheath meningioma
    - Combined hamartoma of the retina and RPE
    - Epiretinal membrane
    - Proptosis, strabismus

DIAGNOSTIC TESTS & INTERPRETATION

Lab

Initial lab tests

Gene sequencing, molecular testing, linkage analysis

Follow-up & special considerations

- For a suspected pheochromocytoma:
  - Plasma catecholamines and free plasma metanephrine
  - 24-hour urine collection to measure urinary free catecholamines (norepinephrine and epinephrine) and their metabolites (normetanephrine, metanephrine, and vanillylmandelic acid)

Imaging

Initial approach

- Radiography
  - Plain films of long bones, spine, and ribs
- MRI/CT
  - NF1 is associated with optic pathway gliomas and astrocytomas. Focal lesions of high signal intensity on T2-weighted MRI are also noted in cerebellar peduncles, basal ganglia, brainstem and optic radiations.
  - Spinal cord tumor, mediastinal mass, deep plexiform neurofibromas, pheochromocytoma
  - MRI using 3D volumetrics is the preferred method for following vestibular schwannoma growth for NF2 (1)[B]

Follow-up & special considerations

- Metaiodobenzylguanidine (MIBG) scintigraphy for pheochromocytoma if MRI/CT is not conclusive
- Positron emission tomography (PET) scan for tumor surveillance
- Gallium-67 scintigraphy for malignant large plexiform neurofibromas
- Electroencephalogram (EEG)

Diagnostic Procedures/Other

- **Neurofibromatosis Type 1**
  - Slit-lamp examination for Lisch nodules
- **Neurofibromatosis Type 2**
  - Dilated fundus examinations for inspection of juvenile cataracts or retinal lesions
  - Brainstem auditory-evoked response (BAER) for early hearing loss

Pathological Findings

- **Neurofibromatosis Type 1**
  - Neurofibromas are composed of well-differentiated tumors that contain spindle-shaped cells, Schwann cells, fibroblasts, and mast cells.
- **Neurofibromatosis Type 2**
  - Tumors of NF2 may consist of Schwann cells, glial cells, or meningeal cells.

DIFFERENTIAL DIAGNOSIS

- **Neurofibromatosis Type 1**
  - Brainstem gliomas
  - Cauda equina and conus medullaris syndromes
  - Low-grade astrocytoma
  - Meningioma
  - NF2
  - Spinal cord hemorrhage/infarction
  - Spinal epidural abscess
  - Legius syndrome (*SPRED1 gene* mutation)
  - McCune-Albright syndrome
- **Neurofibromatosis Type 2**
  - Brainstem gliomas
  - Ependymoma
  - Meningioma
  - NF1

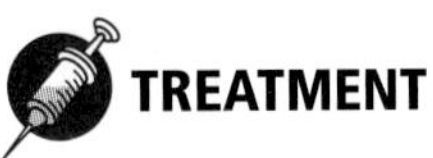

TREATMENT

MEDICATION

- Carboplatin and vincristine for optic nerve gliomas
- Under clinical study are therapeutic uses of erlotinib, bevacizumab, and imatinib mesylate for unresectable, progressive vestibular schwannomas
- Vitamin D supplementation
  - May be of benefit in patients with deficiency or osteopenia

ADDITIONAL TREATMENT

General Measures

- Cutaneous examination for documentation of new neurofibromas or progression of preexisting lesions
- Blood pressure monitoring

Issues for Referral

- Neurology – monitor changes in neurological status
- Ophthalmology – annual eye examinations for detection of optic nerve lesions, resection of orbital plexiform neurofibroma, slit-lamp examination, and dilated fundus examination
- Neurosurgery – resection of spinal cord or brain tumor
- Orthopedic – progressive scoliosis, pseudoarthrosis
- Plastic surgery – resection of neurofibromas
- Geneticist – family planning options and prenatal diagnosis

SURGERY/OTHER PROCEDURES

- **Neurofibromatosis Type 1**
  - Radiotherapy may be utilized in children over 5 years of age as an adjunct or as an alternative to surgery for optic nerve gliomas; however, is generally avoided due to an increased risk of secondary malignancy.
  - Surgical resection is reserved for large tumors causing mass effect or hydrocephalus and optic pathway gliomas confined to the orbit or optic nerve (2)[B].
- **Neurofibromatosis Type 2**
  - Surgical resection and stereotactic radiotherapy are the mainstay of treatment for vestibular schwannomas.
  - Single fraction radiosurgery for spinal cord schwannomas may be used in addition to surgery or as primary therapy.
  - TomoTherapy is able to treat a range of neoplasms using a single helical beam with 360 degrees of rotational radiation.

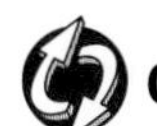

ONGOING CARE

PATIENT EDUCATION

Patients should be made aware of symptoms of worsening vision, tinnitus, hearing loss, or sensory changes that might suggest tumor growth.

PROGNOSIS

- **Neurofibromatosis Type 1**
  - NF1 has a better prognosis due to a lower incidence of CNS tumors than NF2.
  - Clinical manifestations often increase over time with a development in a malignancy or neurological deterioration often ensuing.
  - Due to the malignant transformation of diseased tissues or development of neurofibrosarcoma, patients have a higher mortality/morbidity than the general population. A reduction of life expectancy by up to 15 years may result.
  - 3–15% additional risk of malignant disease during lifetime.
- **Neurofibromatosis Type 2**
  - NF2 is associated with significant morbidity and decreased lifespan.
  - As the tumors themselves are relatively indolent, prompt diagnosis and treatment may improve life expectancy to more than 15 years following diagnosis.

COMPLICATIONS

- **Neurofibromatosis Type 1**
  - Visual loss secondary to optic nerve gliomas
  - Seizures, spinal cord tumors, scoliosis
- **Neurofibromatosis Type 2**
  - Visual loss from optic nerve meningiomas, cataracts, or combined hamartomas of the retina and RPE
  - Hearing loss, tinnitus, seizures

Pregnancy Considerations

- Increase in size of existing neurofibromas and the appearance of new neurofibromas occur commonly in women with NF1 during pregnancy.
- Neurofibromatosis during prenatal period may be diagnosed by:
  - Linkage analysis can track the *NF* genes in a family with multiple affected members to determine which chromosome the fetus received.
  - Gene sequencing to identify specific gene mutation in affected parent. This would permit prenatal diagnosis by amniocentesis or chorionic villus sampling.

REFERENCES

1. Harris GJ, Plotkin SR, Maccollin M, et al. Three-dimensional volumetrics for tracking vestibular schwannoma growth in neurofibromatosis type II. *Neurosurgery* 2008;62(6):1314–1319.
2. Nicolin G, Parkin P, Mabbott D, et al. Natural history and outcome of optic pathway gliomas in children. *Pediatr Blood Cancer* 2009;53(7): 1231–1237.

ADDITIONAL READING

- Lee HH, Lian SL, Huang CJ, et al. Tomotherapy for neurofibromatosis Type 2: Case report and review of literature. *Br J Radiol* 2010;83(988):e74–e78.
- Mukherjee J, Kamnasaran D, Balasubramaniam A, et al. Human schwannomas express activated platelet-derived growth factor receptors and c-kit and are inhibited by Gleevac (Imatinib Mesylate). *Cancer Research* 2009;69(12):5099–5107.
- Plotkin SR, Singh MA, O'Donnell CC, et al. Audiologic and radiographic response of NF2-related vestibular schwannoma to erlotinib therapy. *Nat Clin Pract Oncol* 2008;5(8):487–491.
- Plotkin SR, Stemmer-Rachamimov AO, Barker FG II, et al. Hearing improvement after bevacizumab in patients with neurofibromatosis type 2. *NEJM* 2009;361(4):358–367.

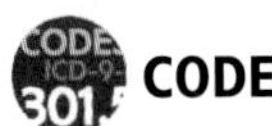

CODES

ICD9

- 216.1 Benign neoplasm of eyelid, including canthus
- 237.9 Neoplasm of uncertain behavior of other and unspecified parts of nervous system
- 237.70 Neurofibromatosis, unspecified

CLINICAL PEARLS

- Neurofibromatosis 1 and 2 are neurocutaneous genetic disorders diagnosed by specific clinical criteria.
- Remember the association between NF and optic nerve glioma, schwannoma, pheochromocytoma, and other tumors.

N

NEUROPROTECTION IN GLAUCOMA

M. Reza Razeghinejad
L. Jay Katz

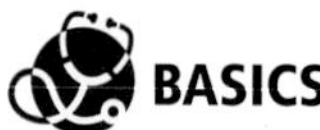

BASICS

DESCRIPTION

Neuroprotection is the use of therapeutic agents to prevent, retard, and in some instances, reverse retinal ganglion cells (RGCs) death in glaucomatous patients.

PATHOPHYSIOLOGY

IOP dependent RGCs loss

- Elevated IOP induces optic neuropathy by:
  - Mechanical theory, posterior bowing of lamina cribrosa, and damaging axon bundles passing through its pores
  - Vascular theory, low perfusion pressure, defined as the difference between systemic blood pressure and IOP
- IOP is no longer regarded as the only causative factor in glaucomatous optic neuropathy because some patients with elevated IOP never develop glaucoma, in normal tension, glaucoma IOP is within normal limit, and some patients continue to progress with controlled low IOP.

Non-IOP dependent RGCs loss

- Excitotoxicity
  - RGCs die by apoptosis (programmed cell death) because of the presence of excessive amounts of glutamate, an excitatory neurotransmitter.
  - Glutamates binds onto postsynaptic receptors, NMDA (N-methyl-d-aspartate) channels, and keeps them open for a long period of time, thereby allowing influx of $Ca2+$ and $Na+$ ions and initiating apoptosis.
- Mitochondrial dysfunction
  - Induced by glaucoma-related stimuli such as tumor necrosis factor and hypoxia
- Oxidative stress
  - Load of reactive oxygen species and lipid peroxides outweigh the antioxidant capacity of cells
- Inflammatory and autoimmune mechanisms
  - Complement system: Several components are upregulated.
  - Heat shock proteins
  - Under physiological conditions act as molecular chaperones and/or have anti-apoptotic activities.
  - Glaucomatous patients have antibodies against HSP.
  - TNF, as a mediator of RGC death is upregulated.
  - Nitric oxide: It is a gaseous second messenger and appears to have physiologic role in optic nerve function. Excessive production of nitric oxide in glaucoma leads to RGCs loss.

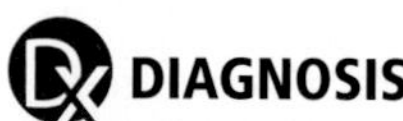

DIAGNOSIS

DIAGNOSTIC TESTS & INTERPRETATION

Imaging

- Establishing neuroprotective effect of drugs is difficult because glaucoma is a slow, progressive disease and the current method of measuring progression, a computerized visual field assessment, is highly variable.
- Optic nerve and nerve fiber layer analyzers (Optical Coherent Tomography, Scanning Laser Polarimetry, and Ophthalmoscopy) may lead to more meaningful assessment.
- Detection of apoptosing retinal cells (DARC), an in vivo method, may become a precise tool to assess the effect of neuroprotective agents.

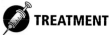

TREATMENT

MEDICATION

- To be deemed a neuroprotective agent should have 4 criteria: (1) Possessing receptors on the optic nerve or retina, (2) Adequate penetration into the vitreous and retina at pharmacologic levels, (3) Triggering intracellular signals that enhance neuronal resistance to apoptosis (4) Demonstration of efficacy in clinical trials.
- No neuroprotectant drug has ever been approved for an optic nerve disorder. Despite successful preclinical cell culture and animal model experiments, most of the phase 2 and virtually all of the phase 3 clinical trials of more than 100 neuroprotective drug candidates have failed to demonstrate efficacy and safety. Following are some of neuroprotectants that are categorized into 2 groups. Promoters of cell survival and inhibitors of cell death.
- **Inhibitors of cell death**
  - **Memantine,** a derivative of amantadine, which was used as an anti-influenza compound. As a NMDA receptor antagonist, is currently the only available clinical glutamate modifier (the first phase 3 trial did not confirm a neuroprotective effect).
  - **Nitric oxidesynthase inhibitors:** Had a neuroprotective effect in animal studies.
  - **Infrared light,** has metabolism-enhancing, antioxidant, and anti-apoptotic properties. A phase 0 clinical trial is currently announced to be in preparation.

- **Vitamin E,** scavenger of peroxyl radicals: Glaucoma patients receiving vitamin E have displayed improved visual fields in some studies.
- **Calciumchannel blockers:** In addition to anti-vasospastic effect, that is an important mechanism in optic nerve damage in some glaucoma patients (i.e., normal tension glaucoma), its topical form may reduce IOP.

• **Promoters of neuronal survival**
- **Brimonidine(α-2 agonist):** Its mechanism of action is similar to an NMDA channel blocker, MK-801. It also causes upregulation of BDNF (brain-derived neurotrophic factor) in the RGCs. Neuroprotective effect in experimental studies, but in clinical trials failed to translate into similar efficacy in humans.
- **Betaxolol(β1-blocker):** Alters excitotoxic/hypoxic pathway to exert its neuroprotective effect. No definite clinical proof for having neuroprotective effect.
- **ExtractGinkgo biloba**, an extract from leaves of Ginkgo biloba, has been effective in models of experimental glaucoma.
- **Neurotrophins,** Nerve growth factor (NGF) and brain-derived neurotrophic factor (BDNF), have been tested extensively in animal studies, both reduce RGCs death. They activate toxic pathways as well as neuroprotective ones.
- **Geranylgeraylacetone,** in animal studies, upregulated HSP-72 expression in RGCs and protected them from glaucomatous damage.
- **Cop-1 (glatiramer acetate; copolymer-1; copax-1):** FDA approved drug for multiple sclerosis. In animal studies, Cop-1 reduced optic nerve damage caused by mechanical injury or intravitreal glutamate injection.
- **Coenzyme Q10,** plays a crucial role in energy production by the mitochondrial electron transport chain. Topical CoQ10 has been effective in experimental glaucoma.

ADDITIONAL READING

- Bessero AC, Clarke PG. Neuroprotection for optic nerve disorders. *Curr Opin Neurol* 2010;23:10–15.
- Sena DF, Ramchand K, Lindsley K. Neuroprotection for treatment of glaucoma in adults. *Cochrane Database Syst Rev* 2010;2:CD006539.
- Cheung W, Guo L, Cordeiro MF. Neuroprotection in glaucoma: Drug-based approaches. *Optom Vis Sci* 2008;85:406–416

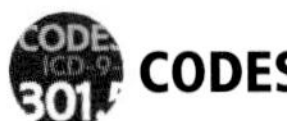

CODES

ICD9

- 365.9 Unspecified glaucoma
- 365.12 Low tension open-angle glaucoma

CLINICAL PEARLS

- No evidence that neuroprotective agents are effective in preventing retinal ganglion cell death, and thus preserving vision in patients with glaucoma has been demonstrated. Long-term randomized clinical trials with long-term follow-up are needed to determine if they may be beneficial in this regard.
- Memantine is the only neuroprotective agent assessed in randomized clinical trials (phase 3) without showing a neuroprotective effect compared to placebo-treated patients.

NEURORETINITIS

David B. Auerbach

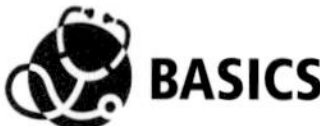

BASICS

DESCRIPTION

Neuroretinitis is a unilateral, or more rarely, bilateral inflammation of the optic nerve and retina with macular exudate formation and associated visual loss. Originally termed "Leber's idiopathic stellate Neuroretinitis," it is now known to have infectious etiologies. Although the most common association in the US is with cat scratch disease, various other causes need to be completely investigated as multiple infectious and inflammatory etiologies exist (1)[A].

EPIDEMIOLOGY

Incidence

- 6 per 100,000 secondary to cat scratch disease
- Cat exposure is seen in 90% of patients who are serology positive for *Bartonella henselae*.

Prevalence

- Exact prevalence remains unknown
- Affects all ages
- No sex predilection
- Right and left eyes equally affected

RISK FACTORS

- May follow a recent upper respiratory viral illness in up to 50% of cases
- Inquire about any recent exposure to cats
- Important to take a sexually transmitted disease history

GENERAL PREVENTION

As disease is idiopathic or secondary to infectious etiology, no general prevention is known.

PATHOPHYSIOLOGY

- Optic nerve edema
- Macular edema with star formation

ETIOLOGY

- Infectious or immune mediated
- May be viral in up to 50% of patients

COMMONLY ASSOCIATED CONDITIONS

Bartonella henselae infection

DIAGNOSIS

HISTORY

- Blurred vision. Visual acuity can range from 20/20 to light perception.
- Usually painless
- Flu-like symptoms
- Regional lymphadenopathy
- Ocular erythema
- Decreased visual field

PHYSICAL EXAM

- Optic disc edema (if bilateral, may be papilledema and neuroimaging and LP may be needed to rule out compressive lesion and/or elevated intracranial pressure).
- Macular star formation (usually starts to appear 2–4 weeks after visual symptoms)
- Regional lymphadenopathy
- Afferent pupillary defect
- Visual field defect (most common is cecocentral, however, arcuate and altitudinal defects can be seen)
- Acquired dyschromatopsia
- Small chorioretinal lesions

DIAGNOSTIC TESTS & INTERPRETATION

Lab

- MRI brain and orbits with and without gadolinium
- *Bartonella henselae* titer
- CBC
- ESR
- ANA
- ACE
- RPR
- Lyme titer
- HIV
- Toxoplasmosis
- Toxocariasis
- Hepatitis B & C antibodies
- Brucellosis
- Epstein Barr titers
- TB skin test
- Leptospirosis

Imaging

Initial approach

- Visual field with central or cecocentral defect
- Fluorescein angiogram shows leakage of disc vessels and late disc staining
- MRI brain and orbits to rule out a compressive lesion

Follow-up & special considerations

Macular exudates usually resolve within a few months but may be present for up to a year.

DIFFERENTIAL DIAGNOSIS
- Cat scratch disease
- Lyme disease
- Lupus
- Sarcoidosis
- Syphilis
- Toxoplasmosis
- Toxocariasis
- Hypertensive retinopathy
- Tuberculosis
- Pseudotumor Cerebri
- Leukemia
- HIV

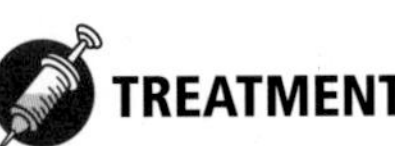

TREATMENT

MEDICATION
First Line
- Continues to be controversial. Usually a benign self-limited condition. Medical therapies may shorten the recovery time.
- All immunocompromised individuals should be treated (A)[2].
- Treat accordingly if any serologic tests are positive.

Second Line
- Doxycycline (3)[A]
- Rifampin
- Azithromycin
- Ciprofloxacin
- Trimethoprim-sulfamethoxazole

ADDITIONAL TREATMENT
Issues for Referral
- Should be evaluated by an ophthalmologist
- Consider neuroophthalmologist and/or retinal specialist.

IN-PATIENT CONSIDERATIONS
Admission Criteria
Treated as an outpatient

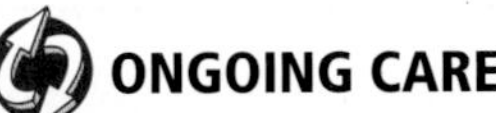

ONGOING CARE

FOLLOW-UP RECOMMENDATIONS
Patient should be seen every 2 weeks for the first 2 months to assess any change in visual function (visual acuity, visual field, color vision, and any change in optic nerve and/or retinal edema)

DIET
Regular diet

PATIENT EDUCATION
If patient is Bartonella positive, education regarding cat handling should be suggested.

PROGNOSIS
- Self-limited in immunocompetent individuals
- Good prognosis

COMPLICATIONS
- Permanent decrease in visual acuity and visual field
- Optic atrophy
- Metamorphopsia
- Dyschromatopsia

REFERENCES

1. Williams N, Miller NR. Neuroretinitis. In: Pepose JS, Holland GN, Wilhelmus KR, editors. *Ocular infection and immunity.* St Louis: Mosby Year Book, 1996:601–608.
2. Cunningham ET, Koehler JE. Ocular bartonellosis. *Am J Ophthal* 2000;130(3):340–349.
3. Ray S, Gragoudas E. Neuroretinitis. *Int Ophthalmol Clin* 2001:41(1):83–102.

ADDITIONAL READING

- Reynolds MG, Holman RC, Curns AT, et al. Epidemiology of cat-scratch disease hospitalizations among children in the United States. *Pediatr Infect Dis J* 2005;24(8):700–704.
- Rost Monahan S. Neuroretinitis: A clinical syndrome of cat-scratch disease. *Clin Eye Vis Care* 2000: 12(3–4):155–159.

CODES

ICD9
- 078.3 Cat-scratch disease
- 363.05 Focal retinitis and retinochoroiditis, juxtapapillary

CLINICAL PEARLS
- No association with multiple sclerosis
- If suspected cat-scratch disease, treat empirically as titers may take about 4–6 weeks to seroconvert.

N

NON-ARTERITIC ANTERIOR ISCHEMIC OPTIC NEUROPATHY (NAION)

Robert J. Granadier

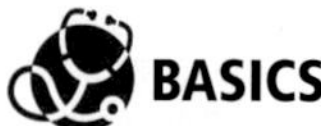

BASICS

DESCRIPTION

Sudden, painless, unilateral visual loss, associated with swelling of the optic disc secondary to vascular insufficiency.

EPIDEMIOLOGY

Incidence

2–10 individuals per 100,000 over 50 years old

Prevalence

1,500–6,000 new cases per year in the US.

RISK FACTORS

- Small vessel disease (1)[B]
- Hypertension
- Diabetes
  - Hypercholesterolemia
  - Migraine
  - Sleep apnea
  - Hypoperfusion
  - Amiodarone
  - Erectile dysfunction medication (unproven)

Genetics

None recognized.

GENERAL PREVENTION

Recommended: Patients who have suffered NAION in one eye should control risk factors and be cautioned in regard to potential nocturnal or anesthesia related hypotension/hypo-perfusion.

PATHOPHYSIOLOGY

Ischemia secondary to vascular insufficiency related to small vessel perfusion at the optic nerve head. (Indirect evidence, no causative factor in a pathologic specimen identified to date).

ETIOLOGY

Anatomic theory: Condition noted to be associated with small, crowded optic disc with small cup to disc ration in fellow eye (so called disc at risk).

COMMONLY ASSOCIATED CONDITIONS

- Diabetes
- Hypertension
- Migraine

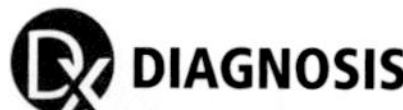

DIAGNOSIS

HISTORY

- Sudden, painless, unilateral vision loss
- Often noted upon awakening

PHYSICAL EXAM

- Decreased visual acuity
- Reduced color vision
- Sluggish pupil with afferent pupillary defect
- Visual field deficit (altitudinal)
- Optic disc edema, segmental with peri-papillary intra-retinal hemorrhage
- Crowded optic disc in fellow eye with small cup to disc ratio, (disc at risk)

ALERT

Must distinguish from arteritic form of ischemic optic neuropathy secondary to giant cell arteritis, because if left untreated, there is a 70% incidence of the second eye being involved within 10–14 days, resulting in bilateral visual loss.

DIAGNOSTIC TESTS & INTERPRETATION

Diagnostic Procedures/Other

- Visual fields: Static or kinetic
- Most frequent visual field defect is an altitudinal loss of the inferior or superior field

Pathological Findings

Ischemic infarction of the retro-laminar optic nerve.

DIFFERENTIAL DIAGNOSIS

- Arteritic anterior ischemic optic neuropathy secondary to GCA, see Alert.
  - Optic neuritis with optic disc swelling
  - Papillophlebitis
  - Amiodarone optic neuropathy

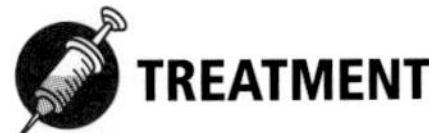

TREATMENT

MEDICATION

None proven.

ADDITIONAL TREATMENT

General Measures

- Blood pressure
- Blood sugar

Issues for Referral

Refer to Internist for general medical evaluation with attention to potential vasculopathic risk factors (2)[B].

Additional Therapies

Prophylactic ASA studied: Unproven (2)[C]

COMPLEMENTARY & ALTERNATIVE THERAPIES

- Anti-Coagulation Studied: Unproven (2)[A]
- Steroids: Studied: Unproven (2)[B]
- Hyperbaric Oxygen: Studied: Unproven (2)[B]

SURGERY/OTHER PROCEDURES

Optic nerve sheath decompression: potentially harmful (3)[A]

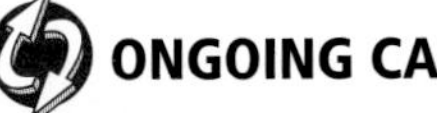

ONGOING CARE

FOLLOW-UP RECOMMENDATIONS

- 1 week, 1 month, 3 months.
- Disc edema resolves over 6–10 weeks.

Patient Monitoring

Uncommon: 24-hour blood pressure monitoring, in individual cases when hypotension is of concern.

PATIENT EDUCATION

Educate patients with respect to general health considerations, and potential risk factors related to individual cases (i.e., erectile dysfunction medication, obstructive sleep apnea).

PROGNOSIS

- Stable visual loss likely in 80–85 %
- Spontaneous recovery of 3 lines of visual acuity approximately 15–20% (3)[A] as high as over 40%. (4)[B]
- Fellow eye risk 15% over 5 years in patients over 50 years. (3)[A]
- Risk moderately increased in younger patients.

REFERENCES

1. Arnold AC. Pathogenesis of nonarteritic anterior ischemic optic neuropathy. *J Neuroophthalmol* 2003; 23(2): 157–163.
2. Atkins EJ, Bruce BB, Newman NJ, et al. Treatment of nonarteritic anterior ischemic optic neuropathy. *Surv Ophthalmol* 2010; 55(1): 47–63.
3. Optic Nerve decompression surgery for nonarteritic anterior ischemic optic neuropathy (NAION) is not effective and may be harmful. The Ischemic Optic NeuropathyDecompression Trial Research Group. *JAMA* 1995; 273(8): 625–632.
4. Hayreh SS. Ischemic optic neuropathy. *Prog Retin Eye Res* 2009; 28(1): 34–62.

ADDITIONAL READING

- Arnold AC. In Miller NR, Newman NJ, Biousse V, et al. Clinical Neuro-Ophthalmology, Ischemic Optic Neuropathy. Vol. 1Philadelphia PA, Lippincott, Williams & Wilkins, ed 6, 2005, 349–384.

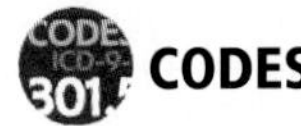

CODES

ICD9

- 377.00 Papilledema, unspecified
- 377.30 Optic neuritis, unspecified
- 377.41 Ischemic optic neuropathy

CLINICAL PEARLS

- Anterior ischemic optic neuropathy should be accompanied by swelling of the visible portion of the intraocular optic nerve or the optic disc. Absence of associated disc swelling should cause one to seek an alternate diagnosis.
- Afferent pupillary defect in the eye of concern may be absent in cases in which the fellow eye has previously sustained optic nerve damage.
- Foster-Kennedy Syndrome: Skull based tumor obstructing the foramen of Monroe must be suspected in patients presenting with optic disc swelling in one eye and optic atrophy in the fellow eye. Once a tumor has been ruled out, the more common diagnosis of pseudo Foster-Kennedy syndrome secondary to remote NAION in the fellow eye and acute NAION in the affected eye may be considered.

NON-GRANULOMATOUS ANTERIOR UVEITIS

Nicole R. Fram
Eliza Hoskins

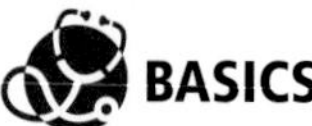

BASICS

DESCRIPTION

- Non-granulomatous anterior uveitis (NGAU) is a broad classification for various inflammatory conditions localized to the iris (iritis), ciliary body (cyclitis), or both (iridocyclitis) that typically present with pain, redness, and photophobia.
  - Etiologies can be infectious or immune-mediated
  - Systemic involvement or isolated to the eye
  - NGAU is characterized by small punctate or stellate keratic precipitates (KP) versus granulomatous anterior uveitis with large greasy mutton fat KP with iris nodules or choroidal granulomas.

EPIDEMIOLOGY

Incidence

- 8–17 cases per 100,000 population (1,2)
- HLA-B27 more common in Caucasian males
- Behçet's disease is more common in Asian and Middle- Eastern males
- Juvenile idiopathic arthritis (JIA) more common in females.

RISK FACTORS

- Trauma
- Genetic predisposition (HLA-B27, HLA-B51)
- Smoking (3)

Genetics

- HLA-B27 (ankylosing spondylitis (AS)), reactive arthritis (formerly Reiter's syndrome), inflammatory bowel disease (IBD), psoriatic arthropathy
- HLA-B51 (Behçet's disease)

GENERAL PREVENTION

No prevention of idiopathic NGAU.

ETIOLOGY

- Idiopathic (50%)
- 30% AS patients have NGAU

COMMONLY ASSOCIATED CONDITIONS

See Review of Systems (ROS).

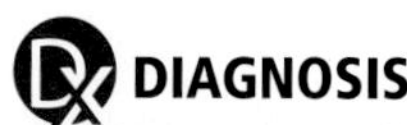

DIAGNOSIS

HISTORY

Targeted history onset, duration, location, quality of symptoms, and associated conditions. Clinical course (acute, chronic, or recurrent) laterality and previous treatments/trauma.

- Standardization of uveitis nomenclature (SUN) (4)
  - Acute: Sudden onset with limited duration.
  - Recurrent: Repeat episodes separated by periods of inactivity without treatment >3 months in duration
  - Chronic: Persistent uveitis with relapse <3 months after discontinuing treatment
- Past medical, social, and family history
  - Infectious disease exposure
  - Autoimmune/Rheumatologic disease
  - STDs/IVDU
  - Medications: Rifabutin, Cidofovir, Prostaglandins
  - Pets: Cats-Toxoplasmosis, puppies-Toxocariasis
  - Family history: HLA-B27
- Review of systems (ROS):
  - Constitutional: Fever, night sweats, chills (Infectious-endogenous endophthalmitis, tuberculosis), weight loss (malignancy)
  - Skin/mucocutaneous: Erythema nodosum (IBD, Behçet's, sarcoid) erythema chronicum migrans (Lyme), polyarteritis nodosa (PAN), aphthous/oral ulcers (Behçet's, herpetic), scaling lesions (psoriasis, reactive arthritis), vitiligo, (Vogt Koyanagi Harada (VKH))
  - Musculoskeletal: Sacroiliitis (ankylosing spondylitis, reactive arthritis, IBD); Monoarticular/pauciarticular arthritis (JIA), fasciitis/tendonitis (reactive arthritis)
  - Respiratory: Asthma, wheezing, shortness of breath, cough (sarcoid, TB, coccidioidomycosis), sinus, and pulmonary disease (Wegener's granulomatosis)
  - Cardiovascular: Pericarditis (reactive arthritis, Lyme), thrombophlebitis (Behçet's), AV block (Lyme)
  - Gastrointestinal: Diarrhea (IBD, reactive arthritis)
  - Genitourinary: Urethritis/circinate balanitis (reactive arthritis, syphilis), epididymitis (reactive arthritis, Behçet's), genital sores/ulcers (syphilis, reactive arthritis, HSV, Behçet), urinary incontinence (Multiple sclerosis (MS)), elevated creatinine, abnormal urinalysis (Tubulointerstitial nephritis and uveitis syndrome (TINU))
  - Hematological: anemia/elevated ESR (TINU)
  - Neurologic: Meningitis (Behçet's, Lyme, sarcoid, VKH), cranial nerve palsies (sarcoid, lyme, lymphoma, MS)

PHYSICAL EXAM

- External: Skin, joints, oral cavity, lymph nodes, neurologic, genitourinary
- Pupils: Irregular/secluded pupil (posterior synechiae), miotic and/or accommodate but don't react to light (syphilis-Argyll Robertson pupil)
- Intraocular pressure:
  - Acute increased IOP: Herpetic (trabeculitis), Fuchs' heterochromic iridocyclitis, Glaucomatocyclitic crisis
- Gonioscopy: Peripheral anterior synechiae (PAS), KP, abnormal angle vessels-"Amsler sign" (Fuchs')
- Eyelids/lashes: Vesicles (HSV), vitiligo (VKH), poliosis (white eyelashes) (VKH)
- Conjunctiva/Sclera: Circumferential ciliary flush, granulomas (sarcoid, TB), papillo-follicular conjunctivitis (reactive arthritis or Reiter's Syndrome) conjunctival dendrites (herpetic), episcleritis/scleritis (IBD, RA, SLE, Wegener's)
- Cornea: Decreased corneal sensation (herpetic), diffuse-stellate KP (Fuchs', herpetic), band keratopathy (JIA, chronic uveitis), stromal edema (herpetic), peripheral ulcerative keratitis (Rheumatoid arthritis (RA), IBD, systemic lupus erythematosus (SLE), Wegener's, PAN)
- Iris/anterior chamber/angle: Posterior synechiae, pupillary membranes, iris nodules (sarcoid-Koeppe-pupillary margin, Busacca-throughout iris), transilluminatory defects (TID's)/atrophic iris (herpetic, UGH), heterochromia (Fuchs'), hypopyon (HLA-B27, Behçet's, Retinoblastoma (Rb), infectious), hyphema (Herpetic, Fuchs', juvenile xanthogranuloma (JXG), Rb, neovascularization of the iris/angle, leukemia)
- Anterior chamber reaction: Grading cell/flare: SUN (1 x1 mm^2 slit beam) (4)
  - Grade 0 (<1 cells)/complete absence
  - Grade 0.5+ (1 – 5 cells)/n/a
  - Grade 1+ (6–15 cells)/Faint
  - Grade 2+ (16–25 cells)/Moderate (iris & lens clear)
  - Grade 3+ (26–50 cells)/Marked (iris & lens hazy)
  - Grade 4+ (>50 cells)/Intense (fibrin, plastic aqueous
- Lens/anterior vitreous: Lenticular precipitates, posterior subcapsular cataracts (chronic inflammation and topical/oral steroids), haptic induced TID's (UGH), retained lens fragment, cyclitic membrane
- Dilated fundus examination: Vitreitis, snowballs, snowbanking (MS), cystoid macular edema (CME), vasculitis (Behçet's), Toxoplasmosis scars, retinal necrosis/whitening (herpetic, acute retinal necrosis (ARN)), choroidal infiltrates (sarcoid, Birdshot, VKH, Dalen-Fuchs' nodules), intraocular foreign body

DIAGNOSTIC TESTS & INTERPRETATION

Lab

Initial lab tests

Workup indicated if bilateral, severe, recurrent/nonresponsive to treatment or guided by History/ROS:

- RPR, FTA-ABS, CXR, ACE, HLA-B27, PPD (or quantiferon if vaccinated), Lyme Ab
  - Target labs according to ROS and anatomic location of inflammation (anterior, intermediate, posterior, panuveitis)
  - Consider ANA, rheumatoid factor if JIA is suspected: Girls: ANA +, RF- and pauciarticular; Boys: HLA-B27+, ANA-, RF-
  - Consider ANCAs, ESR, CRP if associated scleritis and/or peripheral ulcerative keratitis Wegener's/polyarteritis nodosa (PAN), rash (PAN), pulmonary/sinus disease (Wegener's)
  - Consider urinalysis for β_2 microglobulin level, renal biopsy if suspect TINU

Follow-Up & Special Considerations

- Glaucoma
  - Angle closure glaucoma (PAS)
  - Pupillary Block glaucoma (Secluded pupil)
  - Elevated IOP: Steroid induced glaucoma
- Posterior subcapsular cataract
- Cystoid macular edema (CME)

Imaging

- CXR (Sarcoid, TB)
  - Consider CT-chest, pulmonary function tests
- X-ray-sacroiliac joints (HLA-B27, ankylosing spondylitis)
- B scan if there is no view to posterior pole
- Fluorescein angiogram (CME, vasculitis, retinal/choroidal infiltrates)
- OCT for CME monitoring

Diagnostic Procedures/Other

- Anterior chamber/vitreous tap: PCR: herpetic or toxoplasmosis-correlate with serology, Cytology: lymphoma or leukemia
- Conjunctival biopsy (caseating vs. non-caseating granulomas)

Pathological Findings

- Small/medium KP: Neutrophils and lymphocytes
- Large (mutton fat) KP: Macrophages granulomatous
  - Note: Granulomatous disease can present with small/medium KP.

DIFFERENTIAL DIAGNOSIS

- HLA-B27
  - Ankylosing spondylitis
  - Psoriatic arthropathy
  - Inflammatory bowel disease (IBD)
  - Postinfectious, or reactive arthritis (formerly Reiter's syndrome)
- Juvenile idiopathic (rheumatoid) arthritis (JIA)
- Herpetic disease
  - Herpes Simplex virus
  - Varicella Zoster virus
  - Cytomegalovirus
- Glaucomatocyclitic crisis (Posner-Schlossman syndrome)
- Fuchs' heterochromic iridocyclitis
- Behçet's disease
- Tubulointerstitial nephritis and uveitis syndrome (TINU)
- Traumatic iritis
- Lens-associated uveitis
  - Phacolytic
- IOL-associated uveitis: Uveitis, glaucoma, hyphema (UGH)
- Drug induced uveitis
- Lymphoma
- Idiopathic uveitis

NOTE: Syphilis, sarcoidosis, tuberculosis (TB), VKH, and Lyme disease are in the differential diagnosis, but are classified as granulomatous.

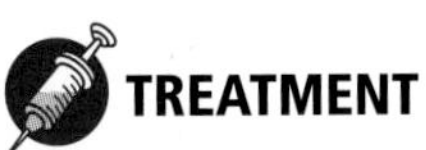

TREATMENT

MEDICATION

First Line

- Topical steroids
  - Prednisolone acetate 1% q 1–2 hour during first week and slowly taper over 4–6 weeks.
  - Difluprednate 0.05% (Durezol) q.i.d = Prednisolone acetate 1% q2h
- Topical cycloplegics (ciliary spasm, prevention of posterior synechiae)
  - Homatropine 5% b.i.d–t.i.d
- Sub-tenons steroid injection for chronic uveitis and/or CME. Consider short-acting prep such as dexamethasone phosphate if steroid response is a concern.
- Oral antiviral if herpetic disease suspected

Second Line

- Oral prednisone (1 mg/kg/d) (max 60–80 mg) do not continue at high dose >1 month. If there is no response after 2–4 weeks or fails a slow taper, steroid sparing immunosuppressive should be considered.
- Calcium 1500 mg and Vitamin D 800 IU (bone density prophylaxis)
- H_2 Blockers (GI prophylaxis)

ALERT

Counsel patients about 1) Cushingoid changes with oral prednisone >5–10 mg/d. 2) Dangers of abrupt discontinuation after adrenal glands have been suppressed. 3) Blood pressure, blood glucose, and cholesterol monitoring every 3 months. 4) Bone mineral density testing if on oral steroids >3 months, then annually. Risk of aseptic necrosis of bone 10–15% if on 60 mg in first month and >20 mg for first 6 months. 5) Children <15 years may have delayed pubertal growth (5).

- Steroid-sparing immunosuppressives if chronic and cannot taper systemic prednisone <10 mg without flare. Rheumatology consult.
  - Antimetabolites: Azathioprine (Imuran), Methotrexate, Mycophenolate mofetil (CellCept)
  - T cell inhibitor: Cyclosporine
  - Biologics (TNF-alpha inhibitors) particularly useful in Ankylosing spondylitis, Behçet's, JIA, or recalcitrant disease

Patients on antimetabolites should be monitored for bone marrow suppression, liver function, and pulmonary function q 3–6 weeks. Patients on cyclosporine should be monitored for nephrotoxicity and hypertension q 3–6 weeks (5). Patients on biologics should be monitored for malignancy, auto-antibodies, sepsis, and infection q 3–6 weeks.

ADDITIONAL TREATMENT

Issues for Referral

- Rheumatology consult (HLA-B27, JIA)
- Gastrointestinal consult (IBD)
- Pulmonary consult (Sarcoid)
- Retina consult (CME, vasculitis, retinal/choroidal infiltrates)
- Glaucoma consult (uncontrolled glaucoma)

SURGERY/OTHER PROCEDURES

- Fluocinolone acetonide intravitreal implant (Retisert) for recalcitrant disease despite maximal oral and topical therapy. (Watch IOP, contraindicated in herpetic disease)
- Filtering procedure for uncontrolled glaucoma

ONGOING CARE

FOLLOW-UP RECOMMENDATIONS

- Weekly exams until AC reaction is controlled and topical steroids are tapered to q.i.d or less.
- If patient is on steroid or steroid-sparing immunosuppressives q 3–6 week, laboratory evaluation. See alerts.

Patient Monitoring

- Intraocular pressure
- Cataract: Special considerations for cataract extraction includes short course of preoperative oral prednisone and intraoperative methylprednisolone.

PROGNOSIS

Depends on etiology and comorbid conditions.

COMPLICATIONS

- Glaucoma: Chronic angle closure, steroid induced glaucoma
- Acceleration of cataract development
- Chronic CME

REFERENCES

1. Darrell RW, Wagener HP, Kurland LT. Epidemiology of uveitis, incidence and prevalence in a small urban community. *Arch Ophthalmology* 1964;68:502–514. [A]
2. London NJ, Rathinam SR, Cunningham ET Jr. The epidemiology of uveitis in developing countries. *Int Ophthalmol Clin* 2010;50(2):1–17. [A]
3. Lin P, Margolis TP, Acharya NR. Cigarette smoking as a risk factor for uveitis. *Ophthalmology* 2010;117(3):585–590. [B]
4. Standardization of Uvelitis Nomenclature (SUN) Working Group. Standardization of uveitis nomenclature for reporting clinical data. Results of the first international workshop. *Am J Ophthalmol* 2005;140:509–516. [A]
5. Jabs DA, Rosenbaum JT, Foster CS, et al. Guidelines for the use of immunosuppressive drugs in patients with ocular inflammation disorders: Recommendations of an expert panel. *Am J Ophthalmol* 2000;130(4):492–513. [A]

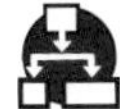

See Also (Topic, Algorithm, Electronic Media Element)

- Granulomatous uveitis
- Intermediate uveitis
- Posterior uveitis

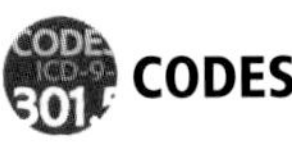

CODES

ICD9

364.00 Acute and subacute iridocyclitis, unspecified

CLINICAL PEARLS

- Uveitis with high IOP: Acute: HSV, VZV, Glaucomatocyclitic crisis, Fuchs' Heterochromia. Chronic: Sarcoid, Toxoplasmosis, TB (PAS related), Schwartz's Disease (Chronic RD), Steroid response
- Uveitis with diffuse KP: Fuchs' Heterochromic iridocyclitis, HSV, VZV, toxoplasmosis
- Uveitis with hypopyon: HLA-B27, Behçet's, JIA, endogenous endophthalmitis

N

NON-PHYSIOLOGIC VISION LOSS

Saunders L. Hupp

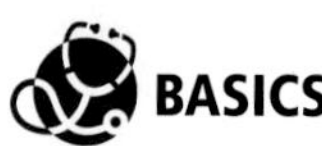

BASICS

DESCRIPTION

- Vision loss in the absence of contributory ocular or neurologic pathology
  - Multiple labels
    - Functional
    - Hysterical
    - Psychosomatic
    - Conversion reaction
    - Munchausen's syndrome
  - May be psychogenic or the result of malingering
    - Malingering symptoms are consciously and voluntarily produced

EPIDEMIOLOGY

Prevalence

- 1–5% of visual problems seen by ophthalmologist 1A, 2A
- Decreased visual acuity most common
  - Most prevalent in children and young adults
  - Psychogenic more common in children and young adults
    - Females > Males
  - Malingerers most often adult males

RISK FACTORS

- Conflict
- Stress
- Anxiety
- Depression
- Secondary gain
- Psychiatric syndrome

PATHOPHYSIOLOGY

- Acuity and visual field decrease
- Ocular motility
  - Spasm of near reflex
  - Convergence insufficiency
  - Horizontal or vertical gaze paralysis
  - Nystagmus
    - Horizontal, vertical, torsional
    - Random saccadic bursts
- Pupil size and reactivity
  - Dilation and tonicity
- Eyelid position
  - Pseudoptosis and blepharospasm
- Corneal and facial sensation
  - Relative anesthesia or hypersensitivity

ETIOLOGY

See Risk Factors 2A

COMMONLY ASSOCIATED CONDITIONS

- See Risk Factors
- Psychiatric syndromes affect approximately one-third patients 2A, 3A
  - Conversion reaction
  - Depression
  - Hypochondriasis
  - Body dysmorphic disorder
  - Somatization disorder

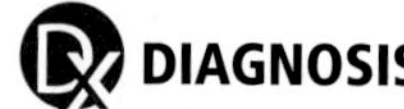

DIAGNOSIS

HISTORY

- Nature of complaint
- Degree of disability
- Affect
- Attitude toward care givers
- Degree of concern toward problem
- Determine motivation for symptoms

PHYSICAL EXAM

- Loss of visual acuity
  - Binocular or monocular
- Loss of visual field
  - Nonspecific constriction most common
  - Central scotomas
  - All types of hemianopias
- Monocular diplopia
  - Not explained by refraction, corneal, or lenticular pathology
  - Images are often equal and separate
- Voluntary nystagmus
  - Rapid to-and-fro movements only able to be sustained for seconds without rest
  - Able to be produced by 5–8% of normal population and may be familial
  - Usually horizontal, but vertical and torsional reported
  - Eyelids open or closed
  - Rarely monocular
  - May occur during normal visual tracking
  - Resemble ocular flutter or opsoclonus but no neurologic pathology
- Convergence loss
  - Often seen with loss of accommodation
- Spasm of the near reflex
  - Convergence, accommodation, and miosis
  - Limitation of abduction

DIAGNOSTIC TESTS & INTERPRETATION

Lab

- Acuity
  - Acuity starting with smallest line
  - Near acuity
  - OKN Drum
  - Mirror test
- Eyes follow tilting mirror
  - Prism dissociation test
- Visual field
  - Goldmann or Tangent Screen
    - Crossing Isopters
    - Target Visual Field 4A
  - Automated
  - Observation
    - Ambulatory ability not consistent with test results

Imaging

Initial approach

- Indicated when acuity not correctable or visual field loss is reproducible
- MRI

Follow-up & special considerations

- Image areas responsible for symptoms
- Functional overlay
  - Present in almost 10% 5A, 6A
  - Symptoms out of proportion to organic pathology

Diagnostic Procedures/Other

- Multi focal ERG 1A
- Visual Evoked Potential 6A

DIFFERENTIAL DIAGNOSIS

- Always consider early or subtle organic disease
  - Macular dystrophies
  - Retinopathy
  - Acute zonal occult outer retinopathy
  - Leber's hereditary optic neuropathy
  - Optic neuritis
  - Paraneoplastic optic neuropathy
  - Occipital epilepsy
  - Atypical migraine aura
  - Infarction, inflammation, or mass lesion

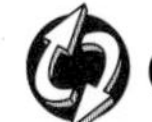

TREATMENT

ADDITIONAL TREATMENT

General Measures

- Reassurance and compassion
- Review exam in a positive manner with patient and family
  - Do not confront suspected malingerer

Issues for Referral

Suspicion of suicide or physical harm to patient or others

Additional Therapies

Psychotherapy

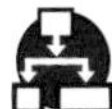

ONGOING CARE

FOLLOW-UP RECOMMENDATIONS

Reevaluate symptoms if persistent or increasing

PROGNOSIS

Resolution occurs in over 50%

REFERENCES

1. Chen CS, Lee AW, Karagiannis A, et al. Practical clinical approaches to functional visual loss. *J Clin Neurosci* 2005;14(1):1–7.
2. Lim SU, Siatkowski RM, Farris BK. Functional visual loss in adults and children. *Opthalmology* 2005;112(10):1821–1828.
3. Taich A, Crowe S, Kosmorsky GS, et al. Prevalence of psychosocial disturbances in children with nonorganic visual loss. *J AAPOS* 2004;8(5): 457–461.
4. Hsu JL, Harley CM, Foroozam R. Target visual field: A technique to rapidly demonstrate nonorganic visual field constriction. *Arch Opthalmol* 2010;128(9):1220–1222.
5. Digre KB, Nakamato BK, Warner JEA, Langeberg WJ, Baggaley SK, Katz BJ: A comparison of idiopathic intracranial hypertension with and without papilledema. *Headache* 2009;49:185–193.
6. Suppiej A, Gaspa G, Cappellari A, et al. The role of visual evoked potentials in the differential diagnosis of functional visual loss and optic neuritis in children. *J Child Neurol* 2011;26(1):58–64.

ADDITIONAL READING

- Slavin ML. The prism dissociation test in detecting unilateral functional vision loss. *J Clin Neuroopthalmol* 1990;10(2):127–130.
- Kathol RG, Cox TA, Corbett JJ, et al. Functional visual loss: I. A true psychiatric disorder? *Psychol Med* 1983;13(2):307–314.
- Beatty S. Non-organic visual loss. *Postgrad Med* 1999;75:201–207.

See Also (Topic, Algorithm, Electronic Media Element)

This is a must for anyone interested in this topic: J Lawton Smith Lecture http://content.lib.utah.edu/cdm4/item_viewer.php?CISOROOT=/EHSL_Lawton_Smith&CISOPTR=153&CISOBOX=1&REC=1

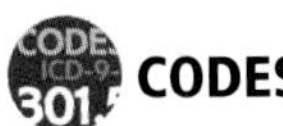

CODES

ICD9

- 369.9 Unspecified visual loss
- 378.83 Convergence insufficiency or palsy
- 379.50 Nystagmus, unspecified

CLINICAL PEARLS

- Watch the patient entering the exam room and navigating around obstacles (stool, phoropter, etc.)

N

NORMAL TENSION GLAUCOMA

Tak Yee Tania Tai
George L. Spaeth

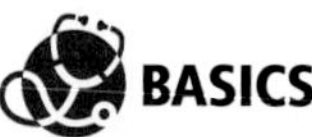

BASICS

DESCRIPTION

Normal tension glaucoma (NTG) is used to describe glaucomatous damage with statistically normal intraocular pressure (IOP).

EPIDEMIOLOGY

Incidence

- There is wide discrepancy in the literature regarding prevalence and incidence of NTG due to inconsistent definitions of the disease, different methods of evaluation of the optic nerve and visual field, and different populations studied.
- NTG is likely an under-reported condition.
- The incidence of chronic open angle glaucoma (COAG) was estimated to be: 0.24% per year in Dalby, Sweden, 0.1% per year in Melbourne, Australia, and 0.55% per year in Barbados.
- NTG accounts for 40–75% of patients with newly diagnosed COAG (1)[B].

Prevalence

- In the Baltimore Eye Survey, prevalence of COAG was: African–Americans 1.23% (40–49 years old) and 11.26% (80 years or older); Caucasians 0.92% and 2.16%, respectively.
  - 16.7% of glaucomatous eyes never had a recorded IOP exceeding 21 mm Hg.
- In 7 regions throughout Japan, the prevalence of NTG in patients older than 40 years is ~2.04%. (2)[B]

RISK FACTORS

- Migraine
- Female gender (3)[A]

Genetics

- The following genes have been reported as causative for NTG; however, the associations between these genes and NTG are either weak, or often not replicated in other populations (4)[B]:
  - Apolipoprotein E
  - Optic atrophy 1
  - Optineurin (associated with a significant fraction of autosomal dominant, NTG cases)
- Other unknown genetic factors likely play a role in the development of NTG.

GENERAL PREVENTION

There is no known prevention of NTG prior to manifestations of the disease.

PATHOPHYSIOLOGY

Retinal ganglion cell damage and death leads to decrease in visual function in patients with glaucoma.

ETIOLOGY

- Intraocular pressure:
  - Studies have shown a significant influence of IOP on the progression of visual field or neuroretinal rim damage.
  - In the Collaborative Normal Tension Glaucoma Study, IOP reduction of at least 30% is significantly associated with protection of visual field and nerve status compared to untreated patients (~20% of treated eyes and ~40% of untreated eyes had glaucomatous progression within 3 years).
- Ocular vascular abnormalities:
  - Drance described 2 forms of NTG – a nonprogressive form perhaps associated with transient vascular compromise, and a more common progressive form possibly due to chronic vascular insufficiency of the optic nerve head (1)[B].

COMMONLY ASSOCIATED CONDITIONS

- Migraine headaches
- Raynaud's phenomenon
- Sleep apnea (1)[B]

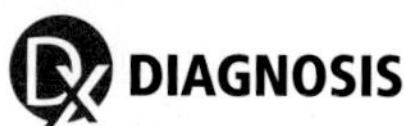

DIAGNOSIS

HISTORY

- Presence, onset, and nature of visual disturbance
- Systemic vascular risk factors such as diabetes and hypertension
- History of ocular trauma or surgeries
- Family history of glaucoma or other optic neuropathies
- Neurological disturbances such as headaches, dizziness, and weakness of extremities

PHYSICAL EXAM

- Check for an afferent pupillary defect.
- Slit-lamp examination of the anterior segment to check for signs of secondary glaucoma, such as iris transillumination defects, pseudoexfoliation material, anterior chamber cell or flare, and signs of prior surgery or trauma
- Gonioscopy
- Direct and indirect stereoscopic slit-lamp biomicroscopy to evaluate the optic nerve head, paying particular attention to:
  - Narrowing of the neuroretinal rim width (relatively narrow rim inferotemporally or superotemporally can indicate glaucomatous damage)
  - Asymmetry in disc cupping
  - Optic disc hemorrhage
  - Optic nerve color
  - Beta zone parapapillary atrophy
  - Loss of retinal nerve fiber layer
  - Acquired pit of the optic nerve head

DIAGNOSTIC TESTS & INTERPRETATION

Lab

Initial lab tests

Lab tests as indicated for clinical suspicion of other or associated conditions.

Follow-up & special considerations

If an oral carbonic anhydrase inhibitor is prescribed for treatment, blood work including CBC and creatinine levels should be obtained.

Imaging

Initial approach

- Optic disc photographs should be obtained to evaluate and follow patients through their course of treatment.
- Other optic nerve head imaging devices are also currently being used for optic nerve head assessment:
  - Scanning laser polarimetry
  - Heidelberg retinal tomography
  - Optical coherence topography

Follow-up & special considerations

Optic disc imaging should be obtained regularly (e.g., annually, or more often if a change in optic disc appearance is suspected) to document and assess the optic nerve head for change.

Diagnostic Procedures/Other

- Visual fields should be obtained at baseline and at regular intervals (e.g., annually, or more often if a change is suspected).
- Diurnal IOP testing may be useful if large IOP fluctuations or periods of IOP spike are suspected.
- Consider neuroimaging for:
  - Loss of central visual acuity or central visual field
  - Acute onset or rapidly progressive visual loss
  - Markedly asymmetric or strictly unilateral optic neuropathy
  - Hemianopic visual field loss
  - Neuroretinal rim pallor (5)[B]

Pathological Findings

Atrophy of the retinal ganglion cell layer can be noted in advanced glaucoma.

DIFFERENTIAL DIAGNOSIS

- Optic nerve anomalies including coloboma, pits, oblique insertion
- Autosomal dominant optic atrophy
- Glaucoma associated with elevated (higher than normal) intraocular pressure – for example, past history of trauma or surgery that may have led to elevated IOP, wide diurnal fluctuation in IOP, and past history of steroid use

- Hemodynamic crisis
- Methyl alcohol poisoning
- Optic neuritis
- Arteritic ischemic optic neuropathy
- Nonarteritic ischemic optic neuropathy
- Compressive lesions of optic nerve and tract
- Traumatic optic neuropathy

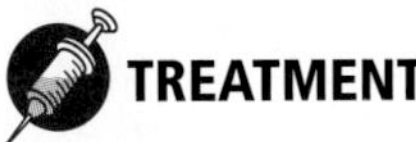

TREATMENT

MEDICATION

First Line

- Prostaglandin agonists (e.g., latanoprost, bimatoprost, travoprost)
- Topical carbonic anhydrase inhibitors (e.g., dorzolamide, brinzolamide)
- Beta-blockers (e.g., timolol, levobunolol) –
- Selective alpha 2 receptor agonists
- Miotics (e.g., pilocarpine)

Second Line

Systemic carbonic anhydrase inhibitors (e.g., methazolamide, acetazolamide).

ADDITIONAL TREATMENT

General Measures

- The goal is to achieve and maintain an intraocular pressure level in which there will presumably be no further optic nerve damage.
- This intraocular pressure level is dynamic and should be reevaluated at each visit – this level is determined by history, examination, and risk factors for progression.
- If the intraocular pressure cannot be maintained low enough to prevent optic nerve damage with noninvasive therapy, glaucoma filtering surgery may be indicated.
- It is important to keep in mind the expense, inconvenience, and side effects of therapy.

Issues for Referral

- Neuro-ophthalmologist – if there is suspicion that the cause of the patient's optic neuropathy or visual field defect is neurological.
- Low-vision specialist – for patients who are functionally inhibited by their quality of vision.

Additional Therapies

Neuroprotective agents are currently being studied for treatment of glaucoma patients.

SURGERY/OTHER PROCEDURES

- Laser procedures, for example, argon laser trabeculoplasty, selective laser trabeculoplasty:
  - Laser procedures have been shown to be effective in lowering intraocular pressure.
  - They should be used with caution in patients with highly pigmented trabecular meshwork.
  - Laser procedures can be considered first line therapy in some patients.
- Filtering procedures:
  - Trabeculectomy
  - Tube shunt implant (e.g., Ahmed, Baerveldt, Molteno)
- Cyclodestructive procedures are not the first operation of choice because of their destructive nature and potential risk of damage to adjacent ocular structures:
  - Endocyclophotocoagulation
  - Laser transscleral cyclophotocoagulation

ONGOING CARE

FOLLOW-UP RECOMMENDATIONS

- Patients are reexamined after starting a new medication or after laser or surgical procedures to evaluate the efficacy.
- If the patient is at high risk for visual loss at their intraocular pressure level, it may be reasonable to recheck the patient within days to ensure that adequate intraocular pressure lowering is achieved with therapy.
- Once the patient has achieved an intraocular pressure level that is at low risk for causing additional glaucomatous damage, they can be reevaluated in 3–6 month intervals.

Patient Monitoring

See "Follow-Up Recommendations" and "Diagnostic Tests and Interpretations" sections.

PATIENT EDUCATION

It is important to counsel patients on the importance of adherence to medical therapy and with ophthalmological follow up for treatment of glaucoma.

PROGNOSIS

- Prognosis of glaucoma depends on the patient's age and rate of progression.
- The prognosis is good if the patient's rate of progression can be slowed to a rate such that they maintain good vision for their lifetime.
- Normal tension glaucoma patients with unilateral field loss are at high risk of developing field damage in the fellow eye (6)[A].

COMPLICATIONS

Uncontrolled glaucoma can lead to loss of vision.

REFERENCES

1. Shields MB. Chapter 9 – Clinical Epidemiology in Glaucoma, and Chapter 11 – Chronic Open-Angle Glaucoma and Normal-Tension Glaucoma. 5th ed, In: Allingham RR, Damji KF, Freedman S, Moroi SE, Shafranov G (eds). Shields' Textbook of Glaucoma, 2005.
2. Dul MW. *Normal Tension Glaucoma*, In: Litwak AB (ed). Glaucoma Handbook, 2001.
3. Drance S, Anderson DR, Schulzer M. Risk factors for progression of visual field abnormalities in normal-tension glaucoma. *Am J Ophthalmol* 2001;131:699–708.
4. Fan BJ, Wang DY, Fan DS, et al. SNPs and interaction analyses of myocilin, optineurin, and apolipoprotein E in primary open angle glaucoma patients. *Mol Vis* 2005;11:625–631.
5. Collignon NJ. Abnormal cupping of the optic disc: Clinical screening before performing a neuroimaging examination. *Bull Soc Belge Ophthalmol* 2006;300:21–23.
6. Fontana L, Armas R, Garway-Heath DF, et al. Clinical factors influencing the visual prognosis of the fellow eyes of normal tension glaucoma patients. *Br J Ophthalmol* 1999;83:1002–1005.

ADDITIONAL READING

- Collaborative Normal-Tension Glaucoma Study Group. Comparison of glaucomatous progression between untreated patients with normal-tension glaucoma and patients with therapeutically reduced intraocular pressures. *Am J Ophthalmol* 1998;126:487–497.

See Also (Topic, Algorithm, Electronic Media Element)

- Primary open angle glaucoma

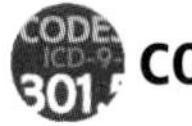

CODES

ICD9

365.12 Low tension open-angle glaucoma

NORRIE DISEASE

Brian J. Forbes
Monica R. Khitri

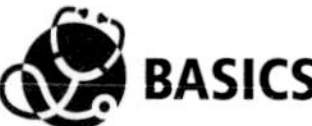

BASICS

DESCRIPTION

- Rare neurodevelopmental disorder of males causing congenital or early infancy blindness from retinal dysplasia, classically characterized by retrolental masses (pseudogliomas) (1)[C]
- Associated with developmental delay, hearing loss, and behavioral abnormalities
- Also known as progressive oculo-acoustico-cerebral degeneration

EPIDEMIOLOGY

- First reported in families from Scandinavia but since reported in almost all ethnic groups
- Affects males predominantly. Very rare female carriers (2)[C]

Incidence

Extremely rare disease that has been reported only in isolated case reports.

RISK FACTORS

Family history of Norrie disease

Genetics

- X-linked recessive disease caused by mutations in the *NDP* gene at Xp11.4
- More than 70 point mutations, chromosomal rearrangements, frame-shift, and splice site mutations described (3)[C]
  - Female carriers may harbor some retinal findings that can range from mild pigmentary changes to retinal detachment, abnormal retinal vasculature, and macular drag. When carrier expression is present, it is usually presumed to be a result of skewed X-chromosome inactivation or chromosomal aberration (2)[C].

GENERAL PREVENTION

- Carrier testing of female relatives can identify individuals at risk of having affected offspring.
- Prenatal testing possible if mutation already identified in an affected family member.

PATHOPHYSIOLOGY

Developmental abnormality of retinal vascularization during embryogenesis causing retinal hypoxia and dysplasia (4)[C]

ETIOLOGY

Norrin, the protein encoded by the *NDP* gene, has a characteristic cysteine knot motif and is involved in Frizzled-dependent signaling cascade important for vascular development and maintenance of the inner ear and retina. Mutations in the *NDP* gene cause aberrant retinal vascularization (4)[C].

COMMONLY ASSOCIATED CONDITIONS

Associated with mental retardation, behavioral disturbances, and sensorineural deafness in 30% cases.

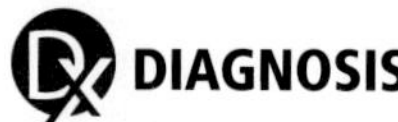

DIAGNOSIS

HISTORY

Family history of Norrie disease, congenital male blindness.

PHYSICAL EXAM

- Classic finding: Yellow–grey, elevated retrolental mass (pseudoglioma) visible through a clear lens. These masses are typically composed of dysplastic retina with unbranched retinal vessels. The peripheral retina may be attached, is usually avascular, and can have pigmentary changes.
- May have mild changes at birth followed by progressive changes though infancy and childhood
- Bilateral, often symmetric, dystrophic changes in the retina including retinal detachments or folds.
- Vitreous hemorrhage
- Iris atrophy, posterior synechiae
- Corneal opacities
- Cataracts
- Can get shallowing of anterior chamber and increased intraocular pressure in later stages (1)[C], (3)[C]

DIAGNOSTIC TESTS & INTERPRETATION

Lab

Initial lab tests

Molecular genetic testing of *NDP* gene mutations can be useful in corroborating diagnosis but cannot definitively exclude disease.

Follow-up & special considerations

- Genetics consult
- Examine mother for evidence of subtle retinal pigmentary changes, retinal folds, peripheral avascular retina.

Imaging

Initial approach

B-scan can be used to characterize the retrolental mass, detect retinal detachments if poor view.

Follow-up & special considerations

Regular ophthalmologic monitoring for glaucoma development, cataracts, retinal detachments, and progression of milder disease.

Diagnostic Procedures/Other

- Audiologic evaluation
- Developmental assessment in early childhood if patient not meeting normal developmental milestones
- Behavioral evaluation as indicated
- Genetic counseling

Pathological Findings
Proliferation of preretinal fibrovascular tissue, retinal detachment and gliosis, disorganized layers of dysplastic retina, defective and dilated retinal vessels (4)[C]

DIFFERENTIAL DIAGNOSIS
- Persistent fetal vasculature syndrome (PFVS)
- Retinopathy of prematurity (ROP)
- Coats disease
- Familial exudative vitreoretinopathy (FEVR)
- Retinoblastoma
- Incontinentia pigmenti
- Isolated or syndromic retinal dysplasia
- Occult child abuse (Shaken baby syndrome)
- Osteopetrosis-pseudoglioma syndrome

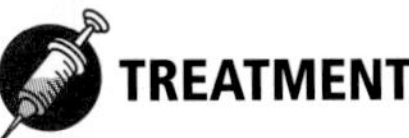

TREATMENT

MEDICATION
- None available to treat the primary disease process
- IOP-lowering agents can be used to treat ocular hypertension should it occur. If anterior chamber shallow and angle closed, the modalities may include peripheral iridectomy, lens extraction, trabeculectomy, glaucoma drainage tube, or cyclodestructive procedures.

ADDITIONAL TREATMENT
General Measures
- Most males with classic phenotypic presentation have complete retinal detachments at birth with little visual potential
- Patients diagnosed without a complete retinal detachment may benefit from surgery and/or laser therapy (1)[C],(3)[C]. Treatment should include ablation of the avascular retina and the vascularized line of demarcation.

Issues for Referral
- Consider audiology and/or ENT referral for patients with hearing loss. Some patients may benefit from hearing aids or cochlear implantation.
- Low vision evaluation and support
- Retinal surgery and/or laser therapy for patients lacking complete retinal detachments.
- Cognitive and behavioral therapies as needed

Additional Therapies
If nonfunctional eye, phthisis bulbi, consider a scleral shell to encourage orbital and periocular tissue growth.

COMPLEMENTARY & ALTERNATIVE THERAPIES
None proven or indicated.

SURGERY/OTHER PROCEDURES
- Repair of retinal detachment, release of retinal traction, ablation of avascular retina, and vascularized demarcation zone (1)[C].
- Glaucoma surgery may be needed if increased intraocular pressure.
- Consider enucleation or evisceration if needed to control pain.

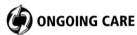

ONGOING CARE

FOLLOW-UP RECOMMENDATIONS
- Regular ophthalmologic examinations as needed to monitor for retinal detachments, cataract, glaucoma.
- Low vision

Patient Monitoring
Behavioral, developmental, psychiatric, and regular audiologic evaluations.

PATIENT EDUCATION
- Genetic counseling
- Low vision evaluation and aids
- Support and education http://www.norries.org/

PROGNOSIS
- Poor visual prognosis, especially if presentation with complete retinal detachments at diagnosis. Often Hand Motion vision or less.
- Many eyes progress to phthisis bulbi.

COMPLICATIONS
- Retinal detachments
- Glaucoma
- Cataracts

REFERENCES

1. Drenser BA, Fecko A, Dailey W, et al. A characteristic phenotypic retinal appearance in Norrie disease. *Retina* 2007;27(2):243–246.
2. Lin P, Shankar SP, Duncan J, et al. Retinal vascular abnormalities and dragged maculae in a carrier with a new NDP mutation (c.268delC) that caused severe Norrie disease in the proband. *J AAPOS* 2010;14:93–96.
3. Wu WC, Drenser K, Trese M, et al. Retinal phenotype-genotype correlation of pediatric patients expressing mutations in the Norrie disease gene. *Arch Ophthalmol* 2007;125(2):225–230.
4. Luhmann UF, Lin J, Acar N, et al. Role of the Norrie disease pseudoglioma gene in sprouting angiogenesis during development of retinal vasculature. *Invest Ophthalmol Vis Sci* 2005;46(9):3372–3382.

ADDITIONAL READING

- http://www.geneclinics.org/profiles/norrie/details.html.

CODES

ICD9
- 743.8 Other specified anomalies of eye, congenital
- 743.56 Other retinal changes, congenital

CLINICAL PEARLS

- Visual prognosis is very limited, and low vision interventions are important in management.
- Examine relatives, males and females, as variable expression can manifest as subtle retinal pathology in older age groups.
- Consider genetic evaluation and counseling.
- Consider audiologic and psychiatric/behavioral consultation.

NYSTAGMUS, ACQUIRED

Sarkis M. Nazarian

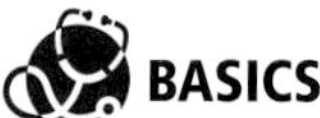

BASICS

DESCRIPTION

- Acquired nystagmus is a repetitive, rhythmic, involuntary oscillation of the eyes, and can be constant, cyclical, or intermittent.
- All nystagmus occurs of a result of the eyes drifting from the desired position of gaze.
- It can be monocular, binocular, or asymmetric (dissociated).
- Nystagmus can be directionally symmetrical with a sinusoidal (pendular) waveform, or it can have a slow drift and a rapid corrective "jerk" component.
- The slow drift can have a linear, exponentially increasing, or exponentially decreasing (decaying) waveform.

EPIDEMIOLOGY

Prevalence

- The prevalence of nystagmus is estimated at 240/100,000 based on a community survey in Leicestershire, UK.

RISK FACTORS

- As acquired nystagmus can occur as a result of a variety of conditions, no specific risk factors can be cited.

Genetics

- A variety of inherited conditions can have nystagmus as part of the spectrum of central nervous system manifestations.

GENERAL PREVENTION

- Prevention measures for acquired nystagmus depend on the specific etiology of the nystagmus.

PATHOPHYSIOLOGY

- Optimal visual acuity requires image motion on retina to be <5 degrees/second. Three main mechanisms hold gaze steady:
  - Vestibulo-ocular reflex
  - Visual fixation
  - Eccentric gaze-holding mechanisms, so-called "Neural integrator."
- Visual fixation has 2 components:
  - Corrective eye movements in response to retinal image drift, and
  - Suppression of unwanted movements that move eyes away from target
- Eccentric gaze-holding mechanisms: The neural integrator is a diffuse system comprising the vestibulocerebellum and cell groups in paramedian tracts, including the medial vestibular nucleus (MVN) and the adjacent nucleus prepositus hypoglossi (NPH) in the medulla for horizontal gaze, and the interstitial nucleus of Cajal (INC) in the midbrain for vertical gaze.
- A pulse of innervation to the extraocular muscles (EOMs) is needed to overcome viscous drag (mediated by burst neurons); a step of innervation to EOMs is needed to overcome elastic restoring forces (mediated by tonic neurons) and keep the eyes from slipping back.
- The saccadic pulse generator for horizontal gaze is located in the ipsilateral paramedian pontine reticular formation (PPRF) in close proximity to the abducens nucleus.
- Ocular motor neurons receive input from both burst and tonic cells in the PPRF neural integrator to achieve correct burst-tonic firing pattern.
- The most common type of pulse-step disorders include mismatch (glissade), where the step is smaller than the pulse, and gaze-evoked nystagmus (due to a variety of toxins, most commonly ethanol), where the step is poorly sustained. Both these conditions lead to nystagmus in eccentric gaze, with slow phases directed toward the primary position.

ETIOLOGY

- Nystagmus can be classified according to the following scheme:
  - **Peripheral vestibular nystagmus:** Benign paroxysmal positional vertigo (BPPV)
  - **Central vestibular nystagmus:** Downbeat, upbeat, and torsional
  - **Nystagmus due to vestibular instability:** Periodic alternating nystagmus (PAN)
  - **Nystagmus caused by disorders of visual fixation:** See-saw nystagmus. Disorders of the anterior visual pathways often cause nystagmus due to both loss of visual motion information that can be used to compensate for drifts of eyes off target, and loss of visual input essential to "calibrate" normal eye movements.
  - **Nystagmus caused by disorders of gaze holding:** Acquired pendular nystagmus, gaze-evoked nystagmus, oculopalatal tremor or "myoclonus."

COMMONLY ASSOCIATED CONDITIONS

- Nystagmus is often accompanied with other neurological findings such as vertigo and ataxia.

DIAGNOSIS

HISTORY

- Acquired nystagmus is accompanied with oscillopsia, or apparent movement of stationary objects. This can become severe enough to degrade visual acuity.

PHYSICAL EXAM

- **Benign paroxysmal positional vertigo (BPPV):**
  - Most commonly due to posterior canal disease
  - Mixed horizontal and torsional nystagmus
  - Waveforms have linear slow phases.
  - Unidirectional, obeys Alexander's law (amplitude greater when eyes turn toward direction of jerk component)
  - Suppressed with fixation, worse under Frenzel glasses
  - Fatigues easily, resolves in days to weeks
- **Downbeat nystagmus:** The vestibulocerebellum inhibits central connections from the anterior canals (which are activated by neck flexion and move eyes up), but not from the posterior canals (which are activated by neck extension and move eyes down).
  - Lesions of the vestibulocerebellum (such as Arnold-Chiari malformation) cause disinhibition of the anterior canal projections, causing eyes to drift upward, and compensatory downward nystagmus to occur.
  - Other etiologies include M.S., medication toxicity (lithium, antiepileptic meds, opioids, amiodarone), deficiency states (B12, thiamine, magnesium), toluene abuse, craniocervical junction pathology (stroke, trauma, or bleed), hydrocephalus, paraneoplastic cerebellar degeneration due to anti-Ta antibody, stiff person syndrome.
  - Cortical projections to vestibulocerebellum are GABAergic, so benzodiazepines can be used (e.g. Clonazepam), as well as baclofen, a GABA-β agonist.
  - 3,4-diaminopyridine (3,4-DAP; amifampridine), a potassium channel blocker, has been shown to suppress downbeat nystagmus. This agent is currently only available in Europe. A related agent, 4-aminopyridine (fampridine, dalfampridine, Ampyra) is now commercially available in the US.
  - Downbeat nystagmus due to Episodic Ataxia type 2, due to a P/Q type calcium channel (CACNL1A4) mutation, responds to acetazolamide.
- **Upbeat nystagmus:** Pathology usually lies in medial medullary tegmentum (nucleus intercalatus).
  - It is caused by M.S., brainstem strokes, cerebellar degenerations, Wernicke's, Behcet's, paraneoplastic, Leber's congenital amaurosis, toxins (organophosphates, anticonvulsants, cyclosporine A), smoking (in the dark only).
- **Torsional nystagmus:** Associated with the ocular tilt reaction and skew deviation. This is a rare condition, and no data on treatment exists.
- **PAN (Periodic alternating nystagmus):**
  - Shifts direction every 80–120 seconds
  - Etiology is similar to that of downbeat nystagmus.
  - Relieved by baclofen, a GABA-β agonist. This has been thought to be due to baclofen's ability to compensate for loss of cerebellar inhibition, but an NMDA effect may also be involved.
- **Disorders of the anterior visual pathways** often cause nystagmus (e.g., see-saw). This is thought to be due to both loss of visual motion information that can be used to compensate for drifts of eyes off target, and loss of visual input essential to "calibrate" normal eye movements.
- **See-saw Nystagmus:** Dysconjugate vertical movements; upward moving eye intorts, downward eye extorts
  - Usually due to parasellar lesions, possibly due to midbrain compression; also, occasionally with congenital chiasm abnormalities.
- **Acquired pendular nystagmus:** Hallmark of M.S. Other etiologies include stroke, bleed, tumor, Pelizaeus Merzbacher disease, mitochondrial disorders, Cockayne syndrome, toluene abuse, adrenoleukodystrophy.
  - May be diagonal, circular, or elliptical.
  - Initially thought to be due to visual deprivation, it is now thought to be due to gaze-holding deficits.
  - GABA and glutamate receptors are thought to be involved.
- **Gaze-evoked nystagmus:** Present in extremes of gaze (except downgaze). It is due to cerebellar dysfunction (in the flocculus and its connections)
  - Most commonly due to sedative–hypnotic drugs.
  - It exhibits decelerating slow phases.

- **Oculopalatal tremor or "myoclonus":** This is another type of acquired pendular nystagmus, vertical-torsional (with unilateral lesions), or vertical (with bilateral lesions).
  - Associated with lesions of the Central Tegmental Tract, which runs from the dentate nucleus to the contralateral red nucleus to the contralateral inferior olivary nucleus ("Mollaret's triangle"); the latter nucleus appears hypertrophic on imaging.
  - Frequency is 1–3 Hz.
  - Often accompanied by tremor of palate of other branchial muscles.

DIAGNOSTIC TESTS & INTERPRETATION

Lab

Initial lab tests

- Routine lab testing is not useful in acquired nystagmus, as history of toxic exposure, physical examination, and imaging are usually sufficient. Urine drug screening and ethanol level are useful in diagnosing intoxications.

Imaging

Initial approach

- Magnetic resonance imaging of the posterior fossa is usually diagnostic. Diffusion-weighted imaging, FLAIR, and post-contrast T1 imaging are most helpful.

DIFFERENTIAL DIAGNOSIS

- **Saccadic intrusions:** These are arrhythmic, chaotic movements made up of saccadic movements only, with and without intervening periods of ocular rest.
  - Saccadic intrusions include square-wave jerks, macrosaccadic oscillations, opsoclonus, and ocular flutter.
- **Superior oblique myokymia:** Intermittent, brief monocular oscillopsia due to small amplitude contraction of the superior oblique.
  - Idiopathic, related to microvascular compression of the trochlear nerve
- **Ocular neuromyotonia:** Episodic monocular deviation caused by overaction of a muscle innervated by the oculomotor nerve, usually adduction, brought on by eccentric gaze.
  - Patients usually have received radiation therapy to the parasellar region.

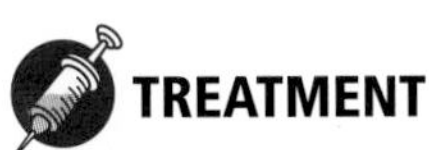

TREATMENT

MEDICATION

First Line

- **Vestibular nystagmus:** Current practice guidelines discourage routine medical therapy, especially with benzodiazepines and antihistamines
- **Downbeat nystagmus:** Clonazepam 0.5–1 mg t.i.d, baclofen 5–10 mg t.i.d, trihexyphenidyl 20–40 mg/d
- **Downbeat nystagmus with episodic ataxia:** Acetazolamide 500–1000 mg/d, dosed b.i.d or t.i.d.
- **Upbeat nystagmus:** Baclofen 5–10 mg t.i.d.
- **Periodic alternating nystagmus:** Baclofen 5–10 mg t.i.d.
- **See-saw nystagmus:** Baclofen 5–10 mg t.i.d, clonazepam 0.5–1 mg t.i.d, gabapentin 1200–2400 mg/d dosed t.i.d or q.i.d.
- **Acquired pendular nystagmus:** Gabapentin 1200–2400 mg/d dosed t.i.d or q.i.d, memantine 20–40 mg/d dosed b.i.d or t.i.d, clonazepam 0.5–1 mg t.i.d, trihexyphenidyl 20–40 mg/d, scopolamine (Transderm Scop) 1.5 mg 3-day patch.
- **Oculopalatal tremor:** Gabapentin 1200–2400 mg/d dosed t.i.d or q.i.d, valproate 10–60 mg/kg daily, and trihexiphenidyl 20–40 mg/d.

Second Line

- **Vestibular nystagmus:** Medications used to treat severe vertigo and nausea due to BPPV include antihistamines, anticholinergics, phenothiazines (promethazine, prochlorperazine), benzodiazepines, and ondansetron. They should not be used for more than 48 hours to prevent delay in healing due to CNS compensation.
- **Downbeat or upbeat nystagmus:** Dalfampridine (Ampyra) 20–30 mg/d dosed b.i.d or t.i.d; amifampridine (Zenas, Firdapse) 40–80 mg/d.
- **See-saw nystagmus:** Ethanol 1.2 mg/kg.
- **Acquired pendular nystagmus:** Cannabis, ethanol 1.2 mg/kg.

ADDITIONAL TREATMENT

General Measures

- Peripheral nystagmus and vertigo due to semicircular canal involvement is usually self-limited. It can be improved by various canal repositioning maneuvers (e.g., Epley and Semont maneuvers).

Additional Therapies

- Base-down prisms can be used for downbeat nystagmus, as it damps with upgaze.
- Retinal image stabilization, which consists of high-negative contact lenses coupled with high-positive spectacle lenses, optically reduces acquired pendular nystagmus amplitude.
- Botulinum A toxin injections in extraocular muscles have been reported to be successful in small case studies, but the potential for side effects (ptosis, vertical deviations, worsening of nystagmus in noninjected eye) have prevented the widespread acceptance of this technique.

COMPLEMENTARY & ALTERNATIVE THERAPIES

- None are effective

SURGERY/OTHER PROCEDURES

- Kestenbaum procedures to move eyes into a position that minimizes the nystagmus can be useful, for example, move eyes up for downbeat nystagmus

ONGOING CARE

PROGNOSIS

- Established nystagmus generally persists, except for BPPV, which is a self-limited condition

ADDITIONAL READING

- Baugh RE, Orvidas L, et al. Clinical practice guideline: benign paroxysmal positional vertigo. *Otolaryngol Head Neck Surg* 2008;139(5 Suppl 4): S47–S81.
- Brandt T, Dieterich M. Vestibular syndromes in the roll plane: topographic diagnosis from brainstem to cortex. *Ann Neurol* 1994;36(3):337–347.
- Hertle RW. Nystagmus in infancy and childhood. *Semin Ophthalmol* 2008;23:307–317.
- Lee AGT, Brazil PW. Localizing forms of nystagmus. Symptoms, diagnosis and treatment. *Curr Neurol Neurosci Rep* 2006;6:414–420.
- Leigh RJ, Tomsak RL. Drug treatments for eye movement disorders. *J Neurol Neurosurg Psychiatry* 2003;74:1–4.
- Leigh RJ, Zee DS. *The Neurology of Eye Movements*, Fourth Edition; New York: Oxford University Press, 2006:475–558.
- McLean RJ, Gottlob I. The pharmacological treatment of nystagmus: A review. *Expert Opin Pharmacother* 2009;10(11):1805–1816.
- Rucker JC. An update on acquired nystagmus. *Semin Ophthalmol* 2008;23;91–97.
- Rucker JC. Pearls: Nystagmus. *Semin Neurol* 2010;30:51–53.
- Sarvananthan N, Surendran M, Roberts EO, et al. The prevalence of nystagmus: The Leicestershire nystagmus survey. *Invest Ophthalmol Vis Sci* 2009;50:5201–5206.
- Straube A, Leigh RJ, Bronstein A, et al. EFNS task force – therapy of nystagmus and oscillopsia. *Eur J Neurol* 2004;11:83–89.

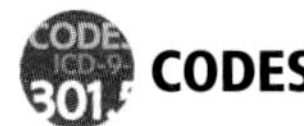

CODES

ICD9

379.50 Nystagmus, unspecified

CLINICAL PEARLS

- Jerk nystagmus can be physiologic, occurs in extreme lateral eye positions, is of low amplitude and high frequency, and resolves when eyes are removed from extreme lateral gaze.
- Acute onset of gaze-evoked or upbeat nystagmus with confusion and ataxia suggests Wernicke's encephalopathy.
- Both peripheral and central vestibular nystagmus worsen when the patient looks in the direction of the fast phase (Alexander's Law).
- Visual fixation suppresses vestibular nystagmus, but worsens infantile nystagmus.
- Jerk nystagmus can be seen with retinal disorders, whereas pendular nystagmus usually is seen with optic nerve disorders.
- Nystagmus associated with visual loss is usually more severe in the eye with worse vision.
- Ophthalmologic examination may reveal a very low amplitude nystagmus, and prolonged observation reveals direction reversal in PAN.

NYSTAGMUS, CONGENITAL

Jing Jin

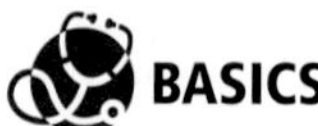

BASICS

DESCRIPTION
Involuntary oscillation of the eyes that may be either motor or sensory in etiology.

EPIDEMIOLOGY
Incidence
Idiopathic motor infantile/congenital nystagmus: 1 in 2,850 (1).

Prevalence
Approximately 0.5%, including those associated with strabismus and other diseases.

RISK FACTORS
- Low vision
  - Strabismus (2)[C]
  - Developmental delay
  - Down, Asperger (2 reported cases), and other syndromes
  - Neurological anomalies
  - Family history of nystagmus

Genetics
- Isolated nystagmus: Autosomal dominant (loci 6p12, 7p11, 13q31–33, 18q22.3–23), autosomal recessive (6p12), and X-linked (locus Xp11.3-11.4; gene FRMD7 at Xq26–q27; gene GPR143 at Xp22.3) (2)[C]
- Genetics of underlying syndrome would otherwise apply.

GENERAL PREVENTION
Genetic counseling

PATHOPHYSIOLOGY
- Low vision results in inability to use visual information to maintain stable fixation.
- Neuronal mechanism of motor nystagmus is a field active research. Currently, there is no unified theory.

ETIOLOGY
- Isolated congenital/infantile motor nystagmus may or may not have genetic etiology.
- Acquired nystagmus
  - Sensory: Vision loss before age 2 years
  - Central nervous system anomalies
  - Degenerative brain disorders, stroke, tumor
  - Vestibular

COMMONLY ASSOCIATED CONDITIONS
- Low vision due to pre-chiasmal pathology (e.g., retinal dystrophy, optic nerve hypoplasia, untreated cataract)
- Albinism
- Central nervous system anomalies or other disorders
- Developmental delay
- Multiple syndromes (e.g., Cornelia de Lange syndrome) and chromosomal aberrations (e.g., trisomy 21)

DIAGNOSIS

HISTORY
- Age of onset. Congenital/infantile nystagmus is usually noticed by parents between 8–12 weeks old and before 6 months of age.
  - Photophobia (e.g., achromatopsia, cone dystrophy, albinism, macular hypoplasia)
  - Poor night vision (e.g., Congenital stationary night blindness [CSNB])
  - Better night than day vision (e.g., achromatopsia)
- History of neurologic signs, brain injury, brain tumor
- Family history
- Medication or illicit drug use

PHYSICAL EXAM
- Systemic and neurology evaluation for anomalies, developmental delay, and hypotonia
- Complete ophthalmologic evaluation to look for
  - Ocular anomalies and media opacities
  - Strabismus (e.g., from poor vision in sensory nystagmus or with infantile esotropia in nystagmus blockage syndrome)
- Evaluation for head positions, null point (may shift over time, e.g., periodic alternating nystagmus)
- Amplitude, frequency, and direction in all gazes
  - Type of nystagmus: Pendular, jerk
  - Amplitude
  - Symmetry
  - Direction (vertical horizontal, see saw, opsoclonus)
  - Changes in character with convergence or monocular viewing
  - Increase beneath closed eyelids – vestibular or brainstem pathology

DIAGNOSTIC TESTS & INTERPRETATION
Lab
- Not required unless systemic disorder which warrants laboratory tests
- If opsoclonus, do urine catecholamines.

Imaging
Initial approach
- Brain MRI in cases of
  - Vertical and asymmetric nystagmus
  - Nystagmus with optic nerve hypoplasia
  - Neurologic signs
  - Unusual patterns of nystagmus (e.g., see saw, opsoclonus – if so, also scan neck and thorax and possibly abdomen for paraspinal neuroblastoma)

Follow-up & special considerations
For progressive neurologic disease

Diagnostic Procedures/Other
- Eye movement recording (3)
- Electrophysiology studies for nystagmus associated with decreased vision without identifiable ocular pathology or suspect CSNB
  - 3-lead visual evoked potentials (VEP) help to establish the diagnosis of albinism

DIFFERENTIAL DIAGNOSIS
- Congenital/infantile nystagmus
- Nystagmus due to vision deprivation before age 2 years
  - Ocular anterior segment pathologies: Corneal opacity, cataract, glaucoma
  - Retinal diseases
  - Optic nerve diseases/congenital anomalies
- Latent nystagmus
  - Usually associated with strabismus
  - Affected by monocular occlusion and reverse direction when the covered eye is changed
- Spasmus nutans
  - Onset during the first year of life in otherwise healthy children
  - Transient high frequency often asymmetric nystagmus with head nodding and abnormal head position
  - Chiasmal, suprachiasmal, or third ventricle gliomas may mimic spasmus nutans.
- Gaze-evoked nystagmus
- Vestibular diseases
- Nystagmus due to brain, brainstem, and cerebellum diseases
  - Trauma
  - Tumor: Glioma, neuroblastoma
  - Inflammation
  - Ischemic
  - Demyelination: Multiple sclerosis
  - Degeneration
  - Malformation
- Toxins and drugs induced oscillations of eyes: Alcohol, lithium, antiseizure medications
- Idiopathic

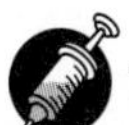

TREATMENT

MEDICATION

- Medical treatment is not usually included in treatment for congenital nystagmus.
- Baclofen and 5-hydroxytryptophan have been tried with limited effect.

ADDITIONAL TREATMENT

General Measures

- Correct refractive error. Contact lens may damp the nystagmus in some patients.
- Obtain ocular alignment by refractive correction, prisms, or surgery – may eliminate manifest latent component.
- Treat amblyopia.
- Photochromic lenses and sun glasses for cone disorders and macular hypoplasia
- Prism
  - Correct face turn.
  - Stimulate fusional convergence: Base out prisms for both eyes.

Issues for Referral

- Genetic counseling for cases with family history, albinism, or other genetic causes
- Low vision
- Neurology referral as needed
- ENT referral in cases of vestibular nystagmus

COMPLEMENTARY & ALTERNATIVE THERAPIES

- Acupuncture
- Biofeedback (4)[C]

SURGERY/OTHER PROCEDURES

- To correct face turn: Transfer the null position into primary gaze – Kestenbaum-Andersen procedure.
- To dampen the movement: Large recession of all 4 horizontal recti
- Artificial divergence surgery to produce a large exophoria that allows the patient to use fusional convergence to dampen the nystagmus (5)[C]

ONGOING CARE

FOLLOW-UP RECOMMENDATIONS

- As needed for monitoring vision, head position, and amblyopia treatment
- As needed for associated ocular, central nervous system, or systemic disease
  - Low vision
- Scheduled ophthalmology evaluation for monitoring and treatment of coexisting ocular condition, strabismus, and amblyopia

Patient Monitoring

School performance and development.

PATIENT EDUCATION

- Genetic counseling where indicated
- Low vision intervention
- Patient support network – American Nystagmus Network, Inc. (ANN) http://www.nystagmus.org/
- Underlying disease specific support groups

PROGNOSIS

- Visual acuity varies and depends on etiology
- Most forms of nystagmus, including congenital/infantile isolated motor nystagmus, dampen with age but rarely resolve.
- Anomalous head positions usually worsen as demand increases with age.

COMPLICATIONS

- Visual blur
  - Only when acquired later in childhood does oscillopsia occur

REFERENCES

1. Stang HJ. Developmental disabilities associated with congenital nystagmus. *J Dev Behav Pediatr* 1991;12(5):322–323.
2. Fingert JH, Roos B, Eyestone ME, et al. Novel intragenic FRMD7 deletion in a pedigree with congenital X-linked nystagmus. *Ophthalmic Genet* 2010;31(2):77–80.
3. Hertle RW, Maldanado VK, Maybodi M, et al. Clinical and ocular motor analysis of the infantile nystagmus syndrome in the first 6 months of life. *Br J Ophthalmol* 2002;86(6):670–675.
4. Sharma P, Tandon R, Kumar S, et al. Reduction of congenital nystagmus amplitude with auditory biofeedback. *J AAPOS* 2000;4(5):287–290.
5. Spielmann A. Clinical rationale for manifest congenital nystagmus surgery. *J AAPOS* 2000;4(2):67–74.

ADDITIONAL READING

- Brodsky MC, Fray KJ. The prevalence of strabismus in congenital nystagmus: The influence of anterior visual pathway disease. *J AAPOS* 1997;1(1):16–19.
- Oetting WS, Armstrong CM, Holleschau AM, et al. Evidence for genetic heterogeneity in families with congenital motor nystagmus (CN). *Ophthalmic Genet* 2000;21(4):227–233.
- Peng Y, Meng Y, Wang Z, et al. A novel GPR143 duplication mutation in a Chinese family with X-linked congenital nystagmus. *Mol Vis* 2009;15:810–814.
- Abadi RV, Bjerre A. Motor and sensory characteristics of infantile nystagmus. *Br J Ophthalmol* 2002:86:1152–1160.
- Blekher T, Yamada T, Yee RD, et al. Effects of acupuncture on foveation characteristics in congenital nystagmus. *Br J Ophthalmol* 1998;82(2):115–120.
- Mezawa M, Ishikawa S, Ukai K. Changes in waveform of congenital nystagmus associated with biofeedback treatment. *Br J of Ophthalmol* 1990;74(8):472–476.

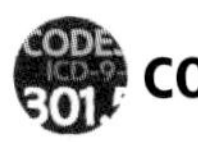

CODES

ICD9

- 379.50 Nystagmus, unspecified
- 379.51 Congenital nystagmus
- 379.56 Other forms of nystagmus

CLINICAL PEARLS

- Review medical and family history.
- Time of onset for infantile/congenital nystagmus is usually 2–3 months and before age of 6 months.
- Search for ocular and optic nerve pathology for nystagmus due to visual deprivation.
- Brain MRI in cases of vertical and asymmetric nystagmus and nystagmus with abnormal optic nerve
- Improve vision through treatment of ocular diseases, correction of refractive error, and amblyopia treatment.
- Surgical intervention for abnormal head position

OCCIPITAL LOBE DISORDERS

Mark L. Moster

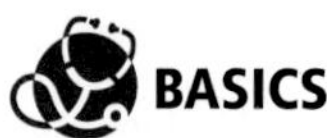

BASICS

DESCRIPTION

Disorders affecting the occipital lobe of the brain, which is almost entirely devoted to visual function

EPIDEMIOLOGY

Varies, depending on the many different causes of occipital involvement

RISK FACTORS

Genetics

Varied, depending on the many different causes of occipital involvement

ETIOLOGY

- Common causes
  - Cerebral infarction
  - Trauma
  - Hemorrhage
  - Tumor
  - Infection
  - Migraine
- Rarer causes
  - Demyelination
  - Posterior reversible encephalopathy syndrome (PRES)
  - Mitochondrial encephalopathy, lactic acidosis, and stroke-like episodes (MELAS)
  - Visual variant of Alzheimer's disease
  - Heidenhain variant of Creutzfeldt–Jakob disease
  - Progressive multifocal leukoencephalopathy

DIAGNOSIS

HISTORY

- Visual blurring on one side of space or if bilateral on both sides of space. Patients may mistakenly believe that it is only blurred in the eye on the side of the visual defect (if they have not occluded one eye to test it).
- Unilateral lesions are occasionally asymptomatic until noted on routine examination.
- Difficulty with locating objects in environment
- Difficulty with identifying colors (*Color Agnosia*).
- Visual hallucinations
  - Phosphenes, photopsias
  - Formed hallucinations
- Visual illusions—inaccurately seeing objects
- Difficulties with reading and writing
- Less commonly
  - Diplopia, polyopia, palinopsia
  - Agnosias—difficulty in identifying objects despite being able to see them

PHYSICAL EXAM

- Homonymous hemianopsia
  - Macular sparing may occur
  - Sometimes sparing the 60–90° region in the temporal visual field (VF) in the contralateral eye
  - Most often congruous
  - Homonymous, congruous central scotomas with occipital tip lesions
- Homonymous quadrantanopsia
- Rarely, a unilateral a contralateral temporal crescent defect between 60 and 90° in the VF with the most anterior occipital lobe lesions
- With bilateral lesions:
  - Bilateral homonymous hemianopic defects
  - Cortical blindness (or cerebral blindness)
- Cortical blindness
  - Normal ocular examination
  - Normal pupillary reaction
  - No visual response, no blink to light or visual threat
  - Most often infarction or prolonged hypotension
- Anton's syndrome
  - Cortical blindness
  - Patient denies blindness
  - Often associated with abnormalities beyond the occipital lobe
- Dyschromatopsia or hemiachromatopsia
- Riddoch phenomenon—patient may perceive a moving object but not a stationary object.
- If occipital visual loss occurs in early life, optic atrophy and pallor may develop due to transsynaptic degeneration

DIAGNOSTIC TESTS & INTERPRETATION

Imaging

- If acute, CT scan to exclude hemorrhage
- Otherwise, MRI scan
- Some patients have occipital patterns of visual loss with normal CT and MRI (e.g., trauma, Alzheimer's). These may be detected with positron emission tomography (PET), single photon emission computed tomography (SPECT), or functional MRI (fMRI) scans.

DIFFERENTIAL DIAGNOSIS

- Lesions of optic tract and parietal and temporal lobe may have similar visual field defects.
  - Other neurologic findings (e.g., aphasia, sensory loss) usually provide localizing value in these cases.
- Patients with cortical blindness may mistakenly be diagnosed with functional visual loss.

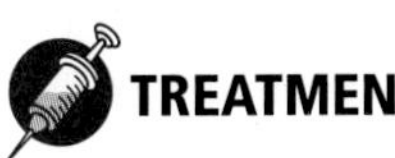

TREATMENT

Treat underlying etiology.

ADDITIONAL TREATMENT

General Measures

- Occupational therapy
  - Strategies for reading
- Saccadic and visual field training
  - These therapies likely help visual function by training the patient to make eye movements toward the VF defect or shift attention to the side of the VF deficit.

Additional Therapies

- Prisms
- Mirrors

SURGERY/OTHER PROCEDURES

- IV or IA thrombolysis for acute infarct
- Neurosurgery for mass lesions
- Radiation for tumors
- Intra-arterial therapy for arteriovenous malformations (AVMs).

IN-PATIENT CONSIDERATIONS

Initial Stabilization

- For infarct—make sure that vitals and metabolic status are stable. Consider thrombolysis if within hours of onset. Consider anticoagulation if high risk for recurrence (e.g., cardiac embolic source).
- For hemorrhage or tumor—stabilize vital signs and monitor and treat for clinically significant mass effect.

Admission Criteria

- If deficit is acute infarct or hemorrhage
- If there is significant mass effect from a structural lesion

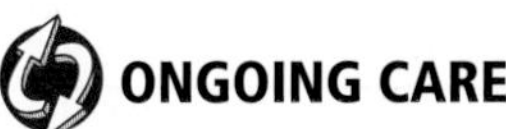

ONGOING CARE

FOLLOW-UP RECOMMENDATIONS

- Varied, depending on etiology
- Counseling the ability to drive
  - Regulations vary by state and country.

ADDITIONAL READING

- Zhang X, Kedar S, Lynn MJ, et al. Homonymous hemianopia in stroke. *J Neuroophthalmol* 2006;26(3):180–183.

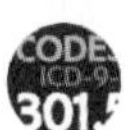

CODES

ICD9

438.7 Disturbances of vision

CLINICAL PEARLS

- Isolated hemianopic defects without other neurologic findings are almost always due to an occipital lesion.
- Patients with hemianopsia may mistakenly believe that the visual loss is only in one eye until it is shown to them by occluding each eye individually.

OCULAR ADNEXAL LYMPHOMA (OAL)

Jurij R. Bilyk
Ann P. Murchison

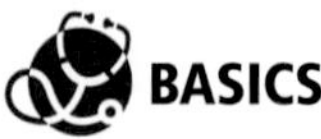

BASICS

DESCRIPTION

- Ocular adnexal lymphoproliferative disease (OALD) represents an amalgam of monoclonal and polyclonal lymphocytic proliferations that involve the ocular adnexa (the eyelids, orbit, conjunctiva, and lacrimal apparatus).
- OALD is further divided into 2 sub-categories:
  - Lymphoid hyperplasia (LH), a polyclonal, T-cell rich proliferation, which may be reactive. A significant percentage of patients with LH will eventually develop systemic lymphoma.
  - Ocular adnexal lymphoma (OAL), a monoclonal, autonomous, self-sustaining lymphocytic malignancy, which is generally of B-cell origin and of the non-Hodgkin type.
  - Idiopathic orbital inflammatory syndrome (IOIS) is *not* in the spectrum of OALD.
- OAL should never be considered a uniform process, but rather a compendium of subtypes of lymphoma, each with its own cytogenetics, therapeutic options, propensity for systemic involvement, and varying prognosis.
- OAL should be classified according to the WHO modifications of the REAL system. The majority of OAL present as 5 subtypes, 3 of which are relatively indolent, and 2 of which are aggressive and potentially fatal (Table 1).

Table 1 Subtypes of OAL

Indolent	Aggressive
Extranodal marginal zone (EMZL)*	Diffuse large B-cell
Follicular cell (Grade I and II)	Mantle cell
Small cell lymphoma (chronic lymphocytic leukemia).	Follicular cell (Grade III)†

*Also known as mucosa-associated lymphoid tissue (MALT) lymphoma.
†Rare in the ocular adnexa.

  - About 50% of all OAL is extranodal marginal zone lymphoma (EMZL)/mucosa-associated lymphoid tissue (MALT).
  - OAL is *not* associated with intraocular lymphoma, which should be considered a form of central nervous system lymphoma.

EPIDEMIOLOGY

Incidence

- 65,000 cases of non-Hodgkin lymphoma (NHL) per year in the US
- OAL occurs in approximately 5% of all NHL cases and accounts for about 10% of all adult orbital tumors. OAL is rare in the pediatric population.
- OALD has no significant gender predilection.
- The mean age at presentation for OAL is about 67 years, but OALD/OAL may occur in any adult age group.

RISK FACTORS

- Autoimmune disease may predispose to the evolution of LH and OAL.
- Chronic immunosuppression increases the risk of NHL in general.
- Higher rate of NHL in HIV-infected patients.

Genetics

No definite genetic predisposition to OALD.

GENERAL PREVENTION

There is no known effective prevention of LH and OAL. Avoidance of chronic immunostimulation (e.g., chronic infection) and chronic immunosuppression (e.g., HIV infection, long term methotrexate therapy for rheumatoid arthritis) may theoretically be protective.

PATHOPHYSIOLOGY

- The pathophysiology of NHL is not clearly understood.
- The specific subtype of NHL typically mimics the clinical behavior of its mature B-cell progenitor. For example, EMZL arising from marginal zone B-cells will behave indolently, whereas mantle cell lymphoma (MCL) will mimic the more aggressive behavior of a mantle zone B-cell.
- Chronic immune stimulation and chronic infection promote an *in situ* evolution of lymphoproliferative disease. Examples of this include the formation of gastric EMZL in patients chronically infected with *Helicobacter pylori* and the proven association between Epstein-Barr virus infection and endemic Burkitt lymphoma.
- Chronic immunosuppression allows for NHL formation, demonstrated by the higher incidence of NHL in HIV infection.

COMMONLY ASSOCIATED CONDITIONS

- Most patients with OALD and OAL have no known associated conditions.
- HIV-infection increases the incidence of NHL.
- Certain autoimmune disease (Sjögren syndrome, possibly rheumatoid arthritis) may increase the risk of NHL.
- Long-term iatrogenic immunosuppression is associated with a higher NHL risk.
- To date, no clear association between OAL and an infectious stimulus has been proven.

DIAGNOSIS

HISTORY

- Most patients with LH and OAL present with slowly progressive, nonspecific symptoms.
- The vast majority of OALD presents without pain. The presence of pain typically signifies an aggressive histopathology.
- Proptosis, ptosis, and eyelid or conjunctival mass are common presenting complaints.
- Diplopia/visual disturbances are infrequent.
- Most patients (78%) have no known history of systemic lymphoma.

PHYSICAL EXAM

- Vision and pupillary examinations are usually normal. Optic neuropathy is uncommon in OALD, and may signify an aggressive histopathology.
- Painless nodularity in the eyelids, conjunctival cul-de-sac, anterior orbit, and lacrimal gland is common. Evert the eyelids to check the tarsal conjunctiva and cul-de-sacs carefully.
- A pink flat or elevated subconjunctival lesion (i.e., "salmon patch") is a common manifestation of LH and OAL.
- Exophthalmos or other globe dystopia may be present, usually without significant external ophthalmoplegia or diplopia.
- Clinically LH and OAL are indistinguishable.

DIAGNOSTIC TESTS & INTERPRETATION

Lab

Initial lab tests

Laboratory testing is usually not helpful. An elevated lactate dehydrogenase may be noted in aggressive or disseminated OAL.

Follow-up & special considerations

Serologic testing is performed after pathologic diagnosis. In general, additional testing includes: CBC with differential, serum lactate dehydrogenase, beta-2-microglobulin, protein electrophoresis, renal and hepatic function, and HIV serology.

Imaging

Initial approach

- CT or MRI of the orbits is performed in all cases of suspected OAL, even with presumed clinically localized conjunctival involvement, since 50% of these patients will have deeper, orbital extension.
- About 50% of OAL lesions mold to the native anatomy and 50% are well-circumscribed.
- Bony erosion and adjacent anatomic spread (paranasal sinuses) are uncommon and suggest aggressive histopathology.

Follow-up & special considerations

- Secondary imaging is necessary for staging.
- In OAL, head and body PET/CT is becoming the imaging modality of choice, both for staging and to monitor response to therapy.
- For LH, PET/CT is usually not approved by insurance carriers and CT or MRI of the neck, thorax, abdomen, and pelvis are performed.
- Depending on the chemotherapeutic regimen planned, cardiac function is typically assessed by multigated acquisition (MUGA) scanning.

Diagnostic Procedures/Other

- For OAL, bone marrow biopsy is usually recommended, at the discretion of the oncologist.
- Lumbar puncture is performed in cases of suspected central nervous system lymphoma, usually seen in conjunction with HIV infection.

Pathological Findings

- For OALD, tissue should be sent for histopathology, immunohistochemistry, and flow cytometry. Additional cytogenetic testing may also be necessary. Correct handling of the excised tissue is important.
  - Histopathology and immunohistochemistry are performed on formalin-fixed tissue.
  - Flow cytometry can only be performed on fresh (non-fixed) tissue. The minimum volume needed for flow cytometry approximates the size of a pea.

DIFFERENTIAL DIAGNOSIS

- Inflammatory conditions (e.g., sarcoidosis, Wegener granulomatosis)
- Metastatic lesions
- Primary conjunctival, eyelid, lacrimal gland (especially pleomorphic adenoma), and orbital lesions
- Sinoorbital aspergillosis

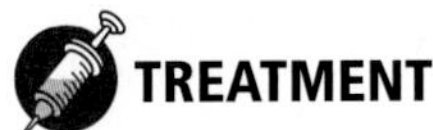

TREATMENT

MEDICATION

- Treatment is highly dependent on several issues:
  - LH is usually treated with a course of oral corticosteroids, and refractory cases with low dose radiotherapy.
  - For OAL, treatment is guided by the subtype of lymphoma.
  - The location of the lesion. In general the best prognosis is for unilateral conjunctival lesions. Negative prognostic features for OAL include location in the eyelids or lacrimal gland, bilateral involvement, bone erosion, and presence of optic neuropathy.
- Localized, indolent disease may be treated with radiotherapy (total dose of 30 Gy).
- Systemic disease or localized, aggressive OAL is typically treated with systemic chemotherapy. The specific protocols are guided by lymphoma subtype, comorbidities, and response to therapy as noted on follow-up PET/CT.
- In cases of localized, indolent OAL in an elderly patient, simple excision and watchful waiting may be all that is necessary.
- Although antibiotic therapy is highly effective in the treatment of *H. pylori*-associated gastric EMZL, there is to date no evidence that any antibiotic regimen is effective for OAL.
- The use of biologics (e.g., rituximab) is increasing, with impressive early results.

ADDITIONAL TREATMENT

General Measures

Long-term follow-up is indicated in all patients with LH or OAL, since both have a risk for subsequent systemic lymphoma development or recurrence.

Issues for Referral

- Patients with LH can be followed by an ophthalmologist, as long as systemic monitoring is performed on a routine and long-term basis.
- Essentially all cases of OAL are referred to an oncologist for staging and therapeutic options.
- Referral to a radiation therapist may be indicated in some cases of LH and OAL.

SURGERY/OTHER PROCEDURES

The goal of surgery is definitive diagnosis. Complete excision is usually unnecessary and not recommended because of increased local morbidity. Correct handling of the tissue specimen is essential (see Pathologic Findings).

IN-PATIENT CONSIDERATIONS

Admission Criteria

As needed for specific chemotherapeutic regimens and for patient comorbidities

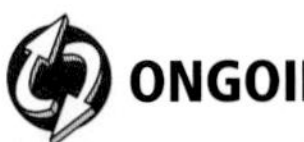

ONGOING CARE

FOLLOW-UP RECOMMENDATIONS

As noted, all patients with LH and OAL must be followed for the long term (years to decades) by the ophthalmologist for local disease monitoring and by an oncologist for systemic monitoring.

Patient Monitoring

- Local monitoring of the ocular adnexa is initially performed every few weeks until response to therapy is noted. Thereafter, patients may be monitored every few months during the first year, and subsequently every 6–12 months.
- Long-term systemic monitoring is indicated for all patients. Typically the oncologist performs serial clinical exams and PET/CT or other imaging modalities.

PATIENT EDUCATION

- Depends on subtype of OALD and staging.
- The patient must understand that even with localized disease or systemic disease with complete therapeutic response, long-term systemic monitoring is mandatory.

PROGNOSIS

- For LH, prognosis is excellent.
- For OAL, prognosis is dependent on multiple factors, including OAL subtype, stage at presentation, and response to therapy (Table 2).

Table 2 **Ten year mortality of OAL subtypes. Note that this data precedes the use of biologics (e.g. rituximab)**

All OAL	20–25%
EMZL	10%
FL*	20–25%
DLBCL	40–45%
MCL	75–100%

*Includes all grades of FL. DLBCL: Diffuse large B-cell lymphoma; EMZL: extranodal marginal zone lymphoma; FL: Follicular cell lymphoma; MCL: Mantle cell lymphoma; OAL: Ocular adnexal lymphoma

COMPLICATIONS

- Local: Recurrence, radiation injury.
- Systemic: Related to chemotherapy and systemic disease.
- Other: Therapeutic failure, disease recurrence, transformation to more aggressive subtype.

ADDITIONAL READING

- Ferry JA, Fung CY, Zukerberg L, et al. Lymphoma of the ocular adnexa: A study of 353 cases. *Am J Surg Pathol* 2007;31:170–184.
- Jaffe ES. The 2008 WHO classification of lymphomas: Implications for clinical practice and translational research. *Hematology Am Soc Hematol Educ Program* 2009:523–531.
- Jakobiec FA. Ocular adnexal lymphoid tumors: progress in need of clarification. *Am J Ophthalmol* 2008;145:941–950.
- Jenkins C, Rose GE, Bunce C, et al. Clinical features associated with survival of patients with lymphoma of the ocular adnexa. *Eye (Lond)* 2003;17:809–820.
- Sullivan TJ, Whitehead K, Williamson R, et al. Lymphoproliferative disease of the ocular adnexa: a clinical and pathologic study with statistical analysis of 69 patients. *Ophthal Plast Reconstr Surg* 2005;21:177–188.
- Sullivan TJ, Valenzuela AA. Imaging features of ocular adnexal lymphoproliferative disease. *Eye (Lond)* 2006;20:1189–1195.

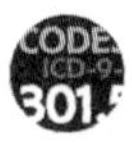

CODES

ICD9

- 190.1 Orbital tumor, malignant
- 200.81 Lymphoma malignant specific

CLINICAL PEARLS

- OALD is a spectrum of lymphoproliferation, from polyclonal LH to monoclonal lymphoma.
- Not all OAL is equal. Certain subtypes are indolent and localized, and others are aggressive and systemic.
- EMZL is the most common form of OAL and generally behaves in an indolent fashion.
- Bilateral OAL is a positive predictive factor for eventual systemic lymphoma.
- Regardless of OALD type, all patients require systemic work-up and long term monitoring.
- The treatment of OALD varies and may include systemic corticosteroids, radiotherapy, chemotherapy, or any combination.
- Biologics may improve OAL survival.

OCULAR HYPERTENSION

Tara A. Uhler

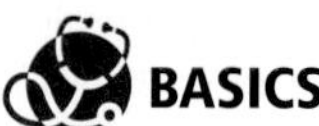

BASICS

DESCRIPTION

Elevated intraocular pressure (IOP >21 mm Hg) with normal anterior chamber angle and anatomy and no evidence of optic nerve or visual field damage

EPIDEMIOLOGY

Incidence

Unknown

Prevalence

4–7% of individuals older than 40 years.

RISK FACTORS

- No specific risk factors identified
- Risk factors for subsequent development of primary open-angle glaucoma include increased age, IOP, cup to disc ratio, and pattern standard deviation (PSD) on visual field testing as well as thinner central corneal thickness (CCT) (1,2)[A].

Genetics

- No specific markers yet identified.
- An association study of Ocular Hypertension Treatment Study (OHTS) participants is underway.

GENERAL PREVENTION

No preventative measures known but routine eye exams result in earlier identification, monitoring, and intervention if glaucomatous damage occurs.

PATHOPHYSIOLOGY

Unknown but may share features with primary open-angle glaucoma

ETIOLOGY

Unknown but may share features with primary open-angle glaucoma

COMMONLY ASSOCIATED CONDITIONS

- Increased CCT
- Primary open-angle glaucoma

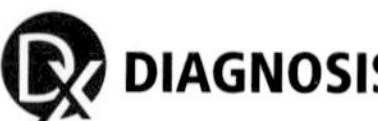

DIAGNOSIS

HISTORY

Asymptomatic

PHYSICAL EXAM

- Elevated IOP with gonioscopically normal anterior chamber angle and anatomy
- No corneal edema, anterior chamber reaction, or conjunctival injection
- No detectable optic nerve or visual field damage

DIAGNOSTIC TESTS & INTERPRETATION

Imaging

Initial approach

Optic nerve head analysis (e.g., Heidelberg retina topography [HRT] or optical coherence tomography [OCT]) will be normal in ocular hypertension but abnormal in primary open-angle glaucoma.

Follow-up & special considerations

Serial evaluation of the optic nerve head is necessary to detect subsequent glaucomatous damage and initiate or alter treatment.

Diagnostic Procedures/Other

- Pachymetry—thinner corneas yield falsely low IOP readings, and thicker corneas yield falsely high IOPs.
- Visual field testing—if abnormal and consistent with optic nerve findings, suspect primary open-angle glaucoma.

Pathological Findings

None—hallmark of ocular hypertension is elevated IOP without detectable damage.

DIFFERENTIAL DIAGNOSIS

- Primary open-angle glaucoma—damage to the nerve and visual field
- Secondary open-angle glaucoma—other associated findings such as inflammation, pigment dispersion, or pseudoexfoliation
- Chronic angle-closure glaucoma—peripheral anterior synechiae and damage to the nerve and visual field

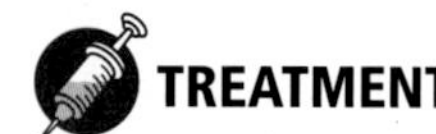

TREATMENT

MEDICATION

First Line

If treatment and not observation is planned, topical prostaglandin analogue or beta-blocker is preferred (3,4)[A].

Second Line

Topical carbonic anhydrase inhibitor or alpha-adrenergic agonist

ADDITIONAL TREATMENT

General Measures

The decision to treat or monitor closely in the absence of glaucomatous damage is complicated and requires discussion with the patient and evaluation of risk factors for open-angle glaucoma.

Additional Therapies

Laser trabeculoplasty is often considered a first-line treatment option or as an adjunct to topical medications.

SURGERY/OTHER PROCEDURES

- Laser trabeculoplasty
- Trabeculectomy if progression and laser or medical therapy insufficient
- Aqueous tube shunt if progression and laser or medical therapy insufficient

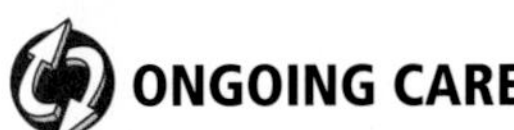

ONGOING CARE

FOLLOW-UP RECOMMENDATIONS

Initially patients, whether treated or not, should be monitored every 3–4 months according to the standard follow-up for primary open-angle glaucoma.

Patient Monitoring

If no damage occurs in the first few years, the frequency of monitoring can be reduced to every 6–12 months.

PATIENT EDUCATION

Patients should understand the importance of monitoring and the increased risk of the development of open-angle glaucoma.

PROGNOSIS

- In 5 years, approximately 10% of untreated patients with ocular hypertension greater than 24 mm Hg will develop glaucoma.
- 4.4% cumulative risk of glaucoma development with treatment group; 9.5% without treatment (3)[A]

COMPLICATIONS

Development of glaucomatous optic nerve and visual field damage

REFERENCES

1. Gordon MO, Beiser JA, Brandt JD, et al. The Ocular Hypertension Treatment Study: Baseline factors that predict the onset of primary open-angle glaucoma. *Arch Ophthalmol* 2002;120(6):714–720; discussion 829–830.
2. Brandt JD SL, Beiser JA, Kass MA, et al. Ocular Hypertension Treatment Study Group. Central corneal thickness in the Ocular Hypertension Treatment Study (OHTS). *Ophthalmol* 2001; 108(10):1779–1788.
3. Mansberger SL, Hughes BA, Gordon MO, et al. Ocular Hypertension Treatment Study Group. Comparison of initial intraocular pressure response with topical beta-adrenergic antagonists and prostaglandin analogues in African American and white individuals in the Ocular Hypertension Treatment Study. *Arch Ophthalmol* 2007;125(4): 454–459
4. Kass MA, Heuer DK, Higginbotham EJ, et al. The Ocular Hypertension Treatment Study: A randomized trial determines that topical ocular hypotensive medication delays or prevents the onset of primary open-angle glaucoma. *Arch Ophthalmol* 2002;120(6):701–713; discussion 829–830.

ADDITIONAL READING

- Kass MA, Gordon MO, Gao F, et al. Ocular Hypertension Treatment Study Group. Delaying treatment of ocular hypertension: The Ocular Hypertension Treatment Study. *Arch Ophthalmol* 2010;128(3):276–287.

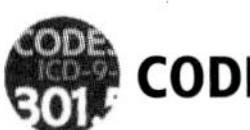

CODES

ICD9

365.04 Ocular hypertension

CLINICAL PEARLS

- Not all patients with ocular hypertension will develop glaucoma.
- The decision to treat will include patient preferences and evaluation of other risk factors for glaucoma.
- Close follow-up will allow earlier identification of progression to glaucoma and earlier intervention or modification of treatment.

OCULAR ISCHEMIC SYNDROME

Eric Chen

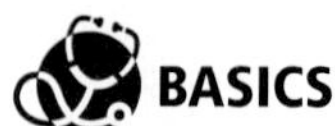

BASICS

DESCRIPTION

- Ocular ischemic syndrome (OIS) refers to anterior and posterior segment signs and symptoms related to chronic ocular hypoperfusion.
- Most common cause is severe carotid occlusive disease.
- The most common symptoms are monocular visual loss and ocular/orbital pain.
- Patients are also at increased risk for cerebral and myocardial infarction.

EPIDEMIOLOGY

Incidence

- Relatively uncommon but probably underdiagnosed
- Estimated at 7.5 cases per million per year

RISK FACTORS

- Males > females 2:1 (atherosclerotic disease)
- Older age: mean 65 years, range 50–80 years
- No racial predilection
- Bilateral involvement in up to 22% of cases

PATHOPHYSIOLOGY

- Decreased vascular perfusion in the presence of poor collateral circulation leads to hypoperfusion of ocular tissues.
- Ischemia and subsequent neovascularization produce ocular signs and symptoms.

ETIOLOGY

- Reduced blood flow to the eye/orbit
  - Most common is severe atherosclerotic disease of carotid vascular system (generally $\geq$90% stenosis), with internal > common > external carotid.
  - 5% lifetime risk for patients with internal carotid artery (ICA) stenosis to develop OIS
  - Less common: ophthalmic artery disease, systemic vasculitis (giant cell arteritis [GCA]), vaso-occlusive disease (i.e., aortic arch syndrome), Takayasu arteritis

COMMONLY ASSOCIATED CONDITIONS

- Systemic vascular disease
  - Systemic arterial hypertension (HTN)
  - Diabetes mellitus (DM)
  - Coronary artery disease (CAD)
  - Previous cerebrovascular accident or transient ischemic attack
  - Peripheral vascular disease

DIAGNOSIS

HISTORY

- Loss of vision
  - Most frequent symptom; present in 70% or above at presentation, absent in less than or equal to 10%
  - Variable in severity and onset—more than 2/3 are less than 20/60 at presentation; most experience vision loss over weeks to months, although some have abrupt vision loss
- Pain—40% present with pain due to increased intraocular pressure (IOP) or ischemia ("ocular angina"—dull, constant ache over the brow)
- Transient vision loss/amaurosis fugax
  - Present in 10–15% of patients
- Afterimages or prolonged recovery of vision after light exposure

PHYSICAL EXAM

- Anterior segment
  - Conjunctival and episcleral injection
  - Corneal edema and/or Descemet's folds
  - Iris atrophy and neovascularization (66%)
  - Anterior and posterior synechiae
  - Fixed and semidilated pupil or afferent pupil defect (APD)
  - Mild iritis in 20% (flare > cell)
  - Cataract
  - Neovascular glaucoma in 1/3 of patients
  - IOP may be low/normal second to decreased ciliary body perfusion.
  - Hypotony can further exacerbate corneal decompensation, cataract, and maculopathy.
- Posterior segment (more frequent)
  - Narrowed retinal arteries
  - Veins dilated but not tortuous
  - Retinal hemorrhages in 80% of patients, mostly dot-blot and in midperipheral retina
  - Microaneurysms common in midperipheral retina; more visible on fluorescein angiogram
  - Spontaneous retinal arterial pulsations
  - Cherry-red spot (12%) from embolic or increased IOP induced occlusion of central retinal artery
  - Cotton–wool spots (6%)
  - Choroidal ischemia and peripheral wedge-shaped chorioretinal atrophy
  - Neovascularization of disc (NVD) in 35%, neovascularization elsewhere (NVE) in 10%
- Orbital infarction syndrome
  - Ischemia of intraocular and intraorbital contents
  - Corneal hypoesthesia, intraocular inflammation, hypotony, ophthalmoplegia, ptosis, proptosis, orbital pain
- Systemic exam
  - Pulses, carotid and cardiac auscultation

DIAGNOSTIC TESTS & INTERPRETATION

Lab

Initial lab tests

- Fluorescein angiography (FA)
  - Delayed or patchy choroidal filling in 60% of patients; most specific FA sign
  - Prolonged arteriovenous transit time in up to 95% of patients; most sensitive
  - Staining of retinal vessels in 85%; arterial more than venous staining
  - Leading edge of arterial dye
  - 15% with macular edema (noncystoid pattern), often with disc leakage
  - Retinal capillary nonperfusion
- Consider ESR or C-reactive protein (CRP) if suspected GCA

Follow-up & special considerations

- Indocyanine green angiography (ICG)
  - Prolonged arm–choroid time; slow intrachoroidal filling time; and watershed zone filling

Imaging

Initial approach

- Carotid Doppler ultrasound
  - Most commonly used noninvasive test shows anatomy and hemodynamics.
  - Reduced peak systolic velocity and increased vascular resistance of end arteries
  - May be limited by complex anatomy, large plaque, calcific shadows, or tortuous vessels
  - Operator and machine dependent

Follow-up & special considerations

- Retrobulbar vessel Doppler
  - May show reversal of ophthalmic artery flow, a highly specific indicator of high-grade ICA stenosis or occlusion
- Magnetic resonance angiography
  - Noninvasive; evaluates anatomy of intracranial vessels and very accurate
  - Limits include claustrophobia, pacemaker, metallic stents, and obesity.
- Carotid angiography
  - Gold standard for imaging cerebrovascular system, but expensive and invasive (risk for cerebral infarction)
  - Perform if surgery a consideration

Diagnostic Procedures/Other

- Electroretinography (ERG)
  - Ischemia of outer and inner retina with decreased amplitude of a and b waves
- Visual-evoked potentials (VEP)
  - Increased latency, decreased amplitude
- Ophthalmodynamometry
  - Decreased ophthalmic and central retinal artery pressure

Pathological Findings

Loss of endothelial cells and pericytes in peripheral retinal vessels can lead to vessel leakage.

DIFFERENTIAL DIAGNOSIS

- Central retinal vein occlusion (CRVO)
  - Dilated and tortuous retinal veins (due to outflow obstruction in CRVO vs. decreased inflow in OIS)
  - Flame-shaped (more superficial) hemorrhages in all 4 quadrants
  - Swollen optic nerve
  - Macular edema is common.
- Diabetic retinopathy
  - Always bilateral, usually symmetric
  - Microaneurysms and dot-blot hemorrhages common in posterior pole as well as midperipheral retina
  - Hard exudates common
  - Rare diabetic papillopathy

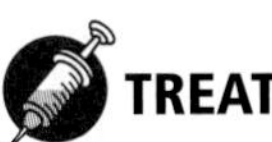

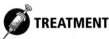

TREATMENT

Goal is to treat the underlying problem (ocular hypoperfusion) and associated ocular complications.

MEDICATION

First Line

- Topical treatment (1)[B]
  - Steroids—reduce inflammation
  - Cycloplegia—stabilize blood–aqueous border
  - IOP-lowering agents that reduce aqueous outflow (beta-blockers, alpha-agonists, or carbonic anhydrase inhibitors)
  - Avoid pilocarpine and prostaglandins (may increase inflammation)
- Intravitreal injections (2)[C]
  - Anti–vascular endothelial growth factor (VEGF) and steroids can be considered to treat macular edema.
  - Anti-VEGF may help with neovascularization.

Second Line

- Panretinal photocoagulation can cause regression of NVD, neovascularization of the iris (NVI), and NVE in 1/3 of cases and can reduce risk of neovascular glaucoma (NVG).
- NVG is often refractory to medical treatment and may require surgery with trabeculectomy, tube shunt, or cycloablation if poor visual prognosis.

ADDITIONAL TREATMENT

General Measures

- Systemic disease must be treated as patients have high risk of vascular death.
  - Treatment of systemic disease: HTN, DM, dyslipidemia, CAD
  - Antiplatelet therapy
  - Lifestyle modification: smoking cessation, healthy diet, weight loss

Issues for Referral

- All patients with OIS should have medical workup by primary care physician.
- Consider consultations from cardiology and neurosurgery.

Additional Therapies

Thrombolytic therapy can be considered in appropriate patients

SURGERY/OTHER PROCEDURES

- Carotid endarterectomy (CEA) (3)[A]
  - CEA and aspirin superior to aspirin alone in preventing stroke in patients with symptomatic/asymptomatic carotid stenosis
  - CEA for symptomatic stenosis of 50–99% if risk of stroke/death is less than 6%
  - CEA for asymptomatic stenosis of 60–99% if risk of stroke/death is less than 3%
  - Effect on visual outcome inconclusive: more beneficial if CEA performed before development of NVG
- Carotid artery stenting
  - Alternative in patients with difficult anatomy or medical conditions that preclude CEA
- Extraintracranial bypass surgery
  - Consider if complete occlusion of ICA or common carotid artery (CCA)

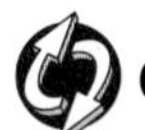

ONGOING CARE

DIET

Low-fat, low-salt, low-sugar diet given other systemic conditions

PROGNOSIS

- Overall visual prognosis is poor.
  - Visual acuity at presentation is an important predictor of final outcomes.
  - Iris neovascularization at presentation associated with poor visual outcome—97% of these eyes have final visual acuity (VA) less than finger counting
- Systemic outcomes
  - Mortality rate 40% at 5 years
    - Cardiovascular disease (myocardial infarction [MI]) accounts of 2/3 for deaths.
    - Cerebral infarcts cause 19% of deaths.
    - Cancer is the 3rd leading cause.
  - Mortality rate is 11% in age- and sex-matched controls.

REFERENCES

1. Mendrinos E, Machinis TG, Pournaras CJ. Ocular ischemic syndrome. *Surv Ophthalmol* 2010; 55(1):2–34.
2. Hazin R, Daoud YJ, Khan F. Ocular ischemic syndrome: Recent trends in medical management. *Curr Opin Ophthalmol* 2009;20(6):430–433.
3. Goldstein LB, Adams R, Alberts MJ, et al. Primary prevention of ischemic stroke: A guideline from the American Heart Association/American Stroke Association Stroke Council: Cosponsored by the Atherosclerotic Peripheral Vascular Disease Interdisciplinary Working Group; Cardiovascular Nursing Council; Clinical Cardiology Council; Nutrition, Physical Activity, and Metabolism Council; and the Quality of Care and Outcomes Research Interdisciplinary Working Group. *Circulation* 2006;113(24):873–923.

ADDITIONAL READING

- Brown GC, Magargal LE. The ocular ischemic syndrome. Clinical, fluorescein angiographic and carotid angiographic features. *Int Ophthalmol* 1988;11(4):239–251.
- Chen CS, Miller NR. Ocular ischemic syndrome: review of clinical presentations, etiology, investigation, and management. *Compr Ophthalmol Update* 2007;8(1):17–28.
- Sivalingam A, Brown GC, Magargal LE, et al. The ocular ischemic syndrome II. Mortality and systemic morbidity. *Int Ophthalmol* 1989;13:187–191.

CODES

ICD9

- 369.8 Unqualified visual loss, one eye
- 379.91 Pain in or around eye

CLINICAL PEARLS

- High level of suspicion as delayed diagnosis can lead to ocular or systemic morbidity/mortality.
- Consider OIS in any older patient with new-onset uveitis or any patient with markedly asymmetric diabetic retinopathy.
- Multidisciplinary approach is needed.

OCULAR SURFACE SQUAMOUS NEOPLASIA (OSSN)

Hyunjin Jane Kim
Carol L. Shields

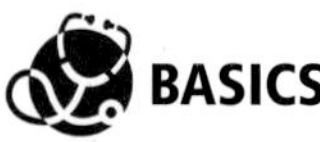

BASICS

DESCRIPTION

- The term "ocular surface squamous neoplasia (OSSN)" describes a spectrum of conjunctival and corneal epithelial dysplasia ranging from conjunctival/corneal intraepithelial dysplasia (CIN) to squamous cell carcinoma (SCC) (1)[A].
  - CIN is analogous to actinic keratosis and does not invade conjunctival substantia propria or corneal Bowman's layer.
    - Mild CIN: partial dysplasia of epithelium.
    - Severe CIN (carcinoma in situ): full-thickness intraepithelial neoplasia.
  - Invasive SCC (when neoplasia breaches the basement membrane) is locally invasive and may metastasize in 1–2%.

EPIDEMIOLOGY

Incidence

- Most common tumor of the ocular surface
  - 0.03/100,000 persons in the U.S. (only of SCC; 18-year period)
  - 0.13/100,000 persons in Uganda (6-year period)
  - 1.9/100,000 persons in Australia (10-year period)

Prevalence

- Ranks among the top three most common ocular surface malignancies with melanoma and lymphoma
- In one pathology series, it was the most prevalent malignancy of the ocular surface at 4% of 2,455 conjunctival lesions in adults.

RISK FACTORS

- Advanced age (>60 years)
- Male
- Smokers
- Light complexion
- Exposure to UV light or petroleum products.
- Human papillomavirus (HPV) 16 and 18 (conflicting data)
- Atopic eczema

Genetics

Expression of aberrant *p53* tumor suppressor gene observed in 73% of ocular surface SCC.

GENERAL PREVENTION

- Smoking cessation
- Protection from the sun

PATHOPHYSIOLOGY

UV-induced mutation or HPV-encoded destruction of *p53* gene

ETIOLOGY

UV light, HPV infection

COMMONLY ASSOCIATED CONDITIONS

- HIV/AIDS
- Immunosuppressed state
- Xeroderma pigmentosum
- Atopic eczema
- Organ transplantation

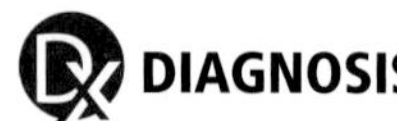

DIAGNOSIS

HISTORY

- Presenting symptoms: ocular irritation
- Ask about history of smoking, sun burns, and chemical exposure.
- Ask about prior eye medications and surgery.
- Ask about systemic conditions.

PHYSICAL EXAM

- Commonly occur in the exposed interpalpebral area at or near the limbus
  - Conjunctival component can be gelatinous, papilliform, or leukoplakic (white due to hyperkeratosis).
  - Corneal component appears as a translucent, gray epithelial sheet with pseudopodia-like margins.
  - Rose bengal staining helps to delineate tumor margins.
- Invasive SCC can be fixed to the underlying tissue and have large feeder vessels, with varying amounts of leukoplakia.
- CIN and SCC cannot be differentiated based on clinical features alone.
- Gonioscopy to evaluate iris and trabecular meshwork
- May be pigmented in patients with dark complexion (2)[C]

DIAGNOSTIC TESTS & INTERPRETATION

Lab

Initial lab tests

HIV test if OSSN present in a young adult.

Follow-up & special considerations

- Gonioscopy to evaluate for invasion of iris and trabecular meshwork through which SCC can access the systemic circulation.
- Uveitis and high intraocular pressure in the setting of known SCC should be considered to have intraocular invasion until proven otherwise.

Imaging

Initial approach

Ultrasound biomicroscopy to estimate the depth of limbal invasion of the SCC.

Follow-up & special considerations

- Two less common but more aggressive variations of SCC are the following:
  - Mucoepidermoid carcinoma: affect the elderly, has yellow mucinous cysts, tendency for intraocular and orbital invasion
  - Spindle cell carcinoma: greater tendency to metastasize

Diagnostic Procedures/Other

- Primary complete excisional biopsy is most appropriate if possible.
- Map biopsy for large and diffuse OSSN in which a plan for topical chemotherapy is considered.
- Some advocate impression cytology to establish the diagnosis.
- Rose bengal staining helps delineate tumor margins.

Pathological Findings

- Mild CIN: partial-thickness replacement of the epithelium by anaplastic cells that lack normal maturation
- Severe CIN: full-thickness replacement of the epithelium by anaplastic cells
- Invasive SCC: anaplastic squamous cells displaying hyperkeratosis and dyskeratosis invading the underlying stroma and adjacent tissues.
  - Mucoepidermoid carcinoma: a malignant epithelial lesion containing both mucinous and epidermoid differentiation, which immunostain for acid mucopolysaccharide and cytokeratin markers, respectively.
  - Spindle cell carcinoma: also known as sarcomatous carcinoma with both epithelial and mesenchymal differentiation, which immunostain for cytokeratin markers and vimentin, respectively.

DIFFERENTIAL DIAGNOSIS

- Benign
  - Conjunctivitis (for diffuse, flat OSSN)
  - Pinguecula, pterygium
  - Papilloma
  - Pyogenic granuloma
  - Nevus
- Malignant
  - Amelanotic melanoma
  - Sebaceous carcinoma
  - Metastasis

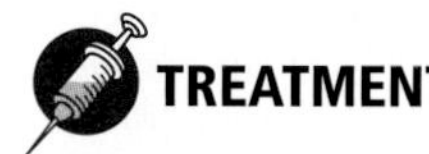

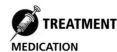

TREATMENT

MEDICATION

Not relevant (complete excision preferred)

ADDITIONAL TREATMENT

General Measures

Complete surgical removal with negative margins is most desirable for tumor removal and diagnostic confirmation.

Issues for Referral

Because of high recurrence after an incomplete removal, early referral to an Ocular Oncology Service may be considered.

COMPLEMENTARY & ALTERNATIVE THERAPIES

- For extensive (>8 mm in basal diameter) or recurrent OSSN, use topical chemotherapeutic as an adjunct to reduce the size and thickness:
  - Mitomycin C (MMC; toxic to ocular surface): 0.4 mg/mL (0.04%) 1 gtt q.i.d.; resolution in 4 months (3)[A], (4,5)[C]
  - 5-Fluorouracil (5-FU; toxic to ocular surface): 10 mg/mL (1%) 1 gtt q.i.d. (6)[C]
  - Interferon α-2b (IFN; follicular conjunctivitis): 1–3 million IU/mL 1 gtt q.i.d.; resolution in 6 months (7)[B]
- Subconjunctival injection of IFN (transient flu-like symptoms)
- Plaque brachytherapy for local recurrence or anterior orbital invasion

SURGERY/OTHER PROCEDURES

- Excisional biopsy for localized OSSN
  - "No touch" technique with alcohol corneal epitheliectomy, partial sclerokeratoconjunctivectomy, and double freeze-thaw cryotherapy (8)[A]
  - Margins: 2–4 mm (greater if suspecting invasive SCC) beyond the clinical margins of the tumor and a thin lamella of the underlying sclera should be removed.
- Excision of larger OSSN requires tissue graft.
- Plaque radiotherapy for local intraocular invasion
- Enucleation for diffuse intraocular invasion
- Eyelid-sparing exenteration for extensive orbital invasion

IN-PATIENT CONSIDERATIONS

Not relevant

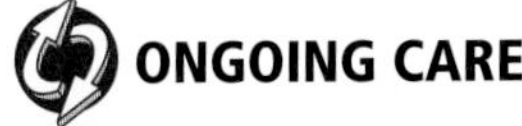

ONGOING CARE

FOLLOW-UP RECOMMENDATIONS

- Long-term follow-up (>10 years) necessary because of high recurrence, but most occur within the first 2 years.
  - Up to 30% with negative surgical margins
  - More than 50% with positive surgical margins
  - Recurrence is now much less with the use of adjunctive topical chemotherapy and IFN.

PATIENT MONITORING

Follow-up every 2–4 months until clinical resolution if using topical agents

DIET

Not relevant

PROGNOSIS

- Overall prognosis is good with extremely rare OSSN-related mortality.
  - Associated with local invasion
- Intraocular invasion via limbal perforating vessels gaining access to Schlemm's canal, trabecular meshwork, anterior chamber, suprachoroidal space, and choroid.
  - Associated with large (>2 cm) OSSN
  - Manifest as uveitis and glaucoma
- Can metastasize to preauricular, submandibular, and cervical lymph nodes; parotid gland; lungs; and bone in advanced disease
- Immunosuppressed patients are at highest risk for lymph node metastasis.

COMPLICATIONS

- Surgical treatment: potential limbal deficiency because of preferential location of OSSN at the limbus, conjunctival scarring, recurrence if multifocal disease unrecognized
- Medical treatment: local toxicity, recurrence due to poor penetration beyond the epithelium

REFERENCES

1. Lee GA, Hirst LW. Ocular surface squamous neoplasia. *Surv Ophthalmol* 1995;39:429–450.
2. Shields CL, Manchandia A, Subbiah R, et al. Pigmented squamous cell carcinoma of the conjunctiva in 5 cases. *Ophthalmology* 2008;115:1673–1678.
3. Hirst LW. Randomized controlled trial of topical mitomycin C for ocular surface squamous neoplasia. *Ophthalmology* 2007;114:976–982.
4. Shields CL, Naseripour M, Shields JA. Topical mitomycin C for extensive, recurrent conjunctival squamous cell carcinoma. *Am J Ophthalmol* 2002;133:601–606.
5. Shields CL, Demirci H, Marr BP, et al. Chemoreduction with topical mitomycin C prior to resection of extensive squamous cell carcinoma of the conjunctiva. *Arch Ophthalmol* 2005;123: 109–113.
6. Yeatts RP, Engelbrecht NE, Curry CD, et al. 5-Fluorouracil for the treatment of intraepithelial neoplasia of the conjunctiva and cornea. *Ophthalmology* 2000;107:2190–2195.
7. Sturges A, Butt AL, Lai JE, et al. Topical interferon or surgical excision for the management of primary ocular surface squamous neoplasia. *Ophthalmology* 2008;115:1297–1302.
8. Shields JA, Shields CL, De Potter P. Surgical management of conjunctival tumors. The 1994 Lynn B. McMahan Lecture. *Arch Ophthalmol* 1997;115:808–815.

ADDITIONAL READING

- Shields CL, Demirci H, Karatza E, Shields JA. Clinical survey of 1643 melanocytic and nonmelanocytic tumors of the conjunctiva. *Ophthalmology* 2004; 111:1747–1754.
- Shields CL, Shields JA. Tumors of the conjunctiva and cornea. *Surv Ophthalmol* 2004;49:3–24.
- Shields JA, Shields CL. Premalignant and malignant lesions of the conjunctival epithelium. In: Eyelid, Conjunctival, and Orbital Tumors. An Atlas and Textbook, 2nd ed. Philadelphia: Lippincott Williams & Wilkins, 2008:284–305.
- Spencer WH. Conjunctiva. In: Spencer WH, ed. *Ophthalmic pathology. an atlas and textbook*, 4th ed. Philadelphia: WB Saunders, 1996:38–125.
- Yanoff M. Conjunctiva. In: Yanoff M, Sassani JW, ed. *Ocular pathology*, 6th ed. Amsterdam, Netherlands: Elsevier, 2009:223–254.

CODES

ICD9

- 190.3 Malignant neoplasm of conjunctiva
- 190.4 Malignant neoplasm of cornea
- 234.0 Carcinoma in situ of eye

CLINICAL PEARLS

- Most common epithelial neoplasm of the cornea and conjunctiva
- Associated with age, sun exposure, smoking, HPV, and immunosuppression
- Clinically appear as a fleshy mass or leukoplakia, usually located at or near the limbus, with feeder vessels and possible corneal involvement
- A complete excision with negative margins preferred, whenever possible
- Adjunctive topical chemotherapy and IFN associated with lower recurrence rate

OCULAR SYPHILIS

Alok S. Bansal
Jeremy D. Wolfe

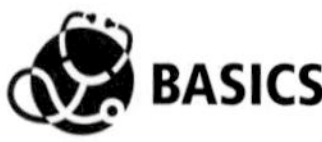

BASICS

DESCRIPTION

- Chronic, multiorgan, systemic bacterial infection caused by spirochete *Treponema pallidum*.
- Responsible for 1–2% of all uveitis cases.
- Ocular syphilis is considered a variant of neurosyphilis (see below).
- Congenital syphilis (systemic findings):
  - Early (<2 years of age): Hepatosplenomegaly, long bone changes, mucocutaneous lesions of buttocks and thighs
  - Late (>2 years of age): Frontal bossing, saddle-nose deformity, saber shins, Hutchinson teeth, deafness
- Acquired syphilis (systemic findings):
  - Primary: Self-limited painless genital chancre
  - Secondary: Maculopapular rash on palms and soles, generalized lymphadenopathy, fever, malaise
  - Early latent (exposure within the last year): Seroreactivity without clinical manifestations
  - Late latent or latent syphilis of unknown duration (exposure >1 year): Seroreactivity without clinical manifestations
  - Tertiary: Gummas, neurosyphilis, cardiovascular abnormalities (aortitis)

EPIDEMIOLOGY

Incidence

- Congenital: 10.1/100,000 in 2008 (1)[A]
  - Increased 23% from 2005
- Primary & Secondary: 15.3/100,000 in 2008
  - Increased 37% from 2005
- Regional: Highest rates (50%) in Southern US
- Age: Highest rates in 20–24 year olds
- 63% of cases in US among men who have sex with men

Prevalence

Due to the rarity of ocular syphilis and incomplete reporting to the CDC, true prevalence data (i.e., total cases) is not well known.

RISK FACTORS

- High-risk sexual behavior
- HIV coinfection
- Intravenous drug abuse

GENERAL PREVENTION

- Prenatal care to prevent congenital syphilis
- Safe sexual practices

PATHOPHYSIOLOGY

- Transmission of acquired syphilis may occur through direct contact with syphilis sore on external genitals, vagina, anus, rectum, or lips and mouth during vaginal, anal, or oral sex.
- Transmission of congenital syphilis occurs by transplacental contact.
- Ocular inflammatory response to infection caused by bacteria *Treponema pallidum*.

ETIOLOGY

Treponema pallidum, spirochete

COMMONLY ASSOCIATED CONDITIONS

- HIV
- Other sexually transmitted diseases

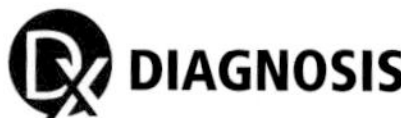

DIAGNOSIS

HISTORY

- Maternal syphilis
- HIV
- High risk sexual behavior
- Pain, redness, photophobia, blurred vision, floaters

PHYSICAL EXAM

- Syphilis may affect any or all ocular structures (2) [A]
- Congenital Syphilis:
  - Early: Chorioretinitis, retinal vasculitis, "salt-and-pepper" retinal pigment mottling
  - Late: Interstitial keratitis with corneal vascularization, ghost vessels
- Acquired Syphilis:
  - Primary: Ocular manifestations rare
  - Secondary: Anterior uveitis (granulomatous or non-granulomatous), iris nodules, scleritis, vitreitis, retinal vasculitis, retinal vascular occlusion, chorioretinitis (focal or multifocal), posterior placoid chorioretinitis, neuroretinitis, exudative retinal detachment, optic neuritis, cranial nerve palsies
  - Latent: Asymptomatic with recurrences
  - Tertiary: Argyll-Robertson pupil (pupil reacts to near target, not to light stimuli), cranial nerve palsies, other ocular findings similar to those with secondary syphilis.

DIAGNOSTIC TESTS & INTERPRETATION

Lab

Initial lab tests

- Non-treponemal: Rapid Plasma Reagin (RPR) or Venereal Disease Research Laboratory (VDRL)
  - Fourfold decrease in antibody titer used to monitor response to therapy
  - False–positives (collagen-vascular disease) and false–negatives (prozone phenomenon)
- Treponemal-specific: Fluorescent treponemal antibody absorption (FTA-ABS) or microhemagglutination-*T. pallidum* (MHA-TP)
  - Remain reactive from time of infection, thus should not be used to monitor therapeutic response.
- Lumbar puncture with cell count, protein, glucose, and CSF-VDRL to evaluate for neurosyphilis.
  - CSF-VDRL is highly specific, but not sensitive
  - 2006 CDC guidelines recommend lumbar puncture in all cases of ocular involvement, although practical indications for lumbar puncture are controversial (3)[A]
  - Isolated syphilitic anterior uveitis without neurologic signs/symptoms may not require lumbar puncture

Follow-up & special considerations

- HIV serology due to high rates of coinfection
- False–positive and false–negative rates of syphilis serologic testing may be higher in HIV patients.

Imaging

Consider MRI for any suspected case of optic nerve involvement and/or neurosyphilis.

Diagnostic Procedures/Other

Lumbar Puncture with CSF-VDRL

Pathological Findings

Corkscrew morphology on darkfield microscopy (not commonly performed).

DIFFERENTIAL DIAGNOSIS

- Ocular syphilis carries a broad differential diagnosis due to its protean manifestations
  - Sarcoidosis
  - Tuberculosis
  - Toxoplasmosis
  - Vogt-Koyanagi-Harada syndrome
  - HLA-B27 associated uveitis
  - Pars planitis
  - Acute retinal necrosis
  - CMV retinitis
  - Fungal endophthalmitis
  - White dot syndromes (e.g., APMPPE)
  - Lyme disease
  - Behçet's disease
  - Diffuse unilateral subacute neuroretinitis
  - Toxocariasis
  - Presumed ocular histoplasmosis

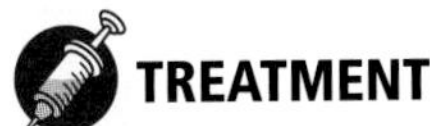

TREATMENT

MEDICATION

First Line

- Congenital: Aqueous crystalline penicillin G 50,000 units/kg/d IV q12 hrs for first 7 days of life, and q8h thereafter for total of 10 days OR Procaine penicillin G 50,000 units/kg/d IM × 10 days (3)[A]
- Primary, secondary, or early latent syphilis: Benzathine penicillin G 2.4 MU IM in single dose (3)[A]
- Late latent or tertiary without evidence of neurosyphilis: Benzathine penicillin G 2.4 MU IM, weekly × 3 doses (3)[A]
- Neurosyphilis: Aqueous penicillin G 3-4 MU IV q4h × 10–14 days OR Procaine penicillin G 2.4 MU IM q day PLUS Probenecid 500 mg PO q.i.d × 10–14 days, followed by Benzathine penicillin G 2.4 MU IM, weekly × 3 doses (3)[A]
- Manage ocular inflammation with cycloplegics, and topical, periocular, and/or oral corticosteroids
- Note: Periocular (depot) steroids should not be employed until other infectious etiologies for inflammation are eliminated from differential diagnosis or identified and treated concurrently.

Second Line

ALERT

- Penicillin Allergy:
  - For congenital syphilis, neurosyphilis, pregnancy, or HIV+, patients should undergo de-sensitization and be treated with penicillin (see above)
  - For primary, secondary, latent, or tertiary syphilis without neurosyphilis, see below:
  - Primary, secondary, or early latent: Doxycycline 100 mg PO b.i.d × 2 weeks OR Tetracycline 500 mg PO q.i.d × 2 weeks (3)[A]
  - Late latent or tertiary without evidence of neurosyphilis: Doxycycline 100 mg PO b.i.d × 4 weeks OR Tetracycline 500 mg PO q.i.d × 4 weeks (3)[A]
  - See also Alternative Therapies.

ADDITIONAL TREATMENT

General Measures

ALERT

- Monitor for Jarisch-Herxheimer reaction:
  - Acute febrile reaction that occurs within 24 hours of treatment due to penicillin-induced spirochete death.
  - Treat with supportive care

Issues for Referral

- Prompt referral to ophthalmologist for any suspected case of intraocular involvement
- Prompt referral to infectious disease specialist for concomitant HIV coinfection
- Prompt referral to neurologist for suspected neurosyphilis

COMPLEMENTARY & ALTERNATIVE THERAPIES

- Bicillin C-R (combination benzathine and procaine penicillin) **should be avoided as alternate treatment** because it contains half the dose of benzathine penicillin G (3)[C].
- Primary, secondary, or early latent: Ceftriaxone 1 gm IM/IV × 8–10 days (3)[C] or Azithromycin 2 gm PO × 1 dose (3)[C]
- Late latent or tertiary without evidence of neurosyphilis: Ceftriaxone (unknown dose or duration) (3)[C]
- Neurosyphilis: Ceftriaxone 2 gm IM/IV × 10–14 days (3)[C]
- Penicillin-allergic patients may exhibit cross-reactivity to ceftriaxone (~10%)
- The use of alternative therapies in HIV+ patients has not been well studied, and should be managed with caution.

ONGOING CARE

FOLLOW-UP RECOMMENDATIONS

- Quantitative non-treponemal (RPR, VDRL) titers should be repeated every 6 months for 2 years (every 3 months for 2 years if HIV+) to monitor for response to treatment (i.e., fourfold decline in titers) (3)[A]
  - Follow either RPR or VDRL because tests are not directly comparable
  - A VDRL titer >1:8 should decline at least fourfold within 1 year of appropriate treatment
  - A VDRL titer <1:8 often does not decrease fourfold
- Consider re-treatment for:
  - Persistent or recurrent signs/symptoms of syphilis
  - Fourfold increase in antibody titers
  - Less than fourfold decrease in antibody titers

PATIENT MONITORING

Serial ophthalmic examinations for resolution of ocular inflammation

PATIENT EDUCATION

- Counseling for safe sexual practices
- Counseling for partners of affected patients

PROGNOSIS

Visual prognosis dependent on severity of ocular inflammation

COMPLICATIONS

- Corneal scarring
- Cataract
- Glaucoma
- Macular Edema
- Retinal detachment

REFERENCES

1. Centers for Disease Control and Prevention. Sexually Transmitted Diseases Surveillance 2008. Atlanta, GA: U.S. Department of Health and Human Services; Nov 2009.
2. Aldave AJ, King JA, Cunningham ET Jr. Ocular syphilis. *Curr Opin Ophthalmol* 2001;12:433–441.
3. Center for Disease Control and Prevention.Workowski KA, Berman SM. Sexually transmitted diseases treatment guidelines 2006. *MMWR Recomm Rep* 2006;55:1–94.

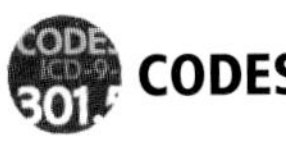

CODES

ICD9

- 091.50 Syphilitic uveitis, unspecified
- 091.51 Syphilitic chorioretinitis (secondary)
- 095.8 Other specified forms of late symptomatic syphilis

CLINICAL PEARLS

- Syphilis should be on the differential diagnosis of any case of intraocular inflammation.
- Ocular syphilis is a manifestation of neurosyphilis.
- Treatment regimen for ocular syphilis should be the same as for tertiary neurosyphilis.
- All patients with syphilis should be tested for HIV.

OPEN-ANGLE GLAUCOMAS

Patrick Tiedeken

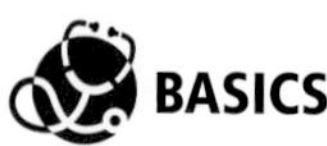

BASICS

DESCRIPTION

- A diverse group of neurodegenerative eye diseases that result in a typical excavated appearance of the optic nerve (ON)
- Associated with midperipheral and central visual field defects with the intraocular pressure (IOP) as a major risk factor
- Glaucomas are divided into open-angle glaucoma (OAG) types if the trabecular meshwork can be visualized, or closed-angle glaucoma if the meshwork cannot be visualized.
- OAG is further subdivided into primary OAG if there are no other ocular or systemic diseases present. Secondary OAG if associated with an ocular cause (i.e., exfoliative or pigmentary glaucoma) or a systemic disease (i.e., amyloidosis).

EPIDEMIOLOGY

Incidence

- 2 million patients in the USA (50% undetected)
- Glaucoma is the second leading cause of blindness in the USA.

Prevalence

10 million patients at risk as ocular hypertensives (elevated IOP with normal ONs and visual fields)

RISK FACTORS

- High IOP (major risk factor)
- Old age
  - 40–49 years = 0.22% prevalence
  - 80 years = 14% prevalence
- African American—3 times increased prevalence (vs. Caucasians) and more severe disease
- Family history (5–19% increased risk)
- Migraine headaches, myopia, hypertension

GENERAL PREVENTION

Screening for glaucoma is most effective if aimed at high-risk groups: elderly and African Americans

PATHOPHYSIOLOGY

- Final pathway is damage to the retinal ganglion cells.
- 1 Million ganglion cells in each ON
- Ganglion cell axon travels from the retina to the lateral geniculate body of the thalamus.
- 2 General theories of glaucoma ON damage: (1) VASCULAR—abnormality of blood flow damages ganglion cells. (2) MECHANICAL—weakness of lamina cribrosa (specialized connective tissue at the level of the ON canal) causes damage to the ganglion cell axons.

ETIOLOGY

- IOP is the most significant and treatable risk factor.
- Degree of glaucomatous ON damage is directly related to the IOP level.
- IOP 25–29 mm Hg = 7% prevalence ON damage.
- IOP 35–39 = 52% prevalence ON damage

ON damage can occur at normal IOP (>21 mm Hg): Baltimore Eye Study demonstrated that 50% of all OAG patients had screening IOPs of <21 mm Hg.

DIAGNOSIS

HISTORY

OAG is a diagnosis based on exam of the ON.

PHYSICAL EXAM

- A dilated stereoscopic exam is the most accurate.
- Important ON findings: large cup/disc ratio (decreased ganglion cell axons), ON asymmetry, progressive cup enlargement, neural rim notching, vertical cup enlargement, regional ON pallor, splinter disc hemorrhage, enlarged ON pit

DIAGNOSTIC TESTS & INTERPRETATION

Visual Field Tests

- Corroborates the clinical exam findings of ON damage (Superior ON damage causes inferior visual field changes.)
- Nonglaucomatous optic neuropathies: lack of correlation of visual field changes with ON damage.
- Glaucomatous optic neuropathies: the site and extent of the disc damage correlates with the severity and location of visual field loss.

Follow-up & special considerations

- Early glaucoma ON damage can have a "normal visual field" (preperimetric glaucoma).
- Postmortem studies showed that 50% of ganglion cells can be lost prior to abnormalities in the visual field.

Imaging

Initial approach

Serial, stereoscopic optic disc photography is the most accurate method of diagnosis and follow-up.

Follow-up & special considerations

Newer imaging techniques may improve clinical assessments (scanning laser polarimetry, confocal scanning laser tomography, optical coherence tomography).

DIFFERENTIAL DIAGNOSIS

- OAG is a diagnosis of exclusion.
- Optic disc pallor in excess of excavation suggests a nonglaucomatous optic neuropathy.
- Nonglaucomatous optic neuropathy may include intermittent angle-closure glaucomas, anterior ischemic optic neuropathies (giant cell arteritis), compressive optic neuropathies, congenital ON colobomas, and dominant ON atrophy.

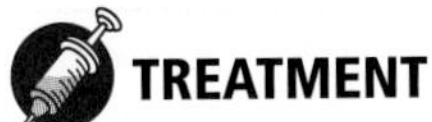

TREATMENT

ADDITIONAL TREATMENT

General Measures

- IOP reduction to prevent further optic disc damage and visual loss is the goal of treatment.
- Treatment options either lower aqueous production or increase aqueous outflow to decrease IOP.
- 3 Main treatment categories:
  - Topical medications (β-blockers, prostaglandins analogs, alpha-agonists, cholinergic agonists, carbonic anhydrase inhibitors [topical or oral])
  - Office laser procedures (laser trabeculoplasty)
  - Operating room incisional surgeries

COMPLEMENTARY & ALTERNATIVE THERAPIES

OAG Treatment Trials

- Studies demonstrating that lowering IOP slowed ON damage
  - **Ocular Hypertensive Treatment Trial**: patients with IOP 24–32 mm Hg with normal ON and visual fields treated with standard medicines versus observation showed 9.5% of observed group versus 4.5% of medically treated group developed OAG (1)[A].
  - **Collaborative Normal Tension Glaucoma Study:** showed that a 30% IOP reduction of an initially normal IOP (<21 mm Hg), prevented or delayed OAG progression in 80% or patients in 5 years (2)[A].
  - **Advanced Glaucoma Intervention Study**: showed that patients with advanced visual field loss who had IOP controlled (<18 mm Hg) 100% of office visits had no progression of visual field loss. Patients with IOP >18 mm Hg at 50% of office visits had significant worsening of visual field (3)[A].
- Studies comparing patient outcomes with different treatment protocols
  - **Glaucoma Laser Trial:** compared argon laser trabeculoplasty with standard topical medicines for lowering IOP in newly diagnosed, untreated OAG patients. 2-year results demonstrated no major differences in terms of visual acuity or visual field changes (4)[A].
  - **Collaborative Initial Glaucoma Treatment Study:** showed that newly diagnosed OAG patients randomized to initial treatment with medications and lasers versus surgical trabeculectomy had similar 5-year visual field outcomes (5)[A].
  - **Tube Versus Trabeculectomy Study:** compared OAG patient outcomes who had prior eye surgery (glaucoma or cataract surgery) and were randomized to glaucoma drainage implant surgery (Baerveldt) or trabeculectomy. The 3-year clinical outcomes were similar (6)[A].

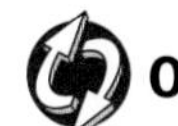

ONGOING CARE

PROGNOSIS

- Patients with worse visual field loss and ON damage at diagnosis have a higher risk of blindness.
- Early diagnosis and effective IOP-lowering treatment are critical to visual field preservation.
- Some patients with OAG progress despite IOP lowering and require more aggressive treatment.
- Close monitoring and follow-up of all patients with OAG are critical to preserve vision.
- Overall quality of life issues are critical to the treatment of patients with glaucoma.

REFERENCES

1. Kass MA, Heur DK, Higginbotham EJ, et al. The Ocular Hypertensive Treatment Study: A randomized trial determines that topical ocular hypotensive medication delays or prevents the onset of primary open-angle glaucoma. *Arch Opthalmol* 2002;120:701–713.
2. The AGIS Investigators. The Advanced Glaucoma Intervention Study (AGIS). The relationship between control or intraocular pressure and visual field deterioration. *Am J Ophthalmol* 2000;130:429–440.
3. Anderson DR, Drance SM, Schulzer M, et al. Natural history of normal-tension glaucoma. Collaborative Normal Tension Study Group. *Ophthalmology* 2001;108:247–253.
4. The Glaucoma Laser Trial Research Group. The Glaucoma Laser Trial (GLT). *Ophthalmology* 1990;97:1403–1413.
5. Lichter PR, Musch DC, Gillespie BW, et al. Interim clinical outcomes in the Collaborative Initial Glaucoma Treatment Study comparing initial treatment randomized to medications or surgery. *Ophthalmology* 2001;108:1943–1953.
6. Gedde S, Schiffman J, Feuer W, et al. Treatment outcomes in the Tube Versus Trabeculectomy Study after one year follow-up. *Ophthalmology* 2007;143:9–22.

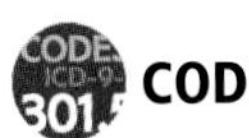

CODES

ICD9

- 365.10 Open-angle glaucoma, unspecified
- 365.11 Primary open angle glaucoma

OPHTHALMIC SARCOIDOSIS

Michael P. Rabinowitz

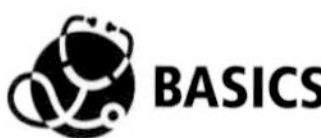

BASICS

DESCRIPTION

- Sarcoidosis is an idiopathic systemic inflammatory disease.
- It most commonly affects eyes, lungs, and skin.
- Up to 80% of patients have ophthalmic involvement.
- Sarcoidosis can affect any part of the eye, orbit, and adnexa.
  - Sarcoidosis may only affect the eye or may affect the eye before or after systemic involvement.
  - Within the eye, the anterior segment is most commonly involved (up to 70%).
  - Within the orbit, the lacrimal gland is most commonly involved (up to 61%).
  - Within the lungs, bilateral symmetric hilar adenopathy is the most common radiographic finding.
  - Skin lesions commonly include erythema nodosum (erythematous tender subdermal nodules) and lupus pernio (purple rash on face).

EPIDEMIOLOGY

- Varies widely with geography
- Can occur in any age, but most common between 20 and 40 years, and rare after 50 years
- More prevalent in women than in men
  - In North America, highest prevalence amongst African Americans: 35.5 cases per 100,000
  - In World, highest prevalence amongst Northern Europeans: up to 60 cases per 100,000
  - Bimodal peaks in Scandinavia: (25–29 years of age and 65–69 years of age)

RISK FACTORS

- African or Northern European extraction
- Although not definitive, environmental triggers such as pesticides and pollutants have been postulated.

Genetics

- May be familial, often minimal concordance
- Association with various HLAs and gene products is a current area of research.
- Two genomewide scans for sarcoidosis loci:
  - White Germans—chromosomes 3p and 6p
  - African Americans—chromosomes 5p and 5q
  - Genes uncovered may be biased by populations studied.

GENERAL PREVENTION

None available

PATHOPHYSIOLOGY

- See pathological findings.
- Impetus of noncaseating granuloma formation remains unknown; likely that some nidus of inflammation, once cleared, triggers an uncontrolled inflammatory cascade.

ETIOLOGY

Unknown, see pathophysiology.

COMMONLY ASSOCIATED CONDITIONS

- Löfgren's syndrome—arthritis, erythema nodosum, and bilateral hilar adenopathy
- Sjögren-like syndrome—keratoconjunctivitis sicca, parotid dysfunction, and lacrimal gland dysfunction
- Erythema nodosum—mostly in women
- Arthritis—rheumatoid or juvenile rheumatoid
- Heerfordt's syndrome—parotid enlargement, anterior uveitis, and cranial nerve palsies
- Blau's syndrome (familial juvenile systemic granulomatosis)—children may present with granulomatous arthritis, skin and eye pathology.
- Hepatitis C—it is possible interferon therapy, and not hepatitis C, is associated with sarcoidosis.

DIAGNOSIS

HISTORY

- Systemic symptoms such as fevers, chills, sweats, and weight loss
- Sarcoidosis most commonly affects the lungs, eyes, and skin. A focused history is therefore targeted toward but not limited to
  - Coughing, wheezing, dyspnea, tachypnea, rashes, skin lesions, and arthritis are common systemic symptoms.
  - Anterior, intermediate, or posterior uveitis: pain, photophobia, floaters, redness, and decreased vision
  - Conjunctival or scleral involvement: pain, redness, pain with motility, and tearing
  - Lid or skin involvement: dry and itchy eyes, and scaling skin
  - Orbital muscle or soft tissue involvement: pain with motility, proptosis, diplopia, decreased vision, and ptosis
  - Lacrimal gland involvement: adnexal tenderness, enlargement, and dry eyes

PHYSICAL EXAM

- Physical exam should be a thorough ophthalmologic evaluation of all aforementioned ocular anatomy.
- Visual acuity, intraocular pressure, visual fields, and extraocular motility should be documented in all patients.
- Anterior slit lamp exam includes evaluation of conjunctival nodules, conjunctivitis, episcleritis, scleritis, lacrimal gland enlargement, dry eyes, corneal edema, keratic precipitates (may be granulomatous, particularly in a triangular distribution on the inferior corneal endothelium), anterior chamber cell and flare, peripheral anterior synechiae, and posterior synechiae.
- Posterior slit lamp and indirect fundus exam should evaluate for peripheral retinal neovascularization, periphlebitis and peripheral retinal vein sheathing (candle-wax drippings), intermediate uveitis, vitritis, cystoid macular edema, optic nerve edema, and Dalen–Fuchs nodules.
- All cranial nerves should be evaluated, particularly cranial nerve VII.
- Glaucoma and cataracts may result and should be followed.
- Optic nerve infiltration should be evaluated with visual acuity, visual fields, color plates, pupillary examination, and neurology consultation to evaluate for neurosarcoidosis.
- Full physical exam should evaluate for tachypnea, arthritis, lymphadenopathy, hepatosplenomegaly, erythema nodosum (most commonly found over shins), and lupus pernio.
- Imaging and further evaluation as below.

DIAGNOSTIC TESTS & INTERPRETATION

Lab

Initial lab tests

- ACE: elevated in 60–90% of patients with active sarcoidosis. Rates tend to be higher in those with active signs and symptoms. ACE may be normal in more than 9% of subjects with active sarcoidosis, and is typically unreliable in children. Furthermore, 17% of normal patients may have elevated ACE levels, and ACE levels may be decreased in those on ACE inhibitors. Sensitivity and specificity of ACE for ophthalmic sarcoidosis range from 70% to 90% in most studies. Although widely used, the sensitivity and specificity therefore make ACE levels a less than ideal screening test.
- Kveim test: splenic tissue from sarcoidosis patient injected into skin of the subject. If granulomas result several weeks later, test is positive (rarely used any longer due to lack of sensitivity/specificity and inherent health risks).
- Thorough workup to evaluate differential diagnosis of above presenting symptoms and signs (see Differential Diagnosis: HLA-B27, rapid plasma reagin (RPR), antinuclear antibody (ANA), Lyme antibodies, rheumatoid factor (RF), ESR, and other target laboratory values may be obtained.
  - Purified protein derivative (PPD) and anergy panel
  - Serum and urine calcium levels, liver function tests, and serum lysozymes are of variable utility without radiographic or histologic evidence of sarcoidosis (see below), although some authors advocate their use.

Follow-up & special considerations

Pulmonary, dermatologic, or neurologic involvement should involve internal medicine, pulmonology, dermatology, and neurologic referral. Further evaluation and treatment, as below, is often performed in conjunction with healthcare practitioners in those fields.

Imaging

Initial approach

Chest X-ray: evaluate for bilateral hilar adenopathy or infiltrates.

Follow-up & special considerations
- Chest CT if X-ray irregular or nonconclusive
- MRI to evaluate neurosarcoidosis if warranted
- Visual fields obtained for optic nerve involvement
- Consider fluorescein angiogram, B-scan ultrasonography, and optical coherence tomography to further evaluate ophthalmic findings (e.g., retinal vasculitis, neovascularization, ischemia, macular edema, vitreitis, scleritis).
- Whole-body gallium scan, when combined with positive ACE, is up to 73% sensitive and 100% specific for sarcoidosis. It has been shown positive in 90% of lacrimal glands of sarcoidosis patients even without clinical changes. A "panda sign" indicates involvement of the lacrimal, parotid, and submandibular glands, and a "lambda sign" connotes perihilar and paratracheal node involvement.

Diagnostic Procedures/Other
- Biopsy is considered if lesions are accessible, and all samples should be examined for typical granulomas with negative special stains (methenamine-silver to rule out tuberculosis and fungal infections, and acid-fast to look for mycobacteria).
- Conjunctiva may be biopsied: yield of blind conjunctival biopsy is 66% in sarcoidosis patients and 80% in those with conjunctival involvement.
- Lacrimal gland biopsy in patients suspected of having lacrimal gland involvement has around a 60% yield.
- Skin lesions may be biopsied: the edges of lesions should be sampled. Erythema nodosum does not contain pathologic changes.
- Bronchoscopy with pulmonary biopsy may be performed with consideration from a pulmonologist and/or cardiothoracic surgeon. See Issues for Referral.

Pathological Findings
Noncaseating granulomas, or congregations of epithelioid cells and macrophages, with negative special stains as above.

DIFFERENTIAL DIAGNOSIS
- May entail any potential etiology of symptoms listed in history
- May entail other causes of granulomatous inflammation including mycobacterial infection as diagnosed by biopsy with special stains
  - Other causes of granulomatous anterior uveitis include syphilis, tuberculosis, sympathetic ophthalmia, trauma, lens-induced iritis, and rarer autoimmune pathologies.
  - Multiple sclerosis, idiopathic cases, Lyme disease, inflammatory bowel disease, toxocariasis, cat scratch disease, and tubulointerstitial nephritis and uveitis syndrome may cause intermediate uveitis.
  - Posterior uveitis may be secondary to white dot syndromes, syphilis, lymphoma, sympathetic ophthalmia, and Vogt–Koyanagi–Harada syndrome.

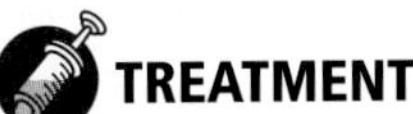

TREATMENT

MEDICATION
First Line
- Anterior uveitis: topical steroids (e.g., prednisolone acetate 1% q.i.d.), cycloplegics (e.g., atropine 1% b.i.d.) to prevent synechiae
- Posterior uveitis: systemic steroids (e.g., prednisone 20–100 mg p.o. daily) with a histamine type 2 receptor blocker or proton pump inhibitor for gastrointestinal prophylaxis. Periocular steroid injections (e.g., 1–4 mg of sub-tenon triamcinolone 40 mg/mL)
- Orbital/neurologic involvement: systemic immunosuppression, usually with corticosteroids initially
  - Majority of sarcoidosis cases regress spontaneously but observation recommended.

Second Line
- High-dose NSAIDs (standard of care in the U.K.).
- Systemic immunomodulators (e.g., methotrexate, cyclosporine, hydroxychloroquine) if steroids failed or poorly tolerated, and referral to uveitis specialist is often necessary.
- Surgical debulking or radiation therapy.
- Cystoid macular edema may be treated with topical NSAIDs (e.g., ketorolac q.i.d.), topical or periocular steroids as above, or systemic immunomodulators as above.
- Orbital and central nervous system disease usually requires systemic steroids or immunomodulators as above.
- Glaucoma should be managed with topical therapy (e.g., alpha agonists such as brimonidine 0.1% or beta blockers such as timolol 0.5%), when possible, with care to avoid prostaglandin analogues (e.g., latanoprost), as they may worsen inflammation.
- Retinal neovascularization may require panretinal photocoagulation.

ADDITIONAL TREATMENT
Issues for Referral
- Referral to an internist is warranted to evaluate possible systemic involvement: studies show between 50% and 91% of patients with primary ophthalmic sarcoidosis manifest systemic signs, and that systemic sarcoidosis may often present with ophthalmic changes.
- Referral to a pulmonologist for bronchoscopy, pulmonary function testing, and biopsy may be warranted, often with the guidance of an internist.
- Immunosuppression, as indicated above, is often coordinated with a primary care practitioner.
- Optic nerve or central nervous system involvement warrants prompt neurology and neuroophthalmology consultation.

SURGERY/OTHER PROCEDURES
See second-line therapy

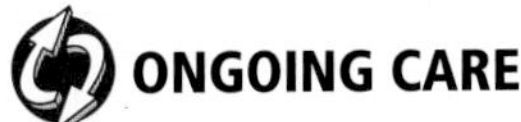

ONGOING CARE

FOLLOW-UP RECOMMENDATIONS
- Manage appropriately to resolution of presenting issue.
- Follow-up intervals depend on severity of inflammation, and patients are usually followed every 1–7 days.
- Steroid doses, whether topical or oral, are adjusted according to response to treatment and are tapered as clinical progress allows.
- Patients treated with oral steroids should be seen by their primary care physicians every 3–6 weeks for general exams and blood work to evaluate blood pressures and blood sugars.
- Quiescent disease is reevaluated every 3–6 months.

ADDITIONAL READING

- Iannuzz MC, Rybicki B, Teirstein AS. Sarcoidosis. *N Engl J Med* 2007;357:2153–2165.
- Obenauf CD, Shaw HE, Sydnor CF, Klintworth GK. Sarcoidosis and its ophthalmic manifestations. *Am J Ophthalmol* 1978;86(5):648–655.
- Bradley D, Baughman RP, Raymond L, Kaufman AH. Ocular manifestations of sarcoidosis. *Semin Respir Crit Care Med* 2002;23(6):543–548.

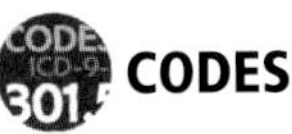

CODES

ICD9
- 135 Sarcoidosis
- 364.11 Chronic iridocyclitis in diseases classified elsewhere

CLINICAL PEARLS
- Sarcoidosis may affect any part of the eye and orbit and should therefore be considered in the differential of many orbital and ocular conditions.
- Anterior uveitis is the most common ophthalmic sign.
- Lacrimal gland involvement is the most common orbital sign.
- Many patients have no previous history of sarcoidosis.

OPTIC DISC COLOBOMA

Michael J. Bartiss

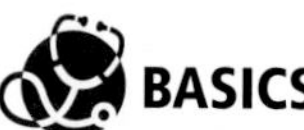

BASICS

DESCRIPTION

- Well defined, white bowl-shaped excavation inferiorly displaced in an enlarged optic disc
- Excavation location reflects position of the embryonic fissure relative to the primitive epithelial papilla
- More involved cases appear as enlargement of the peripapillary area with a deep, central excavation lined by glistening white tissue
- Superior disc typically spared, but occasional involvement of the entire disc occurs
- Defect can extend into the adjacent inferior and nasal choroid and retina
- Iris and ciliary body colobomas can coexist
- Visual acuity is primarily dependent upon integrity of the papillomacular bundle; may be mildly-to-severely decreased
- Visual acuity difficult to predict based on appearance of the disc
- Occur unilaterally and bilaterally with approximately equal frequency
- Occasional orbital cysts can occur with possible communication between the cyst and the excavation

RISK FACTORS

Genetics

- Can be accompanied by CHARGE association (CHD7)
- May arise sporadically or be inherited in an autosomal dominant pattern

GENERAL PREVENTION

Possible genetic counseling and/or prenatal testing (if mutated gene known or syndrome recognized in family)

PATHOPHYSIOLOGY

Neuroimaging demonstrates a crater-like excavation of the posterior globe at its junction with the optic nerve

ETIOLOGY

Thought to result from incomplete or abnormal coaptation of the proximal end of the embryonic fissure

COMMONLY ASSOCIATED CONDITIONS

May be accompanied by multiple systemic conditions such as:

- CHARGE Association
- Walker-Warburg Syndrome
- Goltz Focal Dermal Hypoplasia
- Aicardi Syndrome
- Goldenhar Sequence
- Linear Sebaceous Nevus Syndrome
- Increased risk of acquired visual loss through serous retinal detachment in cases of isolated optic nerve coloboma (versus the typical rhegmatogenous retinal detachments seen in chorioretinal coloboma)
- Microphthalmia may also be present in cases with coexistent chorioretinal involvement

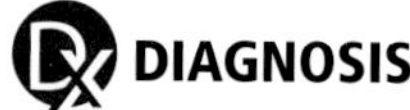

DIAGNOSIS

HISTORY

Congenital defect

PHYSICAL EXAM

- Full ocular examination including careful evaluation of the optic discs and evaluation for concomitant treatable amblyopia
- Systemic examination for other anomalies

DIAGNOSTIC TESTS & INTERPRETATION

Lab

Initial lab tests

None unless associated systemic abnormalities exist

Follow-Up & Special Considerations

Significant risk of acquired visual loss through retinal detachment dictates regular follow up with careful retinal evaluation.

Pathological Findings

Presence of intrascleral smooth muscle oriented concentrically around the distal optic nerve.

DIFFERENTIAL DIAGNOSIS

- Morning Glory Disc Anomaly (funnel-shaped excavation of the posterior fundus that incorporates the optic disc)
- Peripapillary staphyloma (relatively normal appearing disc located in a recess peripapillary excavation)

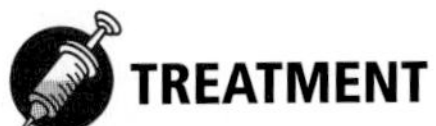

TREATMENT

MEDICATION
No medical treatment for the primary disorder

ADDITIONAL TREATMENT

General Measures
Impact resistant glasses for protection of the non-involved eye if subnormal visual acuity is demonstrated or suspected in the involved eye, or in cases of bilateral involvement.

Issues for Referral
- Low vision evaluation and support as indicated in cases with significant bilateral involvement
- Retinal surgery for detachment

COMPLEMENTARY & ALTERNATIVE THERAPIES
None proven or indicated

SURGERY/OTHER PROCEDURES
- Amblyopia therapy and strabismus surgery as indicated
- Retinal detachment surgery as indicated

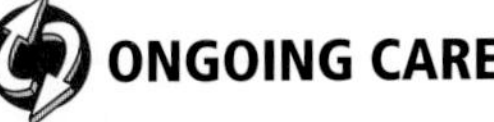

ONGOING CARE

FOLLOW-UP RECOMMENDATIONS
- Regular follow-ups to monitor for evidence of retinal detachment
- As needed for amblyopia and strabismus monitoring and treatment
- Low vision care

Patient Monitoring
- Patient concerns about appearance if significant strabismus is present
- Monitor for possible development of acquired loss of vision from retinal detachment

PATIENT EDUCATION
- Possible genetic counseling in cases with family history of the condition
- Low vision intervention in patients with significant bilateral involvement

PROGNOSIS
- Broad range of best corrected visual acuity
- Relatively high risk of subsequent retinal detachment

COMPLICATIONS
Retinal detachment

ADDITIONAL READING

- Brodsky MC, Baker RS, Hamed LM. *Pediatric Neuro-Ophthalmology*. New York: Springer, 1996:53–55.
- Brown G, Tasman W. *Congenital Anomalies of the Optic Disc*. New York: Grune & Stratton, 1983:128–141.
- Nucci P, Mets MB, Gabianelli EB. Trisomy 4q with morning glory disc anomaly. *Ophthalmic Paediatr Genet* 1990;11(2):143–145.
- Pollack S. The Morning glory disc anomaly; contractile movement, classification, and embryogenesis. *Doc Ophthalmol* 1987;65: 439–460.

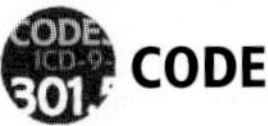

CODES

ICD9
377.23 Coloboma of optic disc

CLINICAL PEARLS

- Work to maximize visual potential, especially in bilateral cases. Difficult to predict eventual best corrected visual acuity based on the appearance of the optic disc.
- Use of a high plus lens to equalize the image size of the iris through spectacle lenses can help to provide a more normal appearance in patients with associated microphthalmia.
- Major ophthalmic concerns include protecting the better seeing eye, monitoring the involved eye for possible treatable overlying amblyopia and strabismus, and monitoring for acquired loss of vision in the involved eye from retinal detachment.
- Significant associated systemic abnormalities include CHARGE association.

OPTIC NERVE CUPPING

Tak Yee Tania Tai
L. Jay Katz

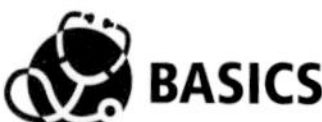

BASICS

DESCRIPTION

- Optic nerve cupping can be physiological.
- Pathological optic nerve cupping is a manifestation of regional ganglion cell death and loss of ganglion cell axons from the optic nerve.
- The majority of eyes with pathologic enlargement of the optic cup have glaucoma (1)[B].
- Distinguishing glaucomatous from nonglaucomatous disc cupping can be difficult—in a retrospective review of optic nerve head photographs, Trobe et al. reported that pallor of the neuroretinal rim is 94% specific in predicting nonglaucomatous cupping while focal or diffuse obliteration of the neuroretinal rim is 87% specific in predicting glaucomatous cupping (2)[B].

EPIDEMIOLOGY

Incidence

- The incidence of pathological nonglaucomatous cupping is unknown.
- The observed 4-year incidence of open-angle glaucoma was 1.2% at ages 40–49 years, 1.5% at ages 50–59 years, 3.2% at ages 60–69 years, and 4.2% in persons aged 70 years or more according to the Barbados Incidence Study of Eye Diseases (1992–1997) (3)[B].

Prevalence

- The prevalence of pathological nonglaucomatous cupping is unknown.
- Approximately 67 million people are affected with glaucoma worldwide, and approximately 2 million people in the U.S. have glaucoma (1 in 136 people) (1)[B].
- In developed countries, probably only half of those with glaucoma have been diagnosed.

RISK FACTORS

- Larger optic discs tend to have larger physiologic cup/disc ratio (4)[A].
- Please refer to the "Differential Diagnosis" section of this chapter.
- Please refer to the "Risk Factors" section of the specific diagnosis responsible for the pathological optic disc cupping.

Genetics

There is some dependence of an individual's physiologic cup/disc ratio on the cup/disc ratio of the parents—multifactorial inheritance is likely (5)[B].

GENERAL PREVENTION

For glaucomatous optic disc cupping: lowering intraocular pressure (IOP)

PATHOPHYSIOLOGY

- Pathologic optic nerve head cupping is a manifestation of retinal ganglion cell death and loss of ganglion cell axons from the optic nerve.
- The primary site of glaucomatous optic nerve damage is thought to be the lamina cribrosa—deformations of the lamina, kinking of nerve fibers, misalignment of laminar pores, blockade of axonal transport; however, the relationship between these findings and glaucomatous damage have not been firmly established (1)[B].
- Other contributing factors may act at the level of the ganglion cell body.

ETIOLOGY

- Elevated IOP
- Ischemia/hypoxia
- Trauma
- Excitotoxicity and aberrant immunity have also been hypothesized to be factors in optic nerve damage (1)[B].

COMMONLY ASSOCIATED CONDITIONS

- Please refer to the "Differential Diagnosis" section of this chapter.
- Please refer to the "Commonly Associated Conditions" section of the specific diagnosis responsible for the pathological optic disc cupping.

DIAGNOSIS

HISTORY

- Presence, onset, and nature of visual disturbance
- Systemic vascular risk factors, such as migraine, Raynaud's diabetes, and hypertension
- History of ocular trauma or surgeries
- Family history of glaucoma or other optic neuropathies
- Neurological disturbances such as headaches, dizziness, and weakness of extremities

PHYSICAL EXAM

- Check for an afferent pupillary defect.
- Slit lamp examination of the anterior segment to check for signs of secondary glaucoma, such as iris transillumination defects, pseudoexfoliation material, anterior chamber cell or flare, and signs of prior surgery or trauma
- Gonioscopy
- Direct and indirect stereoscopic slit lamp biomicrospy to evaluate the optic nerve head, paying particular attention to
  - narrowing of the neuroretinal rim width (relatively narrow rim inferotemporally or superotemporally can indicate glaucomatous damage)
  - asymmetry in disc cupping ($\geq$0.2)
  - optic disc hemorrhage
  - optic nerve color
  - beta zone parapapillary atrophy
  - optic nerve edema
  - loss of retinal nerve fiber layer (focal or diffuse)
- The normal optic disc neuroretinal rim is characteristically broadest inferiorly, followed by superior and nasal rims, and narrowest temporally (ISNT rule).
- An analysis of patients from the Ocular Hypertensive Treatment Study and the European Glaucoma Prevention Study showed that an ocular hypertensive patient's risk of developing glaucoma increased almost 50% for every 0.1 difference between eyes in cup-to-disc ratio (6)[B].
- Staging of the optic disc using Armaly's cup-to-disc ratio is commonly used.
- Spaeth's disc damage likelihood scale directs attention to the narrowest area on the optic disc rim (scale 1–10) (7)[B].

DIAGNOSTIC TESTS & INTERPRETATION

Lab

Initial lab tests

- Lab tests as indicated for suspected cause of pathologic optic disc cupping.
- Please refer to the "Differential Diagnosis" section of this chapter.

Follow-up & special considerations

Follow-up as indicated for the suspected cause of pathologic optic disc cupping

Imaging

Initial approach

- Optic disc photographs should be obtained to evaluate and follow patients through their course of treatment.
- Other optic nerve head imaging devices are also currently being used for optic nerve head assessment in glaucoma:
  - Scanning laser polarimetry
  - Heidelberg retinal tomography
  - Optical coherence topography

Follow-up & special considerations

- Follow-up as indicated for the suspected cause of pathologic optic disc cupping
- If glaucoma is suspected, optic disc imaging should be obtained regularly (e.g., annually, or more often if a change in optic disc appearance is suspected) to document and assess the optic nerve head for change.

Diagnostic Procedures/Other

- Visual fields should be obtained at baseline and at regular intervals (e.g., annually, or more often if a change is suspected).
- Diurnal IOP testing may be useful if large IOP fluctuations or periods of IOP spike are suspected.
- Consider neuroimaging for:
  - Loss of central visual acuity or central visual field
  - Acute onset or rapidly progressive visual loss
  - Markedly asymmetric or strictly unilateral optic neuropathy
  - Hemianopic visual field loss
  - Neuroretinal rim pallor

Pathological Findings

Atrophy of the retinal ganglion cell layer can be noted.

DIFFERENTIAL DIAGNOSIS

- Glaucoma
- Tilted optic nerve insertion
- Coloboma
- Myopic disc
- Posterior staphyloma
- Optic pit
- Hereditary optic neuropathy
- Antecedent optic nerve infarction
- Trauma
- Demyelinating optic neuritis
- Intraorbital and intracranial mass lesions
- Carotid artery fusiform enlargement
- Ischemic optic neuropathy

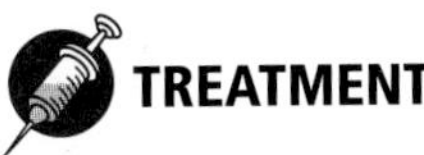

TREATMENT

MEDICATION

First Line

Please refer to the "Treatment" section of the specific diagnosis responsible for pathological optic disc cupping.

Second Line

Please refer to the "Treatment" section of the specific diagnosis responsible for pathological optic disc cupping.

ADDITIONAL TREATMENT

General Measures

Please refer to the "Treatment" section of the specific diagnosis responsible for pathological optic disc cupping.

Issues for Referral

Referral to a neuro-ophthalmologist may be considered if there is suspicion that the cause of the patient's optic neuropathy or visual field defect has a possible neurological etiology.

Additional Therapies

Please refer to the "Treatment" section of the specific diagnosis responsible for pathological optic disc cupping.

COMPLEMENTARY & ALTERNATIVE THERAPIES

Please refer to the "Treatment" section of the specific diagnosis responsible for pathological optic disc cupping.

SURGERY/OTHER PROCEDURES

Please refer to the "Surgery/Other Procedures" section of the specific diagnosis responsible for pathological optic disc cupping.

IN-PATIENT CONSIDERATIONS

Initial Stabilization

Please refer to the "Inpatient Considerations" section of the specific diagnosis responsible for pathological optic disc cupping.

Admission Criteria

Please refer to the "Inpatient Considerations" section of the specific diagnosis responsible for pathological optic disc cupping.

IV Fluids

Please refer to the "Inpatient Considerations" section of the specific diagnosis responsible for pathological optic disc cupping.

Nursing

Please refer to the "Inpatient Considerations" section of the specific diagnosis responsible for pathological optic disc cupping.

Discharge Criteria

Please refer to the "Inpatient Considerations" section of the specific diagnosis responsible for pathological optic disc cupping.

ONGOING CARE

FOLLOW-UP RECOMMENDATIONS

Please refer to the "Ongoing Care" section of the specific diagnosis responsible for pathological optic disc cupping.

Patient Monitoring

Please refer to the "Ongoing Care" section of the specific diagnosis responsible for pathological optic disc cupping.

DIET

Please refer to the "Ongoing Care" section of the specific diagnosis responsible for pathological optic disc cupping.

PATIENT EDUCATION

Please refer to the "Ongoing Care" section of the specific diagnosis responsible for pathological optic disc cupping.

PROGNOSIS

Please refer to the "Ongoing Care" section of the specific diagnosis responsible for pathological optic disc cupping.

COMPLICATIONS

Please refer to the "Ongoing Care" section of the specific diagnosis responsible for pathological optic disc cupping.

REFERENCES

1. Greenfield DS. Glaucomatous versus nonglaucomatous optic disc cupping: clinical differentiation. *Semin Ophthalmol* 1999;14(2): 95–108.
2. Trobe JD, Glaser JS, Cassady J, et al. Nonglaucomatous excavation of the optic disc. *Arch Ophthalmol* 1980;98:1046–1050.
3. Wu SY, Nemesure B, Leske MC. Observed versus indirect estimates of incidence of open-angle glaucoma. *Am J Epidemiol* 2001;153(2):184–187.
4. Hoffmann EM, Zangwill LM, Crowston JG, et al. Optic disc size and glaucoma. *Surv Ophthalmol* 2007;52(1):32–49.
5. Armaly MF. Genetic determination of cup/disc ratio of the optic nerve. *Arch Ophthal* 1967;78:35–43.
6. The Ocular Hypertension Study Group and the European Glaucoma Prevention Study Group. The accuracy and clinical application of predictive models for primary open-angle glaucoma in ocular hypertensive individuals. *Ophthalmol* 2008; 115:2030–2036.
7. Bayer A, Harasymowycz P, Henderer JD, et al. Validity of a new disk grading scale for estimating glaucomatous damage: correlation with visual field damage. *Am J Ophthalmol* 2002;133(6):758–763.

ADDITIONAL READING

- Collignon NJ. Abnormal cupping of the optic disc: clinical screening before performing a neuroimaging examination. *Bull Soc Belge Ophthalmol* 2006;300:21–23.

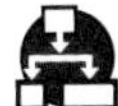

See Also (Topic, Algorithm, Electronic Media Element)

- Glaucoma
- Optic neuritis

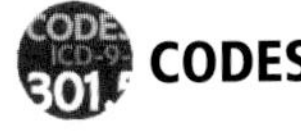

CODES

ICD9

377.14 Glaucomatous atrophy (cupping) of optic disc

OPTIC NERVE HYPOPLASIA

Louis C. Blumenfeld

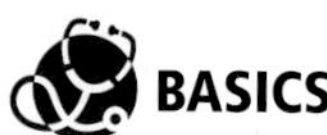

BASICS

DESCRIPTION

- Abnormally small optic nerve; often appears pale or gray in color
  - 80% are bilateral, but may be asymmetric
- Most common congenital optic disc anomaly encountered; it was not widely recognized until the late 1960s

EPIDEMIOLOGY

Incidence

10.9:100,000 (England 2006) (1)

Prevalence

6.3:100,000 (Sweden -1997)

RISK FACTORS

- Maternal use of alcohol, quinine, PCP, LSD, and Dilantin
- Maternal insulin dependent diabetes (associated with subtype – superior segmental optic hypoplasia [topless disc])
- Young maternal age
- Primiparity
- Preterm labor
- Low maternal weight gain
- Gestational vaginal bleeding
- Most factors occur without known predisposing factors

Genetics

- Reported cases of affected siblings are rare
- Subsequent siblings of children with optic nerve hypoplasia are at little additional risk
  - Mutations in HESX1 have been identified in children with sporadic septo-optic dysplasia and pituitary disease
  - Homozygous mutations in the HESX1 gene have been found in 2 siblings with optic nerve hypoplasia, absence of the corpus callosum, and pituitary hypoplasia

GENERAL PREVENTION

There are no known methods of general prevention except for avoidance of known teratogenic agents such as Dilantin, Quinine, PCP, LSD, and alcohol.

PATHOPHYSIOLOGY

- Possible relationship to axon guidance molecules, such as Netrin-1 at the optic nerve head. Similar mechanism may account for other associated CNS abnormalities
- There is also evidence that some cases of optic nerve hypoplasia may result from axonal degeneration (apoptosis)

ETIOLOGY

- Usually unknown
- Teratogenic agents listed under risk factors

COMMONLY ASSOCIATED CONDITIONS

- Septo-optic dysplasia – constellation of optic nerve hypoplasia, absence of the septum pellucidum, and thinning or agenesis of the corpus callosum
- Pituitary – endocrine dysfunction
  - Clinical hypopituitarism in 15%
  - Subclinical endocrinopathy in 72%
    - Growth hormone most common, followed by thyrotropin, corticotrophin, and antidiuretic hormone
- 45% patients have cerebral anomalies such as error in hemispheric migration (schizencephaly, cortical heterotopias) or hemispheric injury (periventricular leukomalacia, encephalomalacia)
- Developmental delay is present in 39% of unilateral optic nerve hypoplasia and 78% of bilateral patients
  - Developmental delay is most highly correlated with corpus callosum hypoplasia and hypothyroidism (2)

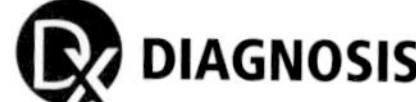

DIAGNOSIS

HISTORY

Bilateral optic nerve hypoplasia often presents with poor vision and nystagmus (often develops at 1–3 months of age). Unilateral optic nerve hypoplasia may present later with strabismus.

PHYSICAL EXAM

- Careful attention to visual acuity, including difference in acuity between the two eyes.
- Range of visual acuity is 20/20 to NLP
- Nystagmus
- Strabismus
- Small optic discs, may be pale or gray in appearance.
- Superior segmental optic nerve hypoplasia (associated with insulin dependent diabetic mothers) may be referred to as topless disc syndrome.
- Double ring sign (larger ring representing sclera canal that surrounds small optic nerve)
- Major retinal vessels may be tortuous

DIAGNOSTIC TESTS & INTERPRETATION

Lab

Initial lab tests

- Endocrine evaluation
  - Fasting morning cortisol and glucose
  - TSH, free T4
  - IGF-1, IGFBP-3
  - Prolactin
  - In children <6 months, luteinizing hormone, follicle stimulating hormone, and testosterone levels should also be checked.

Follow-Up & Special Considerations

- Neonatal jaundice suggests congenital hypothyroidism
- Neonatal seizures suggest congenital panhypopituitarism
- Irreversible adverse effects of hypothyroidism may occur by 15 months of age – Serum TSH levels are helpful for early detection

Imaging

Initial approach

MRI is indicated to evaluate for associated CNS malformations.

Follow-up & special considerations

Posterior pituitary ectopia on MRI is highly associated with anterior pituitary hormone deficiency.

Diagnostic Procedures/Other

Automated visual field testing may be useful, but children are often too young to do this test reliably.

Pathological Findings

Markedly reduced retinal ganglion cells and nerve fiber layer

DIFFERENTIAL DIAGNOSIS

- Optic atrophy
- Ocular albinism
- Optic nerve coloboma

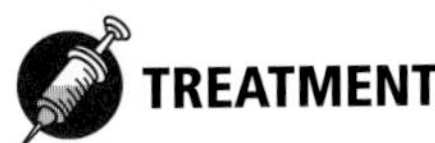

TREATMENT

MEDICATION

No known medical therapy available.

ADDITIONAL TREATMENT

General Measures

- Eyeglasses for protection of the better-seeing eye when asymmetry is present
  - Correction of refractive errors
  - Treatment of possible concurrent amblyopia
  - Surgery for concurrent strabismus or nystagmus may be considered

Issues for Referral

- Pediatric ophthalmology referral to treat any underlying amblyopia and possible surgery for strabismus/nystagmus
- Pediatric neurology referral if evidence of coexisting CNS abnormalities
- Pediatric endocrinology referral to evaluate frequent coexisting endocrinopathies

COMPLEMENTARY & ALTERNATIVE THERAPIES

Stem cell transplantation is not proven to affect visual function in optic nerve hypoplasia

SURGERY/OTHER PROCEDURES

- There is no known useful surgery for optic nerve hypoplasia at this time.
  - Surgery may be considered for coexisting strabismus or nystagmus

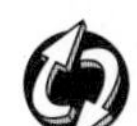

ONGOING CARE

FOLLOW-UP RECOMMENDATIONS

Yearly or more frequent examinations for evaluation and treatment of strabismus, amblyopia, and refractive errors

Patient Monitoring

Patients should be monitored for possible coexisting amblyopia. This may occur as a result of the optic nerve hypoplasia itself or associated refractive errors or strabismus.

PATIENT EDUCATION

Importance of treating any associated conditions, such as amblyopia and the need for low vision assessment and aids should be discussed.

PROGNOSIS

Visual acuity generally remains stable over time. There is some tendency for mild visual improvement with maturity.

COMPLICATIONS

Generally related to associated endocrinopathies and other CNS malformations

REFERENCES

1. Patel I, McNally RJQ, Harrison E, et al. Geographic distribution of optc nerve hypoplasia and septo-optic dysplasia in northwest England. *J Pediatr* 2006;148(1):5–88.
2. [c]Garci-Filion P, Epport K, Nelson M, et al, Neuroradiographic, endocrinologic, and ophthalmic correlates of adverse developmental outcomes in children with optic nerve hypoplasia: A prospective study. *Pediatrics* 2008;121:e653–e659.

ADDITIONAL READING

- Borchert M, Garcia-Filion P. The syndrome of optic nerve hypoplasia. *Curr Neurol Neurosci Rep* 2008; 8:395–403.

CODES

ICD9

377.43 Optic nerve hypoplasia

CLINICAL PEARLS

- Visual acuity does not correlate well to the size of the optic disc.
  - Acuity correlates primarily with integrity of the papillomacular nerve fibers.
- There may be some improvement in visual acuity with patching the fellow eye in asymmetric cases due to component of amblyopia.

OPTIC NEURITIS

Tulay Kansu

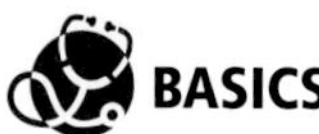

BASICS

DESCRIPTION

- Optic neuritis (ON) is the inflammation of the optic nerve.
- Vision loss is rapid and may be progressive in the first 2–15 days.
- It typically occurs in 1 eye at a time (70%), bilateral occurrence is 30%.
- Optic nerve inflammation and edema at the optic nerve head is termed papillitis.
- If nerve damage is behind the eyeball, it is called retrobulbar neuritis.

Pediatric Considerations

- Optic disc swelling and bilateral disease are more common in children.
- Loss of visual acuity is more severe.
- Recovery of visual acuity is 20/40 or better in 76% of patients.
- Subsequent risk of multiple sclerosis (MS) varies among studies.

Pregnancy Considerations

Management is the same as in the nonpregnant patient.

EPIDEMIOLOGY

- Acute demyelinating ON is the most common cause of unilateral painful visual loss in a young adult.
- Tends to afflict young adults with an average age in their 30s.
- 75% of patients are women.

Incidence

- The annual incidence is 5 per 100,000.
- The incidence is highest in northern countries at higher latitudes.

Prevalence

The prevalence is 115 per 100,000.

RISK FACTORS

- People who are younger than 15 years will acquire the risk of the country to which they migrate.
- 69% of females and 33% of males may develop MS approximately 15 years after the initial attack.

Genetics

No known genetic features of typical ON

PATHOPHYSIOLOGY

An inflammatory process that leads to activation of peripheral T lymphocytes and cause a delayed type of hypersensitivity reaction resulting in demyelination and axonal loss. The recovery can occur with remyelination.

ETIOLOGY

Autoimmune

COMMONLY ASSOCIATED CONDITIONS

Acute demyelinating ON is the initial presentation in approximately 20% of cases of MS.

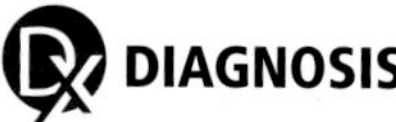

DIAGNOSIS

The diagnosis of ON is usually made on clinical grounds.

HISTORY

- Sudden onset blurred vision, progressive over a few days to 2 weeks
- Pain with eye movement
- Exacerbation of symptoms with increased body temperature (Uhthoff phenomenon)
- Spontaneous improvement starting within 2–3 weeks

PHYSICAL EXAM

- Impaired vision
- Impaired color vision
- Impaired contrast sensitivity
- Visual field defect mostly central scotoma, or any type
- Optic disc normal (65%) or swollen (35%), pale within 4–6 weeks
- Venous sheathing
- Relative afferent pupillary defect (RAPD)
- Pulfrich phenomenon: The course of a pendulum is perceived as an elliptical movement.

DIAGNOSTIC TESTS & INTERPRETATION

Lab

Initial lab tests

- The yield from diagnostic tests is extremely low in a typical case.
- Ancillary investigations should be done for an alternative diagnosis, if there are atypical features.

Follow-up & special considerations

Appropriate test according to the symptom

Imaging

Initial approach

- Brain MRI with contrast
- Look for hyperintense white matter lesions in T2-weighted images and enhancement of the optic nerve.
- Characteristic demyelinating lesions in patients at risk for MS are 3 mm or larger in diameter, ovoid in shape, and located in periventricular areas

Follow-up & special considerations

- Repeat brain MRI in 3–6 months for new lesions
- Spinal MRI for the presence of demyelinating lesions

Diagnostic Procedures/Other

- Visual evoked potentials (VEP)
- Contrast sensitivity
- Optical coherence tomography (OCT)
- Lumbar puncture (LP) for oligoclonal band, IgG
- Neuromyelitis optica (NMO) (aquaporin 4) antibodies in bilateral or recurrent cases

Pathological Findings

The main pathology is the demyelination and axonal injury of the optic nerve fibers. Remyelination occurs during the recovery phase.

DIFFERENTIAL DIAGNOSIS

- Other inflammatory/vasculitic optic neuropathies (sarcoidosis, systemic lupus erythematosus, Sjögren's syndrome, Behçet's syndrome, autoimmune optic neuropathy, chronic relapsing inflammatory optic neuropathy)
- NMO, also known as Devic's disease should be considered if the ON is bilateral, associated with myelitis and/or there is no visual improvement.
- Infectious ON (tuberculosis, syphilis, Lyme disease, viral disease)
- Postinfections, postvaccination, neuroretinitis
- Ischemic ON (arteritic, nonarteritic)
- Compressive ON (pituitary tumors, glioma, meningioma, craniopharyngioma, aneurysm)
- Toxic (methanol)
- Hereditary (Leber's hereditary ON)
- Retinal diseases (central serous retinopathy, big blind spot syndrome)
- Functional visual loss

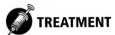

TREATMENT

MEDICATION

First Line

- Corticosteroids are considered for patients with severe visual loss (>20/40) to hasten recovery, but they do not affect the ultimate visual outcome.
- 1 g IV methylprednisolone (MP) per day given for 3 days. An oral taper is not necessary (1).
- Giving oral prednisone alone is contraindicated because of the risk of increasing new attacks.

Second Line

- Treatment with immunomodulators (interferon beta 1a, interferon beta 1b, glatiramer acetate) should be considered for patients with ON whose brain lesions on MRI indicate a high risk of developing clinically definite MS (2).
- Therapies should be individualized and the patient involved in the decision-making process.

ADDITIONAL TREATMENT

General Measures

Review within 1 month is recommended to ensure that vision does not deteriorate after cessation of the treatment.

Pediatric Considerations

- Treatment with IV MP is recommended if visual loss is severe or bilateral.
- Interferon therapy is considered with abnormal MRI of the brain.

Issues for Referral

Neurology consultation for MS evaluation

IN-PATIENT CONSIDERATIONS

Initial Stabilization

IV MP is given as an outpatient.

Admission Criteria

Admission is not necessary for typical ON. Atypical cases can be admitted for work up.

IV Fluids

MP 1 g is given in 500 mL NaCl with slow IV infusion >2 hours.

ONGOING CARE

FOLLOW-UP RECOMMENDATIONS

Follow-up at 1 week, 1 month, 3 months, and then every 6 months for the first 2 years in an asymptomatic patient

PATIENT EDUCATION

Patient should be informed about the disease and the possibility of developing MS.

PROGNOSIS

- Recovery occurs spontaneously within 2–3 weeks in 80%, stabilizing over months to a year.
- 93% had a visual acuity better than 20/40, and 69% had 20/20 vision 1 year following the initial attack (Optic Neuritis Treatment Trial [ONTT])
- The severity of initial visual loss is the only predictor of the final visual outcome.
- Temporal disc pallor develops within 4–6 weeks from the onset and RAPD may disappear when visual recovery is full.
- Anterior optic neuropathy has better prognosis than posterior type.
- 28% and 35% of patients have recurrence of ON within 5 and 10 years, respectively.
- The risk of development of MS after an isolated unilateral ON is 38% at 10 years and 50% at 15 years.
- 75% of female patients and 35% of male patients may ultimately develop MS.
- Treatment does not alter the final visual outcome (3).
- The risk of developing MS is 25% if baseline MRI is normal, and 75% if MRI has one or more MS plaques.

COMPLICATIONS

- Less than 10% of patients may have permanent visual acuity less than 20/40.
- Treatment with IV MP has mainly minor side effects such as transient flushing, a brief disturbance of taste, insomnia, and mild weight gain.
- An anaphylactoid reaction after IV MP treatment has been described in rare cases.

REFERENCES

1. Vedula SS, Brodney-Folse S, Gal RL, Beck R. Corticosteroids for treating optic neuritis. *Cochrane Database Syst Rev* 2007;(1):CD001430.
2. Beck RW, Chandler DL, Cole SR, et al. Interferon beta-1a for early multiple sclerosis: CHAMPS trial subgroup analyses. *Ann Neurol* 2002;51:481–490.
3. Optic Neuritis Study Group. Visual Function 15 years after optic neuritis: a final follow-up report from the Optic Neuritis Treatment Trial. *Ophthalmology* 2008;115:1079–1082.

ADDITIONAL READING

- Abou Zeid N, Bhatti MT. Acute inflammatory demyelinating optic neuritis: evidence-based visual and neurological considerations. *Neurologist* 2008;14:207–223.
- Balcer L. Clinical practice. Optic neuritis. *N Engl J Med* 2006;354:1273–1280
- Shams PN, Plant GT. Optic neuritis: a review. *Int MS J* 2009;16:82–89.

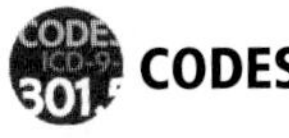

CODES

ICD9

- 377.30 Optic neuritis, unspecified
- 377.31 Optic papillitis
- 377.32 Retrobulbar neuritis (acute)

CLINICAL PEARLS

- The presence of white matter lesions on the initial MRI of the brain is the strongest predictor for the development of MS.
- The 15-year risk of developing MS is 25% with no lesions, 75% with one or more lesions (ONTT).
- Treatment with high-dose IV corticosteroids may accelerate visual recovery but has little impact on long-term visual outcome.
- Giving oral prednisone alone is contraindicated because of the risk of increasing new attacks.
- Disease-modifying drugs should be considered in patients at high risk of developing MS.

ORBITAL CELLULITIS

Scott M. Goldstein

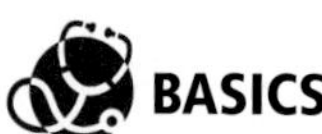

BASICS

DESCRIPTION

Orbital cellulitis is an acute infection of the soft tissue contained within the orbital space. It typically arises from adjacent sinusitis but can also occur from spreading of a superficial skin infection or dacryocystitis, penetrating trauma, extension of endophthalmitis, or endogenous bacteremia.

EPIDEMIOLOGY

Incidence

Orbital cellulitis has an approximate incidence of 3 to 6/1,000,000. It has a higher incidence in blacks than in whites or (1) Hispanics and is slight more common in men than in women. Finally, it is more common in children than in teenagers and adults.

RISK FACTORS

- Sinusitis
- Periocular trauma

PATHOPHYSIOLOGY

- Upwards of 80% of orbital cellulitis infections are the result of a sinus infection spreading into the orbit, typically from ethmoid sinusitis. This is due to the thin bone separating the two spaces and the valveless veins that drain from the sinus through the orbit en route to the cavernous sinus.
- Fungal infections such as mucormycosis and aspergillosis can cause these infections but are much less common.

ETIOLOGY

- The ethmoid, maxillary, and frontal sinuses surround the orbit. Thus infection in these spaces can potentially spread in to the orbit. The sinus is typically a sterile space but with upper respiratory infections, the sinus drainage can be compromised leading to congestion and infection. In children younger than 9 years, these infections are typically monomicrobial aerobic infections, which respond well to antibiotics alone. By the time patients reach their mid teenage years, and beyond, the infection is more typically a polymicrobial aerobe/anaerobe infection requiring more intense antibiotic therapy and more often surgery.
- Common bacteria include coagulase-negative Staphylococcus species, Streptococcus species, and *Staphylococcus aureus*, both Methicillin-susceptible Staphylococcus Aureus (MSSA) and Methicillin-resistant Staphylococcus Aureus (MRSA). In addition, pseudomonas species, *Moraxella catarrhalis*, *Eikenella corrodens*, and various anaerobes can be the culprit.
- In immunocompromised patients and uncontrolled diabetes, do not overlook the possibility of a fungal infection, such as mucormycosis.

COMMONLY ASSOCIATED CONDITIONS

Bacterial sinusitis, fungal sinusitis, pre-septal cellulitis of eyelid, dacryocystitis, orbital trauma

DIAGNOSIS

HISTORY

Patient presents acutely with increasing edema, erythema, and pain around the eye that has occurred over several hours to several days. Many will have a history of underlying sinus disease, an acute respiratory tract infection, skin infection, or recent trauma. They progress to develop decreased motility with double vision (if the eyelids are not swollen shut).

PHYSICAL EXAM

- Erythema and edema of lids and orbit
- Proptosis
- Decreased vision
- Conjunctival injection and chemosis
- Limitation in ocular motility
- Sluggish pupil with possible afferent pupil defect
- Elevated intraocular pressure

DIAGNOSTIC TESTS & INTERPRETATION

Lab

- CBC with white count
- Culture of any discharge
- Blood cultures may be helpful.

Imaging

Initial approach

CT scan of the orbits

Follow-up & special considerations

- Repeat imaging studies are frowned upon as clinical findings and radiologic findings do not progress and regress at the same pace. Rather, the radiologic findings fade much more slowly and may still show inflammation or edema even though the patient is improving.
- MRI/magnetic resonance venography (MRV) can be obtained if cavernous sinus thrombosis is a concern.

Diagnostic Procedures/Other

CT scan is the gold standard.

DIFFERENTIAL DIAGNOSIS

- Preseptal cellulitis
- Orbital inflammatory syndrome
- Dacryoadenitis
- Metastatic tumor
- Herpes zoster ophthalmicus

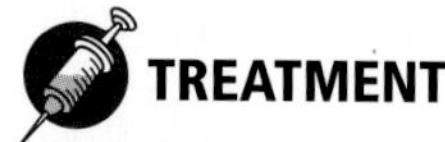

TREATMENT

MEDICATION

First Line

Broad-spectrum IV antibiotics that cover gram positive, gram negative, and anaerobes, especially in patients older than 14 years. These include fortified penicillins, third-generation cephalosporins, fluoroquinolones, or a combination of these medications. Intravenous antibiotic choices would include ampicillin sulbactam, ceftriaxone, aminoglycosides, vancomycin, clindamycin, and fluoroquinolones.

Second Line

Steroid therapy is controversial but can be a helpful adjunct to the antibiotics in reducing swelling and congestion in both the orbit and sinus.

ADDITIONAL TREATMENT

General Measures

Typically admit these patients to the hospital for IV antibiotics, close observation, and possibly surgery. Regular examination of the eye 1–4 times per day depending on the severity to ensure that the vision is not being compromised.

Issues for Referral

The nonophthalmologist can manage this in an inpatient setting, but an ophthalmologist should be involved to monitor the status of the orbit and vision. If sinusitis is the underlying source of infection, ENT surgeons should also be involved.

SURGERY/OTHER PROCEDURES

- The primary source of the infection must be treated. Since 60–80% of orbital cellulitis cases arise from sinus disease, sinus surgery should be included with any plan to surgically treat the orbit.
- An orbitotomy should be considered if there is a frank abscess in the orbit, visual compromise exists, there is an atypical infection, or the patient is not responding to intravenous antibiotic therapy after several days.

IN-PATIENT CONSIDERATIONS

Initial Stabilization

Start IV antibiotic therapy as soon as possible but be aware it typically takes 24–48 hours for the patient to stabilize, especially if they are older than 14 years with a polymicrobial infection.

Admission Criteria

Confirmation of orbital cellulitis as a diagnosis should almost always be treated as an inpatient. Patient needs to be observed closely for evidence of significant visual compromise and posterior intracranial spread of the infection.

Nursing

Check vision and pupils at least once a shift. Warm compresses can help with the infection.

Discharge Criteria

Significant improvement of infection with no further acute threat to the vision.

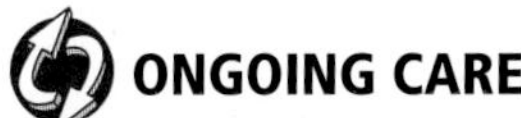

ONGOING CARE

FOLLOW-UP RECOMMENDATIONS

Patients should receive approximately two full weeks of antibiotic therapy total. Thus they should be discharged home on oral antibiotics or with a peripherally inserted central catheter (PICC) line for continued IV antibiotics when indicated.

Patient Monitoring

- Outpatient follow-up within a week of discharge to ensure that the infection is resolving and the vision is stable.
- If there was an associated sinusitis, follow-up with an ENT surgeon is recommended as well.

DIET

Typically not a concern. However, patients with diabetes should have their glucose control optimized as hyperglycemia promotes infection.

PROGNOSIS

Excellent, with today's imaging capabilities, antibiotics, and team approach to managing these patients.

COMPLICATIONS

Blindness, cavernous sinus thrombosis, eyelid necrosis, meningitis, brain abscess, sepsis, death

REFERENCE

1. Rabinowitz MP, Goldstein SM. *Periorbital cellulitis in the early 21st century." Essentials of ophthalmology-oculoplastics & orbit*. New York, NY: Springer Verlag, 2009.

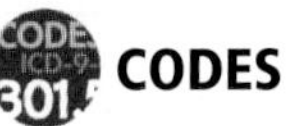

CODES

ICD9

- 375.30 Dacryocystitis, unspecified
- 376.01 Orbital cellulitis
- 473.9 Unspecified sinusitis (chronic)

CLINICAL PEARLS

- It is important to consider MRSA as a cause of infection when choosing appropriate antibiotic therapy.
- CT scan of the orbit and sinus is a very helpful tool when determining the best course of treatment.
- Antibiotics are most effective as single therapy in young children, whereas antibiotics and surgery are more often needed in teenagers and adults.
- MRSA infections of the orbit require aggressive management with appropriate antibiotics and early surgery when indicated.
- Atypical infections, such as orbital cellulitis not arising from the sinus or infections that potentially may spread to adjacent areas (such as frontal sinusitis with orbital involvement and possible intracranial spread) should be treated surgically in a more urgent matter.

ORBITAL HEMORRHAGE

Edward H. Bedrossian, Jr.

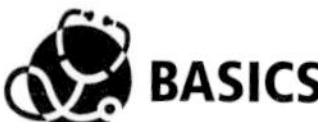

BASICS

DESCRIPTION

An orbital hemorrhage is a hemorrhage within the orbital cavity, bound anteriorly by the orbital septum and canthal tendons.

EPIDEMIOLOGY

Incidence

- Orbital fractures (0.45–0.6%)
- Retrobulbar injections (0.005–0.44%)
- Facial fracture repair (0.24–0.3%)
- Postblepharoplasty (0.005%)
- Endoscopic sinus surgery (0.43%)

RISK FACTORS

- Blunt head/orbital trauma
- Penetrating orbital foreign bodies
- Postseptal eyelid surgery
- Orbital/sinus surgery
- Hypertension
- Anticoagulant medications (aspirin, NSAIDs, warfarin [Coumadin])
- Postoperative Valsalva maneuver (vomit, cough, sneeze)
- Coagulopathy
- Blood dyscrasia (thrombocytopenia, leukemia)
- Cirrhosis

GENERAL PREVENTION

- Preoperative assessment of risk factors
- Meticulous intraoperative hemostasis
- Postoperative patient education and surveillance

PATHOPHYSIOLOGY

- An orbital hemorrhage acts like an expanding space occupying orbital lesion confined by the bony orbital walls and orbital septum.
- As the intraorbital pressure increases, the eye and orbital contents bulge anteriorly to the limit of the orbital septum and canthal tendons (7–8 mm). Beyond that, the optic nerve is maximally stretched, limiting further anterior displacement of the globe.
- Subsequent increases in orbital pressure can produce visual loss by direct optic nerve compression, or more likely, by ischemic optic neuropathy from compression of the central retinal artery, posterior ciliary vessels, and fine pial perforating vessels supplying the retina, choroid, and optic nerve.

ETIOLOGY

- Blunt and penetrating orbital trauma
- Eyelid, orbital, sinus, and lacrimal surgery
- Idiopathic (rare)

COMMONLY ASSOCIATED CONDITIONS

Spontaneous orbital hemorrhage has occurred with

- Orbital lymphangiomas
- Cavernous hemangiomas
- Ophthalmic artery aneurysms
- Hemophilia
- Leukemia
- Vitamin K deficiency
- Anemia
- Hypertension
- Von Willebrand's disease

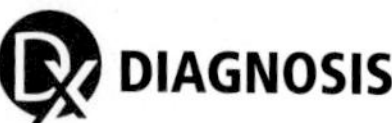

DIAGNOSIS

HISTORY

- Recent trauma to the eye, orbit
- Recent eyelid, lacrimal, orbital, or sinus surgery
- Sudden ocular and orbital pain
- Diplopia
- Nausea/vomiting

PHYSICAL EXAM

Complete ophthalmic exam checking for

- Decreased visual acuity
- Afferent papillary defect
- Limited extraocular motility
- Loss of color vision
- Eyelid ecchymosis
- Progressive proptosis with resistance to retropulsion
- Chemosis
- Diffuse subconjunctival hemorrhage
- Elevated intraocular pressure (IOP)
- Optic disc and retinal pallor
- Central artery pulsations
- Choroidal folds

DIAGNOSTIC TESTS & INTERPRETATION

Lab

Initial lab tests

- CBC & differential
- PT, PTT, platelets

Follow-up & special considerations

Hematology/oncology evaluation if blood dyscrasia

Imaging

Initial approach

- Orbital CT scan (axial and coronal views)
- If vision is threatened, CT scan should be delayed until initial treatment has been instituted (see below).

Diagnostic Procedures/Other

- In spontaneous orbital hemorrhage, consider MRI (using head coils) if suspect vascular malformation or mass.
  - Biopsy of mass if present with spontaneous orbital hemorrhage

Pathological Findings

If spontaneous orbital hemorrhage, biopsy of mass may show vascular anomaly including

- Orbital lymphangiomas
- Cavernous hemangiomas

DIFFERENTIAL DIAGNOSIS

- Orbital cellulitis
- Orbital fractures (floor, medial wall, tripod)
- Ruptured globe
- Subperiosteal hemorrhage
- Optic nerve sheath hemorrhage

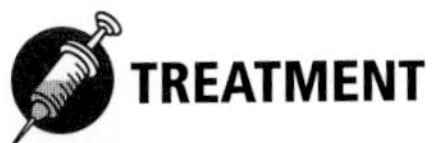

TREATMENT

MEDICATION

- Hyperosmotic agent (mannitol 20% 1–2 g/kg IV over 45 minutes)
  - Acetazolamide 500 mg IV
  - Methylprednisolone 100 mg IV for neuroprotection
  - Topical beta-blocker (timolol $\frac{1}{2}$% q30min × 2)

ADDITIONAL TREATMENT

General Measures

If vision is threatened, then a lateral canthotomy and cantholysis of the inferior and superior lateral canthal tendons should be done at the same time that medical therapy is being instituted and before the patient is sent for the CT scan.

Issues for Referral

- Hematology/oncology, if blood dyscrasia, if spontaneous retrobulbar hemorrhage
  - ENT, if postoperative sinus surgery

Additional Therapies

- Treat underlying blood dyscrasia, if spontaneous orbital hemorrhage
- Orbital exploration to find and ligate bleeder, if patient is postoperative orbital, sinus, lacrimal, or eyelid surgery
- Drain subperiosteal hemorrhage, if present.

SURGERY/OTHER PROCEDURES

- Optic nerve sheath decompression if optic nerve sheath hemorrhage
- Two wall (floor and medial wall) decompressions if the above measures fail.

IN-PATIENT CONSIDERATIONS

Initial Stabilization

Airway, respiration, and circulation (ABCs), in acute trauma

Admission Criteria

- Progressive visual loss
- For IV pulse therapy with corticosteroids

IV Fluids

Methylprednisolone 250 mg q6h for 12 doses

Nursing

Frequent vision checks

Discharge Criteria

Stable vision

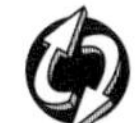

ONGOING CARE

FOLLOW-UP RECOMMENDATIONS

- See patient education
- Hematology/oncology consultation. If spontaneous orbital hemorrhage

Patient Monitoring

For postoperative visual acuities, IOP, motility, pupils, color vision, and external evaluation for proptosis

DIET

Preoperative and postoperative diet: low in garlic ginger, ginseng, ginkgo, high in antioxidants

PATIENT EDUCATION

- Preoperatively, patients should discontinue vitamin E, anticoagulants, antiplatelet agents, and herbal supplements, if medically stable (preinternist). compresses
  - Postoperatively, patients should apply ice. Avoid Valsalva maneuvers (bending, lifting, coughing, sneezing, nose blowing, straining at stool).
  - Seek medical attention stat, if sudden loss of vision, explosive exophthalmos, or severe orbital pain.

PROGNOSIS

- Poor, if visual loss is beyond 100 minutes of acute bleed
- Fair, if above treatment is instituted within 100 minutes of acute bleed

COMPLICATIONS

Loss of vision

ADDITIONAL READING

- Lelli GJ, Lisman RD. Blepharoplasty complications. *Plast Reconstr Surg* 2010;125(3):1007–1017.
- Lewis CD, Perry JD. Retrobulbar hemorrhage: epidemiology/incidence. *Expert Rev Ophthalmol* 2007;2(04):557–570.
- Sullivan TJ, Wright JE. Non-traumatic orbital hemorrhage. *Clin Experiment Ophthalmol* 2000;28(1):26–31.
- Tan JC, Chan EW, Looi A. Bilateral orbital subperiosteal hemorrhage following labor. *Ophthal Plastic Reconstr Surg* 2011;27(3):e59–e63.

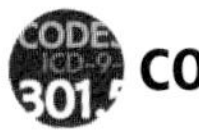

CODES

ICD9

- 376.32 Orbital hemorrhage
- 377.42 Optic nerve sheath hemorrhage
- 871.0 Ocular laceration without prolapse of intraocular tissue

CLINICAL PEARLS

- Most orbital hemorrhages are from trauma or are postoperative lid, orbit, sinus, or lacrimal surgery.
- Prevention depends on careful preoperative, intraoperative, and postoperative management.
- Emergent surgical intervention (lateral canthotomy/cantholysis and wound exploration if necessary) are the definitive treatment.

ORBITAL RHABDOMYOSARCOMA

Sara Lally
Carol Shields

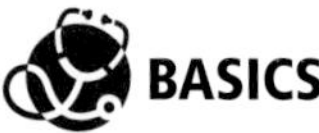

BASICS

DESCRIPTION

- Rhabdomyosarcoma (RMS) is a highly malignant neoplasm that arises from pluripotential cells that demonstrate histopathologic features of striated muscle.
- This tumor can arise in soft tissues throughout the body.
- RMS is the most common primary malignant orbital tumor of childhood.

ALERT
Optional. None.

Geriatric Considerations
Optional field. None.

Pediatric Considerations
Optional field. Rhabdomyosarcoma is more common in the pediatric age group.

Pregnancy Considerations
Optional field. Illicit drug use during pregnancy has been associated with an increased risk of rhabdomyosarcoma.

EPIDEMIOLOGY

Incidence
- 4.3 cases per 1 million children for all cases of RMS
- 5:3 male to female ratio for RMS of the orbit
- No racial predilection

Prevalence
- 350 new cases of systemic RMS per year
- Estimated 25–50 new cases of orbital RMS per year

RISK FACTORS

- Maternal use of marijuana during pregnancy has been found to cause 3-fold increased risk.
- Maternal use of cocaine during pregnancy is associated with 5-fold increased risk.
- Paternal use of marijuana, cocaine, or any recreational drug is associated with 2-fold increased risk.

Genetics
- Sporadic
- RMS has been associated with neurofibromatosis (NF) and Li–Fraumeni syndrome (LFS)

GENERAL PREVENTION
None

PATHOPHYSIOLOGY
In those cases with NF and LFS the *p53* tumor suppressor gene has been identified.

ETIOLOGY
Unknown

COMMONLY ASSOCIATED CONDITIONS
None

DIAGNOSIS

HISTORY
Based on a large review of orbital RMS by Shields et al., the history reveals:

- Mean age at presentation of 10 years
- Acute and subacute painless proptosis in 30%
- Eyelid swelling in 21%
- Conjunctival injection in 9% and edema of the eyelids in 21%
- Symptoms present for a mean of 5 weeks
- Downward and outward displacement of the globe
- Pain and decreased vision are uncommon.
- History of trauma

PHYSICAL EXAM
Based on a comprehensive review of orbital RMS by Shields et al., the findings include the following:

- Orbital mass in 76%
- Conjunctival mass in 12%
- Proptosis in 79%
- Chemosis in 41%
- Eyelid edema in 21%
- Can mimic inflammation

DIAGNOSTIC TESTS & INTERPRETATION

Lab

Initial lab tests
- CBC count with differential to rule out leukemia, infection, and other simulating conditions

Follow-up & special considerations
- Complete systemic workup to evaluate for metastatic disease
- Chest radiograph to rule out lung metastasis, the most common site for RMS metastasis

Imaging

Initial approach
- MRI of orbits
- CT of orbits
  - Round, oval, or irregular mass
  - Well-circumscribed or diffuse
  - Enhances with contrast
  - May have cavities within it
  - Usually in soft tissue
  - Most common site is superonasal in the extraconal space

Follow-up & special considerations
- Patients with RMS need to be followed by a pediatric oncologist as well as an ocular oncologist or ophthalmologist familiar with the disease.

Diagnostic Procedures/Other
- Orbitotomy with intent to remove the malignancy completely intake within its pseudocapsule
- If the tumor is diffuse, enwrapping vital visual structures, then debulking of the tumor without damaging surrounding structures is advised.

Pathological Findings
- Small round blue cells with cross-striations within the cytoplasm representing 4 histological types:
  - Pleomorphic—rarely involves the orbit
  - Embryonal—most common in the orbit
  - Alveolar—poorer prognosis
  - Botryoid—often involves anterior portion of orbit, which appears as grape-like lesion beneath the conjunctiva

DIFFERENTIAL DIAGNOSIS
- Neuroblastoma
- Lymphangioma
- Hemangioma
- Dermoid cyst
- Inflammatory conditions
  - Cellulitis
  - Nonspecific inflammatory diseases

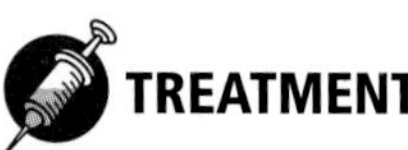

TREATMENT

MEDICATION

First Line
Chemotherapy is delivered by a pediatric oncologist. According to the Intergroup Rhabdomyosarcoma Study Group, the chemotherapy agents include vincristine, actinomycin-D, dactinomycin, cyclophosphomide, ifosfamide, and etoposide.

Second Line
Phase I/II trials include the use of chemotherapy agents such as doxorubicin (Adriamycin), melphalan, methotrexate, topotecan/irinotecan, taxol/docetaxel (Taxotere). These drugs are used alone or in combination with first-line agents.

ADDITIONAL TREATMENT

General Measures

- Refer to pediatric oncologist
- Staging—most orbital disease are group II or group III.
  - Group I—tumor completely resected
  - Group II—microscopic residual
  - Group III—gross residual
  - Group IV—metastasis
- According to Intergroup Rhabdomyosarcoma Study Group IV recommendations
  - Group I is treated with chemotherapy for 32 weeks.
  - Group II is treated with chemotherapy for 32 weeks and orbital radiotherapy (4,140 cGy).
  - Group III is treated with chemotherapy for 52 weeks and orbital radiotherapy (5,040 cGy).

Issues for Referral

Any suspicious orbital lesion in a young patient should raise suspicion and prompt referral to an ocular oncologist.

Additional Therapies

See next item

COMPLEMENTARY & ALTERNATIVE THERAPIES

- Adjuvant chemotherapy
- Orbital radiotherapy
  - Microscopic residual—4,000–4,500 cGy
  - Gross residual—5,000–5,500 cGy

SURGERY/OTHER PROCEDURES

As indicated above, orbitotomy with excisional biopsy complete removal if possible is the first goal of therapy. Then further chemotherapy and radiotherapy depend on the staging.

IN-PATIENT CONSIDERATIONS

Initial Stabilization

Inpatient hospitalization might be necessary for chemotherapy.

Admission Criteria

Inpatient hospitalization might be necessary for chemotherapy.

IV Fluids

May be necessary for inpatient hydration

Nursing

Per floor routine for chemotherapy patients

Discharge Criteria

Once medically stable

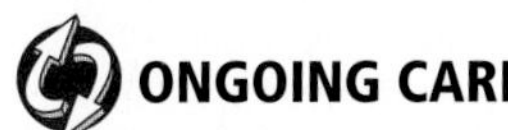

ONGOING CARE

FOLLOW-UP RECOMMENDATIONS

- Every 2–3 months for the first year then every 6 months
  - Repeat imaging every 6 months.

Patient Monitoring

- Watch for radiation side effects to eye and in field of treatment
- Based on a comprehensive review of orbital RMS by Shields et al., the findings include the following:
  - Cataract in 55%
  - Orbital hypoplasia in 24%
  - Dry eye in 36%
  - Chronic keratoconjunctivitis in 9%
  - Retinopathy in 9%
  - Recurrence can occur years after treatment.
  - Late side effects of chemotherapy such as leukemia

DIET

No dietary restrictions

PATIENT EDUCATION

See Additional Readings.

PROGNOSIS

- Historically there was about 30% survival, but with adjuvant radiation/chemotherapy there is a 95% survival rate.
  - Favorable prognosis in orbit because of early presentation and lack of lymphatic drainage

COMPLICATIONS

Side effects of radiation/chemotherapy

REFERENCES

1. Shields CL, Shields JA, Honavar SG, et al. The clinical spectrum of primary ophthalmic rhabdomyosarcoma. *Ophthalmology* 2001;108: 2284–2292.
2. Shields JA, Shields CL, Scartozzi R. Survey of 1264 patients with orbital tumors and simulating lesions: The 2002 Montgomery lecture, part 1. *Ophthalmology* 2004;111(5):997–1008.
3. Hayes-Jordan A, Andrassy R. Rhabdomyosarcoma in children. *Curr Opin Pediatr*. 2009;21(3): 373–378.
4. Shields JA, Shields CL. Rhabdomyosarcoma: Review for ophthalmologist. *Surv Ophthalmol*. 2003; 48(1):39–57.
5. Karcioglu ZA, Hadjistilianou D, Rozans M, et al. Orbital rhabdomyosarcoma. *Cancer Control*. 2004;11(5):328–333.

ADDITIONAL READING

- Shields JA, Shields CL. *Eyelid, conjunctival, and orbital tumors. An atlas and textbook*, 2nd ed. Philadelphia: Lippincott Williams & Wilkins, 2008.

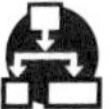

See Also (Topic, Algorithm, Electronic Media Element)

- www.fighteyecancer.com
- www.malignantmelanomainfo.com
- www.retinoblastomainfo.com
- www.eyecancerinfo.com
- www.eyecancerbook.com
- www.etrf.org

CODES

ICD9

190.1 Malignant neoplasm of orbit

CLINICAL PEARLS

- Presentation can mimic inflammation.
- Remove lesion completely if possible.
- Adjuvant chemotherapy and radiation has improved survival to 95%.

ORBITAL TUMORS: CONGENITAL

Linda H. Ohsie
Jacqueline R. Carrasco

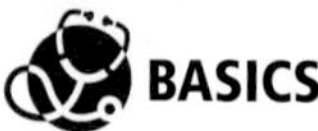

BASICS

DESCRIPTION

- Congenital orbital tumors are typically found at birth or in early childhood.
- The most common congenital orbital tumors are dermoid or epidermoid cysts and teratomas.
  - Orbital dermoid/epidermoid cysts are benign choristomas typically found at the junction of bony sutures (most commonly the frontozygomatic suture).
  - Orbital teratomas are benign germ cell tumors that are a rare cause of proptosis at birth.

EPIDEMIOLOGY

Incidence

- Orbital dermoid/epidermoid cysts (1)[C], (2)[C]
  - Incidence – Most common space-occupying orbital lesion of childhood. May comprise 30–46% of excised orbital tumors in children.
  - Age at diagnosis is most commonly in infants and young children, but may be diagnosed at any age
  - Sex – No predilection
- Teratomas – most commonly found in gonadal tissue, rarely involves the orbit (3)[C]
  - Incidence – Very rare in the orbit
  - Age – Majority present at or shortly after birth
  - Sex – 2:1 Females:Males

RISK FACTORS

None identified

PATHOPHYSIOLOGY

- Orbital dermoid/epidermoid Cysts (1)[C], (2)[C]
  - Arise from embryonic ectoderm that is sequestered between bones along fetal lines of closure
  - Rarely, a dermoid/epidermoid cyst may be completely confined within orbital soft tissues without direct contact with a bony suture
  - There are 3 types identified: Juxtasutural, sutural, and soft-tissue types
- Orbital teratomas (3)[C]
  - Arises from aberrant germ cells and more commonly occurs in the gonads, retroperitoneum, or mediastinum
  - Tumor comprised of mature tissue derivatives from all 3 germ cell layers

COMMONLY ASSOCIATED CONDITIONS

- Orbital dermoid/epidermoid Cysts (1)[C]
  - Occasionally astigmatism
  - Rarely proptosis, diplopia or motility disturbance
  - No association with visual loss or elevation of intraocular pressure
- Orbital teratomas (3)[C]
  - Severe proptosis and expansion of the orbit are common
  - Large masses with severe proptosis may lead to exposure keratopathy, conjunctival keratinization, corneal ulcer formation, and vascular congestion

DIAGNOSIS

HISTORY

- Orbital dermoid/epidermoid cysts (1)[C]
  - Generally asymptomatic unless they increase in size or rupture (spontaneously or with trauma) resulting in an inflammatory reaction and pain
  - Rarely cause proptosis or displacement of the globe
  - Growth of these lesions is typically slow
- Orbital teratomas (3)[C]
  - Rapidly growing proptosis noted at birth or early infancy
  - Typically unilateral

PHYSICAL EXAM

- Orbital dermoid/epidermoid Cysts (1)[C], (2)[C]
  - Frequently presents as painless, subcutaneous mass
  - Typically located in the superotemporal orbital region (frontozygomatic suture), less frequently superonasally
  - On palpation are not fixed to overlying skin – they are partially mobile, smooth, and not tender to touch
  - Do not affect vision or intraocular pressure
- Orbital teratomas (3)[C]
  - Tend to be more common in the left orbit
  - Decreased vision (may be difficult to assess)
  - Proptosis, tight eyelids, and a tense orbit may be present
  - Performing transillumination may illuminate cystic areas within the mass

DIAGNOSTIC TESTS & INTERPRETATION

Imaging

- Orbital dermoid/epidermoid cysts (1)[C]
- Initial approach
  - Orbital CT (with axial and coronal views) or MRI to aid with surgical planning
  - On CT – A round to ovoid lesion with distinct margins. Lumen is usually homogeneous and does not enhance with contrast.
  - On MRI – A round to ovoid lesion with variable amounts of material in the lumen relatively isointense to vitreous on T1- and T2-weighted images. The wall enhances with gadolinium.
- Follow Up & Special Considerations
  - Repeat imaging may be ordered when observing the lesion for growth or for any change in clinical exam
- Orbital Teratomas (3)[C]
- Initial Approach
  - Orbital CT – helpful in detecting calcification characteristic of teratomas which helps to distinguish this from other orbital lesions
  - Both CT and MRI show an enlarged orbit with a multiloculated soft tissue mass
- Follow Up & Special Considerations
  - Repeat imaging should be performed after surgical excision of teratoma

Pathological Findings

- Orbital dermoid/epidermoid cysts (1)[C], (4)[C]
  - Smooth, cystic structure usually white, tan, or yellow in color
  - Cysts typically lined by keratinizing, stratified squamous epithelium
  - Hair shafts, sebaceous glands, sweat glands, and inflammatory cells may also be found in dermoid specimens
  - Histologically, epidermoid cysts have no dermal appendages (2)[C]
- Orbital Teratomas (3)[C], (4)[C]
  - Fleshy pink mass on gross inspection – may have solid and cystic components
  - Histologically contains structures representing all 3 embryonic germ layers: Ectoderm, mesoderm, and endoderm
  - May be partially calcified or ossified

DIFFERENTIAL DIAGNOSIS

- If proptosis is present in an infant or child, these other processes should also be considered.
- Capillary hemangiomas also commonly present as orbital masses manifesting at birth within the first year of life (2)[C], (4)[C]
  - Orbital hemangiomas may produce proptosis or displacement of the globe and can enlarge with crying or Valsalva maneuvers
  - For more information on orbital hemangiomas, please refer to the Orbit/Oculoplastics or Pediatric Section on capillary hemangiomas
- Rhabdomyosarcomas are the most common pediatric malignant orbital tumors (2)[C], (4)[C]
  - Presents with rapid proptosis in the first decade of life, with an average age of 7 years
  - CT imaging shows an irregular tumor with well-defined margins, soft tissue attenuation and there is often bony destruction/erosion.
  - Once a tissue diagnosis is made, systemic survey, including bone marrow biopsy, and staging should be performed
  - Prognosis improved with advancements in systemic chemotherapy and radiation therapy.
- Lymphangiomas are benign congenital vascular malformations that may involve the conjunctiva, eyelids or deep orbit (2)[C], (4)[C]
  - Typically present in the first 2 decades of life
  - May slowly enlarge over years but may also have sudden proptosis from an intralesional hemorrhage
  - For more information on lymphangiomas, please refer to the Orbit/Oculoplastics section on vascular orbital tumors

- Optic nerve gliomas are the third most common orbital tumors in children (2)[C]
  - Most often associated with Neurofibromatosis type I (usually bilateral), but may also occur sporadically
  - Mean age of 8 years at presentation
  - Common presenting symptoms are proptosis and visual changes and may have headache or pain with intracranial extension
  - On CT gliomas appear as a fusiform enlargement of the optic nerve
  - Treatment is surgical excision
- Congenital cystic eye – failure of globe to form during embryogenesis resulting in orbital cysts composed of primitive ocular tissue (2)[C]
- Other considerations:
  - Retinoblastoma with orbital extension
  - Lymphoid tumors
  - Neuroblastoma
  - Melanocytoma
  - Orbital cellulitis
  - Lacrimal mass
  - Dacryops
  - Abscess
  - Parasitic larval cyst
  - Sarcomas
  - Malignant medulloepithelioma
  - Fibrous dysplasia
  - Mucocele
  - Encephalocele
  - Colobomatous cyst

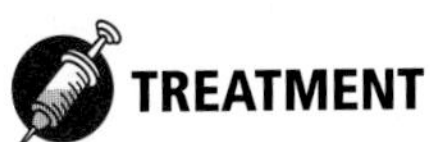

TREATMENT

ADDITIONAL TREATMENT

Issues for Referral

- Orbital dermoid/epidermoid cysts
  - If asymptomatic, patient may follow-up routinely with a general ophthalmologist or pediatric ophthalmologist
  - If large or symptomatic (globe displacement, pain, inflamed), consider referring promptly to an oculoplastic surgeon or pediatric ophthalmologist
- Orbital teratomas
  - If an orbital teratoma is suspected or confirmed by imaging, the patient should promptly be referred to an oculoplastic surgeon or pediatric ophthalmologist for surgical management.

SURGERY/OTHER PROCEDURES

- Orbital dermoid/epidermoid cysts (1)[C], (2)[C], (4)[C]
  - These benign lesions may be observed or excised surgically
  - Surgery may be considered when cosmesis is an issue due to its size or if it is in a location subject to trauma and possible rupture
  - Must consider risk of general anesthesia when pursuing surgical management especially in infants
  - Rupture of the capsule should be avoided during removal of the cyst
- Orbital teratomas (3)[C], (4)[C]
  - Surgical excision/debulking – should aim to preserve the globe and visual function, as well as orbital/facial development and cosmesis
  - Massive teratomas may require treatment with orbital exenteration

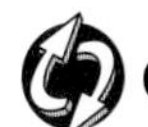

ONGOING CARE

FOLLOW-UP RECOMMENDATIONS

Patient Monitoring

- Orbital dermoid/epidermoid cysts
  - If observation is elected, a general ophthalmologist, pediatric ophthalmologist, or oculoplastic surgeon may follow the patient routinely and also intervene surgically if warranted
  - An oculoplastic surgeon may be most comfortable and experienced in surgically excising orbital dermoid cysts
- Orbital teratomas
  - Needs regular follow-up to detect recurrences or malignant transformation
  - May require further reconstructive procedures after surgical excision or exenteration

PROGNOSIS

- Orbital dermoid/epidermoid cysts (1)[C]
  - Benign lesions
  - Normal vision/ocular development
- Orbital teratomas (3)[C]
  - Benign lesions
  - Rarely malignant
  - If the globe is salvaged, visual prognosis may be poor

COMPLICATIONS

- Orbital dermoid/epidermoid cysts (1)[C]
  - May rupture spontaneously or with trauma resulting in an intense inflammatory reaction resembling orbital cellulitis
  - Very rarely, these cysts may evolve into squamous cell carcinoma
- Orbital teratomas (3)[C]
  - Surgical excision or exenteration may result in loss of vision or loss of the eye

REFERENCES

1. Castillo BV, Kaufman L. Pediatric tumors of the eye and orbit. *Pediatr Clin N Am* 2003;50:149–172.
2. Mehta M, Chandra M, Sen S, et al. Orbital teratoma: A rare cause of congenital proptosis. *Clin Experiment Ophthalmol* 2009;37:626–628.
3. Shields JA, Kaden IH, Eagle RC, et al. Orbital dermoid cysts: Clinicopathologic correlations, classification, and management. The 1997 Josephine E. Schueler Lecture. *Ophthalmic Plast Reconstr Surg* 1997;13:265–276.
4. Volpe NJ, Jakobiec FA. Pediatric orbital tumors. *Int Ophthalmol Clin* 1992;32:201–21.

CODES

ICD9

- 224.1 Benign neoplasm of orbit
- 238.8 Neoplasm of uncertain behavior of other specified sites

CLINICAL PEARLS

- Both orbital dermoid/epidermoid cysts and orbital teratomas are typically benign lesions.
- Orbital dermoids/epidermoids are usually superotemporal, painless subcutaneous masses that do not commonly affect vision or intraocular pressure.
- Orbital teratomas are a rare cause of rapidly growing proptosis in an infant and require prompt referral to an oculoplastic surgeon or pediatric ophthalmologist for management.
- Proptosis in a child must be investigated and always consider rhabdomyosarcoma as possible etiology.

ORBITAL TUMORS: METASTATIC

Rachel K. Sobel
Jacqueline Carrasco

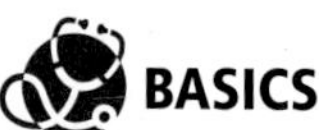

BASICS

DESCRIPTION

- Metastatic orbital tumors are tumors that have spread hematogenously to the soft tissue or bones in the orbit.
- The most common primary sites are breasts in women and lungs in men.
- Other metastases may originate from prostate gland, skin melanoma, gastrointestinal, and kidney cancers.
- Carcinoid tumors of ileal or appendiceal origin usually metastasize to orbit, whereas bronchial carcinoid tumors usually involve the uveal tract.
- Cutaneous melanoma can also metastasize to the orbit.
- Metastatic tumors in children are uncommon and come from adrenal neuroblastoma, Wilms tumors, and Ewing tumor.

EPIDEMIOLOGY

Incidence

Data not available.

Prevalence

Metastatic orbital tumors comprise about 7% of all orbital tumors.

RISK FACTORS

The risk factors for primary neoplasm are also the risk factors for orbital metastasis.

Genetics

- Genetics plays a strong role in many cancers and their ability to metastasize. We have not yet characterized the genes that specifically enable cancers to metastasize to the orbit.
- There is no specific gender predilection.

GENERAL PREVENTION

Prevention and treatment of primary neoplasm helps prevent metastatic orbital tumors.

PATHOPHYSIOLOGY

- Extraocular muscles are often seeded because of their abundant blood supply.
- The bone marrow of the sphenoid bone is also commonly involved because of the high volume of low-flow venous channels in the bone.

ETIOLOGY

See above.

COMMONLY ASSOCIATED CONDITIONS

Not applicable.

DIAGNOSIS

HISTORY

- Average age of presentation is seventh decade in adult cases.
- 25–35% of patients do not have a primary malignancy at the time of ocular presentation.
- Diplopia, pain, and visual loss are most common symptoms.
- Also, ptosis (droopy eyelid), proptosis (bulging eye), eyelid swelling, and palpable mass are common features.

PHYSICAL EXAM

- Clinical presentation can be divided into 3 subcategories:
  - Infiltrative is characterized by motility restriction, resistance to retropulsion, ptosis, and enophthalmos.
  - Mass is characterized by proptosis and often a palpable orbital mass.
  - Inflammatory is characterized by pain, chemosis, erythema, and periorbital swelling.
- Decreased vision can occur from orbital congestion, with optic neuropathy and choroidal folds.
- Enophthalmos is another important diagnostic sign. It comes from tethering and posterior traction on the globe from scirrhous metastasis such as breast or gastrointestinal carcinoma.
- Cranial neuropathies from orbital apex involvement or cavernous sinus involvement are possible.

DIAGNOSTIC TESTS & INTERPRETATION

Lab

Initial lab tests

Patients suspected of having metastatic disease by history and examination should have biopsy before extensive lab testing is performed. However, if inflammatory processes are also in the differential, ACE, p-ANCA, c-ANCA, and PPD may be helpful.

Follow-up & special considerations

Once biopsy results show suspected metastatic disease, prompt referral to a medical oncologist is warranted and further laboratory testing is indicated based upon the individual cancer.

Imaging

Initial approach

CT scan or MRI with contrast can delineate extent of orbital involvement. These images may assist in surgical planning.

Follow-up & special considerations

Medical oncologists coordinate further imaging, including PET scanning and other modalities to determine the involved sites.

Diagnostic Procedures/Other

- Histopathology is necessary to make diagnosis.
  - Incisional biopsy is done when the tumor is infiltrative and/or unable to be completely removed because it is adherent to adjacent vital structures.
  - Excisional biopsy is preferred whenever possible.
  - Fine-needle aspiration biopsy (FNAB) may also be performed. Scirrhous breast carcinoma and gastrointestinal cancer may be dry taps.

Pathological Findings

- Histopathology will be similar to primary neoplasm. Standard hematoxylin and eosin stains can help make the diagnosis.
- Immunohistochemistry, cytopathology, and special stains may aid in distinguishing final pathologic diagnosis, particularly in poorly differentiated specimens.

DIFFERENTIAL DIAGNOSIS
- Inflammatory orbital processes such as sarcoid, TB, and idiopathic orbital inflammation
- Primary orbital tumors, such as ocular adnexal lymphoma, meningioma, or vascular lesions
- Orbital cellulitis
- Thyroid eye disease

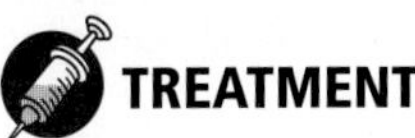

TREATMENT

MEDICATION
Medical treatment, that is, chemotherapy and hormone therapy, varies depending upon the type of primary neoplasm and its stage. External beam radiotherapy if often used as additional therapy.

ADDITIONAL TREATMENT
General Measures
- Treatment is aimed at preserving vision and addressing pain.
- External beam radiotherapy is often first line treatment for local control of orbital tumor.

Issues for Referral
Prompt referral to a medical oncologist is necessary.

COMPLEMENTARY & ALTERNATIVE THERAPIES
Discuss with primary medical oncologist.

SURGERY/OTHER PROCEDURES
Aggressive surgical treatment may rarely be indicated including wide excision or exenteration with radiation depending upon staging and prognosis.

IN-PATIENT CONSIDERATIONS
Initial Stabilization
Typically not indicated.

Admission Criteria
Patients are typically staged as outpatients but may be admitted to the hospital for medical or social indications.

IV Fluids
As needed for associated systemic problems.

Nursing
As needed for associated systemic problems.

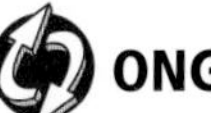

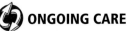

ONGOING CARE

FOLLOW-UP RECOMMENDATIONS
- Close follow-up is indicated to stage patient from a systemic standpoint. Ophthalmic care should be coordinated in a step-wise logical fashion with life-saving treatments.
- Palliative radiotherapy, chemotherapy, and hormone therapy are indicated depending upon the cancer.

PROGNOSIS
- Overall prognosis is poor. It is about 1 year.
- The exception is orbital carcinoid metastases, whose 5-year survival is 72%.
- Survival is short-lived in most cases of metastatic adenocarcinoma.

COMPLICATIONS
Systemic manifestations of metastatic cancer.

ADDITIONAL READING

- Char DH, Miller T, Kroll S. Orbital Metastases: Diagnosis and course. *Br J Ophthalmol*. 1997;81(5): 386–390.
- Ferry AP, Font RL. Carcinoma metastatic to the eye and orbit. I. A clinicopathologic study of 227 cases. *Arch Ophthalmol* 1975;93(7):472–482.
- Goldberg RA, Rootman J. Clinical characteristics of Metastatic Orbital Tumors. *Ophthalmology* 1989;97: 620–624.
- Mehta JS, Abou-Rayyah Y, Rose GE. Orbital carcinoid metastases. *Ophthalmology* 2006;113(3): 466–472.
- Shields JA, Shields, CL, Scartozzi R. Survey of 1264 Patients with Orbital Tumors and Simulating Lesions. *Ophthalmology* 2004;11;997–1008.
- Shields JA, Shields CL. Orbital Metastatic Cancer. In: Shields JA, et al. *Eyelid, Conjunctival, and Orbital Tumors: an Atlas and Textbook. Orbital Metastatic Cancer*. Philadelphia: Lippincott Williams and Wilkins, 2007:728–743.

CODES

ICD9
198.4 Secondary malignant neoplasm of other parts of nervous system

CLINICAL PEARLS

- A quarter of all patients with orbital metastasis do not have a primary diagnoses at the time of presentation.
- An ophthalmologist may therefore be the first to diagnose a serious illness like metastatic cancer. A high index of suspicion and rapid diagnosis is crucial. Prompt referral for systemic work-up can then be pursued.
- Enophthalmos can be the tricky presenting sign of scirrhous breast carcinoma or gastrointestinal cancer. It is often confused with contralateral proptosis.
- Although survival is dismal, local treatment as well as systemic chemotherapy can greatly affect quality of life. Radiotherapy can improve vision.

ORBITAL TUMORS: VASCULAR

Rachel K. Sobel
Jacqueline R. Carrasco

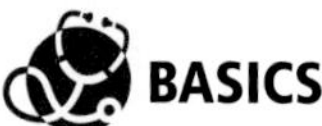

BASICS

DESCRIPTION

- Orbital vascular tumors encompass a wide variety of pathology. They can be subdivided by histopathology and growth characteristics (1).
- Capillary hemangiomas
- Venous vascular malformations (cavernous hemangiomas and orbital varices)
- Venous lymphatic malformations
- Arteriovenous lesions
- Neoplasms (i.e., hemangiopericytoma)
- Orbital vascular tumors may also be classified by hemodynamic characteristics (2)
  - No flow (lymphangioma)
  - Venous flow (varix)
  - Arterial flow (arteriovenous malformation)

EPIDEMIOLOGY

Incidence

- Vasculogenic tumors make up 17% of all orbital tumors (3).
  - Capillary hemangioma (3%)
  - Cavernous hemangioma (6%)
  - Varix 2%
  - Lymphangioma (4%)
  - Hemangiopericytoma (1%)

Prevalence

Unknown

PATHOPHYSIOLOGY

See below

ETIOLOGY

- Capillary hemangiomas: Unknown but current theory is that they are of placental origin and may be either emboli or direct extension of placental tissue.
- Cavernous hemangioma: Some have proposed that these are of venous origin; others theorize that they are low flow arteriovenous malformations. Growth may be mediated by angiogenic or cytokine induced factors due to association between growth of hemangioma and puberty and pregnancy.
- Lymphangioma: A vascular malformation that occurs during embryogenesis from sequestration of lymphatic tissue.
- Varix: Results from presumably a congenital weakness in the postcapillary venous wall, which leads to proliferation of venous elements and massive dilation of the valveless orbital veins.
- Arteriovenous lesions: Derived from multiple congenital microvascular connections between arteries and veins without a capillary bed.
- Hemangiopericytoma: There is controversy as to the existence of these as a distinct entity versus part of the category of solitary fibrous tumors. Thought to be derived from vascular pericytes, contractile. 15% metastasize.

COMMONLY ASSOCIATED CONDITIONS

- Kasabach-Merritt syndrome is a syndrome of platelet entrapment and thrombocytopenia associated with hemangiomas.
- Blue rubber bleb nevus syndrome is associated with multiple cavernous hemangiomas.
- Orbital lymphangiomas have been seen with orbital and intracranial arteriovenous malformations.
- Orbital varices can be associated with defects in orbital bone and cephaloceles.
- PHACE syndrome (posterior fossa brain malformations, large facial hemangiomas, arterial anomalies, cardiac anomalies, and eye abnormalities) is associated with capillary hemangiomas.
- Wyburn-Mason syndrome is associated with arteriovenous malformations.

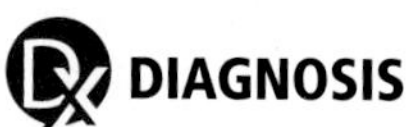

DIAGNOSIS

HISTORY

- Capillary hemangiomas appear in the first few months of life as a soft bluish mass deep to the eyelid. Typically they progress during the first few months of life, then stabilize at 6–12 months, and regress over the next 5–7 years. Often they have accompanying skin changes, "strawberry hemangiomas" that help make the diagnosis. More common in females.
- Cavernous hemangioma is most common in the fifth decade (40s). Patients typically present with unilateral painless proptosis without involution. More common in women.
- Lymphangiomas are probably present at birth but don't become apparent until years later when the lesions abruptly present due to hemorrhage.
- Varix: Presents in young adulthood associated with positional proptosis (worse with Valsalva or bending over).
- Hemangiopericytoma: Mean age of presentation is fifth decade with slowly progressive proptosis, sometimes painful. More common in orbit in males.
- Arteriovenous malformation: These are rare in the orbit. Typically present with periorbital swelling.

PHYSICAL EXAM

- External skin changes
- Ptosis
- Astigmatism
- Amblyopia
- Lagophthalmos/corneal exposure
- Afferent pupillary defect
- Restriction of motility
- Proptosis
- Color vision deficit
- Visual field constriction
- Dilated exam: Choroidal folds
- Glaucoma
- Changes in vascular tumors in size can occur with crying, coughing, and upper respiratory infections due to vascular or lymphatic engorgement.

DIAGNOSTIC TESTS & INTERPRETATION

Imaging

- CT or MRI will help delineate characteristic features of the tumor (4)
  - Capillary hemangioma: Round, ovoid circumscribed mass.
  - Cavernous hemangioma: Round, ovoid mass usually in the muscle cone. May also occur in bone. Progressive accumulation of contrast in late phases due to low flow.
  - Lymphangioma: Chocolate cysts as seen on imaging are hemorrhagic cystic structures. Sometimes these have fluid–fluid levels within the cyst based on different ages of the fluid.
  - Varix: Round or irregular mass that becomes apparent with Valsalva.
  - Hemangiopericytoma: Typically lobulated and well-circumscribed but may have infiltrative margins.
  - Arteriovenous malformation: May need angiographic protocol or traditional angiography to diagnose.

Diagnostic Procedures/Other

Fine needle aspiration or total excision may be necessary if there is diagnostic uncertainty or a concern for malignancy.

Pathological Findings

- Capillary hemangioma: Capillary sized vascular spaces surrounded by proliferating benign endothelial cells.
- Cavernous hemangioma: Dilated congested vascular channels lined by flattened endothelial cells with an intervening fibrous interstitium.
- Lymphangioma: Dilated ecstatic vascular channels filled with clear fluid or blood.
- Varix: Dilated veins with hyalinization and thrombosis.
- Hemangiopericytoma: Staghorn-like capillary spaces lined by proliferating pericytes. One-third are histopathologically consistent with malignancy.
- Arteriovenous malformation: Multiple congenital connections between arteries and veins without a capillary bed.

DIFFERENTIAL DIAGNOSIS

- Orbital tumors (meningioma, glioma)
- Metastatic orbital tumors
- Idiopathic orbital inflammation
- Thyroid-related orbitopathy

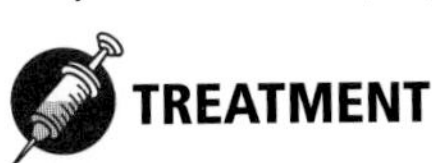

TREATMENT

MEDICATION

First Line

- Capillary hemangiomas: Observation; topical, oral or intralesional corticosteroids; interferon alpha; laser; surgical. A new noninvasive therapy is beta-blocker propanolol (5)[C].
- Cavernous hemangioma: Typically conservative unless unacceptable proptosis or visual deficit makes surgery an option.
- Varix: Surgical excision if unacceptable cosmetic changes or visual compromise.
- Lymphangioma: Observation is typical, but if there is unacceptable proptosis or visual compromise, treatment includes intralesional injection of sclerosing agents (6)[C], carbon dioxide ablation (7)[C], and intralesional injection of steroids. Surgical management is very difficult as it is challenging to remove the entire growth.
- Hemangiopericytoma: Standard treatment is wide surgical excision with postoperative irradiation for incompletely excised tumors.
- Arteriovenous malformation: Embolization and in some cases, surgery.

SURGERY/OTHER PROCEDURES

- Observation is acceptable for vascular tumors that do not cause visual deficit or facial deformity.
- Surgical removal or debulking can be difficult with vascular tumors because of the risk of bleeding.
- Surgical treatment is recommended when the tumor becomes symptomatic, visually or cosmetically.

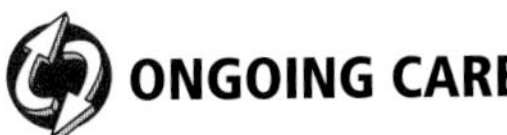

ONGOING CARE

PROGNOSIS

Varies with the type of vascular tumor and its location in the orbit

COMPLICATIONS

Incomplete excision of hemangiopericytoma may lead to malignant transformation.

REFERENCES

1. Mulliken JB, Glowacki J. Hemangiomas and vascular malformations in infants and children. A classification based on endothelial characteristics. *Plast Reconstr Surg* 1982;69(3):412–422.
2. Harris GJ. Orbital vascular malformations: A consensus statement on terminology and its clinical implications. Orbital Society. *Am J Ophthalmol* 1999:127(4):453–455.
3. Shields JA, Shields CL, Scartozzi R. Survey of 1264 patients with orbital tumors and simulating lesions. *Ophthalmology* 2004;111(5):997–1008.
4. Smoker W, Gentry L, Yee N, et al. Vascular lesions of the orbit: More than meets the eye. *Radiographics* 2008;28(1):185–204.
5. Leaute-Labreze C, Dumas de la Roque E, Hubiche T, et al. Propanolol for severe hemangiomas of infancy. *N Engl J Med* 2008; 358(24):2649–2651.
6. Burrows PE, Mason KP. Percutaneous treatment of low-flow vascular malformations. *J Vas Interv Radiol* 2004;15:431–445.
7. Kennerdell JS, Maroon JC, Garrity JA, et al. Surgical management of orbital lymphangioma with the carbon dioxide laser. *Am J Ophthalmol* 1986;102: 308–314.

ADDITIONAL READING

- Shields JA, Shields CL. Orbital vascular and hemorrhagic lesions. In: Shields JA, Shields CL, eds. *Eyelid, conjunctival and orbital tumors*. Philadelphia: Lippincott Williams and Wilkins, 2008:516–553.

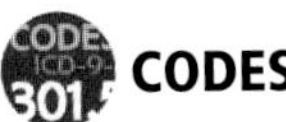

CODES

ICD9

- 224.1 Benign neoplasm of orbit
- 228.09 Hemangioma of other sites
- 456.8 Varices of other sites

CLINICAL PEARLS

- Vascular tumors may be difficult to remove because of their association with blood supply and deep location in the orbit.
- Close observation is an acceptable option until cosmetic deformity or visual compromise occurs.
- Most vascular tumors are not really tumors, but rather malformations.
- Propranolol is an increasingly acceptable noninvasive way to treat infantile capillary hemangiomas.

PAGET'S DISEASE

Lili Grunwald
Lan Chen
Vatinee Bunya

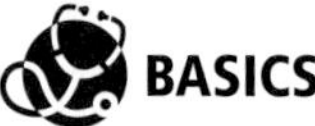

BASICS

DESCRIPTION

- A bone remodeling disorder resulting in increased bone turnover
- Disorganized bone formation and break down impairs integrity of affected bone.
- Often asymptomatic, however can be associated with pathologic fractures, bone deformity, deafness, and cranial nerve compression due to enlarged bones and secondary osteoarthritis.
- Elevated serum alkaline phosphatase (SAP) and abnormal radiography or bone scan
- Ocular manifestations include angioid streaks, orbital involvement of sarcomas, and compressive optic neuropathy.

EPIDEMIOLOGY

Prevalence

- Paget's disease is found in 1–2% of Caucasian adults older than 55 years.
- Prevalence increases with age.
- Up to 15% of patients with Paget's disease have angioid streaks.

RISK FACTORS

- Poorly understood; however, genetic and environmental risk factors - such as viral infection, may have a role.
- Large ethnic and geographic differences in prevalence. It is more common in people of Anglo-Saxon origin.

Genetics

- There appears to be a genetic component.
- Approximately 15% of patients have a positive family history.
- Some families with autosomal dominant inheritance have been described.

GENERAL PREVENTION

No treatment is known to prevent choroidal neovascular (CNV) membranes, which are the most visually significant complications of angioid streaks.

PATHOPHYSIOLOGY

- Focal areas of increased osteoclastic bone resorption with bone marrow fibrosis, increased vascularity of bone, and disorganized bone formation
- Enlarging and abnormally contoured bones that may bow or fracture
- Elevated SAP, normal serum calcium (can be elevated if immobile due to unopposed increased bone resorption)
- Hypercalcemia in an ambulatory patient with Paget's may be due to another cause such as hyperparathyroidism.
- Angioid streaks in the eye occur due to discontinuities in thickened Bruch's membrane.

ETIOLOGY

- Cause unknown
- Viral infection may play a role in the etiology.

COMMONLY ASSOCIATED CONDITIONS

- The most common diseases to be associated with angioid streaks can be remembered with the "PEPSI" mnemonic.
  - P: Paget's disease
  - E: Ehlers–Danlos
  - P: Pseudoxanthoma elasticum (PXE)
  - S: Sickle cell hemoglobinopathy
  - I: Idiopathic

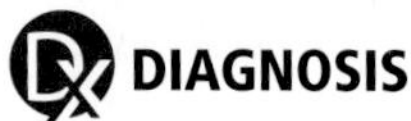

DIAGNOSIS

HISTORY

- Majority are asymptomatic and diagnosed by routine serum chemistry screen with elevated alkaline phosphatase or radiography performed for another reason.
- Bone pain, bowed tibias, fractures, headache, large head, deafness, warmth over affected areas
- Decreased vision, metamorphopsia, scotoma
- Cardiac disease and abnormalities in calcium and phosphate balance can occur.
- Excessive bleeding during orthopedic surgery may occur.

PHYSICAL EXAM

- Systemic features:
  - The most common bones affected by Paget's disease are the flat and long bones including the spine, femur, pelvis, skull, clavicle, and humerus.
  - Bone fractures may occur.
  - Increased incidence of bone tumors, which present with pain or an enlarging mass
  - Cardiac complications due to widespread severe disease causing heart failure, aortic stenosis, and conduction abnormalities
- Ophthalmic features:
  - Angioid streaks: dark red to brown bands irregularly radiating from optic nerves deep to the retina. Usually bilateral
  - Atrophic retinal pigment epithelium (RPE) overlying angioid streaks
  - RPE clumping with focal hyperpigmentation
  - High risk for CNV membranes with RPE detachment or serous and/or hemorrhagic detachments of the retina
  - Peau d' orange is midperipheral RPE mottling sometimes associated with angioid streaks due to Paget's.
  - Compressive optic neuropathy that may cause optic atrophy
  - Orbital soft tissue sarcomas

DIAGNOSTIC TESTS & INTERPRETATION

Lab

Initial lab tests

- Elevated SAP
- Also check serum calcium, albumin, parathyroid hormone, phosphorus, 25-hydroxy vitamin D, and urinary calcium.

Follow-up & special considerations

- Routinely monitor SAP
- Fundus examination may show angioid streaks or CNV.

Imaging

Initial approach

- Radiography shows dense mosaic bones.
- Bone scans are the most sensitive test and can be used to evaluate the extent and activity of disease. Pagetic bone lesions appear as focal areas of increased uptake.

Follow-up & special considerations

- Repeat imaging with change in symptoms.
- CT or MRI if bone pain increased or refractory to treatment

Diagnostic Procedures/Other

- Please refer to the angioid streaks chapter for more details.
- Ophthalmic diagnostic imaging tests for angioid streaks and CNV may include fundus fluorescein angiography (FA), optical coherence tomography (OCT), or indocyanine angiography (ICG).

Pathological Findings

Mosaic pattern of lamellar bone associated with increases in local bone blood flow and in fibrous tissue in adjacent marrow

DIFFERENTIAL DIAGNOSIS

- Osteomalacia
- Hyperparathyroidism
- Vitamin D deficiency
- Malignancy such as multiple myeloma

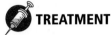

TREATMENT

MEDICATION

First Line

- All medications used to treat Paget's disease of bone are inhibitors of osteoclastic bone resorption.
- Newer-generation nitrogen-containing bisphosphonates are the primary initial agents:
  - Zoledronic acid: 5 mg IV single infusion reference (1)[A]
  - Risedronate: 30 mg orally daily for 2 months
  - Pamidronate: 30 mg IV for 3 days
  - Alendronate: 40 mg daily for 6 months

Second Line

- Simple bisphosphonates:
  - Tiludronate: 400 mg orally daily for 3 months.
  - Etidronate: 200–400 mg orally for 6 months (5 mg/kg of body weight per day)
- Calcitonin (rarely used): Salmon calcitonin 50–100 units subcutaneously daily or 3 times per week.
- Side effects of bisphosphonates at the dosing regimen used in Paget's disease include but are not limited to
  - Influenza-like syndrome
  - Musculoskeletal pain
  - Osteonecrosis of the jaw
  - Dyspepsia or diarrhea
  - Esophagitis
  - Rarely, uveitis and scleritis
- Contraindications to bisphosphonates include impaired renal function, particularly with IV infusion.
- Common side effects of calcitonin include nausea, vomiting, and flushing. Rarely, tachyphylaxis.

ADDITIONAL TREATMENT

General Measures

- NOTE: Bisphosphonates are poorly absorbed orally. They must be taken with water, first thing in the morning, at least 30 min before any food, beverage, or other oral medications. Patients should not lie down during these 30 min.
- If supplemental calcium is taken, it should be separated by at least 2 h from bisphosphonates because calcium can decrease the absorption of bisphosphonates.
- A normal serum 25-hydroxy vitamin D and calcium levels are generally needed before giving bisphosphonates.

Issues for Referral

- Refer to ophthalmology to monitor and treat ocular complications.
- No treatment for angioid streaks
- Treatment options for ocular CNV include the following:
  - Laser coagulation (2)[C]
  - Photodynamic therapy (PDT) (3)[C]
  - Intravitreal antivascular endothelial growth factor (anti-VEGF) therapy such as bevacizumab (4)[C]

Additional Therapies

- Supplemental calcium with vitamin D for patients with Paget's disease, particularly if they are receiving bisphosphonate therapy.
  - Antiresorptive therapy can improve bone pain; however, analgesics and anti-inflammatory medications may also be necessary.

SURGERY/OTHER PROCEDURES

- Orthopedic surgery to manage bony complications
- For planned surgery at an active pagetic site, preoperative medical treatment may possibly decrease perioperative blood loss.

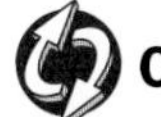

ONGOING CARE

FOLLOW-UP RECOMMENDATIONS

Depends upon severity of systemic and ophthalmic disease

Patient Monitoring

- Amsler grid monitoring for metamorphopsia
- Safety glasses for patient with angioid streaks because of increased risk of choroidal rupture and subsequent subretinal hemorrhage after trauma

PROGNOSIS

Increased risk of osteosarcomas

COMPLICATIONS

- Fractures and skeletal deformities
- Increased risk of hip and knee replacements
- Osteoarthritis
- Bone pain
- Hearing loss
- Spinal stenosis and nerve compression
- Visual loss
- Hypercalcemia possible with immobilization
- Rarely, osteosarcoma, cardiac failure, hydrocephalus, and paraplegia

REFERENCES

1. Reid IR, Miller P, Lyles K, et al. Comparison of a single infusion of zoledronic acid with risedronate for Paget's disease. *N Engl J Med* 2005;353:898–908.
2. Lim JL, Bressler NM, Marsh MJ, et al. Laser treatment of choroidal neovascularization in patients with angioid streaks. *Am J Ophthalmol* 1993;116:414–423.
3. Browning AC, Chung AK, Ghanchi R, et al. Verteporfin photodynamic therapy of choroidal neovascularization in angioid streaks. *One-year results of a prospective case series. Ophthalmology* 2005;112:1227–1231.
4. Sawa M, Fumi G, Motokazu T, et al. Long-term results of intravitreal bevacizumab injection for choroidal neovascularization secondary to angioid streaks. *Am J Ophthalmol* 2009;148:584–590.

ADDITIONAL READING

- Dabbs TR, Skjodt K. Prevalence of angioid streaks and other ocular complications of Paget's disease of bone. *Br J Ophthalmol* 1990;74:579–582.
- Ralston SH, Langston AL, Reid IR. Pathogenesis and management of Paget's disease of the bone. *Lancet* 2008;372:155–163.
- Whyte MP. Paget's disease of bone. *N Engl J Med* 2006;355:593–600.

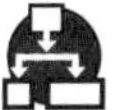

See Also (Topic, Algorithm, Electronic Media Element)

- Angioid streaks

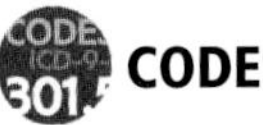

CODES

ICD9

- 363.43 Angioid streaks of choroid
- 731.0 Osteitis deformans without mention of bone tumor

CLINICAL PEARLS

- Features of Paget's disease include the following:
  - Bone pain
  - Pathological bone fractures causing cranial nerve impairment
  - Elevated SAP
  - Abnormal radiography or bone scan
- Bisphosphonates are effective therapeutic agents.

PAPILLEDEMA

Rod Foroozan

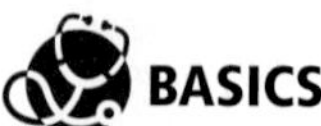

BASICS

DESCRIPTION

Papilledema is defined as optic disc swelling secondary to elevated intracranial pressure. It is typically bilateral but can be asymmetric.

ALERT

Papilledema may be caused by a life-threatening condition including meningitis, mass lesion, hydrocephalus, and cerebral venous sinus thrombosis (CVST).

Pediatric Considerations

Unlike in adults, idiopathic intracranial hypertension (IIH) occurs with equal frequency in prepubescent boys and girls.

Pregnancy Considerations

Treatment with acetazolamide during pregnancy is controversial and generally avoided during the first trimester of pregnancy. Intra-abdominal catheters and CSF diversion procedures may be limited by the growing fetus.

EPIDEMIOLOGY

Incidence

- The incidence and prevalence of all causes of papilledema are difficult to establish.
- IIH, also known as pseudotumor cerebri, is most common in women with obesity between 18 and 45 years of age.
- IIH 1–3 per 100,000 in the general population
- 20 per 100,000 in women with obesity ages 20–40 years
- The incidence of IIH is equal in prepubescent boys and girls.

RISK FACTORS

- Weight gain and obesity predispose to IIH.
- Sleep apnea may increase the risk of papilledema (IIH).
- Some medications (tetracyline, vitamin A, growth hormone) may cause elevated intracranial pressure.
- Hypercoagulability predisposes to CVST.
- Surgical procedures such as internal jugular vein ligation (CVST)

Genetics

- No clear genetic predisposition to papilledema
- Some conditions may have a genetic component (e.g., hyercoagulable disorders predisposing to CVST).
- Some familial reports of IIH

GENERAL PREVENTION

- Weight loss (IIH)
- Serial eye examinations for patients taking medications thought to predispose to elevated intracranial pressure.

PATHOPHYSIOLOGY

- Mostly a mechanical process whereby nerve fibers within the optic nerve are compressed by elevated CSF pressure in the subarachnoid space. This results in blocked axoplasmic flow. As swelling progresses vascular obstruction may occur, with dilation of the retinal venous system.

ETIOLOGY

The compartment surrounding the brain and spinal cord act as a closed system containing neural tissue, CSF, and the vascular system. Alterations in any of these three components may cause elevated intracranial pressure.

COMMONLY ASSOCIATED CONDITIONS

- IIH (most common in ophthalmic practice): The diagnostic criteria for IIH include the absence of a mass lesion on neuroimaging, elevated opening pressure on lumbar puncture, and normal CSF consistency (1)[A].
- Venous obstruction (including CVST), which may cause stroke and death
- Intracranial mass lesion
- Cerebral edema
- Meningitis
- Thickening of the skull and craniosynostosis syndromes
- Hydrocephalus
- Endocrinologic dysfunction
- Spinal cord or choroid plexus tumor (rare)

DIAGNOSIS

HISTORY

- Symptoms related to the underlying cause of papilledema: for example, headache and stiff neck in meningitis, seizures and focal deficits from mass lesion, and stroke related to venous sinus thrombosis
- Symptoms that can be related to elevated intracranial pressure include the following:
  - Headache, often positional and improves in the recumbent position and worsens with the Valsalva maneuver
  - Nausea and vomiting
  - Pulsatile or pulse-synchronous tinnitus or other auditory phenomena likely related to turbulent flow within the cerebral venous sinuses
  - Transient visual obscurations or temporary blackouts of vision lasting seconds, often related to a change in position. They are thought to occur from a transient loss of perfusion due to optic disc swelling.
  - Diplopia occurs most commonly from sixth nerve palsy, which may be unilateral or bilateral. It may also be from comitant esotropia and rarely from third or fourth nerve palsy.

PHYSICAL EXAM

- Visual acuity is generally normal in early papilledema unless there is another abnormality (e.g., choroidal folds).
- Pupils are brisk early on, as the optic neuropathy progresses they may become sluggish and, with asymmetric involvement a relative afferent pupillary defect may be present.
- Color vision is relatively preserved unless central visual function is compromised.
- Visual field defects are nerve fiber bundle type: arcuate defects and enlargement of the blind spot. As optic disc edema progresses central visual function may be lost.
- Optic disc edema is most commonly bilateral but may be asymmetric and rarely unilateral. Grading schemes (e.g., the Frisén staging system) have been proposed to provide a semiquantitative measure of the optic disc edema (2)[C]. Early changes include opacification of the retinal nerve fiber layer, loss of spontaneous venous pulsations, and loss of the normal physiologic cup. Later vascular changes occur with optic disc hemorrhages, cotton wool spots, and retinal and choroidal folds. More severe disc edema may cause retinal vascular occlusions and retinal, subhyaloid, and vitreous hemorrhage.
- Hard exudate may form within the retina in a pattern of a macular star.
- Choroidal folds, typically horizontal and within the macula may cause a reduction in visual acuity.
- Concentric folds around the optic disc (Paton's lines) may occur with optic disc swelling.
- Several changes in the appearance of the optic disc may develop over time, which are not specific for papilledema. Disc pallor occurs and a reduction in the number of optic disc hemorrhages and cotton wool spots can occur. Pseudodrusen (areas of blocked axoplasmic flow that look like optic disc drusen but are not calcium deposits) may develop. Alterations of the retinal pigment epithelium may occur around the optic disc in areas where there was prior swelling or subretinal fluid. Gliosis may develop on the surface of the optic disc. Once it is damaged the optic disc may not swell from papilledema.

DIAGNOSTIC TESTS & INTERPRETATION

Lab

Initial lab tests

- Possible higher prevalence of anemia in IIH
- Coagulopathy may exist in CVST.

Follow-up & special considerations

Can check electrolytes, particularly potassium levels, in patients treated with diuretics

Imaging

Initial approach

- Neuroimaging of the brain is vital. MRI is preferred over CT in most patients. Some recommend magnetic resonance venography (MRV) or computed tomographic venography (CTV) to exclude CVST in all patients with papilledema, particularly in those without a structural lesion who do not fit the typical demographic profile of IIH (3)[B].
- MRV and CTV may show narrowing of the cerebral venous sinuses (which may be a reflection of elevated intracranial pressure).
- Nonspecific imaging findings from elevated intracranial pressure may include an empty sella, increased T2-weighted signal consistent with increased CSF around the optic nerves, posterior bowing of the globes, and enhancement in the area of the optic nerve heads.

Follow-up & special considerations

In atypical patients with papilledema, spinal cord imaging may reveal a tumor or structural abnormality in the region of craniocervical junction.

Diagnostic Procedures/Other

- Ultrasonography (with the 30° test) may be helpful (e.g., rule out optic disc drusen).
- Lumbar puncture may be used to measure the opening pressure and assess CSF consistency.
- Intracranial pressure monitoring may be used to follow and document spikes in CSF pressure.

Pathological Findings
- Optic disc edema with axonal swelling
- Retinal nerve fiber layer thinning

DIFFERENTIAL DIAGNOSIS
- Hypertensive retinopathy
- Optic disc drusen
- Congenitally anomalous optic discs
- Optic disc edema from other causes including ischemic optic neuropathy, inflammatory optic neuropathy (particularly neuroretinitis), and compressive optic neuropathy

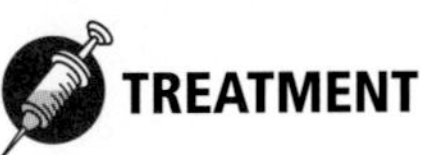

TREATMENT

MEDICATION
First Line
- Acetazolamide
- Corticosteroids to decrease brain edema in patients with mass lesions or cerebral edema
- Corticosteroids have also been used in IIH.
- Anticoagulants for CVST

Second Line
- Furosemide and other diuretics
- Topiramate, both for the headache and to help with appetite suppression in patients with IIH

ADDITIONAL TREATMENT
General Measures
Weight loss for patients with IIH

Issues for Referral
- Neurosurgery for mass lesions and CSF diversion procedures (4)[B]
- Consider hematologic consultation for coagulation disorders in patients with CVST
- Endocrinologic evaluation in some patients (e.g., polycystic ovarian syndrome)

Additional Therapies
- Gastric bypass surgery and ensuing weight loss can lead to an improvement of papilledema in patients with IIH (5)[C].
- Repeated lumbar punctures can be performed as a temporizing measure to lower CSF pressure (e.g., during pregnancy) in patients with IIH.

SURGERY/OTHER PROCEDURES
- Neurosurgery for mass lesions and CSF diversion procedures such as ventriculostomy
- Ventriculoperitoneal and lumboperitoneal shunting
- Surgical intervention is often undertaken after a trial of medical therapy in IIH.
- Optic nerve sheath fenestration, particularly in patients with progressive visual loss despite medical therapy, more marked visual loss, and those without headache as a predominant symptom

IN-PATIENT CONSIDERATIONS
Initial Stabilization
Depending on the cause of papilledema some patients may require hospitalization (e.g., for intravenous antibiotics in meningitis or hydrocephalus with impending brain herniation)

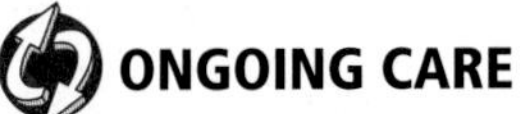

ONGOING CARE

FOLLOW-UP RECOMMENDATIONS
Depending on degree of optic disc edema, visual deficit, and choice of treatment

Patient Monitoring
- Serial eye examinations with visual field assessment should be considered.
- Depending on the cause of papilledema, patients may need to follow with other specialists including neurosurgeons to monitor tumors or shunts, and neurologists to treat headache.

DIET
- Weight loss (often 10–20% of body weight) can cause resolution of optic disc edema in IIH.
- Current clinical trials to determine the efficacy of acetazolamide versus weight loss in IIH.

PATIENT EDUCATION
- Patients should be instructed to return for examination if they develop progressive symptoms including visual loss, headaches, and diplopia.
- Recurrent or progressive papilledema (depending on the etiology) may represent:
  - Tumor growth
  - Recurrent or progressive CVST
  - Progressive optic disc edema from IIH
  - Worsening hydrocephalus

PROGNOSIS
Systemically depends on the cause of the papilledema. Visual outcome depends on the degree of optic disc edema and visual loss at the onset of treatment. Excellent visual prognosis for patients with mild optic disc edema.

COMPLICATIONS
- Fixed visual loss
- Chronic headaches
- Allergic reactions or side effects to medication (particular acetazolamide)
- Complications related to lumbar puncture (bleeding, infection, postspinal headache)
- Complications related to shunts (infection, catheter migration, failure necessitating revision)
- Complications from optic nerve sheath fenestration, including visual loss and diplopia

REFERENCES

1. Friedman DI, Jacobson DM. Diagnostic criteria for idiopathic intracranial hypertension. *Neurology* 2002;59:1492–1495.
2. Scott CJ, Kardon RH, Lee AG, et al. Diagnosis and grading of papilledema in patients with raised intracranial pressure using optical coherence tomography vs clinical expert assessment using a clinical staging scale. *Arch Ophthalmol* 2010;128: 705–711.
3. Lin A, Foroozan R, Danesh-Meyer HV, et al. Occurrence of cerebral venous sinus thrombosis in patients with presumed idiopathic intracranial hypertension. *Ophthalmology* 2006;113: 2281–2284.
4. Binder DK, Horton JC, Lawton MT, et al. Idiopathic intracranial hypertension. *Neurosurgery* 2004;54: 538–551.
5. Fridley J, Foroozan R, Sherman V, et al. Bariatric surgery for the treatment of idiopathic intracranial hypertension. *J Neurosurg* 2010;114(1):34–39.

ADDITIONAL READING

- Foroozan R, Kline LB. *Chapter 3 papilledema. Optic nerve disorders*, 2nd ed. In: Kline LB, Foroozan R, eds. New York, New York: Oxford University Press, 2007:41–64.
- Friedman DI. *Papilledema in Walsh & Hoyt's clinical neuro-ophthalmology*, 6th ed. In: Miller NR, Newman NJ, eds. Philadelphia PA: Lippincott Williams & Wilkins, 2005:237–291.

CODES

ICD9
- 377.00 Papilledema, unspecified
- 377.01 Papilledema associated with increased intracranial pressure

CLINICAL PEARLS

- Papilledema is optic disc edema secondary to elevated intracranial pressure.
- Papilledema may be a marker of a potentially life-threatening disorder including an intracranial mass lesion, hydrocephalus, meningitis, or CVST.
- IIH is the most common cause of papilledema in an ophthalmic practice.

PAPILLEDEMA IN CHILDREN

Robert A. King

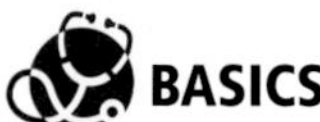

BASICS

DESCRIPTION

Papilledema is bilateral optic nerve swelling from elevated intracranial pressure (ICP).

EPIDEMIOLOGY

Incidence

Related to incidence of underlying cause of raised ICP. In young infants with open sutures, papilledema may not occur.

Prevalence

Unknown

RISK FACTORS

- Hydrocephalus with or without shunting
- Head trauma
- Premature infants with grade 3 or 4 intraventricular hemorrhage
- For pseudotumor cerebri: certain medications (in particular systemic retinoids, steroid withdrawal, growth hormone, tetracycline) and systemic disorders (e.g., Down syndrome, obesity)
- Craniosynostosis syndromes
- Brain tumor

Genetics

No known genetic predisposition

Pediatric Considerations

- Examination may be difficult, so it is imperative to identify those children who may be at risk of having papilledema.
- Papilledema may be absent even in the presence of markedly raised ICP in infants with open sutures or in shaken baby syndrome.

GENERAL PREVENTION

Early recognition and treatment of increased ICP

PATHOPHYSIOLOGY

- Increased ICP is transmitted to the optic nerve causing reduced axoplasmic flow initially causing papilledema and ultimately leading to optic atrophy.
  - Brain tumors, especially infratentorial tumors, cause obstruction of normal intraventricular flow of cerebral spinal fluid (obstructive hydrocephalus).
  - Idiopathic intracranial hypertension (IIH) (pseudotumor cerebri), either primary or secondary, leading to decreased absorption of CSF and subsequent ICP elevation

ETIOLOGY

- Elevated ICP from any cause
- IIH can be either primary or secondary.

COMMONLY ASSOCIATED CONDITIONS

See Risk Factors

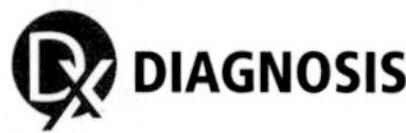

DIAGNOSIS

HISTORY

- Headache; especially those associated with awakening from sleep or awakening in the morning. Headache in a patient with a known cause for high ICP such as hydrocephalus or a teenager taking retinoids for acne is an ominous sign.
  - Transient vision blurring (visual obscuration) lasting for a few seconds occurring several times per day
  - Nausea and vomiting
  - Infants and preverbal children may present with listlessness, irritability, and somnolence

PHYSICAL EXAM

- Normal visual acuity early. Pupils usually normal. Cranial nerves can be affected, especially sixth nerve palsy. When visual acuity is affected, it can be lost quickly. Later or with recurrences (as in shunt malfunctions) vision can be further reduced. Color vision may be affected before visual acuity falls.
- Swollen optic nerve with engorged veins on the optic nerve surface
- Nerve fiber layer edema blurring the disc margin and covering blood vessels
- Peripapillary and disc hemorrhages
- Loss of spontaneous venous pulsations. Venous pulsations are an important observation. When present they indicate normal ICP. When absent they are of no value unless they were present on a prior examination.

DIAGNOSTIC TESTS & INTERPRETATION

Lab

- Lumbar puncture for opening pressure, cells, and protein. Normal opening pressure less than 180 mm Hg CBC count might detect anemia or leukemia.
  - Urinalysis for diabetes insipidus

Imaging

Initial approach

- MRI (preferred) or computerized axial tomography (CAT) scan to rule out intracranial mass and diagnose enlarged ventricles or small ventricles in cerebral edema/pseudotumor
- Optic nerve ultrasound can document swollen nerve sheath and help in diagnosing drusen of the optic nerve head (main cause of pseudopapilledema).

Follow-up & special considerations

- Papilledema may take 4–6 weeks to resolve after ICP normalized.
- Optic atrophy can occur in long term. Follow patients for visual acuity, afferent pupillary defect, and color vision.

Diagnostic Procedures/Other

Visual field may show early defects near or adjacent to the blind spot or enlarged blind spot.

DIFFERENTIAL DIAGNOSIS

- Optic nerve head drusen
- Hyperopic disc
- Optic neuritis in children presents with asymmetric and/or severe vision loss and asymmetric optic nerve swelling. The vision loss is a key difference in presentation of papilledema versus optic neuritis.
- Papillitis (Epstein–Barr virus [EBV] infection, vasculitis, uveitis). Associated with vision loss.

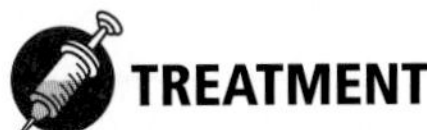

TREATMENT

Determined mostly by the cause of the papilledema. No specific treatment of optic nerve involvement

MEDICATION

- Ventriculoperitoneal shunt for obstructive hydrocephalus or lumboperitoneal shunt is used primarily in IIH.
  - Optic nerve sheath fenestration is used as first line at many centers for IIH.
- Medications also may be used as first-line treatment in IIH. Acetazolamide (Diamox) (10–15 mg/kg divided q.i.d.) and/or prednisone 1 mg/kg and/or diuretic (e.g., furosemide)
  - Repeat lumbar punctures to remove a volume of CSF. Useful in IIH both primary and secondary. Can be curative.
  - Cessation of medication causing IIH might be the primary treatment, for example, in a teenager being treated with retinoids for acne.

ADDITIONAL TREATMENT

Issues for Referral

Headaches with questionable optic nerve exam, especially those accompanied by visual obscuration or reduction in visual acuity, should be seen by ophthalmologist.

IN-PATIENT CONSIDERATIONS

Initial Stabilization

Hospitalization is done as needed by neurosurgery, neurology, or neuro-oncology.

Discharge Criteria

- Follow-up with ophthalmology usually within a few weeks following surgical procedure with shunting or tumor treatment, sooner if vision loss has already occurred.
  - Follow-up sooner and ongoing if cerebral edema is being treated with systemic steroids and tapering or withdrawal is initiated.

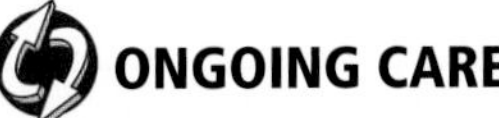

ONGOING CARE

FOLLOW-UP RECOMMENDATIONS

Patients with shunts should have eye exams periodically to document stability of optic nerve appearance and function.

Patient Monitoring

- Visual fields are useful to monitor stability of the optic nerve. Good computerized visual fields are difficult until the child is 8 or 9 years old.
  - Ophthalmic exam should be done periodically. The follow-up ophthalmic exam (along with the visual field) is a front line defense for detecting occult shunt malfunction or early recurrent asymptomatic increased ICP.

DIET

- For IIH in obese children dietary restriction is indicated.
- Vitamin A toxicity may cause IIH.

PATIENT EDUCATION

- Recognizing signs of shunt malfunction
  - Recognizing the need for routine ophthalmology follow-up in patients with shunts including need for yearly visual fields and funduscopic evaluation of optic nerve.

PROGNOSIS

- With normalization of ICP, the prognosis for vision is good.
  - Recurrence of elevated pressure with shunt malfunction could cause vision loss from optic atrophy.

COMPLICATIONS

Recurrence as a result of shunt malfunction or recurrence of any underlying cause of increased ICP is an uncontrolled cause of IIH.

REFERENCES

1. Brodsky M. The swollen optic disc in childhood. In: Brodsky M, ed. *Pediatric neuro-ophthalmology*. Springer, 2010.
2. Taylor D. Optic disc swelling in children. In: Hoyt CS, Taylor D, eds. *Pediatric ophthalmology and strabismus*. Elsevier Saunders, 2005.
3. Sergott RC, Hug D. Pediatric ophthalmology. In: Nelson LB, Olitsky SE, eds. *Harley's pediatric ophthalmology*. Lippincott Williams & Wilkins, 2005.

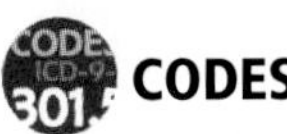

CODES

ICD9

- 377.00 Papilledema, unspecified
- 377.01 Papilledema associated with increased intracranial pressure

CLINICAL PEARLS

- Babies with open fontanelles can develop papilledema but may not.
- Initial evaluation of child with shaken baby syndrome may initially have no optic nerve swelling, which can then develop a few days later when cerebral edema worsens.
- Once an optic nerve develops atrophy, swelling is difficult to detect.

PATTERN DYSTROPHY

John O. Mason, III
Thomas A. Finley

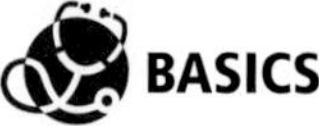

BASICS

DESCRIPTION

- Group of disorders related to macular pigment depositions in the retinal pigment epithelium (RPE) that are usually inherited in an autosomal dominant fashion
- Commonly manifest in the second and third decades of life
- Often found in asymptomatic patients on routine eye exam
- Affected patients may remain asymptomatic until mid- or late-adulthood with presenting symptoms of slightly diminished visual acuity or metamorphopsia.
- Slowly progressive loss of central vision
- Dystrophies may be subdivided into several patterns based on clinical appearance, including the following:
  - Butterfly dystrophy
  - Reticular dystrophy
  - Adult-onset foveomacular vitelliform dystrophy
  - Fundus pulverulentus
  - Multifocal pattern dystrophy simulating fundus flavimaculatus
- Clinical appearance is variable, may progress to another pattern with time, or even display different patterns between the two eyes of a single patient.

EPIDEMIOLOGY

Incidence

- Unknown due to phenotypic variability
  - Males and females affected equally

Prevalence

Unknown due to phenotypic variability

RISK FACTORS

Genetics

- Typically inherited in an autosomal dominant fashion
- Most common genetic association is due to mutations in the RDS/peripherin gene located on the short arm of chromosome 6.
- RDS/peripherin gene codes for a surface glycoprotein expressed in the outer segments of rods and cones.
- More than 90 mutations of the gene are known to exist, resulting in great phenotypic variability.

GENERAL PREVENTION

Genetic counseling

PATHOPHYSIOLOGY

- Various patterns of pigment deposition occur at the level of the retinal pigment epithelium (RPE) in the macula.
- Slow progressive atrophy of the RPE and overlying photoreceptors
- May develop choroidal neovascularization

ETIOLOGY

- The different subdivisions of pattern dystrophy are phenotypic variations of the many mutations that may occur within the RDS/peripherin gene.

COMMONLY ASSOCIATED CONDITIONS

- Most cases are not associated with systemic illness.
- Maternally inherited diabetes and deafness (MIDD) and mitochondrial myopathy, encephalopathy, lactic acidosis, and stroke-like episodes (MELAS) are frequently associated with pattern dystrophy.

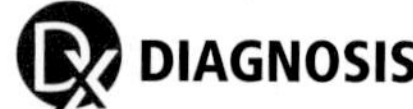

DIAGNOSIS

HISTORY

May be asymptomatic or have complaints of slight decrease in vision or metamorphopsia

PHYSICAL EXAM

- Gray, yellow, or orange pigment accumulations at the level of the RPE in the macula
- Usually symmetric but can show different pigment patterns

DIAGNOSTIC TESTS & INTERPRETATION

Diagnostic Procedures/Other

- Visual fields: normal
- Color vision: normal until late in disease process
- Dark adaptation: normal
- Fluorescein angiography: Hypofluorescence due to pigment figure blocking. Hyperfluorescence due to RPE atrophy associated window defects
- Electroretinogram (ERG): normal
- Electrooculogram (EOG): may show decreased response
- Fundus autofluorescence: fundus may show increased autofluorescence in areas of accumulated lipofuscin, however, may show decreased levels once atrophy of the RPE and overlying photoreceptors develops (1)[C]

Pathological Findings

- Destruction of the RPE and overlying photoreceptor layer with accumulation of lipofuscin within the RPE (2)[C]

DIFFERENTIAL DIAGNOSIS

- Stargardt's disease
- Age-related macular degeneration
- Dominant drusen
- Cone dystrophy
- Benign concentric annular macular dystrophy
- Medication toxicity

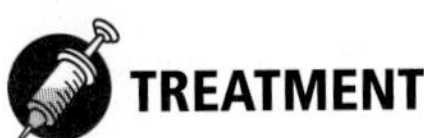

TREATMENT

MEDICATION

No treatment available for Pattern dystrophy (PD)

ADDITIONAL TREATMENT

General Measures

Secondary choroidal neovascular membrane (CNVM) may be treated with photodynamic therapy (PDT) (3)[C] versus vascular endothelial growth factor inhibitors (anti-VEGF) (4)[C] with variable visual results

Issues for Referral

Development of choroidal neovascularization

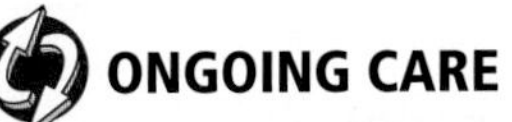

ONGOING CARE

FOLLOW-UP RECOMMENDATIONS

- Annual examination by ophthalmologist
- Low vision evaluation

PATIENT EDUCATION

http://www.nei.nih.gov/resources/eyegene.asp

PROGNOSIS

- Good prognosis for retaining useful vision throughout life
- Most patients retain reading vision in at least one eye through late adulthood.

COMPLICATIONS

- Central visual loss
- Choroidal neovascularization

REFERENCES

1. Schmitz-Valckenberg S, Holz FG, Bird AC, et al. Fundus autofluorescence imaging: review and perspectives. *Retina* 2008;28(3):385–409.
2. Zhang K, Garibaldi DC, Li Y, et al. Butterfly-shaped pattern dystrophy: a genetic, clinical, and histopathological report. *Arch Ophthalmol* 2002; 120(4):485–490.
3. Parodi M, Liberali T, Pedio M, et al. Photodynamic therapy of subfoveal choroidal neovascularization secondary to reticular pattern dystrophy: Three-year results of an uncontrolled, prospective case series. *Am J Ophthalmol* 2006;141(6):1152–1154.
4. Parodi M, Iacono P, Cascavilla M, et al. Intravitreal bevacizumab for subfoveal choroidal neovascularization associated with pattern dystrophy. *Invest Ophthalmol Vis Sci* 2010;51(9): 4358–4361.

ADDITIONAL READING

- Gass J, Donald M. *Stereoscopic atlas of macular diseases: diagnosis and treatment*, Vol. 1, 4th ed. St. Louis, MO: CV Mosby, 1997:1.

CODES

ICD9

362.76 Dystrophies primarily involving the retinal pigment epithelium

CLINICAL PEARLS

- Most commonly an autosomal dominant condition
- Variable pigment deposition at the level of the RPE in the macula
- Slowly progressive loss of central vision
- Monitor for development of CNVM

PEDIATRIC OPTIC NERVE HYPOPLASIA

Jonathan H. Salvin

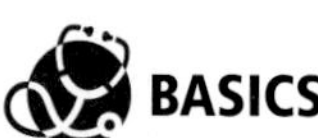

BASICS

DESCRIPTION

- Optic nerve hypoplasia (ONH) is a congenital optic nerve disorder in which the optic nerve is smaller than normal, typically with decreased function.
  - May be unilateral or bilateral
  - Often associated with other CNS, in particular, midline defects (septo-optic dysplasia [SOD], de Morsier's syndrome)

EPIDEMIOLOGY

Incidence

SOD: 2–10 per 100,000 births (1,2)[C]

Prevalence

ONH: 6.3 per 100,000 children (3)[C]

RISK FACTORS

- Fetal alcohol syndrome (4)[C]
  - Maternal drug use (psychopharmaceutical drugs, some anticonvulsants, quinine LSD, and phencyclidine reported)
  - Possibly younger maternal age (5)[C]
  - Premature/postmature birth
  - Infants of diabetic mothers may have hemihypoplasia of the optic nerve.

Genetics

- Most cases sporadic
  - Mutation in *HESX1* (*3p21.1*) identified in SOD, autosomal dominant
  - Duplications of *SOX3* identified in SOD
  - There are numerous ocular (e.g., aniridia) and systemic genetic syndromes (e.g., oculocutaneous albinism) as well as intrauterine infections, which may have ONH as a feature.

GENERAL PREVENTION

- Maternal prenatal care
- Genetic counseling

PATHOPHYSIOLOGY

- Reduced optic nerve fibers
- Poorly understood; possibly related to failed differentiation of retinal ganglion cells or excessive axonal regression during normal optic nerve development

ETIOLOGY

Unknown

COMMONLY ASSOCIATED CONDITIONS

- Decreased visual acuity (ranging to light perception)
- SOD (de Morsier syndrome) (MIM #182230): ONH associated with midline brain defects including absent septum pellucidum, agenesis of corpus callosum, and hypothalamic and pituitary dysfunction. May also have cortical migration defects (e.g., cortical ectopia, pachygyria). Classic de Morsier's syndrome associated with abnormal facies, macrocrania, and large open anterior fontanelle
- Endocrinopathies including hyperprolactinemia, hypothyroidism, adrenal insufficiency, diabetes insipidus, growth hormone deficiency

DIAGNOSIS

HISTORY

- History of poor visual behavior in one or both eyes since birth with/without nystagmus
  - Prenatal history of maternal alcohol/drug use
  - Poor infant growth, neonatal jaundice, hypoglycemia, or seizures suggesting pituitary axis dysfunction

PHYSICAL EXAM

- Complete eye exam with indirect ophthalmoscopy to evaluate optic nerve appearance. May have the appearance of the "double ring sign": a yellow–white ring around the small disc representing the scleral canal that is unfilled due to reduction in optic nerve size
- Increased distance between fovea and temporal optic nerve edge
- May have immature vascular pattern of arcades
- May have foveal hypoplasia
- Nystagmus or strabismus in affected eye(s) may be present.
- May have associated microphthalmia
- Loss of percentiles on growth chart
- May have microcephaly, large anterior fontanel (de Morsier), seizures, developmental delay
- Majority of children, especially with unilateral ONH, will be systemically well, developmentally normal, and with no brain or pituitary involvement.

DIAGNOSTIC TESTS & INTERPRETATION

Lab

Initial lab tests

If abnormal neuroimaging of pituitary or evidence of hormonal signs: thyroid functions (TSH, T3, T4), even if neonatal screen was normal, other serum hormonal screening per endocrinology

Follow-up & special considerations

- Endocrinology evaluation as indicated
- Follow growth charts

Imaging

Initial approach

- MRI of brain and orbits to evaluate intracranial optic nerves and for midline CNS defects (5)[C], cortical migration defects, and pituitary abnormalities including absent pituitary stalk, or ectopic bright spot (displacement of the posterior pituitary up into area of pituitary stalk
- Neuroimaging is an imprecise way of determining optic nerve size or function.

Follow-up & special considerations

Follow development and neurologic signs

Diagnostic Procedures/Other

Referral to endocrinology and neurology as indicated

Pathological Findings

Reduced optic nerve fibers, reduced retinal ganglion cell count, normal outer retinal layers (2)

DIFFERENTIAL DIAGNOSIS

- Optic atrophy
  - High hypermetropia
  - Tilted optic nerve
  - Optic nerve coloboma
  - Peripapillary staphyloma/atrophy

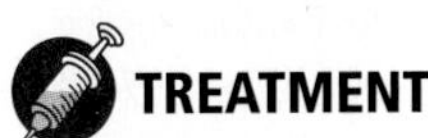

TREATMENT

MEDICATION

Hormonal replacement therapy if needed

ADDITIONAL TREATMENT

General Measures

- Amblyopia treatment especially if asymmetric bilateral or unilateral
- Low vision aids and support
  - Strabismus correction
  - Refractive correction if indicated
  - Protective eyewear if unilateral poor vision

Issues for Referral

- Endocrinology referral for pituitary dysfunction
- Neurology referral if neurologic signs
- Developmental assessment
- Genetics consultation

COMPLEMENTARY & ALTERNATIVE THERAPIES

- None
- NOTE: there is currently no scientific evidence to support the use of stem cell treatment for this disorder.

SURGERY/OTHER PROCEDURES

Strabismus or nystagmus surgery as indicated

IN-PATIENT CONSIDERATIONS

Admission Criteria

Admission rarely indicated but sudden death and severe pituitary dysfunction may occur.

ONGOING CARE

FOLLOW-UP RECOMMENDATIONS

- Ongoing ophthalmologic follow-up for visual evaluation, refractive correction, amblyopia therapy
  - Low vision evaluation as indicated
  - Endocrinology, neurology, and developmental follow-up

PATIENT EDUCATION

- Focus Families: ONH/SOD Information, Education and Support: http://www.focusfamilies.org/

PROGNOSIS

- Visual prognosis variable depending on optic nerve function.
  - Prognosis poorly correlated with optic nerve appearance on physical exam or neuroimaging

COMPLICATIONS

- Potentially significantly decreased visual acuity in affected eye(s)
  - Pituitary axis dysfunction
  - Neurologic sequelae including seizures and developmental delay

REFERENCES

1. Kelberman D, Dattani MT. Genetics of septo-optic dysplasia. *Pituitary* 2007;10:393–407.
2. Patel L, McNally R, Harrison E, et al. Geographical distribution of optic nerve hypoplasia and septo-optic dysplasia in Northwest England. *J Pediatrics* 2006;148:85–88.
3. Ahmad T, Garcia-Filion P, Borchert M, et al. Endocrinological and auxological abnormalities in young children with optic nerve hypoplasia: a prospective study. *J Pediatr* 2006;148:78–84.
4. Zeki S, Dutton G. Optic nerve hypoplasia in children. *Br J Ophthalmol* 1990;74:300–304.
5. Hellstrom A, Wiklund L, Svensson E. The clinical and morphologic spectrum of optic nerve hypoplasia. *J AAPOS* 1999;3:212–220.
6. Brodsky M, Glasier C. Optic nerve hypoplasia: clinical significance of associated central nervous system abnormalities on magnetic resonance imaging. *Arch Ophthalmol* 1993;111:66–74.

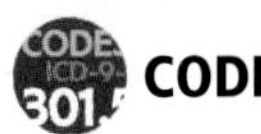

CODES

ICD9

377.43 Optic nerve hypoplasia

CLINICAL PEARLS

- Visual prognosis is variable and cannot be predicted on basis of clinical exam or neuroimaging. Amblyopia therapy should be attempted as this may offer some improvement.
- Prompt referral to endocrinology if clinical or neuroimaging signs of pituitary dysfunction
- Prompt MRI of brain indicated to evaluate for other CNS abnormalities especially in bilateral cases
- Practice patterns vary regarding neuroimaging in unilateral ONH.

PEDICULOSIS

Olga A. Shif
Julie Rosenthal

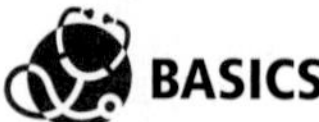

BASICS

DESCRIPTION

- A rare condition associated with infestation of eyelashes and eyebrows by *Phthirus pubis* (crab louse)
- Manifests as irritation and pruritus of eyelid margins
- *P. pubis* is typically transmitted by sexual intercourse with an infested individual or by the transfer of the organism from genital area to the eye by hand, clothing, and bedding.
- System(s) affected: skin/exocrine
- Synonym(s): Pediculosis ciliaris; Pediculosis pubis; Phthiriasis palpebrarum; pubic lice; crabs.

Pediatric Considerations

In children, pediculosis may be an indication of sexual abuse and involvement of social services and/or child protection agency is imperative.

EPIDEMIOLOGY

- Adolescents > Adults > Children
- Male = Female
  - Men tend to have a more extensive infestation due to a greater distribution of body hair.
- Blacks = Whites

Incidence

Estimated 3 million new cases annually in the US.

Prevalence

Approximately 2% of the world population

RISK FACTORS

- Sexual activity, especially in adolescents
- Multiple sexual partners
- Sexual contact with infested individuals or contact with their clothes, towels, and bedding
- Crowded conditions
- Poor personal hygiene

Genetics

No genetic pattern

GENERAL PREVENTION

- Avoidance of sexual contact with infested individuals and their personal items
- Safe sexual practices
- Maintenance of good personal hygiene

PATHOPHYSIOLOGY

- Pubic lice are ectoparasites that feed on human blood by piercing the skin and injecting their saliva.
- Symptoms are a result of a hypersensitivity reaction to louse saliva.

ETIOLOGY

- Infestation with *P. pubis* (pubic louse/crab)
- Rounded, stubby, translucent parasite with 4 of its 6 legs terminating in prominent crab-like claws
- Size 0.8–1.2 mm
- Life cycle = 14 days
- Female louse lays as many as 26 ova
- Nit (louse egg) incubation period = 7 days
- Nymphs (young lice) mature over 14 days.

COMMONLY ASSOCIATED CONDITIONS

- Blepharoconjunctivitis
- Toxic follicular conjunctivitis
- Itching of the skin may lead to secondary bacterial infection.
- 1/3 of individuals may have a concomitant sexually transmitted infection.

DIAGNOSIS

HISTORY

- Complaints of severe itching and burning of the lids, especially at night
- Presence of eye irritation or conjunctival injection
- Itching in and around the pubic area or other areas heavily covered with body hair (1)[C], (2)[C]

PHYSICAL EXAM

- External examination of periorbital region at a slit lamp can demonstrate lice and nits on lids, lashes, and brows unilaterally or bilaterally.
  - Lice: 1–2 mm brownish-gray specks, embedded in eyelid skin
  - Nits: tiny white-gray specks, attached to the lashes or brow hair
- Evidence of follicular conjunctivitis
- Serous crusting and blood-tinged debris may be present on the lids.
- Eyelid edema suggests a severe infestation.
- Skin lesions:
  - Painless blue-gray macules (maculae ceruleae) may be apparent on eyelids and cheeks. These are thought to be breakdown products of heme affected by louse saliva.
  - Small erythematous papules (papular urticaria) are found at feeding sites.
- Enlargement of preauricular and submental nodes may be present on exam (3)[C].

DIAGNOSTIC TESTS & INTERPRETATION

Diagnostic Procedures/Other

Examination of a louse under light microscopy can help confirm identity of the organism if necessary.

P

DIFFERENTIAL DIAGNOSIS
- Seborrheic blepharitis
- Allergic blepharitis
- Herpes simplex blepharitis
- Keratoconjunctivitis sicca
- Demodex folliculorum
- Eyelid malignancies
- Eczema
- Rosacea
- Viral conjunctivitis

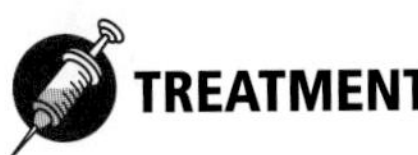

TREATMENT

Mechanical removal of lice and nits

MEDICATION
First Line
- A bland ophthalmic ointment, such as erythromycin, applied to lids and lashes twice daily for 10 days.
- Permethrin 1% cream rinse or pyrethrin with piperonyl butoxide shampoo/mousse
  - Applied to the affected nonocular area and washed off after 10 min (4)[A]

Second Line
- Malathion 0.5% lotion
  - Applied to the nonocular affected area and washed off after 8–12 h (4)[A]
- Lindane 1% shampoo
  - Applied to the nonocular affected area and washed off after 4 min (4)[A]

ADDITIONAL TREATMENT
General Measures
- Bedding and clothing must be decontaminated or kept away from body contact for at least 72 h.
  - Machine wash with water at least 55°
  - Dryer on hot cycle at least 5–10 min

Issues for Referral
- All patients should undergo thorough examination of genital area, even if no symptoms are present.
- Up to 30% of individuals with pediculosis pubis have at least 1 other sexually transmitted infection.
  - Additional testing is highly recommended.

Additional Therapies
- Oral ivermectin should be considered with resistant infestation.
  - 250 μg/kg orally, repeated in 2 weeks (5)[C]

Pregnancy Considerations
Lindane and ivermectin should not be used by pregnant or lactating women due to small possibility of toxicity and side effects (4)[A].

ONGOING CARE

FOLLOW-UP RECOMMENDATIONS
Patients with pubic lice are recommended to notify their sexual partners who also require treatment.

PATIENT MONITORING
Patients should be reexamined for presence of lice/nits after 1 week of treatment.

PATIENT EDUCATION
- Patients should be advised to avoid close bodily contact with others until they and their partners have been fully treated.
- Condoms do not prevent transmission.

PROGNOSIS
- Re-treatment may be necessary if lice or nits are present at follow-up examination.
- Patients who do not respond to initial treatment should be provided with an alternative.

COMPLICATIONS
Secondary bacterial infections

REFERENCES

1. Ngai JW, Yuen HK, Li FC. An unusual case of eye itchiness. *Hong Kong Med J* 2008;14(5):414–415.
2. Turgut B, Kurt J, Catak O, et al. Phthiriasis palpebrarum mimicking lid eczema and blepharitis. *J Ophthalmol* 2009;2009:803951.
3. Thappa DM, Karthikeyan K, Jeevankumar B. Phthiriasis palpebrarum. *Postgrad Med J* 2003;79(928):102.
4. Leone PA. Scabies and pediculosis pubis: An update of treatment regimens and general review. *Clin Infect Dis* 2007;44:S153–S159.
5. Burkhart CG, Burkhart CN. Oral ivermectin for *Phthirus pubis*. *J Am Acad Dermatol* 2004;51(6):1037; author reply 1037–1038.

ADDITIONAL READING

- Centers for Disease Control and Prevention. http://www.cdc.gov
- National Institute of Allergy and Infectious Diseases. http://www.niaid.nih.gov

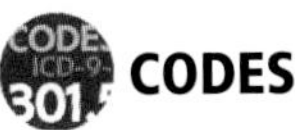

CODES

ICD9
- 132.2 *Phthirus pubis* (pubic louse)
- 372.20 Blepharoconjunctivitis, unspecified
- 372.39 Other conjunctivitis

CLINICAL PEARLS

- Patients with unilateral or persistent blepharitis should be examined closely for nits/lice.
  - If found, further examination is warranted.
- If pediculosis pubis is present in children, appropriate authorities must be alerted, as this may be a harbinger of sexual abuse.
- All partners should undergo concurrent treatment.

PERIOCULAR CAPILLARY HEMANGIOMA

Emily A. DeCarlo
Katherine A. Lane
Christopher B. Chambers

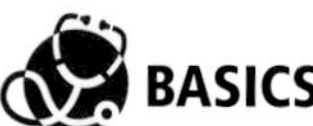

BASICS

DESCRIPTION

- Infantile hemangioma (IH) preferred term
- Benign, high flow, vascular hamartoma
- Classified as superficial or deep
- Superficial lesions present as pink, compressible, circumscribed lesions with cutaneous epithelial involvement.
- Deep lesions involve the subcutaneous tissue and orbit with little epithelial involvement. They are darker purple and can cause proptosis.
- Synonyms: Strawberry hemangioma, strawberry nevus, hemangioblastic hemangioma, benign hemangioendothelioma

Pediatric Considerations

- Concern in children for development of amblyopia secondary to strabismus, ptosis, induced astigmatism
- Evaluate for associated systemic disorders such as Kasabach–Merritt and PHACES.

Pregnancy Considerations

Some believe that capillary hemangiomas (CHs) could represent placental "metastasis."

EPIDEMIOLOGY

Incidence

- The most common benign tumor in pediatric population affect up to 2% of all infants.
  - F:M ratio 3:1–2
  - Multiple gestations and preterm infants have a higher rate (25%) of cutaneous IH (1)[C].
  - Incidence of periocular CH is approximately 1/10 that of systemic IH.
  - 60% occur in the head/neck area and 20% have >1 IH.
  - Account for 5.6% of all pediatric orbital tumors
  - Haik et al. (2)[C] reported a case series of 101 periorbital CHs: 33% had isolated skin lesions, 7% had isolated orbital lesions, the remaining 60% had a combination of both superficial and deep components.

Prevalence

1.1–2.6% of all newborns

RISK FACTORS

- Prematurity
- Multiple gestation
- Advanced maternal age of greater than 30 years
- Low birthweight
- Maternal chorionic villus sampling or amniocentesis

Genetics

- Usually sporadic
- Rarely, heritable infantile CHs have been described.

GENERAL PREVENTION

There are no preventative measures.

PATHOPHYSIOLOGY

- Hamartomatous proliferations of vascular endothelial cells
- Demonstrate a distinct proliferative phase characterized by actively dividing and multiplying endothelial cells, followed by slow involution.

ETIOLOGY

- Unknown, although several theories exist:
  - Placenta-to-embryo embolization
  - Sequestrations of persistent omnipotent angioblasts
  - Abnormal angiogenesis with imbalance angiogenesis and angiostatic factors

COMMONLY ASSOCIATED CONDITIONS

- Subglottic, paratracheal, oral, and nasal IH may coexist with orbital lesions.
  - Potential for respiratory distress, asphyxiation
- Amblyopia secondary to induced astigmatism, anisometropia, strabismus, and occlusion (up to 64%)
- Strabismus is seen in 33% of patients.
- Cutaneous changes after involution: dilated capillaries, skin thinning and pigmentation, residual mass
- **PHACES** syndrome; acronym for **P**osterior fossa brain malformations, **H**emangiomas, **A**rterial cerebrovascular anomalies, **C**ardiovascular anomalies, **E**ye anomalies, **S**ternal defects, or **S**upraumbilical abdominal raphe
  - 20% of infants with large cervicofacial hemangiomas have another associated anomaly in the PHACES syndrome.
  - Eye anomalies in 16% of patients with PHACES (microphthalmos, Horner syndrome, retinal vascular abnormality, optic nerve atrophy, iris hypoplasia, congenital cataracts, sclerocornea, lens coloboma, exophthalmos, strabismus, choroidal hemangioma, congenital 3rd nerve palsy, morning glory deformity, peripapillary staphyloma, and glaucoma)
- **Kasabach–Merritt**, that is, hemangioma thrombocytopenia syndrome
  - Large tumors sequester platelets and consume coagulation factors causing thrombocytopenia
  - Lethal in 10–37% of cases
  - Treatment includes fresh frozen plasma transfusion, supportive care, and lesion resection
- High-output cardiac failure
  - Associated with large visceral IH with abnormal arteriovenous shunts

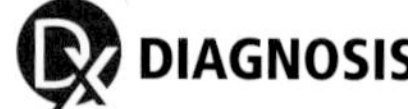

DIAGNOSIS

HISTORY

- 2% of IHs are present at birth; the majority become evident in the first few postnatal weeks.
- Typically described by the parents as a small pink scratch that enlarges and may become a protruding mass
  - This differs from a port-wine stain in Sturge–Weber syndrome, which is present at birth, occurs in the V1 distribution, and does not typically produce mass effect and does not blanch with applied pressure.
- Lesion undergoes rapid expansion after birth, continued expansion up to the first year of life and then begins to involute.
  - Usually the quickly expanding lesions will involute more rapidly than its slower growing counterpart
  - Most show early partial involution by 6–10 months
  - Timing of involution:
    - 30% involute by age 2 years
    - 60% involute by age 4 years
    - 76% involute by age 7 years

PHYSICAL EXAM

- Superficial IHs display classic strawberry red pigmentation that blanch with pressure.
- Deep hemangiomas may have a bluish hue.
- Lesions are soft and compressible.
- May expand when head is held in a dependent position, with crying, or Valsalva
- IH often present at multiple levels.

DIAGNOSTIC TESTS & INTERPRETATION

Imaging

- Gadolinium-enhanced MRI demonstrates extent of orbital lesions.
- Black serpiginous signal voids on T1- and T2-weighted images secondary to high flow rate. T1 lesion is isointense with the brain; T2 lesion is hyperintense.

Diagnostic Procedures/Other

- CT
  - Diffuse homogeneous soft tissue mass with marked enhancement with contrast
- B-scan ultrasound—rarely used
  - Irregular mass blending with normal orbital structures. Shows variable internal reflectivity depending on the structural composition
- Biopsy
  - In cases of rapidly expanding orbital mass
  - Immunohistochemical staining is positive for factor VIII.

Pathological Findings

- Nonencapsulated vascular tumor
- Benign appearing endothelial cells with limited basement membrane, assuming a lobular architecture
- High concentration of mast cells, which may be a stimulus for vessel growth

DIFFERENTIAL DIAGNOSIS

- Capillary vascular malformation (port-wine stain)
  - Present at birth; flat; enlarge proportionately
- Vascular malformation
  - Abnormal aggregates of capillaries, veins, arteries, and lymphatics; no proliferative phase; normal endothelial turnover rate
- Symptoms of rapid orbital growth can mimic:
  - Metastatic neuroblastoma
  - Rhabdomyosarcoma
  - Teratoma
  - Lymphangioma
  - Cavernous hemangioma
- Color change and lesion enlargement with Valsalva seen in CHs can help differentiate these tumors form other lesions.

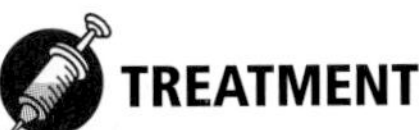

TREATMENT

MEDICATION

Treatment Indications

- Decision to treat periocular hemangiomas is directed by four factors:
  - Location
  - Extent
  - Degree of or potential for amblyopia
  - Presence of systemic hemangiomas
- Secondary indications for treatment include bleeding, obstruction of nasopharyngeal pathways, and the avoidance of possible cutaneous breakdown.

First Line

- Propranolol, oral (3,4)[C]: 2 mg/kg/day divided in 3 doses. This is a new, evolving treatment for select cases.
  - Some advise starting at 0.5 mg/kg/day for 1 week, then 1 mg/kg/day for 1 week if tolerated then maximal dose at 2 to 3 mg/kg/day. If monitoring as inpatient, can increase dose 0.5 mg/kg/day daily to reach maximum dose (3)[C]
  - Some advise maintaining the dose until the tumor is resolved, then slowly taper over 3–6 months to prevent rebound.
  - Possible mechanisms include vasoconstriction, decreased expression of growth factors, and triggering apoptosis of capillary endothelial cells.
  - Do not use during first week of life.
  - Monitor at onset of treatment of systemic hypotension, transient bradycardia, bronchospasm, and hypoglycemia.
  - Higher risk of adverse events in PHACES—cardiac evaluation with echocardiogram is recommended.
- Corticosteroids, systemic or intralesional
  - 80% show 80% shrinkage in 4–6 weeks
  - Systemic oral prednisolone: 1–3 mg/kg/day every morning for 4–6 weeks then taper over 2–4 weeks
    - Monitor every 2–4 weeks (blood pressure, evaluate for infection)
    - Complications include lesion rebound (common), steroid side effects (Cushing syndrome, adrenal suppression, irritability, insomnia)

Second Line

- Intralesional steroid (e.g., betamethasone 6 mg/mL and triamcinolone 40 mg/mL)
  - Complications: retinal artery occlusion, skin depigmentation, fat atrophy, necrosis, hematoma, eyelid necrosis
- Topical corticosteroids (clobetasol propionate 0.05%)
- Timolol maleate 0.5%, topical ophthalmic solution (5)[C]: 2 drops onto the surface of the hemangioma with a gentle spread twice daily. Most appropriate for small hemangiomas.
  - May be effective in very superficial CH
- Now rarely used historical treatments include the following:
  - Interferon alpha-2b daily subcutaneous injection: inhibits angiogenesis
  - External beam radiation therapy: for superficial lesions. Slows angiogenesis and induces involution. Complications include scarring, cataract formation, and tissue atrophy.

ADDITIONAL TREATMENT

General Measures

- Prospective monitoring without treatment in non–sight-threatening cases
- Spontaneous resolution occurs with time

Issues for Referral

- Ophthalmic:
  - Monitoring development of visual acuity
  - Amblyopia occurs in up to 60% with periorbital IH.
  - Treatment often involves spectacle correction and patching of noninvolved eye.
- Dermatologic:
  - Epidermal and subcutaneous hypertrophy may ulcerate, predispose to infection or scarring.

Additional Therapies

- Nd:Yag or argon laser: thermal injury to blood vessels induces involution. Argon absorbed superficially, Nd:Yag penetrates to 5–7 mm.
- May be a useful treatment of residual ecstatic vessels after involution

SURGERY/OTHER PROCEDURES

- Primary excision
  - Well-circumscribed IH may be completely excised.
  - Large, vision-threatening IH may be debulked.
  - May be definitive early treatment and prevent astigmatism and occlusion-related amblyopia
  - Intraoperative bleeding and postoperative ecchymosis are common

ONGOING CARE

FOLLOW-UP RECOMMENDATIONS

- Ophthalmology every 1–3 months if no signs of amblyopia, anisometropia, astigmatism greater than 1.5 diopters, severe proptosis with exposure keratopathy, or total pupillary occlusion
- Dermatology

Patient Monitoring

- Monitor for development of amblyopia.
- Monitor for response to treatment and treatment-related side effects.
- Monitor at home for development of occlusion, strabismus, or proptosis.

PROGNOSIS

- 70–90% show near-complete resolution.
- Cosmetic and visual recovery is excellent if treatment is instituted at an appropriate time and careful attention is paid to the visual development.

COMPLICATIONS

- Amblyopia (deprivation, anisometropic, astigmatic, or strabismic) can develop in 65%
- Strabismus in 30%
- Orbital bony distortion and/or enlargement
- Skin distention, redundancy, or ulceration leading to dermal scarring
- Residual proptosis

REFERENCES

1. Drolet BA, Esterly NB, Frieden IJ. Hemangiomas in children. *N Engl J Med* 1999;341(3):173–181.
2. Haik BG, Jakobiec FA, Ellsworth RM, Jones IS. Capillary hemangioma of the lids and orbit: An analysis of the clinical features and therapeutic results in 101 cases. *Ophthalmology* 1979;86(5): 760–792.
3. Léauté-Labrèze C, Dumas de la Roque E, Hubiche T, et al. Propranolol for severe hemangiomas of infancy. *N Engl J Med* 2008;358(24):2649–2651.
4. Lawley LP, Siegfried E, Todd JL. Propranolol treatment for hemangioma of infancy: Risks and recommendations. *Pediatr Dermatol* 2009;26(5): 610–614.
5. Guo S, Ni N. Topical treatment for capillary hemangioma of the eyelid using β-blocker solution. *Arch Ophthalmol* 2010;128(2):255–256.

ADDITIONAL READING

- Katowitz JA. *Pediatric oculoplastic surgery*. New York: Springer-Verlag, 2002:451–459.
- Tasman W, Jaeger E. *Duane's ophthalmology*. Philadelphia: Lippincott Williams & Wilkins, 2009:Chapter 37.

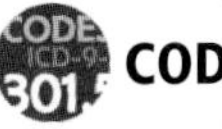

CODES

ICD9

- 228.01 Hemangioma of skin and subcutaneous tissue
- 228.09 Hemangioma of other sites
- 757.32 Vascular hamartomas

CLINICAL PEARLS

- Benign superficial or deep vascular hamartoma
- Potential for amblyopia and/or strabismus
- Treat if amblyopia present or likely, systemic hemangiomas, or large
- Treatments include beta-blockers, steroids, or surgery

PERIPHERAL CORNEAL ULCERS

Stephanie Jones Marioneaux

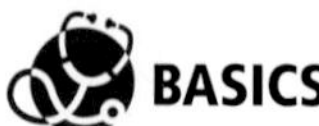

BASICS

DESCRIPTION

- **Noninfectious/immune mediated:** Peripheral cornea is 2 mm from the limbus and is susceptible to vasculitis because of its dependency and proximity to the limbal vascular arcade. Compromised blood flow, immunoglobulin/complement deposition create inflammation, which leads to peripheral ulcerative keratitis (PUK) (1). Necrotizing scleritis can occur with PUK if an aggressive vasculitis exists.
- **Infectious:** Peripheral epithelial defect provides entry of organism.
  - Bacterial: If inferiorly: possible lagophthalmos debilitated state, e.g., *Moraxella* infections (alcoholics) and *Pseudomonas* (hospitalized comatose patients)
  - Fungal: Similar to central ulcers
  - Viral: Herpes simplex—May not be hypesthetic, more refractory to treatment
  - Herpes zoster (2)

EPIDEMIOLOGY

Incidence

Infectious—fungal keratitis 24% (3)

RISK FACTORS

- Connective tissue (CT) diseases/vasculitides: Rheumatoid arthritis, Wegener's granulomatosis, polyarteritis nodosa; eye trauma(ensuing aberrant immune response)
- Debilitated state-chronic lagophthalmos

PATHOPHYSIOLOGY

Systemic CT disease with deposition of immune complexes in limbal vessels that cause inflammation, stimulate complement release with limbal and corneal infiltration by inflammatory cells with ulceration of the cornea and possible sclera.

ETIOLOGY

Systemic immune-mediated limbal vasculitis that leads to peripheral corneal ulceration. Infrequently trauma/surgery (4). Possible autoimmune response to tissue antigens.

COMMONLY ASSOCIATED CONDITIONS

Rheumatoid arthritis, Wegener's granulomatosis, polyarteritis nodosa, CT diseases

DIAGNOSIS

HISTORY

- Red, painful eye with photophobia. Sometimes more severe pain, possible "headache" if scleritis is present
- History of rheumatoid arthritis, Wegener's granulomatosis, polyarteritis nodosa, and other CT diseases. The systemic diseases may not clinically correlate with the severity of the ocular manifestation.
- **Infectious**—Eye trauma, eye rubbing, surgery, lagophthalmos, possible purulent discharge

PHYSICAL EXAM

- **Immune:** Intact overlying epithelium in some cases, concentric immune infiltrates that spread concentrically. Hypopyon rare. Microulcerative: less than 2 clock hours and do not progress centrally. Macroulcerative: greater than 2 clock hours; generally ulceration, both central and circumferential progression; undermined central edge, dense infiltration, epithelial breakdown, and melting. Necrotizing scleritis may occur with corneal perforation. If inferior may suggest a dry eye with lagophthalmos.
- **Infectious:** Epithelial defect that spreads centrally as it worsens. Possible ring corneal infiltrates surround a central infection. Some may advance to perforation if treatment delayed. May have purulent discharge; hypopyon.
- **Viral:** Peripheral dendrites that coalesce, possible stromal infiltrate. If metaherpetic, may result in corneal thinning.

DIAGNOSTIC TESTS & INTERPRETATION

Lab

Initial lab tests

- **Immune:** May not be necessary if Dx of CT disease exists. If suspect Wegener's or polyarteritis: chest X-ray (CXR), U/A, BUN/Cre, antineutrophil cytoplasmic antibodies (ANCAs). Possible CBC, anti-nuclear antibody (ANA), ESR, fluorescent treponemal antibody absorption test (FTAabs), reactive plasma reagin (RPR), hepatitis C serologies, rheumatoid factor (RF). Wegener's/polyarteritis Dx may require a lung or renal biopsy.
- **Infectious:** Corneal scrapings for culture and sensitivities if bacteria or fungus are suspected.
- **Viral:** Immunoassay? Polymerase chain reaction (PCR) for herpes simplex virus (HSV) only if high suspicion and all other studies are negative (5). Viral cultures (Richmond viral transport medium), fluorescent antibody testing (FAB) (No fluorescein stain prior to collection of sample. Fluorescein alters results.) (5)

Follow-up & special considerations

Immune: Consult Rheumatologist or Clinical Immunologist with experience in corneal manifestations of CT disorders.

Imaging

Initial approach

Only if suspect Wegener's or polyarteritis—Chest X-ray

Follow-up & special considerations

Immune/infectious follow-up frequently, daily if necessary, until some improvement, in the event of an impending perforation.

Diagnostic Procedures/Other

Corneal scrapings for culture and sensitivity

Pathological Findings

- Noninfectious—Peripheral inflammation that can progress to corneal melting and perforation.
- Infectious—Can progress to corneal thinning and perforation.

DIFFERENTIAL DIAGNOSIS

- **Immune**—Rheumatoid arthritis, Wegener's granulomatosis, polyarteritis. Mooren's ulcer is diagnosis of exclusion. Herpes zoster virus (HZV) sclerokeratitis: limbal vasculitis and ischemia
- **Infectious**—Bacterial (staph, *B* hemolytic strep, *Pseudomonas*, *Moraxella*, *Neisseria gonorrhoeae*), HSV, herpes zoster ophthalmicus, systemic hepatitis 83–84, chlamydial (trachoma and inclusion conjunctivitis)

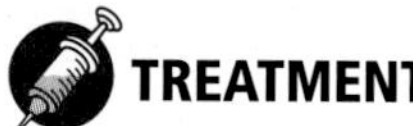

TREATMENT

MEDICATION

First Line

- Immune: Treat underlying disease, suppress inflammation with tectonic support, and promote healing. (Cornea p. 347) Systemic treatment by rheumatologist—corticosteroids and immunosuppressive medications, e.g., methotrexate, cyclosporine, mycophenolate mofetil (CellCept), azathioprine, and cyclophosphamide. Treatment may increase lifespan (6).
- Provide tectonic support via cyanoacrylate adhesive application to the ulcer bed with a bandage soft contact lens. May need a peripheral lamellar keratoplasty. Treat any underlying dry eye: preservative-free tears, punctual plugs/cautery, bandage soft contact lenses with lubrication, and fluoroquinolone antibiotic coverage or partial tarsorrhaphy if partial lid closure. Avoid corticosteroids if inferior and may be associated with a dry eye. May cause corneal melting.

- Infectious:
  - Bacterial: Treat with broad-spectrum antibiotic coverage: Fortified antibiotics or fluoroquinolones. Cultures and sensitivities can guide antibiotic selection.
  - Fungal: Treat with broad-spectrum antifungals—pending cultures/fungal stains or corneal biopsies if necessary
  - Viral: Topical antivirals, PO Acyclovir

Pregnancy Considerations
Immune: Notify rheumatologist before immunosuppressive oral treatments are given.

Second Line
- Immune/infectious: Provide tectonic support if threat of perforation. Tissue glue; peripheral lamellar grafts.
- Immune: Conjunctival resection adjacent to area of peripheral corneal ulceration and thinning

ADDITIONAL TREATMENT
General Measures
Frequent monitoring until stabilized

Issues for Referral
- Impending perforation
- Recalcitrant to treatment with worsening visual prognosis

COMPLEMENTARY & ALTERNATIVE THERAPIES
- Vitamin C—promotes healing
- Fish oil—helps to normalize meibomian gland secretions and stabilize tear film

SURGERY/OTHER PROCEDURES
- Peripheral lamellar keratoplasties
- Tissue glue for focal perforations
- Conjunctival resection

IN-PATIENT CONSIDERATIONS
Initial Stabilization
Infectious: Begin appropriate therapy immediately upon arrival to the hospital.

Admission Criteria
Inability to administer necessary frequent topical medications and requiring IV meds

IV Fluids
Defer to internist/hospitalist

Nursing
Instruct re: proper drop instillation

Discharge Criteria
Stabilization of ulceration

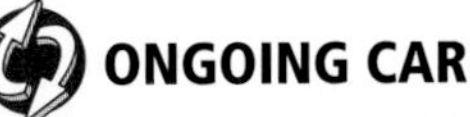

ONGOING CARE

FOLLOW-UP RECOMMENDATIONS
- Immune: Continued follow up with rheumatologist. Careful ophthalmic monitoring with tapering of systemic meds. May require chronic long-term, low-dose maintenance as determined by the rheumatologist.
- Infectious: May need surgery if scarring involves visual axis. Depth of scarring and location will determine necessity for full-thickness or partial-thickness lamellar keratoplasties.

Patient Monitoring
- Immune: Co-management with rheumatologist as determined by response to treatment
- Infectious: According to response to treatment

DIET
No restrictions

PATIENT EDUCATION
Signs and symptoms of peripheral keratitis for earlier diagnosis

PROGNOSIS
Depends on involvement of visual axis and extent of peripheral thinning—induced astigmatism

COMPLICATIONS
Perforation, thinning, severe scarring, possible recurrences for the immune, and herpetic causes

REFERENCES

1. Mondino BJ. Inflammatory diseases of the peripheral cornea. *Ophthalmology* 1988;95: 463–472.
2. Polack FM, Kaufman HE, Newmark E. Keratomycosis: Medical and surgical treatment. *Arch Ophthalmol* 1971;85:410–416.
3. Mondino BJ, Brown SI, Mondzelewski JP. Peripheral corneal ulcers with herpes zoster ophthalmicus. *Am J Ophthalmol* 1978;86:611–614.
4. Akpek E, Demetriades A, Gottsch J. Peripheral ulcerative keratitis after clear corneal cataract extraction. *J Cataract Refract Surg* 2000;26(9): 1424–1427.
5. Tuli SS. Herpetic corneal infections. *Focal Points, AAO* 2008;XXVI(8).
6. Messmer E, Foster CS. Vasculitic peripheral ulcerative keratitis. *Surv Ophthalmol* 1999;43(5): 379–396.

ADDITIONAL READING

- Krachmer JH, Mannis MJ, Holland EJ, eds. *Cornea*, Philadelphia: Elsevier Mosby, 2005.
- Rapuano CJ, Heng W-J. *Corneal atlas & synopsis of clinical ophthalmology Wills Eye Hospital Series*. New York: McGraw-Hill, 2003.
- Zaher SS, Sandinhe T, et al. Herpes simplex keratitis is diagnosed in Rheumatoid arthritis-related peripheral ulcerative keratitis. *Cornea* 2005; 24(8):1015–1017.

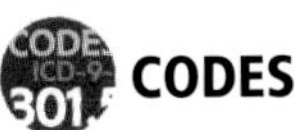

CODES

ICD9
- 370.00 Corneal ulcer, unspecified
- 370.01 Marginal corneal ulcer
- 370.02 Ring corneal ulcer

CLINICAL PEARLS

- Consider the full differential diagnosis in patients with peripheral keratitis even in patients with known collagen vascular diseases, i.e., bacterial, viral, fungal, and immune mediated.
- Co-manage with rheumatologists for systemic agents when indicated.
- Treat aggressively with systemic agents as the occurrence of ulcerative keratitis is associated with a shorter lifespan.
- Immune-mediated PUK does not always appear concomitantly with the systemic exacerbation of the autoimmune disease. Strong clinical suspicion, rather than evidence of systemic exacerbation, should direct you to request rheumatologic assistance in initiating treatment with immunosuppressive treatment.

PERSISTENT FETAL VASCULATURE (PFV)

Raza M. Shah

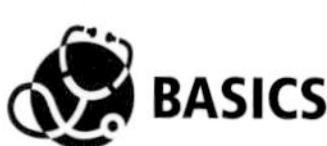

BASICS

DESCRIPTION

- Pathologic entity resulting from failure of the primary vitreous to regress
  - Persistence and/or hypertrophy of the vessels within the primary vitreous can result new vessels in the posterior segment.
  - There are three forms (1)[B]:
    - Anterior: there is a retrolental opacity, cataract, or elongation of the ciliary processes (2)[C].
    - Posterior: optic disc hypoplasia, a stalk emanating from the optic disc, a retinal fold, retinal dysplasia, retinal detachment
    - Combined: Both anterior and posterior manifestations

Pediatric Considerations

Persistent hyperplastic primary vitreous (PHPV), also known as persistent fetal vasculature (PFV), presents during infancy and is a failure of the primary vitreous and its vascular system to regress normally. Infants typically present with microphthalmia, cataracts, and retinal traction or dysplasia.

EPIDEMIOLOGY

PFV is very rare.

RISK FACTORS

No risk factors have been isolated at this point.

Genetics

- Most cases are sporadic.
- It can be inherited as in an autosomal dominant as well as an autosomal recessive (AR) fashion. In one family with AR PFV, a gene was isolated to 10q11–q21.
- *PAX6* gene mutations were detected recently in patients with optic nerve malformations that included PFV.

PATHOPHYSIOLOGY

- As reported by Cloquet in 1818, it occurs because of a failure of the primary vitreous and the hyaloid vascular system to regress (3)[C].
- The primary vitreous forms around the 7th week of life and begins involuting by 20 weeks. These vessels should completely regress by the time of birth. Persistence of these vessels can result in PFV in both the anterior and/or posterior chambers.

ETIOLOGY

Unknown

COMMONLY ASSOCIATED CONDITIONS

- None at this time
- Bilateral PFV with retinal dysplasia can be indistinguishable from Norrie's disease, a condition in which children can also have hearing loss or other CNS problems.

DIAGNOSIS

HISTORY

- Leukocoria in an infant
- The involved eye is often smaller than the other eye, and posterior lens opacity is present.

PHYSICAL EXAM

- No systemic changes are associated.
- It is most often unilateral.
- Cataract, posterior lens opacity, elongated ciliary process, and/or a stalk that extends from the lens posterior to the optic disc.
- The lens itself is clear anteriorly with an opaque posterior surface.
- The pupil may be difficult to dilate because of the anterior tunica vasculosa lentis (TVL).
- Microphthalmia

DIAGNOSTIC TESTS & INTERPRETATION

Lab

None generally necessary

Imaging

- B scan ultrasonography can show a stalk from the posterior pole anteriorly to the lens, microphthalmia and retinal detachment.
- CT scanning also can demonstrate the PFV membrane.
- The absence of calcification on CT scanning is an important point in differentiating PFV from retinoblastoma, as calcification usually can be seen with retinoblastoma.
- MRI is superior to CT in differentiating noncalcified retinoblastoma from PFV.
- Visual evoked potential testing is helpful. If a response is present, surgery for retinal detachment repair might be worthwhile.

Diagnostic Procedures/Other Pathological Findings

PFV in the hyaloid canal

DIFFERENTIAL DIAGNOSIS

- Retinoblastoma
- Congenital cataract
- Norrie disease
- Walker–Warburg syndrome
- Trisomy
- If total retinal detachment and retrolental fibrous tissues are present, familial exudative retinopathy, incontinentia pigmenti, and retinopathy of prematurity should be included.

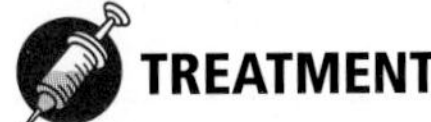

TREATMENT

SURGERY/OTHER PROCEDURES

- The decision to perform surgery may be based on the severity of PFV and whether or not the fundus can be visualized, the presence or absence of retinal detachment, and the degree of cataract.
- Surgery often offers a greater chance of obtaining better visual acuity.
- Patients should be concomitantly treated for amblyopia.

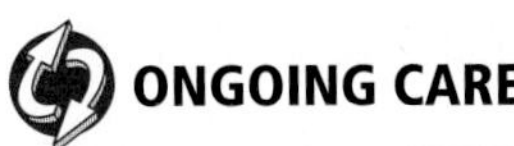

ONGOING CARE

FOLLOW-UP RECOMMENDATIONS

Patients will need monitoring regardless of whether observation or surgical intervention is chosen.

PROGNOSIS

- Prognosis depends on the extent of the membrane as well as the type of PFV.
- In purely anterior PFV, a good visual outcome is achieved when the visual axis is clear and amblyopia therapy are successful.
- Treatment of posterior and combined anteroposterior PFV has a less favorable outcome, with most patients attaining hand motion or light perception.

COMPLICATIONS

- Glaucoma
- Hemorrhage
- Enucleation

REFERENCES

1. Pollard ZF. Persistent hyperplastic primary vitreous: diagnosis, treatment and results. *Trans Am Ophthalmol Soc* 1997;95:487–549.
2. Castillo M, Wallace D, Mukherji S. Persistent hyperplastic primary vitreous involving the anterior eye. *Am J Neuropathol* 1997;18(8):1526–1528.
3. Gulati N, Eagle RC Jr, Tasman W. Unoperated eyes with persistent fetal vasculature. *Trans Am Ophthalmol Soc* 2003;101:59–64.

ADDITIONAL READING

- Capone A, Hartnett M, Trese M. *Persistent fetal vasculature syndrome (persistent hyperplastic primary vitreous). Pediatric retina: Medical and surgical approaches*. Philadelphia: Lippincott Williams & Wilkins, 2005.

CODES

ICD9

743.51 Vitreous anomalies, congenital

CLINICAL PEARLS

- Must be differentiated from retinoblastoma
- Treatment is typically surgical clearing the visual axis and relieving anterior to posterior traction.
- Anisometropic amblyopia often limits visual recovery.
- Retinal dysplasia is found in varying amounts in PFV and can limit visual function and rehabilitation.

PERSISTENT HYPERPLASTIC VITREOUS/PERSISTENT FETAL VASCULATURE

Jeffrey P. Blice

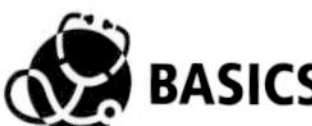

BASICS

DESCRIPTION

- Persistent fetal vasculature (PFV) is usually a nonheritable set of vascular malformations in systemically normal infants.
- Usually unilateral
- Range of anterior segment and posterior segment complications possible
- Manifestations can range from mild to severe.
- Rare, serious congenital malformation syndromes affecting both eyes, the brain, and other parts of the body can also be associated with PFV.
- Persistent hyperplastic primary vitreous (PHPV) is a term describing a subset of clinical findings seen in the retrolental space.

EPIDEMIOLOGY

Uncommon

RISK FACTORS

Most cases are sporadic and not genetically linked. Rare associations exist (see below).

Genetics

- *NDP*-related retinopathies are characterized by a spectrum of fibrous and vascular changes of the retina at birth that progress through childhood or adolescence to cause varying degrees of visual impairment.
- The most severe phenotype is Norrie's disease (ND), characterized by grayish-yellow fibrovascular masses (pseudogliomas). Congenital blindness is almost always present. Developmental delay/mental retardation, behavioral abnormalities, or psychotic-like features can be present. The majority develop sensorineural hearing loss.
- X-linked familial exudative vitreoretinopathy (XL-FEVR), an exudative proliferative vasculopathy characterized by peripheral retinal vascular anomalies with or without fibrotic changes and retinal detachment. Phenotypes can vary within families.
- Retinal dysplasia with changes like PFV can be associated Walker–Warburg syndrome, an autosomal recessive disorder, and with multiple anomalies in trisomy 13.

GENERAL PREVENTION

None

PATHOPHYSIOLOGY

Abnormal regression and persistence of normal embryologic vasculature alters the normal anatomy of the cornea, lens, angle, iris, retina, and/or optic nerve.

COMMONLY ASSOCIATED CONDITIONS

See Genetics

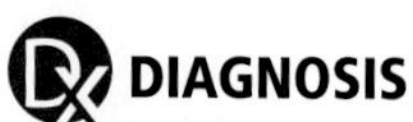

DIAGNOSIS

HISTORY

- Present at birth
- Presents in infancy commonly as leukocoria

PHYSICAL EXAM

Findings vary from case to case. Not all findings are present in all cases. An accumulation of findings make the case for diagnosis.

- Microphthalmia
- Anterior segment findings
  - Microcornea
  - Corneal clouding
  - Persistent pupillary membrane
  - Iridohyaloid blood vessels can lead to dragged ciliary processes, ectropion uvea, and lens subluxation.
  - Persistence of the posterior fetal fibrovascular sheath and retrolental membrane
  - Lens swelling and narrow angle
  - Mittendorf's dot
- Posterior segment findings
  - Vitreous opacities—remnants of regressed vessels
  - Persistent hyaloid artery
  - Bergmeister's papilla with the potential for anomalous optic nerve and macular traction
  - Retinal detachment and folds
  - Macular dysplasia; absence of the foveal pit
  - Optic nerve dysplasia or hypoplasia

DIAGNOSTIC TESTS & INTERPRETATION

Imaging

- B-scan ultrasonography—can be used to identify and document persistent vascular anatomy tractional retinal abnormalities
- CT—Although tractional retinal changes and abnormal ocular anatomy may be visible, excluding the presence of intraocular calcium is most useful when retinoblastoma is a possibility.
- MRI—Can be useful in clarifying CT findings or identifying CNS disease in associated syndromes or disease

Diagnostic Procedures/Other

Fluorescein angiography may be useful in identifying the presence of persistent perfused fetal vessels.

Pathological Findings

Consistent with the spectrum of clinical disease

DIFFERENTIAL DIAGNOSIS

- Retinoblastoma
- Stage V retinopathy of prematurity
- ND
- Trisomy 13
- Congenital subluxation of the lens
- XL-FEVR

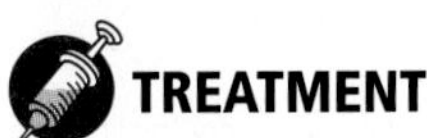

TREATMENT

ADDITIONAL TREATMENT

General Measures

- Mild cases may require no treatment.
- Severe cases can be so severely affected that no surgical treatment is reasonable.
- Patients should be counseled about protective eyewear.

SURGERY/OTHER PROCEDURES

- The decision to perform surgery should be based on the risks, benefits, and visual prognosis as related to the severity of the anatomical abnormalities.
- The surgical approach may require surgical expertise in both the anterior and posterior segments.
- Surgery should be considered for the following complications in eyes with some vision:
  - Recurrent or severe vitreous hemorrhage
  - Progressive retinal detachment
  - Angle closure and ocular hypertension
  - Anterior displacement of the lens or subluxation of the lens

ONGOING CARE

FOLLOW-UP RECOMMENDATIONS

- Ophthalmologist
- Coordinated care with pediatric ophthalmologist and vitreoretinal surgeon may also be necessary.
- Amblyopia and its prevention is a concern in any case with unilateral disease and vision in the affected eye.

PATIENT EDUCATION

- Monocular patients should be counseled to wear protective eyewear.
- Families with rare hereditary forms should receive genetic counseling.

PROGNOSIS

- The prognosis is variable and depends on the severity of the disease. Those patients with milder findings may not warrant any surgical intervention.
- Eyes with less severe disease remain at risk for amblyopia.
- More severe cases may have such advance disease that no treatment is effective.
- Patients with good vision and moderate disease are at risk for progression and complications as outlined below.

COMPLICATIONS

- Corneal clouding
- Progression of cataract
- Glaucoma
- Recurrent vitreous hemorrhage
- Progression of retinal traction and detachment
- Amblyopia

ADDITIONAL READING

- Goldberg MF. Lecture. *Am J Ophthalmol* 1997; 124(5):587–626.
- Gulati N, Eagle RC Jr, Tasman W. Unoperated eyes with persistent fetal vasculature. *Trans Am Ophthalmol Soc* 2003;101:59–64; discussion 64–65.
- Sims KB. NDP-related retinopathies. In: *GeneReviews [Internet]*. Pagon RA, Bird TC, Dolan CR, Stephens K, eds. Seattle, WA) University of Washington, Seattle, 2009.

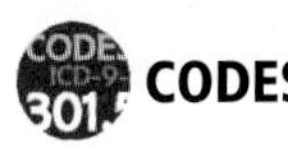

CODES

ICD9

743.51 Vitreous anomalies, congenital

CLINICAL PEARLS

- Usually unilateral
- Microphthalmia, microcornea, cataract, and dragging of ciliary processes are classic findings.
- Surgical choices and prognosis are influenced by status of retinal disease.
- Amblyopia threatens even the best surgical outcomes.

The views expressed in this article are those of the author and do not necessarily reflect the official policy or position of the Department of the Navy, Army, Department of Defense, nor the U.S. Government. I certify that all individuals who qualify as authors have been listed; each has participated in the conception and design of this work, the analysis of data (when applicable), the writing of the document, and the approval of the submission of this version; that the document represents valid work; that if we used information derived from another source, we obtained all necessary approvals to use it and made appropriate acknowledgements in the document; and that each takes public responsibility for it.

PETERS ANOMALY

Tak Yee Tania Tai
Alex V. Levin

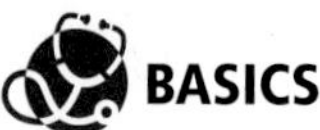

BASICS

DESCRIPTION

- Peters anomaly is characterized by a congenital corneal opacity associated with a posterior defect in Descemet's membrane and endothelium. Although usually central, the opacity may be eccentric.
- Variable degrees of iris and lenticular adherence to the posterior cornea may be present.
- May be isolated or associated with other ocular malformations or systemic syndromes.
- Peters plus syndrome describes the concurrence of Peters anomaly, and short stature, with or without abnormal ears, and occasionally, cleft lip and palate.

EPIDEMIOLOGY

Incidence

Peters anomaly is a rare disease affecting less than 200,000 people in the US.

RISK FACTORS

- Genetic predisposition
- Maternal alcohol intake during pregnancy has been reported as a feature of fetal alcohol syndrome (1)[C].

Genetics

- Most cases are sporadic, but both autosomal recessive and dominant modes of inheritance have been reported.
- Isolated Peters anomaly has been reported with mutations in the following genes: *PAX6* (autosomal dominant), *CYP1B1* (autosomal dominant), *PITX2/RIEG1* (autosomal dominant), *PITX3*, *FOXE3* (autosomal recessive), *NDP* (X-linked recessive), and *FOXC1* (autosomal dominant) (2)[C].
- Reported chromosomal anomalies include ring chromosome 20, trisomy 13, and partial deletion of 11q (3)[C].
- Mutations in *B3GALTL* (13q12.3–13.1) can be associated with Peters plus syndrome, which is inherited in an autosomal recessive manner (2)[C].

GENERAL PREVENTION

Genetic counseling and molecular genetic testing

PATHOPHYSIOLOGY

- Several theories have been implicated:
  - Failure of lens placode invagination from surface ectoderm during weeks 4–7 of gestation
  - Misdirected neural crest migration and abnormal neural crest differentiation (1)[C]

ETIOLOGY

Drug-induced and infectious (congenital cytomegalovirus) etiologies have been implicated, although most cases appear to be genetic or idiopathic (1)[C].

COMMONLY ASSOCIATED CONDITIONS

- Ophthalmologic problems (1)[C]
- Glaucoma occurs in 30–70%
- Microphthalmia occurs in 25–50%
- Iris abnormalities—aniridia, abnormal vascularization, iris coloboma, polycoria, iridocorneal adhesions, microcoria
- Ptosis
- Cataract
- Posterior pole abnormalities—chorioretinal coloboma, staphyloma, retinal dysplasia/dystrophy, persistent ocular fetal vasculature, optic nerve hypoplasia, foveal hypoplasia/aplasia, macular pigment epitheliopathy, macular "coloboma"
- Systemic malformations occur in 60% of cases (1)[C].
- Mental retardation
- CNS malformations
- Craniofacial abnormalities
- Microcephaly
- Seizure disorder
- Autism
- Congenital heart disease
- Genitourinary malformations
- Skeletal abnormalities (Peters plus syndrome)
- Ear defects
- Cleft lip and palate

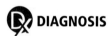

DIAGNOSIS

HISTORY

- Course of pregnancy and birth history
- Family history
- Additional directed questions are necessary for recognition and treatment of associated conditions (see "Commonly Associated Conditions").

PHYSICAL EXAM

- Complete ophthalmological examination with attention to posterior surface of cornea and clarity of visual axis
- Complete neurological and physical exam is necessary to assess for associated conditions (see "Commonly Associated Conditions).

DIAGNOSTIC TESTS & INTERPRETATION

Lab

Initial lab tests

- Peters anomaly is a clinical diagnosis.
- Laboratory studies may be warranted depending on the physical examination.
  - Growth hormone stimulation testing for possibility of a treatable cause of growth delay
  - Thyroid function testing for congenital hypothyroidism
  - Urine and lens for cytomegalovirus, serum titers

Follow-up & special considerations

- Karyotype, microarray, and molecular genetic testing for *B3GALTL* gene when Peters plus syndrome suspected.
- Molecular genetic studies may be performed for isolated Peters anomaly.

Imaging

Initial approach

- Imaging may be performed as necessary for findings on physical examination.
  - Ocular ultrasound for evaluation of ocular structures if no view of posterior segment
  - Ultrasound biomicroscopy or optical coherence tomography can identify posterior corneal defect
  - Echocardiography for congenital heart malformations when indicated
  - Abdominal ultrasound examination for renal anomalies when indicated
  - Cranial imaging for hydrocephalus or structural brain abnormalities where indicated
  - Skeletal survey for Peters plus

Follow-up & special considerations

- Serial plotting of growth and development
- Intense vision follow-up is required to screen for amblyopia and treat accordingly.
- Suggest examination to rule out glaucoma every 6 months as a minimum even if examination under anesthesia required.

Pathological Findings

- Type 1—characterized by central or paracentral corneal opacity with iris strands that arise from the iris collarette and attach to the cornea. Usually unilateral.
- Type 2–includes lens adherence to the posterior cornea, with or without cataract histopathology shows iris stromal fibers attaching to the posterior cornea with an absent Descemet's membrane and endothelium Bowman's layer may appear thickened.

DIFFERENTIAL DIAGNOSIS

- Sclerocornea
- Birth trauma from forceps
- Intrauterine keratitis
- Mucopolysaccharidoses
- Congenital hereditary endothelial/stromal dystrophy
- Corneal dermoid
- Herpes simplex keratitis
- Congenital glaucoma
- Amniocentesis needle corneal perforation
- Covert or overt postnatal trauma

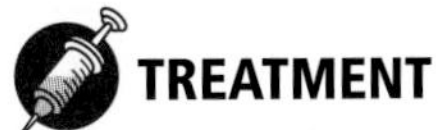

TREATMENT

MEDICATION

Medical treatment of glaucoma

ADDITIONAL TREATMENT

General Measures

The goal of ophthalmological treatment is to maximize vision and minimize amblyopia.

Issues for Referral

- Infant Development Program—appropriate developmental assessment may be helpful if indicated.
- Genetic consultation and counseling—helpful if a heritable disorder is suspected
- Pediatric ophthalmologist—management of amblyopia and refractive error, cataract, and glaucoma
- Cornea specialist—keratoplasty may be indicated.
- Low-vision specialist
- Endocrinologist—if endocrine problems are suspected

Additional Therapies

Additional therapies may be performed as indicated for the associated conditions of Peters anomaly.

SURGERY/OTHER PROCEDURES

- The indication for surgery in patients with Peters anomaly is controversial—considerations include whether monocular or binocular, age, and visual prognosis (1)[C].
- Keratoplasty
  - Optical iridectomy (sector) has been used as an alternative to penetrating keratoplasty.
  - The degree of visual deprivation depends on the size and location of the ocular opacity.
  - When the opacity is small, gradual clearing may occur.
  - When the opacity is dense, and, especially if bilateral, penetrating keratoplasty is likely indicated.
  - This should be considered at age 1–6 months. One must balance high failure rate and technical difficulties if too young versus high amblyopia rate if too old.
  - The probability of first grafts remaining clear for 10 or more years was 35% according to one study (4)[C].
- Glaucoma surgery
  - Multiple procedures and adjunctive medical therapy are often required.
  - Trabeculotomy or goniotomy may be difficult technically and have high failure rates due to maldevelopment of drainage structures.
  - Trabeculectomy and tube implantation may be preferred.
  - Cyclodestructive procedures as last option
- Lensectomy/vitrectomy
  - May be indicated for patients with cataract
  - Lens may spontaneously come out at penetrating keratoplasty.

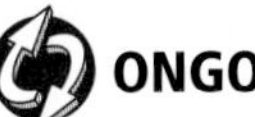

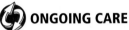

ONGOING CARE

FOLLOW-UP RECOMMENDATIONS

- Regular follow-up care for visual rehabilitation, corneal graft management, and glaucoma management as needed
- Regular follow-up with a pediatrician to manage the patient's other congenital abnormalities as necessary

Patient Monitoring

Patient monitoring as necessary for ophthalmological and associated systemic issues.

PATIENT EDUCATION

- www.pgcfa.org (Pediatric Glaucoma and Cataract Family Association)
- www.rarediseases.org/ (National Organization for Rare Diseases)
- www.petersanomaly.org/ (Peters Anomaly Support Group)

PROGNOSIS

- Systemic prognosis depends on associated systemic problems.
- After penetrating keratoplasty:
  - ~20% of eyes achieve acuities of 20/200 or better.
  - ~40% of eyes achieve light perception (LP) or no light perception (NLP) vision.
  - The remaining eyes achieve 20/300 to hand motion vision (1)[C].
- Prognosis is more promising in bilateral cases.

COMPLICATIONS

Amblyopia and decreased vision or blindness from glaucoma

REFERENCES

1. Yang LLH, Lambert SR. Peters anomaly—A synopsis of surgical management and visual outcome. *Ophthalmol Clin North Am* 2001;14(3):467–477.
2. Gudrun A, Kriek M, Lesnik Oberstein SAJ. Peter's plus syndrome. http://www.ncbi.nlm.nih.gov/mbk1464.
3. Traboulsi EI, Maumenee IH. Peters anomaly and associated congenital malformations. *Arch Ophthalmol* 1992;110:1739–1742.
4. Yang LLH, Lambert SR, Lynn MJ, et al. Long-term results of corneal graft survival in infants and children with Peters anomaly. *Ophthalmology* 1999;106(4):833–848.

ADDITIONAL READING

- Heon E, Barsoum-Homsy M, Cervette L, et al. Peters anomaly. *Ophthalmic Paediatr Genet* 1992;13(2): 137–143.

See Also (Topic, Algorithm, Electronic Media Element)

- OMIM:
  - http://www.ncbi.nlm.nih.gov/omim/604229
  - http://www.ncbi.nlm.nih.gov/omim/261540

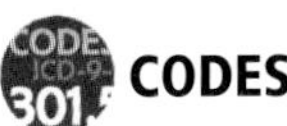

CODES

ICD9

743.44 Specified congenital anomalies of anterior chamber, chamber angle, and related structures

CLINICAL PEARLS

- Peters anomaly is a congenital malformation that may be associated with glaucoma, cataract, and other ocular malformations.
- Peters plus syndrome is characterized by skeletal dysplasia.
- Peters anomaly, especially when bilateral, may be associated with other systemic abnormalities.
- Visual prognosis is guarded and long-term follow-up is required.

PHACOANAPHYLACTIC GLAUCOMA

Rachel M. Niknam

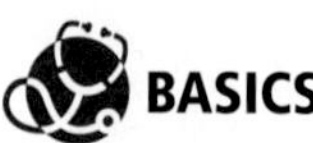

BASICS

DESCRIPTION
A zonular granulomatous-type of inflammation that centers on retained lens material in the involved eye or in the fellow eye.

EPIDEMIOLOGY
- Seen in eyes with traumatic disruption of the lens or that have undergone extracapsular cataract extraction
- Usually seen in the 6th or 7th decade coinciding with the average age of cataract extraction
- Slightly higher male prevalence

GENERAL PREVENTION
Meticulous removal of lens material during cataract extraction

PATHOPHYSIOLOGY
- Disruption of the lens capsule, either traumatic or surgical
- A period of time, wherein there is a sensitization to lens protein that occurs
- A chronic and persistent inflammation then ensues

ETIOLOGY
- Autologous lens protein has been shown to be antigenic.
- Sensitization occurs only when there is a violation of the lens capsule.

COMMONLY ASSOCIATED CONDITIONS
- Glaucoma is related to the accumulation of leukocytes, epithelioid, and giant cells in the trabecular meshwork.
- Lens protein and lens particles may also be found in the trabecular meshwork and may additionally account for the associated glaucoma.

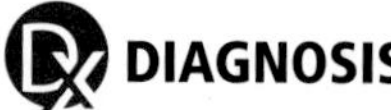

DIAGNOSIS

HISTORY
Prior cataract surgery, lens trauma, or rarely spontaneous rupture of the lens capsule with prolonged period of low-level persistent inflammation.

PHYSICAL EXAM
- Inflammation with associated photophobia and ciliary's injection
- Anterior chamber cell and flare
- The aqueous may contain lens fragments.
- Often mutton-fat keratic precipitates and posterior synechia are present.

DIAGNOSTIC TESTS & INTERPRETATION

Lab

Initial lab tests

Aqueous or vitreous aspiration for histologic examination

Imaging

Initial approach
- B-scan ultrasound to look for retained lens fragments
- Aggressive control of inflammation and intraocular pressure (IOP)

Follow-up & special considerations

Frequent follow-up until definitive treatment is implemented, which involves removal of retained lens material

Diagnostic Procedures/Other
- Histological examination of the surgically removed lens material
- Microscopic examination of aqueous and/or vitreous

Pathological Findings
Polymorphonuclear leukocytes, epithelioid cells, and giant cells in a zonular pattern surrounding a portion of lens material

DIFFERENTIAL DIAGNOSIS
- Phacolytic glaucoma
- Lens particle glaucoma
- Toxic reaction to materials introduced at surgery
- Exacerbation of prior uveitis
- Infection with low virulence organisms, that is, propionibacterium
- Sympathetic ophthalmia

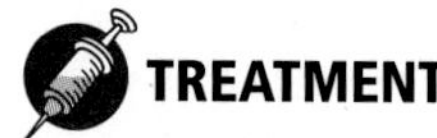

TREATMENT

MEDICATION

First Line
- Topical steroid therapy to reduce inflammation
- Antiglaucoma therapy to control IOP: with hyperosmotics, topical carbonic anhydrase inhibitors, topical beta-blockers and alpha-2 agonists.

ADDITIONAL TREATMENT

Issues for Referral
- If the retained lens material or the traumatic disruption of the lens capsule involves the anterior segment then the anterior segment surgeon should remove the inciting lens material.
- Often the retained lens material is in the vitreous and consultation or referral to a retina surgeon for appropriate removal is suggested.

Additional Therapies
- Once the lens material is removed, the uveitis is usually easier to control and steroid therapy should be tapered.
- IOP control must be monitored as there may be secondary angle closure glaucoma due to synechia formation.

SURGERY/OTHER PROCEDURES
- Surgical removal of retained lens material
- If the IOP remains elevated after surgical removal of lens and if either the secondary open-angle or angle closure glaucoma is uncontrolled then glaucoma filtering surgery is indicated.

IN-PATIENT CONSIDERATIONS
Initial Stabilization
Admission and intravenous mannitol may be necessary to control IOP until definitive surgery.

Discharge Criteria
Once the IOP is controlled the patient may be discharged with close follow-up appointments.

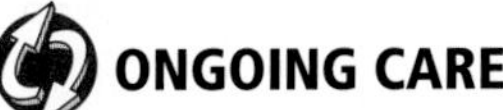

ONGOING CARE

FOLLOW-UP RECOMMENDATIONS
Very close follow-up during the initial postoperative period is warranted to manage the uveitis and IOP.

Patient Monitoring
- Once the IOP and uveitis are controlled lifelong IOP monitoring and treatment are necessary for the secondary open- or closed-angle glaucoma.
- 3–6 month intervals depending on the severity of disease

PATIENT EDUCATION
The physiology of glaucoma and the importance of adherence to medication should be discussed.

PROGNOSIS
The prognosis depends on the severity of the disease upon presentation and the prompt treatment of the uveitis and glaucoma.

COMPLICATIONS
- Vision loss secondary to glaucoma or uveitis, that is, cystoid macular edema
- Surgical complication of vitrectomy or additional anterior segment removal of lens material
- Surgical complications of glaucoma filtering surgery

ADDITIONAL READING

- Allingham RR, Damji KF, Freedman S, et al. *Shields textbook of glaucoma*, 5th ed. 2004, Philadelphia: Lippincott Williams & Wilkins.
- Marak GE Jr. Phacoanaphylactic endophlamitis. *Surv Ophthalmol* 1992;36:5325–5340.
- Epstein DL. Diagnosis and management of lens-induced glaucoma. *Am Acad Ophthalmol* 1982;89(3):227–230.

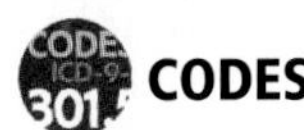

CODES

ICD9
- 365.59 Glaucoma associated with other lens disorders
- 365.62 Glaucoma associated with ocular inflammations

CLINICAL PEARLS

Suspect in patients with persistent low level uveitis after cataract extraction

PHACOLYTIC GLAUCOMA

Rachel M. Niknam

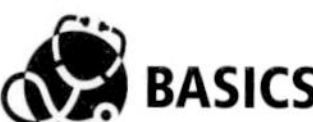

BASICS

DESCRIPTION
Sudden onset of open-angle glaucoma secondary to leakage of soluble lens proteins from an intact mature cataractous lens.

EPIDEMIOLOGY
- More common in underdeveloped countries where patients with cataract tend to present late.
- Cataract either mature (white) or hypermature (liquid cortex and free-floating nucleus)

RISK FACTORS
Elderly patient with advanced cataract

GENERAL PREVENTION
Removal of cataract before it has advanced or liquefaction has occurred.

PATHOPHYSIOLOGY
- Macrophagic response to heavy molecular weight (HMW) lens proteins that have leaked from a hypermature cataract
- Obstruction of the trabecular meshwork with HMW proteins that have leaked from the mature cataract
- Macrophages distended with engulfed lens material are found in the trabecular meshwork; however, it is now largely believed that the HMW proteins are the cause of a high intraocular pressure (IOP). The macrophagic response is associated but not causative of the glaucoma.

ETIOLOGY
Mature cataract or hypermature cataract, which is leaking HMW lens protein through an intact capsule.

COMMONLY ASSOCIATED CONDITIONS
- Uveitis is associated with the leakage of lens protein.
- Open-angle glaucoma is related to the obstruction of the trabecular meshwork by HMW lens proteins.

DIAGNOSIS

HISTORY
- Hypermature cataract with elevated IOP and white material in the anterior chamber
- History of gradually diminishing vision over months or years and recent red, painful eye

PHYSICAL EXAM
- Usually unilateral
- Redness, pain
- Elevated IOP
- Diffuse corneal edema
- Intense cell and flare in the anterior chamber
- Iridescent or hyperrefringent particles in both lens and aqueous
- White material aggregates in the anterior chamber. In the presence of a mature cataract
- Keratic precipitates are not seen.
- Fellow eye usually has a deep chamber and a mature cataract.

DIAGNOSTIC TESTS & INTERPRETATION

Lab

Initial lab tests

Aqueous aspiration for histologic examination

Imaging

Initial approach
- B-scan ultrasound to ensure that there is no other concomitant ocular pathology
- Aggressive control of inflammation and IOP

Follow-up & special considerations

Frequent follow-up until definitive treatment is implemented, which involves removal of the inciting cataract.

Diagnostic Procedures/Other
Needle aspirate of the anterior chamber fluid and examination of the sample for macrophages laden with eosinophilic lenticular material.

DIFFERENTIAL DIAGNOSIS
- Phacoanaphylactic glaucoma
- Lens particle glaucoma
- Exacerbation of prior uveitis
- Endophthalmitis

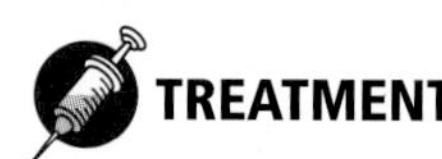

TREATMENT

MEDICATION

First Line
- Topical steroid therapy to reduce inflammation
- Antiglaucoma therapy to control IOP: with hyperosmotics, topical carbonic anhydrase inhibitors, topical beta-blockers, and alpha-2 agonists

ADDITIONAL TREATMENT

Issues for Referral
Retina consultation and referral may be necessary, if there is associated cystoid macular edema related to the uveitis.

Additional Therapies
- Once the cataract is removed, the uveitis is usually easier to control and steroid therapy should be tapered.
- IOP must be monitored and treatment instituted if open-angle glaucoma persists.

SURGERY/OTHER PROCEDURES
- Surgical removal of the inciting cataract, the source of the HMW proteins, and wash out of proteinaceous material from the anterior chamber
- Most often cataract removal is curative and no further surgery is needed.
- If the IOP remains elevated after surgical removal of the cataract and open-angle glaucoma is uncontrolled then glaucoma filtering surgery may be indicated.

IN-PATIENT CONSIDERATIONS
Initial Stabilization
Admission and intravenous mannitol may be necessary to control IOP until definitive surgery.

Discharge Criteria
Once the IOP is controlled, the patient may be discharged with close follow-up appointments.

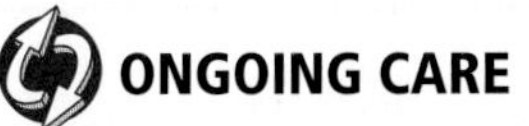

ONGOING CARE

FOLLOW-UP RECOMMENDATIONS
Very close follow-up during the initial postoperative period is warranted to manage the uveitis and IOP.

Patient Monitoring
- Once the IOP and uveitis are controlled lifelong IOP monitoring and treatment are necessary for open-angle glaucoma.
- 3–6-month intervals depending on the severity of disease

PATIENT EDUCATION
The physiology of glaucoma and the importance of adherence to medication should be discussed.

PROGNOSIS
- Eyes with poor vision, even light perception without projection, often obtain good vision after treatment.
- The prognosis depends on the prompt treatment of the uveitis and glaucoma.

COMPLICATIONS
- Vision loss secondary to glaucoma or uveitis, that is, cystoid macular edema
- Surgical complications of complex cataract surgery and/or glaucoma filtering surgery

ADDITIONAL READING

- Allingham RR, Damji KF, Freedman S, et al. *Shields textbook of glaucoma*, 5th Ed. Philadelphia: Lippincott Williams & Wilkins, 2004.
- Ellant JP, Obstbaum SA. Lens-induced glaucoma. *Ophthalmology* 1992;81:317–338.
- Epstein DL. Diagnosis and management of lens-induced glaucoma. *Am Acad Ophthalmol* 1982;89(3):227–230.

CODES

ICD9
- 364.3 Unspecified iridocyclitis
- 365.11 Open-angle glaucoma
- 365.51 Phacolytic glaucoma

CLINICAL PEARLS

Suspect in patients with mature, white, or liquefied cataract

PHACOMORPHIC GLAUCOMA

Rachel M. Niknam

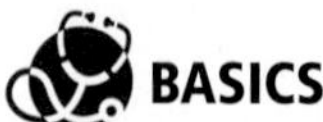

BASICS

DESCRIPTION

Swelling of a cataractous lens causing a pupillary block mechanism of angle closure.

EPIDEMIOLOGY

- Elderly patient with advanced cataract
- More common in underdeveloped countries where patients with cataract tend to present late

RISK FACTORS

Shallow anterior chamber—the shorter axial length of the globe and greater axial lens thickness predispose an eye to phacomorphic glaucoma

GENERAL PREVENTION

- Prophylactic laser iridotomy
- Cataract extraction

PATHOPHYSIOLOGY

- The mechanism of phacomorphic glaucoma is that of angle-closure glaucoma from a relative pupillary block.
- As the cataract advances, the lens assumes a greater thickness and curvature to the anterior surface. This causes a shallow anterior chamber as well as greater iridolenticular touch.
- Aqueous fluid continues to be produced causing a rise in the posterior chamber pressure causing the lens iris diaphragm to move forward furthering the rise in intraocular pressure (IOP).
- If the anterior forces are sufficient, the iris will contact the peripheral cornea and an acute angle closure will occur.

ETIOLOGY

- Mature cataract
- Traumatic cataract
- Lens swelling from systemic medications
  - Diuretics
  - Hemorrhagic fever with renal syndrome
- Miotics constrict the pupil resulting in zonule laxity and forward movement of the lens.

COMMONLY ASSOCIATED CONDITIONS

- Hyperopia
- Miotics—increase zonular laxity causing forward movement of the lens
- Anticholinergics and sympathomimetics cause the pupils to dilate increasing iridolenticular touch especially in the mid dilated state.

DIAGNOSIS

HISTORY

- History of gradually diminishing vision over months or years and recent red, painful eye accompanied with headache, halos around lights, and nausea or vomiting
- History of previous subacute attacks usually at night or in dim illumination.

PHYSICAL EXAM

- Redness
- Diffuse corneal edema
- Shallow anterior chamber
- Mature cataract
- Angle closure
- Elevated IOP
- Cell and flare in the anterior chamber
- Fellow eye usually has a somewhat deeper chamber and a mature cataract as well

DIAGNOSTIC TESTS & INTERPRETATION

Imaging

B-scan ultrasound to ensure that there is no mass or other ocular pathology posterior to the lens.

Initial approach

Aggressive control of inflammation and IOP in preparation for laser or surgical iridectomy

Follow-up & special considerations

- Frequent follow-up and IOP management until definitive treatment is implemented
- Laser iridotomy may close secondary to the subluxated lens, and the preferred definitive treatment is removal of the inciting cataract.

DIFFERENTIAL DIAGNOSIS

- Angle closure secondary to intraocular tumors
- Lens particle glaucoma
- Phacolytic glaucoma
- Uveitic glaucoma

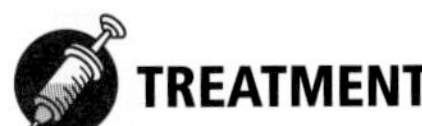

TREATMENT

MEDICATION

- Antiglaucoma therapy to control IOP: with hyperosmotics, topical carbonic anhydrase inhibitors, topical beta-blockers and alpha-2 agonists; topical steroid therapy to reduce inflammation
- Laser iridotomy
- Surgical iridectomy

ADDITIONAL TREATMENT

General Measures

Definitive treatment: Removal of the mature cataract

Issues for Referral

- Uncontrolled open-angle glaucoma or closed-angle glaucoma may necessitate glaucoma filtering surgery.
- Chronic angle-closure glaucoma may persist if there is synechial closure of the angle.
- Alternatively open-angle glaucoma may be present as a result of prior angle closure resulting in a reduction in outflow facility of the trabecular meshwork.

Additional Therapies

Once the cataract is removed IOP must be monitored and treatment instituted if glaucoma persists.

SURGERY/OTHER PROCEDURES

- Most often cataract removal is curative and no further surgery is needed.
- If the IOP remains elevated after surgical removal of the cataract and glaucoma is uncontrolled then glaucoma filtering surgery may be indicated.

IN-PATIENT CONSIDERATIONS

Initial Stabilization

Admission and IV mannitol may be necessary to control IOP until definitive surgery

Discharge Criteria

Once the IOP and inflammation is controlled, the patient may be discharged with close follow-up appointments.

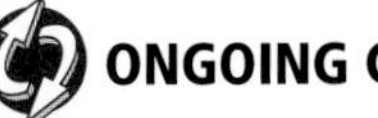

ONGOING CARE

FOLLOW-UP RECOMMENDATIONS

Very close follow-up during the initial postoperative period is warranted to manage the IOP and inflammation.

Patient Monitoring

- Once the IOP is controlled, lifelong IOP monitoring and treatment are necessary for glaucoma.
- 3–6-month intervals depending on the severity of disease

PATIENT EDUCATION

The physiology of glaucoma and the importance of adherence to medication should be discussed.

PROGNOSIS

- Eyes with poor vision, even light perception, often obtain good vision after treatment.
- The prognosis depends on the prompt treatment of glaucoma and success of the, often difficult, cataract surgery.

COMPLICATIONS

- Vision loss secondary to glaucoma
- Vision loss secondary to surgical complications either from the complex cataract surgery (i.e., zonular dialysis, iris prolapse, vitreous loss, or corneal endothelial injury) or from glaucoma filtering surgery

ADDITIONAL READING

- Allingham RR, Damji KF, Freedman S, et al. *Shields textbook of glaucoma*, 5th ed. Philadelphia: Lippincott Williams & Wilkins, 2004.
- Lee SJL, Lee CKL, Kim WS. Long-term therapeutic efficacy of phacoemulsification with intraocular lens implantation in patients with phacomorphic glaucoma. *J Cataract and Refract Surg* 2010;36: 783–789.
- Ellant JP, Obstbaum SA. Lens-induced glaucoma. *Ophthalmology* 1992;81:317–338.
- Epstein DL. Diagnosis and management of lens-induced glaucoma. *Am Acad Ophthalmol* 1982;89(3):227–230.

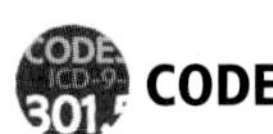

CODES

ICD9

Lens-induced angle closure one must use the primary diagnosis of cataract either:

- 365.20 Primary angle-closure glaucoma, unspecified
- 365.59 Glaucoma associated with other lens disorders

CLINICAL PEARLS

- Suspect in patients with mature cataract and hyperopia

PHLYCTENULAR KERATOCONJUNCTIVITIS

Vasudha A. Panday

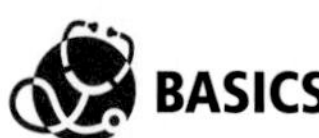

BASICS

DESCRIPTION

- Uncommon, usually unilateral, affects conjunctiva and/or cornea
- Seen more commonly in children and young adults
- Due to type IV hypersensitivity reaction to microbial agents
- Pinkish-white nodule at limbus involving conjunctiva and/or cornea

EPIDEMIOLOGY

Incidence

60–70% female

Prevalence

Unknown

RISK FACTORS

Blepharitis

Genetics

None

GENERAL PREVENTION

Treat blepharitis: lid scrubs

PATHOPHYSIOLOGY

Delayed type hypersensitivity to bacterial antigen

ETIOLOGY

- Staphylococcal infection
- Tuberculosis
- *Chlamydia*, *Candida*, *Coccidioides*

COMMONLY ASSOCIATED CONDITIONS

Blepharitis

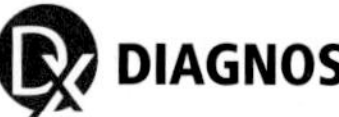

DIAGNOSIS

HISTORY

- Pain, photophobia, tearing, foreign body sensation, redness
  - If cornea involved, symptoms more severe

PHYSICAL EXAM

- Conjunctival phlycten: small, round, elevated, yellow to white nodule near limbus
- Corneal phlycten: starts at limbus, can extend onto cornea, may have associated epithelial defect

DIAGNOSTIC TESTS & INTERPRETATION

Lab

Chest X-ray (CXR), purified protein derivative (PPD) if suspicious of tuberculosis (1)[C]

Imaging

CXR, PPD in suspicious cases

Diagnostic Procedures/Other

Corneal cultures if infectious keratitis suspected (1)[C]

Pathological Findings

Histopathology shows that nodules are composed of lymphocytes, histiocytes, and plasma cells.

DIFFERENTIAL DIAGNOSIS

- Rosacea keratitis
- Inflamed pinguecula
- Limbal herpes keratitis
- Microbial keratitis
- Nodular episcleritis

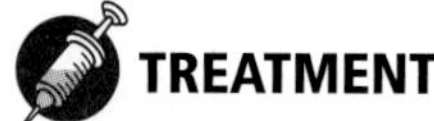

TREATMENT

MEDICATION

First Line

Treat underlying blepharitis: lid scrubs, artificial tears, antibiotic ointment (erythromycin or bacitracin) 4 times a day

Second Line

- Short course of topical steroid–antibiotic combination 4–6 times a day
- Systemic tetracycline 250 mg q.i.d. for 2–4 weeks (2)[C]
- Topical metronidazole
- Topical antibiotics if bacterial keratitis suspected

Geriatric Considerations

Side effects of long-term topical steroid use include cataract formation and glaucoma.

Pediatric Considerations

Tetracycline contraindicated in children. Substitute erythromycin 250 mg q.i.d.

Pregnancy Considerations

- Tetracycline contraindicated in pregnant or nursing women. Substitute erythromycin 250 mg q.i.d.
- Steroids are class C and of unknown safety in lactation.

ADDITIONAL TREATMENT

General Measures

Treat tuberculosis

Issues for Referral

Recurrent or causing corneal scarring

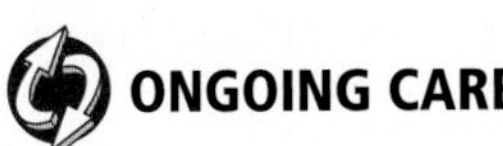

ONGOING CARE

FOLLOW-UP RECOMMENDATIONS

- Mild cases will resolve in 2–4 weeks.
- Follow patient weekly.

PATIENT MONITORING

If cornea involved, monitor for scarring or epithelial defect leading to melting.

PATIENT EDUCATION

Long-term treatment of blepharitis with lid scrubs, artificial tears, and ointment to prevent recurrence

PROGNOSIS

Overall good; if severe, may have residual corneal scarring leading to decreased vision.

COMPLICATIONS

Corneal scarring, decreased vision

REFERENCES

1. Robin JB, Schanzin DJ, Verity SM, et al. Peripheral cornea disorders. *Surv Ophthalmol* 1986;31:1–36.
2. Abu el-Asrar AM, Tabbara KF. Tetracycline treatment of phlyctenulosis. *Ophthalmology* 1994;101:1161–1162.

ADDITIONAL READING

- Mozayeni RM, Lam S. Phlyctenular keratoconjunctivitis and marginal staphylococcal keratitis. In: *Cornea: fundamentals, diagnosis, and management*, Krachmer JH, Mannis MJ, Holland EJ, eds. Vol. 1. Philadelphia: Elsevier Mosby, 2005: 1235–1240.

See Also (Topic, Algorithm, Electronic Media Element)

Blepharitis

CODES

ICD9

370.31 Phlyctenular keratoconjunctivitis

CLINICAL PEARLS

- Delayed type hypersensitivity reaction to bacterial antigen
- Can involve conjunctiva or cornea
- Treatment of underlying blepharitis will help resolve lesion in many cases.
- Corneal involvement can lead to scarring and decreased vision in severe cases.

PIGMENTARY GLAUCOMA

Shelly R. Gupta
Jonathan S. Myers

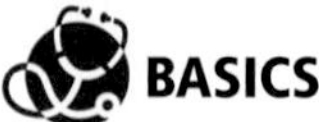

BASICS

DESCRIPTION
- Pigment dispersion syndrome (PDS) is a disorder characterized by the release of pigment particles from the pigment epithelium of the iris. These pigment particles are carried by the aqueous humor and deposited on the structures of the anterior segment.
- Pigmentary glaucoma (PG) is a secondary open-angle glaucoma, occurring in one third of patients with PDS. Released iris pigment interferes with trabecular meshwork function, leading to elevated intraocular pressure (IOP) and an optic neuropathy.

EPIDEMIOLOGY
Incidence
- Approximately one third of patients with PDS will go on to develop PG over 15 years.
- Conversion from the syndrome to glaucoma is less frequent as age increases into the 40s and 50s, and in some cases, the glaucoma may regress over time.

Prevalence
- Constitutes 1–2.5% of all glaucoma seen in most Western countries
- Can be detected as early as the mid-teen years of life
- Peak prevalence 3rd and 4th decades of life

RISK FACTORS
- Most often seen in young adults—can be diagnosed in adolescents and in older individuals
- Caucasians—rarely seen in Asians and African Americans
- Male gender—possibly due to increased chamber depth as compared with females
- Myopia—present in 80% of individuals with PDS

Genetics
PDS is thought to be autosomal dominant with incomplete penetrance. At least one genetic locus has been identified on chromosome 7q.

PATHOPHYSIOLOGY
- Mechanical:
  - A posterior bowing of the peripheral iris induces recurrent contact between the iris pigment epithelium and the lens zonules, leading to a dispersion of pigment.
    - Posterior iris bowing may be from a posterior iris insertion to the sclera, a concave profile in the setting of a deeper than normal anterior chamber, and/or a floppy iris stroma.
    - A posteriorly directed pressure gradient can trigger this phenomenon, such as blinking or reverse pupillary block seen with iris–lens contact, accommodation, and exercise.
  - Long anterior zonular fibers inserted onto the central lens capsule may also cause mechanical disruption of the pigment epithelium at the central iris, leading to pigment dispersion.
- Genetic and environmental conditions leading to weakness of the iris pigment epithelium.
- As affected individuals age, many patients experience a decrease in pigment dispersion.
  - Increased pupillary miosis and cataract formation cause an increase in relative pupillary block. This permits accumulation of aqueous within the posterior chamber and increases the distance between the zonule fibers and the iris.

ETIOLOGY
- Certain conditions have been found to exacerbate the dispersion of pigment:
  - Accommodation, jarring physical exercise, emotional stress, and naturally occurring or drug-induced mydriasis

COMMONLY ASSOCIATED CONDITIONS
- PDS
- Myopia

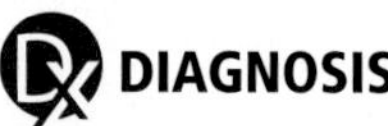

DIAGNOSIS

HISTORY
- Like many open-angle glaucomas, PG is usually asymptomatic. Thus, diagnosis is often made on routine exam.
- Most often bilateral in nature
- Conditions triggering an acute dispersion of pigment (exercise, accommodation, prolonged dark environment, etc.), can lead to an acute rise in IOP, with resultant symptoms.
  - Haloes around lights, ocular pain, and blurred vision from corneal edema

PHYSICAL EXAM
- On slit lamp exam, pigment may be seen on numerous structures throughout the anterior ocular segment.
  - Increased anterior chamber depth with visible melanin granules in the aqueous
  - Aqueous convection currents cause released pigment to deposit in a vertical fashion, slightly decentered inferiorly, on the corneal endothelium (*Krukenberg spindle*). The pigment is then phagocytized by corneal endothelial cells. This spindle is neither pathognomonic nor invariably present.
  - Radial midperipheral slit-like iris defects seen on retroillumination or transillumination—corresponds to location of iris–zonule contact (best seen using a small slit beam, in a dark room, prior to patient dilation)
  - Open anterior chamber angle with increased pigmentation of the trabecular meshwork 360° and pigment deposition anterior to Schwalbe's line (*Sampaolesi's line*), in the inferior 180°
  - Pigment inside a glaucoma filtering bleb
  - Pigment deposition in circumferential iris furrows. This can lead to iris heterochromia if the disease is asymmetric between the two eyes (with the darker iris being the more affected side).
  - Anisocoria—larger pupil is on the side with the greater iris transillumination.
    - Combination of iris heterochromia and anisocoria may mimic Horner syndrome.
  - Pigment deposition on the posterior lens surface at the site of zonular attachments (*Zentmayer's ring* or *Scheie's line*)
  - Pigment granules on the lens zonular fibers and equatorial region seen in mydriasis
    - In contrast to pseudoexfoliation glaucoma, this pigment deposition does not seem to lead to zonular weakness.
- A concave appearance of the peripheral iris seen on slit lamp exam and gonioscopy.
- On peripheral retinal examination, lattice degeneration or retinal breaks may be seen.

DIAGNOSTIC TESTS & INTERPRETATION
Imaging
Initial approach
- Ultrasound biomicroscopy (UBM) analysis (optional)—provides high-resolution imaging of anterior and posterior chamber anatomy.
  - Concave profile of the peripheral iris with iridozonular contact
  - Reverse pupillary block
  - Longer than usual radial iris length leading to iris flattening on the anterior lens surface (iridolenticular contact)
  - Increased anterior chamber depth
  - Posterior iris insertion
- Slit lamp optical coherence tomography (optional)—may be used to assess the parameters of the anterior chamber and angle dimensions.

Diagnostic Procedures/Other
- Gonioscopy—increased pigmentation of the anterior chamber angle 360°
- Transillumination/retroillumination—visualize midperipheral iris defects
- Diurnal curve measurements—diurnal curve fluctuations are thought to occur more often in PG and can lead to acute symptomatic elevations in IOP.

Pathological Findings
- Pigment and debris in the trabecular meshwork cells.
  - Trabecular meshwork cells engulf the pigment and eventually detach from the trabecular beams, leading to sclerosis and eventual fusion of the intratrabecular spaces.
- The cul-de-sacs, which normally terminate in aqueous channels, are reduced, contributing to increased resistance to aqueous outflow.
- Atrophy and hypopigmentation of the iris pigment epithelium
- Hyperplasia of the iris dilator muscle

DIFFERENTIAL DIAGNOSIS
- Pseudoexfoliation glaucoma—differs by pseudoexfoliative material on the anterior lens and pupillary border. No myopic predilection, older age, and 50% of cases are unilateral. Iris transillumination characteristically begins at the pupillary border rather than the midperiphery. Darker and less homogenous pigment deposition in meshwork.
- Primary open-angle glaucoma with increased trabecular meshwork pigmentation. Often see patchy pigment band in angle, older age.

P

- Cysts of the iris and ciliary body, typically unilateral
- Pigmented neoplasms of the iris–ciliary body complex—will not see Krukenberg spindle or midperipheral transillumination defects. May see narrowing of the angle at the area of neoplasm.
- Iris chafing syndrome—misplacement of posterior chamber intraocular lens leading to haptics rubbing the posterior iris
- Uveitis—careful examination for keratic precipitates on corneal endothelium and lack of pigment deposition on other anterior segment tissues, greater pigmentation inferiorly
- Previous surgery or trauma—obtain thorough history. Iris transillumination, if present, usually more confluent and/or segmental.

TREATMENT

MEDICATION

First Line

- Medical therapy directed at lowering IOP:
  - Aqueous suppressant drops—beta-blockers, α-agonist, carbonic anhydrase inhibitors
  - Aqueous outflow enhancing drops—prostaglandin analogues
    - Iris surface color change seen with the use of prostaglandin analogues is due to increased melanin production by iris melanocytes. This is not known to affect the iris pigment epithelium or result in increased pigment dispersion.

Second Line

- Cholinergic agents (pilocarpine)—lowers IOP by both increasing aqueous outflow at the trabecular meshwork and by pulling the iris away from zonular fibers, leading to reduced pigment release.
  - Pilocarpine has been found to be effective in inhibiting exercise-induced pigment dispersion and resultant increase in IOP.
  - Especially in young patients, miotics may induce headaches, blurred vision, or increase the risk of retinal detachment.
  - In this setting, thymoxamine, an α-adrenergic antagonist that constricts the pupil without inducing a myopic shift, may be considered. Note: Thymoxamine is not available in all parts of the world.
  - Ocusert, a low-dose pilocarpine, has also been found to provide enough miosis to create pupillary block, without the disabling adverse effects.
  - Note: Headaches, myopic shift, and the risk of retinal detachment limit the use of pilocarpine in this condition.
- Laser trabeculoplasty
  - Laser treatment is effective but not always lasting. Treatment effect may be reduced in degree or duration in younger patients. Energy must be reduced as high TM pigment absorption of laser energy may lead to IOP spikes.

ADDITIONAL TREATMENT

Issues for Referral

- In cases of uncertain diagnosis, referral to a glaucoma specialist is indicated.
- Consider referral to a retinal specialist for dilated peripheral retinal exam if concerns arise for retinal degeneration or retinal detachment.

SURGERY/OTHER PROCEDURES

- Surgery is indicated when maximal medical therapy fails and there is concern for optic nerve damage.
  - Laser trabeculoplasty—often requires lower laser power (ALT: 200–600 mW, SLT: 0.4–0.7 mJ), as the increased trabecular meshwork pigment absorbs energy readily.
  - Laser peripheral iridotomy—relieves reverse pupillary block and may reduce iris chafe and pigment release (remains controversial).
- Incisional surgery is indicated when both medications and laser fail to control IOP.
  - Filtering surgery—use antimetabolites cautiously as patients may be young and myopic, thus more prone to hypotony maculopathy.

ONGOING CARE

FOLLOW-UP RECOMMENDATIONS

- PDS—periodic evaluation for the development of PG
- PG—follow-up is similar to other types of open-angle glaucoma.
  - IOP measurement before and after dilation
  - Visual field testing
  - Evaluation of optic nerve appearance
  - Pachymetry—to measure central corneal thickness
  - Gonioscopy—to access the degree and progression of trabecular pigmentation
- Dilated exam of peripheral retina—increased incidence of myopia, peripheral retinal degeneration, and risk of retinal detachment
- Visual field and optic nerve status evaluation or imaging yearly

Patient Monitoring

- Annually in pigment dispersion; every 3–6 months in PG. Increased frequency depending on the severity of the disease.
- Frequency of follow-up may decrease with aging if pigment liberation ceases or trabecular pigmentation begins to diminish.

PATIENT EDUCATION

- Educate patients on the importance of long-term follow-up and treatment to prevent irreversible optic neuropathy and associated vision loss.
- Signs and symptoms of acute IOP elevation–haloes around lights, blurry vision, ocular pain
- Warning signs and symptoms of retinal detachment, including flashes, floaters, and decrease in vision

PROGNOSIS

- Prognosis is good with regular follow-up and careful control of IOP.
- Uncontrolled disease can lead to elevated IOP, optic nerve cupping, and visual field loss.
- Success rates of filtering surgery are similar to other forms of open-angle glaucoma at comparable age levels.
- Over time, a "burn out," phase often occurs—pigment begins clearing from the iris surface, trabecular meshwork, corneal endothelium, iris defects disappear, and IOP decreases. Visual field and optic nerve appearance stabilize.
  - As the pigment clears from the trabecular meshwork, the pigment band is darker superiorly more than inferiorly (pigment reversal sign).
  - May be attributable to age-related increase in axial length of the lens, which pulls the peripheral iris away from the zonules
  - This phase does not occur invariably, most patients require lifelong therapy.

COMPLICATIONS

Patients have a higher incidence of lattice degeneration, retinal breaks, and rhegmatogenous retinal detachment. Retinal detachment may occur in as many as 6–7% of individuals.

Geriatric Considerations

This condition most typically manifests in early to mid adulthood.

Pediatric Considerations

This condition is very uncommon at ages below 20 years.

Pregnancy Considerations

Most medications used to treat PG are pregnancy class C: studies have shown risks to the fetus in animal models.

REFERENCES

1. Sugar HS, Barbour FA. Pigmentary glaucoma: a rare clinical entity. *Am J Ophthalmol* 1949;32:90.
2. Campbell DG. Pigmentary dispersion and glaucoma. A new theory. *Arch Ophthalmol* 1979;97(9):1667–1672.
3. Migliazzo CV, Shaffer RN, Nykin R, et al. Long-term analysis of pigmentary dispersion syndrome and pigmentary glaucoma. *Ophthalmology* 1986;93:1528.
4. Lichter PR, Shaffer RN. Diagnostic and prognostic signs in pigmentary glaucoma. *Trans Am Acad Ophthalmol Otolaryngol* 1970;74(5):984–998.
5. Campbell DG, Schertzer RM. Pathophysiology of pigment dispersion syndrome and pigmentary glaucoma. *Curr Opin Ophthalmol* 1995;6(2):96–101.

ADDITIONAL READING

- Ritch R, Barkana Y. Glaucoma, pigmentary, eMedicine, Feb 17 2010.http://emedicine.medscape.com/article/1205833-overview.
- Shaaraway TM, et al. *Pigmentary glaucoma*, Vol. 1. Saunders Elsevier Limited, 2009;29:349–360.
- Shields MB, Allingham RR, et al. *Shields' textbook of glaucoma*. 5th ed. Philadelphia: Lippincott Williams & Wilkins, 2005;17:303–311.
- Stamper RL, Lieberman MF, Drake MV. *Becker-Shaffer's diagnosis and therapy of the glaucomas*, 8th ed. St. Louis, MO: Mosby Elsevier, 2009;18:266–268.

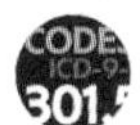

CODES

ICD9

365.13 Pigmentary open-angle glaucoma

CLINICAL PEARLS

- Typical patient: young, myopic, male
- "Burn out," phase of PG may be mistaken for normal tension glaucoma. Older patients who have optic nerve cupping, visual field loss, and normal IOP may have had PG and elevated IOP in the past.

PLAQUENIL TOXICITY/DRUG TOXICITIES

Jared D. Peterson

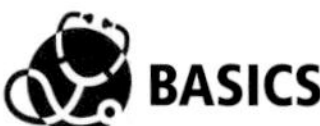

BASICS

DESCRIPTION

- Chloroquine and hydroxychloroquine (HCQ) (Plaquenil), drugs used to treat malaria and various dermatologic and inflammatory conditions - such as lupus and rheumatoid arthritis, can cause a maculopathy.
- Because of a lesser degree of retinotoxicity, HCQ has largely replaced chloroquine in the United States.

EPIDEMIOLOGY

Incidence

- Reported anywhere from 0 to 4%, with most reports citing an incidence of less than 1%
- Less than 50 cases reported from 1960 to 2005 (1)

RISK FACTORS

- Daily dose
  - This is the most important risk factor. Nearly all reports of toxicity have occurred in those taking greater than 6.5 mg/kg/day of HCQ and greater than 3 mg/kg/day of chloroquine (2).
- Duration of treatment
  - Reports of retinal toxicity at doses lower than 6.5 mg/kg/day have occurred almost universally in patients with more than 5 years of continuous usage (2).
- Age
  - Malfunction of retinal pigment in the elderly may result in reduced drug clearance with increased accumulation (1).
  - One case series of 47 patients showed that none of 9 patients younger than 60 years manifested retinopathy, whereas 13 patients older than 60 years did (3).
- Obesity
  - Antimalarials do not accumulate in fat, which is why ideal body weight should be used in calculating dosages.
- Hepatic/renal failure
  - Both chloroquine and HCQ are cleared via hepatic and renal pathways, with failure of either system potentially resulting in toxicity.
- Cumulative dose
  - Initially believed to be the most important risk factor but there are reports of patients with no retinopathy despite very high cumulative doses of drug (3).

GENERAL PREVENTION

Absolute prevention requires avoidance of the drug; however, risk is extremely low when taking appropriate doses.

PATHOPHYSIOLOGY

- The mechanism of maculopathy is not well understood; however, it is known that both agents bind to melanin in the retinal pigment epithelium (RPE) (2), where they affect RPE metabolism, including its function of scavenging shed outer photoreceptor segments. This may in turn lead to photoreceptor degeneration.
  - HCQ demonstrates less ocular toxicity due to the presence of the hydroxyl group, which renders it less able to traverse the blood–retinal barrier (1).

ETIOLOGY

Use of chloroquine or HCQ

COMMONLY ASSOCIATED CONDITIONS

In addition to retinopathy, these drugs are associated with intraepithelial corneal deposits, ciliary body involvement with impaired accommodation, and cataracts. These are less common with HCQ compared with chloroquine.

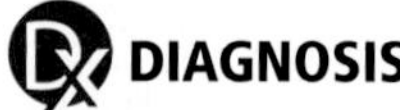

DIAGNOSIS

HISTORY

Symptoms can range anywhere from severe to asymptomatic. Most patients describe: decreased vision, blurry vision, difficulty reading, missing central vision, glare, light flashes, or metamorphopsia (1).

PHYSICAL EXAM

- Visual field testing
  - Central visual field testing is the most important test for early diagnosis as functional loss in the area around the macula may appear prior to funduscopic changes.
  - Defect begins as paracentral scotoma that may progress to confluence as a pericentral ring scotoma "bull's eye" and finally a central scotoma.
  - Peripheral loss occurs in advanced stages.
- Visual acuity testing
  - Acuity defect does not typically manifest until a central scotoma occurs.
- Funduscopic examination
  - In early, "premaculopathy" stages, the earliest visible signs of toxicity may include macular stippling and loss of foveal reflex.
  - True maculopathy shows hyperpigmentation of the macula surrounded by a clear zone of depigmentation, which is surrounded by another ring of hyperpigmentation, giving the classic "bull's eye" appearance.
  - More extensive damage may show diffuse RPE atrophy over the entire fundus as well as vascular attenuation and disk pallor (1).
  - Findings are almost always bilateral and symmetric.
- Funduscopic photography is used to document fundus appearance for later comparison.
- Color vision is not usually affected until later in disease course. Baseline screening of males is helpful to discern preexisting color deficits.

DIAGNOSTIC TESTS & INTERPRETATION

Imaging

Fluorescein angiography may not be helpful early as in early toxicity the subtle macular changes precede angiographic alterations (1).

Diagnostic Procedures/Other

- Electrophysiologic testing
  - Electroretinogram (ERG) and electrooculogram (EOG) will show abnormalities in late toxicity and are helpful to assess extent of damage but have little role in screening for early toxicity.
  - Multifocal ERG (mfERG) is newer technology that may be better able to detect a bull's eye maculopathy; however, its role as a screening test remains unclear (2).
  - Optical Coherence Tomography (OCT) can demonstrate "flying saucer" sign.

Pathological Findings

- Widespread destruction of rods/cones and the outer nuclear layer, with relative foveal sparing
- Migration of pigment from the RPE in the form of large pigment-laden cells has been reported in both the inner (4) and the outer (5) nuclear layer.
  - Arteriolar narrowing in more advanced stages

DIFFERENTIAL DIAGNOSIS

- HCQ toxicity must be distinguished from cone dystrophy, cone-rod dystrophies, Stargardt's disease, chronic macular hole, neuronal ceroid lipofuscinosis, and fenestrated sheen macular dystrophy.
- Premaculopathy must be distinguished from age-related macular degeneration (ARMD).

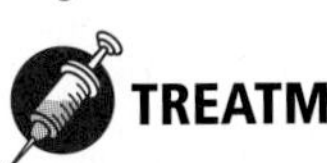

TREATMENT

ADDITIONAL TREATMENT

General Measures

- Cessation of the offending agent is critical. However, cessation of HCQ should be performed in conjunction with the internist or rheumatologist.
- Use ideal instead of actual body weight in calculating daily dose requirement.
- Ideal body weight for males = 50 kg + 2.3 kg/inch over 5 ft. For females = 45.5 kg + 2.3 kg/inch over 5 ft (1).

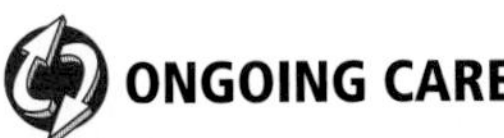

ONGOING CARE

FOLLOW-UP RECOMMENDATIONS

- The American Academy of Ophthalmology (AAO) prepared a consensus recommendation as follows (2):
  - Within the first year of beginning therapy, all patients should have a baseline examination that includes visual acuity testing, dilated examination of cornea/retina, as well as central visual field testing using either red Amsler grid or Humphrey Visual Field 10-2 perimetry. Color vision testing, fundus photography, fluorescein angiography, and multifocal ERG are considered optional. Autofluorescence testing was not widely available but may also be considered.
  - Each patient should be risk stratified as either high risk or low risk. A patient is high risk if they have: (1) a daily dose exceeding above recommendations, (2) duration of use more than 5 years, (3) obesity, (4) renal or liver disease, (5) concomitant retinal disease, or (6) age above 60 years.
  - Low-risk patients (no risk factors) should be screened at least once from age 20–29 years, at least twice from age 30–39 years, every 2–4 years for age 40–64 years, and every 1–2 years for 65 years and older. Exams should include dilated corneal/retina exams and Amsler grid or Humphrey 10-2 fields. Other tests are optional at the discretion of the physician.
  - High-risk patients should be screened annually. Exams should include the same components as in low-risk patients.
  - Patients can be given Amsler grids to use at home and all patients should be instructed to return if they note any change in vision.
  - Any patient with early toxicity should discuss drug cessation. Any patient with findings that may indicate early toxicity should be seen again in 3 months for reevaluation.

PATIENT EDUCATION

- Patient counseling is imperative.
  - Antimalarials are typically prescribed by nonophthalmologists, so patients may not be fully informed of the ocular risk at the onset of treatment. It is important to emphasize that, although rare, retinopathy is a real and potentially devastating entity.
  - Once retinopathy is suspected, a frank discussion regarding risks/benefits of continuing versus stopping the drug is important.
  - Even with drug cessation, the majority of cases show persistence or even worsening of visual symptoms.

PROGNOSIS

- Depends on the severity of the retinopathy at the time of medication cessation. If stopped in premaculopathy stages, reversal is possible and visual prognosis is good.
- If true retinopathy exists, it will likely remain stable or can continue to progress.

COMPLICATIONS

Impaired vision

REFERENCES

1. Yam JCS, Kwok AKH. Ocular toxicity of hydroxychloroquine. *Hong Kong Med J* 2006;12(4):294–304.
2. Marmor M, Carr R, Easterbrook M, et al. Recommendations on screening for chloroquine and hydroxychloroquine retinopathy. *Ophthalmology* 2002;109:1377–1382.
3. Johnson MW, Vine AK. Hydroxychloroquine therapy in massive total doses without retinal toxicity. *Am J Ophthalmol* 1987;104(2):139–144.
4. Bernstein HN, Ginsberg J. The pathology of chloroquine retinopathy. *Arch Ophthalmol* 1964;71:238–245.
5. Wetterholm DH, Winter FC. Histopathology of chloroquine retinal toxicity. *Arch Ophthalmol* 1964;71:82–87.

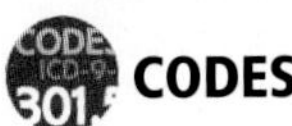

CODES

ICD9

362.55 Toxic maculopathy of retina

CLINICAL PEARLS

- Risk factors are (1) daily dose greater than 3 mg/kg of chloroquine or greater than 6.5 mg/kg of HCQ, (2) duration of treatment more than 5 years, (3) age above 60 years, (4) obesity, (5) hepatic/renal failure, (6) baseline retinal disease
- Symptoms include decreased vision, blurry vision, difficulty reading, missing central vision, glare, light flashes, and metamorphopsia.
- The classic funduscopic finding is a bilateral bull's eye maculopathy.
- Central visual field testing is the most important test for detecting early functional loss.
- If the drug is stopped in the premaculopathy stages, there is a chance of recovery; however, most patients do not recover vision or even progressively worsen after drug cessation.

PLATEAU IRIS GLAUCOMA

Arun Prasad

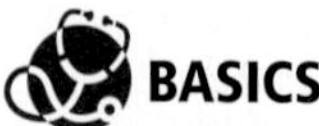

BASICS

DESCRIPTION

- A condition that predisposes to acute or chronic angle-closure glaucoma in which pupillary block is not the primary mechanism of angle closure
- Should be suspected when the central anterior chamber depth appears normal and the iris plane flat, whereas the peripheral iris is sharply convex with an anterior iris apposition, as seen on gonioscopy
- Because of angle crowding, an eye with plateau iris is predisposed to angle closure, even if there is a patent peripheral iridotomy (PI).

EPIDEMIOLOGY

Prevalence

A study in 2007 that used ultrasound biomicroscopy (UBM) to assess the presence of plateau iris found a prevalence of 32.3% in a cohort of primary angle-closure suspects.

RISK FACTORS

Patients with plateau iris tend to be female and younger (30s–50s). They also tend to be less hyperopic than those with pupillary block angle closure, and they often have a family history of angle-closure glaucoma.

PATHOPHYSIOLOGY

- Anteriorly positioned ciliary processes that push the peripheral iris anteriorly, causing angle crowding
- A component of pupillary block may be present.
- In plateau iris *configuration*, acute angle-closure glaucoma develops from only a mild degree of pupillary block; a PI is curative.
- In plateau iris *syndrome*, there is no component of pupillary block; plateau iris syndrome is present when the angle closes and intraocular pressure (IOP) rises after dilation in the absence of phacomorphic glaucoma.

ETIOLOGY

- Idiopathic
- Hyperopia is not as common in plateau iris as it is in angle closure due to pupillary block; one should consider the diagnosis of plateau iris if angle closure occurs in a younger patient with myopia.
- Peripheral iris or ciliary body cysts can cause a plateau-like iris configuration.

DIAGNOSIS

PHYSICAL EXAM

- Gonioscopy or an angle imaging technique such as UBM is necessary for diagnosis.
- The *double hump* sign seen on compression gonioscopy is strongly correlated with the presence of plateau iris.
- Relying solely on the Van Herick method of determination of angle depth will cause the examiner to miss the plateau iris configuration.
- Work-up should include slit lamp examination to check for the presence of a patent PI, IOP measurement, gonioscopy with compression, undilated optic nerve evaluation, angle imaging if available.

DIAGNOSTIC TESTS & INTERPRETATION

Imaging

- UBM
- Anterior segment optical coherence tomography (AS-OCT)

DIFFERENTIAL DIAGNOSIS

- Acute angle-closure glaucoma associated with pupillary block: decreased central anterior chamber depth, convex iris appearance
- Aqueous misdirection: diffuse shallowing of the anterior chamber, especially after cataract or glaucoma surgery
- Phacomorphic glaucoma: closure of the angle due to a large, intumescent cataract

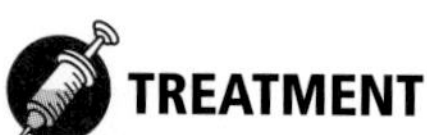

TREATMENT

MEDICATION

Pilocarpine 0.5–1% t.i.d. to q.i.d. may be used long term if plateau iris syndrome is diagnosed.

SURGERY/OTHER PROCEDURES

- If acute angle-closure glaucoma is present, break the attack medically. If an attack cannot be controlled medically, a surgical peripheral iridectomy may need to be done emergently. (See section on Acute angle-closure glaucoma.)
- If an attack can be broken medically, a laser PI should be done within 3 days. 1 week later, repeat gonioscopy and perform a dilation challenge test by instilling a weak mydriatic such as tropicamide 0.5%. If angle closure occurs and the IOP increases, plateau iris *syndrome* is present. Treatment with argon laser peripheral iridoplasty (ALPI) will flatten and thin the peripheral iris. As an alternative to ALPI, one could consider long-term treatment with pilocarpine (see above) (4)[C].
- If angle closure is not present, a laser PI should be performed to relieve the pupillary block component.

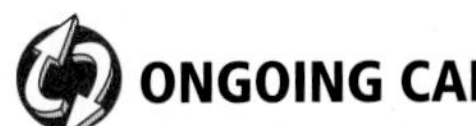

ONGOING CARE

FOLLOW-UP RECOMMENDATIONS

- If a PI has been performed for acute angle-closure glaucoma, reevaluate in 1 week, 1 month, and 3 months.
- If plateau iris configuration is present, follow-up should be done every 6 months.

Patient Monitoring

- Gonioscopy should be performed every 6 months to monitor the angle, looking for any evidence of new peripheral anterior synechiae (PAS) or if further angle narrowing has occurred, as ALPI can be done in these situations. If the angle continues to become more narrow or if more PAS form despite a patent PI, treat as chronic angle-closure glaucoma. (See section on Chronic angle-closure glaucoma.)
- In addition to gonioscopy, measure the IOP, and ensure that the PI is patent. Evaluation of the optic disc should be done.
- Every 2 years, perform dilation to ensure that the PI is adequate to prevent angle closure.
- Although ALPI is very effective in treating plateau iris syndrome and the effect maintained over several years in most patients, a small number of patients may need retreatment with ALPI.

COMPLICATIONS

Despite measures to deepen the angle recess, chronic angle closure may develop and may necessitate filtration surgery.

ADDITIONAL READING

- Crowston JG, Medeiros FA, Mosaed S, et al. Argon laser iridoplasty in the treatment of plateau-like iris configuration as result of numerous ciliary body cysts. *Am J Ophthalmol* 2005;139(2):381–383.
- Kiuchi Y, Kanamoto T, Nakamura T. Double hump sign in indentation gonioscopy is correlated with presence of plateau iris configuration regardless of patent iridotomy. *J Glaucoma* 2009;18(2): 161–164.
- Kumar RS, Baskaran M, Chew PT, et al. Prevalence of plateau iris in primary angle closure suspects: an ultrasound biomicroscopy study. *Ophthalmology* 2008;115(3):430–434.
- Ritch R, Tham CC, Lam DS. Argon laser peripheral iridoplasty (ALPI): an update. *Surv Ophthalmol* 2007;52(3):279–288.
- Ritch R, Tham CC, Lam DS. Long-term success of argon laser peripheral iridoplasty in the management of plateau iris syndrome. *Ophthalmology* 2004;111(1):104–108.

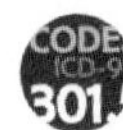

CODES

ICD9

364.82 Plateau iris syndrome

CLINICAL PEARLS

- The diagnosis of plateau iris can be made only by gonioscopy and/or anterior segment imaging.
- Consider plateau iris when a younger myope presents with angle closure.
- Remember the distinction between plateau iris *configuration* and plateau iris *syndrome*.
- ALPI is very effective in treating plateau iris syndrome.

POLYMYALGIA RHEUMATICA

Joshua J. Ney
Erin M. Ney
Lan Chen
Susan Hoch
Vatinee Y. Bunya

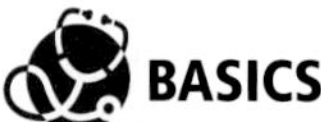

BASICS

DESCRIPTION

- Polymyalgia rheumatica (PMR) is a disease characterized by pain and stiffness of the proximal muscles and joints, primarily the shoulders, hip girdles, neck, and torso.
- Occurs in people aged 50 years and older
  - Characterized by bilateral aching and morning stiffness (lasting 30 min or more) persisting for at least 1 month
  - Also can be associated with fever, malaise, anorexia, and weight loss. Erythrocyte sedimentation rate (Westergren) is increased to 40 mm/h or more.
- Thought to be on the same clinical spectrum with giant cell arteritis (GCA, also known as temporal arteritis)

EPIDEMIOLOGY

Incidence

- Varies geographically; annual incidence ranges from 13 to 113 per 100,000 between Italy and Norway, respectively.
- In Olmsted County, Minnesota, the annual incidence was 54.8 per 100,000 population aged 50 years and older.
- Higher incidence in women and Caucasians

Prevalence

Prevalence increases with increasing age

RISK FACTORS

See "Genetics" and "Commonly Associated Conditions"

Genetics

- No definitive inheritance pattern
- Associated with HLA-DR4 and HLA-DRB1, both of which have been implicated in GCA

GENERAL PREVENTION

Awareness of the overlap between PMR and GCA, with prompt diagnosis and treatment of GCA to prevent permanent visual loss (see "Commonly Associated Conditions")

PATHOPHYSIOLOGY

- Idiopathic chronic inflammatory syndrome characterized by synovitis and bursitis
- Associated with IL-6 upregulation

ETIOLOGY

There have been no causative agents identified.

COMMONLY ASSOCIATED CONDITIONS

- GCA
  - Vasculitis of large and medium-sized vessels characterized by headache, jaw claudication (pain with chewing), scalp tenderness particularly over temporal arteries, palpable cord-like temporal artery, and visual disturbances
  - Visual phenomenon include amaurosis fugax, anterior ischemic optic neuropathy, diplopia, central retinal artery occlusion, optic chiasm, and retrochiasmal vascular damage.
  - 15% of patients with PMR develop GCA
  - 40–50% of patients with GCA have PMR

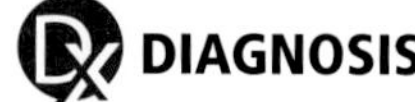

DIAGNOSIS

HISTORY

- Pain and stiffness of at least 4 weeks duration
  - Joints involved include neck, shoulders, low back, hips, thighs, and trunk.
  - Pain is usually symmetrical.
- Weight loss
- Anorexia
- Malaise
- Headache, scalp tenderness, acute visual loss

PHYSICAL EXAM

- Decreased range of motion in involved joints
- Muscle strength is normal, although testing may be limited by pain.
- Occasionally patients will have diffuse edema of hands and feet.
- If GCA is suspected, perform complete ophthalmic examination including visual acuity, pupils, color plates, visual fields, and dilated fundus examination.
  - Optic nerve evaluation often reveals pale, edematous disc sometimes with flame hemorrhages.
  - Fundus examination may reveal central retinal artery occlusion and evidence of arteritis (vascular sheathing).

DIAGNOSTIC TESTS & INTERPRETATION

Lab

Initial lab tests

- ESR
  - Greater than 40 mm/h; values can exceed 100 mm/h
- Elevated C-reactive protein (CRP)
- Normal values for both ESR and CRP are much less common, occurring in only 1.2% with PMR and/or GCA.
- Platelets: an acute phase reactant, can have thrombocytosis with GCA

Follow-up & special considerations
ESR and CRP levels should be monitored to gauge treatment efficacy and diagnose recurrence.

Diagnostic Procedures/Other
- Temporal artery biopsy
  - Obtain if there are any visual disturbances or signs or symptoms consistent with GCA.
  - If GCA is clinically suspected, do not defer treatment to attain biopsy specimen.
  - Perform the biopsy within 1 week of initiating high-dose corticosteroid treatment (see "Inpatient Considerations"), although positive biopsy results can be seen up to 1 month after treatment.

DIFFERENTIAL DIAGNOSIS
- Rheumatoid arthritis
- Fibromyalgia
- Polymyositis
- Bursitis & tendinitis
- Malignancy
- Hypothyroidism
- Infection: endocarditis

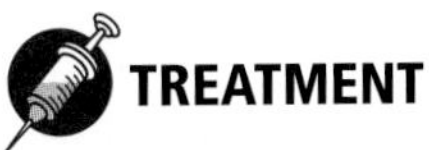

TREATMENT

MEDICATION
First Line
- Prednisone
  - No proven efficacious dose, initial goal of therapy is symptom control.
  - Usually responds to oral prednisone 7.5–20 mg/day. The initial dose of prednisone needed to alleviate musculoskeletal symptoms associated with GCA is higher at 50–60 mg/day.

Second Line
- Methotrexate
  - Can be used in patients with glucocorticoid-induced side effects
  - Dosage of 10 mg with 1 mg of folinic acid supplementation (1)

IN-PATIENT CONSIDERATIONS
Admission Criteria
- Admit if the patient has vision loss or amaurosis fugax as could be GCA and may require IV methylprednisolone.
  - While in hospital arrange for temporal artery biopsy.

IV Fluids
Typical methylprednisolone dose is 250 mg IV q6h × 12 doses then switch to oral prednisone 80–100 mg daily

Discharge Criteria
After completion of IV steroid course and temporal artery biopsy

ONGOING CARE

FOLLOW-UP RECOMMENDATIONS
- Primary care doctor
- Rheumatologist
- Ophthalmologist for evaluation and work-up of GCA

Patient Monitoring
- Prednisone should be tapered slowly once symptom control has been achieved.
  - Once a daily dose of less than 5–10 mg is achieved, reduction should not exceed 1 mg/month.
- While on prednisone, blood pressure, glycemic control, and need for calcium and vitamin D supplementation and gastric acid suppression should be evaluated by primary care physician.
- ESR and CRP should be checked, if there is clinical evidence of recurrence.

PATIENT EDUCATION
- The Arthritis Foundation (http://www.arthritis.org)
- The American College of Rheumatology (www.Rheumatology.org)

PROGNOSIS
- Generally self-limited course over months to a year
  - Most patients can be tapered off glucocorticoids

COMPLICATIONS
Developing GCA

REFERENCE

1. Caporali R, Cimmino MA, Ferraccioli G, et al. Prednisone plus methotrexate for polymyalgia rheumatica: a randomized, double-blind, placebo-controlled trial. *Ann Intern Med* 2004;141:493–500.

ADDITIONAL READING

- Salvarani C, Cantini F, Boiardi L, et al. Polymyalgia rheumatica. *Best Pract Res Clin Rheumatol* 2004;18:705–722.
- Frearson R, Cassidy T, Newton J. Polymyalgia rheumatica and temporal arteritis: Evidence and guidelines for diagnosis and management in older people. *Age Ageing* 2003;32:370–374.

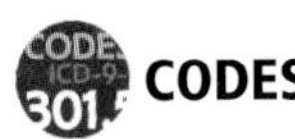

CODES

ICD9
- 362.34 Transient retinal arterial occlusion
- 377.41 Ischemic optic neuropathy
- 725 Polymyalgia rheumatica

CLINICAL PEARLS
- Proximal muscle tenderness and stiffness in patients older than 50 years
- High ESR and CRP
- Association with GCA
- Good response to prednisone

POSNER–SCHLOSSMAN SYNDROME (GLAUCOMATOCYCLITIC CRISIS)

Geoffrey P. Schwartz

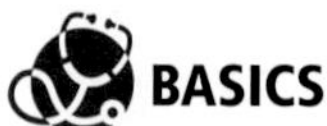

BASICS

DESCRIPTION

- Posner–Schlossman syndrome, also known as glaucomatocyclitic crisis, is a form of open-angle glaucoma characterized by self-limited recurrent episodes of marked elevation in intraocular pressure (IOP) associated with nongranulomatous anterior uveitis. It is typically unilateral, with attacks lasting a few hours to several weeks. Mild to no discomfort. Optic nerve damage and visual field damage may occur from repeated attacks (1)[C].

EPIDEMIOLOGY

Typically affects patients between 20 and 50 years of age. Rare cases have been reported in adolescence and patients older than 60 years.

Incidence

- No study in the US
- 0.4 (per 100,000) in Finland

Prevalence

- No study in the US
- 1.9 (per 100,000) in Finland

RISK FACTORS

See "Etiology."

ETIOLOGY

Unclear, however significantly elevated levels of several entities have been found in the aqueous humor of patients during recurring attacks of Posner–Schlossman syndrome and normalize between episodes:

- Cytomegalovirus (CMV)
- Herpes simplex virus (HSV)
- Prostaglandins
- Associations with HLA-Bw54
- Associations with peptic ulcer disease

COMMONLY ASSOCIATED CONDITIONS

Unclear. See "Etiology"

DIAGNOSIS

HISTORY

The patient presents complaining of mild discomfort and blurring of vision or colored halos in 1 eye. However, there may be no pain despite high IOP. The eye is not red and typically looks normal to the patient or the casual observer. Recurrent attacks lasting several hours to 1 month, but rarely over 2 weeks, may occur. Patients have a variable clinical course; some have many recurrences over many years, whereas others have 1 or 2 episodes in their lives.

PHYSICAL EXAM

- On external examination, the eye is quiet and typically looks normal.
- The conjunctiva is white.
- Elevated IOP develops 1–2 days prior to anterior inflammation and keratic precipitates.
- The corneal endothelium develops fine stellate keratic precipitates, nonpigmented, typically distributed over the inferior part of the cornea, ranging from 1 to 20 in number.
- The anterior chamber shows very mild aqueous cell and flare not in proportion to the degree of IOP elevation.
- The IOP elevation is greater than 30, usually in the range of 40–60 mm Hg, much greater than would be expected given the mild degree of inflammation.
- Microcystic corneal edema may or may not be present.
- The iris may be slightly dilated, but peripheral anterior synechiae and posterior synechiae do not develop.
- Rarely, iris heterochromia may occur, with the affected eye being lighter in color, due to stromal atrophy from repeated inflammation.
- Gonioscopy reveals an open angle that may show keratic precipitates on the trabecular meshwork.
- Examination of the lens and fundus are normal.

DIAGNOSTIC TESTS & INTERPRETATION

Gonioscopy to rule out acute angle closure glaucoma.

Lab

Posner–Schlossman syndrome is a clinical diagnosis, there are no laboratory tests.

Imaging

Optic nerve imaging with either stereo disc photographs, Heidelberg retinal tomography (HRT), or optical coherence tomography (OCT) should be obtained to document the current optic nerve status, and to have a baseline to look for future damage to the optic nerve.

Diagnostic Procedures/Other

Humphrey visual field (HVF) testing to determine loss of a patient's visual field.

Pathological Findings

Repeated episodes may lead to optic nerve damage.

DIFFERENTIAL DIAGNOSIS

- Acute angle-closure glaucoma
- Chronic angle-closure glaucoma
- Fuchs heterochromic iridocyclitis
- Nongranulomatous anterior uveitis
- Inflammatory open-angle glaucoma
- Pigmentary glaucoma
- Neovascular glaucoma
- Herpes simplex and herpes zoster keratouveitis

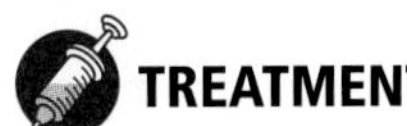

TREATMENT

MEDICATION

Topical steroids to control the inflammation and topical glaucoma drops to control the elevated IOP are usually used together to control the acute attack. The steroids are tapered off and glaucoma medications stopped as the inflammation resolves and IOP normalizes (2)[C].

First Line

- Topical steroids: Prednisolone acetate 1% q.i.d.
- Topical glaucoma drops: Beta-blockers (timolol 0.5% b.i.d.), and/or alpha-agonists (brimonidine 0.2%, 0.15%, 0.1% b.i.d./t.i.d.), and/or carbonic anhydrase inhibitor (dorzolamide 2% b.i.d./t.i.d.)

Second Line

- Topical NSAIDs (diclofenac 0.1% q.i.d. or equivalent),
- Oral NSAIDs—indomethacin 75–150 mg PO q.d. (3)[C]
- Oral carbonic anhydrase inhibitors—acetazolamide 250 mg PO b.i.d. to q.i.d. as tolerated
- Note: all of the above can be used as first-line treatment as well, depending on how the patient responds.

ADDITIONAL TREATMENT

Issues for Referral

Ophthalmologist for proper monitoring and treatment

SURGERY/OTHER PROCEDURES

Glaucoma filtering procedures such as trabeculectomy and tube shunts are rarely needed (4)[C].

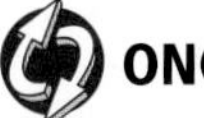

ONGOING CARE

FOLLOW-UP RECOMMENDATIONS

Patient Monitoring

- Every few days until the IOP improves then weekly until the episode resolves and the patient is tapered off the medications appropriately.
- Monitor with a complete ophthalmic examination and appropriate optic nerve imaging and visual field assessment as circumstances dictate, every 6 months initially to yearly if stable.

PATIENT EDUCATION

- Stress the recurrent nature of the disorder.
- The importance of proper monitoring of this condition as it can silently lead to optic nerve damage with possible visual impairment. Loss of vision can be permanent.
- Monitoring is important because the patient may not know that they are sustaining damage to the optic nerve. The patient experiences no or mild symptoms, and will not experience changes in their vision until a significant portion of the optic nerve is damaged.

PROGNOSIS

- Good, if properly diagnosed, treated and followed.
- Vision should be uncompromised throughout the patient's lifetime.
- However, it can be easily overlooked in an emergency department or primary care giver setting. Optic nerve damage and visual field changes can be significant and are usually permanent.

REFERENCES

1. Posner A, Schlossman A. Syndrome of unilateral recurrent attacks of glaucoma with cyclitic symptoms. *Arch Ophthal* 1948;39(4):517–535.
2. Moorthy RS, Mermoud A, Baerveldt G, et al. Glaucoma associated with uveitis. *Surv Ophthalmol* 1997;41:361–394.
3. Masuda K, Izawa Y, Mishima SS. Prostaglandins and glaucomato-cyclitis crisis. *Jpn J Ophthalmol* 1975;19:368.
4. Dinakaran S, Kayarkar V. Trabeculectomy in the management of Posner-Schlossman syndrome. *Ophthalmic Surg Lasers* 2002;33(4):321–322.

CODES

ICD9

- 364.00 Acute and subacute iridocyclitis, unspecified
- 364.22 Glaucomatocyclitic crises
- 365.10 Open-angle glaucoma, unspecified

CLINICAL PEARLS

- The eye is quiet looking with very mild symptoms and inflammation despite a significantly elevated IOP.
- Easily overlooked in an emergency department and primary care setting

POSTERIOR EMBRYOTOXON

M. Reza Razeghinejad
Alex V. Levin

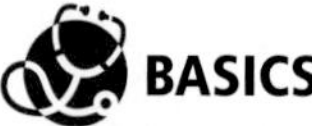

BASICS

DESCRIPTION

Posterior embryotoxon (PE) is a thickened and anteriorly displaced Schwalbe's line. The PE may be discontinuous. Schwalbe's line is the circumferential collagenous band at the junction of Descemet's membrane and the trabecular meshwork.

EPIDEMIOLOGY

Prevalence

- Its prevalence among normal population is 8–15%.
- It is almost an obligatory feature of the Axenfeld–Rieger spectrum and is seen in 80% of patients with Alagille syndrome.

RISK FACTORS

- Patients with Alagille or Axenfeld–Rieger are at particular risk.
- PE is a congenital malformation without risk factor for acquisition.

Genetics

- Most cases are not inherited and not heritable.
- Both patterns of autosomal dominant (more common) and recessive isolated PE have been reported.
- Otherwise, genetics parallels any associated syndrome (e.g., Axenfeld–Rieger and Alagille autosomal dominant).

ETIOLOGY

Schwalbe's line, trabecular meshwork, and Descemet's membrane are derivatives of neural crest. PE develops when neural crest migration and differentiation in this region of the eye is disrupted, presumably due to defective genetic instruction. For example, *JAG1*, the gene, which when mutated causes Alagille type 1 (MIM 118450), encodes a protein, NOTCH1, which is involved with pathways that determine cell fates in early development.

COMMONLY ASSOCIATED CONDITIONS

Ocular

- Few iris strands bridging the angle and attaching to the PE, cornea plana, corectopia, polycoria, aniridia, megalocornea, glaucoma, and unspecified anterior segment dysgenesis.

Systemic

- Alagille syndrome (arteriohepatic dysplasia), is a rare genetic disorder with autosomal dominant transmission. Types 1 and 2. Ophthalmologist may be asked to assist in the diagnosis of this syndrome.
  - Hepatic manifestations:
    - Most often presents within the first 3 months of life
    - Ranges from jaundice, mild cholestasis, and pruritus to progressive liver failure
  - Cardiac manifestations:
    - Ranges from benign heart murmurs to significant structural defects occur in 90–97%.
    - Pulmonic stenosis is the most common cardiac finding (67%).
  - Ophthalmologic manifestations
    - PE (78–89%), iris abnormalities (45%), diffuse fundus hypopigmentation (57%), speckling of the retinal pigment epithelium (33%), and optic disc anomalies (76%) including optic disc drusen (94%) and papilledema
    - Visual acuity is usually not significantly affected.
  - Skeletal manifestations,
    - The most common radiographic finding is butterfly vertebrae (33–87%)
    - Most common in the thoracic vertebrae
  - Facial features
    - Almost always present and include a prominent forehead, deep set eyes with moderate hypertelorism, pointed chin ("triangular facies"), and saddle or straight nose with a bulbous tip.
- Axenfeld–Rieger spectrum
- 22q11.2 deletion syndrome
- Noonan syndrome
- Aarskog (facial–digital–genital) syndrome

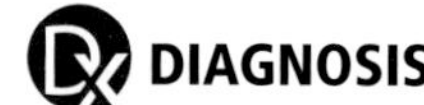

DIAGNOSIS

HISTORY

- May be history of at-risk associated disorders in family, especially if autosomal dominant
- May be history of glaucoma in family without known associated disorders or diagnoses

PHYSICAL EXAM

- Slit lamp examination:
  - A glass-like hyaline membrane, sharply defined and concentric, on the inner surface of cornea, may be discontinuous, located 0.5–2 mm anterior to the posterior limbus. May not be visible without gonioscopy.
  - Translucent posterior corneal surface between the PE and the limbus.
  - The ring in many cases does not extend for a full 360°. More often temporally than nasally.
  - May or may not have iridocornea strands attached to the PE
- Gonioscopy:
  - Required if PE suspected and not visible at slit lamp

DIAGNOSTIC TESTS & INTERPRETATION

Lab

Initial lab tests

None required unless multisystem involvement suggests PE as part of a syndrome (e.g., liver function tests if suspect Alagille syndrome).

Follow-up & special considerations

- Risk for glaucoma in patients without iridocorneal adhesion is unknown. Ophthalmic follow-up suggested.
- PE accompanied with iris attachment should be followed for early glaucoma detection.
  - Examine siblings, offspring, and parents where possible to identify others who may be at glaucoma risk.

Imaging

High-resolution anterior segment optical coherence tomography (OCT) or ultrasound biomicroscopy may be helpful. Usually not required.

Initial approach

- Full ophthalmic examination with particular attention to possibility of glaucoma
- Review of systems to identify other possible syndromic findings.

Pathological Findings

- Hypertrophy or thickening and anterior displacement of Schwalbe's line, in cross-section appears as a collagenous condensation.
- Thin Descemet's membrane and endothelium on either side of Schwalbe's line.

DIFFERENTIAL DIAGNOSIS

- Peripheral corneal endothelial or inner stromal opacification or deposition.
- Iridocorneal adhesion from other causes (e.g., peripheral anterior synechia)
  - Surgical wounds (in particular stepped self-sealing wounds as in temporal cataract extraction) or external trauma

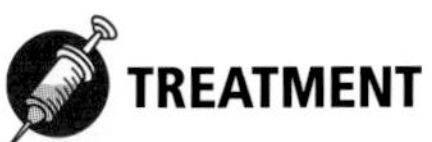

TREATMENT

MEDICATION

First Line

Treat glaucoma when identified.

Second Line

Treat associated syndromic abnormalities as indicated.

ADDITIONAL TREATMENT

Issues for Referral

- Genetics consultation if associated with systemic syndromes or other malformations
- Glaucoma referral as needed

SURGERY/OTHER PROCEDURES

- No surgery indicated or available to alleviate PE. Surgery if focuses on treatment of associated glaucoma if fails medical treatment
  - No indication to lyse iridocorneal strands

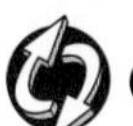

ONGOING CARE

FOLLOW-UP RECOMMENDATIONS

- Follow for early identification and treatment of glaucoma.
- PE associated with any ocular or systemic problems should be followed for those conditions.

PATIENT EDUCATION

Pediatric Glaucoma and Cataract Family Association (www.pgcfa.org).

PROGNOSIS

No known increased or decreased risk for adverse outcome secondary to glaucoma.

ADDITIONAL READING

- Rennie CA, Chowdhury S, Khan J, et al. The prevalence and associated features of posterior embryotoxon in the general ophthalmic clinic. *Eye (Lond)* 2005;19(4):396–399.
- Krantz ID, Piccoli DA, Spinner NB. Alagille syndrome. *J Med Genet* 1997;34:152–157.
- Burian HM, Braley AE, Allen L. External and gonioscopic visibility of the ring of Schwalbe and the trabecular zone; an interpretation of the posterior corneal embryotoxon and the so-called congenital hyaline membranes on the posterior corneal surface. *Trans Am Ophthalmol Soc* 1954–1955;52:389–428.

CODES

ICD9

- 377.21 Drusen of optic disc
- 743.43 Other congenital corneal opacities
- 743.44 Specified congenital anomalies of anterior chamber, chamber angle, and related structures

CLINICAL PEARLS

- Isolated PE is a common dominantly inherited ocular finding that may be associated with Axenfeld–Rieger spectrum or Alagille syndrome.
- Glaucoma risk should always be recognized except in Alagille syndrome where there does not appear to be a glaucoma risk.

POSTERIOR POLYMORPHOUS CORNEAL DYSTROPHY

Daniel Warder
Edward Moss
Stephanie Baxter

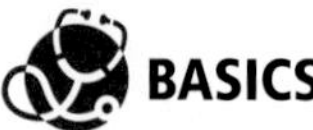

BASICS

DESCRIPTION

- Posterior polymorphous corneal dystrophy (PPMD or PPCD) is an inherited corneal disorder characterized by alterations in Descemet's membrane and corneal endothelium, typically bilaterally but often asymmetric.
- Many patients with PPMD are asymptomatic. The clinical course varies from slowly progressive to aggressive disease, which may lead to vision-threatening complications necessitating surgical intervention.

Pediatric Considerations

- Consider investigating for PPMD in children with strong family history.
- In some rare cases, stromal and epithelial edema may be present at birth, with the possibility of anterior corneal scarring.

ALERT
Failure to treat advanced, vision-threatening cases in children may result in form-deprivation amblyopia.

EPIDEMIOLOGY

Incidence

Very rare, with exact incidence and prevalence unknown

RISK FACTORS

Genetics

- Autosomal dominant inheritance, with multiple genetic loci identified:
- PPCD 1—20p11.2-q11.2—unknown gene
- PPCD 2—1p34.3-p32.3—collagen type VIII alpha 2 (COL8A2)
- PPCD 3—10p11.2—two-handed zinc finger homeodomain transcription factor 8 (ZEB1)

PATHOPHYSIOLOGY

Abnormalities in Descemet's membrane and in endothelial cells result in posterior corneal pathology such as vesicular lesions, band lesions, and irregular opacities. These may cause symptoms or interfere with the visual axis.

ETIOLOGY

Remains unknown.

COMMONLY ASSOCIATED CONDITIONS

- Glaucoma
  - Glaucoma is reported in cases of PPMD with peripheral anterior synechiae (PAS) as well as with open angles.
- Case reports document PPMD in association with keratoconus, keratoglobus, Terrien's marginal degeneration.

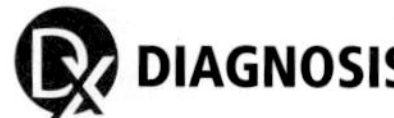

DIAGNOSIS

HISTORY

- Usually asymptomatic; however more severe cases may present with photophobia, foreign body sensation, and/or decreased visual acuity due to stromal and epithelial edema secondary to endothelial decompensation.
- Family history should be assessed.

PHYSICAL EXAM

The following may be observed on slit lamp biomicroscopy:

- Individual or grouped corneal vesicles seen at the level of Descemet's membrane, with or without characteristic "halo"
- Polymorphous or linear posterior corneal opacities ("railroad tracks")
- Descemet's membrane thickening in sheets and bands, sometimes with focal protrusion through the endothelium
- Corneal stromal and epithelial edema usually absent, however may develop in advanced cases
- Iridocorneal adhesions or PAS
- Elevated intraocular pressure (IOP)
- Findings are typically bilateral; however, there may be a marked asymmetry between eyes, and occasionally may present unilaterally.

DIAGNOSTIC TESTS & INTERPRETATION

Lab

No lab investigations are currently available for the diagnosis of the condition.

Imaging

Initial approach

PPMD can usually be diagnosed clinically based on slit lamp examination, without the need for further diagnostic tests.

Follow-up & special considerations

- Confocal microscopy can demonstrate characteristic changes of PPMD, thus aiding in its diagnosis (1)[C]. This modality is potentially useful when slit lamp biomicroscopic view of posterior cornea is obscured by stromal edema.
- Specular microscopy may be useful in identifying the characteristic vesicular changes and to help differentiate PPMD from other posterior corneal dystrophies (1)[C].

Diagnostic Procedures/Other

- Tonometry is important because of the association of PPMD with glaucoma.
- Pachymetry can be useful to indirectly measure and follow endothelial function.
- Examination of family members may be useful in establishing pedigree and confirming diagnosis.

Pathological Findings

- Irregular thickening of posterior collagenous layer of Descemet's with focal protrusion through the endothelial cell layer.
- Interspersed atrophic and normal corneal endothelium.
- Multiple layers of endothelial cells, with ultrastructural features of typical epithelial cells (such as tonofilaments, cytokeratin, desmosomes, and abundant microvilli), present histologically as stratified squamous epithelium.

DIFFERENTIAL DIAGNOSIS

- Iridocorneal epithelial (ICE) syndrome
  - useful differentiating factors: PPMD is generally nonprogressive and familial, unlike ICE
- Fuchs' endothelial dystrophy
- Early-onset congenital hereditary endothelial dystrophy—in the rare cases that present at birth
- Tears in Descemet's membrane

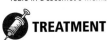

TREATMENT

MEDICATION

- Hypertonic saline drops can be used to prevent and treat corneal edema.
- IOP-lowering drops should be used in cases with associated glaucoma.

SURGERY/OTHER PROCEDURES

- Penetrating keratoplasty (PK) has been the treatment of choice in advanced PPMD.
- Descemet's stripping endothelial keratoplasty (DSEK) is gaining popularity in treating posterior corneal pathologies, and it has proven effective in cases of advanced PPMD (2)[C], (3)[C])
- Laser and aqueous filtration procedures may be indicated in cases associated with refractory glaucoma.

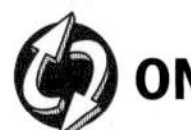

ONGOING CARE

PROGNOSIS

- Usually asymptomatic or only slowly progressive and therefore only rarely requires surgical intervention.
- Glaucoma and iridocorneal adhesions are associated with poor PK outcomes.

REFERENCES

1. Szaflik JP, Ko-Codzieiska U, Udziela M, et al. Posterior polymorphous dystrophy—Changes in corneal morphology in confocal microscopy. *Klin Oczna* 2008;110:252–258.
2. Chen ES, Terry MA, Shamie N, et al. Descemet-stripping automated endothelial keratoplasty—Six-month results in a prospective study of 100 eyes. *Cornea* 2008;27:514–520.
3. Basak SK. Descemet stripping and endothelial keratoplasty in endothelial dysfunctions: Three-month results in 75 eyes. *Ind J Ophth* 2008;56:291–296.

ADDITIONAL READING

- Laganowski HA, Sherrard ES, Kerr Muir MG. The posterior corneal surface in posterior polymorphous dystrophy: A specular microscopical study. *Cornea* 1991;10:224–232.
- Weiss JS, Moller HU, Lisch W, et al. The IC3D classification of the corneal dystrophies. *Cornea* 2008;27(Suppl 2):S1–S42.

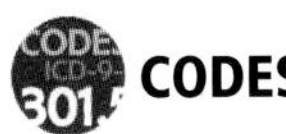

CODES

ICD9

371.58 Other posterior corneal dystrophies

CLINICAL PEARLS

- PPMD is a rare condition.
- Most affected patients are asymptomatic.
- Be sure to screen for glaucoma.
- Consider DSEK for patients who are visually symptomatic requiring intervention.

POSTERIOR STAPHYLOMA

Michael J. Bartiss

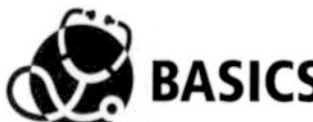

BASICS

DESCRIPTION

- Rare, typically unilateral anomaly characterized by a deep fundus excavation surrounding the optic disc
- Optic disc appears at the bottom of excavation.
- Optic disc may appear normal or demonstrate temporal pallor.
- Walls and margins of excavation demonstrate atrophic pigmentary changes in the choroid and retinal pigment epithelium.
- May contain contractile elements
- Visual acuity is typically significantly reduced, although cases with normal visual acuity have been reported.
- Affected eyes typically emmetropic or slightly myopic
- Centrocecal scotomas frequently occur in affected eyes with decreased vision.
- Not associated with glial or vascular abnormalities of the disc

RISK FACTORS

Genetics

Sporadic

PATHOPHYSIOLOGY

Staphylomatous defect surrounding the optic disc

ETIOLOGY

Development of the optic disc (around 4 months gestation) thought to be completed prior to the onset of the development of the staphylomatous process (which occurs around 5 months gestation)

COMMONLY ASSOCIATED CONDITIONS

- Nystagmus, strabismus, head turn
- Some unilateral cases associated with contralateral congenital ocular abnormality

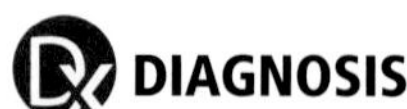

DIAGNOSIS

HISTORY

Congenital defect

PHYSICAL EXAM

- Full ocular examination including careful evaluation of the optic discs and evaluation for concomitant treatable amblyopia
- Careful evaluation of the contralateral eye

DIAGNOSTIC TESTS & INTERPRETATION

Pathological Findings

Presence of contractile elements reported

DIFFERENTIAL DIAGNOSIS

- Morning glory disc anomaly (funnel-shaped excavation of the posterior fundus that incorporates the optic disc)
- Optic disc coloboma (deep excavation occupying most of the disc, typically sparing the superior aspect)

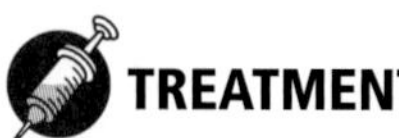

TREATMENT

MEDICATION

No medical treatment of the primary disorder

ADDITIONAL TREATMENT

General Measures

Impact resistant glasses for protection of the noninvolved eye if subnormal visual acuity is demonstrated or suspected in the involved eye, or in cases of bilateral involvement.

Issues for Referral

- Low vision evaluation and support as indicated in cases with significant bilateral involvement
- Retinal surgery for detachment

COMPLEMENTARY & ALTERNATIVE THERAPIES
None proven or indicated

SURGERY/OTHER PROCEDURES
- Amblyopia therapy and strabismus surgery as indicated
- Retinal detachment surgery as indicated

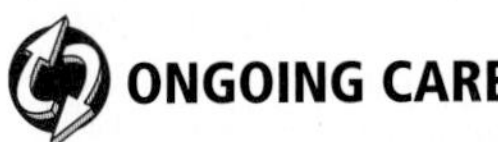

ONGOING CARE

FOLLOW-UP RECOMMENDATIONS
- Increased risk of acquired visual loss via retinal detachment dictates regular follow-up with careful retinal evaluation
- As needed for amblyopia and strabismus monitoring and treatment
- Low vision care if appropriate

Patient Monitoring
- Psychosocial concerns about appearance if significant strabismus is also present
- Monitor for possible development of acquired loss of vision from retinal detachment.

PATIENT EDUCATION
Low vision intervention in patients with significant bilateral involvement

PROGNOSIS
- Broad range of best corrected visual acuity
- Relatively high risk of subsequent retinal detachment

COMPLICATIONS
Retinal detachment

ADDITIONAL READING

- Nucci. Paulo in ophthalmic genetics. 1990;11(2): 143–145.
- Brodsky MC, Baker RS, Hamed LM. *Pediatric neuro-ophthalmology*. New York: Springer, 1996:41, 55, 177, 413.
- Pollack S. The morning glory disc anomaly; contractile movement, classification, and embryogenesis. *Doc Ophthalmol* 1987;65:439–460.
- Brown G, Tasman W. *Congenital anomalies of the optic disc*. New York: Grune & Stratton, 1983:178–183.

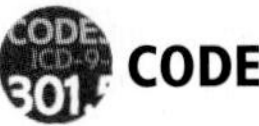

CODES

ICD9
- 368.41 Scotoma involving central area
- 377.49 Other disorders of optic nerve
- 379.12 Staphyloma posticum

CLINICAL PEARLS

- Work to maximize visual potential, especially in bilateral cases
- Protective eyewear in unilateral cases

POSTERIOR VITREOUS DETACHMENT

Brian P. Connolly

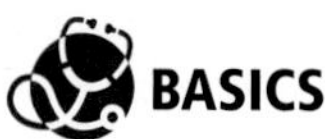

BASICS

DESCRIPTION

- A posterior vitreous detachment (PVD) is the physical separation of the cortical vitreous from the internal limiting membrane (ILM) of the retina.
- With improved imaging modalities such as high-resolution optical coherence tomography (OCT), earlier stages of structural partial PVD are readily detectable before symptoms occur and before a complete PVD is present.

EPIDEMIOLOGY

Incidence

- The incidence of PVD increases with age.
- Although some estimates have indicated that 50% of phakic eyes have PVD by the age of 50 years, this has been somewhat disputed in autopsy studies.

RISK FACTORS

- Increasing age.
- Axial myopia
- Trauma
- Inflammation
- Pseudophakia
- Aphakia
- Prior surgeries (especially cataract extraction complicated by vitreous loss)
- Vitreous hemorrhage

Genetics

- Axial myopia (caused by both genetic and environmental factors) correlates with an earlier onset of vitreous liquefaction and PVD.
- An earlier onset of PVD and PVD-related complications are seen in Stickler's and Marfan's syndromes due to anomalous collagen metabolism.

PATHOPHYSIOLOGY

- Liquefaction of the vitreous gel is clinically evident as optically empty vacuoles within the vitreous cavity. This may be accompanied by coalescence of collagen fibrils into visible strands, which may be visualized ophthalmoscopically.
- Decreased strength of the vitreoretinal interface is also believed to precipitate PVD.

ETIOLOGY

- Vitreous liquefaction is detectable from early childhood and increases with age.
- Significant vitreous liquefaction together with loss of cohesion of the vitreoretinal interface combine to facilitate PVD formation.
- In the earliest stages of a PVD, the vitreous and the retina gradually separate. This process often starts in the macular region, but often spares the fovea until a later stage.
- Once the posterior vitreous face degrades sufficiently, liquefied vitreous can pass abruptly through even a minute defect in the posterior vitreous face into the subhyaloid space and this is known as an acute PVD (2).
- In areas where the ILM is especially thin (i.e., optic nerve, foveola, vitreous base, retinal vessels), the vitreoretinal interface is especially strong. These areas are often the last to separate from the hyaloid face.
- A Weiss ring is a clinical sign that confirms separation of the vitreopapillary junction, and it typically confirms the completion of the PVD.

COMMONLY ASSOCIATED CONDITIONS

- Early-stage PVD
  - Epiretinal membrane
  - Macular microhole
  - Foveal red spot
  - Idiopathic macular hole
  - Pseudooperculum
  - Inner lamellar macular hole
  - Vitreofoveal traction (traction cystoid macular edema)
  - Vitreomacular traction syndrome
  - Traction diabetic macular edema
  - Myopic traction maculopathy
  - Neovascular age-related macular degeneration
  - Vitreopapillary traction syndrome
- Late-stage (complete) PVD
  - Retinal or optic disc hemorrhage
  - Vitreous hemorrhage
  - Retinal tear
  - Rhegmatogenous retinal detachment (1)

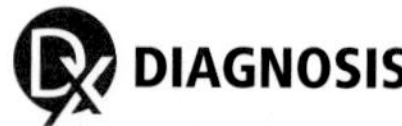

DIAGNOSIS

- Ophthalmoscopy
  - Visible Weiss ring seen with slit lamp biomicroscopy or with indirect ophthalmoscopy.
  - Apparent separation of the vitreous from the posterior pole without the presence of a Weiss ring may be misleading and may simply represent vitreous schisis.
- Ancillary testing
  - Spectral domain OCT nicely visualizes the posterior hyaloid face in PVD.
  - Ultrasonographic confirmation of detachment of the peripheral vitreous together with the presence of a Weiss ring is also confirmatory of PVD in equivocal cases and is used to confirm onset of PVD for research purposes.
  - Vitreous hemorrhage and/or the presence of pigment within the vitreous are highly predictive of a retinal tear (70%).

HISTORY
- Patients with early PVD can present with photopsias as the vitreous gradually separates from the retina.
- Patients with a personal or family history of retinal tears or detachments merit especially careful examination as they have an increased risk of tears being present.

PHYSICAL EXAM
- Indirect ophthalmoscopy with scleral depression
- Slit lamp biomicroscopy
- Contact lens biomicroscopy
  - Goldman 3 mirror lens
  - Widefield contact lens

DIAGNOSTIC TESTS & INTERPRETATION
Diagnostic Procedures/Other
- Ultrasonography
  - B-scan ultrasonography should be considered in cases where media opacity precludes an adequate clinical examination.
  - B-scans are also used in the context of clinical trials to accurately document the presence or absence, as well as stage, of PVD.
- OCT
  - OCT (especially spectral domain OCT) can be used to document the presence or absence *and* the progression of early PVD.

Pathological Findings
After PVD, up to 44% of patients at autopsy have been demonstrated to have residual hyalocytes present on the macular surface.

DIFFERENTIAL DIAGNOSIS
See "Associated Conditions."

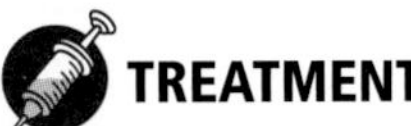

TREATMENT

ADDITIONAL TREATMENT
General Measures
Careful extended ophthalmoscopy should be performed in those patients who report symptoms of PVD or who are noted to have a PVD.

SURGERY/OTHER PROCEDURES
- For uncomplicated PVD, no treatment is necessary.
- When a retinal tear or detachment is present, prompt treatment is imperative.
- Rarely, pars plana vitrectomy may be offered to alleviate severe PVD-related symptoms; however, this is the exception.

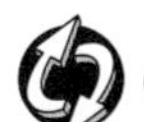

ONGOING CARE

FOLLOW-UP RECOMMENDATIONS
- Prompt evaluation by an ophthalmologist or optometrist when symptoms of acute PVD occur
- Prompt referral to an ophthalmologist skilled in the treatment of retinal tears and/or detachments in the event that one is detected

PATIENT EDUCATION
- After an acute PVD, patients are often significantly bothered by floaters and flashes. It is often reassuring to let patients know that symptoms will typically lessen within months.
- Patients should be educated to report the symptoms of a retinal tear or detachment should they occur.

PROGNOSIS
- After an uncomplicated PVD, the prognosis is excellent.
- In some cases, as in eyes with vitreomacular traction, visual acuity may improve.
- After a complicated PVD (i.e., with a retinal break), there is an elevated risk of additional tears occurring.
- When a complicated PVD occurs in one eye, the fellow eye has a higher risk of complications from PVD likely due to the nature of the vitreoretinal interface.

COMPLICATIONS
- Retinal tears
- Rhegmatogenous retinal detachment
- See Commonly Associated Conditions above

REFERENCES

1. Foos RY, Wheeler NC. Vitreoretinal juncture. Synchysis senilis and posterior vitreous detachment. *Ophthalmology* 1982;89(12):1502–1512.
2. Johnson MW. Posterior vitreous detachment: evolution and complications of its early stages. *Am J Ophthalmol* 2010;149(3):371–382 e1.

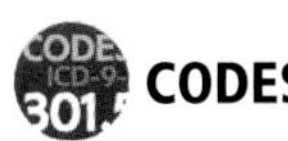

CODES

ICD9
379.21 Vitreous degeneration

CLINICAL PEARLS

- The presence of a vitreous hemorrhage and/or pigmented clumps with PVD is highly suspicious for retinal tears and should prompt careful examination.
- A Weiss ring provides clinical confirmation of complete PVD.

PREGNANCY AND OPHTHALMIC DISEASE

Chirag P. Shah

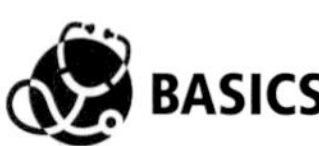

BASICS

DESCRIPTION

- Various ophthalmic conditions are associated with or exacerbated by pregnancy.
  - Refractive changes: transient loss of accommodation; increased corneal thickness, edema, and curvature; decreased corneal sensitivity
  - Preeclampsia or pregnancy-induced hypertension (PIH): marked by hypertension, proteinuria, peripheral edema. Eclampsia also includes seizures. Symptoms include headache and blurred vision. Hypertension can lead to cortical blindness.
  - HELLP syndrome: hemolysis, elevated liver enzymes, and low platelet counts. Occurs in 10% of patients with severe PIH.
  - Occlusive vascular disease: due to the hypercoagulable state of pregnancy. Can lead to artery or vein occlusions, disseminated intravascular coagulopathy (DIC), and thrombotic thrombocytopenia purpura (TTP; thrombus formation, hemolytic anemia, thrombocytopenia, neurologic changes, fever, renal dysfunction). Ocular DIC has widespread small vessel thrombosis, particularly in the choroid.
  - Amniotic fluid embolism: can occur during labor, delivery, or the immediate postpartum period from particulate matter from the amniotic fluid entering the maternal circulation. It can cause cardiopulmonary failure, as well as central retinal artery occlusion, and is associated with 80% mortality.
  - Purtscher-like retinopathy: within 24 hours of birth, usually associated with late complications such as preeclampsia, pancreatitis, TTP.
  - Meningioma of pregnancy: meningiomas can grow aggressively during pregnancy. May regress postpartum.
  - Diabetic retinopathy and diabetic macular edema: tends to progress during pregnancy usually with varying degrees regression postpartum. No risk of diabetic retinopathy with gestational diabetes. Nonproliferative diabetic retinopathy (NPDR) progresses in up to 50%. Proliferative diabetic retinopathy (PDR) progresses rapidly.
  - Central serious chorioretinopathy (CSCR): associated with pregnancy, as well as increased endogenous or exogenous cortisol
  - Pituitary apoplexy: preexisting pituitary adenomas can enlarge during pregnancy. Apoplexy is the acute expansion of a pituitary adenoma due to infarction or hemorrhage. Leads to acute headache, nausea, visual field loss (bitemporal hemianopia), limitation of extraocular motility (due to involvement of cranial nerves III, IV, and VI, in the cavernous sinus), and/or Horner syndrome. Sheehan syndrome is pituitary apoplexy of a nontumorous pituitary gland, presumably due to postpartum arterial spasm of arterioles supplying the anterior pituitary and its stalk.

EPIDEMIOLOGY

Prevalence

Preeclampsia occurs in 5% of pregnancies, typically after 20 weeks of gestation and in primigravidas (first pregnancy).

RISK FACTORS

- PIH risk factors: first and multifetal pregnancies, extremes of maternal age, mothers with vascular disease
- DIC risk factors: complicated abortions, abruptio placenta, severe preeclampsia, and retained dead fetus.
- Diabetic retinopathy: increased risk of progression if longer duration of preexisting diabetes, poorer glycemic control before and during pregnancy, rapid normalization of glucose levels during pregnancy, severity of retinopathy at conception, and presence of concomitant hypertension.

GENERAL PREVENTION

Prenatal care to monitor for hypertension, hyperglycemia, and proteinuria

PATHOPHYSIOLOGY

- Serous retinal detachments in PIH is felt due to choroidal ischemia.
- Cortical blindness in PIH is due to cerebral arteriolar vasospasm and cerebral edema.
- Purtscher-like retinopathy is due to complement-induced granulocyte aggregation and vascular occlusion.
- It is unclear why diabetic retinopathy accelerates during pregnancy.

DIAGNOSIS

HISTORY

- History of hypertension or diabetes?
- Blurred vision, distortion, micropsia, photopsias, floaters, visual field loss, headache, fluctuating vision?
- Seizures, increased urinary frequency, peripheral edema?
- History of corticosteroid use?
- Nausea or ocular paresis?

PHYSICAL EXAM

- Complete ophthalmic examination, including vital signs (particularly blood pressure), pupils, visual fields, color plates, gonioscopy (if PDR), optic nerve assessment, and dilated fundus examination.
  - Preeclampsia or PIH: findings are related to HTN, including retinal hemorrhages, nerve fiber layer infarcts, exudation, serous retinal detachment (in 1% of preeclamptic and 10% of eclamptic patients), focal arteriolar narrowing and spasm, optic nerve edema, nonarteritic ischemic optic neuropathy, and bilateral occipital lobe infarcts (preeclampsia/eclampsia hypertensive posterior encephalopathy syndrome [PEHPES])
  - HELLP: bilateral serous retinal detachment, subretinal yellow–white opacities, vitreous hemorrhage
  - Occlusive vascular disorders: retinal artery and vein occlusions, nerve fiber layer infarcts, retinal hemorrhage and exudation, Purtscher-like retinopathy with multiple nerve fiber layer infarcts around the optic nerve associated with TTP
  - Ocular DIC: hemorrhage, tissue necrosis, serous retinal detachments, underlying retinal pigment epithelium (RPE) alterations
  - Purtscher-like retinopathy: widespread nerve fiber layer infarcts with or without hemorrhage
  - Diabetic macular edema: cystic macular edema in foveal region often associated with microaneurysms and hard exudates
  - NPDR: dot-blot retinal hemorrhages, microaneurysm, venous beading, exudation, macular edema, intraretinal microvascular abnormalities
  - PDR: NPDR plus neovascularization of optic nerve, elsewhere in the retina, iris, or angle
  - CSCR: serious retinal detachment without hemorrhage, subretinal exudation is more common (90%) than in nonpregnant females (<20%), RPE irregularities

DIAGNOSTIC TESTS & INTERPRETATION

Lab

Initial lab tests

- Urinalysis for proteinuria
- Electrolytes
- CBC
- PT/PTT

Follow-up & special considerations

- Ophthalmic examination warranted if patient experiences visual symptoms
- Gestational diabetes: no risk of retinopathy during pregnancy; routine ophthalmic examination not needed
- None or minimal NPDR: minimal to no progression during pregnancy; ophthalmic examination first and third trimester
- Mild to moderate NPDR: progression in up to 50% during pregnancy; ophthalmic examination every trimester
- High-risk NPDR: progression in up to 50% during pregnancy; monthly ophthalmic examination
- PDR: tends to progress rapidly during pregnancy; monthly ophthalmic examination (1)[A]

Imaging

- If PEHPES is suspected, check brain MRI. Findings include bilateral occipital lobe lesions (identical to nonobstetric hypertensive encephalopathy)
- If pituitary apoplexy suspected, emergently check brain MRI. Hemorrhage within the sella is isointense or hypointense on T1-weighted images within first 3–5 days. In nonhemorrhagic (ischemic) pituitary apoplexy, MRI reveals an enlarged pituitary gland bulging under the optic chiasm with peripheral enhancement surrounding a hypointense gland (pituitary ring sign).
- If meningioma is suspected, check MRI of brain and/or orbits.

Diagnostic Procedures/Other

- OCT to evaluate for CSCR or macular edema
- Intravenous fluorescein dye crosses the placenta and is present in breast milk for at least 76 h. No additional adverse effects have been noted in pregnant women nor teratogenic or embryogenic effects in animal studies. Most vitreoretinal specialists would avoid fluorescein angiograms in pregnant women unless necessary for a sight threatening condition (e.g., choroidal neovascularization).
- Indocyanine green (ICG) dye does not cross the placenta and it is unknown if it's found in breast milk. ICG has been used for nanophthalmic conditions in pregnant woman without adverse effect on mother or fetus. Most vitreoretinal specialists would avoid ICG angiography in pregnant women unless necessary.

DIFFERENTIAL DIAGNOSIS

For PEHPES: posterior circulation stroke, intracranial venous thrombosis due to coagulation disorder, migraine, intracranial hemorrhage, infectious cerebritis or meningitis, tumor with hemorrhage, atypical seizure, demyelination.

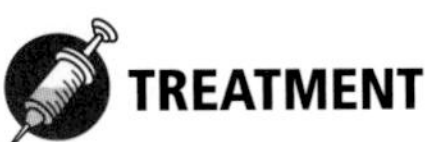

TREATMENT

MEDICATION

- Avoid prescribing new glasses until several weeks postpartum given the shifting refraction during pregnancy
- For preeclampsia, eclampsia, or PIH, treat electrolyte imbalances and hypertension, and deliver baby

ADDITIONAL TREATMENT

General Measures

- Treat PDR with panretinal photocoagulation (PRP) and follow monthly. Consider earlier PRP for severe pre-PDR.
- Observe diabetic macular edema; it often resolves postpartum.
- Consider caesarian section in PDR to prevent risk of vitreous hemorrhage during Valsalva.
- CSCR usually resolves spontaneously.

Issues for Referral

- Internal medicine for hypertension and hyperglycemic control
- Endocrinology for hyperglycemic management and for pituitary apoplexy
- Neurology for seizures with eclampsia, for neurologic findings with meningiomas, and for PEHPES.
- Neurosurgery for pituitary apoplexy
- Ophthalmologist or vitreoretinal specialist for diabetic retinopathy, diabetic macular edema, CSCR, Purtscher's retinopathy.

SURGERY/OTHER PROCEDURES

Neurosurgical transsphenoidal surgical decompression of pituitary apoplexy.

IN-PATIENT CONSIDERATIONS

Initial Stabilization

- Control blood pressure in PIH
- Medically stabilize patients with pituitary apoplexy, administer high-dose corticosteroids, evaluate pituitary hormones, electrolytes, and glucose, administer appropriate endocrinologic replacement therapy, consider neurosurgical transsphenoidal surgical decompression.

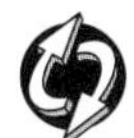

ONGOING CARE

DIET

Healthy, well-balanced diabetic diet for patients with diabetes.

PATIENT EDUCATION

Contact your obstetrician or seek emergency care if you experience visual changes, blurred vision, visual field loss, double vision, headache, nausea/vomiting, or seizures.

PROGNOSIS

- Perinatal mortality rate with PIH is 13–30%. Causes of death include pulmonary edema, CNS hemorrhage, or cardiac, liver, or renal failure.
- Vascular changes seen in PIH resolve postpartum. Permanent visual change is unusual.
- Serous retinal detachment seen in PIH usually resolves postpartum. Visual acuity may be affected by RPE changes.
- CSCR usually resolves but may recur postpartum or during a subsequent pregnancy.
- High likelihood of postpartum regression in diabetic retinopathy changes that occur during pregnancy

COMPLICATIONS

- Decreased visual acuity
- Visual field loss
- Ophthalmoplegia
- Vitreous hemorrhage
- Tractional retinal detachment
- Neovascular glaucoma

REFERENCE

1. Chew EY, Mills JL, Metzger BE, et al. Metabolic control and progression of retinopathy. The diabetes in early pregnancy study. National Institute of Child Health and Human Development Diabetes in Early Pregnancy Study. *Diabetes Care* 1995;18:631–637.

ADDITIONAL READING

- Schultz KL, Bimbaum AD, Goldstein DA. Ocular disease in pregnancy. *Curr Opin Ophthalmol* 2005;16:308–314.
- Sheth BP, Mieler WF. Ocular complications of pregnancy. *Curr Opin Ophthalmol* 2001;12: 455–463.

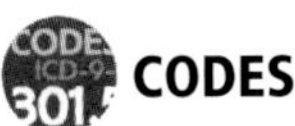

CODES

ICD9

- 642.60 Eclampsia complicating pregnancy, childbirth or the puerperium, unspecified as to episode of care
- 367.51 Paresis of accommodation
- 368.8 Other specified visual disturbances

CLINICAL PEARLS

- Pregnancy can precipitate or exacerbate several conditions that affect vision.
- Progression of diabetic retinopathy during pregnancy can show variable amounts of regression postpartum.
- Pituitary apoplexy is an endocrine and neurosurgical emergency.
- Preeclampsia or PIH is relatively common (5% of pregnancies) and can lead to various ophthalmic and neurologic findings.
- Prenatal care is important to monitor for hypertension, hyperglycemia, and proteinuria.

PRESBYOPIA

Bruce J. Markovitz

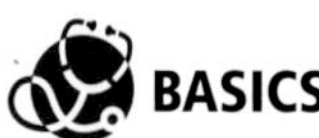

BASICS

DESCRIPTION

Presbyopia, literally "old eyes," is the condition where the ability to see clearly at near is lost due to the gradual loss of accommodation in the aging eye.

EPIDEMIOLOGY

Incidence

100% of population older than 50 years with average age of onset at 45 years.

Prevalence

38% of U.S. population (115 million people).

GENERAL PREVENTION

No evidence that onset of presbyopia can be prevented or delayed with exercises, lenses, vitamins, or diet.

PATHOPHYSIOLOGY

Accommodative amplitude (AA) gradually decreases from childhood to adulthood. From approximately 12 diopters (D) at age 10 years to 10 D at 20 years, 8 D at 30 years, 5 D at 40 years, 2 D at 50 years, and 1 D at 60 years (1), (2), (3)[C].

ETIOLOGY

- Helmholtz theory of accommodation—The long accepted hypothesis, published in 1855, attributes increased focusing power of the lens during accommodation to relaxation of the zonules during ciliary body contraction allowing the lens to assume a more spherical shape. At rest, the ciliary body ring expands increasing zonular tension on the lens equator flattening the lens and decreasing the power for distance vision. Presbyopia is attributed to the hardening of the crystalline lens with age preventing it from changing shape.
- Schachar theory of accommodation—Introduced in 1992, attributes accommodation to relaxation of the anterior and posterior zonules, but **increased** equatorial zonular tension during ciliary body contraction resulting in peripheral flattening and central steepening of the lens. Presbyopia is attributed to the gradual equatorial growth of the lens with aging effectively decreasing the working distance of the ciliary body (4).

DIAGNOSIS

HISTORY

Patients complain of gradual onset of blurred near vision, especially with small print, dim lighting, after prolonged near work or when fatigued. May also note difficulty changing focus from near to far. The classic complaint is "my arms are not long enough to read anymore."

PHYSICAL EXAM

- Distance and near acuity depends on presence of any refractive error.
  - Emmetropes (patients with no refractive error) and corrected ametropes (patients with refractive error)—clear distance vision with blurred near vision
  - Myopes—clear near vision at a near point determined by the amount of myopia
  - Hyperopes—better distance vision than near vision
  - Myopic astigmatism—may have some improvement in near vision over distance vision

DIAGNOSTIC TESTS & INTERPRETATION

Diagnostic Procedures/Other

- Goal is to determine the amount of plus power, the "add," over the distance correction needed to give comfortable clear near vision.
- Age-appropriate adds: Near adds are commonly prescribed without clinical measurement. Prescribing the average add power appropriate for the patient's age will usually allow clear comfortable near vision for most patients. As a rule, patients are more comfortable with an add that is undercorrected compared with an add that is overcorrected. When prescribing age-appropriate adds consider the patient's habitual near add and any symptoms. The following is a guide for prescribing age-appropriate adds:

40–45	1.00–1.50
45–50	1.50–1.75
50–55	1.75–2.00
55–60	2.00–2.25
60–65	2.25–2.50
65	2.50

- Near refraction: With near test card at habitual reading distance and distance refraction in place the amount of plus power needed for clear near vision is determined. Range of clear near vision can also be measured and adjusted as needed. More plus moves focus closer, but collapses range of clear near vision. Reducing plus moves near point further away and expands range of clear vision.
- Fused Jackson cross cylinder (JCC) test: With distance correction in place and near target of vertical and horizontal crossed lines at habitual reading distance, JCC lenses introduced binocularly with red axis vertical. Add plus lenses +0.50 D greater than expected age-appropriate add. Patient should report vertical lines are darkest. Reduce plus until reversal and horizontal lines darkest. Midpoint where lines are equal is the amount of plus needed in combination with patient's accommodation that places focus on target.
- Measuring AA:
  - Push up method—Measured monocularly with distance correction in place. Near point of clear vision is determined and converted to diopters ($D = 1/M$)
  - Minus lens to blur—Monocularly with distance correction in place and near card at 40 cm, minus lenses slowly added until 20/40 line blurs. Amount of minus added, +2.5 D for accommodating to 40 cm, equals AA

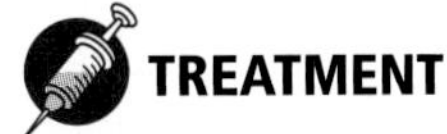

TREATMENT

MEDICATION

First Line

- As a rule, one half of AA can be used comfortably for extended periods. Total amount of plus power needed to read is determined by the patient's working distance, usually 40 cm (16"), requiring +2.50 D of power. When AA drops below 5 D, presbyopic symptoms can occur and additional plus power will be needed for near work. For example, if AA is 3 D then 1.5 D can be comfortably provided toward the 2.50 D needed for extended reading. Theoretically, a +1.00 D add together with +1.50 D accommodation would provide the +2.50 D needed to allow comfortable extended near work. This additional plus power can be provided in several ways:
- Glasses:
  - Over-the-counter readers—Good for patients without significant astigmatism or anisometropia.
  - Single vision near Rx—For patients with good distance vision or unable to adjust to bifocals. Calculated by adding the distance Rx and near add together.
  - Bifocals—Advantage of allowing clear distance and near vision without two pairs of glasses. Even advantageous for emmetropes allowing clear distance vision without need to remove reading Rx.
  - Lined bifocal—One near focal power limits intermediate vision. Cosmetically less desirable.
    - Progressive bifocal—Add power increases gradually from distance to full near power at bottom. Provides clear vision at all distances. Cosmetically more acceptable. Can be harder to adjust to, especially for previous lined bifocal wearers. Expensive.

Second Line

- Contacts:
  - Monovision—Dominant eye corrected for distance and nondominant eye corrected for near. Compromised clarity and depth perception. High percentage of failures.
  - Bifocal contacts—Compromised clarity and depth perception. High percentage of failures although improved newer lens designs result in greater number of satisfied patients.

SURGERY/OTHER PROCEDURES

- All surgical options for presbyopia correction require careful patient selection and patient education.
  - LASIK: Monovision correction possible in previously successful monovision contact lens wearers or after successful monovision trial (5)[C].
  - Intraocular lenses: With cataract surgery patients have multiple options for presbyopic correction
    - Monovision—For previously successful monovision contact lens wearers traditional IOLs can be used to achieve monovision correction.
    - Multifocal and accommodating IOLs—Clear distance, intermediate, and near vision possible. Some dissatisfied patients require lens exchange. Significant cost to patient (6)[C].
- Scleral expansion bands: Increases distance from ciliary body to lens equator to reverse effect of presbyopia. Inconsistent results. Not generally accepted.

ONGOING CARE

PROGNOSIS

Once presbyopic symptoms begin, the process progresses until all accommodation is lost, usually above 65 years of age. At this point, a full add of +2.50 is required for the average reading distance of 40 cm. Adds greater than +2.50 will only decrease the working distance and should not be used unless a reading distance of less than 40 cm is desired due to acuity less than 20/40, occupational needs, or patient has a shorter habitual reading distance.

REFERENCES

1. Donders FC. Accommodation and refraction of the eye. *The New Society. London* 1864:204–215.
2. Duane A. Studies in monocular and binocular accommodation with their clinical applications. *Am J Ophthalmol* 1922;5:865.
3. Chattopadhyay DN, Seal GN. Amplitude of accommodation in different age groups and age of onset of presbyopia in Bengalese population. *Indian J Ophthalmol* 1984;32:85–87.
4. Schachar RA. Cause and treatment of presbyopia with a method for increasing the amplitude of accommodation 1992;24(12):445–447, 452.
5. Farid M, Steinert RF. Patient selection for monovision refractive surgery. *Curr Opin Ophthalmol* 2009;20(4):251–254.
6. Buznego C, Trattler WB. Presbyopia-correcting intraocular lenses. *Curr Opin Ophthalmol* 2009;20(1):13–18.

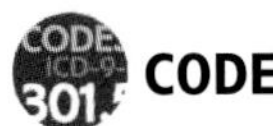

CODES

ICD9

367.4 Presbyopia

CLINICAL PEARLS

- Accommodative demand is greater for myopes in contact lenses than in glasses. A prepresbyope able to read with their glasses may have presbyopic symptoms in contacts. Opposite is true with hyperopes.
- Do not add an additional +0.25 D to desired add for progressive lenses. This practice was popular in the past when it was difficult for patients to get the full reading power at bottom of progressive segment. Improved progressive lens designs with larger full power reading area at bottom have eliminated the need for this practice.
- Any near testing must be done prior to dilation. An obvious but often forgotten point.

PRESEPTAL CELLULITIS

Anthony W. Farah
Alan R. Forman

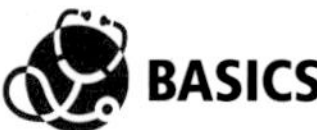

BASICS

DESCRIPTION

- An infection of the eyelid and surrounding skin anterior to the orbital septum. By definition, the infection does not involve intraorbital tissue.
- Synonym: Periorbital cellulitis

ALERT

Exclude orbital involvement early in the evaluation. In preseptal cellulitis, vision and ocular motility are normal with absence of both proptosis and pain with motion. The distinction is important as orbital cellulitis can be a vision and life-threatening infection.

Pediatric Considerations

- Preseptal cellulitis can lead to visual impairment in very young children if prolonged eyelid edema leads to occlusion amblyopia.
- If physical exam is difficult, imaging may be required to rule out orbital cellulitis. After trauma, if the eye cannot be adequately examined, an exam under anesthesia is mandatory to rule out a ruptured globe.
- Ask about vaccinations, especially *Haemophilus influenzae* type B.

EPIDEMIOLOGY

- Predominantly affects the pediatric age group
  - Most younger than 5 years; mean age is 21 months (1)
- Occurs more commonly in the winter months
- No known predilection for gender or race

RISK FACTORS

- Adjacent infection or trauma (see "Etiology")
- Sinusitis
- Surgical procedure near the eyelid
- Oral procedures
- Poorly controlled diabetes mellitus
- Immunocompromised patients

GENERAL PREVENTION

- Childhood vaccination for *H. influenzae* type B
- Proper detection and early treatment of sinus, dental, ear, and other adjacent infections

PATHOPHYSIOLOGY

- Preseptal cellulitis is an infection anterior to the orbital septum. The orbital septum largely prevents the spread of infection to the orbit and CNS. Any preseptal infection can extend back into the orbit.
- Routes of infection include direct inoculation from trauma or the spread of an adjacent infection.
- *Streptococcus pneumoniae* is the most frequent pathogen associated with sinus infection while *Staphylococcus aureus* and *Streptococcus pyogenes* predominate when infection arises from local trauma.

ETIOLOGY

- Adjacent infection
  - Most commonly from the spread of infection from paranasal sinuses
  - Other infectious sources include hordeolum, acute chalazion, dacryocystitis, dacryoadenitis, teeth or gums, or impetigo
- Trauma
  - Insect or animal bites, lacerations, puncture wounds, or retained foreign bodies
- Causative organisms
  - The most common bacterial agent identified in children is *S. pneumoniae* followed by *S. aureus* and *S. pyogenes*.
  - Prior to introduction of the *H. influenzae* type B vaccine, *H. flu* was the most common cause of preseptal and orbital cellulitis.
  - With a human or animal bite, suspect anaerobic, non-spore–forming bacteria
  - Polymicrobial infections are more common in older patients (>15 years) and in open wounds.
  - Methicillin-resistant *S. aureus* (MRSA) must be considered in at-risk populations, especially with trauma.
  - Fungi (mucormycosis, aspergillosis) possible in immunocompromised patients
  - Clostridial gas gangrene if soil contamination

COMMONLY ASSOCIATED CONDITIONS

- A concurrent or recent upper respiratory tract infection (URI), especially sinusitis (2)
- Chronic staphylococcal blepharitis
- Anthrax and smallpox vaccinations have rarely been linked to preseptal cellulitis (3).

DIAGNOSIS

HISTORY

- Recent trauma, surgery, or nearby infection
- Recent URI, sinus infection, or ear infection
- Pain with eye movement or change in vision
- Constitutional symptoms (e.g., fever, nausea)
- Vaccination status (especially *H. Flu* type B)
- Prior cancer diagnosis

PHYSICAL EXAM

- Vital signs
- Comprehensive ocular examination
  - Note any restrictions of ocular motility or proptosis, suggesting an orbital process.
  - Record visual acuity, pupillary reaction, eye pressure, and optic nerve head appearance.
- Palpate the periorbital area and the head and neck lymph nodes.
- Note any tenderness, swelling, warmth, redness, or discoloration of the eyelid.
- Assess for neurological deficits.
- Check for meningeal signs.
- Thorough examination of the globe is required in all patients with any history of trauma to rule out a ruptured globe.

DIAGNOSTIC TESTS & INTERPRETATION

Lab

Initial lab tests

- In all cases, obtain a culture and Gram stain of any open wound or drainage.
- In severe cases or with constitutional symptoms, obtain a CBC count with differential, two sets of blood cultures, and CT scan (see "Imaging").
- If patient exhibits CNS signs, obtain CSF after an intracranial mass is ruled out.

Follow-up & special considerations

If patient deteriorates clinically, consider orbital cellulitis and hospital admission.

Imaging

Initial approach

- CT scan, with contrast if possible, of the brain and orbits (axial and coronal views) in any one of the following scenarios:
  - Possible orbital involvement or proptosis
  - A history of significant trauma
  - Concern of an orbital or intraocular foreign body
  - There is high suspicion for subperiosteal abscess/paranasal sinusitis/cavernous sinus thrombosis/cancer.

Follow-up & special considerations

Consider ordering a repeat or initial CT scan if the patient does not improve in 24–48 h with appropriate antibiotic therapy or if the patient begins to clinically deteriorate

DIFFERENTIAL DIAGNOSIS

- Orbital cellulitis
- Allergic edema of eyelids
- Viral conjunctivitis
- Erysipelas
- Necrotizing fasciitis (*Gr A Beta hemolytic Strep*)
- Cavernous sinus thrombosis
- Herpes simplex or herpes zoster blepharitis
- Idiopathic orbital inflammatory syndrome
- Other possibilities: thyroid eye disease, leukemic infiltrates, blepharochalasis, and autoimmune inflammatory disorders

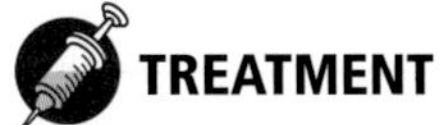

TREATMENT

MEDICATION

First Line

- Hospitalize patients younger than 1 year.
- Milder cases of preseptal cellulitis in adults and children older than 1 year with no signs of systemic toxicity, adequate vaccination status, and who are reliable for follow-up visits can be managed on an outpatient basis (4)[C]. Initial daily follow-up is required (see "Follow-up Recommendations")
  - Amoxicillin/clavulanate (e.g., Augmentin) can be used in children and adults.
    - For children, 20–40 mg/kg/day PO t.i.d. For adults, 500 mg PO q8h
  - Trimethoprim/sulfamethoxazole (e.g., Bactrim) should be considered in MRSA suspected infections or in penicillin allergic patients.
    - For children, dosage is 8–12 mg/kg/day trimethoprim with 40–60 mg/kg/day sulfamethoxazole PO b.i.d.
    - For adults, 160–320 mg trimethoprim with 800–1,600 mg sulfamethoxazole PO, b.i.d.. Doxycycline is an alternative in nonpregnant adults only (100 mg PO, b.i.d.)
  - Recommended duration of broad-spectrum oral antibiotics is 7–10 days (5)[C].

Second Line

- For children or adults with penicillin allergies, trimethoprim/sulfamethoxazole can be substituted (see "First Line" for dosing)
- For adults only, moxifloxacin (400 mg PO daily) can be substituted.

ADDITIONAL TREATMENT

General Measures

- Hot compresses
- Incision and drainage of localized eyelid abscess if present (see "Surgery")

Issues for Referral

- Ophthalmology consultation is advised for moderate to severe cases and all pediatric cases.
- ENT consultation is suggested for medical and surgical treatment of sinusitis.

Additional Therapies

If patient is on broad-spectrum antibiotics and flocculence or abscess detected, then low-dose, short-duration adjunct corticosteroids can be given in the absence of retained foreign body.

SURGERY/OTHER PROCEDURES

- A lid abscess may complicate preseptal cellulitis and can be surgically drained in an outpatient setting with alert cooperative patients.
  - Pus obtained from wounds or abscess cavities: directly inoculate onto blood agar, chocolate agar, and an anaerobic medium

IN-PATIENT CONSIDERATIONS

Initial Stabilization

- Patients with severe cases or less than 1 year of age should be initially managed as an orbital cellulitis with a CT scan, IV broad-spectrum antibiotics, and hospital observation (6)[B].
  - IV antibiotic choices include ampicillin/sulbactam or ceftriaxone. Consider local trends in antimicrobial therapy. If MRSA is suspected or if patient is allergic to penicillin, consider vancomycin.
  - Choice of specific IV antibiotic depends on the results of Gram stain and culture.

Admission Criteria

- Children younger than 1 year (6)[B]
- Orbital cellulitis is suspected
- Patient appears toxic
- Patient may be noncompliant with outpatient treatment or follow-up
- Clinical deterioration or no noticeable improvement after 48 h of oral antibiotics

Nursing

- Continue monitoring vitals and symptoms.
- Alert physician if patient develops worsening signs of toxicity, orbital involvement, changes in visual acuity, or neurological signs.

Discharge Criteria

- IV antibiotics can be switched to comparable oral antibiotics and monitored on an outpatient basis after significant improvement is observed.
- Patient should be afebrile for a minimum of 24 h before switching to oral antibiotics or afebrile for 48 h if blood cultures were positive.

ONGOING CARE

FOLLOW-UP RECOMMENDATIONS

- Daily outpatient visits are necessary until consistent improvement is demonstrated, then followed every 2–7 days until total resolution.
- Cell phone photographs may be useful during this period for monitoring.

Patient Monitoring

Observe for signs of worsening infection, orbital cellulitis, and/or systemic toxicity

PATIENT EDUCATION

Patients are advised to receive immediate care if they experience systemic toxicity, worsening visual acuity, or pain with eye movements.

PROGNOSIS

Prognosis for complete recovery is excellent in patients identified and treated promptly.

COMPLICATIONS

- Infection may spread along tissue planes and progress to orbital cellulitis, subperiosteal abscess, orbital abscess, intracranial infection, and cavernous sinus thrombosis.
- Immunocompromised patients are more likely to develop potentially fatal fungal infections and should be monitored more aggressively.

REFERENCES

1. Sadovsky R. Distinguishing periorbital from orbital cellulitis. *Am Fam Physician* 2003;67:1327.
2. Babar TF, Zaman M, Khan MN, et al. Risk factors of preseptal and orbital cellulitis. *J Coll Physicians Surg Pak*. 2009;19(1):39–42.
3. Sobol AL, Hutcheson KA. Cellulitis, preseptal. *eMedicine*, April 2008.
4. Starkey CR, Steele RW. Medical management of orbital cellulitis. *Pediatr Infect Dis J* 2001;20:1002.
5. Howe L, Jones NS. Guidelines for the management of periorbital cellulitis/abscess. *Clin Otolaryngol Allied Sci* 2004;29:725.
6. Uzcategui N, Warman R, Smith A, et al. Clinical practice guidelines for the management of orbital cellulitis. *J Pediatr Ophthalmol Strabismus* 1998;35:73.

ADDITIONAL READING

- Ehlers JP, Shah CP, eds. *The Wills eye manual: Office and emergency room diagnosis and treatment of eye disease*, 5th ed. Philadelphia, PA: Lippincott Williams & Wilkins, 2008:139–141.
- Tasman W, Jaeger EA, eds. *Duane's ophthalmology*, 15th ed. Philadelphia, PA: Lippincott Williams & Wilkins, 2009: Volume 2, Chapter 34; Volume 4, Chapter 25.

See Also (Topic, Algorithm, Electronic Media Element)

- Orbital cellulitis

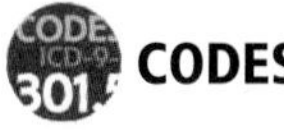

CODES

ICD9

- 373.2 Chalazion
- 373.11 Hordeolum externum
- 376.01 Orbital cellulitis

CLINICAL PEARLS

- Preseptal cellulitis should be distinguished from orbital cellulitis early in patient evaluation. If the distinction is unclear, a CT scan should be done to rule out orbital involvement.
- Broad-spectrum oral antibiotic therapy covering gram-positive organisms can be provided on an outpatient basis provided that the patient is older than 1 year, has had adequate immunizations, has no signs of systemic toxicity, and is considered reliable for daily follow-up visits.
- Patients younger than 1 year or with signs of severe preseptal cellulitis or systemic toxicity should be managed as an inpatient with a CT scan and IV broad-spectrum antibiotics.

PRESUMED OCULAR HISTOPLASMOSIS SYNDROME

Anita P. Schadlu
Ramin Schadlu

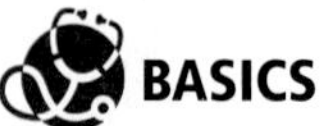

BASICS

DESCRIPTION

- Presumed ocular histoplasmosis syndrome (POHS) is an inflammatory condition associated with systemic infection by the fungus *Histoplasma capsulatum*. It may be unilateral or bilateral.
  - POHS is most common in the Ohio and Mississippi River valleys, where *H. capsulatum* is endemic.

Geriatric Considerations

Elderly patients with coexisting age-related macular degeneration should be monitored closely due to the increased risk of choroidal neovascular membrane (CNVM).

EPIDEMIOLOGY

Incidence

Incidence of new cases of POHS is difficult to determine but has been approximated at 2 per 100,000 per year in an endemic area.

Prevalence

- The prevalence ranges from 1.6% to 5.3% in endemic areas based on epidemiologic data from the 1960s and 1970s.
- In endemic regions, up to 70% of the population demonstrate exposure to *H. capsulatum* and react positively to histoplasmin antigen skin testing (1).

RISK FACTORS

- Exposure to *H. capsulatum* is the major risk factor for developing POHS.
  - 4.4% of those who are skin test positive to *H. capsulatum* have clinical findings consistent with POHS (1).

Genetics

The HLA subtypes DRw2 and B7 have been associated with POHS. This suggests that POHS is possibly an immune-mediated response to an infectious trigger (1).

GENERAL PREVENTION

Avoiding exposure to *H. capsulatum* by avoiding sites of possible contamination such as excavation sites, old buildings being demolished, bird habitats, and bat-infested caves may prevent infection.

PATHOPHYSIOLOGY

- Focal infection of the choroid with *H. capsulatum* and/or a chronic reaction to immunogenic remnants of the organism causes the choroidal lesions in POHS.
  - Very little pathologic evidence exists implicating *H. capsulatum* in POHS.

ETIOLOGY

- *H. capsulatum* has been implicated by epidemiologic studies and antigen skin testing in the U.S.
- However, a study in the Netherlands found no immunologic evidence to support a relationship between the clinical findings of POHS and *H. capsulatum* or other endemic organisms (2).

COMMONLY ASSOCIATED CONDITIONS

CNVM, which can be vision threatening

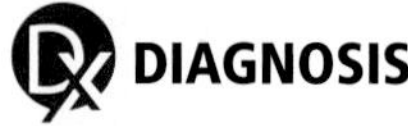

DIAGNOSIS

HISTORY

- Patients are typically young or middle-aged and may be asymptomatic.
- Patients should be questioned about time spent in endemic areas.

PHYSICAL EXAM

- POHS may be unilateral or bilateral.
- The classic findings for POHS are as follows:
  - Multiple, focal, discrete, atrophic choroidal scars in the macula or periphery (termed "punched-out" lesions or "histo spots") can result from previous choroiditis or CNVM.
    - Linear atrophic lesions may also be seen ("histo streaks").
  - Peripapillary atrophy (chorioretinal atrophy adjacent to the optic nerve)
  - No cellular reaction in the anterior chamber or vitreous cavity
- Active and/or regressed CNVM may be seen in association with POHS. A fibrovascular disciform scar may also be seen as a remnant of prior CNVM.
  - The development of CNVM is more likely in eyes with macular "histo spots."
- Active areas of choroiditis may be seen.

DIAGNOSTIC TESTS & INTERPRETATION

Lab

- Laboratory testing is not generally indicated in patients with POHS, since it is a clinical diagnosis.
- Skin testing with histoplasmin antigen is generally no longer performed.
- In patients with ocular disease only, serum and/or urine antigen testing for *H. capsulatum* is unlikely to yield positive results.
- Serum antibodies to *H. capsulatum* can be detected in patients with a history of exposure to the organism.

Imaging

Initial approach

- Imaging tests are indicated to confirm the presence of CNVM.
  - Fundus photographs
  - Fluorescein angiogram
  - Ocular coherence tomography
  - Indocyanine green angiography

Follow-up & special considerations

Patients with POHS should be followed at least yearly for early detection of CNVM.

Pathological Findings

One study detected products of *H. capsulatum* DNA via polymerase chain reaction in 1 eye with POHS (3).

DIFFERENTIAL DIAGNOSIS

- Multifocal choroiditis with panuveitis
  - Clinically similar to POHS but can be differentiated by the presence of a cellular reaction.
- Pathologic myopia
- Age-related macular degeneration
- Angioid streaks
- Idiopathic CNVM
- Other fungal choroiditis
- Bacterial choroiditis
- Viral choroiditis

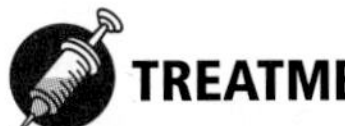

TREATMENT

MEDICATION

- Medication is not indicated for most cases of POHS.
- Patients with choroiditis may be treated with oral or periocular steroid.

ADDITIONAL TREATMENT

Issues for Referral

- Patients with any suspicion of CNVM should be evaluated by a retinal specialist.
  - Immunocompromised patients may develop disseminated histoplasmosis. Such cases should be referred to an infectious disease specialist.

Additional Therapies

- Thermal laser has been shown to be beneficial in CNVM secondary to POHS (1)[A].
  - However, thermal laser to subfoveal or juxtafoveal lesions can cause a central scotoma, so alternative therapies should be explored.
- Photodynamic therapy can be beneficial for treatment of CNVM due to POHS. Patients typically require only 1 or 2 treatments and have good 2-year maintenance of treatment benefit (4)[A].
- Intravitreal bevacizumab has resulted in an increase in vision in 71% of eyes treated for CNVM due to POHS. Intravitreal bevacizumab should be considered especially in patients with subfoveal CNVM in whom other treatment modalities may lead to central scotoma (5)[A].

SURGERY/OTHER PROCEDURES

- In patients with extension of peripapillary CNVM into the subfoveal space, pars plana vitrectomy with removal of the CNVM may be beneficial. In a retrospective review, 15/17 patients had stabilization or improvement of their vision after a year or more (6)[B].
- The submacular surgery trial found that there was a benefit to surgery in patients with vision worse than 20/100, but this was before anti-VEGF therapy. There was a 58% recurrence rate.

IN-PATIENT CONSIDERATIONS

Initial Stabilization

In patients with disseminated histoplasmosis, a complete medical evaluation to determine organ involvement should be performed. Intravenous antifungals should be initiated.

Admission Criteria

Disseminated histoplasmosis may occur in immunocompromised patients. These patients require hospitalization and aggressive management.

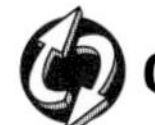

ONGOING CARE

FOLLOW-UP RECOMMENDATIONS

Patients need regularly scheduled follow-up visits at least yearly. In patients with evidence of previous or active CNVM, more frequent follow-up is indicated.

Patient Monitoring

Patients should monitor their central vision daily with an Amsler grid. Any changes should be evaluated immediately.

PATIENT EDUCATION

Patients should be educated on the need for regular follow-up and daily Amsler grid monitoring.

PROGNOSIS

Visual prognosis can be good, as long as glaucoma and any posterior segment complications are controlled.

COMPLICATIONS

Permanent visual loss can occur secondary to CNVM.

REFERENCES

1. Prasad AG, Van Gelder RN. Presumed ocular histoplasmosis syndrome. *Curr Opin Ophthalmol* 2005;16:364–368.
2. Ongkosuwito JV, Kortbeek LM, Van Der Lelij A, et al. Aetiological study of the presumed ocular histoplasmosis syndrome in the Netherlands. *Br J Ophthalmol* 1999;83:535–539.
3. Spencer WH, Chan CC, Shen DF, et al. Detection of *Histoplasma capsulatum* DNA in lesions of chronic ocular histoplasmosis syndrome. *Arch Ophthalmol* 2003;121:1551–1555.
4. Postelmans L, Pasteels B, Coquelet P, et al. Photodynamic therapy for subfoveal classic choroidal neovascularization related to punctate inner choroidopathy (PIC) or presumed ocular histoplasmosis-like syndrome (POHS-like). *Ocul Immunol Inflamm* 2005;13:331–333.
5. Schadlu R, Blinder KJ, Shah GK, et al. Intravitreal bevacizumab for choroidal neovascularization in ocular histoplasmosis. *Am J Ophthalmol* 2008;145:875–878.
6. Almony A, Thomas MA, Atebara NH, et al. Long-term follow-up of surgical removal of extensive peripapillary choroidal neovascularization in presumed ocular histoplasmosis syndrome. *Ophthalmology* 2008;115:540–545.
7. Hawkins BS, Bressler NM, Bressler SB, et al. Submacular Surgery Trials Research Group. Surgical removal versus observation for subfoveal choroidal neovascularization, either associated with the ocular histoplasmosis syndrome or idiopathic I. Ophthalmic findings from a randomized clinical trial: Submacular Surgery Trial Group H Trial: SST Report No. 9. *Arch Ophthalmol* 2004;122(11): 1597–1611.

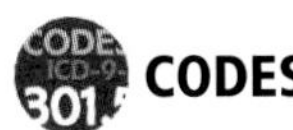

CODES

ICD9

379.8 Other specified disorders of eye and adnexa

CLINICAL PEARLS

- POHS is an ocular syndrome based on clinical findings. Linkage to *H. capsulatum* is controversial.
- CNVM is the primary cause of visual loss in POHS.
- Except early in inoculation, patients will not have noticeable intraocular inflammation.

PRIMARY OPTIC NERVE SHEATH MENINGIOMA (ONSM)

Matthew D. Kay

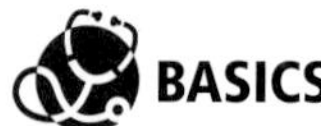

BASICS

DESCRIPTION

Tumor of perioptic meningeal sheath producing a compressive optic neuropathy

EPIDEMIOLOGY

Incidence

- Represent approximately 1–2% of all meningiomas
- Represent approximately 1.5% of all orbital tumors
- 94% unilateral
- Childhood through 8th decade with mean age of 41 years
  - Female:Male 3:2
  - Site of origin: 92% intraorbital optic nerve (ON); 8% optic canal

RISK FACTORS

Neurofibromatosis type 2 (NF2) is present in 9% of optic nerve sheath meningioma (ONSM) patients.

Genetics

Disorder localized to chromosome 22 if related to NF2

PATHOPHYSIOLOGY

Chronic compression of the ON by enveloping tumor or ischemic change secondary to compromised blood supply related to compression of the pial vasculature, central retinal vein, or central retinal artery

ETIOLOGY

Tumor arising from the meningothelial "cap cells" of the arachnoid villi along the intraorbital and canalicular portions of the ON

COMMONLY ASSOCIATED CONDITIONS

NF2 (9%)

DIAGNOSIS

HISTORY

Painless progressive generally unilateral visual loss ± transient visual obscurations lasting seconds, proptosis (59%), and/or diplopia (47%)

PHYSICAL EXAM

- Demonstrates features of an optic neuropathy: decreased visual acuity; decreased color vision; nerve fiber bundle-type visual field defect; afferent pupillary defect if unilateral or asymmetric ON involvement
- ON may appear normal, pale, or edematous based upon the location of tumor with anterior involvement producing ON edema while posterior orbital and canalicular lesions generally demonstrate either a normal ON appearance or ON pallor.
- Optociliary shunt vessels in 30% of patients

DIAGNOSTIC TESTS & INTERPRETATION

Imaging

Initial approach

- MRI orbits with and without contrast including T1-weighted postcontrast images with fat suppression: coronal images demonstrate the ON to be a hypodense area surrounded by the tumor that appears as an enhancing thin, fusiform, or globular ring of tissue.
- MRI demonstrates characteristic features generally sufficient to establish diagnosis.
- Precontrast CT images may demonstrate calcifications in the tumor in some cases, whereas postcontrast CT may demonstrate "tram-track" sign.

Follow-up & special considerations

Serial MRI orbits q6–18 months unless change in visual function prompts earlier reevaluation.

Diagnostic Procedures/Other

- Biopsy rarely indicated given characteristic radiographic features, but can be performed if MRI and clinical features are unclear.
  - If biopsy is performed, it should be limited to the dural sheath and subdural tissue and should not involve the ON per se.

Pathological Findings

- Two histological patterns: meningothelial pattern with polygonal cells separated by vascular trabeculae; transitional pattern with spindle- or oval-shaped cells arranged in concentric whorl formation
  - Psammoma bodies are more common in transitional pattern.

DIFFERENTIAL DIAGNOSIS

- ON glioma
- Optic perineuritis
- Metastatic infiltration
- Sarcoidosis
- Lymphoma

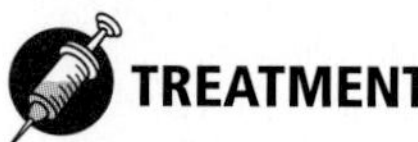

TREATMENT

ADDITIONAL TREATMENT

General Measures

Conformal 3-dimensional external beam radiation therapy should be performed in patients with evidence of progressive visual loss on serial clinical exams and visual field studies or if significant visual loss at presentation (1).

Issues for Referral

Radiation oncology consultation for radiation therapy

SURGERY/OTHER PROCEDURES

Complete resection of ON and tumor up to chiasm via craniotomy is reserved for patients with severe visual loss and intracranial extension (rarely indicated).

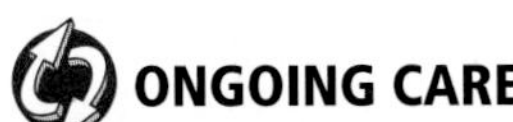

ONGOING CARE

FOLLOW-UP RECOMMENDATIONS

Call for visual changes

Patient Monitoring

- Serial clinical exams with formal perimetry should be performed q3–6 months initially if being observed without radiation therapy unless subjective visual changes prompt earlier reevaluation, with decreasing frequency thereafter based upon clinical course.
- Serial MRI or orbit CT scans should be obtained q6–18 months unless change in visual function prompts earlier reevaluation; it may be more frequent when initially diagnosed.

PATIENT EDUCATION

Inform of the benign nature of tumor with generally favorable prognosis for stabilization or improvement of visual function with radiation therapy if administered.

PROGNOSIS

Favorable prognosis for stabilization or improvement of visual function (94%) with radiation therapy

COMPLICATIONS

- Potential for radiation optic neuropathy or radiation retinopathy if treated with radiation therapy (rare with above protocol)
- Blindness if ONSM remains untreated or if attempt surgical excision

REFERENCES

1. Turbin RE, Thompson CR, Kennerdell JS, et al. A long-term visual outcome comparison in patients with optic nerve sheath meningioma managed with observation, surgery, radiotherapy, or surgery and radiotherapy. *Ophthalmology* 2002;109:890–900.
2. Andrews DW, Faroozan R, Yang BP, et al. Fractionated stereotactic radiotherapy for the treatment of optic nerve sheath meningiomas: Preliminary observations of 33 optic nerves in 30 patients with historical comparison to observation with or without prior surgery. *Neurosurgery* 2002; 51:890–904.

ADDITIONAL READING

- Cockerham KP, Kennerdell JS, Maroon JC, et al. Tumors of the meninges and related tissues: Meningiomas and sarcomas. In: Miller NR, Newman NJ, eds., *Walsh and Hoyt's Clinical Neuro-ophthalmology*. 6th Ed. 2005:1502–1507.
- Dutton JJ. Optic nerve sheath meningiomas. *Surv Ophthalmol* 1992;37:167–183.
- Miller NR. New concepts in the diagnosis and management of optic nerve sheath meningioma. *J Neuro-ophthal* 2006;26(3):200–208.

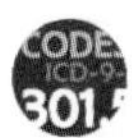

CODES

ICD9

- 225.1 Benign neoplasm of cranial nerves
- 225.2 benign neoplasm of meninges
- 377.49 Other disorders of optic nerve

CLINICAL PEARLS

- Triad of progressive visual loss, optic atrophy, and optociliary shunt vessels, albeit not pathognomonic, is highly suggestive of an ONSM.

P

PROLIFERATIVE DIABETIC RETINOPATHY

Brett J. Rosenblatt

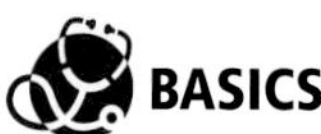

BASICS

DESCRIPTION

Proliferative diabetic retinopathy (PDR) is characterized by the growth of fibrovascular tissue due to chronic, poorly controlled diabetes. PDR includes preretinal neovascularization, vitreous hemorrhage, traction retinal detachment, and secondary rhegmatogenous retinal detachment.

EPIDEMIOLOGY

Incidence

About 50% of patients with PDR will progress to legal blindness without treatment (1)[A].

Prevalence

Overall, 5% of patients with diabetes have PDR. Approximately 29% of patients who have had type 1 diabetes for greater than 15 years have PDR, compared with 16% of patients with type 2 diabetes for a similar duration.

RISK FACTORS

- Longer duration of diabetes
- Poor glycemic control
- Hypertension
- Pregnancy

GENERAL PREVENTION

- Optimizing blood pressure and blood glucose levels
- Routine eye exams and timely laser treatment

PATHOPHYSIOLOGY

- Accumulated capillary damage including endothelial proliferation, loss of pericytes, and capillary closure leading to retinal ischemia
- Local vascular and fibrovascular proliferation mediated by growth factors (e.g., vascular endothelial growth factor)

COMMONLY ASSOCIATED CONDITIONS

- Diabetic nephropathy and neuropathy
- Cardiovascular disease
- Macular edema and ischemia

DIAGNOSIS

HISTORY

- Determine onset of diabetes, duration and degree of glycemic control
- History of hypertension
- Previous laser treatment
- Pregnancy status
- Symptoms:
  - Acute vision loss preceded by extensive floaters suggests vitreous hemorrhage or retinal detachment.
  - Pain and redness of the eye may be due to neovascular glaucoma.
  - Gradual loss of vision with macular ischemia, edema, or tractional retinal detachment

PHYSICAL EXAM

- Anterior segment exam: iris or angle neovascularization, hyphema, posterior synechiae
- Elevated intraocular pressure
- Posterior exam: vitreous hemorrhage, neovascularization of the disc (fibrous proliferation typically arising from optic disc and extending along major retinal vessels), and neovascularization elsewhere, both grow from the retinal surface into the vitreous and can lead to vitreous hemorrhage and/or tractional retinal detachments.

DIAGNOSTIC TESTS & INTERPRETATION

Lab

- HbA1c, CBC, blood pressure
- Consider Hgb electrophoresis
- Carotid ultrasound
- Pregnancy test

Imaging

- Fluorescein angiography identifies areas of nonperfusion and neovascularization.
- Optical coherence tomography can assess macular edema.
- Ultrasound if vitreous hemorrhage

DIFFERENTIAL DIAGNOSIS

- Sickle cell retinopathy
- Ocular ischemia (carotid stenosis)
- Radiation retinopathy
- Retinal vein occlusion
- Hypertensive retinopathy
- Coats disease
- Occlusive vasculitis
- Talc retinopathy

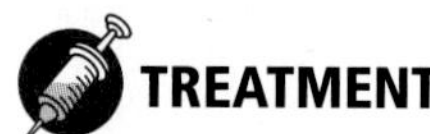

TREATMENT

MEDICATION

- Consider antivascular endothelial growth factor medications (bevacizumab, ranibizumab) for control of neovascularization (2)[C].
- Topical glaucoma drops or oral acetazolamide to control eye pressure

ADDITIONAL TREATMENT

General Measures

Laser Photocoagulation

- Pan-retinal photocoagulation (PRP) if high-risk characteristics are present:
- Neovascularization associated with vitreous or preretinal hemorrhage or disc neovascularization larger than one-third disc area are high-risk characteristics and these patients should have PRP (3)[A].

SURGERY/OTHER PROCEDURES

Consider vitrectomy for nonclearing vitreous hemorrhage (>3 months duration), and tractional or rhegmatogenous retinal detachment or dense premacular hemorrhage.

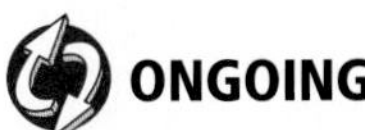

ONGOING CARE

FOLLOW-UP RECOMMENDATIONS

Patients require very close monitoring until the disease is brought under control.

PATIENT MONITORING

Every 3 months until the disease is stable

PATIENT EDUCATION

Glycemic control. Exercise, weight management, blood pressure control, and close monitoring by internist/endocrinologist

PROGNOSIS

- Improved prognosis with early detection and treatment
- PRP reduces risk of severe vision loss by 50%.
- Macular detachments or severe macular ischemia leads to severe vision loss.

COMPLICATIONS

Retinal detachment, retinal ischemia, neovascular glaucoma

REFERENCES

1. Diabetic Retinopathy Study Research Group. Photocoagulation treatment of proliferative diabetic retinopathy. *Ophthalmology* 1978;85:82–106. [A]
2. Avery RL, Pearlman J, Pieramici DJ, et al. Intravitreal bevacizumab (Avastin) in the treatment of proliferative diabetic retinopathy. *Ophthalmology* 2006;10:1695–1705. [C]
3. Early Treatment Diabetic Study Group. Early Photocoagulation for diabetic retinopathy report 9. *Ophthalmology* 1991;98:766–785. [A]

CODES

ICD9

- 250.50 Diabetes mellitus with ophthalmic manifestations, type II or unspecified type, not stated as uncontrolled
- 362.02 Proliferative diabetic retinopathy

CLINICAL PEARLS

- Prompt PRP can prevent blindness.
- Keeping the head elevated and limiting activity may allow vitreous hemorrhage to clear faster.

PSEUDOEXFOLIATION SYNDROME

Andrea Knellinger Sawchyn
George L. Spaeth

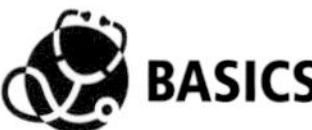

BASICS

DESCRIPTION

- A systemic disorder characterized by the deposition of a fibrillar material on the lens, ciliary epithelium, zonules, iris, and corneal endothelium, which may be associated with the development of open- or closed-angle glaucoma
- In the U.S., approximately 40% of patients with pseudoexfoliation syndrome (PXS) develop pseudoexfoliation glaucoma (PXG).
- Differentiated from true exfoliation (capsular delamination seen in individuals exposed to infrared radiation)

EPIDEMIOLOGY

Incidence

- Varies depending on country, ethnicity, and age
- In the U.S., the incidence of PXS has been estimated to be 25.9 per 100,000, but varies by age (1)[C]:
  - 40–49 years old: 2.8 per 100,000
  - ≥80 years old: 205.7 per 100,000
- In the U.S., the incidence of PXG is 9.9 per 100,000, but also varies by age (1)[C]:
  - 40–49 years old: 0.6 per 100,000
  - ≥80 years old: 114.3 per 100,000

Prevalence

- Varies depending on location and ethnicity
- In the Framingham Eye Study, the rate of PXS was 0.6% for ages 52–64 years and 5.0% for ages 75–85 years.
- In some Scandinavian countries, PXG may account for more than 50% of open-angle glaucoma.

RISK FACTORS

- Age (more common >60 years)
- Female
- Scandinavian descent
- Family history

Genetics

- Strong familial association
- Multiple modes of inheritance (including autosomal dominant, autosomal recessive, X-linked, and maternal inheritance patterns) have been described.
- Some studies suggest that polymorphisms in the lysyl oxidase-like 1 (*LOL1*) gene (which is involved in the synthesis and maintenance of elastic fibers) is associated with pseudoexfoliation (2)[B].
- Polymorphisms in the clusterin gene may be a risk factor for pseudoexfoliation.
- Role of genetic testing is not clear.

GENERAL PREVENTION

No known modes of prevention

PATHOPHYSIOLOGY

- Several mechanisms of pathogenesis have been proposed:
  - Elastic microfibril hypothesis: pseudoexfoliation material accumulates due to excessive synthesis of elastin fibrils.
  - Pseudoexfoliation material may be composed of basement membrane proteoglycans and may accumulate due to abnormal metabolism of glycosaminoglycans in the iris.
  - Overexpression of transforming growth factor $\beta 1$ and an imbalance between matrix metalloproteinases and tissue inhibitors of matrix metalloproteinases probably contribute to the pathogenesis.
- Glaucoma may be the result of accumulation of the fibrillar material in the juxtacanalicular tissue.
- Accumulation of the pseudoexfoliation material in Schlemm's canal may lead to narrowing or collapse of this structure, also contributing to elevated intraocular pressure (IOP).

ETIOLOGY

- The exact etiology has not been elucidated.
- See Pathophysiology section for current hypotheses.

COMMONLY ASSOCIATED CONDITIONS

- Cataract
- Open or closed angle glaucoma
- Hyperhomocysteinemia
- Cardiovascular disease
- Sensorineural hearing loss

DIAGNOSIS

HISTORY

Generally asymptomatic

PHYSICAL EXAM

- Usually bilateral but frequently asymmetric
- Flakes of pseudoexfoliation material and pigment on the corneal endothelium
- Pseudoexfoliation material is seen on the anterior lens capsule in a characteristic pattern: central plaque of pseudoexfoliation material surrounded by a clear zone surrounded by a peripheral zone of pseudoexfoliation material.
- Nuclear opacities
- Pseudoexfoliation material deposits on and weakens the lens zonules, leading to phacodonesis and lens subluxation.
- Pseudoexfoliation flakes on the pupillary margin.
- Moth-eaten transillumination defects near the pupillary margin
- Iridodonesis
- Loss of pupillary ruff
- Poor mydriasis
- Increased pigmentation of the trabecular meshwork
- Sampaolesi's line (undulating line of pigment anterior to Schwalbe's line)
- Zonular laxity may lead to a closed angle and shallow anterior chamber depth.
- Glaucomatous optic cupping may be present
- Elevated IOP
- Mild anterior chamber flare
- On fluorescein angiography, iris vessels often leak.

DIAGNOSTIC TESTS & INTERPRETATION

Lab

Consider checking plasma homocysteine levels (hyperhomocysteinemia has been detected in 27.1% of patients with PXG) (3)[B].

Imaging

Initial approach

- Optic nerve photos
- Optic nerve imaging (confocal scanning laser ophthalmoscopy, scanning laser polarimetry, or optical coherence tomography)

Follow-up & special considerations

Repeat optic disc photos or imaging every 1–2 years.

Diagnostic Procedures/Other

- Visual fields should be obtained every 1–2 years (or more frequently if indicated by rate of glaucomatous progression).
- A-scan or IOLMaster axial length measurements and corneal curvature measurements for those undergoing cataract surgery.
- Pachymetry to assess central corneal thickness

Pathological Findings

- Eosinophilic pseudoexfoliation material is found on the anterior lens capsule, zonules, anterior and posterior surfaces of the iris, ciliary body epithelium, corneal endothelium, and incorporated into the trabecular meshwork.
- Elastin and tropoelastin are present by immunoelectron microscopy.
- Pseudoexfoliation material has been found in other ocular (conjunctiva, posterior ciliary vessels), periocular (eyelid skin, extraocular muscles, orbital septa) and extraocular (heart, lungs, liver, kidney, gallbladder, and cerebral meninges) sites (4)[B].

DIFFERENTIAL DIAGNOSIS

- True exfoliation (see Description)
- Primary amyloidosis
- Pigmentary dispersion syndrome/glaucoma
- Uveitic glaucoma
- Chronic angle-closure glaucoma

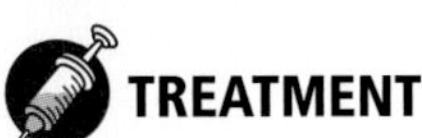

TREATMENT

MEDICATION

First Line

- Observation may be appropriate, if there are no signs of ocular hypertension or glaucoma.
- When ocular hypertension is present, close observation is warranted. As the course of PXS from normal IOP to ocular hypertension to glaucoma can be rapid, initiation of IOP-lowering treatment may be indicated.
- When signs of glaucoma are present, treatment (medications, laser, or surgery) should be initiated. Medications include the following:
  - Topical prostaglandin analogues (e.g., travoprost, latanoprost, bimatoprost)
  - Topical beta-blockers (e.g., timolol, betaxolol)
  - Topical alpha$_2$-agonists (e.g., brimonidine)
  - Topical carbonic anhydrase inhibitors (e.g., dorzolamide, brinzolamide)
  - Fixed combination meds (e.g., dorzolamide/timolol, timolol/brimonidine)

Second Line

Oral carbonic anhydrase inhibitors (e.g., acetazolamide, methazolamide)

ADDITIONAL TREATMENT

Issues for Referral

- Consider referral to an experienced anterior segment surgeon for cataract extraction if zonular laxity is present.
- Consider referral to a glaucoma specialist when indicated.

SURGERY/OTHER PROCEDURES

- Laser trabeculoplasty can be highly effective, but the duration of effectiveness may be short compared with primary open angle glaucoma (POAG).
- Cataract extraction when lenticular opacities are visually significant (be prepared to use iris expansion techniques due to poor mydriasis and consider use of a capsular tension ring; extracapsular cataract extraction is indicated in some cases). NOTE: Pseudoexfoliation does not resolve following cataract extraction (5)[B].
- Trabecular aspiration has been described but has not been well studied.
- Trabeculectomy with mitomycin-C
- Tube shunt
- Cyclophotocoagulation may be considered when other medical and surgical treatments fail.

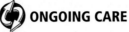

ONGOING CARE

FOLLOW-UP RECOMMENDATIONS

- Patients with PXS should be seen for a full exam annually to monitor for signs of glaucoma and/or lens subluxation.
- Patients with PXG should be seen every 3–12 months depending on disease severity.

DIET

Consider folate and vitamin B_{12} supplementation if hyperhomocysteinemia is present.

PROGNOSIS

- Variable
- Greater diurnal IOP variation in PXG compared with POAG
- PXG is often more difficult to treat than POAG.
- When PXG progresses, it often progresses more rapidly than POAG.

COMPLICATIONS

- Lens subluxation
- Glaucomatous visual field loss
- Corneal decompensation

REFERENCES

1. Karger RA, Jeng SM, Johnson DH, et al. Estimated incidence of pseudoexfoliation syndrome and pseudoexfoliation glaucoma in Olmsted County, Minnesota. *J Glaucoma* 2003;12:193–197.
2. Challa P. Genetics of pseudoexfoliation syndrome. *Curr Opin Ophthalmol* 2009;20:88–91.
3. Clement CI, Goldberg I, Healey PR, et al. Plasma homocysteine, MTHFR gene mutation, and open angle glaucoma. *J Glaucoma* 2009;18:73–78.
4. Streeten BW, Li ZY, Wallace RN, et al. Pseudoexfoliation fibrillopathy in visceral organs of a patient with pseudoexfoliation syndrome. *Arch Ophthalmol* 1992;110:1757–1762.
5. Shingleton BJ, Crandall AS, Ahmed II. Pseudoexfoliation and the cataract surgeon: preoperative, intraoperative, and postoperative issues related to intraocular pressure, cataract, and intraocular lenses. *J Cataract Refract Surg* 2010;36:702.

ADDITIONAL READING

- Ritch R, Schlotzer-Schrehardt U. Exfoliation syndrome. *Surv Ophthal* 2001;45:265–315.
- Shlotzer-Schrehardt U, Naumann GO. Ocular and systemic pseudoexfoliation syndrome. *Am J Ophthalmol* 2006;141:921–937.

CODES

ICD9

- 365.52 Pseudoexfoliation glaucoma
- 366.11 Pseudoexfoliation of the lens capsule

CLINICAL PEARLS

- PXS, which is more common after the age of 60 years, is characterized by deposition of fibrillar material on the anterior lens capsule, zonules, iris, and corneal endothelium. These changes may be minimal. Iris and angle changes are important in making the diagnosis of pseudoexfoliation.
- PXG may develop in up to 40% of individuals with PXS.
- Cataract extraction can be complicated by poor mydriasis and loose zonules.
- IOP control in PXG can be more challenging than in POAG.

PSEUDOPAPILLEDEMA

Saunders L. Hupp

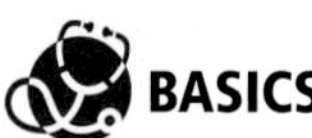

BASICS

DESCRIPTION

Optic disc elevation unrelated to increased intracranial pressure (ICP)

EPIDEMIOLOGY

Incidence

0.3–2.4% (1)[A]

Prevalence

- 3.4–4.9/1000 clinically, up to 20.4/1000 in autopsy studies (2)[A], (3)[A]
- 75% bilateral (1)[A]
  - males = females
  - Less prevalent in African Americans

RISK FACTORS

Hyperopes and myopes equally affected

Genetics

- Drusen are transmitted as autosomal dominant.
  - Rarely visible in an infant, drusen enlarge and calcify with age.

PATHOPHYSIOLOGY

- Elevation and crowding of the optic nerve axons not associated with ICP.
  - drusen, collections of a mucoprotein matrix, most often concentrated in the nasal portion of the disc
  - remnants of hyaloid system remain with gliosis and/or traction on the axons
  - crowding due to a small cup
  - tilted disc due to angle of optic nerve entry into eye
  - retained myelin
  - metastatic or primary tumors of the optic nerve
  - scleral infiltration

ETIOLOGY

Drusen are the result of extracellular deposition of axoplasmic material either from mechanical interruption of axonal transport or from axonal degeneration (2)[A].

COMMONLY ASSOCIATED CONDITIONS

- Optic nerve buried or superficial drusen
- Down's syndrome
- Alagille syndrome (arteriohepatic dysplasia)
- Kenny syndrome (hypocalcemic dwarfism)
- Linear nevus sebaceous syndrome
- Leber's hereditary optic neuropathy

DIAGNOSIS

HISTORY

- Usually asymptomatic with no visual complaints
  - Rarely, brief transient visual obscurations
  - Visual field or central acuity loss if associated with complications (see below)
  - Presence of hypertension, neurologic symptoms (especially headache), and fever

PHYSICAL EXAM

- Visual acuity
- Color vision
- Pupil exam
  - Afferent defect often accompanies complications (see below).
  - Not diagnostic
- Measure blood pressure
- Dilated fundus exam
  - Disc vessels usually clearly visible
    - Rarely may be obscured by gliosis or myelin
    - No hyperemia or dilated capillaries
  - Elevation greatest in center of disc from which central vessels emerge and is confined only to disc
  - Absence of exudates
  - Absence of venous congestion
  - Anomalously elevated disc has no physiologic cup and is usually small.
  - Presence of superficial drusen
  - Disc may be tilted.
  - Spontaneous venous pulsations may or may not be present.
  - Congenitally anomalous vessels may be present.
- Family members may have anomalous discs and drusen.

DIAGNOSTIC TESTS & INTERPRETATION

Lab

- Usually not indicated
- If Leber's hereditary optic neuropathy suspected, arrange genetic analysis.

Imaging

Stereo disc photos

Diagnostic Procedures/Other

- Visual field
  - Peripheral defects develop in 21% of patients with buried drusen and 71% with visible drusen (4)[A].
    - Nerve fiber bundle defects
    - Concentric constriction
    - Enlargement of blind spot
- B-scan ultrasonography
  - Buried drusen exhibit high reflectivity
- CT
  - Calcifications in disc
- Fluorescein angiography
  - Drusen autofluorescence
  - True papilledema exhibits late dye leakage and capillary dilation
- Optical coherence tomography (1)[A], (2)[A]
- Pathological findings
  - Usually none, invasive procedures not indicated

DIFFERENTIAL DIAGNOSIS

- Optic neuritis
- Posterior scleritis
- Toxoplasmosis
- Idiopathic intracranial hypertension
- Ischemic optic neuropathy
  - Anterior
  - Giant cell arteritis
- Compressive optic neuropathy
- Optic nerve infiltrates
- Papilledema
- Sarcoidosis
- Optic nerve tumors
- Papillitis
- Leber's hereditary optic neuropathy

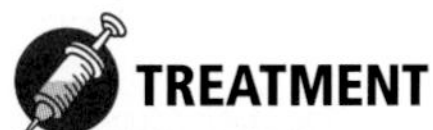

TREATMENT

MEDICATION

Drusen alone need no medical therapy.

ADDITIONAL TREATMENT

General Measures

Patient education (see below)

Issues for Referral

- Choroidal neovascular membrane
  - May require laser photocoagulation or use of antivasogenic drugs
- Nonarteric ischemic optic neuropathy
  - Optimize cardiovascular status
  - Treat even borderline ocular hypertension

IN-PATIENT CONSIDERATIONS

Initial Stabilization

- Evaluate for the presence of severe hypertension and acute neurologic signs and symptoms.
- Measure visual acuity.
- Rule out true papilledema.

Admission Criteria

- Severe hypertension
- Acute visual loss
  - Giant cell arteritis in the elderly
    - Elevated sedimentation rate and or C-reactive protein
- Papilledema

Discharge Criteria

- Vital signs stable
- Acute visual loss static or transient
- Absence of papilledema
- Ophthalmology follow-up

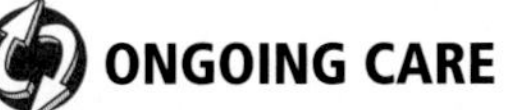

ONGOING CARE

FOLLOW-UP RECOMMENDATIONS

Annual exam unless complications (see below)

Patient Monitoring

- Physical exam (see above)
- Visual field exam

PATIENT EDUCATION

- Patient and family should be able to relate history of pseudopapilledema to future caregivers.
  - Provide disc photo

PROGNOSIS

Usually very good

COMPLICATIONS

- Peripapillary or disc hemorrhage
  - Most patients retain normal or near-normal vision.
- Peripheral visual field loss in 71–75%
- Loss of central vision
  - Acute and nonprogressive
  - Usually preceded by progressive peripheral field loss
  - A diagnosis of exclusion
- Nonarteritic ischemic optic neuropathy
- Retinal artery or vein occlusion
- Transient visual loss
  - Rarely may be a harbinger of retinal vascular occlusion
- Peripapillary subretinal neovascularization

REFERENCES

1. Johnson LN, Diehl ML, Hamm CW, et al. Differentiating optic disc edema from optic nerve head drusen on optical coherence tomography. *Arch Ophthalmol* 2009;127(1):45–49.
2. Yi K, Mujat M, Sun W, et al. Imaging of optic nerve head drusen: improvements with spectral domain optical coherence tomography. *J Glaucoma* 2009;18(5):373–378.
3. Grippo TM, Shihadeh WA, Schargus M, et al. Optic nerve head drusen and visual field loss in normotensive and hypertensive eyes. *J Glaucoma* 2008;17(2):100–104.
4. Katz BJ, Pomeranz HD. Visual field defects and retinal nerve fiber layer defects in eyes with buried optic nerve drusen *Am J Ophthalmol* 2006;141(2): 248–253.

ADDITIONAL READING

- The Neuro-ophthalmology Virtual Education Library http://library.med.utah.edu/NOVEL/
  - Search both pseudopapilledema and optic disc drusen

CODES

ICD9

- 377.21 Optic nerve drusen
- 377.24 Pseudopapilledema

CLINICAL PEARLS

- Examine family members

PTERYGIUM

Peter R. Laibson

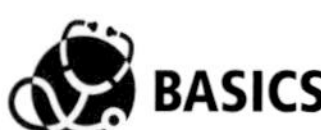

BASICS

DESCRIPTION

A pterygium is a benign, limbal, epithelial, wing-shaped, degenerative growth, mostly nasally, that migrates onto the cornea from the conjunctiva and may cause visual distortion or loss of vision if it progresses into the visual axis. It is treated by surgical removal when vision is threatened or if it is a cosmetic problem. Recurrence of the pterygium can be an issue after surgical removal (1).

EPIDEMIOLOGY

- More prevalent in outdoor workers exposed to highly reflective surfaces such as water and sand
- Encountered in latitudes less than 30°, due to ultraviolet (UV) light exposure
- Chemical exposure, excessive dust, wind, and ethnicity have been linked to pterygium formation and growth.
- Genetic considerations and the presence of human papillomavirus may be linked in some cases to pterygium formation (2).

Pediatric Considerations

Usually not seen in children and teenagers, due probably to cumulative exposure to UV light

RISK FACTORS

- Presence of pinguecula
- Exposure to UV light commonly in those living within 30° of the equator
- Wind
- Dust

Genetics

May be a factor but not yet delineated

GENERAL PREVENTION

Use of sun block, UV protective glasses, and hat when exposed to excessive and reflective sun

PATHOPHYSIOLOGY

Actinic degeneration of sensitive limbal stem cells probably in genetically predisposed individuals.

COMMONLY ASSOCIATED CONDITIONS

- Pingueculum
- None beyond the corneal surface

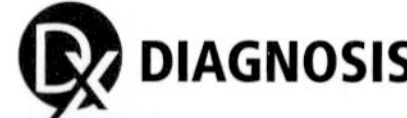

DIAGNOSIS

HISTORY

- Redness nasally usually, but occasionally temporally
- Distorted or reduced vision as pterygium grows toward the visual axis
- Slight irritation as pterygium advances onto the cornea

PHYSICAL EXAM

- Early, small whitish elevated nodule at 9 o'clock limbus
- Later, wing-like growth of fibrovascular tissue extends onto the cornea from nasal limbus mostly.
- May reach and cross visual axis in worst cases
- Hemorrhage from leaking capillaries at pterygium head indicates activity
- Iron line (Stocker's line) at pterygium head indicates inactivity

DIAGNOSTIC TESTS & INTERPRETATION

Diagnostic Procedures/Other

Biopsy not indicated

DIFFERENTIAL DIAGNOSIS

- Pseudopterygium—conjunctival adherence to the cornea due to inflammation or trauma
- Dermoid of the limbus
- Squamous cell carcinoma (rare)

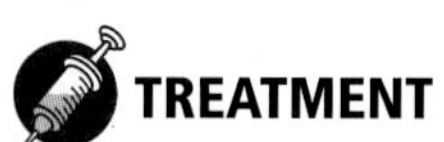

TREATMENT

MEDICATION

- None for prevention or treatment
- Astringents or vasoconstrictors to reduce redness, but limit use

SURGERY/OTHER PROCEDURES

- Surgical removal of pterygium when it threatens vision or becomes a cosmetic problem
- Removal of pterygium from cornea and conjunctiva with dissection of subconjunctival fibrovascular tissue
- Placement of conjunctival autograft (CAG) from the 12 o'clock position of same eye

- Mitomycin C application before placement of cag when appropriate
- Suture cag into position or use tissue adhesives. If conjunctiva must be spared, use amniotic membrane tissue as transplant (3).
- Mitomycin C should be used judiciously (4).

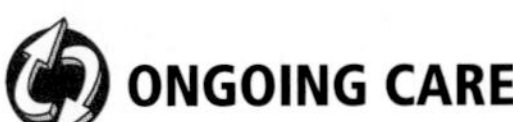

ONGOING CARE

FOLLOW-UP RECOMMENDATIONS

- Topical steroids must be used postoperatively for at least 6 months in tapering dosage to prevent recurrent pterygium (5).

REFERENCES

1. Chang RI, Ching ST. Corneal and conjunctival degenerations. In: *Cornea*. Krachmer JH, Mannis MJ, Holland EJ, eds. Philadelphia: Elsevier Mosby, 2005:1001–1002.
2. Hsiao C, Lee B, Ngan K, et al. Presence of human papillomavirus pterygium in Taiwan. *Cornea* 2010;29:123–127.
3. Kucukerdonmez C, Akova YA, Altinors DD. Comparison of conjunctival autograft with amniotic membrane transplantation for pterygium surgery. *Cornea* 2007;26:407–413.
4. Young AL, Tam PMK, Leung GYS, et al. Prospective study on the safety and efficacy of combined conjunctival rotational autograft with intraoperative 0.02% mitomycin C in primary pterygium excision. *Cornea* 2009;28:166–169.
5. Kandavel R, Kang JJ, Memarzadeh F, et al. Comparison of pterygium recurrence rates in Hispanic and White patients after primary excision and conjunctival autograft. *Cornea* 2010;29: 141–145.

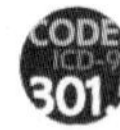

CODES

ICD9

- 224.3 Benign neoplasm of conjunctiva
- 372.40 Pterygium, unspecified

CLINICAL PEARLS

- Most pterygium can be observed at first. If there is progressive growth, they should be surgically removed before coming close to the visual axis.

PTOSIS

Katherine A. Lane

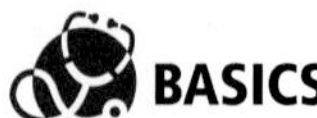

BASICS

DESCRIPTION
- Drooping of the upper eyelid
  - May be congenital or acquired
  - May cause blurred vision or loss of visual field

EPIDEMIOLOGY
Unknown

RISK FACTORS
See associated conditions

Genetics
- Most commonly idiopathic
- May be inherited as autosomal dominant trait
- Familial occurrences suggest that genetic or chromosomal defects are likely, although yet unknown.

PATHOPHYSIOLOGY
- Aponeurotic: levator stretching or dehiscence (1)
- Myogenic: primary or secondary levator and/or Muller's muscle abnormality
- Neurogenic: damage to nerves innervating the levator and/or Muller's muscle
- Mechanical
- Traumatic: damage to eyelid retractors

ETIOLOGY
- Congenital:
  - Myogenic: levator dysgenesis
  - Blepharophimosis
  - Neurogenic: synkinetic, Horner's syndrome, cranial nerve (CN) III palsy
- Acquired:
  - Aponeurotic: normal aging changes, repetitive trauma in patients who rub eyes, contact lens wearers, patients with previous intraocular surgery
  - Myogenic: myasthenia gravis, chronic progressive external ophthalmoplegia (CPEO), myotonic dystrophy, oculopharyngeal dystrophy
  - Neurogenic: CN III palsy, Horner's syndrome
  - Mechanical
  - Traumatic: history of eyelid laceration with levator transection, contusion injury to the levator
  - Reactive: due to ocular or orbital inflammation

COMMONLY ASSOCIATED CONDITIONS
- CN III palsy
  - Congenital, compressive, vasculopathic, traumatic
- Horner's syndrome
- Myasthenia gravis
- Other: Marcus Gunn jaw winking syndrome, ophthalmoplegic migraine, multiple sclerosis

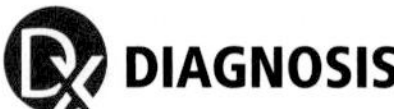

DIAGNOSIS

HISTORY
- Determine the onset and duration of ptosis.
- History of surgery in either eye?
- Symptoms of ocular irritation?
- Orbital or eyelid trauma?
- Variability with fatigue?
- Associated with headache or neck pain?
- Associated diplopia?
- History of autoimmune disease (lupus, Sjögren's syndrome)?

PHYSICAL EXAM
- Visual acuity
- External
  - Position of upper and lower eyelid margins (primary, up and down gaze)
  - Levator function
  - Presence and position of eyelid crease
  - Amount of dermatochalasis, position of eyebrows
  - Preexisting eyelid scars
  - Evert upper eyelid
  - Orbital exam: palpable masses or proptosis?
- Pupils
  - Irregular, miosis or mydriasis
- Motility
  - Ductions and versions
  - Bell's phenomenon
  - Strabismus or diplopia
- Anterior segment
  - Conjunctival inflammation, filtering blebs
  - Tear film
  - Keratopathy
  - Anterior segment inflammation
- Retina
- Pigmentary changes

DIAGNOSTIC TESTS & INTERPRETATION

Lab
Acetylcholine receptor antibody testing and/or edrophonium chloride (Tensilon) testing under monitored conditions are recommended in cases of suspected myasthenia gravis.

Imaging
- Suspected orbital mass: orbital CT or MRI
- Painful Horner's syndrome: rule out carotid artery dissection with emergent CT/CT angiography (CTA) or MRI/magnetic resonance angiography (MRA) of the head/neck.
- CN III palsy (partial or pupil involving): rule out intracranial aneurysm with emergent CT/CTA, MRI/MRA, or angiography.

Diagnostic Procedures/Other
- Visual fields to determine functional impact
- Clinical photographs
- Ice test
  - Improvement of ptosis with ice suggests myasthenia gravis.
- Cocaine and/or hydroxyamphetamine tests
  - In cases of suspected Horner's syndrome
- Single fiber electromyography (EMG)
  - In cases of suspected myasthenia gravis

Pathological Findings
- Congenital ptosis
  - Underdeveloped levator muscle, may be infiltrated by fatty tissue
- Aponeurotic ptosis
  - Thinning, lengthening, and/or disinsertion of the levator aponeurosis from the tarsal plate
- Myogenic ptosis
  - Ragged red fibers in CPEO

DIFFERENTIAL DIAGNOSIS
- Contralateral upper lid retraction
- Ipsilateral exophthalmos
- Small globe: microphthalmos, phthisis bulbi
- Dermatochalasis
- Brow ptosis
- Eyelid edema

TREATMENT

MEDICATION
- Myasthenia gravis: treatment of primary disorder will improve ocular symptoms
  - Pyridostigmine, prednisone, intravenous immunoglobulin (IVIG), steroid-sparing agents

ADDITIONAL TREATMENT
General Measures
- Observation
- Management of chalazion and eyelid and/or orbital neoplasms with excision
- Treatment of ocular irritation in reactive ptosis
- Traumatic ptosis should be observed for spontaneous improvement for at least 6 months.

Issues for Referral
- Congenital ptosis
  - Referral to pediatric ophthalmologist for monitoring/management of possible amblyopia and/or strabismus
- Neurogenic ptosis
  - Referral to neuro-ophthalmologist, neurologist, and/or neurosurgeon

COMPLEMENTARY & ALTERNATIVE THERAPIES
Taping and eyelid crutches attached to glasses

SURGERY/OTHER PROCEDURES
- External levator resection/advancement
- Internal levator resection
- Frontalis sling procedure: for patients with poor levator function

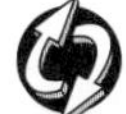

ONGOING CARE

FOLLOW-UP RECOMMENDATIONS
See issues for referral.

Patient Monitoring
Congenital ptosis: see issues for referral.

PROGNOSIS
Dependent of etiology

COMPLICATIONS
- After surgical repair:
  - Orbital hemorrhage
  - Under-/overcorrections
  - Eyelid asymmetry
  - Infection
  - Dry eye syndrome
  - Corneal exposure/lagophthalmos

REFERENCE

1. Frueh BR. The mechanistic classification of ptosis. *Ophthalmology* 1980;87:1019–1021.

ADDITIONAL READING

- Holds JB, Anderson RL. Blepharoptosis, Ch. 12. In: *Color atlas of ophthalmic surgery- Vol. 6. Oculoplastic surgery.* David T, Tse MD, eds. Philadelphia, PA: J.B. Lippincott Co, 1992:151–174.
- Jeffrey A. Nerad. Evaluation and treatment of the patient with ptosis, Ch. 7. In: *Oculoplastic surgery: The requisites in ophthalmology.* Krachmer JH, Series ed. St. Louis, MO: Mosby, 2001:157–192.

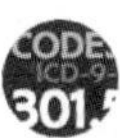

CODES

ICD9
- 374.32 Myogenic ptosis
- 374.33 Mechanical ptosis
- 743.61 Congenital ptosis of eyelid

CLINICAL PEARLS

- All cases of acute onset ptosis require a thorough motility and pupil exam to rule out associated neurological conditions.
- Ptosis exam pearls:
  - Aponeurotic:
    - Moderate ptosis, high eyelid crease, good levator function (10–15 mm), may worsen in downgaze.
- Myogenic:
  - Decreased levator function (>10 mm), weak or absent eyelid crease
  - Congenital cases have demonstrated lagophthalmos in downgaze.
- Neurogenic:
  - CN III palsy: complete ptosis, exotropia/hypotropia, and/or dilated pupil
  - Horner's syndrome: subtle upper and lower eyelid ptosis, miosis, regional anhidrosis; congenital cases may have iris heterochromia.
  - Myasthenia gravis: variable ptosis, worsens with fatigue; often associated with diplopia
- Mechanical:
  - Foreign body in superior fornix, eyelid edema, inflammation, lesion/neoplasm, giant papillary conjunctivitis, ocular irritation
- Traumatic:
  - Evidence of previous trauma, decreased levator function, and/or eyelid retraction

PTOSIS-CONGENITAL

Barry N. Wasserman
Alex V. Levin

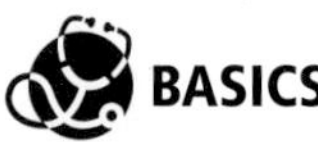

BASICS

DESCRIPTION
- Child born with drooping eyelid toward or into the visual axis
- May be unilateral or bilateral

EPIDEMIOLOGY
Unreported.

RISK FACTORS
- Family history
- Birth trauma

Genetics
- Mostly unknown
- Reported genomic loci include 8q21.11–q22.1 (1), 1p32–1p34.1 (autosomal dominant), and Xq24–27.1 (X linked recessive)
- Associated with many genetic syndromes (e.g., Cornelia de Lange, Turner syndrome, craniofacial disorders)
- One of the cardinal features of blepharophimosis syndrome (congenital ptosis, epicanthus inversus, horizontal shortening of palpebral fissures), autosomal dominant, FOXL2 gene (3q22), may be associated with female infertility, also a locus at 7q34.

GENERAL PREVENTION
- Genetic counseling where appropriate
- Otherwise no specific intervention

PATHOPHYSIOLOGY
Dysgenesis of levator palpebrae muscle: Decreased contractile force of the levator muscle.

ETIOLOGY
Usually idiopathic, possible genetic factors.

COMMONLY ASSOCIATED CONDITIONS
- Marcus-Gunn Jaw Wink phenomenon (2%)
- Amblyopia
- Strabismus
- Chin lift
- Brow lift
- Refractive error (myopia or astigmatism)

DIAGNOSIS

HISTORY
- Onset from birth
- May be symmetric or asymmetric,
- May range from less than a millimeter to complete closure.
  - Possible chin up position to view straight ahead.
  - Inquire about lagophthalmos when sleeping.

PHYSICAL EXAM
- Visual acuity testing to reveal amblyopia secondary to obstruction of the visual axis or induced aniso-astigmatism
- Child may have chin up position, particularly if ptosis is bilateral and in the visual axis.
  - Evaluate ocular motility for possible cranial nerve III palsy, or double elevator palsy.
  - Absent upper lid skin crease if severe
  - Evaluate pupils and lower lid position to rule out Horner syndrome and mydriasis of cranial III palsy.
  - Cycloplegic refraction to uncover induced astigmatism, myopia, and anisometropia
  - Measure interpalpebral fissure height, margin reflex distance, and maximal levator function if possible.
  - Anterior segment evaluation to reveal iris heterochromia of Horner syndrome.
- Check for "reversal" of ptosis in downgaze. Congenital myogenic ptotic eyelids are typically short. Downgaze may reveal lower eyelid on normal side.
  - Evaluate eyelid position while child is drinking from bottle or chewing for Marcus-Gunn Jaw-Wink phenomenon.
  - Full systemic examination for malformation is indicative of an associated systemic syndrome.

DIAGNOSTIC TESTS & INTERPRETATION

Lab

Initial lab tests
- None
- Electrocardiography in cases of suspected chronic progressive ophthalmoplegia

Follow-up & special considerations
- Consider genetic testing if blepharophimosis syndrome suspected.
- Anti-acetylcholine receptor antibody titers in cases of suspected myasthenia gravis.

Imaging

Initial approach
Usually none required.

Follow-up & special considerations
Consider neuroimaging in cases of suspected cranial nerve III palsy, double elevator palsy, Horner syndrome, and tumor.

Diagnostic Procedures/Other
B scan ultrasound may be useful if lid mass suspected.

Pathological Findings
- Fibrous and adipose tissues replace normal muscle fibers in the muscle belly.
- Lack of normal muscle fibers with some changes to extracellular matrix
- Amorphous extracellular material stained positively for collagen type III and fibronectin (2).

DIFFERENTIAL DIAGNOSIS
- Cranial nerve III palsy
- Horner syndrome
  - Double elevator palsy
  - Hypotropia
  - Congenital fibrosis of extraocular muscles
  - Rarely myasthenia gravis, myotonic dystrophy, chronic progressive external ophthalmoplegia, birth trauma, orbital tumors
  - Blepharophimosis syndrome
  - Pseudoptosis in cases of microphthalmia or enophthalmos

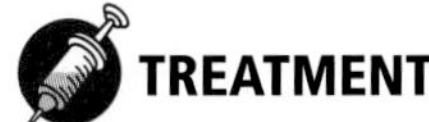

TREATMENT

MEDICATION

First Line

None.

Second Line

May need ocular lubrication (e.g., artificial tear ointment), especially as child gets older, if significant corneal exposure due to lagophthalmos when sleeping.

ADDITIONAL TREATMENT

General Measures

- Glasses for refractive error
- Patching or atropine penalization for amblyopia as needed
- Taping lid shut at night may be helpful in cases of significant lagophthalmos while sleeping particularly if corneal exposure develops.
- If secondary, then treatment of primary disorder (e.g., strabismus surgery for hypotropia)

Issues for Referral

- If considering cranial nerve III palsy, Horner syndrome, chronic progressive ophthalmoplegia, consult pediatric neurologist or neuro-ophthalmologist.
  - Genetic counseling if indicated

SURGERY/OTHER PROCEDURES

- Surgery when amblyopia likely or for significant chin up position
  - If poor levator muscle function (usually <4 mm), frontalis suspension surgery
  - When adequate levator muscle function, levator resection surgery

IN-PATIENT CONSIDERATIONS

Discharge Criteria

Usually same day surgery with discharge when stable post anesthesia.

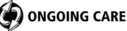

ONGOING CARE

FOLLOW-UP RECOMMENDATIONS

- Observation may be indicated in mild congenital ptosis cases when there is no obstruction of the visual axis, induced refractive error, or anomalous head position. Continued follow-up indicated to monitor for amblyopia.
- If diagnosed in infancy, follow up when child is sitting up to evaluate ptosis, visual axis, and anomalous head position.
  - Repeat pupil, motility, and cycloplegic refraction for changes.
- If surgery performed
- Usually 4–7 days postoperative
  - Follow up at 1 and 4 months, then every 6 months.
  - Recurrence of ptosis may require repeated surgeries over years.

Patient Monitoring

Must monitor for recurrent ptosis, induced astigmatism, amblyopia, and anomalous head position (3).

PATIENT EDUCATION

- Patients and or parents need to understand recurrence of ptosis and need for continued follow up to screen for amblyopia and refractive error.
- http://www.mdjunction.com/congenital-ptosis

PROGNOSIS

Excellent with consistent follow-up care.

COMPLICATIONS

- Amblyopia if significant ptosis is not addressed. (4)
  - Recurrent ptosis may occur at any time.
  - Infections or granulomas can occur in the early postoperative period following frontalis sling surgery, and may require return to operating room for incision and drainage, and systemic antibiotics.
  - Lid asymmetry may require repeat surgery.
  - Exposure keratopathy in some cases of lagophthalmos

REFERENCES

1. Nakashima M, Nakano M, Hirano A, et al. Genome-wide linkage analysis and mutation analysis of hereditary congenital blepharoptosis in a Japanese family. *J Hum Genet* 2008;53(1):34–41.
2. Clark BJ, Kemp EG, Behan WM, et al. Abnormal extracellular material in the levator palpebrae superioris complex in congenital ptosis. *Arch Ophthalmol* 1995;113(11):1414–9.
3. Berry-Brincat A, Willshaw H. Paediatric blepharoptosis: A 10-year review. *Eye* 2009;23(7): 1554–9.
4. Oral Y, Ozgur OR, Akcay L, et al. Congenital ptosis and amblyopia. *J Pediatr Ophthalmol Strabismus* 2010;47(2):101–4.

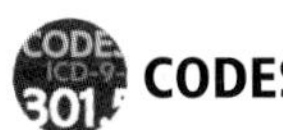

CODES

ICD9

- 743.61 Congenital ptosis of eyelid
- 743.62 Congenital deformities of eyelids

CLINICAL PEARLS

- Old photos may reveal chronicity of ptosis and torticollis, or variability in cases of myasthenia gravis.
- Check for Bell's phenomenon to assess risk of exposure keratopathy secondary to lagophthalmos post surgery.
- Consider neurologic causes in differential diagnosis.
- Monitor throughout the first decade for amblyopia, refractive error, and chin up head position.
- In bilateral cases, chin up head position does not prove the absence of amblyopia.

PUPILLARY BLOCK GLAUCOMA

Tak Yee Tania Tai
L. Jay Katz

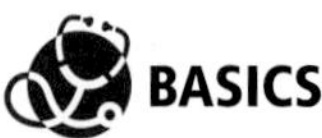

BASICS

DESCRIPTION

- Pupillary block is the most common mechanism responsible for angle closure.
- It is caused by increased resistance to flow of aqueous from the posterior chamber to the anterior chamber.

EPIDEMIOLOGY

Incidence

- The incidence of pupillary block increases with age and is greater in females.
- Angle closure peaks in incidence between 55 and 70 years of age (1)[A].

Prevalence

- About 22 million people worldwide are affected with primary angle-closure glaucoma (PACG).
- About 90% of patients with angle closure have relative pupillary block as the underlying mechanism (2)[A].
- The prevalence of PACG in the European population is approximately 0.1%.
- The prevalence of PACG is higher in Asians, Eskimos (~0.5% of population, ~2–3% of those older than 40 years), and Inuits (1)[A].

RISK FACTORS

- Increasing age
- Asian, Eskimo, or Inuit ethnicities
- Female gender
- Hyperopia
- Spherophakia
- Lens dislocation
- Chronic anterior uveitis
- May be precipitated by topical mydriatics, miotics (rarely), systemic anticholinergics, accommodation, and dim illumination (3)[A]

Genetics

There is heritability in angle-closure glaucoma; however, specific genes have not been identified.

GENERAL PREVENTION

Laser peripheral iridotomy (LPI) is the standard treatment for prevention of angle closure in eyes with occludable angles due to pupillary block (3)[A].

PATHOPHYSIOLOGY

- Increase in resistance to aqueous flow from the posterior chamber to the anterior chamber
- The resulting increase in intraocular pressure (IOP) leads to retinal ganglion cell damage.

ETIOLOGY

- Aqueous is produced into the posterior chamber and normally flows between the posterior surface of the iris and the anterior lens capsule (in phakic eyes) or intraocular lens (in pseudophakic eyes) or hyaloid face (in aphakic eyes).
- Relative resistance to flow of aqueous from the posterior to anterior chamber is usually present; however, the resistance may increase when channel becomes more narrow or longer (e.g., posterior movement of iris insertion, anterior movement of lens, extreme miosis, increase of lens size).
- Increased pressure differential between the posterior and anterior chamber leads to convexity of iris and apposition of iris to trabecular meshwork, leading to decreased aqueous outflow and increased IOP (1)[A].
- Posterior synechiae resulting from inflammation can also lead to pupillary block.

COMMONLY ASSOCIATED CONDITIONS

- Hyperopia
- Pseudoexfoliation
- Spherophakia
- Intumescent cataract
- Nanophthalmos
- Retinopathy of prematurity
- Ciliochoroidal expansion syndromes
- Lens subluxation (e.g., Marfan's syndrome, homocystinuria) (2)[A]

DIAGNOSIS

HISTORY

- Symptoms of eye pain, blurry vision, or haloes in vision
- Family history
- History of retinal problems
- Recent laser treatment or surgery
- Medications

PHYSICAL EXAM

- Check for an afferent pupillary defect or nonreactive pupil.
- Slit lamp exam of anterior segment: presence of anterior chamber cell or keratic precipitates, anterior chamber depth, presence of a cataract, lens position, presence of glaukomflecken, posterior synechiae, and corneal edema
- Gonioscopy. indentation with 4-mirror lens
- Early peripheral anterior synechiae (PAS) superiorly
- IOP
- Examination of the fundus looking for signs of central retinal vein occlusion, hemorrhage, optic nerve cupping, or uveal effusion

DIAGNOSTIC TESTS & INTERPRETATION

Lab

Lab tests as indicated for clinical suspicion of associated conditions

Imaging

Ultrasound biomicroscopy or optical coherence tomography in dark and light conditions may be indicated if diagnosis or etiology of apparent pupillary block is uncertain.

Diagnostic Procedures/Other

- Provocative tests for pupillary block have high false-positive and false-negative rates. These tests include the following:
  - Prone darkroom test
  - Pharmacologic dilation of pupil (3)[A]

Pathological Findings

- Apposition of the peripheral iris and trabecular meshwork
- Glaukomflecken—patchy anterior subcapsular opacities, foci of anterior subcapsular epithelial cell necrosis, associated with severe elevation of IOP

DIFFERENTIAL DIAGNOSIS

- Causes of open-angle glaucoma
- Neovascular or inflammatory glaucoma
- Choroidal swelling or detachment
- Medication-induced narrow angles
- Posterior segment tumor
- Aqueous misdirection syndrome
- PAS

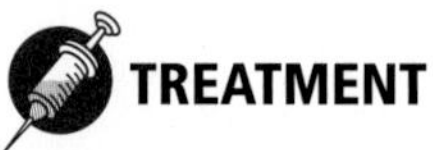

TREATMENT

MEDICATION

First Line

- Prostaglandin agonists (e.g., latanoprost, bimatoprost, travoprost)
- Beta-blockers (e.g., timolol, levobunolol)
- Selective alpha-2 receptor agonists (e.g., brimonidine)
- Topical carbonic anhydrase inhibitors (e.g., dorzolamide, brinzolamide)
- Systemic carbonic anhydrase inhibitors (e.g., methazolamide, acetazolamide)
- Intravenous mannitol

Second Line

Miotics (e.g., pilocarpine)—may be ineffective during acute attack due to pressure-induced ischemia of their iris—may be used after IOP has been reduced to break pupillary block.

ADDITIONAL TREATMENT

General Measures

- Lower the IOP with medical treatment first, if possible.
- A paracentesis may be performed to lower the IOP.
- If the cornea remains cloudy, topical glycerin can be used to temporarily clear the cornea for laser therapy.
- Definitive management requires peripheral laser iridotomy or surgical iridectomy, or lens extraction and/or filtering procedure.

Issues for Referral

Inability to lower the IOP to a safe level using medical or laser therapy may require referral to a glaucoma specialist for surgical intervention.

Additional Therapies

Corneal indentation with a soft instrument may lower the IOP during an acute pupillary block attack by forcing aqueous into the peripheral anterior chamber, temporarily opening the chamber angle and allowing aqueous outflow (3)[A].

P

COMPLEMENTARY & ALTERNATIVE THERAPIES

Argon laser peripheral iridoplasty may be helpful in cases of acute pupillary block glaucoma where corneal edema, shallow anterior chamber, or marked inflammation renders an LPI unfeasible or unsafe, or in cases that are unresponsive to LPI by drawing the peripheral iris away from the anterior chamber angle and allowing aqueous flow and decrease of IOP (4)[A].

SURGERY/OTHER PROCEDURES

- In acute pupillary block angle-closure glaucoma—perform LPI if possible, and safe to do so.
- Surgical peripheral iridectomy may be performed if a laser iridotomy is not possible.
- If pressure remains elevated despite laser iridotomy or peripheral iridectomy and medications, filtering surgery (trabeculectomy) and/or cataract extraction may be necessary.
- Cataract extraction alone may be performed to lessen pupillary block in nonacute cases with little PAS or in cases of pupillary block due to lens subluxation or spherophakia.

IN-PATIENT CONSIDERATIONS

Initial Stabilization

See medical management above.

Admission Criteria

Inability to lower the IOP to a safe level acutely using either medical or laser therapy

IV Fluids

- Diamox and/or mannitol if necessary to lower IOP
- IV fluids may be necessary, if patient is vomiting actively.

Nursing

No special recommendations

Discharge Criteria

Successful lowering of IOP to a safe level

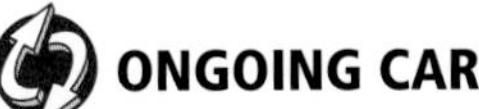

ONGOING CARE

FOLLOW-UP RECOMMENDATIONS

- Follow-up is variable and depends on the therapeutic modality used and the level of IOP at discharge.
- LPI should be performed if the anterior chamber angle is occludable in the contralateral eye at a follow-up visit.

Patient Monitoring

Sequential gonioscopy on follow-up visits should be performed to assess for progressive narrowing of the angle or PAS.

PATIENT EDUCATION

- Patients at risk of pupillary block or angle closure should be educated on the signs and symptoms of an acute angle closure attack (e.g., acute eye pain and blurry vision, seeing haloes), and counseled to seek ophthalmological attention immediately if these symptoms occur.
- Family members should be examined.

PROGNOSIS

- LPI is not reliably protective against chronic angle closure—in a study of LPI in Asian eyes, 100% had resolution of acute attack after LPI; however, 58.1% subsequently developed elevated IOP requiring treatment and 32.7% required trabeculectomy for pressure control (5)[B].
- The failure of LPI to prevent recurrent IOP elevation has been correlated with the amount of PAS present in these eyes.
- Progression of angle closure and PAS may continue after successful LPI.

COMPLICATIONS

- Glaucoma
- Loss of vision
- Acute angle closure

REFERENCES

1. Tarongoy P, Ho CL, Walton DS. Angle-closure glaucoma: The role of the lens in the pathogenesis, prevention, and treatment. *Surv Ophthalmol* 2009;54(2):211–225.
2. Ritch R, Chang BM, Liebmann JM. Angle closure in younger patients. *Ophthalmology* 2003;110(10): 1880–1889.
3. Shields MB. Pupillary-block glaucoma, Chap. 12. In: *Shields' textbook of glaucoma*. Allingham RR, Damji KF, Freedman S, et al. eds, 5th ed, 2005.
4. Lam DS, Lai JS, Tham CC, et al. Argon laser peripheral iridoplasty versus conventional systemic medical therapy in treatment of acute primary angle-closure glaucoma: A prospective, randomized, controlled trial. *Ophthalmology* 2002;109(9):1591–1596.
5. Aung T, Ang LP, Chan S, et al. Acute primary angle-closure: Long-term intraocular pressure outcome in Asian eyes. *Am J Ophthalmol* 2001; 131(1):7–12.

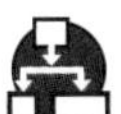

See Also (Topic, Algorithm, Electronic Media Element)

- Plateau iris

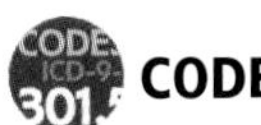

CODES

ICD9

365.61 Glaucoma associated with pupillary block

CLINICAL PEARLS

- Indentation gonioscopy is essential in evaluating narrow angles.
- In eyes with narrow angles, PAS are found most commonly in the superior quadrant.

PURTSCHER'S RETINOPATHY

Andre J. Witkin
Sunir J. Garg

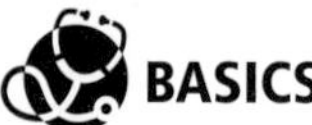

BASICS

DESCRIPTION

- An acute, usually bilateral, patchy, posterior retinal whitening due to crush injuries of the body, or from systemic diseases such as pancreatitis
- Visual acuity is commonly affected but often improves somewhat over time.

EPIDEMIOLOGY

Incidence

Very rare eye disease (probably ∼1/1,000,000)

RISK FACTORS

- In 1910, Dr. Otmar Purtscher initially described bilateral patchy retinal whitening with hemorrhage in a patient who had sustained severe head trauma.
- Purtscher's retinopathy also occurs following severe chest trauma and with long bone fractures.
- Similar findings have also been described in a variety of systemic diseases (see list under "Commonly Associated Conditions"), which have sometimes been referred to as Purtscher's-like retinopathy.

PATHOPHYSIOLOGY

- Experimental data suggest that Purtscher's retinopathy is likely a microembolic phenomenon.
- Possible activation of complement with secondary granulocytic reaction.
- The embolic particles may consist of fat, air, or fibrin. Disseminated intravascular coagulation may be another cause.
- Sparing of larger retinal vessels suggests involvement of precapillary arterioles.

ETIOLOGY

- Typically, Purtscher's retinopathy occurs in association with severe head, chest, or long bone trauma.
- However, systemic medical conditions (see below under "Commonly Associated Conditions") may also cause retinopathy identical to that caused by severe distant trauma; this has sometimes been referred to as "Purtscher-like retinopathy"

COMMONLY ASSOCIATED CONDITIONS

- Severe head, chest, or long bone trauma
- Acute pancreatitis
- Systemic lupus erythematosus
- Scleroderma
- Dermatomyositis
- Fat embolism syndrome
- Amniotic fluid embolism
- Chronic renal failure
- Childbirth
- Cryoglobulinemia
- Hemolytic uremic syndrome/thrombotic thrombocytopenic purpura

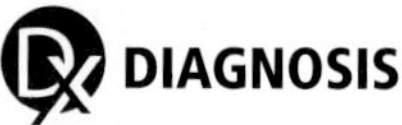

DIAGNOSIS

HISTORY

- Acute painless vision loss that occurs 1–2 days after trauma.
- Usually bilateral, although it may be asymmetric.
- Vision loss ranges from very mild to very severe.
- History of direct ocular trauma should be excluded.

PHYSICAL EXAM

- Typically, multiple areas of polygonal retinal whitening are seen between the retinal arterioles and venules (*Purtscher Flecken*).
- Cotton wool spots may also be seen in one or both eyes.
- The lesions are posterior to the equator.
- Minimal retinal hemorrhages are seen.
- No emboli are visible in retinal vessels.
- Late in the disease course, patients may develop disk pallor, attenuation of the retinal arterioles, alterations of the retinal pigment epithelium, and nerve fiber layer dropout.

DIAGNOSTIC TESTS & INTERPRETATION

Lab

- Typically, Purtscher's retinopathy is associated with bodily trauma.
- However, the eye findings may be the first manifestation of underlying systemic illness, for which a systemic work-up may be warranted.

Imaging

- Fluorescein angiography (FA) typically shows multiple areas of small arteriolar occlusion and capillary dropout (nonperfusion), with late leakage in areas of retinal whitening.
- Optical coherence tomography (OCT) initially shows swelling of the nerve fiber layer, followed by thinning of the inner retina.

Pathological Findings

Findings on pathology are likely similar to those found in cotton wool spots, including retinal capillary obliteration and distension of the nerve fiber layer (cytoid bodies).

DIFFERENTIAL DIAGNOSIS

- Branch or central retinal artery occlusion
- Commotio retinae
- Valsalva retinopathy
- Shaken baby syndrome
- Terson's syndrome
- Blood dyscrasias
- Fat embolism syndrome
- HIV retinopathy
- Interferon retinopathy
- Lupus retinopathy

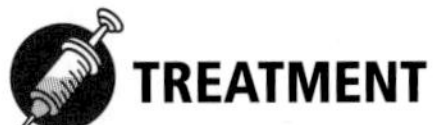

TREATMENT

MEDICATION

- No treatments are recommended to treat Purtscher's retinopathy.
- Any underlying systemic disease, however, should be treated to prevent further retinal damage.

ADDITIONAL TREATMENT

Issues for Referral

- Because of the array of systemic diseases that are associated with Purtscher's retinopathy, referral is dependant on the systemic condition responsible for the ocular findings.
- Collaboration with a trauma specialist, internal medicine, gastroenterology, nephrology, or rheumatology may be warranted.
- If visual acuity loss is profound, eventual referral to a low vision specialist can be beneficial.

ONGOING CARE

FOLLOW-UP RECOMMENDATIONS

- Extent of visual recovery may be related to duration of retinal whitening.
- In patients with shorter duration of retinal whitening, visual acuity has been shown to improve.
- Patients with longer-standing retinal whitening have a more dismal visual prognosis.

Patient Monitoring

- If an active systemic illness is the cause of the retinopathy, patients should be examined at close intervals to assess if there is worsening of the retinopathy.
- Subsequently, patients may be monitored at longer intervals.

PATIENT EDUCATION

Patients should be aware that loss of visual acuity is often longstanding; however, vision loss typically does not worsen.

PROGNOSIS

Prognosis for visual recovery is guarded, although the disease is typically acute and nonprogressive.

COMPLICATIONS

Optic nerve damage may be present to varying degrees and manifests on fundus examination as optic atrophy later in the disease course.

ADDITIONAL READING

- Bhan K, Ashiq A, Aralikatti A, et al. The incidence of Purtscher retinopathy in acute pancreatitis. *Br J Ophthalmol* 2008;92(1):151–153.
- Agrawal A, McKibbin M. Purtscher's retinopathy: epidemiology, clinical features and outcome. *Br J Ophthalmol* 2007;91(11):1456–1459.
- Agrawal A, McKibbin MA. Purtscher's and Purtscher-like retinopathies: a review. *Surv Ophthalmol* 2006;51(2):129–136.
- Holak HM, Holak S. Prognostic factors for visual outcome in Purtscher retinopathy. *Surv Ophthalmol* 2007;52(1):117–118; author reply 118–119.

CODES

ICD9

- 360.43 Hemophthalmos, except current injury
- 362.83 Retinal edema

CLINICAL PEARLS

- Acute bilateral disease causing patchy whitening of the posterior inner retina
- Typically caused by distant and severe head, chest, or long bone trauma
- Identical findings have also been reported in association with a variety of other systemic illnesses, most commonly pancreatitis.
- Visual acuity typically affected, but the degree of loss is variable.

RADIATION KERATOPATHY

David R.P. Almeida
Kelly D. Schweitzer
Stephanie Baxter

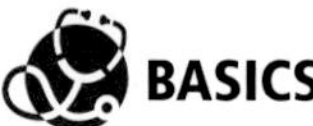

BASICS

DESCRIPTION

- The cornea absorbs the majority of ultraviolet (UV) (10–8 m) and X-ray (10–10 m) energy in the radiation spectrum.
- Acute or chronic damage may occur to all corneal layers (epithelium, stroma, endothelium) in a cumulative fashion secondary to photochemical reactions, heat, structural changes, or metabolic disturbance.
- It is often the earliest cause of vision loss post-periocular radiation therapy.

EPIDEMIOLOGY

Incidence

- Photokeratitis secondary to UV radiation is uncommon.
- Radiation keratopathy secondary to X-ray radiation is rare.

Prevalence

Unknown

RISK FACTORS

- Sun exposure, especially at high altitudes, without protective eyewear
- Occupational exposure (e.g., welder)
- Ocular, CNS, head and neck neoplasm treated with radiation therapy >60 Gy
- Preexisting ocular surface disease or a denervated cornea

Genetics

No specific genetic association

GENERAL PREVENTION

- Protective eyewear and limited UV exposure time
- Ocular considerations in the radiation treatment plan including ocular and lacrimal gland shielding are critical in the prevention of radiation keratopathy.

PATHOPHYSIOLOGY

- Radiation generates highly reactive free radicals which inhibit mitosis, damage cellular DNA, and render the cell incapable of repair and replication leading to cell death.
- Free radicals are produced directly by electrons from the radiation source or indirectly by electrons from the irradiated tissues.

ETIOLOGY

- Photokeratitis secondary to UV radiation (e.g., solar exposure or reflection, welder's or carbon arcs, tanning beds, lightning sparks)
- Brachytherapy: Direct irradiation secondary to radiation therapy of intraocular tumors
- Indirect irradiation within the field of external beam radiation (X-ray teletherapy) for paranasal sinus tumors, eyelid lesions, or CNS neoplasms
- The above may result in direct injury to the cornea or indirect injury due to tear film abnormalities secondary to lacrimal and meibomian gland dysfunction, or conjunctival goblet cell loss.

COMMONLY ASSOCIATED CONDITIONS

- Pinguecula, pterygium
- Spheroidal degeneration
- Hyperkeratosis
- Endothelial dystrophy
- Squamous metaplasia, carcinoma
- Epidermoid carcinoma of the bulbar conjunctiva associated with UV radiation

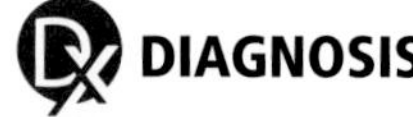

DIAGNOSIS

HISTORY

- Eliciting an accurate history on timing, type, and duration of radiation exposure and on ocular protection is key.
- Ocular pain and irritation, redness, foreign-body sensation, photophobia, and tearing
- May be associated with decreased visual acuity
- Symptoms develop ~6–12 h after UV exposure or hours-to-years after radiation therapy exposure.

PHYSICAL EXAM

- Diffuse epithelial erosions
- Frank epithelial defects
- Filamentary keratitis secondary to epithelial toxicity
- Stromal edema from loss of epithelium or from endothelial dysfunction
- Stromal ulceration from direct toxicity to keratocytes (more frequent at high radiation does >60 Gy over 6 weeks)
- Endothelial granules and keratic precipitates
- Anterior chamber flare and cell
- Corneal opacification, neovascularization, keratinization, thinning or perforation in advanced cases

DIAGNOSTIC TESTS & INTERPRETATION

Imaging

Accurate clinical drawings combined with anterior segment photographs to assess for progression of disease and response to treatment

Diagnostic Procedures/Other

- Pachymetry could be considered to monitor corneal thickness in both edematous and thinned corneas.
- If infectious corneal ulceration is suspected, corneal scraping for culture and sensitivity may be required.

Pathological Findings
- Involutional atrophy of meibomian and lacrimal glands post periocular radiation treatment
- Conjunctival goblet cell loss and squamous metaplasia

DIFFERENTIAL DIAGNOSIS
- Trauma
- Exposure keratopathy
- Dry eye syndrome
- Topical drug toxicity

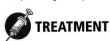

TREATMENT

MEDICATION
First Line
- Aggressive lubrication (q1–2h) with preservative-free tears and ointment recognizing that the irradiated cornea has a poor capacity to heal
- Topical antibiotic drops (t.i.d.–q.i.d.) combined with ointment at bedtime
- Cycloplegia
- Bandage contact lens or pressure patch in patients with significant loss of epithelium
- Prompt diagnostic and therapeutic measures for infected corneal ulcers
- Eye protection for the affected and unaffected eye

Second Line
Oral analgesics

ADDITIONAL TREATMENT
Issues for Referral
- Nonhealing epithelial defects
- Infected corneal ulcers
- Advanced corneal scarring
- Corneal thinning or perforation

SURGERY/OTHER PROCEDURES
- If risk of perforation or severe corneal changes occur due to tear film abnormalities, conjunctival flaps or amniotic membrane grafting may be considered.
- Limbal stem cell transplantation may be considered with persistent evidence of limbal stem cell deficiency.

IN-PATIENT CONSIDERATIONS
Admission Criteria
- If the patient is unable to meet the significant demands of ocular lubrication due to physical or cognitive deficits, admission is required.
- Severe corneal ulceration may require admission.

Nursing
Hospital care staff must be informed of the importance regarding intensive ocular lubrication treatment regimens.

Discharge Criteria
An established care system that is capable of meeting the treatment plan demands

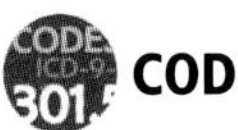

ONGOING CARE

FOLLOW-UP RECOMMENDATIONS
After acute stabilization, regularly scheduled follow-ups post-treatment are necessary to diagnose late ocular surface changes if history of large doses of radiation.

PATIENT EDUCATION
- Emphasis on preventative strategies to avoid re-injury
- Commitment to lifetime maintenance treatment for radiation therapy-induced keratopathy
- Emphasis on eye protection with unilateral loss of vision to protect a well-seeing eye

PROGNOSIS
- It depends on the type and extent of radiation injury and use of ocular and lacrimal gland shielding.
- UV injury prognosis is generally excellent.

COMPLICATIONS
- Limbal ischemia and limbal stem cell deficiency
- Nonhealing epithelial defect or ulceration
- Secondary infectious keratitis
- Panophthalmitis
- Corneal vascularization, opacification, perforation, lipid infiltration
- Neurotrophic and exposure keratopathy from cranial nerve 5 and 7 dysfunction

R

ADDITIONAL READING

- Barabino S, et al. Radiotherapy-induced ocular surface disease. *Cornea* 2005;24(8):909–914.
- Cullen A. Photokeratitis and other phototoxic effects on the cornea and conjunctiva. *Int J Toxicol* 2001;21:455–464.
- Kwok SK, et al. An analysis of the incidence and risk factors of developing severe keratopathy in eyes after megavoltage external beam irradiation. *Ophthalmology* 1998;105:2051–2055.

CODE ICD-9 301.

CODES

ICD9
- 940.4 Other burn of cornea and conjunctival sac
- 990 Effects of radiation, unspecified

CLINICAL PEARLS
- Proper documentation of whether the protective eyewear was worn at the time of injury is necessary for legal and workmen's compensation cases.
- Progression of corneal injury can be extensive so close follow-up (24–48 h) is warranted early until full extent of injury is ascertained.
- Commitment to ophthalmologic follow-up and maintenance treatment can prevent or minimize many long-term radiation problems.

RADIATION OPTIC NEUROPATHY

Matthew D. Kay

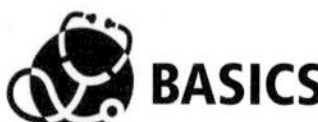

BASICS

DESCRIPTION

Acute onset of visual loss which may be unilateral or bilateral in an individual with a history of having undergone radiation therapy usually for tumors involving or in close proximity to the optic apparatus (i.e., optic nerve, chiasm, or tract), including the orbit, parasellar region, and paranasal sinuses

ALERT

Acute onset of unilateral or bilateral visual loss in a patient with a history of radiation therapy to regions involving or adjacent to the optic apparatus (e.g., eye, optic nerve, optic chiasm, optic tract, paranasal sinuses, sella/parasellar regions) should prompt urgent referral to an ophthalmologist or a neuro-ophthalmologist in order to evaluate for the potential benefit of hyperbaric oxygen therapy and to exclude alternative etiologies (e.g., recurrent tumor) that warrant treatment to preserve or restore visual function.

EPIDEMIOLOGY

Incidence

- If <5,000 cGy total dose, radiation optic neuropathy (RON) rare
- If 5,000–6,000 cGy total dose, 5% 10-year actuarial risk of RON
- Majority of cases occur within 3 years of radiation therapy with a peak of 1.5 years.

Prevalence

Unknown, but extremely rare

RISK FACTORS

- Radiation therapy to regions involving or adjacent to the optic apparatus
- Patients with diabetes mellitus or who have received adjunctive chemotherapy may be at higher risk for developing RON.

GENERAL PREVENTION

- Limiting dosimetry of fractionated radiation therapy when possible to fractions of ≤200 cGy and total dosage to ≤5,400 cGy
  - "Safe dose" of gamma knife radiosurgery adjacent to optic apparatus unclear but estimated around 8,000–10,000 cGy

PATHOPHYSIOLOGY

Unclear whether primary insult is secondary to radiation vasculitis or direct parenchymal injury to the optic apparatus secondary to the effects of radiation therapy or a combination of these two mechanisms

ETIOLOGY

Adverse effects of radiation either directly on the optic apparatus or on its vascular supply

COMMONLY ASSOCIATED CONDITIONS

Tumors (malignant or benign) in regions involving or adjacent to the optic apparatus

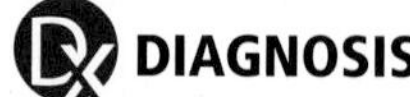

DIAGNOSIS

HISTORY

- Progressive painless unilateral or bilateral visual loss over the course of several weeks
- History of undergoing radiation therapy to anatomic regions involving or adjacent to the optic apparatus
- Second eye involvement, if it occurs, generally develops within few weeks of initial eye onset.

PHYSICAL EXAM

- Demonstrates features of an optic neuropathy: Decreased visual acuity (usually severe); decreased color vision; nerve fiber bundle-type visual field defects though may have temporal defects or homonymous defect if involvement of the optic chiasm or tract, respectively; afferent pupillary defect if unilateral or asymmetric optic nerve involvement
- Affected optic nerve usually normal in appearance or pale from prior compression by radiated lesion; occasionally edematous (if anterior optic nerve involved)
- Optic nerve pallor develops within 6–12 weeks if not present at onset from prior compression
- Possible concurrent radiation retinopathy

R

DIAGNOSTIC TESTS & INTERPRETATION

Imaging

- MRI orbits through chiasm with and without contrast with post-contrast fat suppressed images:
  - MRI demonstrates segmental enhancement of the involved optic nerve(s), chiasm, or tract(s) which may be overlooked as involvement may be limited to a single acquired image slice.

Diagnostic Procedures/Other

Lumbar puncture to be considered to evaluate for meningeal carcinomatosis and serologic testing for paraneoplastic syndrome if MRI not typical for RON

Pathological Findings

Ischemic demyelination, reactive astrocytosis, endothelial hyperplasia, obliterative endarteritis, and fibrinoid necrosis of optic nerves

DIFFERENTIAL DIAGNOSIS

- Infiltrative optic neuropathy secondary to malignancy
- Compression of optic apparatus secondary to recurrent tumor or radiation-induced parasellar tumor
- Meningeal carcinomatosis with optic nerve involvement if history of malignancy
- Toxic optic neuropathy secondary to chemotherapy if previously administered
- Paraneoplastic optic neuropathy or retinopathy if history of malignancy
- Arachnoiditis

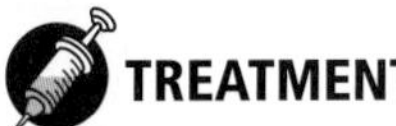

TREATMENT

ADDITIONAL TREATMENT

General Measures

- No therapy of uniformly accepted efficacy
- Hyperbaric oxygen therapy of potential benefit in selected cases though efficacy remains controversial

Nursing

Appropriate precautions for a blind patient in setting of bilateral visual loss if the patient admitted to hospital or other in-patient care facility

ONGOING CARE

FOLLOW-UP RECOMMENDATIONS

Referral for low vision evaluation and blind services if severe bilateral visual loss

Patient Monitoring

Serial clinical and visual field studies at a frequency determined by an ophthalmologist or a neuro-ophthalmologist

PATIENT EDUCATION

- Explain poor visual prognosis and lack of proven effective therapy for condition
- Instruct to call immediately for any visual changes

PROGNOSIS

Generally poor with most affected eyes having visual acuity <20/200 and 45% of eyes with no light perception in spite of attempts at therapeutic intervention

COMPLICATIONS

Permanent unilateral or bilateral blindness

ADDITIONAL READING

- Arnold AC. Ischemic optic neuropathy. In: Miller NR, Newman NJ, eds. *Walsh and Hoyt's clinical neuro-ophthalmology*, 6th ed. Philadelphia: Lippincott Williams Wilkins, 2005:374–376.
- Levy RL, Miller NR. Hyperbaric oxygen therapy for radiation-induced optic neuropathy. *Ann Acad Med Singapore* 2006;35:151–157.

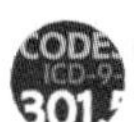

CODES

ICD9

377.34 Toxic optic neuropathy

CLINICAL PEARLS

- Acute onset of painless unilateral or bilateral visual loss in an individual with a history of radiation therapy to regions involving or adjacent to the optic apparatus should prompt strong consideration of RON if recurrent tumor excluded by brain and orbital imaging studies.

RADIATION RETINOPATHY

Chris S. Bergstrom

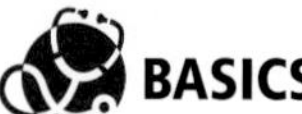

BASICS

DESCRIPTION

- Radiation retinopathy is a delayed onset, chronic, progressive, occlusive vasculopathy of the retinal circulation resulting from previous radiation treatment to the eye, orbit, head, or neck.
  - It can be divided into nonproliferative and proliferative retinopathy.

EPIDEMIOLOGY

Incidence

- Varies by total radiation dose, mode of delivery (brachytherapy vs. external beam), fraction size, and isotope.
- Rare when dose is <40 Gy.
- Incidence peaks 2–3 years post radiation exposure.

Prevalence

Depends on the length of follow-up

RISK FACTORS

- Diabetes
- Chemotherapy
- High dose per fraction

PATHOPHYSIOLOGY

Loss of retinal capillary endothelial cells leading to vascular incompetence and eventually occlusion and nonperfusion.

ETIOLOGY

Radiation induced free radical formation causing direct damage to endothelial cells. Radiation induced damage to cellular chromosomal DNA.

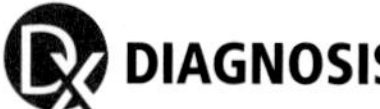

DIAGNOSIS

HISTORY

Previous radiation treatment to the eye, orbit, head, or neck.

PHYSICAL EXAM

- Capillary dilation
- Telangiectasias
- Microaneurysm
- Cotton wool spots
- Macular edema
- Intraretinal hemorrhages
- Lipid exudates
- Vascular sheathing
- Neovascularization of the retina, disc, or iris
- Vitreous hemorrhage
- Retinal detachment

DIAGNOSTIC TESTS & INTERPRETATION

Lab

- Careful slit lamp examination for anterior segment neovascularization
- Tonometry and gonioscopy to monitor neovascular glaucoma

Diagnostic Procedures/Other

- Diagnosis is usually made clinically.
- Fluorescein angiography may show microaneurysms, telangiectasias, capillary nonperfusion, neovascularization, and cystoid macular edema.
- Optical coherence tomography may demonstrate cystoid macular edema.

DIFFERENTIAL DIAGNOSIS

Diabetic retinopathy, hypertensive retinopathy, arteriole obstruction, venous occlusions, ocular ischemia syndrome

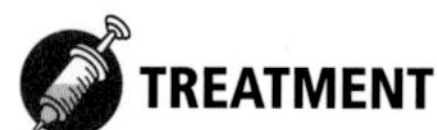

TREATMENT

ADDITIONAL TREATMENT

General Measures

- Loss of visual function due to nonperfusion is irreversible and permanent.
- Focal or grid laser treatment may be beneficial for vision loss associated with macular edema. Panretinal photocoagulation is indicated for optic nerve, retinal, or anterior segment neovascularization.

Additional Therapies

Anti-VEGF (bevacizumab or ranibizumab) therapy for macular edema or neovascularization may provide short-term benefit.

COMPLEMENTARY & ALTERNATIVE THERAPIES
- Monocular precautions
- Polycarbonate lenses

SURGERY/OTHER PROCEDURES
Vitrectomy surgery for patients with vitreous hemorrhage or retinal detachment.

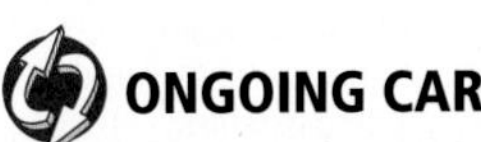

ONGOING CARE

FOLLOW-UP RECOMMENDATIONS
An ophthalmologist should be consulted every 3–6 months.

Patient Monitoring
Monitor visual acuity, IOP, slit lamp exam, and dilated fundus exam for neovascular complications.

PROGNOSIS
Radiation retinopathy is a slowly progressive condition that often leads to irreversible vision loss.

COMPLICATIONS
- Visual loss
- Neovascular glaucoma

ADDITIONAL READING

- Archer DB, Amoaku WM, Gardiner TA. Radiation retinopathy – clinical, histopathological, ultrastructural and experimental correlations. *Eye* 1991;5:239–251.
- Gunduz K, Shields CL, Shields JA, et al. Radiation retinopathy following plaque radiotherapy for posterior uveal melanoma. *Arch Ophthalmol* 1999;117:609–614.
- Monroe AT, Bhandare N, Morris CG, et al. Preventing radiation retinopathy with hyperfractionation. *Int J Radiat Oncol Biol Phys* 2005;61:856–864.

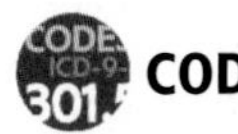

CODES

ICD9
- 362.10 Background retinopathy, unspecified
- 362.15 Retinal telangiectasia
- 362.29 Other nondiabetic proliferative retinopathy

RECURRENT CORNEAL EROSION SYNDROME

Harminder S Dua
Dalia G. Said

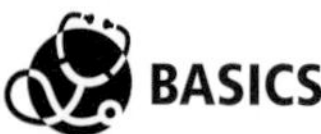

BASICS

DESCRIPTION

Recurrent corneal erosion syndrome (RCES) is characterized by episodes of spontaneous breakdown of the corneal epithelium associated with symptoms ranging from ocular discomfort to severe pain. It is usually unilateral and is associated with awakening from sleep. It may be primary or secondary.

EPIDEMIOLOGY

Incidence

The incidence is unknown as the milder forms of the condition may go undiagnosed.

Prevalence

The disease is reported to occur more commonly in women, is more in the third and fourth decades, and is bilateral in 10% of cases.

RISK FACTORS

- Tiredness, menstruation, menopause, and alcohol intake are aggravating factors.
- Nocturnal lagophthalmos
- Trauma
- Corneal dystrophies
- Diabetes

Genetics

- A familial tendency has been reported among patients with map dot fingerprint epithelial basement membrane dystrophy (EBMD).
- A dominant inheritance has been reported to occur in 3% of cases in one study.

GENERAL PREVENTION

Avoidance of eye injury by wearing protective eyewear during activities such as gardening

PATHOPHYSIOLOGY

- Tear hypotonicity and corneal epithelial edema are implicated.
- Increased activity of matrix metalloproteinases (MMP-2 and -9) resulting in enzymic dissolution of epithelial anchoring structures including hemidesmosomes and anchoring filaments (1)[C].
- Abnormal basement membrane, abnormal or deficient hemidesmosomes, defective anchoring system, and accumulation of collagenous debris between and beneath epithelial cells result in easy slippage or tearing of the basal cells from the underlying connective tissue.
- Ocular saccades associated with rapid eye movement phase of sleep can exert shearing forces on the loose or poorly attached epithelium causing erosions to occur, the pain thus waking the patient, which is subtly different from experiencing pain on waking or eye opening.
- The relative reduced tear secretion during sleep may contribute by inducing greater friction between the apposing conjunctival and corneal epithelia on eye lid opening.

ETIOLOGY

- Primary: These include conditions that affect the basement membrane of the corneal epithelium.
  - EBMD of which map dot fingerprint dystrophy (MDF) is the most common. Reis Bucklers and Thiel-Behnke dystrophy.
  - Stromal dystrophies such as granular and lattice dystrophy
  - Idiopathic
- Secondary: Trauma to the corneal surface with organic matter such as twigs, leaves, paper and finger nails is the commonest cause of RCES.

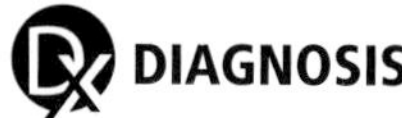

DIAGNOSIS

HISTORY

- Corneal trauma, which may be some time in the past.
- Recurrent attacks of pain, redness, photophobia, and watering which may last from a few minutes to several days. The frequency and intensity of episodes can be variable in the same patient.
- The frequency of episodes (number of times in a day, week, or month); duration of pain (minutes, hours, or days) and intensity of pain (on a scale of 1 = slight discomfort to 10 = severe pain) should be recorded in all cases. This helps in monitoring response to treatment and progression.

PHYSICAL EXAM

- Lid edema
- Conjunctival injection
- Impaired vision
- Cornea:
  - Tear film debris and reduced tear break-up time
  - Intraepithelial and subepithelial microcysts
  - Punctate erosions staining with fluorescein (microform erosions)
  - Large epithelial defects staining with fluorescein (macroform erosions) with the surrounding hazy loose epithelium
  - A tag of epithelium attached to one edge of a frank defect
  - Features of underlying dystrophy, e.g., fingerprint lines, maps, and dots; granular stromal deposits and lattice lines
  - Very often areas of EBMD changes, loose epithelium, epithelial detachment and intraepithelial cysts present as "negative fluorescein staining." These are dark areas (where the tear film is deficient or breaks instantaneously) seen after instilling fluorescein dye and visualized with cobalt blue light.
  - A frank erosion or epithelial defect (staining positively with fluorescein) is often surrounded by an area of negative staining, which indicates the full extent of the defective epithelium.
  - Most of the erosions occur in the lower third to half of the cornea. Following trauma, the erosions tend to recur at the same site but primary RCES may recur at different sites.
  - Subtle corneal changes are best visualized by retroillumination or indirect illumination on the slit lamp.

DIAGNOSTIC TESTS & INTERPRETATION

Imaging

In vivo confocal microscopy can be used to demonstrate features of the underlying pathology, but these are not specific to RCES. For example, intraepithelial cysts, deposits in basal epithelial cells, subbasal microfolds, reduplicated basement membrane, damaged subbasal nerves, and altered morphology of anterior stroma can be seen in MD without erosions.

Diagnostic Procedures/Other

Diagnosis is essentially based on history and clinical features. Specific lab or other tests are not required.

Pathological Findings

- Histopathology:
  - Epithelium: Intercellular edema, accumulation of connective tissue debris, flattening of basal cells, intraepithelial polymorphonuclear cells, intraepithelial cysts containing cellular debris, and degenerating cells
  - Hemidesmosomes: Abnormal morphology; reduced in number. Deficient anchoring fibrils
  - Basement membrane: Discontinuous and fragmented, multilaminar reduplication with extensions into the epithelial cell layers
  - Collagenous debris interposed between basal epithelial cells and Bowman's zone.

DIFFERENTIAL DIAGNOSIS

- Meesmann's corneal dystrophy: Intermittent rupture of epithelial microcysts as they reach the surface of the cornea, causing symptoms.
- Bullous keratopathy: Rupture of fluid filled epithelial vesicles or bullae can cause pain.
- Band keratopathy: When the calcific plaques are thick and erode through the epithelium, the eye becomes symptomatic.
- Salzmann's nodular degeneration: The nodules often sit proud of the tear film causing poor wetting of the surface epithelium which is prone to breakdown and become symptomatic.
- Eyelid abnormalities: Trichiasis and tarsal concretions that have eroded through the covering epithelium can cause repeated mechanical abrasions of the cornea.
- Meibomian gland dysfunction and dry eyes.
- Ocular surface syndrome: Following photorefractive keratectomy or LASIK. Usually attributed to aberrant re-innervation with tear film instability and punctuate keratitis.
- Viral keratitis: A few cases of recalcitrant RCES have eventually manifested clinical features of herpes simplex viral keratitis. This association is known but unexplained.
- Multiple corneal foreign bodies: Following blast injury, insect hair, leather fibres (snooker or pool cue injury). The embedded foreign particles may intermittently make their way to the corneal surface and extrude causing "foreign body sensation" and irritation.

- Systemic conditions such as epidermolysis bullosa and Juvenile X-linked Alport's syndrome have inherent basement membrane abnormality that makes the epithelium vulnerable to repeated breakdown.
- Munchhausen syndrome: Self-inflicted trauma to the cornea.

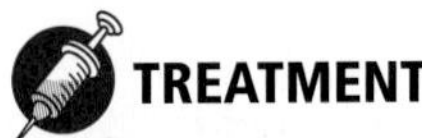

TREATMENT

MEDICATION

- Simple conservative measures such as eye padding and use of lubricating drops, gels, and ointment help to provide relief from symptoms and prevent or reduce occurrence of erosions in most cases. The regular use of ointment, immediately before going to sleep is beneficial.
- Eyelid margin cleansing helps if associated with blepharitis.

ADDITIONAL TREATMENT

General Measures

- When the above conservative measures provide partial relief or none at all, a therapeutic extended wear (bandage) contact lens should be considered. It provides symptomatic relief and encourages healing of the epithelium by affording projection against the rubbing action of the lids. The lens can be changed daily, weekly, or monthly depending on the patient's preference, environmental pollution, and prevailing practice. It should be used for at least 6–8 weeks to allow for remodeling of the basement membrane and consolidation of hemidesmosomal attachments.
  - The eye should be examined within 24–48 h to ensure that the lens does not tighten on the eye. This can cause exacerbation of pain, corneal edema, and sloughing of the epithelium due to hypoxia.
  - Use of ointment should be avoided whilst using the contact lens.

Issues for Referral

RCES not responding to the above measures necessitating surgical intervention

Additional Therapies

- Sodium chloride 2% drops or 5% ointment helps to dehydrate the epithelium.
- Oral tetracyclines (e.g., doxycycline 100 mg b.i.d.) as a metalloprotease inhibitor. This provides additional benefit in cases with posterior blepharitis and rosacea.
- Autologous serum eye drops in recalcitrant cases to facilitate closure of epithelial defects and afford lubrication.

SURGERY/OTHER PROCEDURES

- The area of positive and negative fluorescein staining should be treated:
  - Superficial keratectomy, mechanical debridement, or diamond burr polishing of the loose epithelium and affected area.
  - Anterior stromal puncture: Multiple punctures through the affected epithelium into Bowman's zone/superficial stroma with a 23–25 gauge needle. This can also be achieved with a Nd:YAG laser. Can leave behind tiny scars and affect vision if in the visual axis.
  - Phototherapeutic keratectomy: With the excimer laser ablating the epithelium and 5–7 μm of Bowman's zone. Can induce a hyperopic shift especially if it has to be repeated.
  - Alcohol delamination: With 18–20% ethanol applied to the affected area for 30 s with the help of a hollow cylindrical well (e.g., optical zone marker) of appropriate diameter. The sheet of epithelium removed can be used for histological examination (2)[B].
- Postoperatively a Bandage Contact Lens (BCL) may be applied for 1 or 2 weeks and the eye treated with antibiotic and lubricant drops. Regular instillation of eye ointment before sleeping may have to be continued for a while.

ONGOING CARE

PATIENT EDUCATION

Instructions should be given to maintain therapeutic contact lens hygiene, to avoid eye rubbing, and excessive alcohol intake.

PROGNOSIS

Most patients achieve symptomatic relief and freedom from recurrence with conservative and/or surgical management. Reported success rate is between 80 and 90%.

COMPLICATIONS

- Secondary bacterial infection: Corneal ulcer or abscess. The risk is higher with use of a therapeutic extended wear contact lens. Can also occur following an interventional procedure.
- Localized corneal stromal haze related to the wound healing response associated with persistent and recurrent epithelial breakdown.

REFERENCES

1. Das S, Seitz B. Recurrent corneal erosion syndrome. *Surv Ophthamol* 2008;53:3–15.
2. Dua HS, Lagnado R, Raj D, et al. Alcohol delamination of the corneal epithelium: An alternative in the management of recurrent corneal erosions. *Ophthalmology* 2006;113:404–411.

ADDITIONAL READING

- Ewald M, Hammersmith KM. Review of diagnosis and management of recurrent erosion syndrome. *Curr Opin Ophthalmol* 2009;20:287–291.

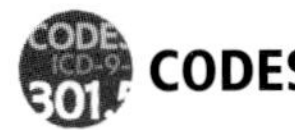

CODES

ICD9

- 371.23 Bullous keratopathy
- 371.42 Recurrent erosion of cornea
- 371.51 Juvenile epithelial corneal dystrophy

CLINICAL PEARLS

- Keep anesthetic drops away from reach of patients: Use of topical anesthesia helps with clinical examination of acute episodes, but the instant relief provided may tempt patients to "acquire" anesthetic agents and use them indiscriminately.
- Consider preservative-free lubricants and antibiotics to treat acute episodes and for prophylaxis, if required over a prolonged duration.
- When managing episodes with therapeutic extended wear contact lenses consider use of antibiotic (preservative-free) prophylaxis in the presence of epithelial defects.
- In some patients, RCES episodes are distinctly related to alcohol intake the previous night.
- Be wary of the occasional case manifesting a dendritic ulcer of disciform keratitis (herpes simplex keratitis) during the course of follow-up.

RED EYE IN CHILDREN

Judith B. Lavrich

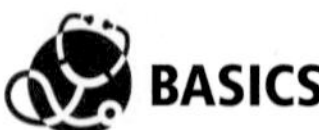

BASICS

DESCRIPTION

The appearance of redness on the surface of the eye resulting from enlargement and dilation or leakage of the blood vessels of the conjunctiva or episclera

EPIDEMIOLOGY

Prevalence

Depends on the etiology of the red eye

RISK FACTORS

- Blepharitis
- Trauma
- Systemic disease (e.g., iritis, chicken pox lesion of conjunctiva, episcleritis/scleritis)
- Contact lens wear
- Loss of protective ocular factors: tear film, corneal sensation, intact corneal epithelium, etc.
- Infection
- Exposure to noxious chemical by direct contact or airborne dispersion

Genetics

Most entities are not genetic unless there is an underlying systemic disorder with genetic influence (e.g., iritis due to arthritis)

GENERAL PREVENTION

- Eye protection for any high-risk activity, especially sports involving balls
- Excellent hygiene when inserting and removing contact lenses from the eye
- Not wearing contact lenses while sleeping and removal immediately upon discomfort
- Routine follow-up with contact lens provider to check fit and ocular surface health
- Screening eye examinations for those at risk of ocular complications (e.g., screen for iritis in juvenile idiopathic arthritis)
- Avoid contact with conjunctivitis and if contact occurs, frequent hand washing

PATHOPHYSIOLOGY

- Blepharitis—disorder of the Meibomian glands of lids leads to suboptimal flow with ocular surface desiccation and/or overgrowth of *Staphylococcus epidermidis* with hypersensitivity reaction of conjunctiva and cornea
- As the cornea has no blood vessels of its own, when it becomes infected, the surrounding blood vessels enlarge and bring immunomodulators to help fight the infection.
- Infection or inflammation of the conjunctiva or episclera results in blood vessel engorgement.
- Inflammation inside the eye results in "limbal flush", an engorgement of the circumcorneal vessels.
- Small conjunctival vessels are sensitive to increased blood pressure and microvascular disease causing them to burst and leak blood under the outer membrane of the eye (subconjunctival hemorrhage).
- With overwear and poor fit, contact lenses can decrease the oxygenation of the cornea creating inflammation.
- Cavernous fistula can result in conjunctival vascular engorgement (and "corkscrew vessels") due to a resistance to venous return and/or increased perfusion pressure.

ETIOLOGY

- Blepharitis
- Disorders of the lashes: trichiasis, lice
- Subconjunctival hemorrhage—trauma or anticoagulation/platelet disorders, strangulation/asphyxia (consider child abuse), Valsalva maneuver, hypertension, and diabetes (all uncommon causes in children)
- Conjunctivitis—viral, bacterial, allergic, or toxic
- Corneal abrasion/foreign body
- Corneal infection: Bacterial, herpes, varicella,
- Iritis—idiopathic, traumatic, or due to systemic disease (juvenile idiopathic arthritis, sarcoidosis, tuberculosis, inflammatory bowel disease, Kawasaki – see chapter)
- Trauma
- Contact lens: keratitis, hypoxia, infectious corneal ulcer, damaged contact lens, etc.

COMMONLY ASSOCIATED CONDITIONS

- Eye pain
- Reduced vision if cause is corneal or intraocular
- Photophobia
- Itchy lids (e.g., allergy, blepharitis)

DIAGNOSIS

HISTORY

- How long has red eye been present (acute vs. chronic)
- History of eye trauma (foreign body, traumatic iritis)
- Past ocular history
  - Previous eye surgery making the eye more susceptible to trauma or infection
  - Contact lens wearer
- Past medical history—rosacea associated with blepharitis, recent herpes simplex infection, chicken pox, underlying malignancy or immunosuppression, arthritis, inflammatory bowel disease, or fever
- Exposure to foreign bodies, individuals with conjunctivitis, toxins that irritate the eyes, or chemical splash
- Ocular symptoms:
  - Eye pain—describe location, duration, and intensity
  - Foreign body sensation in eyes
  - Discharge from eye—purulent (bacterial), clear or mucous (viral or allergic), stringy white (allergic), or tearing (herpes simplex, corneal ulcer, acute iritis)
  - Eye irritation/itching
  - Visual loss/blurred vision
  - Triad of eye pain, light sensitivity, and blurred vision suggest more serious ocular involvement

PHYSICAL EXAM

- Detailed eye examination including dilated fundus view, especially if decreased vision or trauma
  - Visual acuity in both eyes. Reduced visual acuity may suggest corneal etiology or iritis.
  - Check pupillary size and shape. Mid-dilated pupil in iritis. An irregular pupil may suggest trauma, posterior synechiae of iritis, or and intraocular foreign body.
  - Inspect the lids for any crusting, lice, or redness of the lid margin. Look under the upper and lower eyelids for foreign bodies, fine follicles indicating viral infection, and papillae/edema suggesting allergic conjunctivitis.
  - Note location of redness and characterize discharge
  - Fluorescein staining of cornea for abrasion, ulceration, and dendrites of herpes
  - Tonometry
  - Assess the red reflex. If abnormal, may suggest globe rupture or hyphema.
- Physical examination
  - Preauricular lymph nodes (viral conjunctivitis)
  - Other signs of trauma (consider child abuse)
  - Stiff or tender joints (juvenile idiopathic arthritis)
  - Abdominal tenderness
  - Other infection in immunosuppression

DIAGNOSTIC TESTS & INTERPRETATION

Lab

- Bacterial culture of eye discharge if copious
- If iritis is suspected:
  - CBC with differential, ESR, ANA, ACE level (sarcoidosis), RPR, serum calcium, and rheumatoid factor
  - Urinalysis
  - PPD
  - Lyme titers
  - See uveitis chapter for further evaluation

Imaging

- If suspecting globe rupture or intraocular foreign body—CT of orbits
- Chest radiograph if suspecting iritis

DIFFERENTIAL DIAGNOSIS

- Acute conjunctivitis—viral, bacterial, allergic, or toxic
- Blepharitis
- Subconjunctival hemorrhage
  - Consider nonaccidental trauma with bilateral subconjunctival hemorrhages in infants, especially in those with facial petechiae. May be secondary to asphyxia/strangulation or severe chest compression (1)[C].
- Iritis
- Trauma
- Corneal or intraocular foreign body
- Corneal ulceration or infection
- Contact–lens induced keratitis

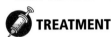

TREATMENT

MEDICATION

First Line

- Blepharitis—consider topical erythromycin ointment
- Allergic conjunctivitis—topical antihistamines and mast cell stabilizers
- Viral conjunctivitis—artificial tears for symptomatic relief; some authors have suggested topical antibiotics, if severe, to prevent secondary bacterial infection (2)[C].
- Bacterial conjunctivitis—topical antibiotics (see chapter)
- Corneal infection
  - Bacterial infiltrate—consider scraping and culture before treatment with fortified and high-dose topical antibiotics (see chapter)
  - Herpes simplex dendrite—topical and/or systemic antivirals
  - Do not use topical steroids
- Iritis—topical steroids and cycloplegia, treat secondary glaucoma
- Hyphema—topical steroids and cycloplegic glaucoma medication if needed. Eye shield and avoidance of antiplatelet medication to prevent secondary bleed. (see chapter)

Second Line

- Systemic antibiotics may be needed if periocular or orbital infection
- Systemic steroids or immunosuppressive agents may be needed in iritis (see chapter)

ADDITIONAL TREATMENT

General Measures

Cool compresses are helpful for symptomatic relief

Issues for Referral

- As appropriate for underlying systemic disease
- To child-protective agency if concern of possible abuse

Additional Therapies

- Baby shampoo eyelash scrubs for blepharitis
- Warm compresses may also be helpful
- Massage for nasolacrimal duct obstruction (see chapter on 'Nasolacrimal Duct Obstruction, Adults')

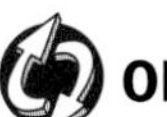

ONGOING CARE

FOLLOW-UP RECOMMENDATIONS

- Because of high potential for visual loss and other complications, serial follow-up for corneal disease and iritis
- If contact lens related, do not restart contacts until seen by provider

Patient Monitoring

By ophthalmologist for chronic eye disease (e.g., iritis, herpes simples keratitis)

PATIENT EDUCATION

- Promote appropriate eye protection for sports
- Baby shampoo eyelash scrubs for blepharitis

PROGNOSIS

- Excellent if appropriate treatment instituted
- Depends on etiology

COMPLICATIONS

- Corneal disease: perforation, scar, and amblyopia
- Trauma—blood staining of cornea, amblyopia, optic atrophy, and glaucoma
- Iritis—glaucoma, cataract, band keratopathy, and recurrence

REFERENCES

1. Spitzer SG, Luorno J, Noël LP. Isolated subconjunctival hemorrhages in nonaccidental trauma. *J AAPOS* 2005;9:53–56.
2. Kuo SC, Shen SC, Chang SW, et al. Corneal superinfection in acute viral conjunctivitis in young children. *J Pediatr Ophthalmol Strabismus* 2008;45:374–376.

ADDITIONAL READING

- Greenberg MF, Pollard ZF. The red eye in childhood. *Pediatr Clin North Am* 2003;50:105–124.
- Levin AV. Eye emergencies: Acute management in the pediatric ambulatory setting. *Pediatr Emerg Care* 1991;7:367–377.
- Sethuraman R, Kamat D. The red eye: Evaluation and management. *Clin Pediatr (Phila)* 2009;48: 588–600.
- Teoh DL, Reynolds S. Diagnosis and management of pediatric conjunctivitis. *Pediatr Emerg Care* 2003;19:48–55.

CODES

ICD9

- 372.30 Conjunctivitis, unspecified
- 373.00 Blepharitis, unspecified
- 379.93 Redness or discharge of eye

CLINICAL PEARLS

- Triad of 'red flag' symptoms—eye pain, reduced vision, and photophobia—indicate more serious ocular involvement.
- Red eye in a patient who wears contact lenses may be corneal ulceration requiring urgent care.

REFRACTIVE ERROR (MYOPIA, HYPEROPIA, ASTIGMATISM)

Bruce J. Markovitz

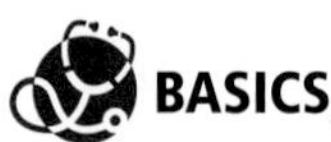

BASICS

DESCRIPTION

- Refractive error exists when parallel light rays from a distant object do not come to focus on the retina of an unaccommodating eye. In refractive error the focusing power of the unaccommodating eye does not match its axial length.
- Myopia: The focusing power is very strong and the image of a distant object is focused in front of the retina.
- Hyperopia: The focusing power (cornea and lens) is insufficient to bring parallel light rays to focus on the retina in the unaccommodated eye and the distant object is focused behind the retina.
- Astigmatism: The curvature of the corneal surface is not spherical. In regular astigmatism one meridian has a maximal curvature while the meridian 90° away has a minimum curvature. (Explain to patients as a circle cut from the side of a football compared to the side of a basketball.) In an eye with astigmatism, light rays from an object are focused with an amount of power determined by which meridian of the cornea they pass through. Irregular astigmatism is a pathologic condition most commonly associated with keratoconus or corneal scarring where the principal meridians are not 90° apart.

EPIDEMIOLOGY

Incidence

Clinically significant refractive error increases with age. ~5% of children 0.5 to 6 years of age need glasses (1). 50% of the U.S. population 20 years and older require correction (2).

Prevalence

- Of the 50% of those aged 20 and older in the USA requiring correction
- Myopia 33.1%
- Hyperopia 3.6%
- Astigmatism 36.2%

RISK FACTORS

Genetics

Strong heritability. Up to 90% in twin studies (3)

GENERAL PREVENTION

Many theories have been advanced to suggest environmental factors involved in myopia development and progression from increased reading and near work to use of children's night-lights. Some suggest accommodative exercise, under-correcting myopes, or use of plus lenses for reading. None are generally accepted.

PATHOPHYSIOLOGY

Most refractive error (between –4.00 and +4.00) occurs in eyes with axial length and focal power considered within normal range. Greater refractive error is usually associated with abnormal axial length.

COMMONLY ASSOCIATED CONDITIONS

- High myopia:
  - Down's syndrome
  - Stickler's syndrome
  - Ehlers–Danlos syndrome
  - Retinopathy of prematurity
  - Marfan's syndrome
  - Weill Marchesani syndrome

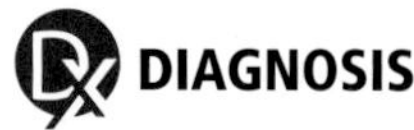

DIAGNOSIS

HISTORY

- Symptoms depend on the type and degree of error and patient age. Any refractive error can cause headaches and asthenopia (eye strain). Specifically:
  - Myopia: Distance blur, clearer at near. (The higher the myopia the more distance is blurred and the closer is the near focus.)
  - Hyperopia: Distance is clearer than near. (Hyperopia can be corrected by accommodation.) If accommodative amplitude is greater than degree of hyperopia, distance and near vision may be clear. In older patients, especially if presbyopic, or high degrees of hyperopia, both distance and near are blurred.
  - Astigmatism: Distance and near blur.

PHYSICAL EXAM

- Distance and near unaided acuity will usually suggest type of error.
- Improvement with pinhole indicates that decreased vision is refractive as opposed to other pathology.
- Uncorrected hyperopia can be associated with esotropia (accommodative esotropia), especially with high degrees of hyperopia or high AC/A ratio.

DIAGNOSTIC TESTS & INTERPRETATION

Diagnostic Procedures/Other

- Subjective refraction: Using a phoropter or loose trial lenses various lens combinations are introduced before the eye to determine the prescription giving best-corrected visual acuity (BCVA). Starting point is usually the habitual prescription or determined by an objective test such as follows:
  - Retinoscopy
  - Automated refractor
  - Keratometry – measures corneal curvature allowing an estimate of the astigmatic error
- Jackson cross cylinder (JCC) test: Used to subjectively measure the axis and power of the astigmatic error. A JCC is a spherocylindrical lens with spherical equivalent power of plano.
- Manifest refraction: A "dry" refraction performed without drops. More natural state of the eye, but the patient can accommodate causing overcorrection of myopes and under correction of hyperopes. The amount of hyperopia found with a dry refraction is the "manifest hyperopia."
- Cycloplegic refraction: A "wet" refraction done with cycloplegic drops such as cyclopentolate or tropicamide which paralyzes the ciliary body preventing accommodation. Not the normal physiologic state of the eye. The additional hyperopia uncovered with a wet refraction is the "latent hyperopia."

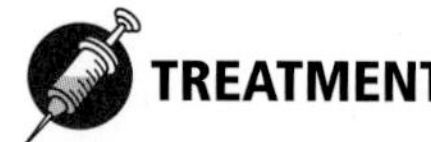

TREATMENT

ADDITIONAL TREATMENT

General Measures

- Correcting myopia: A patient with myopia can generally be given the least minus power while still maintaining BCVA. With manifest refraction must be careful not to over minus young myopes who can accommodate and "eat minus." Accommodation makes an image appear smaller and darker, and may be erroneously perceived as clearer. With cycloplegic refraction –0.25 D can be added to adjust for return of ciliary body tone (4)[C].
- Correcting hyperopia: A happy patient with uncorrected hyperopia without complaints of blur, fatigue, or headaches may not yet need correction. If symptomatic, can generally be given maximum plus power that still maintains BCVA found by manifest refraction. Amount of latent hyperopia to be corrected depends on age, symptoms, and needs. As a rule, up to half of accommodative amplitude can be used for extended periods comfortably. As accommodative amplitude decreases with age more plus will be needed to maintain comfortable vision even though total amount of hyperopia present remains unchanged. Children with esotropia should be given full cycloplegic refraction. If reducing plus, must reduce plus equally in each eye to keep accommodation balanced.

- Correcting astigmatism: Children need full astigmatic correction to prevent amblyopia. They will usually adapt to large amount of new astigmatic correction (5)[C]. Adults are less adaptable. If no previous cylinder correction has been worn glasses may be rejected. New oblique cylinder is especially hard to accept. If wearing cylinder correction, difficulty may be experienced in adapting to increased power or axis change. If reducing cylinder power found on refraction in order to increase chance of acceptance, the spherical equivalent should be maintained.

SURGERY/OTHER PROCEDURES

- Laser correction: Lasik and PRK for correcting up to ~10 D of myopia, 6 D of hyperopia, and 4 D of astigmatism
- Intrastromal corneal rings: Used to correct mild to moderate degrees of myopia to approximately 3 D and astigmatism up to 1 D. Advantage of being reversible.
- Clear lens extraction and phakic IOLs: Alternative to laser correction for high degrees of refractive error or thin corneas.

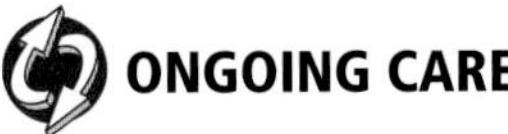

ONGOING CARE

FOLLOW-UP RECOMMENDATIONS

- If glasses rejected:
  - Verify glasses made to prescription
  - Check patient and spectacle PD
  - Check frame fit looking for vertex distance, position of optic centers, pantoscopic and face form tilt
  - Double check refraction especially if prescribed from cycloplegic
  - Remake Rx closer to habitual
  - Decrease or eliminate cylinder power
  - Rotate axis closer to habitual or toward 90/180

PROGNOSIS

- Myopia generally progresses through teenage years and then stabilizes. Later, myopic shift can occur as nuclear sclerosis develops.
- Hyperopia generally lessens through childhood, but hyperopic symptoms can develop as greater near demands are placed on school children and as accommodative amplitude decreases into adulthood.
- Astigmatism generally changes less through the years. There is a slow increase in with-the-rule astigmatism in the aging eye.

COMPLICATIONS

- Myopia:
  - Retinal detachment
  - Posterior vitreous detachment
  - Open angle glaucoma
  - Myopic degeneration with choroidal neovascular membrane
- Hyperopia:
  - Amblyopia
  - Strabismus
  - Narrow angle glaucoma
- Astigmatism:
  - Keratoconus
  - Amblyopia

REFERENCES

1. Giordano L, Friedman DS, Repka MX, et al. Prevalence of refractive error among preschool children in an urban population: the Baltimore Pediatric Eye Disease Study. *Ophthalmology* 2009;116(4):739–746.
2. Vitale S, Ellwein L, Cotch MF, et al. Prevalence of refractive error in the United States, 1999–2004. *Arch Ophthalmol* 2008;126(8):1111–1119.
3. Lopes MC, Andrew T, Carbonaro F, et al. Estimating heritability and shared environmental effects for refractive error in twin and family studies. *Invest Ophthalmol Vis Sci* 2009;50126–50131.
4. Milder B. Prescribing glasses for myopia. *Ophthalmology* 1979;86(5):706–712.
5. Harvey EM, Dobson V, Clifford-Donaldson CE, et al. Optical treatment of amblyopia in astigmatic children: the sensitive period for successful treatment. *Ophthalmology* 2007;114(12): 2293–2301.

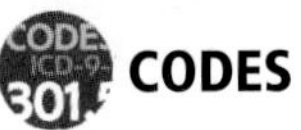

CODES

ICD9

- 367.0 Hypermetropia
- 367.1 Myopia
- 367.20 Astigmatism, unspecified

CLINICAL PEARLS

- As a rule, for adults, anisometropia over 2.00 D in glasses is not tolerated due to unequal retinal image size. (Children may tolerate much greater amount.) Contact lenses greatly reduce minification and magnification effects allowing large anisometropic corrections such as those needed in monocular aphakia.

REIS-BUCKLERS CORNEAL DYSTROPHY

Mark M Fernandez
Terry Kim

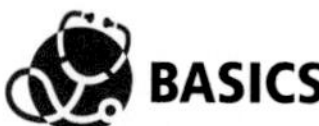

BASICS

DESCRIPTION

- An autosomal dominant dystrophy of Bowman's layer (CDB) of the cornea; Reis-Bucklers (RBCD) or CDB-1 is linked to the BIGH3 gene on chromosome 5q31 (1)[B]. It is associated with specific mutations of the TGFBI protein: Arg124leu[2] and, less typically, Gly23asp.
- Alternate names: Corneal dystrophy of Bowman's layer type 1 (CDB-1) and granular dystrophy type III.

Pediatric Considerations

Onset of symptoms is typically at 4–5 years of age and may include photophobia, eye rubbing, tearing, or other signs of ocular surface discomfort.

EPIDEMIOLOGY

Incidence

The incidence of Reis-Bucklers corneal dystrophy (RBCD) is rare, with most cases occurring in families with a known mutation in chromosome 5q31. The exact incidence and prevalence are unknown.

RISK FACTORS

Patients with specific mutations of TGFI are at risk of RBCD. This is an inheritable condition.

Genetics

As in "Description" above; autosomal dominant

GENERAL PREVENTION

No method of prevention exists; therapy is supportive and targeted at reducing ocular surface disease.

PATHOPHYSIOLOGY

Superficial ring-shaped deposits in the central cornea are composed of fibrocellular material which is further composed of mutated transforming growth factor-beta induced protein. These localize to Bowman's layer. Recurrent erosions lead to stromal scarring by young adulthood.

ETIOLOGY

See "Description" and "Pathophysiology."

COMMONLY ASSOCIATED CONDITIONS

RBCD has no known systemic associations. Other conditions resulting in mutations of the BIGH3 gene include Thiel-Behnke dystrophy (CDB-2), lattice dystrophy, and Avellino dystrophy.

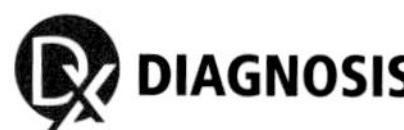

DIAGNOSIS

HISTORY

- Family history of early onset ocular surface disease or known mutation in the BIGH3 gene.
- Recurrent epithelial erosions which last from days to weeks during childhood; patients experience symptomatic improvement in pain by young adulthood with decreased vision due to superficial stromal scarring.
- During acute attacks, symptoms include pain, hyperemia, and photophobia.

PHYSICAL EXAM

- Slit lamp biomicroscopy reveals multiple bilateral, central, reticular, honeycomb-shaped opacities within Bowman's layer early in life. As patients reach adulthood, gray-white opacities become interspersed and the anterior corneal surface becomes irregular (2)[B].
- The cornea's appearance by broad-beam illumination is said to resemble "curdled milk."
- The corneal appearance by optical cross section shows fibrillar projections from Bowman's layer into the epithelium.
- Retroillumination of the cornea reveals a frosted glass appearance.

DIAGNOSTIC TESTS & INTERPRETATION

Lab

Genetic testing for known BIGH3 mutations including Arg124leu and Gly23asp, in combination with pedigree analysis, supports the diagnosis of Reis-Bucklers dystrophy. Electron microscopy is also diagnostic (see below).

Imaging

The appearance of RBCD using in vivo confocal imaging has been characterized (3)[B]; however, this is not a commonly utilized modality for diagnosis.

Pathological Findings

- Masson's trichrome stain of histopathologic specimens shows red deposits in the anterior cornea with disruption of Bowman's layer (1)[B].
- Transmission electron microscopy (TEM) of specimens in RBCD shows lamellated deposits parallel to collagen fibers in the anterior cornea. TEM is required to distinguish RBCD, or CDB-1, from Thiel-Behnke corneal dystrophy, or CDB-2. In contrast to RBCD, corneas with Thiel-Behnke dystrophy show arcuate, rounded fibers termed "curly fibers" (4)[B]. The slit lamp biomicroscopic appearances of CDB-1 and CDB-2 can be indistinguishable.

DIFFERENTIAL DIAGNOSIS

- Thiel-Behnke corneal dystrophy (CDB-2)
- Granular corneal dystrophy
- Epithelial basement membrane dystrophy
- Lattice dystrophy
- Meesmann's corneal dystrophy
- Subepithelial mucinous corneal dystrophy
- Herpetic keratitis

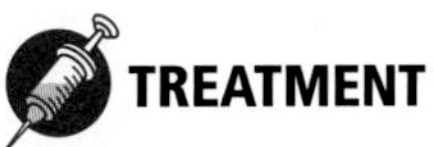

TREATMENT

MEDICATION

Lubrication (artificial tears, lubricating ointments applied 3–6 times per day) [B].

ADDITIONAL TREATMENT

General Measures

- Bandage contact lenses may be utilized for symptomatic relief of epithelial erosions [B].
- Topical antibiotic prophylaxis (during episodes of epithelial erosions)
- Topical corticosteroid medication (to avoid or minimize corneal scarring)

Issues for Referral

Stromal scarring with poor visual acuity or persistent surface disease can be addressed by a corneal specialist using the surgical options below.

SURGERY/OTHER PROCEDURES

- Phototherapeutic keratectomy (PTK) treats superficial scarring and anterior surface irregularity [B]. Recurrence of deposits has been reported at 58% (5)[B]. Intraoperative administration of mitomycin-C has been proposed as a way to slow the recurrence of TGFBI deposition, with encouraging results 1 year after surgery (6)[B].
- Epithelial debridement or superficial keratectomy can be utilized when excimer laser PTK is unavailable [B].
- Deep lamellar keratoplasty or penetrating keratoplasty are infrequently indicated. The rate of recurrence is estimated at 17.5% at 5 years in corneal dystrophies of Bowman's layer, which includes RBCD [B].

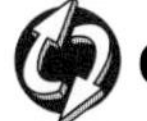

ONGOING CARE

FOLLOW-UP RECOMMENDATIONS

Patient Monitoring

- Patients should be monitored closely during episodes of recurrent erosion to avoid microbial ulcers and control pain.
- Patients should also be monitored for decreased vision due to the corneal opacities, irregular surface, and stromal scarring.

PROGNOSIS

The natural history of RBCD involves recurrent corneal erosions starting at the 4th year of life with scarring and decreased vision that continues to progress in the 2nd, 3rd, and 4th decades. RBCD recurs quickly in penetrating keratoplasty (averaging 2 years in one study) as well as in PTK. Best-corrected visual acuity is limited by corneal scarring.

COMPLICATIONS

- Microbial infection: Monitor patients closely during episodes of corneal erosion and consider antimicrobial prophylaxis.
- Corneal scarring: Monitor patients for scarring and consider topical corticosteroids as treatment.

REFERENCES

1. Klintworth GK. Corneal dystrophies. *Orphanet J Rare Dis* 2009;4:7
2. Rice NSC, et al. Reis-Bucklers' dystrophy: A clinico-pathological study. *Br J Ophthalmol* 1968;52:577–603.
3. Kobayashi A, Sugiyama K. In vivo laser confocal microscopy findings for Bowman's layer dystrophies (Thiel-Behnke and Reis-Bucklers corneal dystrophies). *Ophthalmology* 2007;114:69–75.
4. Dighiero, et al. Histological phenotype-genotype correlation of corneal dystrophies associated with eight distinct mutations in the TGFBI gene. *Ophthalmology* 2001;108:818–823.
5. Dinh R, et al. Recurrence of corneal dystrophy after excimer laser phototherapeutic keratectomy. *Ophthalmology* 1999;106:1490–1497.
6. Miller A, et al. Prevention of recurrent Reis-Bucklers dystrophy following excimer laser phototherapeutic keratectomy with topical mitomycin-C. *Cornea* 2004;23:732–735.

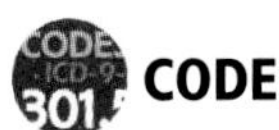

CODES

ICD9

371.52 Other anterior corneal dystrophies

CLINICAL PEARLS

- RBCD or CDB-1 is distinguished from Thiel-Behnke, or CDB-2 by its appearance on electron microscopy. Both conditions are associated with mutations of BIGH3; however, CDB-1 is associated with arg123leu while CDB-2 is associated with arg555gln. Thiel-Behnke corneal dystrophy typically has a later onset and a lower rate of recurrence following penetrating keratoplasty or phototherapeutic keratectomy.
- RBCD is a disease of the anterior cornea, specifically Bowman's layer that can result in decreased vision due to the corneal opacities, irregular surface, and stromal scarring.
- RBCD has a high rate of recurrence following penetrating keratoplasty and phototherapeutic keratoplasty.

REITER'S SYNDROME (REACTIVE ARTHRITIS)

Allen Chiang

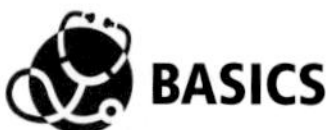

BASICS

DESCRIPTION

- Reiter's syndrome, also referred to as reactive arthritis (ReA), is a rheumatoid factor (RF) seronegative spondyloarthropathy with associated ocular inflammation that is precipitated by genitourinary or gastrointestinal infections.
  - Classic triad of sterile arthritis, urethritis, and conjunctivitis

EPIDEMIOLOGY

- It is the most common inflammatory polyarthritis in young men.
- Incidence is about 3.5 cases per 100,000 per year.
  - Epidemiologic studies differ in reported prevalence and incidence rates of causative agents, perhaps due to true epidemiologic variation, selection bias, or sampling errors (1)[B].
- Frequency of HLA-B27 in ReA is 70–90% (of the seronegative spondyloarthropathies, only ankylosing spondylitis has a higher frequency of HLA-B27 positivity).

RISK FACTORS

- HLA-B27
- HIV:
  - Prevalence of reactive arthritis may be significantly increased in those with HIV; in sub-Saharan Africa it is 12 times higher (2)[B].

GENERAL PREVENTION

- Measures to prevent genital and sexually transmitted disease:
  - Chlamydia is the most common cause of reactive arthritis in Western countries (42–69%) (3)[B].
- Measures to prevent gastrointestinal infection:
  - Enteric bacteria such as shigella, salmonella, campylobacter, and *Ureaplasma urealyticum* are common pathogens worldwide.

PATHOPHYSIOLOGY

- The pathogenesis involves an exaggerated immune response to bacterial antigens.
- Post-urogenital ReA:
  - Chlamydia takes on a "persistent state" within host tissues, an alternative life cycle that avoids host immune response (3)[B].
  - Interferon (IFN)-γ concentration is lower in HLA-B27-positive patients, contributing to persistence of infected cells which act as depots stimulating sustained inflammation.
- Post-enteric ReA:
  - Degraded particles of the bacterial envelope alone may persist in host tissues, creating long-lasting immune response.

ETIOLOGY

An immunologic response to an infectious organism in an individual with genetic predisposition (~75% are HLA-B27-positive) (4)[B]

COMMONLY ASSOCIATED CONDITIONS

See "General Prevention."

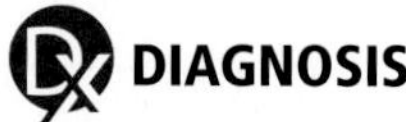

DIAGNOSIS

- Ophthalmic manifestations (60%) (5)[B]:
  - Conjunctivitis (a feature of early disease)
  - Non-granulomatous anterior uveitis (NGAU) in 20–40%; typically unilateral (7% bilateral) (3)[B]
  - Keratitis (4%)
  - Cystoid macular edema (rare)
  - Multifocal choroiditis (rare)

HISTORY

- Symptoms generally appear within 1–3 weeks from the inciting genitourinary or gastrointestinal infection:
  - Mild constitutional symptoms such as low-grade fever and malaise
  - Urogenital: Dysuria, frequency, discharge
  - Musculoskeletal: Myalgias (early), swelling and pain of the large joints
  - Ophthalmic: Decreased vision, pain, injection, photophobia

PHYSICAL EXAM

- Asymmetric, acute oligoarthritis affecting large joints
- Periostitis
- Sacroiliitis
- Mucocutaneous lesions:
  - Circinate balanitis, cervicitis, or painless oral ulcers
- Keratoderma blennorrhagicum

DIAGNOSTIC TESTS & INTERPRETATION

Lab

- CBC
- Erythrocyte sedimentation rate
- C-reactive protein
- Urethra, cervix, or throat cultures
- Chlamydia PCR
- HIV
- HLA-B27 genetic marker

Imaging

MRI of large joints

Diagnostic Procedures/Other

- Synovial joint fluid aspiration (classically culture negative)

DIFFERENTIAL DIAGNOSIS

- Ankylosing spondylitis
- Inflammatory bowel disease-associated arthritis
- Psoriatic arthritis
- Gonococcal arthritis
- Lyme disease
- Systemic lupus erythematosus
- Rheumatoid arthritis
- Juvenile rheumatoid arthritis (Still's disease)
- Gouty arthritis

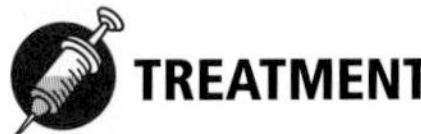

TREATMENT

MEDICATION

First Line

- If still present, treat the inciting infection with appropriate antibiotic therapy.
- Topical uveitis treatment:
  - Prednisolone acetate 1%, 1 drop q1–2 hours (slow taper over several weeks)
  - Scopolamine hydrobromide 0.25% (or similar cycloplegic agent) 1 drop b.i.d.–t.i.d.
- NSAIDs: Indomethacin SR 75 mg PO b.i.d.–t.i.d.

Second Line

- Disease-modifying antirheumatic drugs (DMARDs) for chronic arthritis
  - Sulfasalazine 1 g PO b.i.d.–t.i.d.
  - Oral corticosteroids
  - Methotrexate 7.5–15 mg PO per week
  - Azathioprine 100–150 mg PO daily
  - Biologics (anti-TNF agents) such as infliximab (Remicade) and adalimumab (Humira) (1)[C]

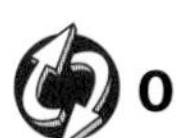

ONGOING CARE

FOLLOW-UP RECOMMENDATIONS

- Ophthalmologist
- Rheumatology consultation
- Primary care physician
- Physical therapist

PATIENT EDUCATION

- The Spondylitis Association of America (http://www.spondylitis.org)

PROGNOSIS

- Recurrent NGAU may lead to vision loss if not properly monitored and treated.
- Reactive arthritis may be self-limited, episodic and relapsing, or chronic and progressive (2)[B].
  - Self-limited form resolves over 3–12 months.
  - 15–50% of patients develop recurrent bouts of arthritis (more common in Chlamydia-associated cases).
  - 15–30% develop chronic arthritis.
  - 10% of those with chronic disease develop cardiac complications such as aortic regurgitation and pericarditis.

COMPLICATIONS

- Vision loss
- Chronic arthritis
- Cardiac manifestations

REFERENCES

1. Colmegna I, Espinoza LR. Recent advances in reactive arthritis. *Curr Rheumatol Rep* 2005; 7(3):201–207.
2. Khan MA. Update on spondyloarthropathies. *Ann Intern Med* 2002;136(12):896–907.
3. Gerard HC, Whittum-Hudson JA, Carter JD, et al. The pathogenic role of *Chlamydia* in spondyloarthritis. *Curr Opin Rheumatol* 2010;22(4): 363–367.
4. Tay-Kearney ML, Schwam BL, Lowder C, et al. Clinical features and associated systemic diseases of HLA-B27 uveitis. *Am J Ophthalmol* 1996;121: 47–56.
5. Lee DA, Barker SM, Su WPD, et al. The clinical diagnosis of Reiter's syndrome: Ophthalmic and non-ophthalmic aspects. *Ophthalmology* 1986;93:350–356.

ADDITIONAL READING

- Braun J, Sieper J. Early diagnosis of spondyloarthritis. *Nat Clin Pract Rheumatol* 2006;2(10):536–545.

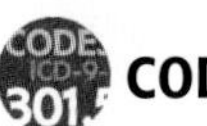

CODES

ICD9

- 099.3 (Reiter's syndrome); use additional codes for associated manifestations:
  - Reiter's disease
    - 364.3 Unspecified iridocyclitis
    - 372.33 Conjunctivitis in mucocutaneous disease

CLINICAL PEARLS

- Reiter's syndrome, or reactive arthritis (ReA), comprises sterile arthritis, urethritis, and conjunctivitis. It is uncommon for all features of the classic triad to be simultaneously present.
- Chlamydia is the most common etiologic agent of ReA in Western countries.
- Conjunctivitis is an early feature that may be missed if patients present later; uveitis is the more serious ocular manifestation and requires continued follow-up.

RELATIVE AFFERENT PUPILLARY DEFECT (RAPD)

Stephen Best

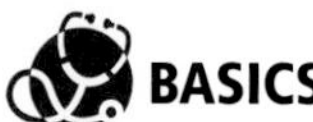

BASICS

DESCRIPTION
- Different response of one pupil compared with the contralateral pupil when stimulated by a bright light. It is a sign that can be seen in a large variety of disease entities.
- Previously known as the Marcus–Gunn pupillary phenomenon.

Geriatric Considerations
Cataract (commonly seen in geriatric patients) does not cause a relative afferent pupillary defect (RAPD).

Pediatric Considerations
Absolute indication of pathology involving the afferent visual pathway especially in preverbal patients

Pregnancy Considerations
Meningiomas and pituitary tumors occur or increase in size with increased frequency during pregnancy resulting in RAPD

EPIDEMIOLOGY

Incidence
Not applicable

Prevalence
Relates to the prevalence of afferent visual system disease in the particular population

RISK FACTORS
Depends on underlying pathology

Genetics
- Most inherited retinal conditions are less likely to cause an RAPD unless there exists considerable asymmetry of involvement of one eye compared with the other.
- Mitochondrial disease such as Leber's hereditary optic neuropathy may present asymmetrically or with one eye involved prior to the contralateral eye.

PATHOPHYSIOLOGY
- Decreased amount of light transmitted along one side of the anterior visual pathway
- Pathology resulting in loss of function within the afferent visual pathway, which may include the retina, optic nerve head, optic nerve, chiasm, and the anterior optic tract proximal to the lateral geniculate body
  - Media opacity within the eye such as cataract will not cause an RAPD. Dense, extensive anterior chamber or vitreous hemorrhage produce RAPD

ETIOLOGY
- Optic neuropathy of any etiology if unilateral or asymmetric
- Extensive retinal involvement from multiple causes

COMMONLY ASSOCIATED CONDITIONS
- Demyelinating disease (multiple sclerosis)
- Hypertension
- Diabetes
- Giant cell arteritis
- Optic nerve/chiasmal compression
- Nonarteritic anterior ischemic optic neuropathy (NAION)

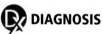

DIAGNOSIS

HISTORY
- Unilateral vision loss
- Unilateral loss of brightness
- Unilateral loss of color perception or desaturation of color
  - Pain associated with eye movement in optic neuritis
  - Various visual field defects

PHYSICAL EXAM
- Patient asked to distance fixate preferably in dim ambient light conditions
- A bight light source is directed at the right eye
- The direct ipsilateral pupillary response is observed (pupil should constrict)
- The consensual contralateral pupillary response in the left eye is observed (pupil should also constrict)
- The light is now directed at the left eye (swinging flashlight test), and both the direct and consensual pupillary reflexes are observed.
- When an RAPD is present the pupil on the affected side will dilate more (pupillary escape)
  - Subjective grading by the examiner often ranging from "trace" or ±, through +1 to +4
  - Objective measurement using a neutral density filter to quantitate
  - Subjective impression of brightness differential can be asked of the patient
  - Advanced objective measurements with pupillometry devices but less often used clinically

DIAGNOSTIC TESTS & INTERPRETATION

Imaging

Initial approach

- An RAPD infers objective evidence of pathology of the anterior visual pathways. If there is no explanation from the ophthalmic examination, neuroimaging is mandatory.
- MRI with fat suppression and gadolinium of the orbits and brain is considered the minimum work-up.

Follow-up & special considerations

- Exclude other associated intracranial abnormalities such as demyelinating plaques
  - Adequate consultation with neuroradiology is highly recommended.

Diagnostic Procedures/Other

- Automated visual field analysis of both eyes looking for topographical patterns of vision loss
- Complete ophthalmic examination including measurement of intraocular pressure and dilated retinal examination
  - CBC count with ESR and CRP in patients older than 60 years or if other symptoms or signs of giant cell arteritis (GCA)

Pathological Findings

Depends on underlying pathology

DIFFERENTIAL DIAGNOSIS

- Retinal disorders
- Optic neuropathy
- Chiasmal disease
- Optic tract lesions

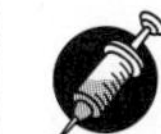

TREATMENT

MEDICATION

Depends on the underlying pathology

ADDITIONAL TREATMENT

Issues for Referral

Refer to neuroophthalmology if the cause or treatment of the cause is in doubt

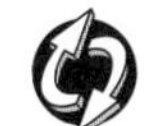

ONGOING CARE

FOLLOW-UP RECOMMENDATIONS

Depends on underlying pathology

REFERENCES

1. Levatin P. Pupillary escape in disease of the retina or optic nerve. *Arch Ophthalmol* 1959;62: 768–779.
2. Danesh-Meyer HV, Papchenko TL, Savino PJ, et al. Brightness sensitivity and color perception as predictors of relative afferent pupillary defect. *Invest Ophthalmol Vis Sci* 2007;48:3616–3621.

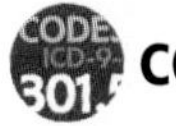

CODES

ICD9

- 379.23 Vitreous hemorrhage
- 379.49 Other anomalies of pupillary function
- 742.8 Other specified congenital anomalies of nervous system

CLINICAL PEARLS

- An RAPD is a "red flag" objective indication of pathology involving the afferent visual pathway that requires explanation!
- Cataract alone will not cause an RAPD.

R

RETINA COATS' DISEASE

Jerry A. Shields
Carol L. Shields

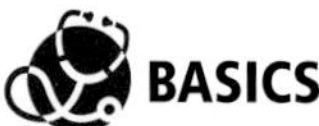

BASICS

DESCRIPTION
- Nonhereditary condition
- Unilateral
- Retinal telangiectasia
- Retinal exudation
- Exudative retinal detachment
- Classification proposed by Shields et al:
  - Stage 1. Retinal telangiectasia (T)
  - Stage 2. T + and exudation (E)
  - Stage 3. T + E + subretinal fluid (F)
  - Stage 4. T + E + F + neovascular glaucoma (G)
  - Stage 5. T + E + F + G + phthisis bulbi

ALERT
Any child with an abnormal pupillary reflex should have a fundus examination to rule out Coats' disease.

Geriatric Considerations
Coats' disease occurs almost exclusively in young patients under the age of 10 years. It is rare to diagnose this condition in the elderly.

Pediatric Considerations
Coats' disease occurs primarily in children at approximately of 2–11 years of age and rarely is related to systemic conditions.

EPIDEMIOLOGY
Unknown

RISK FACTORS
None.

Genetics
No proven genetic defect.

PATHOPHYSIOLOGY
- Idiopathic congenital retinal telangiectasia.
- Affects temporal retina most often but can be 360 degrees in the fundus.
- Progressive retinal and subretinal exudation.
- Exudative retinal detachment

COMMONLY ASSOCIATED CONDITIONS
- None in true unilateral Coats' disease
- In cases of bilateral exudative retinopathy that resemble Coats' disease (but not true Coats' disease), one must consider a list of systemic conditions including IRVAN syndrome, familial exudative vitreoretinopathy, dyskeratosis congenital, retinopathy of prematurity, facioscapulohumeral dystrophy, turner syndrome, incontinentia pigmenti, neurofibromatosis, kabuki makeup syndrome, and others.

DIAGNOSIS

HISTORY
- Blurred vision
- Yellow or white pupillary reflex
- Strabismus

PHYSICAL EXAM
- The following data is based on an analysis in 150 consecutive cases by Shields et al.
- Symptoms include
  - Decreased visual acuity in 43%
  - Strabismus in 23%
  - Leukocoria in 20%
  - Pain in 3%
  - Heterochromia in 1%
  - Nystagmus in 1%
  - No symptoms in 8%
- Findings include
  - Telangiectasia in 100%
  - Retinal exudation in 99%
  - Exudative retinal detachment in 81%
  - Retinal hemorrhage in 13%
  - Retinal macrocyst in 11%
  - Vasoproliferative tumor in 6%
  - Neovascularization of disc in 2%
  - Neovascularization of retina in 1%
  - Neovascularization of iris in 8%
  - Corneal edema in 3%
  - Anterior chamber cholesterol in 3%

DIAGNOSTIC TESTS & INTERPRETATION

Lab

Initial lab tests
No lab abnormalities except in older patients, check blood cholesterol, and lipids.

Follow-up & special considerations
- If bilateral involvement, evaluate patient for related syndromes as previously mentioned.
- Treat all leaking telangiectasia

Imaging

Initial approach
- Fundus photography to document the retinal findings.
- Ocular ultrasonography to confirm retinal detachment.
- Fluorescein angiography to identify leaking telangiectasia.
- Optical coherence tomography to study the macular region for edema or fluid.

Follow-up & special considerations
- Repeat fundus photography at each visit.
- Repeat fluorescein angiography if subretinal fluid or exudation detected.
- Repeat optical coherence tomography for macular findings.

Diagnostic Procedures/Other Pathological Findings
- Peripheral retinal telangiectasia
- Retinal detachment
- Retinal and subretinal exudation
- Cholesterol clefts in subretinal space
- Advanced cases show neovascular glaucoma

DIFFERENTIAL DIAGNOSIS
- Retinoblastoma
- Retinal hemangioblastoma
- Retinal vasoproliferative tumor
- Persistent hyperplastic primary vitreous
- Rhegmatogenous retinal detachment
- Radiation retinopathy
- Hypertensive crisis

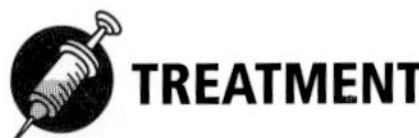

TREATMENT

MEDICATION

First Line

Management depends on stage of disease.

- No medication necessary
- Laser photocoagulation
- Cryotherapy

Second Line

- Intravitreal bevacizumab
- Intravitreal triamcinolone
- Subtenons triamcinolone
- Antiglaucoma medications if necessary

ADDITIONAL TREATMENT

General Measures

- Laser photocoagulation
- Cryotherapy

Issues for Referral

Any child with suspected Coats' disease should be referred for management by a qualified specialist.

Additional Therapies

- Medical treatment for secondary glaucoma
- Cataract extraction if necessary
- Vitrectomy with repair retinal detachment

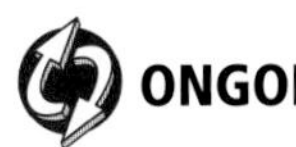

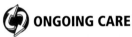

ONGOING CARE

FOLLOW-UP RECOMMENDATIONS

- The patient should be reassessed every 2–4 months following treatment.
- At each reassessment, a judgment on the status of the retina will be made and the need for further treatment. In general, this condition requires at least 3 extensive treatments to quiet the leakage.
- All examinations are best performed under anesthesia, especially if the child is under 4 years of age.
- When 4 years old or older, office exams can be considered.

Patient Monitoring

- Check retina status long-term twice yearly for life.
- Return for examination if visual acuity decreases.

PATIENT EDUCATION

- www.fighteyecancer.com
- www.eyecancer.info
- www.eyetumor.org
- www.eyecancerbook.com
- www.etrf.org
- www.choroidmelanoma.com

PROGNOSIS

- The systemic prognosis is unaffected by this ophthalmic condition.
- The visual prognosis with stage of disease, based on an analysis of 150 consecutive eyes. Below is the risk for poor visual outcome of 20/200 or worse:
  - Stage 1 – 0%
  - Stage 2 – 50%
  - Stage 3 – 70%
  - Stage 4 – 100%
  - Stage 5 – 100%

COMPLICATIONS

- Retinal detachment
- Cataract
- Chronic pain
- Phthisis bulbi

ADDITIONAL READING

- Shields JA, Shields CL, Honavar S, et al. Coats' disease. Clinical variations and complications of Coats' disease in 150 cases. The 2000 Sanford Gifford Memorial Lecture. *Am J. Ophthalmol* 2001;131:561–71.
- Shields JA, Shields CL, Honavar SG, et al. Classification and management of Coats' disease. The 2000 Proctor lecture. *Am J Ophthalmol* 2001;131:572–83.
- Shields JA, Shields CL. Lesions that can simulate retinoblastoma. In: Shields JA, Shields CL (eds). *Intraocular tumors, an atlas and textbook*, 2nd ed. Philadelphia: Lippincott, Williams and Wilkins, 2008:364–365.

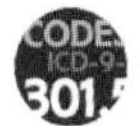

CODES

ICD9

- 361.2 Serous retinal detachment
- 362.12 Exudative retinopathy
- 362.15 Retinal telangiectasia

CLINICAL PEARLS

- Coats' disease can simulate retinoblastoma
- Typical features can assist in diagnosis
- Visual prognosis good if discovered early before macular exudation.

RETINA RETINOBLASTOMA

Carol L. Shields
Jerry A. Shields

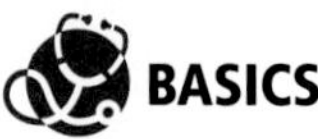

BASICS

DESCRIPTION

- Eye cancer of children
- Tends to manifest between 6 months and 3 years of age
- Accounts for 4% of all childhood malignancies
- Can occur in one (unilateral) or both (bilateral) eyes
- Can have a sporadic or familial tendency
- Can be germline or somatic mutation
- Appears as a white mass within the retina, best seen on dilated eye examination
- In more advanced stages can present with white pupil (leukocoria), red eye, or glaucoma
- International Classification of Retinoblastoma (RB) includes
  - Group A – RB <3 mm
  - Group B – RB >3 mm or in the macula or with clear subretinal fluid
  - Group C – RB with subretinal or vitreous seeds <3 mm from tumor
  - Group D – RB with subretinal or vitreous seeds >3 mm from tumor
  - Group E – extensive RB fill >50% globe or with hemorrhage or iris neovascularization

ALERT
Any child with leukocoria (white pupil) or strabismus (drifting eye) should have a dilated examination by a qualified ophthalmologist to evaluate for fundus abnormalities, particularly malignancies such as retinoblastoma.

Geriatric Considerations

The intraocular scar from this malignancy should be followed for life. More important consideration in the older population with retinoblastoma is the risk for second cancers in those with germline mutation.

Pediatric Considerations

Retinoblastoma nearly always manifests in children, usually those under age 3 years.

Pregnancy Considerations

If a pregnant woman has a family history of retinoblastoma, then the fetus should be imaged with ultrasonography at 8-month gestation in utero to evaluate the eyes. If retinoblastoma is detected, then early but safe delivery can be considered.

EPIDEMIOLOGY

Incidence

1/15,000 newborn infants

Prevalence

Retinoblastoma develops in 5,000 children worldwide and 300 children in the USA annually.

RISK FACTORS

There is no known cause for Rb1 mutation.

Genetics

- In 1971, Knudson "2 hit" hypothesis for the development of retinoblastoma was proposed.
- In 1980, research confirmed that both alleles of retinoblastoma gene (RB1) at chromosome 13q14 locus were mutated in retinoblastoma.
- Currently, there are arguments that genomic instability and aneuploidy are likely responsible for the genesis of Rb.

GENERAL PREVENTION

- For patients with known germline mutations, there are several methods of prevention, including the following:
  - Avoid having children.
  - Use donor germ cells to avoid transmission of the genetic defect.
  - In vitro fertilization with preimplantation genetic sampling at the 8-cell morula stage for the Rb gene can identify affected individuals. Those not affected can be implanted.
- For patients with somatic mutations, the defect does not transmit to future generations but it is important to examine the eyes of all children within 2 weeks from birth.

PATHOPHYSIOLOGY

Some authorities believe that retinoblastoma develops from an undifferentiated cell or a retinal progenitor cell whereas others believe that a fully differentiated horizontal cell of the retina is the cell of origin.

ETIOLOGY

The etiology for retinoblastoma is a genetic mutation on chromosome 13q14 in all cells in the body in germline retinoblastoma and in only the tumor in somatic retinoblastoma.

COMMONLY ASSOCIATED CONDITIONS

- 13q syndrome:
  - This syndrome is related to the phenotypic abnormalities from the mutated portion of chromosome 13.
  - Features include microcephaly, broad nasal bridge, hypertelorism, microphthalmos, epicanthus, ptosis, micrognathia, short neck, low set ears, facial asymmetry, anogenital malformations, hypoplastic thumbs and toes, mental and psychomotor retardation.

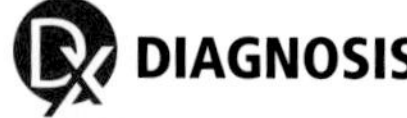

DIAGNOSIS

HISTORY

- The infant or toddler gives no history
- The parent might note leukocoria or strabismus

PHYSICAL EXAM

- The most common sign is the white pupil (leukocoria) in an otherwise quiet comfortable eye.
- The second most common sign is crossed eye (strabismus) where the eye drifts inward or outward.
- Red eye
- Bulging eye
- Droopy eyelid (ptosis)

DIAGNOSTIC TESTS & INTERPRETATION

Lab

Complete blood count

Imaging

Initial approach

- Ultrasonography to confirm the mass, retinal detachment, and calcification
- Fundus photography to document tumor size and location
- Intravenous fluorescein angiography to document blood supply to the tumors
- Brain and orbit magnetic resonance Imaging to rule out extraocular spread and rule out pinealoblastoma

Follow-up & special considerations

Monitor monthly for tumor regression then slowly increase the interval between visits if all malignancy stable.

Diagnostic Procedures/Other

Do not perform fine needle aspiration biopsy as this could seed the tumor.

Pathological Findings

- Gross findings:
  - Chalky white friable tumor
  - Dense foci of calcification
  - Retinal detachment
  - Scleral, optic nerve, or epibulbar invasion
- Microscopic findings:
  - Small to medium sized round neuroblastic cells with large hyperchromatic nuclei and scanty cytoplasm
  - Well or poorly differentiated cells
  - Growth patterns:
    - Exophytic – growth underneath the retina
    - Endophytic – growth superficial to the retina in the vitreous
    - Intraretinal – growth within the retina
    - Diffuse – flat infiltration

DIFFERENTIAL DIAGNOSIS
- Coats disease
- Persistent hyperplastic primary vitreous
- Retinal astrocytic hamartoma
- Retinal astrocytoma
- Combined hamartoma of the retina and retinal pigment epithelium
- Retinal detachment
- Familial exudative vitreoretinopathy
- Cataract
- Glaucoma

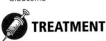

TREATMENT

MEDICATION
- Intravenous chemoreduction consisting of vincristine, carboplatin, and etoposide followed by thermotherapy or cryotherapy
- Intraarterial chemotherapy with melphalan

ADDITIONAL TREATMENT
General Measures
- If group A, treat with laser photocoagulation or cryotherapy
- If group B, treat with chemoreduction or plaque radiotherapy
- If group C, treat with chemoreduction
- If group D or E, treat with chemoreduction or enucleation
- Note that intraarterial chemotherapy can be substituted for intravenous chemoreduction in certain select cases.

Issues for Referral
All children with retinoblastoma should be referred to and managed at retinoblastoma centers of excellence. There are perhaps only 6 such centers in the USA.

SURGERY/OTHER PROCEDURES
- Enucleation for advanced tumors or massive tumor recurrence
- Plaque radiotherapy for smaller tumors or tumor recurrence
- External beam radiotherapy

IN-PATIENT CONSIDERATIONS
Initial Stabilization
Ophthalmic treatment is outpatient.

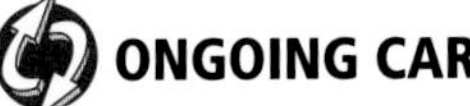

ONGOING CARE

FOLLOW-UP RECOMMENDATIONS
- If germline mutation, then mag resonance imaging of the eye and brain to rule out pinealoblastoma or related brain tumor and lifelong follow-up for second malignancies
- If somatic or germline mutation:
  - Fundus examination with treatment every month until the retinoblastoma is completely regressed and stable for 3 months; then slowly increase the interval of the follow-up to every 2 months, then every 3 months, and so on.

Patient Monitoring
Examination under anesthesia until age 4 years for the eyes, and evaluation by pediatric or adult oncology for life.

PATIENT EDUCATION
- www.fighteyecancer.com
- www.eyecancer.info
- www.eyetumor.info
- www.eyecancerbook.com
- www.eyeretinoblastoma.com
- www.retinoblastomainfo.com
- www.etrf.org

PROGNOSIS
- In developed countries, prognosis has improved from 5% survival in the early 1900s to 50% in the 1930s to 98% currently.
- In undeveloped countries prognosis currently remains approximately 50% survival, likely related to delay in diagnosis.

COMPLICATIONS
- Vision loss
- Loss of the eye
- Dry eye
- Retinal atrophy
- Retinal detachment
- Glaucoma
- Cataract
- Facial deformity
- Second cancers

ADDITIONAL READING

- Hungerford JL, Toma NM, Plowman PN, et al. External beam radiotherapy for retinoblastoma: I. Whole eye technique. *Br J Ophthalmol* 1995;79: 109–111.
- Kivela T. Trilateral retinoblastoma: A meta-analysis of hereditary retinoblastoma associated with primary ectopic intracranial retinoblastoma. *J Clin Oncol* 1999;17:1829–1837.
- Roarty JD, McLean IW, Zimmerman LE. Incidence of second neoplasms in patients with retinoblastoma. *Ophthalmology* 1988;95:1583–1587.
- Shields CL, Au A, Czyz C, et al. The International Classification of Retinoblastoma predicts chemoreduction success. *Ophthalmology* 2006;113(12):2276–2280.
- Shields CL, Honavar SG Meadows AT, et al. Chemoreduction plus focal therapy for retinoblastoma: Factors predictive of need for treatment with external beam radiotherapy or enucleation. *Am J Ophthalmol* 2002;133:657–664.
- Shields CL, Shields JA. Basic understanding in the current classification and management of retinoblastoma. *Curr Opin Ophthalmol* 2006;17(3): 228–234.
- Shields JA, Shields CL. Management and prognosis of retinoblastoma. *Intraocular tumors: A text and atlas*. Philadelphia: WB Saunders 1992:377–392.
- Shields JA, Shields CL. Retinoblastoma. In: Shields JA, Shields CL, eds. *Atlas of intraocular tumors*. Philadelphia: Lippincott Williams Wilkins 1999:207–232.
- Shields CL, Shields JA, Cater J, et al. Plaque radiotherapy for retinoblastoma: Long term tumor control and treatment complications in 208 tumors. *Ophthalmology* 2001;108:2116–2121.
- Toma NM, Hungerford JL, Plowman PN, et al. External beam radiotherapy for retinoblastoma: II. Lens sparing technique. *Br J Ophthalmol* 1995;79:112–117.

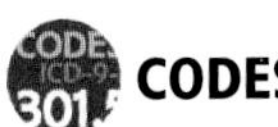

CODES

ICD9
190.5 Malignant neoplasm of retina

CLINICAL PEARLS

- Any child with leukocoria or strabismus should be evaluated by an experienced ophthalmologist familiar with retinoblastoma.
- Chemotherapy has become the most common method for management.
- Enucleation is still a powerful method of tumor control and life salvage.

RETINAL BREAK

Caroline Baumal

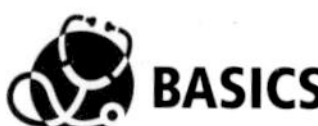

BASICS

DESCRIPTION
- A full thickness defect in the neurosensory retina.
- May be round/oval (retinal hole), horseshoe shaped (retinal tear), irregularly shaped or semicircular/ adjacent to the ora serrata (dialysis).
- Location usually in peripheral retina, although may occur anywhere.
- A retinal break may allow vitreous fluid to pass through the break into the subretinal space leading to rhegmatogenous retinal detachment (RRD) with potential for severe visual loss.
- The etiology, underlying risk factors and shape of the retinal break may increase the risk of progression of a retinal tear to RRD.
- A retinal break does not produce visual loss (exception is a macular hole), but the vitreous hemorrhage or retinal detachment occurring secondarily lead to the loss of vision.

EPIDEMIOLOGY
Incidence
- Incidence of retinal breaks is 6–11% in adult eyes at autopsy.
- Incidence of retinal tears in eyes with symptomatic posterior vitreous detachment (PVD) is 8.2% (1).
- 1.8% of patients develop a retinal tear that was not visualized on initial examination but was noted with follow-up.
- Features associated with delayed-onset diagnosis or development of retinal break associated with PVD include vitreous hemorrhage at initial examination, hemorrhage in the peripheral retina at initial examination, or new symptoms.
- Annual incidence of retinal detachment is 12 per 100,000 per year.

Prevalence
Prevalence of retinal break ranges from 6 to 14%.

RISK FACTORS
- Myopia
- Increased age
- Lattice degeneration
- PVD
- History of intraocular surgery, including cataract surgery
- Trauma
- History of retina break or RRD in the contralateral eye
- Family history
- Stickler syndrome

Genetics
- Genetic syndromes that predispose to myopia or collagen abnormalities may be a risk factor for retinal break.
  - These include Stickler's syndrome, Marfan's syndrome, Wagner's syndrome, Ehlers–Danlos syndrome, and homocystinuria.

GENERAL PREVENTION
- Development of PVD is not preventable.
- In most cases progression of PVD to retinal break is not preventable.
- Laser prophylaxis to retinal lesions that predispose to retinal breaks may seal the area and prevent development of retinal detachment.
- Prompt recognition of symptoms of PVD and assessment may prevent the progression of retinal break to retinal detachment.

PATHOPHYSIOLOGY
Retina breaks develop either secondary to peripheral retina stretching and atrophy near the ora serrata (retinal hole) or due to PVD with vitreous traction (horseshoe-shaped tear, operculated hole, dialysis)

COMMONLY ASSOCIATED CONDITIONS
- Myopia
- Lattice degeneration
- See risk factors

DIAGNOSIS

HISTORY
- Symptoms of PVD with attention to photopsia, floaters, visual field disturbance, reduced visual acuity
- Family history
- Prior eye trauma
- Myopia
- History of intraocular surgery, including cataract surgery

PHYSICAL EXAM
- Examination of the peripheral retinal with scleral depression and assessment of the vitreous
- Features may include:
  - Retinal hole – round or oval
  - Horseshoe-shaped tear – tip of the tear is pointed toward the optic nerve, may be an associated bridging vessel
  - Retinal dialysis – may have pigment along its edge if there is associated avulsion of the vitreous base and trauma
- Changes in adjacent retina such as lattice degeneration or pigmentary change
- Peripheral retinal abnormalities
- Pigmented cells in the vitreous (aka tobacco dust, Schafer's sign)
- Vitreous traction
- Vitreous hemorrhage
- PVD with Weiss ring

DIAGNOSTIC TESTS & INTERPRETATION
Imaging
B-scan ultrasound may demonstrate retinal break if cloudy media obscure visualization of the retina such as with vitreous hemorrhage

Pathological Findings
Full thickness defect in the neurosensory retina

DIFFERENTIAL DIAGNOSIS

- Chorioretinal atrophy or scar
- Pars plana cyst
- Enclosed oral bay
- Meridional folds
- Vitreoretinal tuft
- Peripheral cystoid degeneration

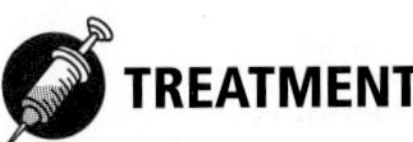

TREATMENT

ADDITIONAL TREATMENT

General Measures

- Goal is to treat retinal breaks that are at a high risk of progression to RRD, thus preventing any secondary visual loss.
- Observation may be recommended when the risk of progression to RRD is extremely low (2) as in the following situations: Asymptomatic retinal holes that do not have vitreoretinal traction, round holes with operculum (relieved vitreous traction) and atrophic round holes, atrophic holes within an area of lattice that is self-sealed by pigment.

Additional Therapies

- Treatment with laser or cryotherapy creates a firm chorioretinal adhesion in the attached retina immediately adjacent to and surrounding the retinal tear.
- Treatment of peripheral breaks should extend anteriorly up to the ora serrata and to completely around the entire break or dialysis.
- Laser prophylaxis to areas of thin retina may be considered in eyes with an increased risk of development in retinal tear or RRD.
- Cryotherapy may be used as an alternative to laser in eyes with cloudy media, if the laser cannot reach the oral serrata, or if the laser is not available.

SURGERY/OTHER PROCEDURES

- May be indicated if media opacity such as asteroid hyalosis, vitreous hemorrhage, or cataract precludes viewing of the retina for laser/cryotherapy or if RRD develops.
- This may include pneumatic retinopexy, vitrectomy, or scleral buckling procedure.

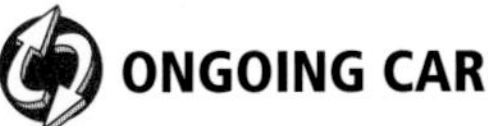

ONGOING CARE

FOLLOW-UP RECOMMENDATIONS

There is an increased risk of retinal break in the same or contralateral eye.

PATIENT EDUCATION

- Individuals at an increased risk of retinal break/detachment should notify their ophthalmologist promptly if they develop or note a change in symptoms such as floaters, photopsia, visual field defect, or reduced acuity.
- Myopic individuals who undergo refractive surgery should be aware of the fact that they remain at a risk of retinal beaks and RRD.

PROGNOSIS

Treatment is usually uncomplicated with a high rate of successfully sealing the break and preventing retinal detachment.

COMPLICATIONS

- Progression of retinal tear to RRD despite the fact that laser/cryotherapy may occur on occasion (3).
- Most common cause of failure is inadequate treatment of the anterior extent of tear. Continued vitreous traction can extend the tear beyond the treated area, allowing fluid to leak into the subretinal space with RRD. Also, continued vitreous traction may produce new tears.
- Vitreous hemorrhage.
- Epiretinal membrane formation may develop after PVD, and it does not appear to have an increased incidence after laser photocoagulation.

REFERENCES

1. Coffee RE, Westfall AC, Davis GH, et al. Symptomatic posterior vitreous detachment and the incidence of delayed retinal breaks: Case series and meta-analysis. *Am J Ophthalmol* 2007;144:409–413.
2. Byer NE. What happens to untreated asymptomatic retinal breaks, and are they affected by posterior vitreous detachment? *Ophthalmology* 1998;105:1045.
3. Mastropasqua L, Carpineto P, Ciancaglini M, et al. Treatment of retinal tears and lattice degeneration in fellow eyes in high risk patients suffering retinal detachment: A prospective study. *Br J ophthalmol* 1999;83;1046.

ADDITIONAL READING

- American Academy of Ophthalmology. Preferred Practice Patterns. Posterior Vitreous Detachment, Retinal Breaks, and Lattice Degeneration PPP, September 2008

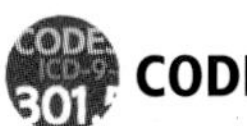

CODES

ICD9

- 361.30 Retinal defect, unspecified
- 361.31 Round hole of retina without detachment
- 361.32 Horseshoe tear of retina without detachment

CLINICAL PEARLS

- Vitreous or retinal hemorrhage at initial examination and new symptoms are associated with delayed-onset diagnosis of retinal break associated with PVD.

RETINAL HEMORRHAGES

Brian J. Forbes
Kathleen Romero
Alex V. Levin

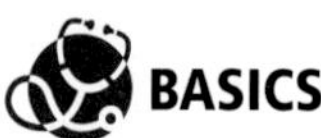

BASICS

DESCRIPTION

- RH may occur on the surface or just below the retina (preretinal or subretinal), or they may be found within the retinal layers. Intraretinal hemorrhages include those in the nerve fiber layer (flame, splinter) or RH deep in retinal tissue (dot, blot).
- Intraretinal and preretinal hemorrhages may have white centers, a nonspecific finding found in virtually any cause of RH.

ALERT
Child abuse should be considered in the diagnosis of retinal hemorrhage (RH) in any child <5 years old.

EPIDEMIOLOGY

Incidence

- Hemorrhage is seen in ~85% of shaken baby syndrome (SBS)/Abusive head trauma (AHT) victims.
- Hemorrhage can be seen in over 40% of children after birth in the first 24 h of life.
- Newborn RH are seen most often with vacuum-assisted delivery followed by forceps delivery, with the lowest incidence in C-section delivery.

RISK FACTORS

- Trauma: Abusive head trauma (AHT), direct orbital/ocular injury, birth process, accidental
- Infection: Bacterial endocarditis, sepsis, meningitis, CMV retinitis, toxoplasmosis, malaria
- Intracranial: Papilledema, arteriovenous malformation (AVM), ruptured aneurysm
- Systemic disease: Hemolytic uremic syndrome, vasculitis, diabetes (post pubertal only), sickle cell, hypertension (acute on chronic, older children only)
- Coagulopathies: Including thrombocytopenia, severe anemia, leukemia, factor deficiencies, protein C/S deficiency, vitamin K deficiency
- Cardiopulmonary: Carbon monoxide poisoning, hypoxia, hypotension, ECMO
- Metabolic/endocrine: Hypo/hypernatremia, galactosemia, glutaric aciduria type 1

Genetics

Genetic retinal disease may be associated with RH: Norrie disease, Coats disease, juvenile X-linked retinoschisis, von Hippel Lindau.

GENERAL PREVENTION

- Control of systemic diseases
- Child abuse prevention

PATHOPHYSIOLOGY

- AHT: Repetitive acceleration–deceleration with or without impact causing vitreo-retinal traction is a major factor. Modulating factors may include hypoxic ischemic injury, increased venous pressure, and/or disruption of autonomic supply to the retinal vessels.
- Increased intracranial pressure, intracranial hemorrhage, blunt trauma, occlusive thrombi in retinal veins, leaky vessels, and infection.

ETIOLOGY

- Hemorrhage originates from retina or choroid.
- It depends on a causative agent.

COMMONLY ASSOCIATED CONDITIONS

- AHT, accidental trauma
- Multiple systemic and retinal diseases

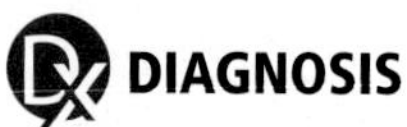

DIAGNOSIS

HISTORY

- Any history of trauma (trauma to orbit, head trauma), fussy irritable child, increased/abnormal bruising, bleeding
- Newborn
- Investigate for related systemic diseases
- Spotted vision, decreased vision in older verbal children

PHYSICAL EXAM

- Complete eye evaluation including visual acuity if age appropriate, visual fields, indirect ophthalmoscopy.
- Describe RH: Types, patterns, distribution, and number
- Use detailed descriptions, both words and careful drawings. Photography not required but may be useful.
- Pharmacologic dilation of pupils is essential when possible.

DIAGNOSTIC TESTS & INTERPRETATION

Lab

Initial lab tests

CBC with differential, PT, aPTT/INR

Follow-up & special considerations

- If possible, in case of trauma, consider liver function tests, amylase/lipase.
- If there is any concern about coagulopathy, consider vWF, ristocetin cofactor, platelet function, Factors VII, VIII, XII, and XVIII. D-dimer, fibrinogen.
- If there is any concern about vasculitis/hemoglobinopathy, consider ANA, ESR, ACE, serum Ca, sickle cell electrophoresis.
- If possible conduct the glutaric aciduria test for urine organic acids.

Imaging

- Retinal photography if possible
- OCT if available
- Possible role for ultrasound if view of retina obscured
- Skeletal survey and bone scan if there is any concern about abusive injury, CT/MRI head for intracranial bleed

Diagnostic Procedures/Other

Indirect ophthalmoscopy required for full retinal view.

Pathological Findings

- Traumatic retinoschisis (most often subinternal limiting membrane blood) has particular diagnostic significance in recognizing SBS/AHT.
- RH in AHT (present in two thirds of cases) are often described as diffuse, extensive, multilayered RH extending to ora serrata, although some cases may have milder RH in the posterior pole.
- Additionally, there are reports of diffuse, extensive RH with leukemia, fatal head crush injury, newborns, and fatal motor vehicle accidents.
- Hemorrhages associated with other systemic conditions and accidental head injury are usually few in number and confined to the posterior pole; subretinal hemorrhage is extremely rare is these circumstances and retinoschisis is not reported (although sub-ILM hemorrhage can be seen in leukemia).

DIFFERENTIAL DIAGNOSIS
- Inflicted AHT
- Accidental head trauma
- Neonatal birth trauma
- Hematologic malignancies
- Collagen vascular disease, vasculitis
- Coagulopathies
- Retinal hemangioma
- Prolonged cardiopulmonary resuscitation: Causing only mild RH in posterior pole
- AVM rupture: Case reports
- Galactosemia
- Glutaric aciduria type I
- Malaria
- Carbon monoxide poisoning
- Hyper/hyponatremia

ALERT
Extensive intraocular hemorrhage in young infants in the setting of acute brain injury, and in the absence of a history of severe accidental trauma or underlying medical cause, must be considered to be nonaccidental injury until otherwise proven.

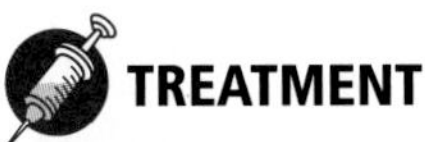

TREATMENT

MEDICATION
Treat underlying condition.

ADDITIONAL TREATMENT

General Measures
- Management of acute intraocular hemorrhage is primarily supportive.
- Gradual resolution is generally seen usually without significant retinal or visual sequelae.
- Report suspected child abuse to child protective services.

Issues for Referral
- Retinal surgery may be indicated for vitreous hemorrhage or macular retinoschisis:
  - Hematology referral if possible leukemia or coagulopathy
  - Infectious disease referral if there is any concern of infection

Additional Therapies
- With prolonged vitreous hemorrhage, intrafoveal hemorrhage, or hemorrhage in front of the fovea, young children have a risk of deprivational amblyopia. Patching the better eye may be needed to treat amblyopia after the hemorrhage resolves.
- In newborns vitamin K can correct clotting deficiency.
- Fresh frozen plasma, cryoprecipitate, packed RBC transfusion may be needed for a low platelet count or bleeding disorder.
- Laser therapy for diabetic retinopathy, retinopathy of prematurity may be given.

SURGERY/OTHER PROCEDURES
- Surgery is rarely indicated.
- Surgical intervention to remove blood within a traumatic schisis cavity is controversial and difficult.
- Young children: Significant nonresolving vitreous hemorrhage lowers threshold for early surgical treatment (vitrectomy).

IN-PATIENT CONSIDERATIONS
Hospitalization and management based on a causative agent or underlying disease.

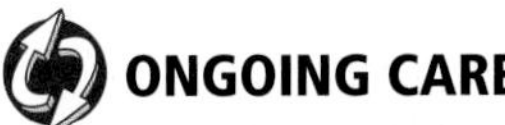

ONGOING CARE

FOLLOW-UP RECOMMENDATIONS
- Depends on severity and pathology of RH
- None needed for newborns
- Often follow-up in 1 month if RH not impacting vision
- Those with acute disease, retinoschisis, or foveal involvement may warrant more frequent monitoring

Patient Monitoring
Close monitoring and observation especially those with large/visually significant RH

PATIENT EDUCATION
Child safety counseling if accident

PROGNOSIS
- Resolution is generally seen without significant retinal or visual sequelae from the RH.
- Birth RH: Flame-shaped RH are typically resolved within 1 week and dot/blot RH usually within 1 month.
- Poor prognostic factors: Severity of intraocular hemorrhage, the presence of macular retinoschisis lesions, and the presence of pupillary abnormalities all predict worse outcome in abusive head injury.

COMPLICATIONS
- Perimacular folds
- Amblyopia and strabismus
- Retinal detachment
- Vision loss
- Neurologically devastated children who have suffered from AHT can have retinal scarring, optic atrophy, and cortical visual impairment.

ADDITIONAL READING

- Forbes BJ, Christian CW, Jukins AR, et al. Inflicted childhood neurotrauma (shaken baby syndrome). *J Pediatr Ophthalmol Strabismus* 2004;41(2):80–88.
- Levin AV. Retinal hemorrhages: Advances in understanding. *Pediatr Clin North Am* 2009;56(2):333–344.
- Kathi M. Review of Retinal Hemorrhages. Child Abuse Identification Toolkit for Professionals Online. 1999–2010, Cincinnati Children's Hospital Medical Center.

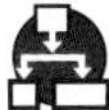

See Also (Topic, Algorithm, Electronic Media Element)

- See also Child Abuse Section, Leukemia, Coagulopathies, Retinal Detachment, Congenital retinopathies

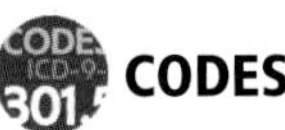

CODES

ICD9
- 361.10 Retinoschisis, unspecified
- 362.81 Retinal hemorrhage
- 995.55 Shaken baby syndrome

CLINICAL PEARLS
- RH in newborns typically resolve in 1 week from birth, and only in extremely rare cases can intraretinal RH can last more than 1 month.
- RH generally are present and regress, it is extremely uncommon to see the progression of RH.
- More widespread hemorrhage is more often seen in AHT, hematologic malignancies and can be seen with newborn delivery.
- Physicians must report reasonable suspicion of abuse to child protective services. Abuse need not be proven.

RETINAL MACROANEURYSM

Allen Chiang
Carl D. Regillo

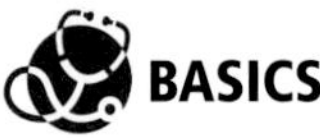

BASICS

DESCRIPTION
- Acquired retinal macroaneurysms are focal saccular or fusiform dilations of retinal arterioles within the first three orders of branching of the arteriolar system:
  - Typically located at arteriovenous crossings or arteriolar bifurcations
  - The superotemporal arteriole is the most commonly reported site of involvement (due to its proclivity for visual impairment).

EPIDEMIOLOGY
- Macroaneurysms may be bilateral in one-fifth of patients.
- Multiple macroaneurysms may be present in about 10% of patients.

RISK FACTORS
- Systemic hypertension (75%)
- Atherosclerotic cardiovascular disease
- Hyperlipidemia
- Age (most patients > 60 years)
- Sex (60–80% female)
- Retinal vein occlusions (12× higher prevalence of macroaneurysm in area drained by occluded vein)

GENERAL PREVENTION
Strict medical management of systemic hypertension

PATHOPHYSIOLOGY
- Inelasticity of retinal arterioles secondary to the effects of aging, hypertension, and atherosclerotic disease predisposes to dilatation and formation of a macroaneurysm, of which there are 2 classical types (2)[C].
  - Saccular (group 1): Characterized by acute decompensation with a variable degree of intraocular hemorrhage
  - Fusiform (group 2): Characterized by chronic exudation of plasma constituents

ETIOLOGY
See "Risk Factors."

COMMONLY ASSOCIATED CONDITIONS
See "Risk Factors."

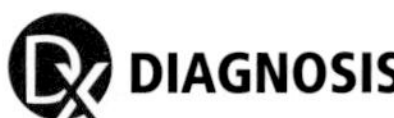

DIAGNOSIS

HISTORY
- Painless vision loss; onset may be acute or subacute depending on the type of macroaneurysm.
  - Macroaneurysms without any exudation or hemorrhage are asymptomatic and usually found incidentally.

PHYSICAL EXAM
- Macroaneurysm is evident on clinical ophthalmoscopic exam; pulsatile flow may be observed.
- Multiple macroaneurysms may be present on rare occasion.
- Serous retinal detachment, lipid exudation, and/or macular edema may be present.
- Hemorrhage may occur at various levels:
  - Subretinal and subretinal pigment epithelium
  - Intraretinal
  - Preretinal
  - Vitreous

DIAGNOSTIC TESTS & INTERPRETATION

Imaging
- Fluorescein angiography (FA):
  - Focal, uniform filling in the early arterial phase
  - Leakage of surrounding dilated capillaries
- Indocyanine green (ICG) angiography:
  - Useful for establishing the diagnosis in the setting of sub- or premacular hemorrhage; longer wavelength
- Optical coherence tomography:
  - May be useful in cases with chronic exudation to track changes

Diagnostic Procedures/Other
Check blood pressure

Pathological Findings
- Gross: Distention of the retinal arteriole
- Microscopic: Fibroglial proliferation, deposits of hemosiderin, lipoidal exudates, extravasated blood

DIFFERENTIAL DIAGNOSIS
- Retinal vascular abnormalities and diseases:
  - Diabetic retinopathy
  - Retinal capillary hemangioma
  - Retinal venous occlusive disease
  - Retinal telangiectasis
  - Retinal cavernous hemangioma
  - Hemorrhagic pigment epithelial detachment of age-related macular degeneration
  - Polypoidal choroidal vasculopathy

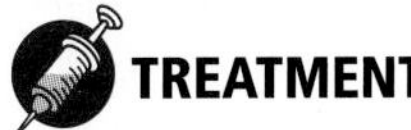

TREATMENT

Observation hemorrhage or in the absence of vision loss

SURGERY/OTHER PROCEDURES

- Laser photocoagulation (2–4)[B]:
  - For exudation that threatens or involves the fovea in the absence of hemorrhage that would preclude laser
  - Low intensity, longer duration argon green or yellow laser to microvascular changes surrounding the leaking aneurysm
  - Direct treatment of the aneurysm remains controversial (may in theory result in vitreous hemorrhage or branch retinal artery occlusion and distal ischemia).
- Pars plana vitrectomy:
  - To clear vitreous hemorrhage
  - For recent (<1 week) massive subfoveal hemorrhage, surgical evacuation with subretinal injection of tissue plasminogen activator has been described.

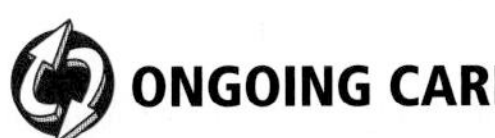

ONGOING CARE

FOLLOW-UP RECOMMENDATIONS

- Retina specialist
- Primary care physician for evaluation and management of associated systemic risk factors (See "Risk Factors")

PATIENT EDUCATION

Macroaneurysm: eMedicine Ophthalmology (http://emedicine.medscape.com/article/1224043-overview)

PROGNOSIS

- The visual prognosis may be variable (2)[B]:
  - Macular hemorrhage or chronic edema may result in decreased visual acuity.
  - Spontaneous thrombosis and involution may occur, leaving a vessel kink overlying a pseudodisciform plaque.
  - Artery may in some cases return to normal.

COMPLICATIONS

- Vision loss related to the following:
  - Macular scarring secondary to hemorrhage or chronic edema
  - Vitreous hemorrhage
  - Retinal detachment

REFERENCES

1. Panton RW, Goldberg MF, Farber MD. Retinal artery macroaneurysm: Risk factors and natural history. *Br J Ophthalmol* 1990;74(10):595–600.
2. Abdel-Khalek MN, Richardson J. Retinal macroaneurysm: Natural history and guidelines for treatment. *Br J Ophthalmol* 1986;70(1):2–11.
3. Brown DM, Sobol WM, Folk JC, et al. Retinal arteriolar macroaneurysms: Long term visual outcome. *Br J Ophthalmol* 1994;78:534–538.
4. Rabb MF, Gagliano DA, Teske MP. Retinal arterial macroaneurysms. *Surv Ophthal* 1988;33:73–96.

ADDITIONAL READING

- Tan CS, Au Eong KG. Surgical drainage of submacular hemorrhage from ruptured retinal arterial macroaneurysm. *Acta Ophthalmol Scand* 2005;83(2):240–241.

CODES

ICD9

- 362.13 Changes in vascular appearance of retina
- 362.15 Retinal telangiectasia
- 362.30 Retinal vascular occlusion, unspecified

CLINICAL PEARLS

- The superotemporal artery is the most commonly reported site of involvement.
- ICG angiography may be very helpful in establishing the diagnosis in the presence of significant hemorrhage.

R

RETINAL MICROANEURYSMS

Dan Montzka

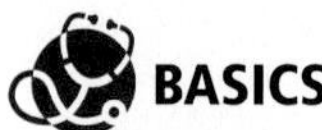

BASICS

DESCRIPTION

Retinal microaneurysms are focal dilations of retinal capillaries that appear as tiny red dots in the retina on ophthalmoscopy. They are most commonly found in the macula and posterior pole but may be found in the peripheral retina. They are an indicator of retinal microvascular disease. Microaneurysms may be an isolated finding but are typically found in association with other microvascular abnormalities such as cotton wool spots, retinal hemorrhages, alterations in vessel caliber, telangiectasias, lipid exudates, and retinal edema. The location and associated findings are important indicators of the underlying disorder.

EPIDEMIOLOGY

Incidence

- In diabetics diagnosed before age 30, the prevalence of retinopathy in persons who had diabetes for <5 years was 17% and it increased to 97.5% in persons who had diabetes for 15 or more years (1).
- In diabetics diagnosed after the age of 30, the prevalence of retinopathy in persons who had diabetes for <5 years was 28.8% and it increased to 77.8% in persons who had diabetes for 15 or more years (2).

Prevalence

In nondiabetics, the prevalence of retinopathy found to be 9.8% in persons over 49 years and was significantly related to the presence and severity of hypertension (3).

RISK FACTORS

- Diabetes
- Hypertension
- Abdominal obesity

PATHOPHYSIOLOGY

Damage to retinal capillary pericytes results in weakness and subsequent dilation and saccular outpouching of capillary walls. Microaneurysms are typically found in the inner nuclear layer (4). They may rupture resulting in retinal hemorrhage or leak leading to retinal edema.

ETIOLOGY

- Increased levels of blood glucose
- Retinal ischemia
- Chronic inflammation

COMMONLY ASSOCIATED CONDITIONS

- Diabetic retinopathy
- Hypertensive retinopathy
- Retinal vein occlusions:
  - Central retinal vein occlusion (CRVO)
  - Branch retinal vein occlusion (BRVO)

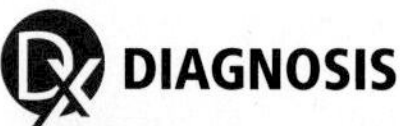

DIAGNOSIS

HISTORY

- Microaneurysms are often asymptomatic but may lead to central visual loss or metamorphopsia due to progressive macular edema from chronic leakage. More commonly, microaneurysms are found in association with other retinal vascular abnormalities such as hemorrhage, macular edema, or capillary nonperfusion that commonly cause visual symptoms.
- Microaneurysms may be the earliest detectable sign of diabetic retinopathy.
- In a chronic retinal vein occlusion, microaneurysms may be the only persistent finding once the retinal hemorrhages and edema have resolved.

PHYSICAL EXAM

On direct or indirect ophthalmoscopy, microaneurysms appear as pin-point red dots. It may be difficult to distinguish them from dot retinal hemorrhages without the help of retinal angiography. Typically, microaneurysms are found in the macula and posterior pole when associated with diabetic retinopathy or retinal vein occlusions. When found in the peripheral retina, less common diagnoses such as chronic lymphoma or sickle cell retinopathy should be considered. Red free filters can be used to enhance the visibility of microaneurysms relative to retinal pigmentary changes on ophthalmoscopy.

DIAGNOSTIC TESTS & INTERPRETATION

Lab

Initial lab tests

Evaluation for diabetes and hypertension. See "Differential diagnosis" for additional testing.

Follow-up & special considerations

Depends on the associated condition

Imaging

- Fundus photography (color and red free)
- Fluorescein angiography:
  - Very useful in differentiating microaneurysms from small dot retinal hemorrhages
  - Early phase of angiogram: Appears as hyperfluorescent dot
  - Late phase: Hyperfluorescent dot begins to fade, may find surrounding faint hyperfluorescence indicating leakage
- Optical coherence tomography (OCT)

DIFFERENTIAL DIAGNOSIS
- Diabetic retinopathy
- Retinal vein occlusions
- Hypertensive retinopathy
- Radiation retinopathy
- Idiopathic parafoveal telangiectasia
- HIV
- Sickle cell retinopathy
- Chronic hyperviscosity syndromes (e.g., chronic lymphoma)

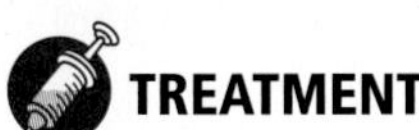

TREATMENT

MEDICATION

First Line
Control of underlying disorder such as diabetes or hypertension

Second Line
See treatment of commonly associated conditions.

ADDITIONAL TREATMENT

Issues for Referral
Refer for evaluation of risk factors or for specific treatment of associated conditions by the specialist.

SURGERY/OTHER PROCEDURES
Direct focal laser photocoagulation of microaneurysms when macular edema affects or threatens vision. Fluorescein angiography is often used to guide treatment. Caution must be exercised when treating juxtafoveal aneurysms since this may result in pericentral scotomas.

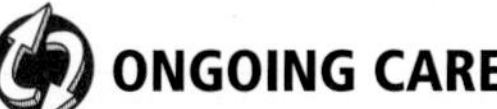

ONGOING CARE

FOLLOW-UP RECOMMENDATIONS
Depends on the underlying condition

Patient Monitoring
Self-testing using an Amsler grid blurred vision or metamorphopsia may be useful in following progression or response to treatment.

PATIENT EDUCATION
Depends on risk factors and associated condition

PROGNOSIS
Depends on the associated condition

COMPLICATIONS
See "Commonly associated conditions."
Microaneurysms may cause loss of vision resulting from leakage and macular edema.

REFERENCES

1. Klein R, Klein B, Moss SE, et al. The Wisconsin epidemiologic study when age at diagnosis is 30 years or more. *Arch Ophthalmol* 1984;102(4): 527–532.
2. Klein R, Klein B, Moss SE, et al. The Wisconsin epidemiologic study when age at diagnosis is less than 30 years. *Arch Ophthalmol* 1984;102(4): 520–526.
3. Yu T, Mitchell P, Berry G, et al. Retinopathy in older persons without diabetes and its relationship to hypertension. *Arch Ophthalmol* 1998;116:83–89.
4. Moore J, Bagley S, Ireland G, et al. Three dimensional analysis of microaneurysms in the human diabetic retina. *J Anat* 1999;194:89.

ADDITIONAL READING

- van Leiden HA, Dekker JM, Moll AC, et al. Risk factors for incident retinopathy in a diabetic and nondiabetic population. *Arch Ophthalmol* 2003;121:245–251.

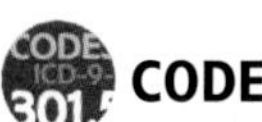

CODES

ICD9
- 362.14 Retinal microaneurysms nos
- 362.81 Retinal hemorrhage
- 362.83 Retinal edema

RETINAL VASCULAR TUMORS

Emil Anthony T. Say
Carol L. Shields

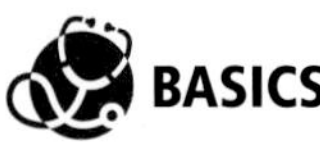

BASICS

DESCRIPTION

- Retinal vascular tumors are uncommon and diverse hamartomas or malformations of the neurosensory retina.
- They may have systemic associations involving the central nervous system (CNS) and other organs that may be life-threatening.
- They may be familial or sporadic.
- Types (and synonyms):
  - Retinal hemangioblastoma (RHB, capillary hemangioma, angiomatosis retinae)
  - Retinal cavernous hemangioma (RCH)
  - Retinal racemose hemangioma (RRH, congenital arteriovenous anastomoses, cirsoid aneurysm, arteriovenous aneurysms)
  - Retinal vasoproliferative tumor (VPT; see the chapter on this topic)

ALERT
Retinal vascular tumors are associated with both vision-threatening and life-threatening conditions.

Pediatric Considerations

Genetic testing and systemic work-up is advised for affected patients.

Pregnancy Considerations

Genetic counseling is recommended for affected pregnant women

EPIDEMIOLOGY

Incidence

- RHB: Incidence is unknown; however, its associated syndrome, von Hippel–Lindau's disease (VHL), occurs in 1 in 40,000 live births.
- In a report by Singh, Shields, and Shields, a solitary RHB in a young patient ($\leq$10 years) is associated with 45% risk for VHL compared to 0.5% when diagnosed in older patients (61–70 years) (see "Additional reading" below).
- RCH: Incidence of RCH is unknown.
- RRH: Incidence of RRH is unknown.

Prevalence

- RHB: Prevalence unknown
- RCH: Prevalence unknown
- RRH: Prevalence unknown
- No definite racial or gender predilections for any retinal vascular tumor

RISK FACTORS

None

Genetics

- RHB: Currently accepted mechanism follows Knudson's two-hit hypothesis affecting the VHL gene (chromosome 3p25–26)
- RCH: Two-hit mechanism in the cerebral cavernous malformation (CCM) gene on chromosome 7q11.2–q21
- RRH: No genetic mutation

GENERAL PREVENTION

None

PATHOPHYSIOLOGY

- RHB: VHL gene is a tumor suppressor gene that controls proliferation of blood vessels and mutation causes elevation of hypoxia inducible factor (HIF) and vascular endothelial growth factor (VEGF) with formation of hemangioblastomas in the brain and retina.
- RCH: Mutation in the CCM gene leads to loss or decreased expression of CCM protein and malformation of endothelial cells in utero.
- RRH: Characterized by congenital arteriovenous malformations (AVMs) without capillary interposition producing turbulent blood flow and dilation of blood vessels.

ETIOLOGY

- RHB: Sporadic or germline mutation in the VHL gene leads to formation of hemangioblastomas.
- RCH: Sporadic or germline mutation in the CCM gene leads to cavernous malformations.
- RRH: It is presumably caused by a local defect in maturation of retinal mesenchyme that gives rise to vascular tissue at the 7th week of gestation.

COMMONLY ASSOCIATED CONDITIONS

- RHB: VHL disease
  - Autosomal dominant inheritance
  - Associated with RHB (57%), cerebellar hemangioma (55%), spinal cord hemangioma (14%), renal cell carcinoma (24%), and pheochromocytoma (19%)
- RCH: Familial cavernous malformation (FCM)
  - Autosomal dominant inheritance
  - Cavernous malformations in the brain, skin, and retina (RCH)
- RRH: Congenital retinocephalic (CRC) vascular malformation syndrome (Wyburn–Mason or Bonnet–Dechaume–Blanc syndrome)
  - Unilateral, progressive, and nonhereditary
  - AVMs involving the skin, brain, and retina (RRH)

DIAGNOSIS

HISTORY

- RHB: Asymptomatic early but may cause severe pain and blindness from neovascular glaucoma when advanced
- RCH: Mostly asymptomatic and are detected only during routine examination
- RRH: Presents as a unilateral blind eye in 48% when associated with CRC but are mostly asymptomatic when isolated
- Family history is extremely important, especially in cases of RHB and RCH, to rule out familial disease or germline mutation.

PHYSICAL EXAM

- Retinal hemangioblastoma (RHB):
  - Orange-red circumscribed retinal lesion typically with dilated feeder vessels
  - Peripheral (85%) or juxtapapillary (15%)
  - May be associated with localized or remote retinal exudation, retinal detachment, glial proliferation with traction detachment, macular pucker, twin vessels, or neovascular glaucoma
- Retinal cavernous hemangioma (RCH)
  - Dark-red, grapelike, saccular aneurysms
  - May occur in the retina or optic disc
  - May be associated with overlying fibrosis with macular traction, vitreous hemorrhage, and vascular occlusion
  - Not associated with leakage and exudation
- Retinal racemose hemangioma (RRH)
  - Dilated arteriovenous communications without capillary interposition
  - Extensive retinal involvement in cases with systemic associations and localized or sectorial involvement when isolated
  - Rarely located in the macula
  - May be associated with neovascular glaucoma, vitreous hemorrhage, vascular occlusion, and conjunctival injection
  - Not associated with leakage and exudation
  - Pulsating exophthalmos or visual field defects when AVMs are present in the orbit or visual pathway, respectively

DIAGNOSTIC TESTS & INTERPRETATION

Lab

Initial lab tests

Genetic testing to rule out systemic disease

Follow-up & special considerations

- Genetic counseling is recommended when germline mutations are found.
- Patients with systemic associations should be promptly referred to a pediatric oncologist, oncologist, neurologist, or neurosurgeon.

Imaging

Initial approach

- Fluorescein angiography (FA) is most helpful:
  - RHB (peripheral): Rapid filling of dilated feeder arteriole in arterial phase, intrinsic fine capillaries, with prominent draining vein and leakage on later films
  - RHB (juxtapapillary): Diagnosis is established by the fine vascular pattern visualized on the angiogram
  - RCH: Slow filling of the aneurysms with hyperfluorescent caps superiorly and hypofluorescence inferiorly due to settling of red blood cells under the supernatant plasma, typically without leakage of dye
  - RRH: Rapid filling of high-flow retinal AVMs with adjacent capillary dropout

Follow-up & special considerations

- Asymptomatic patients with exudates or retinal detachment threatening vision should be followed closely and offered treatment.
- Early treatment is needed for symptomatic patients.
- Frequency of follow-up is determined by severity of the condition and degree of visual impairment.

Diagnostic Procedures/Other
- MRI, MRA, CTA, or angiography may be required to rule out associated systemic disease.

Pathological Findings
- RHB: Composed of capillary-sized blood vessels with normal endothelium, vacuolated stromal cells, and gliosis (1)
- RCH: Dilated, thin-walled blood vessels, with interconnections and an intact endothelium (1)
- RRH: Dilated retinal vessels sometimes occupying the entire retinal thickness causing cystic degeneration and attenuation of the adjacent retinal tissue (1)

DIFFERENTIAL DIAGNOSIS
- Choroidal melanoma
- Choroidal granuloma
- Circumscribed choroidal hemangioma
- Retinal macroaneurysm
- Retinoblastoma
- Coats' disease

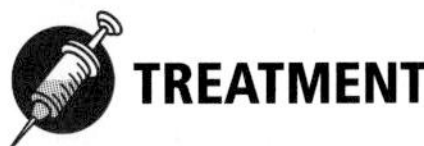

TREATMENT

MEDICATION
See "General measures" below.

ADDITIONAL TREATMENT
General Measures
- Retinal hemangioblastoma (RHB):
  - May be observed if small or juxtapapillary, if it is not visually threatening, or if the patient is asymptomatic (2)[C]
  - Laser photocoagulation or photodynamic therapy preferred for posterior RHB and cryotherapy when more anterior (2)[C]
  - Plaque radiotherapy reserved for more advanced RHB (2)[C]
- Retinal cavernous hemangioma (RCH):
  - Mostly nonprogressive and do not require treatment (1,4,5)[C]
- Retinal racemose hemangioma (RRH):
  - Mostly nonprogressive and do not require treatment (1,6)[C]

Issues for Referral
- Treatment should usually be performed by a retina specialist or an ocular oncologist.
- Patients with positive genetic analyses or imaging tests should be promptly referred to a neurologist, neurosurgeon, or pediatric oncologist.

Additional Therapies
- Retinal surgery is required for persistent vitreous hemorrhage or retinal detachment (1)[C].
- Enucleation may be needed for blind and painful eyes with no potential for vision (1)[C].
- Associated hemorrhage, vascular occlusion, or neovascularization requires appropriate treatment with laser, cryopexy, or retinal surgery (1,4–6)[C].

COMPLEMENTARY & ALTERNATIVE THERAPIES
- RHB: Transpupillary thermotherapy, external or proton beam radiotherapy, and local or systemic anti-VEGF therapy have been used for RHB, but efficacy is inconclusive and role is still uncertain (1–3)[C].
- RCH: There is no proven treatment (1)[C].
- RRH: There is no proven treatment (1)[C].

SURGERY/OTHER PROCEDURES
- RHB: Resection and ligature of feeder vessels has been reported but is technically difficult (2)[C]
- RCH: No surgical reports
- RRH: No surgical reports

IN-PATIENT CONSIDERATIONS
Outpatient management

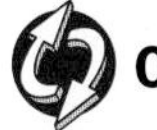

ONGOING CARE

FOLLOW-UP RECOMMENDATIONS
- Outpatient care for photocoagulation, photodynamic therapy, or cryotherapy
- In-patient or outpatient for plaque radiotherapy, vitrectomy, or enucleation

Patient Monitoring
- 6-month follow-ups are recommended for most patients.
- Follow more closely when vision is threatened.

DIET
No restrictions

PATIENT EDUCATION
- Advice regarding implications of genetic analysis and systemic associations
- Genetic counseling is essential
- Use of the Amsler grid for self-monitoring of visual changes for early diagnosis and treatment

PROGNOSIS
- Retinal hemangioblastoma (RHB):
  - 40% of affected eyes have vision $<$20/200.
  - Worse when tumors are larger ($>$ 4 mm), juxtapapillary, or multiple.
  - Enucleation may be required in 6% of eyes.
- Retinal cavernous hemangioma (RCH):
  - Most patients maintain good vision.
  - Progressive growth is rare.
- Retinal racemose hemangioma (RRH):
  - NLP in 48% if cerebral AVMs are present
  - Vision $\geq$20/50 in 56% in isolated cases

COMPLICATIONS
Loss of vision or globe, and even death when systemic associations are not detected.

REFERENCES

1. Heimann H, Damato B. Congenital vascular malformations of the retina and choroid. *Eye* 2010;24:459–467.
2. Singh AD, Shields CL, Shields JA. Von Hippel–Lindau disease. *Surv Ophthalmol* 2001;46: 117–142.
3. Wong WT, Chew EY. Ocular von Hippel–Lindau disease: Clinical update and emerging treatments. *Curr Opin Ophthalmol* 2008;19:213–217.
4. Messmer E, Laqua H, Wessing A, et al. Nine cases of cavernous hemangioma of the retina. *Am J Ophthalmol* 1983;95:383–390.
5. Gass JDM. Cavernous hemangioma of the retina. *Am J Ophthalmol* 1971;71:799–814.
6. Schmidt D, Pache M, Schumacher M. The congenital unilateral retinocephalic vascular malformation syndrome (Bonnet–Dechaume–Blanc syndrome or Wyburn–Mason syndrome): Review of the literature. *Surv Ophthalmol* 2008;53:227–249.

ADDITIONAL READING

- Singh AD, Shields JA, Shields CL. Solitary retinal capillary hemangioma. Hereditary (von Hippel–Lindau disease) or nonhereditary? *Arch Ophthalmol* 2001;119:232–234.

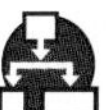

See Also (Topic, Algorithm, Electronic Media Element)
- www.fighteyecancer.com
- www.eyecancerinfo.com
- www.eyecancerbook.com
- www.etrf.org
- www.genetests.org
- www.ncbi.nlm.nih.gov/omim

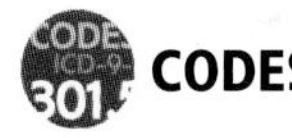

CODES

ICD9
- 228.03 Hemangioma of retina
- 743.58 Vascular anomalies, congenital
- 757.32 Vascular hamartomas

CLINICAL PEARLS
- Retinal vascular tumors have associated life-threatening systemic conditions that require proper imaging tests and genetic analysis.
- RHB often have dilated feeding arterioles and draining veins, with remote macular edema.
- RCH are grape-like aneurysms that are often nonprogressive and do not require treatment.
- RRH are dilated AVMs of the retina and occasionally involve the orbit and visual pathway.

RETINAL VASOPROLIFERATIVE TUMOR

Emil Anthony T. Say
Carol L. Shields

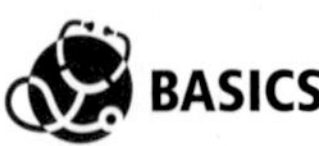

BASICS

DESCRIPTION

- Vasoproliferative tumors of the retina (VPT) are benign vascular lesions located in the sensory retina.
- They are nonfamilial.
- In a series of 103 patients, Shields and associates reported that the patients were classified as follows (2):
  - Primary or idiopathic (74%)
  - Secondary (26%)
- In the same series, they may also be subclassified as follows:
  - Solitary (78%)
  - Multiple (15%)
  - Diffuse (7%)
- Other synonyms for VPT are as follows:
  - Presumed acquired retinal hemangioma
  - Angiomatous mass
  - Peripheral retinal telangiectasia
  - Angioma/hemangioma-like mass
  - Reactionary retinal glioangiosis

ALERT
Retinal vasoproliferative tumor can produce extensive retinal exudation and lead to blindness.

EPIDEMIOLOGY

- Predominantly affects older patients (mean age = 40 years)
- No gender or racial predilection

Incidence

- Represent 1% of all pseudomelanomas
- True incidence is unknown

Prevalence

Unknown

RISK FACTORS

Unknown

Genetics

No definite genetic association

PATHOPHYSIOLOGY

- Precise pathogenesis is presently unclear.
- Current hypothesis is reactive pigment epithelial and vascular proliferation or reactive gliosis secondary to a variety of underlying disease processes.

ETIOLOGY

- Primary cases are idiopathic.
- Secondary cases are associated with the following:
  - Intermediate uveitis (28%)
  - Retinitis pigmentosa (21%)
  - Toxoplasmic retinitis (7%)
  - Toxocariasis (7%)
  - Retinochoroidal coloboma (7%)
  - Traumatic chorioretinopathy (7%)

COMMONLY ASSOCIATED CONDITIONS

- Systemic hypertension (14%)
- Hypercholesterolemia (6%)
- Neurofibromatosis (2%)

DIAGNOSIS

HISTORY

- Blurred vision and/or floaters are common presenting symptoms.
- Photopsias and visual field defects are other possible initial symptoms.
- The disease may be asymptomatic (19%).

PHYSICAL EXAM

- Visual acuity and laterality:
  - Better than 20/40 in up to 50%
  - Most cases are unilateral
  - Can be bilateral in 40% of secondary cases
- Appearance:
  - Yellowish to yellow-red in color
  - Mostly solitary and small (<5 mm)
  - Non- or mildly dilated, nontortuous feeding artery and vein
- Location:
  - Mostly inferotemporal
  - Located between equator and ora serrata
- Associated slit lamp findings:
  - Elevated intraocular pressure
  - Anterior vitreous cells
  - Posterior synechiae
  - Cataract
- Associated vitreoretinal findings:
  - Intraretinal/subretinal exudation
  - Intraretinal/subretinal blood
  - Vitreous hemorrhage
  - Retinal pigment epithelial proliferation
  - Preretinal fibrosis
  - Macular edema
  - Epiretinal membrane
  - Exudative retinal detachment

DIAGNOSTIC TESTS & INTERPRETATION

Lab

Initial lab tests

- Genetic testing is generally not indicated unless von Hippel–Lindau (VHL) disease is considered.
- Toxoplasma titers (Ig G and Ig M)
- Toxocara titers (Ig G and Ig M)
- Systemic work-up to rule out other causes of uveitis
- Lipid profile (cholesterol, HDL, LDL, triglycerides)

Follow-up & special considerations

Positive genetic testing results for VHL should prompt systemic evaluation for associated CNS or kidney disease.

Imaging

Initial approach

- Patients with associated retinitis pigmentosa need additional visual field testing and electroretinogram (ERG).
- Fluorescein angiography:
  - Rapid early filling, fine intrinsic capillary network, and late leakage
- Ultrasonography:
  - Difficult due to peripheral location
  - Medium to high internal reflectivity
  - Acoustic solidity without choroidal excavation
- Indocyanine green angiography:
  - intratumoral vascularization and late diffuse hyperfluorescence

Follow-up & special considerations

- Asymptomatic patients with exudates or retinal detachment threatening vision should be followed closely and offered treatment.
- Early treatment is needed for symptomatic patients.
- Frequency of follow-up is determined by severity of the condition and degree of visual impairment.

Diagnostic Procedures/Other

Systemic evaluation and genetic testing for VHL disease can be performed when diagnosis is in doubt.

Pathological Findings

Irvine and co-workers reported on the histopathological findings of patients who underwent an excisional biopsy of VPT lesions describing the presence of benign glial cell proliferation and secondary vasoproliferation, with perivascular lymphocytes, and adjacent fibrinous, lipid, and serous exudate (6).

DIFFERENTIAL DIAGNOSIS
- Retinal hemangioblastoma (RHB)
- Choroidal melanoma
- Peripheral exudative hemorrhagic chorioretinopathy (PEHCR)
- Retinal cavernous hemangioma (RCH)
- Choroidal granuloma

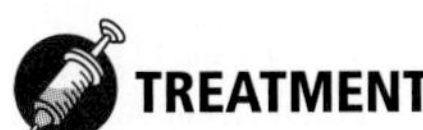

TREATMENT

MEDICATION
See "General measures" below.

ADDITIONAL TREATMENT
General Measures
- Asymptomatic patients are observed (1,2)[C].
- Symptomatic patients with macular edema, retinal detachment, or exudation threatening vision are generally treated.
- Cryotherapy is preferred since most are peripherally located (1,2)[C].
- Laser photocoagulation or photodynamic therapy can be considered when posterior in location (1,2)[C].
- Plaque radiotherapy can be used for advanced cases and large tumors measuring more than 2.5 mm in thickness, as reported by Cohen and colleagues (3)[C].
- The role of antivascular endothelial growth factors is not known, but this class of medications is often used.
- Intravitreal or subtenon's triamcinolone is used to reduce macular edema.

Issues for Referral
Treatment is usually performed by a retina specialist or an ocular oncologist.

Additional Therapies
- Retinal detachment surgery for more extensive involvement (1,2)[C]
- Enucleation for blind painful eyes from neovascular glaucoma (2)[C]

COMPLEMENTARY & ALTERNATIVE THERAPIES
- Photodynamic therapy and transpupillary thermotherapy are recent modalities shown to be beneficial for some patients (4,5)[C].
- Adjunctive intravitreal bevacizumab (Avastin) injection is used in certain cases to reduce exudation and leakage (3)[C].
- Intravitreal or subtenon's triamcinolone has also been used in association with cryotherapy in cases with concomitant macular edema.

SURGERY/OTHER PROCEDURES
Local resection may be performed in selected cases, although technically difficult to perform [C].

IN-PATIENT CONSIDERATIONS
Outpatient management

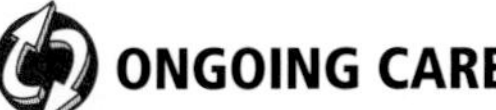

ONGOING CARE

FOLLOW-UP RECOMMENDATIONS
- Outpatient care for photocoagulation, photodynamic therapy, or cryotherapy
- In-patient or outpatient for plaque radiotherapy, vitrectomy, or enucleation

Patient Monitoring
- 6-month follow-ups are recommended for most patients.
- Follow more closely with lesions threatening vision.

DIET
No restrictions

PATIENT EDUCATION
- Advice control of blood pressure and cholesterol for primary cases
- Individualized patient education for secondary cases based on cause
- Use of the Amsler grid for self-monitoring of visual changes for early diagnosis and treatment

PROGNOSIS
Good, patients maintain functional vision in majority of cases.

COMPLICATIONS
Loss of vision or globe

REFERENCES

1. Shields JA, Decker WL, Sanborn GE, et al. Presumed acquired retinal hemangiomas. *Ophthalmology* 1983;90:1292–1300.
2. Shields CL, Shields JA, Barrett J, et al. Vasoproliferative tumors of the ocular fundus. Classification and manifestations in 103 patients. *Arch Ophthalmol* 1995;113:615–623.
3. Cohen VML, Shields CL, Demirci H, et al. Iodiine I 125 plaque radiotherapy for vasoproliferative tumors of the retina in 30 eyes. *Arch Ophthalmol* 2008;126(9):1245–1251.
4. Blasi MA, Scupola A, Tiberti AC, et al. Photodynamic therapy for vasoproliferative retinal tumors. *Retina* 2006;26:404–409.
5. Nomura Y, Tamaki Y, Tsuji H, et al. Transpupillary thermotherapy for vasoproliferative retinal tumor. *Retinal Cases and Brief Reports* 2009;3:358–360.
6. Irvine F, O'Donnell N, Kemp E, et al. Retinal vasoproliferative tumors. Surgical management and histological findings. *Arch Ophthalmol* 2000;118:563–569.

ADDITIONAL READING

- Barbezetto IA, Smith RT. Vasoproliferative tumor of the retina treated with PDT. *Retina* 2003;23(4):565–567.
- Heimann H, Bornfeld N, Vij O, et al. Vasoproliferative tumours of the retina. *Br J Ophthalmol* 2000;84(10):1162–1169.

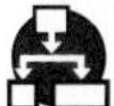

See Also (Topic, Algorithm, Electronic Media Element)
- www.fighteyecancer.com
- www.malignantmelanomainfo.com
- www.retinoblastomainfo.com
- www.eyecancerinfo.com
- www.eyecancerbook.com
- www.etrf.org

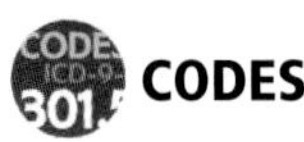

CODES

ICD9
- 362.13 Changes in vascular appearance of retina
- 362.15 Retinal telangiectasia

CLINICAL PEARLS
- Yellow to yellow-red mass of the retina associated with non- to minimally dilated feeding retinal artery and vein
- Mostly small, solitary, and located inferotemporally
- Nonfamilial and idiopathic in majority of cases
- Most patients do not need treatment.

RETINAL/CHOROIDAL COLOBOMA

Raza M. Shah

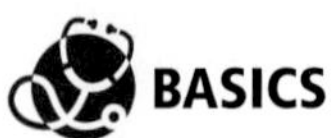

BASICS

DESCRIPTION

Developmental defect is caused by defective closure of the embryonal fissure. Its effect on vision varies depending on the size and location of the defect (1)[B].

Pediatric Considerations

In children, colobomas are associated with other significant comorbid conditions. Specifically, 80–90% of children diagnosed with CHARGE (acronym for a group of developmental abnormalities) have a coloboma.

Pregnancy Considerations

Pregnant mothers with a coloboma have a slightly increased risk of having children with a coloboma, but the condition has not proven to be fatal.

EPIDEMIOLOGY

Incidence

Rare condition occurring in only 0.14% of the general population

Prevalence

Estimated prevalence of coloboma (all types) is 1 per 10,000. More specific epidemiology for choroidal coloboma is not currently available (2)[B].

RISK FACTORS

Risk factors for colobomas include consanguineous parents, positive family history, vitamin A deficiency, and second-born child.

Genetics

- Can be associated with mutations in the PAX-2 gene as part of the renal-coloboma syndrome (3)[B].
- An irregular autosomal dominant inheritance pattern is found in many of these patients.

PATHOPHYSIOLOGY

A typically bilateral birth defect resulting from failed closure of the embryonic optic fissure/cup, during the 6th week of gestation

ETIOLOGY

Unknown. It is postulated that a genetic predisposition is the underlying cause.

COMMONLY ASSOCIATED CONDITIONS

- Iris coloboma
- Retinal detachment
- Microphthalmos
- Microcornea
- Cataract
- Lens coloboma
- Optic pit
- Various systemic birth defects:
  - It is often found in several congenital syndromes, including CHARGE syndrome (Goldenhar, Schmid–Fraccaro, Joubert, Mohr-Clausen, and Aicardi syndromes).

DIAGNOSIS

HISTORY

- The effects on vision differ depending on the size and location of the coloboma.
- Is there a change in vision?
- Does the patient notice visual field loss?
- If the vision loss or peripheral field loss is recent, there may be a recent retinal detachment.
- Are other family members affected?
- Is there any history of renal, genitourinary, growth, palate, or hearing difficulties?

PHYSICAL EXAM

- As there may be malformations in other parts of the body (CHARGE syndrome), patients should be checked for coloboma of the eye, heart defects, atresia of the nasal choanae, retardation of growth, genitourinary abnormalities, and ear abnormalities.
- Findings on funduscopic exam may range from very mild, small white lesions on the inferior optic disc to a large defect, which extends from the optic disc to the anterior segment.
- Rarely, a normal portion of the fundus is located between the defects ("bridge" coloboma).
- Patients may have a coexisting iris coloboma (which is what prompted the initial visit to the ophthalmologist).

DIAGNOSTIC TESTS & INTERPRETATION

Lab

None is generally necessary as it is a clinical diagnosis.

Imaging

- Funduscopic and complete physical examination typically elicits the features of choroidal coloboma.
- B-scan ultrasonography and/or CT scan (none usually needed) can be used to show a small, disorganized globe (microphthalmia) with a retroocular cyst that is connected to the vitreous humor inferiorly.
- Neuroimaging can be used to elicit midline developmental defects.
- Optical coherence tomography can demonstrate the transition from normal retina to intercalary membrane and subretinal fluid (4)[C].

Pathological Findings
- The choroidal coloboma shows an absence or atrophy of choroid and an absence of retinal pigment epithelium (RPE) with atrophic and gliotic retina:
  - The RPE tends to be hyperplastic at the edge of the defect.
  - The sclera in the region is usually thinned and may be cystic; the cystic space is often filled with proliferated glial tissue.

DIFFERENTIAL DIAGNOSIS
- Trauma
- Chorioretinal scar
- Toxoplasmosis
- Aicardi's syndrome
- Goldenhar syndrome
- Staphyloma
- North carolina macular dystrophy

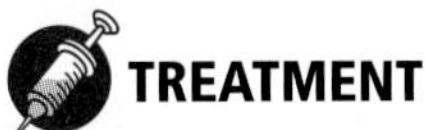

TREATMENT

ADDITIONAL TREATMENT
General Measures
- Consider systemic evaluation for chromosomal abnormality
- Treatment of refractive error and amblyopia, if present
- Low Vision (vision rehabilitation) services, if indicated

SURGERY/OTHER PROCEDURES
If a patient develops a rhegmatogenous retinal detachment, vitrectomy with laser and intraocular gas or silicone oil tamponade is indicated.

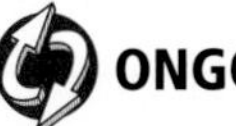

ONGOING CARE

FOLLOW-UP RECOMMENDATIONS
Patients will need periodic follow-up with a retina specialist and/or pediatric ophthalmologist.

PROGNOSIS
- Foveal involvement is an important predictor of visual acuity.
- Even patients with very large colobomas may have good vision is the macular architecture is normal.

COMPLICATIONS
- Amblyopia
- Refractive error
- Choroidal neovascularization
- Retinal detachment (later in life)

REFERENCES

1. Schubert H. Structural organization of choroidal colobomas of young and adult patients and mechanism of retinal detachment. *Trans Am Ophthalmol Soc* 2005;103:457–472.
2. Schubert HD. Choroidal coloboma. *Ophthalmology* 2007;114(12):2369.
3. Eccles MR, Schimmenti LA. Renal-coloboma syndrome: A multi-system developmental disorder caused by PAX2 mutations. *Clin Genet* 1999;56:1–9.
4. Gopal L. A clinical and optical coherence tomography study of choroidal colobomas. *Curr Opin Ophthalmol* 2008;19:249–254.

ADDITIONAL READING

- Daufenbach D, Ruttum M, Pulido J, et al. Chorioretinal colobomas in a pediatric population. *Ophthalmology* 1998;105:1455–1458.
- Yanoff Y, Sassani J. *Congenital and developmental defects of the pigment epithelium. Ocular pathology.* In: Myron Yanoff, ed. China: Mosby Elsevier, 2009.

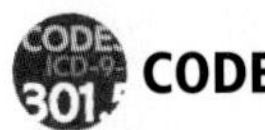

CODES

ICD9
743.52 Fundus coloboma

CLINICAL PEARLS
- Patients may have other concomitant syndromes.
- The colobomas may be very small and involve only a portion of the optic disc, or may involve most of the retina.
- The sclera is generally visible through the defect.

RETINITIS PIGMENTOSA

M. Rasouli
Sunir J. Garg

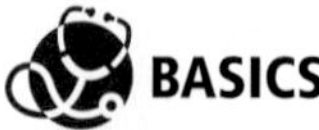

BASICS

DESCRIPTION

- Group of hereditary, progressive retinal diseases that result in the degeneration of rod (mainly) and cone photoreceptors; the degeneration starts in the mid-periphery and advances toward the macula.
- Significant phenotypic and genotypic diversity

EPIDEMIOLOGY

Incidence

- N/A

Prevalence

- 1 in 3,000—5,000 persons

RISK FACTORS

- None

Genetics

- 60% of affected people have associated genetic mutations
- Inherited forms could be autosomal dominant (30–40%), autosomal recessive (50–60%), or X-linked (5–15%).
- Even with the same genotype, patients can present with different manifestations.
- In non-syndromic retinitis pigmentosa (RP), more than 45 genes/loci have been isolated
- Most common genes (30% of RP cases):
  - Rhodopsin gene (RHO): 25% of autosomal dominant RP
  - USH2A gene: 20% of recessive disease
  - RPGR gene: 70% of X-linked RP

GENERAL PREVENTION

- Controversial: Use of dark glasses to slow progression of retinal damage.

PATHOPHYSIOLOGY

- Primary degeneration of rod photoreceptors, and secondary degeneration of cone photoreceptors.
- The exact mechanism has not been established.

ETIOLOGY

- Genetic inheritance in 60%

COMMONLY ASSOCIATED CONDITIONS

- 20–35% of cases are associated with non-ocular disease (about 30 syndromes)
- Usher's Syndrome (10–20% of RP cases): Congenital or early deafness followed by RP in teenage years
- Bardet-Biedel syndrome (5% of RP cases): RP, obesity present in childhood, renal failure, hypogonadism, polydactyly, mental retardation, or mild psychomotor delay.

DIAGNOSIS

HISTORY

- Variable; some have symptoms starting in childhood, while others have symptom onset during young adulthood.
- Nyctalopia (night blindness) is the most common symptom and presents earlier in autosomal recessive form; median age of onset 24 years.
- Constricted mid-peripheral visual fields in early adulthood, which leads to tunnel vision in advanced cases.
- Although many patients have good central acuity for decades, a number eventually develop significant vision loss.
- Photophobia, especially in diffuse light (e.g., overcast days) – difficulty with reading, due to the narrow window between too much and insufficient light.
- Photopsia (35%) – late sign

PHYSICAL EXAM

- Anterior segment
  - Posterior subcapsular cataract (50%)
- Posterior segment
  - Waxy pallor of the optic nerve head
  - Attenuated retinal vessels
  - Retinal hypo- and hyper-granularity
  - Bone spicule formation around intraretinal vessels (mid to far periphery)
  - Cystoid macular edema
  - Optic nerve head drusen (10%)
  - Vitreous cells
- Sectoral RP: Variant of RP; only 1 or 2 quadrants are affected
- Color vision testing can be normal, or show blue cone dysfunction in advanced RP (acquired tritanopia)
- Decreased contrast sensitivity (Pelli-Robson chart)

DIAGNOSTIC TESTS & INTERPRETATION

Lab

Initial lab tests

- Genetic tests, if available

Follow-up & special considerations

- N/A

Imaging

Initial approach

- Optical coherence tomography (OCT) is useful to measure retina thickness, assess the photoreceptor layer, and to assess the presence and degree of cystoid macular edema.

Follow-up & special considerations

- OCT imaging in subsequent follow-ups.

Diagnostic Procedures/Other

- Electroretinogram (ERG) is critical to confirm the diagnosis and assess degree of visual impairment: Diminuted a- and b-wave amplitude and delayed timing during scotopic and photopic conditions are seen even in early stages.
- Visual field tesing initially shows patchy loss of peripheral vision; progresses to mid-peripheral field loss; in advanced cases, only far peripheral and central island of vision remains ("tunnel vision"). Goldmann (kinetic) perimetry is more useful to assess peripheral vision changes.

Pathological Findings

- Rod and cone degeneration
- Bone spicule pattern is due to hyperplasia and migration of RPE cells into the neurosensory retina in response to photoreceptor cell loss.
- Waxy pallor of the nerve: Indicates axonal loss and overlying gliosis

DIFFERENTIAL DIAGNOSIS

- Leber congenital amaurosis – when visual loss is present from birth or first 5 years of life.
- Cancer/melanoma associated retinopathy
- Congenital stationary night blindness
- Fundus albipunctatus
- Vitamin A deficiency
- Congenital infections: Rubella, syphilis
- X-linked disorders: Choroideremia, ocular albinism
- Mitochondrial disease: Kearns-Sayre syndrome
- Gyrate atrophy
- Retinoschisis
- Hereditary vitreoretinopathies: Familial exudative vitreoretinopathy, Wagner disease, Stickler syndrome
- Inflammatory disorders: Birdshot choroidoretinopathy, serpiginous retinopathy, multifocal placoid pigment epitheliopathy, sarcoidosis
- Maculopathies: Stargardt disease, Cone dystrophies, Sorsby disease

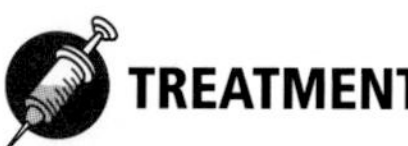

TREATMENT

MEDICATION

First Line

- Vitamin A Palmitate 15,000 units daily
- Omega 3 fatty acids (1400 mg daily)
- Lutein 12 mg daily

ALERT

- If prescribing high dose Vitamin A, need to monitor serum levels for retinol, triglyceridemia, and liver enzymes.

Second Line
- Macular edema and subsequently visual acuity may improve with 3–4 months of chronic topical or oral carbonic anhydrase inhibitors.

ADDITIONAL TREATMENT
General Measures
- Family surveys are recommended
- Genetic counseling

Issues for Referral
- Referral to low vision rehabilitation clinics
- Referral to institutions that introduce coping strategies with loss of vision and help patients obtain new professional skills

Additional Therapies
- Currently various modes of therapy are being explored including: Gene therapy, stem cell transplantation, implanted retinal electrical devices

COMPLEMENTARY & ALTERNATIVE THERAPIES
- Yellow–orange spectacles could help minimize photophobia

SURGERY/OTHER PROCEDURES
- Phacoemulsification and intraocular lens implantation for cataract

IN-PATIENT CONSIDERATIONS
Initial Stabilization
- N/A

Admission Criteria
- N/A

IV Fluids
- N/A

Nursing
- N/A

Discharge Criteria
- N/A

ONGOING CARE

FOLLOW-UP RECOMMENDATIONS
- Regular 6–12 month follow-up examinations

Patient Monitoring
- Follow disease progression by regular evaluation of visual acuity, visual fields, and ERG

DIET
- Foods high in omega 3 fatty acids and dark green leafy vegetables.
- Avoid high dose Vitamin E supplements (400 IU/day)

PATIENT EDUCATION
- Genetic testing is important to determine prognosis and to understand risk to offspring
- Patients should be reassured that most activities of daily living can be performed even with only 50 degrees of central vision and low ERG amplitudes
- Controversy regarding antenatal diagnosis – could be performed in families with severe or early-onset RP.
- Significant role of psycho-social counseling in various stages of the disease and corresponding loss of function.

PROGNOSIS
- The condition is progressive; 2.6–13.5% loss of visual field and 8.7–18.5% loss of ERG amplitude per year
- Prognosis for visual acuity is quite variable; some retain good central visual acuity with advanced RP, while others have early loss of acuity.
- The genetic cause is usually a good predictor of severity – X-linked RP is more severe in early stages of disease.
- In cases of complete central vision loss, most patients retain light perception from peripheral visual field.

COMPLICATIONS
- Macular edema and subsequently visual acuity may improve with 3–4 months of chronic topical or oral carbonic anhydrase inhibitors.
- Inflammation is often mild and does not require treatment.

ADDITIONAL READING

- Hartong DT, Berson E, Dryja TP. Retinitis pigmentosa. *Lancet* 2006;368:1795—1809.
- Hamel C. Retinitis pigmentosa.*Orphanet J Rare Dis*. 2006;1:40.
- Bhatti, MT. Retinitis pigmentosa, pigmentary retinopathies, and neurologic diseases. *Curre Neuroly Neurosci Rep*. 2006;6:403–413.
- Daiger SP, Bowne SJ, Sullivan LS. Perspective on genes and mutations causing retinitis pigmentosa. *Arch Ophthalmol*. 2007;125:151–158.
- Berson EL, Rosner B, Sandberg MA, et al. A randomized trial of vitamin A and vitamin E supplementation for retinitis pigmentosa. *Arch Ophthalmol*. 1993;111(6):761–772.
- Berson EL, Rosner B, Sandberg MA, et al. Further evaluation of docosahexaenoic acid in patients with retinitis pigmentosa receiving vitamin A treatment: Subgroup analyses. *Arch Ophthalmol* 2004;122(9): 1306–1314.
- Berson EL, Rosner B, Sandberg MA, et al. Clinical trial of lutein in patients with retinitis pigmentosa receiving vitamin A. *Arch Ophthalmol*. 2010; 128(4):403–411.
- Genead MA, Fishman GA. Efficacy of sustained topical dorzolamide therapy for cystic macular lesions in patients with retinitis pigmentosa and usher syndrome. *Arch Ophthalmol*. 2010;128(9): 1146–1150.

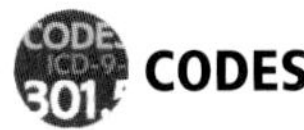

CODES

ICD9
362.74 Pigmentary retinal dystrophy

CLINICAL PEARLS
- RP is a genetically diverse group of diseases that manifest differently in different patients.
- Vitamin supplementation can prolong useful vision in these patients by decades.
- Earlier vision rehabilitation programs should be considered.

RETINOPATHY OF PREMATURITY

Eugene Milder
Richard Kaiser

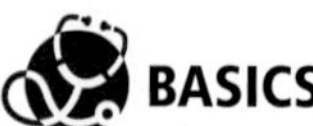

BASICS

DESCRIPTION

Retinopathy of prematurity (ROP) is a potentially blinding proliferative vascular retinopathy which is associated with prematurity and low birth weight and can cause lifelong ocular morbidity.

EPIDEMIOLOGY

Incidence

1,300 cases of visual loss from ROP per year in the USA

RISK FACTORS

- Low birth weight (<1,500 g)
- Prematurity (<30 weeks EGA)
- Complicated clinical course
- Prolonged supplemental oxygen

Genetics

Sporadic

GENERAL PREVENTION

Avoid excessive oxygen therapy using blood gas monitoring

PATHOPHYSIOLOGY

Normal retinal vascular development is arrested by premature birth. Peripheral retinal ischemia leads to release of vascular growth factors. Retinal and extraretinal neovascular proliferation occurs. Advanced proliferative disease can bleed, cause traction, and can lead to a retinal detachment and blindness.

COMMONLY ASSOCIATED CONDITIONS

With premature birth:

- Myopia
- Strabismus
- Cataract
- Retinal detachment
- Glaucoma

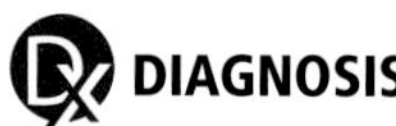

DIAGNOSIS

HISTORY

- Birth weight and EGA
- Neonatal clinical course

PHYSICAL EXAM

- Dilated stereoscopic fundus exam:
  - Dilated fundus exams for neonates 1,500 g or less, 28 weeks EGA or less, or any neonate 2,000 g or less felt to be at high risk.
  - First exam should be at 4–6 weeks of life, or at 31–33 weeks EGA, whichever is later.
- Staging of ROP
- Location:
  - Zone I: A circle of the retina centered at the optic disc with a radius twice the distance from the disc to the fovea
  - Zone II: The area of the retina beyond zone I within a circle centered at the optic disc with a radius equal to the distance from the disc to the nasal ora serrata
  - Zone III: A crescent of the retina outside of zone II in the far periphery which is widest at the temporal retina
- Severity:
  - Stage 1: Demarcation line between vascularized and nonvascularized retina
  - Stage 2: Demarcation ridge
  - Stage 3: Ridge with extraretinal fibrovascular proliferation
  - Stage 4: Subtotal retinal detachment (4A: extrafoveal, 4B: fovea involved)
  - Stage 5: Total retinal detachment
- Plus: Plus disease is defined as dilation and tortuosity of retinal vessels, vitreous haze and iris vessel engorgement
- Type 1 ROP (treatment recommended within 72 h):
  - Zone I, stage 3, or any stage with plus
  - Zone II, stage 2 or 3 with plus
- Type 2 ROP (no treatment recommended, close follow-up)
  - Zone I, stage 1 or 2 without plus
  - Zone II, stage 3 without plus

DIAGNOSTIC TESTS & INTERPRETATION

DIFFERENTIAL DIAGNOSIS

- Familial exudative vitreoretinopathy
- Retinoblastoma
- Incontinentia pigmenti
- Persistent fetal vasculature
- Norrie's disease

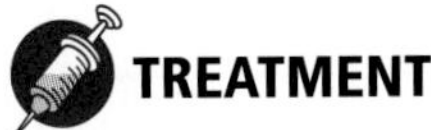

TREATMENT

MEDICATION

First Line

Laser photocoagulation of the avascular retina

Second Line

Cryotherapy ablation of the avascular retina

SURGERY/OTHER PROCEDURES

Retina surgery for retinal detachment

Nursing

Bradycardia and apnea can occur during the eye exam and laser treatment of neonates. Close nursing and respiratory supervision is essential for safety during examinations and treatments.

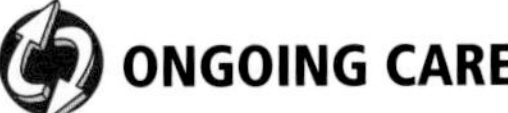

ONGOING CARE

FOLLOW-UP RECOMMENDATIONS

- Examination twice a week for type 2 ROP
- Examination once a week for borderline type 2 ROP
- Examination every 2 weeks for low-risk patients

PATIENT EDUCATION

Educate parents about lifelong morbidity of ROP and the need for close follow-up with ophthalmology.

ADDITIONAL READING

- Cryotherapy for Retinopathy of Prematurity Cooperative Group. Multi-center trial of cryotherapy for retinopathy of prematurity: Ophthalmological outcomes at 10 years. *Arch Ophthalmol* 2001;119: 1110–1118.
- Early Treatment for Retinopathy of Prematurity Cooperative Group. Revised indications for treatment of retinopathy of prematurity: Results of the early treatment of retinopathy of prematurity randomized trial. *Arch Ophthalmol* 2003;121: 1684–1696.
- Tasman W, Patz A, McNamara JA, et al. Retinopathy of prematurity: The life of a lifetime disease. *Am J Ophthalmol* 2006;141:167–174.

CODES

ICD9

- 362.20 Retinopathy of prematurity, unspecified
- 362.84 Retinal ischemia

RHEGMATOGENOUS RETINAL DETACHMENT

Deepak P. Grover
Sunir J. Garg

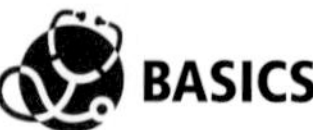

BASICS

DESCRIPTION

- A rhegmatogenous retinal detachment (RRD) occurs as a result of a retinal break or tear that allows fluid to enter the subretinal space and separate the retina from the underlying retinal pigment epithelium (RPE).
- It is the most common type of RD.

EPIDEMIOLOGY

Incidence

- 12 cases per 100,000 population annually in the USA
- Varies amongst different ethnicities from 4 to 12 cases per 100,000
- Appears to be more common in males than in females, and in persons aged 40–70 years

Prevalence

45 cases per 15,000 population or 0.3% in the USA

RISK FACTORS

- Axial myopia
- Lattice degeneration
- Aphakia or pseudophakia
- Prior intraocular surgery
- RRD in the fellow eye
- Trauma
- Family history of a RD
- Familial conditions:
  - Stickler syndrome, Marfan's syndrome, homocystinuria and Ehlers–Danlos
- Inflammatory or infectious conditions:
  - Pars planitis
  - Acute retinal necrosis syndrome
  - Cytomegalovirus retinitis in AIDS patients
  - Ocular toxoplasmosis

Genetics

No specific genetic mutations have been associated with a RRD.

GENERAL PREVENTION

- Controversy exists over prophylactically treating asymptomatic retinal tears and/or lattice degeneration, which may predispose one to a RRD, with laser photocoagulation or cryotherapy reduces the risk of RD formation.
  - An asymptomatic patient with lattice degeneration has a low risk of a RD and may be observed without treatment (1)[A].
  - A myopic, pseudophakic patient with lattice degeneration with a history of a RRD in the fellow eye should strongly be considered for prophylactic treatment.

PATHOPHYSIOLOGY

- Vitreoretinal traction is responsible for a RRD. With aging, the vitreous liquefies, and a posterior vitreous detachment (PVD) often occurs. A PVD usually occurs without complication. Occasionally, strong vitreoretinal adhesions are present and the occurrence of a PVD can lead to a retinal break.
- A retinal break allows vitreous fluid to enter through it, separating the retina from the RPE.

ETIOLOGY

- Retinal breaks are not uncommon. They typically occur with greater frequency in patients with myopia, ocular trauma, developmental or degenerative retinal abnormalities, and pseudophakic patients.
- Certain conditions may predispose one to the formation of a premature PVD (e.g., trauma) and potentiate the formation of a retinal tear.

COMMONLY ASSOCIATED CONDITIONS

- Myopia
- Lattice degeneration
- Stickler syndrome
- Marfan syndrome
- Homocystinuria
- Ehlers–Danlos

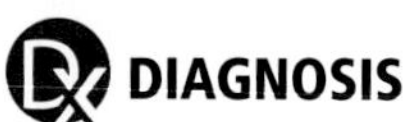

DIAGNOSIS

HISTORY

- Flashes and floaters:
  - Patients with retinal tears or breaks may notice flashes and floaters.
  - Small, peripheral RDs may be asymptomatic or present only with flashes and floaters.
- Visual field defect:
  - A progressive loss of visual field is a common complaint. May progress to a loss of central vision as subretinal fluid encroaches into the macula. A description of a dark shadow or curtain blocking the vision may be given.

PHYSICAL EXAM

- Acute RD:
  - Retinal tear or break, horseshoe tear:
    - Horseshoe, or flap, tear
    - A small, pinpoint hole may be found at the vitreous base with pseudophakic RDs
    - Of all RRDs, 50% have more than one break
    - Of all breaks, 60% are located in the upper temporal quadrant, 15% in the upper nasal quadrant, 15% in the lower temporal quadrant and 10% in the lower nasal quadrant.
  - Loss of retinal transparency, convex, corrugated appearance
  - The RD may undulate with eye movement
  - Cell and flare in the anterior chamber
  - Pigmented granules in the vitreous (tobacco dusting or Shaffer sign)
  - The intraocular pressure is usually lower in the eye with a RD compared to the fellow eye; however, infrequently, it may be higher.
- Chronic RD:
  - May appear transparent
  - May not undulate with eye movement
  - Intraretinal cysts, subretinal fibrosis, and demarcation lines are common findings.
    - A demarcation line of linear pigment may be deposited at the junction of attached and detached retina.
  - Anterior uveitis, rubeosis iridis, cataract, retinal neovascularization

DIAGNOSTIC TESTS & INTERPRETATION

Imaging

Initial approach

- Ultrasonography:
  - A-scan ultrasound:
    - Retinal tissue will show a large spike
  - B-scan ultrasound:
    - Helpful if media opacity precludes a complete ophthalmoscopic exam

Follow-up & special considerations

- Fluorescein angiography (FA):
  - Helpful in diagnosing cystoid macular edema, which may be a complication during the postoperative course of surgery.
- Optical coherence tomography (OCT):
  - Helpful in revealing subretinal fluid. Especially beneficial in eyes with complete retinal reattachment but incomplete visual acuity recovery.
- Electroretinogram (ERG):
  - ERG is useful in differentiating a RD from a thickened posterior hyaloid. If the retina is intact, an ERG signal should be obtained.

Diagnostic Procedures/Other

- Slit lamp exam to detect anterior uveitis, cataract, or vitreous pigmented granules
- Indirect ophthalmoscopy with scleral depression for examining the retina for a RD or retinal tear
- Contact lens examination in conjunction with slit lamp exam for small peripheral retinal breaks

Pathological Findings

- With an acute RD, as the neurosensory retina separates from the RPE, the photoreceptors are separated from their choroidal blood supply. This can lead to degeneration of the photoreceptor outer segments. With successful reattachment surgery, these outer segments may reform.
- With a chronic RD, the photoreceptor layer becomes atrophic. Furthermore, intraretinal cysts and with subretinal fibrosis may form.

DIFFERENTIAL DIAGNOSIS

- Senile retinoschisis
- Serous (exudative) RD
- Tractional RD
- Choroidal detachment
- Acute retinal necrosis

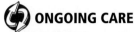

TREATMENT

ADDITIONAL TREATMENT

Issues for Referral

Vitreoretinal specialist – laser and surgical treatment

SURGERY/OTHER PROCEDURES

The goal of surgery is to approximate and seal all the breaks. Closure of the breaks occurs with bringing the edges of the tear into contact with the underlying RPE and then sealing it. Approximating the 2 edges may be accomplished by pushing the detached retina toward the eye wall (pneumatic retinopexy, or vitrectomy) or bringing the eye wall closer to the detached retina (scleral buckle). Sealing of the breaks is then accomplished by creating adhesions between the choroid and detached retina (laser photocoagulation, cryotherapy).

- Laser photocoagulation:
  - May be used to prevent the progression of the detachment by creating a "scarred" barrier with laser burns.
  - Limited in that photocoagulation cannot seal a retinal tear in the presence of subretinal fluid; therefore, it is seldom used as sole management for RD.
- Cryotherapy:
  - May be used alone, or in conjunction with another repair modality, in treating a break with shallow subretinal fluid around it.
  - Limited in cases where large amount of subretinal fluid is present.
- Pneumatic retinopexy:
  - Greatest benefit in a phakic patient with a single, superior retinal break, and without other retinal pathology.
  - The retinal break is tamponaded with an intravitreal gas bubble.
  - After resolution of the subretinal fluid, either laser photocoagulation or cryotherapy may be applied to seal the break.
- Scleral buckle:
  - A flexible silicone band or sponge is permanently sutured onto the sclera, indenting it, to relieve vitreoretinal traction on the retinal break.
  - Cryotherapy or photocoagulation may then be applied.
  - Injection of intravitreal gas may also be used.
  - Success rates of 95% may be achieved.
- Vitrectomy (2)[A]:
  - Especially useful for RDs with posterior breaks, proliferative vitreoretinopathy, or vitreous hemorrhage.
  - Common technique used for primary RD with or without a scleral buckle.
  - Mechanism allows for a direct release of vitreoretinal traction.
  - Intravitreal gas or silicone oil may be used to tamponade the retina in addition to the application of cryotherapy or photocoagulation.

IN-PATIENT CONSIDERATIONS

Initial Stabilization

Prior to reattachment surgery for a RRD, patients should rest as much as possible.

Admission Criteria

Most vitreoretinal surgery is performed on an outpatient basis.

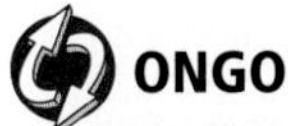

ONGOING CARE

FOLLOW-UP RECOMMENDATIONS

- Following surgical retinal repair, the patient will be instructed to maintain a certain head position for several days following surgery.
- Following surgery, a topical antibiotic is given for 7–10 days, a topical steroid for 1 month, and a cycloplegic agent for 1 month.
- The intraocular pressure is monitored during the postoperative course.

PATIENT EDUCATION

- Provide a patient with a PVD or risk factors for a RD with warning signs of flashes and floaters.
- Warn the patient of the risk of a RD in the fellow eye if one eye has experienced a RRD.
  - Up to 10–15% in phakic eyes
  - Up to 25–40% in aphakic or pseudophakic eyes
- If performing cataract surgery or YAG capsulotomy, warn the patient of the risk of a RD.

PROGNOSIS

- Most RDs, if left untreated, progress causing permanent deterioration of central vision. The final visual potential is dependent on whether the macula is "off" (separated from the RPE). Once the macula is detached, the photoreceptors begin to degenerate.
  - The most important factor affecting postoperative visual acuity is the preoperative visual acuity.
  - If a macula "off" detachment is operated within 72 h from presentation, the patient's visual prognosis is more favorable.
- Chronic, asymptomatic RD may not require treatment if stable.
- After successful reattachment, recovery may take months; however, central vision may never recover even with adequate treatment.
- Of the eyes that are successfully reattached, 50% obtain a final visual acuity of 20/50 or better.

COMPLICATIONS

- Proliferative vitreoretinopathy – the most common reason for surgical failure
- Cystoid macular edema
- Rubeosis iridis

REFERENCES

1. Wilkinson C. Interventions for asymptomatic retinal breaks and lattice degeneration for preventing retinal detachment. *Cochrane Database Syst Rev* 2005(1):CD003170.
2. Arya AV, Emerson JW, Engelbert M, et al. Surgical management of pseudophakic retinal detachments: A meta-analysis. *Ophthalmology* 2006;113(10): 1724–1733.

ADDITIONAL READING

- Albert DM, Miller JW. *Principles and practice of ophthalmology*, 3rd ed. Philadelphia, PA: Saunders Elsevier, 2008.
- Gass JD. *Stereoscopic atlas of macular diseases*, 4th ed. Mosby: St. Louis, MO, 1997.
- Henrich PB, Priglinger S, Klaessen D, et al. Macula-off retinal detachment–a matter of time? *Klin Monbl Augenheilkd* 2009;226(4):289–293.
- Ross WH, Stockl FA. Visual recovery after retinal detachment. *Curr Opin Ophthalmol* 2000;11(3):191–194.
- Ryan SJ. *Retina*, 4th ed. Mosby: St. Louis, MO, 2006.
- Wolfensberger TJ, Gonvers M. Optical coherence tomography in the evaluation of incomplete visual acuity recovery after macula-off retinal detachments. *Graefes Arch Clin Exp Ophthalmol* 2002;240(2):85–89.

CODES

ICD9

- 361.00 Retinal detachment with retinal defect, unspecified
- 361.30 Retinal defect, unspecified

CLINICAL PEARLS

- Flashes, floaters, and a visual field defect, with or without complaints of a dark shadow or curtain veil, are symptoms of a RRD.

RUBELLA (GERMAN MEASLES)

Donelson Manley
Chirag P. Shah

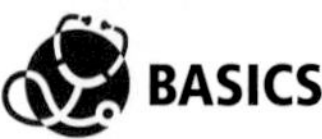

BASICS

DESCRIPTION

- Rubella is a worldwide contagious viral infection best known for its distinctive red rash.
- It is also known as German measles because it was first described by German physicians.
- After an incubation period of 14–21 days, rubella causes a flu-like disease. A pink or light red rash appears on the face that spreads to the trunk and limbs and usually fades after 3 days. This is why it is often called the 3-day measles.
- There may be a low-grade fever, lymphadenopathy, joint pain, headache, and conjunctivitis.
- It is a common childhood illness and is usually mild. Complications are rare.
- It is transmitted by airborne droplets from the upper respiratory tract of an infected individual.
- Rubella can affect individuals of any age.
- The virus can pass though the pregnant woman's bloodstream to infect her fetus, causing congenital rubella syndrome.

EPIDEMIOLOGY

- A person can transmit the disease from 1 week before the rash until 1–2 weeks after the rash disappears.
- After infection there is usually a lifelong immunity.
- There is no carrier state and the virus exists entirely in active human cases.
- Rubella has an incubation period of 2–3 weeks.
- Risk of congenital rubella syndrome is greater with more severe consequences if maternal infection occurs in the first trimester (>50% risk). The risk decreases during the subsequent trimesters.
- The virus may persist in infected infants and may be a source of infection to other infants and to pregnant female contacts.

RISK FACTORS

- Not being vaccinated against rubella
- Exposure to active rubella virus

GENERAL PREVENTION

- The measles-mumps-rubella (MMR) vaccine is usually given to children before they reach school age and is highly effective in preventing rubella.
- Women who are of childbearing age can be tested to see if they have immunity to rubella. If they are not immune they can be vaccinated. Women who are pregnant should not be vaccinated, nor should those who are immunocompromised.

ETIOLOGY

Caused by the rubella virus, a togavirus that is enveloped and has a single stranded RNA genome.

COMMONLY ASSOCIATED CONDITIONS

Findings of congenital rubella syndrome include:

- Miscarriage or stillbirth, prematurity, low birth weight
- Cataracts
- Congenital heart defects (ventricular septal defects, patent ductus arteriosus, pulmonic stenosis, coarctation of the aorta)
- Deafness
- Ear infection (otitis media)
- Encephalitis
- Growth retardation
- Mental retardation in 10–20%
- Microcephaly
- Transient arthritis in adolescents and adults
- Hepatitis
- Hepatosplenomegaly
- Thrombocytopenia
- Obstructive jaundice
- Radiolucent bone disease
- Pigmentary retinopathy with salt-and-pepper changes
- Glaucoma
- Purpura
- Diabetes mellitus in 20% of adults
- Thyroid dysfunction in 5%
- Progressive panencephalitis
- Non-affective psychosis

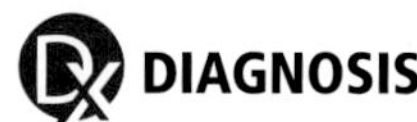

DIAGNOSIS

HISTORY

Exposure to someone with rubella

PHYSICAL EXAM

- External examination including skin to identify characteristic rash
- Prenatal screening with ultrasound, amniocentesis, cordocentesis, or chorionic villous sampling
- Ultrasound assesses for fetal hydrops, bowel hyperechogenicity, and intrauterine growth retardation.

DIAGNOSTIC TESTS & INTERPRETATION

Diagnostic Procedures/Other

- Nasal or throat swab for viral culture and rubella serology. The presence of IgM antibodies along with, or a short time after, the characteristic rash confirms the diagnosis.
- Serological investigation typically employs enzyme-linked immunosorbent assays (ELISA), hemoagglutination inhibition test (HI), or the immunofluorescent antibody assay (IFA)

- **Centers for Disease Control classification criteria for congenital rubella syndrome:**
  - Congenital rubella syndrome case: Infants that present one or, in the majority of cases, more than one of these following clinical signs or symptoms:
    - Cataracts/congenital glaucoma, congenital heart disease (most commonly patent ductus arteriosus or peripheral pulmonic stenosis), hearing impairment, pigmentary retinopathy.
    - Purpura, hepatosplenomegaly, jaundice, microcephaly, developmental delay, meningoencephalitis, radiolucent bone disease.
  - Suspected case: Clinical signs are evident but without the satisfactory criteria to be defined as a probable case.
  - Probable case: A case without laboratory confirmation, that has any of the 2 findings listed in category 1 of the clinical description or one finding from category 1 and one from 2, and lacks evidence of any other etiology.
  - Confirmed case: Clinical evidence and laboratory confirmation.
  - Infection only: Laboratory evidence of infection, without any clinical symptoms or signs.

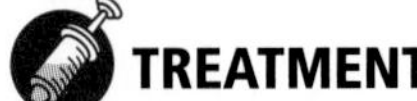

TREATMENT

ADDITIONAL TREATMENT

General Measures

- There is no specific treatment for rubella. Supportive treatment as needed.
- Immune globulin therapy to exposed mothers does not prevent fetal rubella infection.

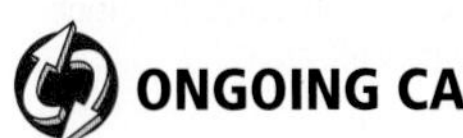

ONGOING CARE

FOLLOW-UP RECOMMENDATIONS

Based on degree and nature of manifestations

PROGNOSIS

- Acquired rubella is usually a mild infection without sequelae.
- Congenital rubella syndrome is chronic and incurable; many its manifestations, such as cataract and diabetes, can be treated.

ADDITIONAL READING

- CDC. MMWR rubella and congenital rubella syndrome, United States,1994–1997. *MMWR Morb Mortal Wkly Rep* 1997;46(16):350–354.
- De Santis M, Cavaliere AF, Straface G, et al. Rubella infection in pregnancy. *Reprod Toxicol* 2006;21(4): 390–398.
- Richardson M, Elliman D, Maguire H, et al. Evidence base of incubation periods, periods of infectiousness and exclusion policies for the control of communicable diseases in schools and preschools. *Pediatr Infec Dis J* 2001;20(4):380–391.
- Siegel M, Fuerst HT, Guinee VF. Rubella epidemicity and embryopathy. Results of a long-term prospective study. *Am J Dis Child* 1971;121(6):469–473.

CODES

ICD9

- 056.79 Rubella with other specified complications
- 647.50 Rubella of mother, complicating pregnancy, childbirth, or the puerperium, unspecified as to episode of care
- 771.0 Congenital rubella

CLINICAL PEARLS

- Risk of congenital rubella syndrome is greater with more severe consequences if maternal infection occurs in the first trimester (>50% risk).
- Ocular manifestations of congenital rubella syndrome include cataracts, pigmentary retinopathy, and glaucoma.

SALZMANN'S NODULAR DEGENERATION

Christopher J. Rapuano

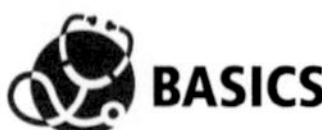

BASICS

DESCRIPTION

Salzmann's nodules are creamy white, occasionally with a yellow or blue-tinged, smooth, elevated lesion(s) on the surface of the cornea.

EPIDEMIOLOGY

Incidence

- Uncommon but exact incidence is unknown
- Tends to occur in middle age

Prevalence

Much more prevalent in women than in men

RISK FACTORS

- Ocular surface inflammation, such as from meibomian gland dysfunction (MGD), dry eye syndrome (DES), phlyctenular keratitis, vernal keratoconjunctivitis, trachoma, interstitial keratitis, and trauma, such as long-term contact lens wear
- Most commonly idiopathic

GENERAL PREVENTION

Treat underlying conditions

ETIOLOGY

Thought to be related to low-grade chronic inflammation

COMMONLY ASSOCIATED CONDITIONS

- See risk factors above.
- Salzmann's has also been associated with epithelial basement membrane dystrophy and after corneal surgery.

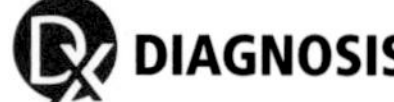

DIAGNOSIS

HISTORY

- Generally asymptomatic
- May have symptoms of foreign body sensation, pain, redness, and tearing
- As nodules reach toward the visual axis, the vision may be mildly to moderately affected.

PHYSICAL EXAM

- Slit lamp examination reveals single or multiple, elevated creamy, yellow- or blue-white corneal nodules.
- Although typically located in the corneal periphery or midperiphery, the nodules may also be paracentral or central.

DIAGNOSTIC TESTS & INTERPRETATION

Imaging

Initial approach

Not required if vision is unaffected

Follow-up & special considerations

Consider corneal topography to evaluate for irregular astigmatism if there are visual complaints.

Pathological Findings

- Collagen plaques with hyaline between epithelium and Bowman's layer
- Bowman's layer may be missing or damaged underlying the lesion.

DIFFERENTIAL DIAGNOSIS

- Climatic droplet keratopathy
- Corneal amyloidosis
- Corneal keloid

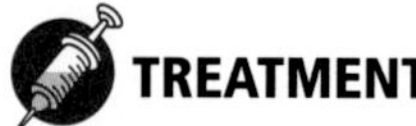

TREATMENT

MEDICATION

First Line

- If asymptomatic, no treatment is required.
- To decrease the risk of progression, underlying conditions can be treated.
- MGD and DES should be treated if present.
- Proper contact lens fit, wearing schedule, and care should be evaluated.

Second Line

Foreign body sensation or pain is treated with increased lubrication with artificial tears, gels and ointments, cyclosporine 0.05% drops, and punctal plugs.

ADDITIONAL TREATMENT

General Measures

Salzmann's nodules may remain stable for years or may slowly progress.

Issues for Referral

When discomfort or visual symptoms are not responding to conservative medical therapy, referral to a corneal specialist may be warranted.

Additional Therapies

A rigid gas permeable or hybrid contact lens may occasionally be useful in improving vision in patients with irregular astigmatism, who are not good candidates for surgical excision of the nodule(s).

SURGERY/OTHER PROCEDURES

- Surgical excision of the nodules is recommended when comfort or vision symptoms are not relieved by medical therapy.
- Excision can often be accomplished by simple removal with a blade, being careful not to incise into Bowman's layer.
- Excimer laser phototherapeutic keratectomy (PTK) is often used to remove these lesions.
- Recurrences of the nodules after excision may be reduced with the use of intraoperative mitomycin C.
- Rarely, a lamellar or penetrating keratoplasty is required for severe disease or multiple recurrences.

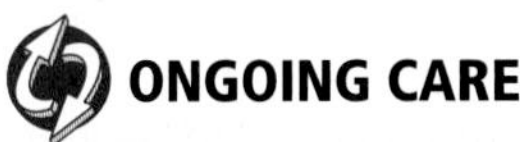

ONGOING CARE

FOLLOW-UP RECOMMENDATIONS

- Asymptomatic patients are generally seen every year.
- Symptomatic patients are seen more frequently based on their symptoms.
- Patients are seen every few days after surgical excision to make sure that the cornea is healing well.

PATIENT EDUCATION

Patients should return to their eye doctor should they develop pain or decreased vision.

PROGNOSIS

- Very good
- Lesions are often stable for many years, also they may slowly enlarge.
- Lesions may recur after surgical excision; repeat excision is often successful.

COMPLICATIONS

Patients may develop epithelial defects or recurrent erosions related to the nodules, which could become infected.

ADDITIONAL READING

- Farjo AA, Halperin GI, Syed N, et al. Salzmann's nodular corneal degeneration clinical characteristics and surgical outcomes. *Cornea* 2006;25:11–15.
- Das S, Link B, Seitz B. Salzmann's nodular degeneration of the cornea A review and case series. *Cornea* 2005;24:772–777.
- Bowers PJ, Price MO, Zeldes SS, et al. Superficial keratectomy with mitomycin-C for the treatment of Salzmann's nodules. *J Cataract Refract Surg* 2003;29:1302–1306.
- Marcon AS, Rapuano CJ. Excimer laser phototherapeutic keratectomy retreatment of anterior basement dystrophy and Salzmann's nodular degeneration with topical mitomycin C. *Cornea* 2002;21:828–830.

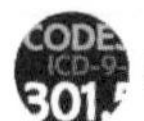

CODES

ICD9

371.46 Nodular degeneration of cornea

CLINICAL PEARLS

- Salzmann's nodular degeneration is not rare, especially among middle-aged women.
- Salzmann's nodular degeneration should be considered in anyone with creamy white, yellow, or bluish, smooth, elevated corneal nodule(s).
- Medical treatment is often successful for lesions causing foreign body sensation, but surgical excision is generally required for patients with frank pain (rare) or decreased vision (common).
- Although surgical excision is quite successful, nodules may recur.
- Any nodules causing significant irregular astigmatism should be removed prior to cataract surgery to obtain the most accurate keratometry readings.

SARCOIDOSIS

Wayne R. Lo

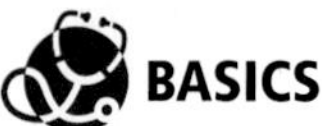

BASICS

DESCRIPTION

- Sarcoidosis is a multisystem granulomatous disease of unknown etiology.
- Organs most commonly affected are the lungs, thoracic lymph nodes, skin, and central nervous system.
- Ocular involvement occurs in 10–50% of sarcoid patients. It may involve the orbit, anterior or posterior segment, or optic nerve.

EPIDEMIOLOGY

Incidence

- Substantial variation exists across ethnic groups and regions for systemic disease.
  - 35–80 per 100,000 in African Americans
  - 3–10 per 100,000 in European Americans
  - 15–20 per 100,000 in Northern Europeans
  - 1–5 per 100,000 in Southern Europeans
  - 1–2 per 100,000 in Japanese
- Ocular sarcoidosis can occur at any time, may predate systemic findings, and is found in
  - 10% of American patients
  - 50% of European patients
  - 50–90% of Japanese patients

RISK FACTORS

- African Americans are 3–10 times more likely than whites to develop sarcoid.
- The highest prevalence is in 25–50 year olds.

Genetics

- Siblings have a 5 times increased risk of developing sarcoidosis.
- *HLA-DRB1* has been associated with susceptibility to sarcoidosis.

PATHOPHYSIOLOGY

Biopsy of affected tissues reveals noncaseating granulomatous inflammation.

ETIOLOGY

- No definite etiology has been identified. An abnormal immune response after exposure to minerals, organic substances, or fragments of infectious agents has been proposed as a cause.
- Macrophages, possibly in response to an inciting agent, release cytokines to recruit T-helper lymphocytes. The activated lymphocytes and macrophages are responsible for granuloma formation.

COMMONLY ASSOCIATED CONDITIONS

- Heerfordt syndrome: uveitis preceding parotid gland enlargement and disc edema
- Löfgren syndrome: erythema nodosum, bilateral hilar adenopathy, and arthralgias

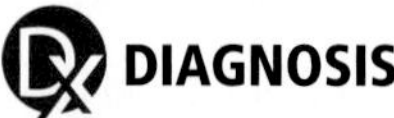

DIAGNOSIS

HISTORY

- Ocular pain, photophobia, floaters, diplopia, and decreased vision may be present, although many patients are asymptomatic.
- Systemic symptoms include shortness of breath, fever, arthralgias, and skin nodules.

PHYSICAL EXAM

Several ocular signs may be present:

- Mutton-fat keratic precipitates and/or iris nodules (Koeppe/Busacca)
- Trabecular meshwork nodules and/or tent-shaped peripheral anterior synechiae
- Vitreous opacities displaying snowballs/strings of pearls
- Multiple chorioretinal peripheral lesions (active and/or atrophic)
- Nodular and/or segmental periphlebitis (candlewax drippings) and/or retinal macroaneurysm in an inflamed eye
- Optic disc nodule/granuloma and/or choroidal nodules
- Conjunctival nodules
- Lacrimal gland enlargement, often resulting in dry eye
- Proptosis may result from orbital involvement with a mass lesion.
- Diplopia may result from either cranial nerve involvement or an orbital mass lesion.
- Findings are typically bilateral though occasionally unilateral or asymmetric.

DIAGNOSTIC TESTS & INTERPRETATION

Lab

- Elevated serum angiotensin-converting enzyme (ACE) levels are found in 60–90% of patients with active sarcoidosis.
- Elevated serum lysozyme may be useful in children when ACE levels are less reliable.
- Purified protein derivative (PPD) with anergy panel may help distinguish sarcoidosis from tuberculosis. Up to 50% of sarcoidosis patients are anergic and have no response to PPD or controls.
- Abnormal liver enzyme tests

Imaging
- Chest X-ray is abnormal in 90% of sarcoidosis patients, typically revealing bilateral and symmetric hilar adenopathy or infiltrates.
  - Chest CT is superior to X-ray and may be useful in patients with atypical clinical or radiographic examinations.

Diagnostic Procedures/Other
- Although definitive diagnosis requires a positive biopsy, the presumptive diagnosis is often made with positive lab tests and imaging.
  - For inconclusive cases, biopsy sites include nodular lesions of the skin and conjunctiva, or the lacrimal gland.
- Whole-body gallium scans often show inflammation in areas such as the lungs, lacrimal glands, and parotid glands. A positive gallium scan and elevated ACE level is 73% sensitive and 100% specific for sarcoidosis.
- Negative testing or biopsy in a patient with high suspicion may warrant referral to a pulmonologist for pulmonary function tests or lung biopsy.

Pathological Findings
Noncaseating epithelioid cell granulomas

DIFFERENTIAL DIAGNOSIS
- Ocular sarcoidosis may masquerade as many uveitic disorders, including
  - Syphilis
  - Tuberculosis
  - Toxoplasmosis
  - Multiple sclerosis
  - Lyme disease
  - Vogt–Koyanagi–Harada syndrome
  - Birdshot chorioretinopathy
  - Intraocular lymphoma
  - Sympathetic ophthalmia
  - Multifocal choroiditis
- Orbital sarcoidosis may resemble
  - Dacryoadenitis
  - Orbital or lacrimal gland tumors
  - Orbital pseudotumor
  - Lipogranulomas
  - Wegener granulomatosis

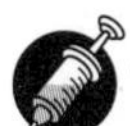

TREATMENT

MEDICATION
First Line
- Topical, periocular, or systemic corticosteroids
- Cycloplegia

Second Line
Patients requiring chronic treatment may benefit from nonsteroidal immunosuppressive agents (e.g., methotrexate, cyclosporine, azathioprine, infliximab), prescribed in conjunction with a uveitis specialist or rheumatologist.

ADDITIONAL TREATMENT
Issues for Referral
- Pulmonologist for lung involvement
- Rheumatologist or uveitis specialist for chronic immunosuppressive therapy

SURGERY/OTHER PROCEDURES
Secondary cataract and glaucoma may require cataract extraction or filtering surgery.

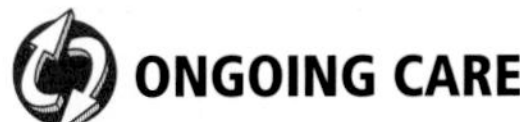

ONGOING CARE

FOLLOW-UP RECOMMENDATIONS
- Routine examination with an ophthalmologist for recurrence of inflammation
- Primary care or pulmonologist for systemic manifestations

PATIENT EDUCATION
Foundation for Sarcoidosis Research (http://www.stopsarcoidosis.org/)

PROGNOSIS
More than 50% retain normal visual acuity, although 5% have severe bilateral visual loss of less than 20/120. Vision loss stems from posterior uveitis, glaucoma, and macular edema.

COMPLICATIONS
- Chronic uveitis
- Cystoid macular edema
- Secondary cataract
- Secondary glaucoma

REFERENCES

1. Margolis R, Lowder CY. Sarcoidosis. *Curr Opin Ophthalmol* 2007;18:470–475.
2. Bonfioli AA, Orefice F. Sarcoidosis. *Semin Ophthalmol* 2005;20:177–182.
3. Herbort C, Rao N, Mochizuki M, et al. International criteria for the diagnosis of ocular sarcoidosis: Results of the First International Workshop on Ocular Sarcoidosis (IWOS). *Occ Imm Inflam* 2009;17(3):160–169.

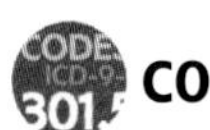

CODES

ICD9
- 135 Sarcoidosis
- 379.24 Other vitreous opacities

SCHNYDER'S CORNEAL DYSTROPHY (SCD)

Jayrag A. Patel

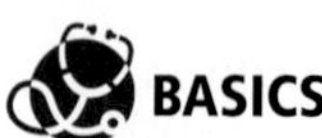

BASICS

DESCRIPTION

Schnyder's corneal dystrophy (SCD) is a rare bilateral condition characterized with slowly progressive abnormal deposition of lipids in the cornea.

EPIDEMIOLOGY

Incidence

- Unknown
- Worldwide largest pedigree (>200 patients with SCD) has a Swede-Finn heritage.

RISK FACTORS

Genetics

- Defective gene localized to short arm of chromosome 1, at 1p34–36 (1)[A].
  - Mutations in the UbiA prenyltransferase domain containing protein 1 (*UBIAD1*) gene have been identified in 28 unrelated families with SCD to date (2,3) [A].

PATHOPHYSIOLOGY

- Related to a primary corneal lipid metabolism disorder
- Deposition of phospholipid, unesterified cholesterol, and cholesterol esters in Bowman's membrane and corneal stroma

ETIOLOGY

Rare autosomal dominant condition

COMMONLY ASSOCIATED CONDITIONS

- Hypercholesterolemia
- Hypertriglyceridemia
- Xanthelasma
- Genu valgum (rare)

DIAGNOSIS

HISTORY

- Symptoms of glare from late teenage years
- Visual acuity only affected in severe cases and worse in photopic conditions

PHYSICAL EXAM

- Central ring-shaped or disciform gray opacities in the anterior stroma, which may consist of fine polychromatic crystals. A crystalline variety in up to 46% of affected individuals (4)[A].
- Diffuse progressive stromal haze can be seen in patients older than 40 years old.
  - Corneal arcus develops later with age.
  - Progressive decrease in corneal sensation may occur over lesions.

DIAGNOSTIC TESTS & INTERPRETATION

Lab

Initial lab tests

Perform fasting cholesterol and triglyceride tests as they may be abnormal.

Follow-up & special considerations

Genetic testing will reveal mutations in *UBIAD1* gene in affected individuals.

Imaging

Initial approach

None

Follow-up & special considerations

Confocal microscopy

Diagnostic Procedures/Other

Characteristic histopathologic features in host corneal button after penetrating keratoplasty

Pathological Findings

- Histopathology: Oil-red-O positive lipid material in stroma, unesterified and esterified cholesterol in Bowman's layer and stroma (5)[A]
- Confocal microscopy: Needle-shaped or rectangular crystals may be seen in the anterior stroma.

DIFFERENTIAL DIAGNOSIS

- Cystinosis
- Bietti's peripheral crystalline dystrophy
- Infectious crystalline keratopathy
- Gout
- Multiple myeloma
- Hodgkin's disease
- Waldenström's macroglobulinemia
- Benign monoclonal gammopathy
- Plant sap injury
- Tangier disease
- Lecithin–cholesterol acyltransferase deficiency

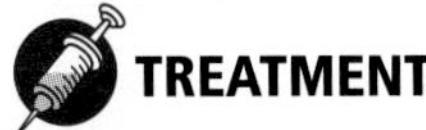

TREATMENT

MEDICATION
Lipid lowering agents if abnormal lipid profile

SURGERY/OTHER PROCEDURES
- If cornea opacity is severely debilitating vision then corneal transplantation is needed (lamellar or full thickness).
- Excimer laser phototherapeutic keratectomy (PTK) for removal of superficial pathology causing glare

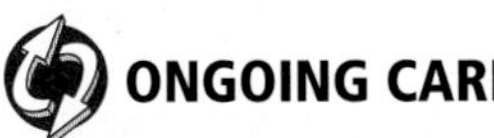

ONGOING CARE

FOLLOW-UP RECOMMENDATIONS
Every 6 months

Patient Monitoring
Visual acuity, glare symptoms

DIET
Control diet to maintain normal lipid profile.

PATIENT EDUCATION
Condition is slowly progressive and hereditary.

PROGNOSIS
- SCD can be diagnosed easily during the first decade, but patients with SCD sine crystals may be harder to diagnose and so be delayed up to the fourth decade.
- Visual acuity remains good usually and may not necessitate corneal transplantation.
- Haze may progress as well as reduced corneal sensation.

COMPLICATIONS
Recurrence of dystrophy may occur in corneal graft or after PTK, but rare.

REFERENCES

1. Orr A, Dube MP, Marcadier J, et al. Mutations in the *UBIAD1* gene, encoding a potential prenyltransferase, are causal for Schnyder crystalline corneal dystrophy. *PLoS ONE* 2007;2(1):e685.
2. Weiss JS, Kruth HS, Kuivaniemi H, et al. Mutations in the *UBIAD1* gene on chromosome short arm 1, region 36, cause Schnyder crystalline corneal dystrophy. *Invest Ophthalmol Vis Sci* 2007; 48(11):5007–5012.
3. Kobayashi A, Fujiki K, Murakami A, et al. In vivo laser confocal Microscopy findings and mutational analysis of Schnyder's crystalline corneal dystrophy. *Ophthalmology* 2009;116:1029–1037.
4. Weiss JS. Visual morbidity in thirty three families with Schnyder's crystalline corneal dystrophy. *Trans Am Ophthalmol Soc* 2007;105:616–648.
5. Rodrigues MM, Kruth HS, Krachmer JH, et al. Unesterified cholesterol in Schnyder's corneal crystalline dystrophy. *Am J Ophthalmol* 1987;104(2):157–163.

ADDITIONAL READING

- Bron AJ. Corneal changes in the dislipoproteinaemias. *Cornea* 1989;8(2):135–140.
- Weiss JS. Schnyder's dystrophy of the cornea: A Swede-Finn connection. *Cornea* 1992;11(2): 93–101.

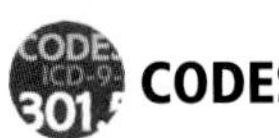

CODES

ICD9
371.56 Other stromal corneal dystrophies

CLINICAL PEARLS
- Check for associated systemic lipid abnormality
- Crystals not necessarily seen
- Visual acuity usually remains good

SCLERITIS

David Fintak

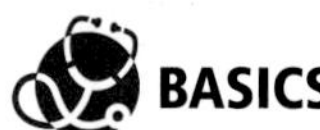

BASICS

DESCRIPTION

A rare condition characterized by inflammation and necrosis of the sclera. Classification:

- Anterior (93–98%)
  - Diffuse (40–64%)
    - Widespread inflammation of anterior segment
  - Nodular (22–45%)
    - Immovable inflamed nodule
  - Necrotizing (13–26%)
    - With inflammation (10–23%)
    - Extreme pain. "Bluish sclera" due to necrosis, thinning, and increased transparency of sclera
    - Without inflammation (3–4%)
    - "Scleromalacia perforans." Asymptomatic
  - Posterior (2–7%)
  - Associated with pain, tenderness, restricted motility, choroidal detachment, exudative retinal detachment, and disc swelling

EPIDEMIOLOGY

Prevalence

- Approximately 6 cases per 100,000
- No racial predilection
- Female to male ratio—1.6:1

PATHOPHYSIOLOGY

- Histopathology may show granulomatous or nongranulomatous inflammation, vasculitis, and necrosis.
  - Antigen–antibody complexes and/or T cells have been implicated.

ETIOLOGY

- Noninfectious
  - Connective tissue diseases (e.g., rheumatoid arthritis, Wegener's granulomatosis, spondyloarthropathies, systemic lupus erythematosus), sarcoidosis, status postocular surgery, gout
- Infectious
  - Herpes zoster, syphilis, tuberculosis, other bacteria (e.g., *Pseudomonas* in cases of scleral ulceration, *Proteus* associated with scleral buckle), foreign body

Although most scleral inflammation is noninfectious, bacterial or fungal organisms such as *Pseudomonas* and *Aspergillus* may cause a severe scleritis that is difficult to treat.

DIAGNOSIS

HISTORY

- Patients typically complain of deep and boring pain that often awakens them from sleep.
  - May radiate to forehead, brow, or jaw
- Onset of red eye and decrease in vision may be acute or gradual in onset.
- Recurrences are common.
- Elicit history of any pertinent underlying medical problems (e.g., rheumatoid arthritis).

PHYSICAL EXAM

- Examine the sclera in all fields of gaze.
- Slit lamp evaluation for any areas of avascularity or thinning
- Check for corneal or anterior chamber involvement.
- Dilated fundus exam to rule out posterior involvement.
- Phenylephrine 2.5% test—place a drop in the affected eye and reexamine the vascular pattern in 10–15 minutes. No significant change should occur in scleritis.

DIAGNOSTIC TESTS & INTERPRETATION

Lab

Initial lab tests

CBC, rapid plasma reagin (RPR), fluorescent treponemal antibody absorption (FTA-ABS), serum antineutrophil cytoplasmic antibody (ANCA)

Follow-Up & Special Considerations

Rheumatoid factor and/or human leukocyte antigen (HLA)-B27—in presence of polyarthritis or spondyloarthropathy

Imaging

Initial approach

Chest X-ray (CXR)—to evaluate for tuberculosis and sarcoidosis

Follow-up & special considerations

Radiograph of sacroiliac joints—if ankylosing spondylitis is suspected

Diagnostic Procedures/Other

- Purified protein derivative (PPD) with anergy panel
- B-scan ultrasound—positive "T" sign in posterior scleritis

DIFFERENTIAL DIAGNOSIS

- Anterior scleritis
  - Episcleritis
    - Sclera not involved, pain and associated symptoms mild if any, blood vessels tend to blanch with phenylephrine
    - Posterior scleritis
  - Amelanotic choroidal melanoma
  - Vogt–Koyanagi–Harada syndrome

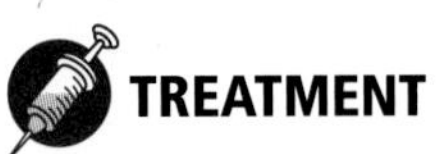

TREATMENT

MEDICATION

- Diffuse and nodular scleritis (depending on disease severity)
  - NSAIDs (e.g., ibuprofen 400–600 mg p.o. q6h, naproxen 250–500 mg q12h)
  - Prednisone 60–100 mg q.d. for 1 week followed by slow taper
  - Immunosuppressive therapy (e.g., methotrexate, azathioprine, cyclosporine, cyclophosphamide, infliximab, mycophenolate mofetil)
- Necrotizing scleritis
  - Prednisone and immunosuppressives as above
- Posterior scleritis
  - NSAIDs, prednisone, or immunosuppressives as above
- Infectious
  - Use appropriate topical and systemic antimicrobials

ALERT
Topical steroids are ineffective.
Subtenon/subconjunctival steroids are relatively contraindicated.

ADDITIONAL TREATMENT

General Measures

Eye protection recommended for patients with significant thinning and risk of perforation

SURGERY/OTHER PROCEDURES

- Rarely necessary
  - Scleral patch grafting for impending/overt scleral perforation

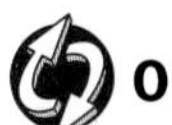

ONGOING CARE

FOLLOW-UP RECOMMENDATIONS

- Depends on the degree of inflammation and scleral thinning
- Decreased pain is a sign of treatment response.

PROGNOSIS

Recurrences are common.

COMPLICATIONS

Scleral perforation

REFERENCES

1. Watson PG, Hayreh SS. Scleritis and episcleritis. *Br J Ophthalmol* 1976;60:163–191.
2. Jabs DA, Mudun A, Dunn JP, et al. Episcleritis and scleritis: Clinical features and treatment results. *Am J Opththalmol* 2000;130:469–476.

ADDITIONAL READING

- Ryan SJ.HintonDR, SchachatAP, et al., eds. *Retina*. 4th ed. St. Louis, MO: Mosby, 2006:1731–1748.

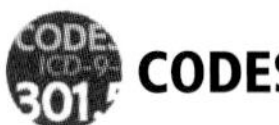

CODES

ICD9

- 379.00 Scleritis, unspecified
- 379.06 Brawny scleritis
- 379.07 Posterior scleritis

SEROUS (EXUDATIVE) RETINAL DETACHMENT

Deepak P. Grover
Sunir J. Garg

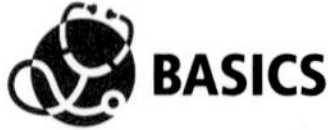

BASICS

DESCRIPTION

- Serous retinal detachment (SRD) is an elevation of the retina due to accumulation of fluid in the subretinal space and is not associated with traction or retinal hole or tear.
- An SRD is not due to a retinal break, as is the case in rhegmatogenous RD (RRD).

EPIDEMIOLOGY

Incidence

- A wide range exists depending on etiology.
  - An incidence of SRD as high as 32% has been found for women with severe preeclampsia or eclampsia, with the majority of these resolving within 1 week.
  - 60% of cases of optic disc pits may be complicated by SRD.

RISK FACTORS

- Underlying vasculitis or autoimmune disease
- Trauma
- Acquired immunodeficiency syndrome
- Chronic or malignant hypertension
- Renal disease
- Coagulopathy
- Neoplastic disorder
- Ocular surgery

PATHOPHYSIOLOGY

- Normally, there is a flow of fluid from the vitreous cavity, through the retina, to the hyperosmolar choroid. In addition, the retinal pigment epithelium (RPE) actively pumps ions and fluid from the retina and subretinal space into the choroid.
- A breakdown of the normal inner (retinal vascular endothelial cells) or outer blood–retinal barrier (RPE) will allow for exudation. In addition, any process that affects the choroidal vascular permeability may lead to an SRD.

ETIOLOGY

- Inflammatory
  - Scleritis
  - Vogt–Koyanagi–Harada (VKH) disease
  - Sympathetic ophthalmia
  - Orbital inflammatory syndrome
  - Lymphomatoid granulomatosis
  - Infectious retinochoroiditis
    - Toxoplasmosis
    - Syphilis
    - Lyme
    - Cat scratch disease
    - Cytomegalovirus (CMV) retinitis
    - Tuberculosis
  - Vasculitis/autoimmune
    - Lupus
    - Wegener's granulomatosis
    - Sarcoidosis
    - Inflammatory bowel disease
    - Polyarteritis nodosa
- Vascular
  - Retinal vein occlusion
  - Coats' disease
  - Retinal capillary hemangioma
  - Malignant hypertension
  - Preeclampsia/eclampsia
  - Disseminated intravascular coagulation
  - Renal disease
    - Renal failure
    - Lupus nephritis
    - Crescentic membranous nephropathy
    - Goodpasture's syndrome
    - IgA nephropathy
- Neoplastic
  - Choroidal melanoma, osteoma, hemangioma, or metastasis
  - Primary intraocular lymphoma
  - Retinoblastoma
- Iatrogenic
  - Scleral buckling
  - Excessive photocoagulation
- Miscellaneous
  - Bullous central serous choroidopathy
  - Uveal effusion syndrome
  - Nanophthalmos
  - Coloboma of the optic nerve
  - Familial exudative vitreoretinopathy
  - Topical prostaglandin use

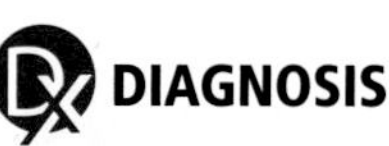

DIAGNOSIS

HISTORY

- A progressive, fluctuating loss of peripheral vision with a variable course is common. The fluid shifts with head position.
- Pain and a red eye may be present in inflammatory conditions (e.g., scleritis).
- A white pupillary reflex (leukocoria) may be noticed in a child with retinoblastoma.

PHYSICAL EXAM

- Dome-shaped elevation of the retina with transparent and smooth retinal walls, as opposed to the corrugated folds in RRD
- The subretinal fluid shifts according to head position.
- Associated signs:
  - Signs of inflammation:
    - Conjunctival injection and chemosis
    - Cell and flare in the anterior chamber
    - Vitreous cells
    - Retinal vascular sheathing
  - Dilated telangiectatic vessels
  - Retinal exudates
  - Solid tumor

DIAGNOSTIC TESTS & INTERPRETATION

Lab

Initial lab tests

Directed according to clinical presentation

- Complete metabolic panel
- PT, PTT, fibrinogen, antithrombin III, factors V and VII
- Inflammatory workup
  - Antinuclear antibodies
  - Antineutrophil cytoplasmic antibodies
  - Erythrocyte sedimentation rate
  - Rheumatoid factor
  - Angiotensin-converting enzyme
- Infectious
  - CBC with differential
  - Lyme titers
  - Venereal Disease Research Laboratory (VDRL) test and fluorescent treponemal antibody (FTA) test
  - Toxoplasma titers
  - CMV titers
  - Bartonella henselae and quintana titers
  - Purified protein derivative (PPD) placement

Imaging

Initial approach

- Ultrasonography
  - A-scan ultrasound
    - Retinal tissue will show a large spike.
    - Short axial length is indicative of nanophthalmos.
  - B-scan ultrasound
    - Helpful in cases in which the retina is not able to be visualized due to media opacity
    - Thickened sclera or choroid may be seen in scleritis, orbital inflammation, or VKH.
    - Calcification suggests retinoblastoma.

Follow-up & special considerations

- Fluorescein angiography (FA)
  - May reveal source of subretinal fluid and the nature of the defect causing it
- Optical coherence tomography (OCT)
  - Helpful in evaluating subretinal fluid

Diagnostic Procedures/Other

- Check blood pressure
- Slit lamp exam in detection of uveitis or vitritis
- Indirect ophthalmoscopy with scleral depression to rule out a retinal tear/RRD

Pathological Findings

- As the neurosensory retina separates from the RPE, the photoreceptors lose part of their blood supply and may degenerate.
- With a chronic RD, intraretinal cysts, RPE proliferation, and massive leakage into the retina and subretinal space occur.
- In an acute case of VKH syndrome, an eosinophilic exudate containing proteinaceous material is found in the subretinal space.
- The subretinal fluid in Coats' disease contains high levels of protein, albumin, and cholesterol.

DIFFERENTIAL DIAGNOSIS

- Retinoschisis
- RRD
- Tractional RD
- Choroidal detachment

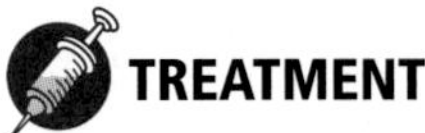

TREATMENT

MEDICATION

Treat the underlying condition

ADDITIONAL TREATMENT

General Measures

- Intravitreal injection of bevacizumab for SRD has been demonstrated to show a significant reduction in central foveal thickness and subretinal fluid with improved visual acuity (1)[B].
- Intravitreal injection of triamcinolone acetonide is an effective treatment of SRD in patients with central retinal vein occlusion (2)[B].

Issues for Referral

- Vitreoretinal specialist—laser and surgical treatment
- Immunologist or rheumatologist—when immunosuppressive therapy is considered.

SURGERY/OTHER PROCEDURES

Must be tailored toward the underlying condition

- Tumors (e.g., choroidal melanoma)
  - External beam radiation
  - Brachytherapy with plaque
  - Photodynamic therapy for choroidal hemangioma
- Vascular abnormalities (e.g., Coats' disease)
  - Laser photocoagulation
  - Cryotherapy
  - Vitrectomy
- Congenital abnormalities
  - Nanophthalmos
    - Vortex vein decompression with scleral windows and suprachoroidal fluid drainage
  - Optic pits or colobomas
    - Laser photocoagulation
    - Vitrectomy
- Central serous chorioretinopathy
  - Laser photocoagulation

IN-PATIENT CONSIDERATIONS

Initial Stabilization

Prior to surgery for SRD, patients should rest as much as possible.

Admission Criteria

Most vitreoretinal surgery is performed on an outpatient basis.

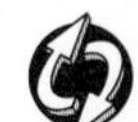

ONGOING CARE

PROGNOSIS

Depends on the underlying cause

- SRD secondary to preeclampsia or eclampsia usually resolves without any long-term complications.
- In patients with central serous chorioretinopathy, 15% have a visual acuity of 20/200 or worse.
- The SRD associated with optic pits has a poor prognosis secondary to the development of cystoid macular edema that may form.
- In Coats' disease, 75% of treated patients show an improvement or stabilization of vision from baseline; whereas, 30% of untreated patients may have stabilization (3)[B].

COMPLICATIONS

- Neovascular glaucoma
- Choroidal neovascularization
- Phthisis bulbi

REFERENCES

1. Song JH, Bae JH, Rho MI, et al. Intravitreal bevacizumab in the management of subretinal fluid associated with choroidal osteoma. *Retina* 2010;30(6):945–951.
2. Karacorlu M, Karacorlu SA, Ozdemir H, et al. Intravitreal triamcinolone acetonide for treatment of serous macular detachment in central retinal vein occlusion. *Retina* 2007;27(8):1026–1030.
3. Shields JA, Shields CL. Review: Coats disease: The 2001 LuEsther T. Mertz lecture. *Retina* 2002;22(1): 80–91.

ADDITIONAL READING

- McDonald HR, Schatz H, Johnson RN. Treatment of retinal detachment associated with optic pits. *Int Ophthalmol Clin* 1992;32(2):35–42.
- Ozdemir H, Karacorlu M, Karacorlu S. Serous macular detachment in central retinal vein occlusion. *Retina* 2005;25(5):561–563.
- Saito Y, Tano Y. Retinal pigment epithelial lesions associated with choroidal ischemia in preeclampsia. *Retina* 1998;18(2):103–108.
- Wang M, Munch IC, Hasler PW, et al. Central serous chorioretinopathy. *Acta Ophthalmol* 2008;86(2): 126–145.

CODES

ICD9

- 361.2 Serous retinal detachment
- 362.42 Serous detachment of retinal pigment epithelium

CLINICAL PEARLS

- In the case of SRD, it is imperative to obtain a good history and targeted review of system survey looking for underlying etiology.
- It is critical to rule out a retinal break in the case of an RRD as the management will be different.

Pregnancy Considerations

- Preeclampsia and SRD
  - In preeclampsia, there is intense vasoconstriction of the choroidal arterioles, leading to choroidal ischemia and RPE infarction. The outer blood–retinal barrier is broken down causing an increase in vascular permeability.
  - After delivery, the subretinal fluid is absorbed by the RPE pump, and the SRD usually resolves without any long-term complications.
  - In severe eclampsia, however, there may be extensive RPE necrosis, which may prevent the visual acuity from returning to baseline.

SERPIGINOUS

Avni Vyas

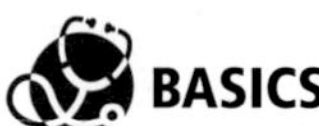

BASICS

DESCRIPTION

Typically a bilateral, chronic, recurrent inflammation of the retinal pigment epithelium (RPE), choriocapillaris, and choroid

EPIDEMIOLOGY

Incidence

- Rare. The incidence and prevalence are not well-established.
- Most reports suggest that cases of serpiginous choroiditis constitute less than 5% of cases of posterior uveitis. Prevalence may be higher in India as one Indian study reported that serpiginous choroiditis made up 19% of all cases of posterior uveitis (1)[A].
- Tends to occur in healthy young to middle-aged adults, more commonly males
- No racial or familial predisposition exists.

RISK FACTORS

No known risk factors

Genetics

One Finnish study suggests that HLA-B7 is more prevalent among patients with serpiginous choroiditis.

PATHOPHYSIOLOGY

Chronic, recurrent inflammation of the RPE, choriocapillaris, and choroid

ETIOLOGY

Unknown

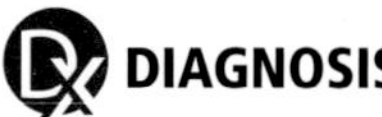

DIAGNOSIS

HISTORY

- Typically presents with unilateral vision loss, distortion, or scotoma. In the majority of cases, both eyes will eventually be affected.
- The disease course is chronic and progressive with recurrences in both eyes.

PHYSICAL EXAM

- Anterior segment exam usually appears quiet with no inflammation.
- Dilated exam classically shows subretinal lesions, which originate in the peripapillary region and spread centrifugally in a serpentine pattern. Macular and amphigenous variants of lesions also exist (see below).
- The visual outcome is related to the proximity of the lesions to the fovea and to the development of choroidal neovascularization.
  There are three main variants:
- Classic (peripapillary geographic)
  - Accounts for 80% of cases
  - Lesions begin as creamy subretinal infiltrates in the peripapillary region and spread centrifugally in a serpentine pattern.
  - Active lesions will resolve in 6–8 weeks (with or without treatment), resulting in atrophy of the affected choroid and RPE.
  - Recurrences generally occur at the edges of old scars and continue to spread in a serpentine pattern. Recurrences occur at variable intervals ranging from months to years.
  - Studies have suggested that the final visual acuity is less than 20/200 in up to 25% of treated eyes.
- Macular
  - Clinical and angiographic features are similar to classic serpiginous except that the lesions begin in the macula and are not continuous with the optic nerve.
  - Visual prognosis is worse than classic serpiginous because of earlier foveal involvement and higher risk of choroidal neovascularization.
- Atypical variants
  - Amphigenous—There is a subset of patients initially diagnosed with acute posterior multifocal placoid pigment epitheliopathy (APMPPE) who eventually developed serpiginous choroiditis. These patients tend to have less foveal involvement.
  - Relentless placoid chorioretinitis—There is a subset of patients with clinical features similar to amphigenous; however, the lesions affect the entire retina from the posterior pole to the periphery.

DIAGNOSTIC TESTS & INTERPRETATION

Lab

None

Imaging

- Fluorescein angiography (FA) and indocyanine green angiography(ICGA)
  - Active lesions (generally at the edges of older lesions) show early hypofluorescence and late staining on FA.
  - Old, atrophic lesions show early hypofluorescence and progressive hyperfluorescence at the margins with late staining of the underlying sclera on FA.
  - ICGA, which focuses on choroidal circulation, shows hypofluorescence of the lesions.
  - The reason for hypofluorescence of the lesions on FA and ICGA is not entirely known. Possible reasons include choroidal nonperfusion or blockage of perfusion by inflammatory cells.

- Visual fields
  - Visual field testing demonstrates scotomata corresponding to the lesions, which may become less dense over time.

DIFFERENTIAL DIAGNOSIS

- APMPPE
- Toxoplasmosis
- Tuberculosis
- Multifocal choroiditis
- Choroidal ischemia
- Sarcoidosis
- Syphilis

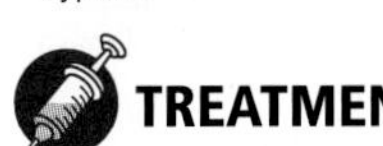

TREATMENT

MEDICATION

Many treatment regimens have been used but given the rarity of the disease and the chronic nature, there is limited data on long-term efficacy.

- Corticosteroids
  - Systemic, peribulbar, and intravitreal steroids are effective in treating active lesions and reducing the period of active disease (2)[A].
  - Relapses are common during steroid tapers or after steroids are stopped.
- Immunomodulatory agents
  - Various agents including methotrexate, cyclosporine A, azathioprine, and mycophenolate mofetil have been used for long-term management in steroid-dependent or resistant cases with good results. Some patients experience recurrences with tapering of immunosuppressive medications (3)[A].
  - Alkylating agents (cyclophosphamide and chlorambucil) were shown to be effective in managing serpiginous choroiditis. However, their use in the current management of this condition is limited by potentially severe adverse effects.

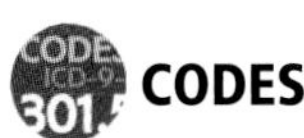

ONGOING CARE

FOLLOW-UP RECOMMENDATIONS

- Frequent follow-up is necessary to diagnose and treat recurrences or choroidal neovascularization.
- Patients should be instructed to call for worsening of vision, metamorphopsia, or new scotomas.

PROGNOSIS

- The disease process is chronic and progressive with multiple recurrences.
- Visual prognosis is guarded due to possible scarring/atrophy of the fovea and secondary choroidal neovascularization.

COMPLICATIONS

- The most common complication of serpiginous choroiditis is choroidal neovascularization, which occurs in 13–35% of patients.
- Reported complications include branch retinal vein occlusion, periphlebitis, pigment epithelial detachment, serous retinal detachment, cystoid macular edema, optic disc neovascularization, subretinal fibrosis, and anterior uveitis.

REFERENCES

1. Lim WK, Buggage RR, Nussenblatt RB. Serpiginous choroiditis. *Surv Ophthalmol* 2005;50:231–244.
2. Akpek EK, Ilhan-Sarac O. New treatments for serpiginous choroiditis. *Curr Opin Ophthalmol* 2003;14(3):128–131.
3. Akpek EK, Baltatzis S, Yang J, et al. Long-term immunosuppressive treatment of serpiginous choroiditis. *Ocul Immunol Inflamm* 2001;9:153–167.

CODES

ICD9

- 363.8 Other disorders of choroid
- 363.20 Chorioretinitis, unspecified

CLINICAL PEARLS

- Aggressive management of serpiginous choroiditis is critical to prevent significant vision loss.

SEVENTH CRANIAL NERVE PALSY

Scott Uretsky

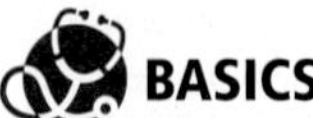

BASICS

DESCRIPTION

- The facial nerve is the VII cranial nerve.
  - Innervation:
    - Muscles of facial expression
    - Sympathetic efferents to lacrimal and salivary glands
    - Sensory afferents from tongue, external ear, and palate
    - Taste afferents from anterior two-thirds of tongue
  - Motor dysfunction causes ipsilateral facial paralysis
- Bell's Palsy (*Idiopathic*): Most common cause of unilateral facial paralysis
  - Acute to subacute (hours to days) onset of unilateral upper and lower facial weakness with variable symptoms of hyperacusis, dysgeusia, and dysfunctional lacrimation and salivation.
- Initial determinations:
  - Peripheral versus central
  - Accompanying clinical signs and symptoms indicating a non-idiopathic etiology
    - Non-isolated & central VII nerve palsy requires work-up

ALERT

Bilateral facial nerve palsy and concomitant additional cranial neuropathies require special attention.

EPIDEMIOLOGY

Incidence

11–40/100,000 per year (1)[A]; more common ages 15–45 years

Prevalence

None recently reported

RISK FACTORS

Bell's Palsy: Pregnancy, diabetes, influenza, upper respiratory infection

Genetics

- Bell's Palsy: Sparse reports of familial cases
- Mobius syndrome: Congenital facial diplegia + variable abducens nerve palsy; sporadic
- Myotonic dystrophy: Autosomal dominant trinucleotide (CTG) repeat expansion on 19q13.3

PATHOPHYSIOLOGY

Supranuclear, nuclear, infranuclear/peripheral dysfunction of the facial nerve

ETIOLOGY

Bell's Palsy: Idiopathic, possible viral-associated inflammation and/or demyelination

COMMONLY ASSOCIATED CONDITIONS

None known; see risk factors.

DIAGNOSIS

HISTORY

- Bell's Palsy: Isolated, acute to subacute onset of unilateral upper and lower facial weakness with variably manifested hyperacusis, dysgeusia, and dysfunctional lacrimation and salivation
  - Assess: Dysarthria, dysphagia, change of hearing and taste, ear and eye pain, diplopia, vertigo, ataxia, gait dysfunction, limb weakness, rashes, facial numbness, and pain
    - Myasthenia Gravis (MG): Variable ptosis and diplopia, fatigable extremity weakness
    - Demyelination/multiple sclerosis (MS): History of prior focal neurological deficits
    - Guillain-Barré Syndrome (GBS): Preceding GI or upper respiratory infection
  - Additional history: Trauma, neoplasia, ischemia, demyelinating disease
    - Guides appropriate work-up for secondary causes
  - Pain is atypical for Bell's Palsy
    - Consider Ramsay-Hunt Syndrome: HZV with vesicular eruption
  - Systemic symptoms

PHYSICAL EXAM

- Determine if palsy is central or peripheral and if palsy exists in isolation
  - At rest: Note asymmetry of muscle tone, blink pattern, widened palpebral fissure, flattened nasolabial fold, and lagophthalmus
- Motor activity: Smile and forced eyelid closure
  - Note decreased function on affected side; Bell's phenomenon
  - Asses forehead/frontalis function
    - Ask patient to raise/furrow eyebrows and brow
    - Central palsies do not affect function of forehead/frontalis; peripheral palsies do
- Examine corneal sensation and reflex
- Examine other cranial nerves: V, VI, and VIII are of particular importance for anatomic localization.
- Examine for long tract signs, for example, extremity weakness.

DIAGNOSTIC TESTS & INTERPRETATION

Lab

Initial lab tests

Serum glucose, syphilis serology, CBC, Lyme titer, ACE, HgbA1c

Follow-up & special considerations

Consider: ESR, CRP, ANA, anti-acetylcholine receptor Abs, mono spot test, ANCA, HIV, CSF analysis, serology/stool culture for *C. jejuni*

Imaging

Initial approach

- MRI is modality of choice to rule out secondary causes except in trauma cases (CT)
- Presentations requiring imaging
  - Slow or insidious onset of palsy
  - Central and bilateral nerve palsies
  - Multiple cranial neuropathies
  - Associated hearing loss and vertigo
  - Attention: Ischemia (diffusion weighted images), masses, CP angle, pachymeningeal enhancement (sarcoid), meningoencephalitis (Lyme), skull base, and brainstem

Follow-up & special considerations

Disease specific for secondary causes

Diagnostic Procedures/Other

- EMG: GBS & MG; include repetitive stimulation, consider single fiber EMG
- CSF: Pleocytosis (infectious/inflammatory), albuminocytologic dissociation (GBS), Lyme, Ig index and oligoclonal bands (MS), ACE (sarcoid) and infectious work-up as appropriate
- Edrophonium test and Ice test (MG)
- Chest x-ray (sarcoid related adenopathy)

Pathological Findings

Mobius syndrome: Aplasia/hypoplasia of cranial nerve nuclei

DIFFERENTIAL DIAGNOSIS

- Infectious, inflammatory/demyelinating, infiltrative, neoplastic/metastatic, compressive, traumatic, and idiopathic
  - Supranuclear: Ischemia, mass lesion
  - Nuclear: Pontine glioma, ischemia, hemorrhage, demyelination, vascular lesions
  - Infranuclear
    - Cerebellopontine (CP) angle: Acoustic schwannoma, meningioma, choleastoma, glomus jugulare tumor (can involve cranial nerves VII – XII)
    - Temporal bone/Skull base: Osteopetrosis, trauma, masses, Ramsay-Hunt syndrome, hemangioma, naso-pharyngeal carcinoma
    - Subarachnoid space: Carcinomatous meningitis, GBS, TB, sarcoid, Lyme
  - Other: MG, syphilis, parotid tumors, amyloid, sarcoma, diabetic mononeuropathy, HIV, lymphoma/leukemia, demyelination/MS, Paget's disease, arteriovenous malformation
- Bilateral VII Nerve palsy: Lyme disease, sarcoidosis, carcinomatous or infectious meningitis, GBS/Miller Fisher Syndrome, myasthenia gravis, leprosy, leukemia/lymphoma

Pediatric Considerations

- Acute otitis media

TREATMENT

MEDICATION

- Bell's Palsy: Antiviral agents (most commonly acyclovir or valacyclovir)
  - Incomplete facial motor function recovery at 1 year:
    - Antivirals versus (vs.) placebo: No significant difference: Relative Rate (RR): 0.88 (1)[A]
    - Antivirals and corticosteroids versus placebo: Significantly better outcomes: RR: 0.56 (1)[A]
    - Adverse events (antivirals vs placebo): No significant differences: RR: 1.06
    - Conclusions: Antivirals versus placebo: Do not enhance complete functional recovery (high quality); antivirals versus corticosteroids: Significantly less likely to produce complete recovery (moderate quality) (1)[A]
- Bell's Palsy: Corticosteroids
  - Incomplete facial motor function recovery $\geq$6 months:
    - Corticosteroids 23%, Placebo 33%; RR 0.71 (2)[A]
    - Motor synkinesis was significantly reduced with corticosteroids versus placebo: RR 0.6 (2)[A]
    - Conclusion: Evidence reveals significant benefit from corticosteroids (2)[A]
- Recommendations
  - Early initiation of corticosteroids is of benefit:
    - Sullivan et al. (3)[A]: Prednisolone 25 mg b.i.d for 10 days
    - Engstrom et al. (4)[A]: Prednisolone 60 mg daily $\times$ 5 days followed by 10 mg/day taper over 5 days
    - Antiviral therapy has no proven benefit; some practitioners recommend use in *severe or complete* palsies.

ADDITIONAL TREATMENT

General Measures

- Ophthalmic concerns: Prevention of exposure keratitis and corneal injury
  - Lubrication: Artificial tears, methylcellulose-based ointment, eye patching, and/or moisture chamber qhs.
  - Surgical management required with potential or ongoing corneal injury.

Issues for Referral

- Corneal exposure
- Acute nerve trauma or transection: Consider primary neurorrhaphy

COMPLEMENTARY & ALTERNATIVE THERAPIES

Acupuncture and physical therapy lack adequate evidence.

SURGERY/OTHER PROCEDURES

- Facial nerve decompression lacks sufficient evidence (5)
- Surgical management: Corneal sequela
  - Gold weight implant (upper lid) or tarsorrhaphy
    - For incomplete eyelid closure
    - Prevents and treats corneal injury

ONGOING CARE

FOLLOW-UP RECOMMENDATIONS

- Idiopathic/uncomplicated cases: 1–2 weeks, thereafter as appropriate.
- Corneal exposure requires ophthalmic monitoring.
  - *Corneal status dictates frequency:* Initial daily follow-up required for corneal breakdown or ulceration.

Patient Monitoring

Diabetics: Serum glucose monitoring during steroid therapy.

PATIENT EDUCATION

Prevention and symptoms of corneal injury

PROGNOSIS

- Bell's Palsy: Functional recovery excellent in $>$80%
  - Improved functional outcomes with incomplete palsies and early onset recovery ($<$3 weeks)
  - More complete palsies: Higher likelihood of incomplete recovery and aberrant regeneration
  - Poorer prognosis: Hyperacusis, decreased tearing, hypertension, age $>$60 years, diabetes, psychiatric disease, pregnancy
- Recovery dependent on site and extent of nerve injury
- EMG and nerve conduction studies: Preservation of motor amplitudes indicates axonal continuity and suggests good prognosis for recovery.

Pediatric Considerations

- Neoplastic and congenital etiologies associated with incomplete recovery

COMPLICATIONS

- Aberrant regeneration resulting in: Motor Synkinesis or Crocodile Tears
- Hemifacial Spasm
- Treatment: Chemodenervation with botulinum toxin

REFERENCES

1. Lockhart P, Daly F, Pitkethly M, et al. Antiviral treatment for Bell's palsy (idiopathic facial paralysis). *Cochrane Database Syst Rev* 2009; (4): CD001869. [A]
2. Salinas RA, Alvarez G, Daly F, et al. Corticosteroids for Bell's palsy (idiopathic facial paralysis). *Cochrane Database Syst Rev* 2010;(3):CD001942. [A]
3. Sullivan FM, Swan IRC, Donnan PT, et al. Early treatment with prednisolone or acyclovir in Bell's Palsy. *N Engl J Med* 2007;357:1598–1607. [A]
4. Engstrom M, Berg T, Stjernquist-Desatnik A, et al. Prednisolone and valaciclovir in Bell's palsy: A randomised, double-blind, placebo-controlled, multicentre trial. *Lancet Neurol* 2008;7:993–1000. [A]
5. Grogan P, Gronseth GS. Practice parameter: Steroids, acyclovir, and surgery for Bell's Palsy (an evidence-based review): Report of the Quality Standards Subcommittee of the AAN. *Neurology* 2001;56: 830–836.

ADDITIONAL READING

- Wang CH, Chang YC, Shih HM, et al. Facial palsy in children: Emergency department management and outcome. *Pediatr Emerg Care* 2010;26:121–125.
- Gilchrist JM. Seventh cranial neuropathy. *Semin Neurol*, 2009;29:5–13.
- Hazin R, Azizzadeh B, Bhatti, MT. Medical and surgical management of facial nerve palsy. *Curr Opin Ophthalmol* 2009;20:440–450.
- Rahman I, Sadiq SA. Ophthalmic management of facial nerve palsy: A review. *Surv Ophthalmol* 2007;52:121–144.

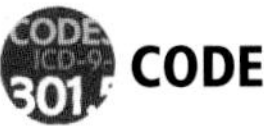

CODES

ICD9

- 351.0 Bell's palsy
- 351.8 Other facial nerve disorders
- 351.9 Facial nerve disorder, unspecified

CLINICAL PEARLS

- Differentiate central versus peripheral palsies
- Bell's Palsy treatment: Oral corticosteroids for 10 days $\pm$ antivirals for severe/complete palsies.
- Corneal health and protection must be monitored closely.

SJÖGREN'S SYNDROME

Apurva Patel
Frederick B. Vivino
Vatinee Y. Bunya

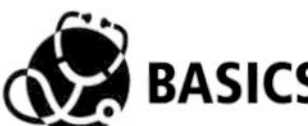

BASICS

DESCRIPTION

- Sjögren's syndrome is a chronic autoimmune disorder in which the body mistakenly attacks its own exocrine tear and salivary glands, leading to dry mouth (xerostomia) and dry eyes (keratoconjunctivitis sicca).
- In addition, patients can have systemic features involving multiple systems throughout the body including the skin, lungs, liver, kidneys, gastrointestinal tract, vasculature, blood, and nervous system.

EPIDEMIOLOGY

Incidence

Not well-defined.

Prevalence

- 1.3 million patients with primary Sjögren's in US (range 0.4–3.1 million)
- Prevalence rate 0.43% (0.13–1%)

RISK FACTORS

- Females are affected 9 times more frequently than males.
- Onset usually fourth to sixth decade of life.

Genetics

Familial predisposition possible, but no single gene has yet been identified.

PATHOPHYSIOLOGY

Lymphocytic infiltration and destruction of the lacrimal and salivary glands likely triggered by a viral and/or environmental cue in a genetically susceptible individual.

ETIOLOGY

Exact etiology unknown.
Commonly Associated Conditions

- Systemic lupus erythematosus, rheumatoid arthritis, mixed connective tissue disease, systemic sclerosis, autoimmune thyroid disease, autoimmune liver disease, inflammatory muscle disease, and leukocytoclastic vasculitis.
- When sicca symptoms (dry eyes and mouth) develop in patients with established connective tissue disease, the diagnosis is considered secondary Sjögren's syndrome.
- About 5% of patients develop non-Hodgkin B-cell lymphoma within 10 years of diagnosis.

DIAGNOSIS

HISTORY

- Symptoms of dry eye (burning, stinging, gritty feeling, artificial tear use)
- Symptoms of dry mouth
- History of rheumatic symptoms or severe fatigue

PHYSICAL EXAM

- Visual acuity
- Lid exam looking for coexisting meibomian gland disease or blepharitis
- Tear break-up time, abnormal if <10 seconds
- Staining of conjunctiva and cornea with lissamine green or rose bengal (note rose bengal may cause stinging and is less well-tolerated than lissamine green)
- Staining of conjunctiva and cornea with fluorescein
- Schirmer's test
  - Abnormal if unanesthetized and ≤ 5 mm at 5 minutes
  - Unanesthetized test measures basal and reflex tear secretion
  - With topical anesthetic, test measures basal tear secretion

DIAGNOSTIC TESTS & INTERPRETATION

Lab

Initial lab tests

- Autoantibodies
- Anti-Ro/SS-A or Anti-La/SS-B positive in 40–60% of patients with primary Sjögren syndrome
- ANA and RF-positivity may be seen in up to 90%

Follow-up & special considerations

Low complement C4 and cryoglobulins may be markers for lymphomas.

Imaging

- No ophthalmic diagnostic imaging indicated.
- Nuclear medicine salivary scintigraphy is useful in evaluation of xerostomia

Diagnostic Procedures/Other

- American–European Consensus Group Diagnostic Criteria (1)[C]
- 6 criteria:
  - Symptoms of aqueous tear insufficiency (dry eye for 3 months, foreign body sensation, artificial tear use $> 3 \times$ /d)
  - Oral symptoms (dry mouth for 3 months, swollen salivary glands, need to drink liquids to swallow food)
  - Ocular signs (unanesthetized Schirmer's test ≤ 5 mm at 5 minutes, rose bengal staining >4 on van Bijsterveld scale),
    - Van Bijsterveld scale sums amount of rose bengal staining in: Nasal conjunctiva, Temporal conjunctiva, and cornea. Each area is assigned a staining score of 0–3. Sum of scores equals total score (maximum score of 9).
  - Oral signs (abnormal salivary scintography, parotid sialography, or unstimulated salivary flow <1.5 mL in 15 minutes)
  - Minor salivary gland biopsy showing ≥ 1 conglomeration of >50 mononuclear cells in 4 mm^2 of glandular tissue.
- Autoantibodies: Positive anti-Ro/SS-A or anti-La/SS-B
- Primary Sjögren's syndrome is diagnosed in previously healthy individuals with sicca symptoms which arise de novo.
- Diagnosis of primary Sjögren's requires at least 4 positive criteria, one of which has to be histopathology or serum autoantibodies.
- Diagnosis of secondary Sjögren's requires at least 1 sicca symptom, an established connective tissue disease diagnosis, plus 3 signs of Sjögren's (see criteria 3–5 above).

Pathological Findings

- Lacrimal gland biopsy shows focal and/or diffuse lymphocytic infiltration. Advanced disease can show fibrous or fatty replacement of glandular structures.
- Labial salivary gland biopsy shows similar changes and is less invasive than lacrimal biopsy.

DIFFERENTIAL DIAGNOSIS

- Age-related or medication-induced dry eye and dry mouth.
- Thyroid eye disease
- Lacrimal infiltrative disease (amyloidosis, sarcoidosis, lymphoma)
- Other causes of ocular irritation (blepharitis, eyelid malposition, trichiasis)
- Hypovitaminosis A
- Other causes of dry mouth (e.g., mouth-breathing, radiation-induced xerostomia)

TREATMENT

MEDICATION

First Line

- Artificial tears (preservative-free if used more than 4x/day)
- Topical cyclosporine 0.05–1% 1 drop OU 2x/day (2)[A]
- Cyclosporine drops often burn on instillation; this usually improves with continued use.
- 10% N-acetylcysteine 1 drop 4x/day for filamentary keratitis.

Second Line

- Topical steroids (monitor for intraocular pressure elevation and cataract formation)
- Topical autologous serum drops
- Systemic immunomodulatory therapy including oral steroids, hydroxychloroquine, azathioprine, cyclophosphamide, methotrexate, and IV rituximab are used for systemic disease. Usually managed in consultation with a rheumatologist.
- Muscarinic agonists (pilocarpine PO 5 mg 3–4x/day or cevimeline 30mg PO 3x/day)

ALERT

Avoid prescribing medications with anti-cholinergic side effects that can exacerbate sicca symptoms.

ADDITIONAL TREATMENT

General Measures

- Humidified air
- Fish oil or flaxseed oil supplements
- Treat meibomian gland disease if present
- Warm compresses to eyelids twice daily for 5–10 minutes.
- Clean eyelid margin daily with commercial eyelid scrub or cotton swab moistened with baby shampoo and water.

Issues for Referral

- An ophthalmologist should be involved at baseline for evaluation of ocular criteria and then every 4–6 months, or more frequently as needed if dry eye symptoms and signs are uncontrolled with artificial tears.
- Refer patients with rheumatic symptoms and/or systemic disease to a rheumatologist.
- Refer pregnant patients who are anti-Ro/SS-A positive to a perinatologist for high-risk obstetric care.

COMPLEMENTARY & ALTERNATIVE THERAPIES

According to some studies, acupuncture may provide relief of rheumatic and/or sicca symptoms.

SURGERY/OTHER PROCEDURES

- Punctal occlusion or cautery
- Lateral tarsorrhaphy in severe cases

IN-PATIENT CONSIDERATIONS

Initial Stabilization

Inpatient admission usually unnecessary except for severe systemic disease.

ONGOING CARE

FOLLOW-UP RECOMMENDATIONS

- Follow every 4–6 months or more frequently depending on severity of disease.
- Warn patients of signs and symptoms of microbial keratitis, as there is a higher risk with corneal epithelial breakdown.
- Contact lenses may be worn with close observation once corneal epithelium is healed. Newer contact lenses designed for patients with dry eyes should be considered.

DIET

Omega-3 fatty acids have been shown to be beneficial in dry eye syndromes in general, and may be helpful in Sjögren's syndrome.

PATIENT EDUCATION

- Patients should understand that Sjögren's syndrome is most often a chronic condition whose symptoms are treatable, but not curable. Dry eye and dry mouth symptoms are usually manageable with medications. Follow-up with a rheumatologist and an ophthalmologist are important in maintaining systemic health and eye health.
- The Sjögren's Syndrome Foundation may be a useful resource for patients. www.sjogrens.org

PROGNOSIS

- Significant reduction but not always elimination of ocular symptoms with therapy as above.
- Systemic manifestations and lymphomas are treatable when diagnosed early.
- Mortality increased in lymphoma patients but equivalent to non-Sjögren's patients with lymphoma.

COMPLICATIONS

- Corneal surface breakdown causing corneal ulceration, scarring.
- Increased prevalence of lymphoma (5%).
- 25% of patients have extraglandular involvement (can be of any organ system).

Pediatric Considerations

Sjögren's syndrome may occur in children (about 300 reported cases) and most commonly presents as recurrent parotitis without sicca symptoms.

Pregnancy Considerations

Mothers who are anti-Ro/SS-A positive may give birth to infants with the neonatal lupus syndrome and should be followed by a perinatologist.

REFERENCES

1. Vitali C, Bombardieri S, Jonsson R, et al. Classification criteria for Sjögren's syndrome: A revised version of the European criteria proposed by the American–European Consensus Group. *Ann Rheum Dis* 2002;61:558–664.
2. Barber LD, Pflugfelder SC, Tauber J, et al. Phase III safety evaluation of cyclosporine 0.1% in ophthalmic emulsion administered twice daily to dry eye disease patients for up to 3 years. *Ophthalmology* 2005;112(10):1790–1794.

ADDITIONAL READING

- Kassan SS, Moutsopoulos HM. Clinical manifestations and early diagnosis of Sjögren syndrome. *Arch Intern Med* 2004;164:1275–1284.
- Foulks GN. Treatment of dry eye disease by the non-ophthalmologist. *Rheum Dis Clin North Am* 2008;34:987–1000.

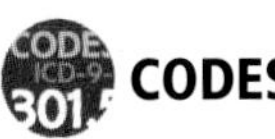

CODES

ICD9

710.2 Sicca syndrome

CLINICAL PEARLS

- There is a wide spectrum of dry eye disease, which can make distinguishing Sjögren's syndrome patients from other dry eye patients challenging. Consider the diagnosis in any patient with symptoms of dry eye and dry mouth, or with refractory or severe dry eye disease. Multidisciplinary evaluation is helpful in making the diagnosis of Sjögren's syndrome.
- The dry eye symptoms of Sjögren's syndrome dry eye can be well-managed with a regimen of lubricants, anti-inflammatory drops, and punctal occlusion or cautery. Some patients will require systemic medications and close collaboration with a rheumatologist to achieve symptom relief.
- Dry eye symptoms are a common presenting complaint to the ophthalmologist. Given the rate of undiagnosed Sjögren's syndrome (estimated at 50%), the ophthalmologist should be mindful of the diagnosis in all dry eye patients and make referrals to other healthcare providers as appropriate.

Note: Grade A recommendation for use in dry eye of any etiology, with a large fraction having Sjögren's syndrome. Grade B recommendation for use in dry eye due to Sjögren's specifically.

SOLAR RETINOPATHY

Gary Shienbaum

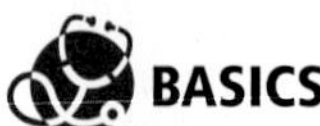

BASICS

DESCRIPTION

Phototoxicity of the retinal pigment epithelium (RPE) and photoreceptor layers in the fovea due to exposure to sunlight.

EPIDEMIOLOGY

Incidence

Uncommon, but clusters of cases appear around eclipses

RISK FACTORS

- Eclipse watching, sun gazing, sunbathing
- Emmetropia/low hypermetropia, aphakia
- Vocation (e.g., aviation, military [e.g., aircraft reconnaissance], astronomy)
- Photosensitizing medications (e.g., tetracyclines), mydriatics, hallucinogenic drugs (e.g., LSD)

GENERAL PREVENTION

Protective shading (e.g., hats, visors, filtering lenses/sunglasses)

PATHOPHYSIOLOGY

- Photochemical damage: resulting from the nonthermal effects of visible spectrum short wavelength (i.e., blue) light and ultraviolet radiation to the RPE and photoreceptor layers.
- Sun exposure is thought to cause thermal damage. Light absorption by the RPE results in a rise in temperature of the surrounding tissues. The exposure also causes formation of reactive oxygen species.

ETIOLOGY

See "Risk Factors" and "Pathophysiology."

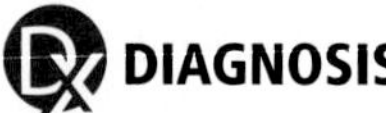

DIAGNOSIS

HISTORY

- Unprotected solar eclipse viewing, sun gazing (i.e., related to religious rituals, psychiatric illnesses, hallucinogenic drugs), sunbathing, vocational exposure (e.g., aviation, military service, astronomy)
- Decreased visual acuity, central/paracentral scotomata, dyschromatopsia, and metamorphopsia can occur following prolonged sun exposure.
- Typically bilateral

PHYSICAL EXAM

- Early:
  - Yellow–white spot in the fovea
    - Can have surrounding granular gray pigmentation.
- Late:
  - The acute findings resolve in several weeks. In the chronic stage, there is a variable appearance to the fovea (ranging from a normal appearance to a pigmentary disturbance or a pseudolamellar hole appearance).
  - A red, sharply demarcated, cyst-like lesion may persist.
  - Eyes with better initial visual acuities are more likely to have unremarkable funduscopic examinations at follow-up.

DIAGNOSTIC TESTS & INTERPRETATION

Imaging

- Fluorescein angiography:
  - Variable; may be unremarkable; window defects seen later in disease course.
- Optical coherence tomography:
  - Acute findings:
    - Hyporeflectivity at the level of the RPE/photoreceptor layer
    - Associated hyperreflectivity of the injured neurosensory retina has been described.
  - Chronic/late findings:
    - Central defect (hyporeflectivity) at the level of the photoreceptor inner segment–outer segment junction
    - Foveal atrophy

Pathological Findings

- Concentrated in foveal and parafoveal regions
  - Photoreceptors: swelling of outer segments, fragmentation of lamellae, mitochondrial swelling within the inner segments, nuclear pyknosis, and atrophy have been described.
  - RPE: irregular pigmentation/depigmentation and atrophy can occur.

DIFFERENTIAL DIAGNOSIS

- Macular hole
- Idiopathic macular telangiectasia type 2
- Cone dystrophy
- Age-related macular degeneration

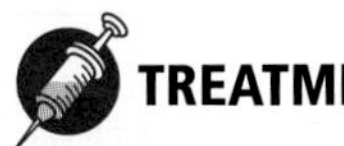

TREATMENT

None

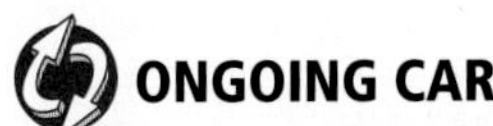

ONGOING CARE

FOLLOW-UP RECOMMENDATIONS

Monthly for the first few months, then as needed.

PATIENT EDUCATION

See "General Prevention."

PROGNOSIS

- Eyes with better visual acuities on initial examination tend to recover more vision.
- Central/paracentral scotomata can persist, despite improvement in visual acuity.
- Long-term significant reduction in visual acuity is rare.

REFERENCES

1. Yannuzzi LA, Fisher YL, Krueger A, et al. Solar retinopathy: A photobiological and geophysical analysis. *Trans Am Ophthalmol Soc* 1987;85:120–158.
2. Hope-Ross MW, Mahon GJ, Gardiner TA, et al. Ultrastructural findings in solar retinopathy. *Eye* 1993;7:29–33.
3. Garg SJ, Martidis A, Nelson ML, et al. Optical coherence tomography of chronic solar retinopathy. *Am J Ophthalmol* 2004;137:351–354.
4. Wu J, Seregard S, Algvere PV. Photochemical damage of the retina. *Surv Ophthalmol* 2006;51:461–481.
5. Jain A, Desai RU, Charalel RA, et al. Solar retinopathy: Comparison of optical coherence tomography (OCT) and fluorescein angiography (FA). *Retina* 2009;29:1340–1345.

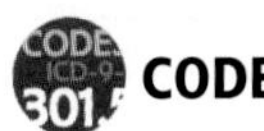

CODES

ICD9

363.31 Solar retinopathy

CLINICAL PEARLS

- Solar retinopathy can occur after prolonged sun exposure, and commonly clusters around natural phenomenon such as eclipses.
- Most patients retain good vision over time.

S

STARGARDT DISEASE

Christopher J. Brady

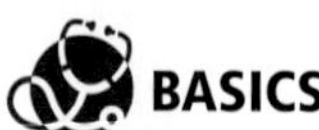

BASICS

DESCRIPTION

- The most common form of juvenile macular degeneration
- Causes vision loss in the first or second decade of life
- "Fundus flavimaculatus" is the descriptive term given to the retinal appearance often found with this condition. The term is usually synonymous with Stargardt disease, although some authors reserve this term for only those patients with the classic retinal appearance or patients with later onset disease.

EPIDEMIOLOGY

Prevalence

1/8,000–1/10,000

RISK FACTORS

- Usually autosomal recessive
- Classic disease linked to mutations in *ABCR* (also called *ABCA4*) on chromosome 1p13–p21.
- More than 400 sequence variations have been described.
- Mutations in this gene are also linked to autosomal recessive cone-rod dystrophy and retinitis pigmentosa.
- Autosomal dominant Stargardt-like diseases caused by mutations on chromosomes 13q, 6q, and 4p.

GENERAL PREVENTION

Genetic counseling may be of value to some families, but there are no strategies for prevention.

PATHOPHYSIOLOGY

- The *ABCR* gene codes for an ATP-binding cassette known as Rim protein (RmP) involved in vitamin A metabolism.
- Vitamin A is used by rod and cone photoreceptors in the outer retina.
- It is thought that *ABCR* mutations interfere with transport of vitamin A between the photoreceptors and underlying retinal pigment epithelium (RPE).
- Leads to a build-up of lipofuscin in RPE cells.
- The disease affects the macula and fovea preferentially due to the high concentration of photoreceptors in the area of central fixation.

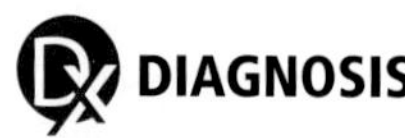

DIAGNOSIS

HISTORY

Patients describe slowly progressive vision loss. There may be affected siblings, although strong family history is uncommon given autosomal recessive inheritance.

PHYSICAL EXAM

- The fundus exam may appear completely normal. For this reason, some patients are suspected of malingering.
- Typical retinal changes are usually bilateral and include the following:
  - Nonspecific foveal RPE mottling, which may take on a "beaten bronze" appearance.
  - Ill-defined, yellow-white deep retinal "flecks" at the level of the RPE, referred to as "pisciform" for their fish-like shape.
  - More advanced disease may have an atrophic macula with a "bull's eye" or geographic atrophy appearance.

DIAGNOSTIC TESTS & INTERPRETATION

Lab

Genetic testing is generally not performed for this condition given the large size of the *ABCR* gene and the diversity of known mutations.

Diagnostic Procedures/Other

- Intravenous fluorescein angiography (IVFA) often reveals a "dark choroid," in which retinal blood vessels are highlighted against a hypofluorescent background due to the accumulation of lipofuscin the RPE cells. This sign is highly specific for this condition, but the absence of this sign does not exclude the diagnosis.
- Fundus autofluorescence photography often reveals hypoautofluorescence at the level of fovea corresponding to RPE atrophy. This is usually surrounded by small flecks of hyperautofluorescence, which may outnumber those flecks seen clinically.
- IVFA may also reveal hyperfluorescent flecks corresponding to RPE atrophy, which may become confluent in advanced disease.
- Full-field ERG (electroretinogram) is usually normal but the photopic (bright-adapted) ERG may be slightly abnormal. Multifocal ERG may show decreased amplitudes corresponding to central vision.
- EOG (electrooculogram) may be slightly abnormal in advanced cases.

Pathological Findings

- Light microscopy reveals a loss of photoreceptors and RPE cells.
- RPE cells in the posterior pole are also irregular in size and shape with intracytoplasmic PAS-positive granules of lipofuscin.

DIFFERENTIAL DIAGNOSIS
- Fundus albipunctatus: flecks in the midperipheral retina, nonprogressive congenital night blindness
- Retinitis punctata albescens: similar appearance to fundus albipunctatus with severe, progressive vision loss
- Drusen: Small yellow-white spots in macula. Usually develop later in life. Hyperfluorescent on IVFA.
- Cone or cone-rod dystrophy: Can present with "bull's eye" maculopathy. Significant color vision loss, abnormal ERG.
- Chloroquine/hydroxychloroquine toxicity: Can present with "bull's eye" maculopathy
- Batten disease and Spielmeyer–Vogt syndrome: Autosomal recessive lysosomal storage disease. Can produce "bull's eye" maculopathy.
- Functional vision loss: Normal exam and testing. Special techniques can unmask better vision than claimed.

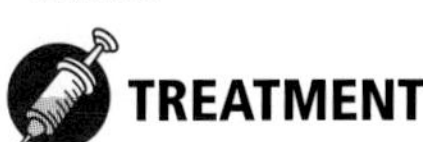

TREATMENT

MEDICATION
- There are no treatments for this disease. Low vision referral may be of great value. UV protection is generally recommended.
- As the genetics are further understood, this disease may be amenable to gene therapy.

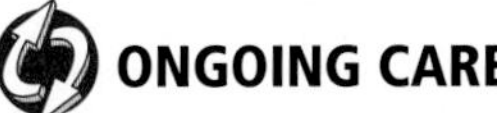

ONGOING CARE

FOLLOW-UP RECOMMENDATIONS
- Ophthalmologic exams
- Low vision
- Services for the blind
- Fundus autofluorescence photography may be of value in assessing disease activity.

PATIENT EDUCATION
- http://www.macular.org/stargardts.html
- http://www.lowvision.org/stargardts.htm

PROGNOSIS
- Stargardt disease is a chronic disease with poor visual prognosis.
- Once visual acuity drops below 20/40 it tends to decrease rapidly, then stabilize near 20/200.

COMPLICATIONS
Central vision loss

REFERENCES

1. Boon CJ, Jeroen Klevering B, Keunen JE, et al. Fundus autofluorescence imaging of retinal dystrophies. *Vision Res* 2008;48:2569–2577.
2. Koenekoop RK. The gene for Stargardt disease, ABCA4, is a major retinal gene: a mini-review. *Ophthalmic Genet* 2003;24:75–80.
3. Walia S, Fishman GA. Natural history of phenotypic changes in Stargardt macular dystrophy. *Ophthalmic Genet* 2009;30:63–68.
4. Westerfeld C, Mukai S. Stargardt's disease and the ABCR gene. *Semin Ophthalmol* 2008;23:59–65.

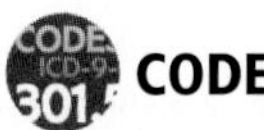

CODES

ICD9
- 362.75 Other dystrophies primarily involving the sensory retina
- 362.76 Dystrophies primarily involving the retinal pigment epithelium

CLINICAL PEARLS
- Most common juvenile macular dystrophy
- Autosomal recessive inheritance
- Vision usually stabilizes around 20/400
- No treatments available, potential gene therapy in the future
- Low vision referral of value

STEROID-INDUCED GLAUCOMA

Robert J. Goulet, III
Anand Mantravadi

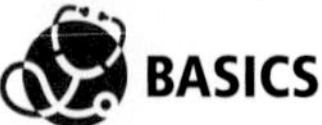

BASICS

DESCRIPTION
Steroid-induced glaucoma is a secondary open-angle glaucoma that results after the use of local or systemic corticosteroids. Intraocular pressure (IOP) increase results from decreased aqueous humor outflow facility. Glaucomatous optic neuropathy can then develop from this ocular hypertension.

EPIDEMIOLOGY
Incidence
- Incidence of IOP rise varies with route of administration, formulation of medication, and total cumulative dose.
- 5% of people treated with topical steroids for 4–6 weeks show an IOP rise of ≥16 mm Hg, 30% show an IOP rise of 6–15 mm Hg
- Intravitreal > periocular > topical > systemic
- Intravitreal triamcinolone acetonide (4 mg)—14.6–44.6%
- Prednisolone acetate (1%)—6.7%
- Loteprednol etabonate (0.2 and 0.5%)—1.7%
- Case reports with inhaled, intravenous, oral, and topical corticosteroid use

Prevalence
Unknown

RISK FACTORS
- Diagnosis of primary open-angle glaucoma
- First-degree relative with primary open-angle glaucoma
- High baseline IOP
- Traumatic angle recession
- High myopia
- Connective tissue disease
- Type 1 diabetes mellitus
- Children
- Elderly

Genetics
- No clear genetic component
- Myocilin may be overexpressed by meshwork cells when exposed to steroids and myocilin gene mutations have been associated with juvenile and adult-onset glaucomas.

GENERAL PREVENTION
- Be aware of those populations at risk.
- Limit exposure to necessary corticosteroids.
- Use formulations less likely to cause IOP rise.

PATHOPHYSIOLOGY
- Decreased aqueous humor outflow facility
- Possible architectural changes of the trabecular meshwork (i.e., actin crosslinking)
- Possible deposition of material in the trabecular meshwork (i.e., glycosaminoglycans)
- Possible decreased phagocytic function of trabecular meshwork cells with decreased ability to remove material accumulated in the meshwork

ETIOLOGY
Unknown

COMMONLY ASSOCIATED CONDITIONS
Any requiring use of corticosteroids

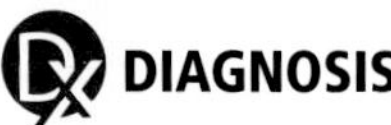

DIAGNOSIS

HISTORY
- Patient being treated with topical or systemic corticosteroids. Do not forget to inquire about depositions (intravitreal, periocular) or inhalational, intranasal, or dermatologic formulations. Attempt to identify those patients that are at higher risk of developing elevated IOP with steroid use.
- Presentation may be within 1 week of initiating therapy but may be delayed up to years later.
- Typical time to presentation for ophthalmic drop formulations is 3–8 weeks

PHYSICAL EXAM
- IOP elevated from baseline
- If asymmetric optic nerve damage exists, there may be a relative afferent pupillary defect
- Slit lamp exam will likely be within normal limits or no change from patient baseline
- Gonioscopy will be consistent with patient baseline
- Examination of the optic nerve may show evidence of typical glaucomatous damage (diffuse narrowing of the neuroretinal rim, focal notches, disc hemorrhage). Prior glaucomatous damage makes the nerve more susceptible to further damage at lower IOP increases for shorter durations.

DIAGNOSTIC TESTS & INTERPRETATION
Imaging
Optic nerve head imaging (i.e., confocal scanning laser ophthalmoscopy) or retinal nerve fiber layer imaging (optical coherence tomography or scanning laser polarimetry) may be used in conjunction with optic nerve exam to evaluate for glaucomatous damage.

Diagnostic Procedures/Other
- Standardized visual fields should be obtained to assess for evidence of glaucomatous functional deficits.
- Pachymetry

Pathological Findings
None

DIFFERENTIAL DIAGNOSIS
- Primary open-angle glaucoma
- Uveitic glaucoma

TREATMENT

MEDICATION

First Line

- Cessation of steroids if possible. Tapering to a lower dose can ultimately result in reduction in pressure.
- Beta-adrenergic antagonists (topical)
  - Timolol maleate 0.25–0.5%, one drop daily or b.i.d.
  - Betaxolol 0.25%, one drop b.i.d.
- Alpha2-adrenergic agonists (topical)
  - Brimonidine tartrate 0.15%, one drop b.i.d. or t.i.d.
- Carbonic anhydrase inhibitors (topical)
  - Dorzolamide 2.0%, one drop b.i.d. or t.i.d.
  - Brinzolamide 1%, one drop b.i.d. or t.i.d.
- Prostaglandin analogues/prostamides (topical)
  - Latanoprost 0.005%, one drop qHS
  - Travoprost 0.004%, one drop qHS
  - Bimatoprost 0.03%, one drop qHS
- Combinations (topical)
  - Dorzolamide/timolol maleate 2%/0.5%, one drop b.i.d.
  - Brimonidine tartrate/timolol maleate 2%/0.5%, one drop b.i.d.

Second Line

- Carbonic anhydrase inhibitors (systemic)
  - Acetazolamide 125–250 mg po b.i.d. to q.i.d.
  - Acetazolamide sequels 500 mg po b.i.d.
  - Acetazolamide (parenteral) 500 mg IV once daily or 5–10 mg/kg q6–8h
  - Methazolamide 50–100 mg po b.i.d. to t.i.d.
- Hyperosmotic agents
  - Mannitol 20% solution, 0.5–2 mg/kg IV infused over 30–60 minutes (20% solution has 20 g per 100 mL)

ADDITIONAL TREATMENT

Additional Therapies

Selective laser trabeculoplasty (SLT) may be effective in some patients. One must consider the potential for IOP rise after SLT and the urgency in which the patient's IOP must be lowered.

SURGERY/OTHER PROCEDURES

- Trabeculectomy with antifibrotic agents (mitomycin C)
- Aqueous drainage device implantation (Baerveldt shunt, Ahmed valve, Molteno implant, etc.)

ONGOING CARE

FOLLOW-UP RECOMMENDATIONS

- Patients should be followed closely after the administration of steroids, especially those receiving intravitreal, periocular, and topical formulations.
- Appropriate follow-up has been suggested to be 2 weeks after steroids are administered. Patients determined to be at higher risk should be examined sooner and more often (after 1, 4, and 8 weeks).
- Generally, lowering IOP below 30 mm Hg is a reasonable goal for individuals without optic nerve damage.
- Preexisting or newly diagnosed glaucomatous damage to the optic nerve warrants more aggressive treatment. In general, IOP should be maintained at or below target IOP as determined in glaucoma patients before starting steroids.

Patient Monitoring

- Serial examinations in which visual function, IOP, and optic nerve are evaluated
- Repeat visual fields as necessary

PATIENT EDUCATION

Patients should be counseled on their risk of IOP rise and the potential of irreversible vision loss via optic nerve damage before implementation of therapy.

PROGNOSIS

Prognosis depends on level of IOP rise and amount of optic nerve damage. With regular monitoring and appropriately aggressive therapy, loss of visual function can frequently be avoided.

COMPLICATIONS

- Visual field constriction
- Vision loss

S

REFERENCES

1. Spaeth GL, de Barros M, Fudemberg S.*Retina* 2009;29(8):1057–1061.
2. Jones R III, Rhee D.*Curr Opin Ophthalmology* 2006;17(2):163–167.
3. Stamper R, Lieberman M, Drake M.*Becker-Shaffer's diagnosis and therapy of the glaucomas*. 270–271.

CODES

ICD9

365.31 Corticosteroid-induced glaucoma, glaucomatous stage

STEVENS–JOHNSON SYNDROME

Bhairavi V. Kharod

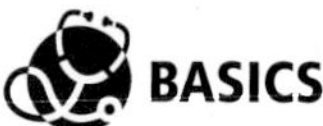

BASICS

DESCRIPTION

- Stevens–Johnson syndrome (SJS) was first described in 1922.
- SJS is a rare life-threatening immune complex–mediated hypersensitivity reaction in which the skin and mucous membranes are severely affected.
- SJS is often referred to as erythema multiforme major or bullous erythema multiforme.

EPIDEMIOLOGY

Incidence

- The reported annual incidence of SJS is approximately 3 cases per million persons per year.
- In the US, approximately 300 new cases of SJS are reported each year.

Prevalence

The prevalence of SJS is reported to be less than 200,000 persons in the US population.

RISK FACTORS

- Immunocompromised status, including malignancies, chronic viral infections with Epstein–Barr virus (EBV) and HIV, systemic lupus erythematosus, and other chronic rheumatologic diseases are considered risk factors.
- Radiation therapy and ultraviolet (UV) light are also considered possible risk factors.
- Previous history of SJS is considered a risk factor for further episodes.

Genetics

Certain HLA subtypes are currently being researched for possible associations with SJS. In some studies, HLA-B12 has been shown to increase susceptibility to SJS.

GENERAL PREVENTION

Early diagnosis, treatment, and supportive therapy are essential to prevent life-threatening complications and permanent damage from SJS.

PATHOPHYSIOLOGY

- SJS is an immune complex–mediated hypersensitivity reaction.
- Cell death causes separation of the epidermis from the dermis.

ETIOLOGY

- Although the cause of SJS may not be determined in some case, it is most often a response to medication, infection, or illness.
- SJS is idiopathic in approximately 50% of the cases.
- The leading cause of SJS is the use of antibiotics and sulfa drugs. Some of the common medications that cause SJS include allopurinol, diclofenac, isotretinoin, fluconazole, penicillins, barbiturates, sulfonamides, phenytoin, and azithromycin.
- Infectious causes of SJS include herpes simplex virus, EBV, influenza, mumps, histoplasmosis, and cat scratch fever.
- Certain lymphomas and carcinomas have also been reported to be the inciting factors for SJS.
- In some studies, herbal supplements containing ginseng have been shown to cause SJS as a rare side effect. Others report cocaine as a possible cause.

COMMONLY ASSOCIATED CONDITIONS

SJS can involve the mucous membrane and skin of multiple organs. Significant involvement of ocular, nasal, oral, vaginal, urethral, gastrointestinal, and respiratory tract mucous membranes can occur over the course of the disease. Necrosis of mucous membranes, especially respiratory and gastrointestinal membranes, may occur over the course of the disease. This can lead to significant morbidity and may lead to death.

DIAGNOSIS

HISTORY

- SJS often begins with flu-like symptoms. Patients may often experience fever, malaise, cough, sore throat, headache, and burning eyes for a few days. Mucocutaneous lesions develop abruptly.
- Patients with oral involvement may complain of severe pain that leads to inability to eat or drink.
- Patients with genitourinary tract involvement may present with dysuria or inability to void.

PHYSICAL EXAM

- Ophthalmic findings:
  - Conjunctivitis of the eyes is reported in approximately 30%.
  - Conjunctival scarring, including symblepharon formation may occur.
  - Pseudomembranes may form on palpebral conjunctiva.
  - Dry eyes and trichiasis are chronic **sequelae**.
  - Corneal neovascularization, corneal scarring, anterior uveitis, panuveitis, and severe visual impairment may occur.
- Systemic findings:
  - Patients may often get tongue and facial swelling.
  - Oral ulcers are common, but ulcers of genital and anal areas may also occur.
  - Skin involvement may start with hives and pain. A red or purple skin nonpruritic rash develops and spreads within hours to days. Papules, vesicles, or bullae may form leading to sloughing of the epidermis. The typical skin lesion of SJS is target shaped. Most commonly affected areas are the palms, soles, dorsum of the hands, and extensor surfaces.
  - Denuded skin may develop a secondary infection.

DIAGNOSTIC TESTS & INTERPRETATION

Lab

- Although SJS may often be medication induced, it is important to rule out infectious etiologies and malignancies.
- Blood and urine cultures should be done in cases where an infectious cause is suspected.
- Sputum cultures should be done in patients with a high index of suspicion for Mycoplasma pneumoniae.
- HIV and EBV testing should be done in patients suspected of these diseases.
- CBC count and workup of malignancy should be performed.
- A tissue biopsy is performed in many cases.

Imaging

Imaging is rarely required, except in cases where a malignancy is suspected.

Pathological Findings

- Biopsy specimens typically show full thickness necrosis of epidermis and minimal dermal inflammatory cell infiltration. The dermal infiltrate is superficial and mostly perivascular.
- Histologic changes in the epidermal–dermal junction range from vacuolar alteration to subepidermal blisters.
- Apoptosis of keratinocytes is also observed.

DIFFERENTIAL DIAGNOSIS

- Erythema multiforme minor (involvement of skin only. SJS, or erythema multiforme major, is defined as involvement of both skin and mucous membranes. SJS is often referred to as bullous erythema multiforme.)
- Drug rash
- Thermal burns
- Paraneoplastic pemphigus
- Toxic shock syndrome
- Ocular cicatricial pemphigoid
- Toxic epidermal necrolysis (TEN) (SJS and TEN are considered similar except for their distribution. SJS is defined as <10% of body surface area involvement. TEN is defined by >30% of body surface area involvement. Involvement of 15–30% of body surface area is considered SJS–TEN overlap.)

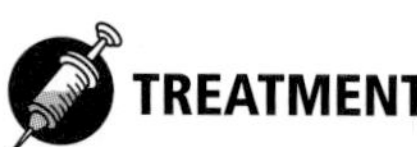

TREATMENT

MEDICATION

First Line

- SJS is a dermatologic emergency that requires hospitalization, often in an intensive care unit or burn unit.
- Often the first and most important step in treating SJS is to discontinue any offending medications.
- Supportive care is a crucial part of treating SJS. Because skin loss can lead to significant loss of body fluid, fluid replacement is essential. A nasogastric tube may be needed for enteral feedings.
- Ophthalmic care should include a thorough eye exam. If a patient has conjunctivitis, pseudomembranes, or other ocular surface disease, topical steroids should be used judiciously. Pseudomembranes should be peeled. Symblepharon should be lysed using a blunt instrument such as a glass rod. A symblepharon ring should be placed to avoid further symblepharon formation. Oral or intravenous corticosteroids should be considered in patients with ocular disease. Patients with uveitis should be treated with steroids.

Second Line
- Skin lesions should be cleaned thoroughly and protected from secondary infections.
- Patients with SJS often have severe pain from mucocutaneous lesions and should be given adequate pain control.
- Intravenous steroids are used by many in acute SJS. In cases of recalcitrant SJS, intravenous immunoglobulin has been proposed by some to be beneficial.
- Cyclophosphamide may be used in chronic conditions.
- Patients on steroids should be placed on gastrointestinal prophylaxis and should be considered at risk for bone mass loss.

ADDITIONAL TREATMENT
General Measures
- Early diagnosis and treatment are crucial to decreasing morbidity and mortality in patients with SJS.
- Patients should be monitored closely to avoid sepsis, shock, and organ failure.

Issues for Referral
Dermatologists and ophthalmologists are consulted for patients with SJS. Specialists are consulted according to the organs involved.

IN-PATIENT CONSIDERATIONS
Initial Stabilization
- SJS is a medical emergency that can rapidly evolve into shock and end-organ damage/failure.
- Treatment should focus on eliminating the underlying cause, controlling symptoms, and minimizing complications.

Admission Criteria
Patients with SJS can rapidly develop shock and end-organ failure and should be monitored very closely.

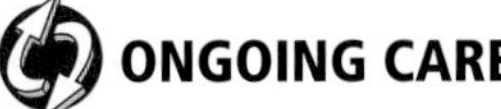

ONGOING CARE

FOLLOW-UP RECOMMENDATIONS
- Patients have to be monitored very closely in the initial stages of SJS.
- Patients should be monitored closely by an ophthalmologist as symblepharon formation, trichiasis, corneal neovascularization, and scarring can develop.

Patient Monitoring
- CBC count should be performed weekly for the first 1–2 months in patients on oral cyclophosphamide to evaluate for leukopenia.
- Urinalysis should be performed periodically to evaluate for hemorrhagic cystitis.

DIET
Many patients have difficulty swallowing in the initial stages of SJS secondary to involvement of the gastrointestinal tract. Enteral feeding may be required until the patient can tolerate oral feedings.

PATIENT EDUCATION
- Patients should be advised of the inciting factor (medication, infection, etc.) and should be told to avoid the inciting factor.
- Patients should be informed of the increased risk of SJS with the use of certain medications.

PROGNOSIS
The mortality in patients with SJS correlates to the body surface area involved. If less than 10% of the body surface is denuded, the mortality rate is approximately 1–5%. If more than 30% of the body surface is denuded, the mortality rate increases to more than 25%.

REFERENCES

1. Wetter DA, Camilleri MJ. Clinical, etiologic, and histopathologic features of Stevens-Johnson syndrome during an 8-year period at Mayo Clinic. *Mayo Clin Proc* 2010;85(2):131–138.
2. Sotozono C, Ueta M, Kinoshita S. Systemic and local management at the onset of Stevens-Johnson syndrome and toxic epidermal necrolysis with ocular complications. *Am J Ophthalmol* 2010; 149(2):354.
3. Knowles S, Shear NH. Clinical risk management of Stevens-Johnson syndrome/toxic epidermal necrolysis spectrum. *Dermatol Ther* 2009;22(5):441–451.
4. Struck MF, Hilbert P, Mockenhaupt M, et al. Severe cutaneous adverse reactions: emergency approach to non-burn epidermolytic syndromes. *Intensive Care Med* 2010;36(1):22–32. Epub 2009 Sep 29.

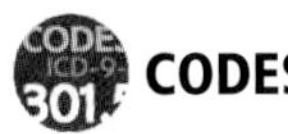

CODES

ICD9
- 372.30 Conjunctivitis, unspecified
- 372.64 Scarring of conjunctiva
- 695.13 Stevens-Johnson syndrome

CLINICAL PEARLS

- SJS is a mucocutaneous disease that can affect multiple organs.
- Drugs, especially sulfa drugs, antiepileptics, and antibiotics, are the most common causes.
- SJS can cause severe morbidity and mortality if left untreated.

STICKLER SYNDROME

Scott E. Olitsky
Erin D. Stahl

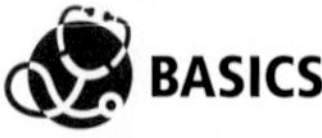

BASICS

DESCRIPTION

Constellation of findings including particular vitreous abnormalities, high myopia, and retinal detachment

EPIDEMIOLOGY

Incidence

1 in 7,500–9,000 newborns

RISK FACTORS

Genetics

- Type 1: STL1 (classic, membranous vitreous) 12q13.11–13.2, *COL2A1* gene, autosomal dominant
- Type 2: STL2 (+/- ocular, beaded vitreous) 1p21, *COL11A1*, autosomal dominant
- Type 3: STL3 (nonocular) 6p21.3, *COL11A2*, autosomal dominant
- Autosomal recessive form with ocular involvement, 6q13, *COL9A1*
- Mutations in *COL11A2* also cause variants: Weissenbacher–Zweymuller syndrome (neonatal form with distinctive skeletal findings), Marshall syndrome (short stature, hearing loss), Marshall/Stickler

GENERAL PREVENTION

- Genetic counseling and/or prenatal testing (if mutation in family known)
- Fetal facial abnormalities may be detected by ultrasound in the second trimester (1).

PATHOPHYSIOLOGY

Defect in collagen biosynthesis collagen types 2, 9, and 11 expressed in vitreous. *COL2A1* mutations must involve exon 2 for eye involvement as this exon is not incorporated in nonocular tissues.

COMMONLY ASSOCIATED CONDITIONS

- Ocular
  - Myopia (90%) (2), with or without pathologic myopia
  - Vitreous condensation (membranous, beaded, veils)
  - "Optically empty" vitreous
  - Retinal detachment (60%) (2)
  - Glaucoma
  - Cataract (usually peripheral cortical wedge)
  - Radial retinal lattice
  - Rare: retinal degeneration
- Nonocular
  - Hearing loss (70%) (2)
  - Facial abnormalities (midline clefting, Pierre Robin sequence, bifid uvula) (84%) (2)
  - Mitral valve prolapse
  - Arthritis, large joints (90%) (2)
  - Slender extremities, long fingers, and normal/tall height

DIAGNOSIS

HISTORY

Family and patient history of high myopia, retinal detachment, arthritis, cleft palate, hearing loss

PHYSICAL EXAM

- Full ocular examination including attention to vitreous abnormalities at slit lamp (veils [best by indirect ophthalmoscopy], beading, membranes optical clarity)
  - Cycloplegic refraction
  - Peripheral retinal examination looking for perivascular lattice-like degeneration and retinal breaks
  - Intraocular pressure (IOP) measurement and optic nerve examination
  - Physical exam with attention to joint dysfunction, abnormal facial features, hearing, clefting of palate/uvula, and heart murmur

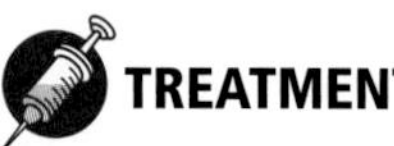

TREATMENT

MEDICATION

- None for the primary disorder but may need treatment for secondary concerns such as glaucoma
- Avoid miotics to avoid additional strain on the peripheral vitreoretinal interface.

ADDITIONAL TREATMENT

General Measures

- Refractive correction, treatment of amblyopia (if present), low vision aids if necessary
- Educate patient on warning signs and symptoms of retinal detachment.
- Every 6 months to yearly full ocular examination with dilated fundus exam, optic nerve evaluation, refraction, and IOP measurement

SURGERY/OTHER PROCEDURES

- Surgical repair of retinal detachment—retinal detachment may reveal multiple severe retinal breaks, prompt referral to retinal specialist is necessary.
- Prophylactic retinopexy, if indicated
- Cataract extraction—NOTE: elevated risk for postoperative retinal detachment
- Medical/surgical treatment of glaucoma

ONGOING CARE

FOLLOW-UP RECOMMENDATIONS

- Educate patient on the need for routine (every 6 months to yearly) ophthalmologic examination to detect retinal breaks.
- Prompt evaluation should symptoms of impending retinal detachment occur (floaters, photopsia, vision changes)
  - Genetics consult
  - Maxillofacial assessment for midline clefting if suspected
  - Rheumatology consult if joint disease present
  - Audiology for hearing testing
  - Examine parents/siblings (3)

PATIENT EDUCATION

- Educate on the signs and symptoms of retinal detachment and the need for prompt examination if these occur.
- Some ophthalmologists may recommend avoidance of direct contact sports such as boxing and wrestling to reduce the risk of retinal detachment (no clear data, practice patterns vary).
- Consider recommendation against refractive surgery as tissue response is unknown and may have thinner central cornea thickness.
- May benefit from protective eyewear when engaging in other sports
- Genetic counseling
- Family support network http://www.sticklers.org/sip2

PROGNOSIS

- Risk for retinal detachment is greater than 50%.
- Morbidity most common from visual dysfunction, 4% blind (1)
- Visual acuity depends on incidence of retinal detachment and success in surgical management.
- Decreased visual acuity may also occur due to refractive amblyopia if refractive error is not corrected.

COMPLICATIONS

- Retinal detachment
- Glaucoma
- Cataract

REFERENCES

1. Parke DW. Stickler syndrome: clinical care and molecular genetics. *Am J Ophthalmol* 2002;134(5):746–748.
2. Stickler GB, Hughes W, Houchin P. Clinical features of hereditary progressive arthro-ophthalmology (Stickler syndrome): a survey. *Genetics Med* 2001;3(3):192–196.
3. Snead MP, Yates JR. Clinical and molecular genetics of Stickler syndrome. *J Mol Genet* 1999;36:353–359.

ADDITIONAL READING

- http://ghr.nlm.nih.gov/condition = sticklersyndrome.

CODES

ICD9

- 367.1 Myopia
- 379.29 Other disorders of vitreous
- 759.89 Other specified congenital anomalies

CLINICAL PEARLS

- High risk for retinal detachment
- Consider genetics consult and counseling.
- Examine parents/siblings for vitreoretinal abnormalities.
- Educate patient and family on signs and symptoms of retinal detachment.
- Stress importance of regular ocular examination.

S

STURGE–WEBER SYNDROME

Jason Hsu

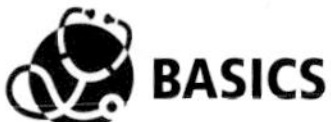

BASICS

DESCRIPTION

- Sturge–Weber syndrome (SWS), also called encephalotrigeminal angiomatosis, is a congenital dermato-oculo-neural syndrome.
  - Cutaneous nevus flammeus in distribution of trigeminal nerve branches
  - Ipsilateral glaucoma and diffuse choroidal hemangioma may occur.
  - Ipsilateral meningeal hemangiomatosis

EPIDEMIOLOGY

- Frequency is estimated at 1 in 50,000 live births
- No apparent gender or racial predilection

RISK FACTORS

Genetics

- Typically sporadic with no genetic inheritance pattern
- Rare familial clusters reported but inheritance pattern unclear

ETIOLOGY

Embryonal developmental anomaly due to errors in mesodermal and ectodermal development

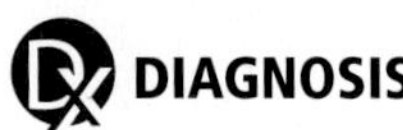

DIAGNOSIS

- Ophthalmic features:
  - Diffuse choroidal hemangioma (50% of patients) ipsilateral to facial nevus flammeus characterized by a much more saturated reddish appearance compared with contralateral eye ("tomato-catsup fundus")
  - Retinal vascular tortuosity and serous retinal detachment may occur.
  - Telangiectasia of conjunctival and episcleral vessels
  - Glaucoma (up to 70% of patients) ipsilateral to facial nevus flammeus especially when eyelids are involved may result from elevated episcleral venous pressure, angle malformation, or both.
  - Buphthalmos may result in cases of congenital glaucoma.
  - Iris heterochromia
  - Anisometropic amblyopia
- Cutaneous features:
  - Facial nevus flammeus ("port-wine stain"): unilateral flat to thickened zone of dilated telangiectatic cutaneous capillaries appearing light pink to deep purple in coloration
  - Involves region innervated by first branch (most common), first and second branches, or all three branches (least common) of trigeminal nerve
  - Localized hypertrophy of ipsilateral nasal and buccal mucosa may occur.
- CNS features:
  - Ipsilateral leptomeningeal hemangiomatosis
  - May be associated with cortical atrophy, seizures (80% of patients), recurrent stroke-like episodes, and developmental delay
  - Recurrent headaches (30–50% of patients), contralateral hemiparesis, hemiplegia, and hemianopsia may also occur.

DIAGNOSTIC TESTS & INTERPRETATION

Diagnostic Procedures/Other

- MRI (preferred modality) or CT scans of the brain may be used to detect leptomeningeal hemangiomatosis, which is present from birth.
  - Granular calcification of parenchymal brain tissue adjacent to cortical atrophy can often be seen on CT scan.
- Ultrasonography: B-scan mode shows generalized choroidal thickening; A-scan demonstrates high internal reflectivity.

Pathological Findings

- Facial nevus flammeus: dilated telangiectatic cutaneous capillaries in the dermis lined by single layer of endothelial cells
- Diffuse choroidal hemangioma:
  - Cavernous vascular channels lined by mature endothelial cells and supported by thin intervascular fibrous septa
  - May contain small, capillary-type vessels
  - Terminate indistinctly in periphery without sharp margins
  - Fibrous transformation of retinal pigment epithelium and calcification may occur.
  - Sensory retina overlying hemangioma often thickened and cystic

DIFFERENTIAL DIAGNOSIS

- Klippel–Trenaunay–Weber syndrome: characteristics of SWS plus port-wine stains of extremities and hemihypertrophy of soft and bony tissues
- Beckwith–Wiedemann syndrome: facial port-wine stain, macroglossia, omphalocele, visceral hyperplasia with severe hypoglycemia due to pancreatic islet cell hyperplasia

TREATMENT

- Facial nevus flammeus: dermatologic vascular-specific pulsed-dye laser therapy
- Diffuse choroidal hemangioma: treatment usually considered when associated with macular edema or serous retinal detachment
  - Photodynamic therapy
  - Low-dose radiation therapy (external beam, proton beam, plaque radiotherapy, gamma knife radiotherapy, stereotactic radiotherapy)
- Glaucoma: topical drops
  - First line: beta-blocker
  - Second line: carbonic anhydrase inhibitor
  - Third line: prostaglandin analog
  - If medical therapy fails, see "Surgery/Other Procedures"
- CNS manifestations:
  - Seizures treated with anticonvulsants
  - Aspirin may be beneficial in patients with recurrent stroke-like episodes
    - Use with caution in children as aspirin use is associated with Reye syndrome
    - Varicella and annual influenza immunizations recommended to lower risk of Reye syndrome

ADDITIONAL TREATMENT

General Measures

- Address refractive error with glasses or contact lens.
- Treat amblyopia, which is typically anisometropic due to glaucoma-induced myopia.

SURGERY/OTHER PROCEDURES

- Subtotal hemispherectomy has been performed for intractable seizures or progressive mental deterioration.
- Trabeculectomy, aqueous tube shunt procedure, goniotomy, trabeculotomy, laser trabeculoplasty, or cyclodestructive procedures may be necessary to manage glaucoma if topical therapy is inadequate.
- Strabismus surgery as needed following completion of amblyopia therapy.

ONGOING CARE

FOLLOW-UP RECOMMENDATIONS

- Ophthalmologist
- Neurologist
- Neurosurgeon if intractable seizures
- Dermatologist

Patient Monitoring

See "Follow-up"

PATIENT EDUCATION

- Sturge–Weber Foundation (http://www.sturge-weber.org)
- Sturge–Weber Syndrome Community (http://www.swscommunity.org)

PROGNOSIS

Life expectancy appears to be significantly reduced especially in patients with profound mental retardation and intractable seizures compared with those with more limited disease.

COMPLICATIONS

- Visual loss due to amblyopia, glaucoma, or serous retinal detachment
- Progressive mental deterioration
- Seizures

ADDITIONAL READING

- Oakes WJ. The natural history of patients with the Sturge-Weber syndrome. *Pediatr Neurosurg* 1992;18:287–290.
- Patrianakos TD, Nagao K, Walton DS. Surgical management of glaucoma with the Sturge-Weber syndrome. *Int Ophthalmol Clin* 2008;48:63–78.
- Singh AD, Kaiser PK, Sears JE. Choroidal hemangioma. *Ophthalmol Clin N Am* 2005;18:151–161.
- Sullivan TJ, Clarke MP, Morin JD. The ocular manifestations of the Sturge-Weber syndrome. *J Pediatr Ophthalmol Strabismus* 1992;29:349–356.

CODES

ICD9

- 228.09 Hemangioma of other sites
- 362.17 Other intraretinal microvascular abnormalities
- 759.6 Other congenital hamartoses, not elsewhere classified

CLINICAL PEARLS

- Suspect glaucoma when the port-wine stain involves the eyelids.
- Neuroimaging should be performed especially in patients with choroidal hemangiomas since leptomeningeal hemangiomas are almost always present in these cases.

SUBCONJUNCTIVAL HEMORRHAGE

Steven J. Kanoff

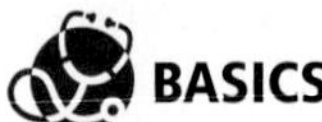

BASICS

DESCRIPTION

Blood that is under the conjunctiva. This can be spontaneous, associated with incidental trauma or obvious trauma, or recurrent, which may be associated with underlying systemic disease.

RISK FACTORS

Antiplatelet therapy, anticoagulant therapy, hypertension, diabetes mellitus, coughing, sneezing, emesis, straining (constipation), bleeding diathesis (thrombocytopenia, impaired clotting, coagulopathy), conjunctivitis (viral).

PATHOPHYSIOLOGY

Extravasation of blood from conjunctival blood vessels.

ETIOLOGY

Incidental or obvious trauma, blood dyscrasias, viral infection.

COMMONLY ASSOCIATED CONDITIONS

Hypertension, diabetes mellitus, blood dyscrasias.

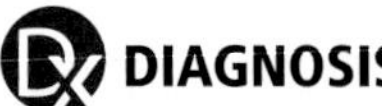

DIAGNOSIS

HISTORY

Patient or bystander usually notes red eye. The patient presents with a painless red eye unless associated with trauma. Question the patient about nose bleeds, spontaneous/easy bruising.

PHYSICAL EXAM

Blood under and/or in the conjunctiva. If concerned about associated bleeding problems do a thorough retinal examination.

DIAGNOSTIC TESTS & INTERPRETATION

Lab

If recurrent subconjunctival hemorrhages consider workup of coagulation system.

Imaging

None, unless degree of trauma justifies this

Diagnostic Procedures/Other

If associated with trauma, a complete eye examination is necessary to rule out ocular pathology.

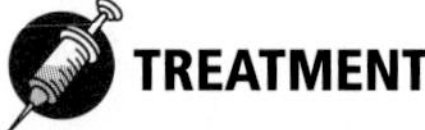

TREATMENT

MEDICATION

None.

ADDITIONAL TREATMENT

General Measures

Reassurance that hemorrhage will clear usually by 2 weeks.

Issues for Referral

Bleeding diathesis

Additional Therapies
If elevated subconjunctival hemorrhage adjacent to the limbus, use frequent artificial tears every 2 h and lubricating ointment at bedtime to try to prevent delle formation.

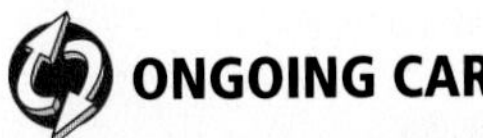

ONGOING CARE

FOLLOW-UP RECOMMENDATIONS
None unless associated ocular pathology from trauma or to monitor delle status

PROGNOSIS
Excellent

COMPLICATIONS
None

ADDITIONAL READING

- American Academy of Ophthalmology Basic and Clinical Science Course. Section 8, 2006–2007, 90–91.
- Mimura T, Usui T, Yamagami S, et al. Recent causes of subconjunctival hemorrhage. *Ophthalmologica* 2009;224(3):133–137.
- Ehlers JP, Shah CP, (eds). *The Wills Eye Manual*, 5th Ed. Philadelphia: JB Lippincott Publisher, 2008: 112–113.

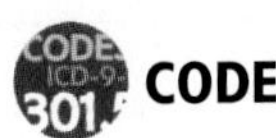

CODES

ICD9
372.72 Conjunctival hemorrhage

SUPERIOR LIMBIC KERATOCONJUNCTIVITIS (SLK)

Nicole R. Fram

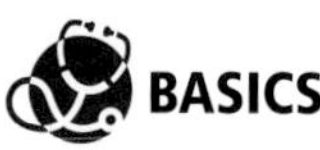

BASICS

DESCRIPTION

- Ocular surface disorder is characterized by foreign body sensation, pain out of proportion to exam, and photophobia. The presentation is typically bilateral and frequently asymmetrical.
- Classic signs include superior bulbar conjunctival staining and injection, redundant superior bulbar conjunctiva, velvety fine papillary reaction of the superior palpebral/tarsal conjunctiva, superior corneal epithelial keratitis, and/or mucous filaments.

EPIDEMIOLOGY

Incidence

About 50–65% of patients with superior limbic keratoconjunctivitis (SLK) have underlying thyroid disease (1,2)

RISK FACTORS

- Keratoconjunctivitis sicca (KCS)
- Thyroid disease
- Cosmetic contact lenses induced (CL-SLK)
- Thimerosal

Genetics

No familial association

PATHOPHYSIOLOGY

Chronic and recurrent clinical course

ETIOLOGY

- Unknown: Mechanical versus autoimmune
- Possibly related to dry eye, autoimmune disease, or superior conjunctivochalasis
- Female:male 3:1
- Mean age 50 years
- Increased incidence in thyroid disease, hyperparathyroidism, and KCS (3)

COMMONLY ASSOCIATED CONDITIONS

- Thyroid disorder
- KCS
- Filamentary keratitis

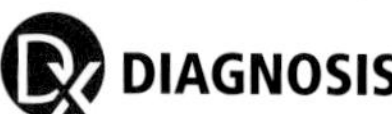

DIAGNOSIS

HISTORY

Targeted history onset, duration, location, quality of symptoms, and associated conditions. History of thyroid disease, KCS, and contact lens wear

PHYSICAL EXAM

- **External exam:** look for symptoms of thyroid eye disease and inflammatory ptosis
- Decreased Schirmer's test, decreased tear lake, increased mucus production in advanced cases
- **Eyelids:** tight upper lids, eversion of upper lid velvety fine papillary reaction of palpebral/tarsal conjunctiva
- **Conjunctiva/sclera:** sectoral superior bulbar and limbal conjunctival injection, redundant superior conjunctiva, lissamine green/rose bengal staining of superior bulbar conjunctiva (keratinization)
- **Cornea:** superior punctate epithelial keratitis, mucus filaments superiorly
- Remainder of anterior and posterior segment exams is typically unremarkable.

DIAGNOSTIC TESTS & INTERPRETATION

Lab

- Thyroid function tests
- Consider parathyroid function tests

Diagnostic Procedures/Other

- Lissamine green/rose bengal will stain keratinized or denuded epithelium.
- Demonstrate redundant superior conjunctiva by topically anesthetizing the eye, having the patient look down and slide the superior conjunctiva with a cotton tip applicator onto the superior cornea. This should not be feasible in a normal eye.

Pathological Findings

- Keratinized conjunctival epithelium with polymorphonuclear leukocytes (PMNs)
- Palpebral/tarsal conjunctival cells with lymphocytes and plasma cells on Giemsa scrapings

DIFFERENTIAL DIAGNOSIS
- Allergic
  - Seasonal allergic conjunctivitis
  - Vernal keratoconjunctivitis
  - Atopic keratoconjunctivitis
  - Giant papillary keratoconjunctivitis (GPC)
- Contact lens–related keratoconjunctivitis
- KCS
- Filamentary keratitis
- Mucus fishing syndrome
- Topical medication toxicity

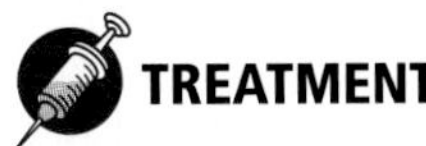

TREATMENT

MEDICATION
First Line
- Silver nitrate 0.5–1% solution to anesthetized superior palpebral and bulbar conjunctiva. Irrigate ocular surface thoroughly after 1 minute to neutralize the silver nitrate exposure.
- Can repeat in 4–6 weeks if necessary

ALERT
Do not use silver nitrate sticks or solid applicators, as this can result in a severe chemical damage to the cornea and sclera.

Second Line
Surgical removal of superior conjunctiva and Tenon's capsule from 10 o'clock to 2 o'clock and extending back from the limbus 5–8 mm. No need to cover or suture conjunctiva (4).

COMPLEMENTARY & ALTERNATIVE THERAPIES
- Filamentary keratitis may respond to N-acetylcysteine 10% topically or temporary bandage contact lens.
- Topical cyclosporine A (0.5%) (5)
- Topical vitamin A (retinol palmitate)
- Topical steroids
- Mast cell stabilizing drops
- Autologous serum
- Punctal occlusion

SURGERY/OTHER PROCEDURES
- Thermocauterization
- Supratarsal triamcinolone injection (3 mg/0.3 cc) with 27 gauge needle (2)

ALERT
Watch for intraocular pressure (IOP) elevation with supratarsal triamcinolone injection. Contraindicated in patients with glaucoma.

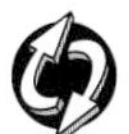

ONGOING CARE

FOLLOW-UP RECOMMENDATIONS
Patient Monitoring
- Monitor IOP if patient is maintained on topical steroids or has received supratarsal triamcinolone injection.
- Monitor for chemical injury or stem cell dysfunction after silver nitrate treatment.

PROGNOSIS
Disease is characterized by frequent remission and exacerbations.

REFERENCES

1. Kadrmas EF, Bartley GB. Superior limbic keratoconjunctivitis. A prognostic sign for severe Graves ophthalmopathy. *Ophthalmology* 1995;102:1472–1475.
2. Shen Y-C, Wang CY, Tsai HY, et al. Supratarsal triamcinolone injection in the treatment of superior limbic keratoconjunctivitis. *Cornea* 2007;26(4): 423–426.
3. Theodore FH. Comments on findings of elevated protein-bound iodine in superior limbic keratoconjunctivitis: I. *Arch Ophthalmol* 1968;79:508.
4. Sun YC, Hsiao CH, Chen WL, et al. Conjunctival resection combined with tenon layer excision and the involvement of mast cells in superior limbic keratoconjunctivitis. *Am J Ophthalmol* 2008; 145:445–452.
5. Perry HD, Doshi-Carnevale S, Donnenfeld ED, et al. Topical cyclosporine A 0.5% as a possible new treatment for superior limbic keratoconjunctivitis. *Ophthalmology* 2003;110:1578–1581.

ADDITIONAL READING

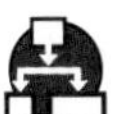

See Also (Topic, Algorithm, Electronic Media Element)

Conjunctivitis

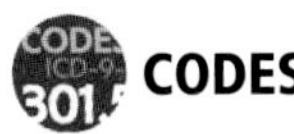

CODES

ICD9
- 370.40 Keratoconjunctivitis, unspecified
- 370.49 Other keratoconjunctivitis, unspecified

CLINICAL PEARLS

- SLK triad: Redundant superior bulbar conjunctiva with sectoral staining, "velvety" fine papillary superior tarsal conjunctiva, superior corneal filaments
- Associate with thyroid disease

S

SYMPATHETIC OPHTHALMIA

P. Kumar Rao

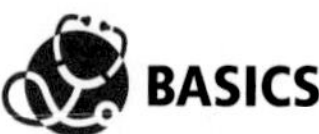

BASICS

DESCRIPTION

- Typically it is a bilateral granulomatous panuveitis that occurs following penetrating injury or surgery to one eye.
- Although the trauma occurs in only one eye, the uveitis involves both eyes. The traumatized eye is commonly referred to as the "inciting" or "exciting" eye and the contralateral eye is known as the "sympathizing" eye.

EPIDEMIOLOGY

Incidence

Incidence of the disorder following trauma or surgery is very rare, occurring in 0.19% of cases following trauma and 0.007% of cases following ocular surgery.

RISK FACTORS

Occurs following penetrating injury or surgery to the eye.

Genetics

HLA-11, DR4/DRw53, DR4/DRw3, DRB1*04, DQA1*03, and DQB1*04 have been identified in some patients.

GENERAL PREVENTION

- The avoidance of trauma
- Enucleation (removal) of a blind eye within 14 days of the trauma may prevent the development of sympathetic ophthalmia.

PATHOPHYSIOLOGY

Histological findings are the same in exciting and sympathizing eyes. Findings include a diffuse granulomatous inflammation consisting of lymphocytes (predominantly T-cells) and epithelioid cells within the uveal tract. Epithelioid cells may contain pigment. Multinucleated giant cells may also be present. In addition, clusters of epithelioid cells may accumulate between the retinal pigment epithelium and Bruch's' membrane. These clusters may appear yellow clinically and are known as Dalen–Fuchs nodules.

ETIOLOGY

Many studies reveal a role for T-cell mediated inflammation directed against uvea–retina proteins.

COMMONLY ASSOCIATED CONDITIONS

Trauma

DIAGNOSIS

HISTORY

- A history of trauma or surgery occurring prior to the onset of inflammation is critical to making the diagnosis.
- There is no specific laboratory test to confirm the diagnosis.
- Patients often complain of pain, redness, photophobia, and blurred vision.

PHYSICAL EXAM

- Exciting eye
- Photophobia, decreased vision, and keratic precipitates on endothelium may be seen.
- Sympathizing eye
- Symptoms are variable and may be insidious or rapid in onset. Mild anterior or posterior uveitis, ciliary flush, keratic precipitates, pain, photophobia, increased lacrimation, and blurred vision may occur.
- Both eyes
- Ciliary injection, partially dilated–poorly responsive pupil, thickened iris, clouding of vitreous, papillitis, generalized retinal edema, Dalen-Fuchs nodules (small, yellow, deposits beneath retinal pigment epithelium), peripheral choroiditis, exudative retinal detachments, and choroidal granulomas have been described.

DIAGNOSTIC TESTS & INTERPRETATION

Imaging

Fluorescein angiography reveals multiple hyperfluorescent dots at the level of the RPE that may persist in to the late phase of angiogram. Coalescence of the dye from these foci may occur in areas of exudative retinal detachment. A pattern similar to multiple evanescent white dot syndrome—early hypofluorescence followed by dye leakage in a wreath-like pattern in the venous phase has also been described.

Pathological Findings

A diffuse granulomatous inflammation consisting of lymphocytes (predominantly T-cells) and epithelioid cells within the uveal tract. Giant cells may also be present. The choriocapillaris and retina are usually not involved.

DIFFERENTIAL DIAGNOSIS

- Sarcoidosis
- Tuberculosis
- Vogt–Koyanagi–Harada syndrome

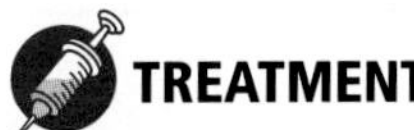

TREATMENT

MEDICATION

First Line

Oral (1 mg/kg/day) or pulse dose corticosteroids have a rapid onset of action. However, patients who need more than 10 mg of prednisone daily to control their inflammation will require steroid-sparing agents as high-dose steroids cannot be used for long periods of time without severe side effects.

Second Line

Enucleation of the traumatized eye within 2 weeks of injury may prevent development of sympathetic ophthalmia. Removal of the traumatized eye after SO develops is controversial.

ADDITIONAL TREATMENT

General Measures

Steroid-sparing agents such as mycophenolate mofetil, azathioprine, cyclosporine, tacrolimus, and anti-TNF inhibitors have all been used with some success.

Issues for Referral

A multidisciplinary team may be required to manage the various systemic effects of steroid-sparing therapies (immunosuppression).

SURGERY/OTHER PROCEDURES

- Laser photocoagulation can be used for retinal neovascularization and does not produce postoperative inflammation.
- Fluocinolone acetonide implantation (Retisert) may help control inflammation in some patients.

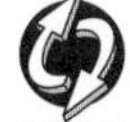

ONGOING CARE

FOLLOW-UP RECOMMENDATIONS

Patients will need very close monitoring until the disease is brought under control. Patients will need continuous follow-up with other specialists as needed.

PROGNOSIS

A majority of patients treated with corticosteroids/immunosuppression can maintain a vision of 20/60 or better.

COMPLICATIONS

- Bilateral vision loss due to ocular inflammation
- Anterior uveitis can cause cataract formation or glaucoma. Posterior segment inflammation can result in macular and peripheral retinal scaring and choroidal detachment.

REFERENCES

1. Galor A, Davis JL, Flynn HW Jr, et al. Sympathetic ophthalmia: incidence of ocular complications and vision loss in the sympathizing eye. *Am J Ophthalmol* 2009;148(5):704–710.
2. Reynard M, Riffenburg RS, Maes EF. Effects of corticosteroid treatment and enucleation on the visual prognosis of sympathetic ophthalmia. *Am J Ophthalmol* 1983;96:290–294.
3. Rao NA, Robin J, Hartmann D, et al. The role of penetrating wound in the development of sympathetic ophthalmia: experimental observations. *Arch Ophthalmol* 1983;101: 102–104.

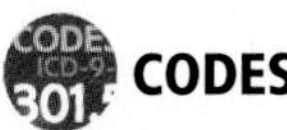

CODES

ICD9

- 360.11 Sympathetic uveitis
- 360.12 Panuveitis

CLINICAL PEARLS

- A history of ocular trauma in a patient with panuveitis should raise the suspicion for sympathetic ophthalmia.
- Aggressive treatment to control the inflammation is critical to prevent blindness.

SYSTEMIC LUPUS ERYTHEMATOSUS (SLE)

Melissa D. Neuwelt

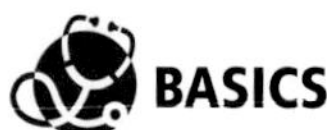

BASICS

DESCRIPTION

- Multisystem autoimmune disease
- Chronic course with relapses and remissions
- Organ systems most frequently involved: skin, joints, kidneys, blood, and CNS
- Diverse manifestations in eye:
  - Discoid lesions of eyelids
  - Keratoconjunctivitis sicca (dry eye)
  - Episcleritis
  - Scleritis
  - Cranial neuropathy
  - Optic neuropathy
  - Retinal vasoocclusive disease
  - Choroidopathy
  - Antimalarial drug toxicity

EPIDEMIOLOGY

Incidence

- Approximately 250,000 people have systemic lupus erythematosus (SLE) in the US (1)[B]
- Up to 1/3 of patients with SLE have ocular manifestations.
  - Ocular surface disease: up to 30%
  - Retinal manifestations: 3–30% (depends on systemic disease activity)
  - Optic nerve involvement: 1%

RISK FACTORS

- Gender: female 9:1
- Age: peak incidence 2nd–4th decade
- Race: African-American and Asian descent
- Family history
- Environmental factors: hormones, sunlight
- Drug-induced lupus: procainamide, hydralazine, quinidine, chlorpromazine, methyldopa, isoniazid

Genetics

- Twin studies support genetic predisposition.
- Linkage studies have identified many candidate genes, particularly on chromosome 1q
- Associated with *HLA-A1*, *HLA-B8*, and *HLA-DR3*

PATHOPHYSIOLOGY

- Autoimmunity may be triggered by autoantigen exposure during apoptosis.
  - Autoantibody production
  - Immune complex deposition
- Lupus retinopathy associated with immune complex–mediated arteriolar occlusion and thrombosis

COMMONLY ASSOCIATED CONDITIONS

- Secondary Sjögren's syndrome
- Antiphospholipid antibody (APA) syndrome (found in 77% of SLE patients with retinal or optic nerve disease vs. 29% of other SLE patients) (2)[B]

DIAGNOSIS

SLE is diagnosed by at least 4 of the 11 following American College of Rheumatology (ACR) criteria:

- Malar rash
- Discoid rash
- Oral ulcers
- Arthritis
- Serositis (pleuritis, pericarditis)
- Renal disorder (proteinuria or cellular casts)
- CNS disorder (seizures, psychosis)
- Hematologic disorder (anemia, leucopenia, thrombocytopenia, lymphopenia)
- Immunologic disorder
  - Antidouble-stranded DNA (anti-dsDNA)
  - APAs
  - Anti-Sm
  - False-positive RPR or VDRL
- Antinuclear antibody (ANA) positive

HISTORY

- Photophobia
- Redness
- Pain
- Diplopia
- Floaters
- Visual decline

PHYSICAL EXAM

- Ocular adnexa—edema, mass, proptosis
- Motility—myositis, cranial neuropathy, intranuclear ophthalmoplegia
- Eyelids—discrete, scaly lesions (discoid lupus)
- Conjunctiva—inflammation (noninfectious conjunctivitis)
- Sclera
  - Episcleritis (superficial, blanches with topical phenylephrine)
  - Scleritis (deep, does not blanch with topical phenylephrine, nodular or diffuse, anterior or posterior)
- Cornea
  - Reduced tear film, punctate keratopathy, filaments (dry eye, Sjögren's syndrome)
  - Interstitial keratitis (rare)
  - Peripheral ulcerative keratitis (rare)
  - Vortex keratopathy (verticillata)
    - Associated with antimalarial drug use
    - Rarely visually significant
    - Reversible with cessation of treatment
- Anterior chamber
  - Cell and flare (iritis)
  - Hypopyon uveitis (rare)
- Lens (cataract)
  - Especially posterior subcapsular
  - Associated with chronic steroid use
- Vitreous—inflammation (posterior uveitis)
- Retina
  - Lupus retinopathy
    - Cotton–wool spots (nerve fiber layer infarcts)
    - Intraretinal hemorrhages
    - Microaneurysms
    - Exudates
    - Vascular tortuosity
  - Vasoocclusive retinopathy (more severe)
    - Capillary nonperfusion
    - BRVO, CRVO, BRAO, CRAO
    - Neovascularization of disc and retina
    - Vitreous hemorrhage
    - Traction retinal detachment
  - Choroid
    - Uveal effusion
    - Serous retinal detachment
    - Choroidal infarction
    - Choroidal neovascular membrane
  - Optic nerve
    - Neuropathy
    - Neuritis
    - Papilledema (intracranial hypertension)
  - CNS
    - Intranuclear ophthalmoplegia
    - Retrochiasmal infarcts

DIAGNOSTIC TESTS & INTERPRETATION

Lab

Initial lab tests

- Anti-dsDNA (highly specific)
- ANA (sensitive)
- CBC

Follow-up & special considerations

- Other autoantibodies
  - APA (anticardiolipin and lupus anticoagulant)
  - Anti-Ro
  - Anti-La
  - Anti-c1q
  - Anti-Sm
  - Anti-nucleosome
  - Anti-N-methyl-d-aspartic acid (NMDA)
  - Anti-alpha actinin

Imaging

Initial approach

- Fluorescein angiography to assess retinal and choroidal circulation
  - ICG to assess choroidal circulation
  - OCT to assess for macular edema or serous retinal detachment
  - B-scan ultrasonography to assess vitritis and for retinal detachment

Follow-up & special considerations
Retinal vasculitis is associated with CNS lupus involvement. Consider CNS imaging with MRI/magnetic resonance angiography (MRA) to evaluate for thrombotic events.

Pathological Findings

- Biopsies of eyelid lesions show immunoglobulin deposition at the junction of epidermis and dermis on immunohistochemical staining.
- Orbital and adnexal involvement can also be confirmed by biopsy.

DIFFERENTIAL DIAGNOSIS

- Discoid lupus on the eyelids should be distinguished from blepharitis.
- Optic neuritis in SLE can resemble demyelinating disease but is often more severe.
- Lupus retinopathy resembles diabetic and hypertensive retinopathy.
- Patients with SLE on immunosuppressive therapy often present with new ocular complaints. It is important to rule out an infectious etiology before continuing or accelerating immunosuppressive therapy. Consider:
  - Herpetic retinitis (herpes simplex virus [HSV], herpes zoster virus [HZV], cytomegalovirus [CMV])
  - Tuberculosis
  - Toxoplasmosis
  - Lyme disease

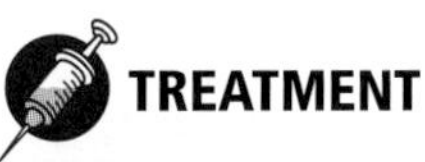

TREATMENT

MEDICATION

First Line

- Artificial tears for episcleritis, dry eye
- Oral prednisone for more severe ocular manifestations: 1–2 mg/kg/day

Second Line

- Nonsteroidal anti-inflammatory drugs (NSAIDs)
- Antimalarials:
  - Chloroquine
  - Hydroxychloroquine
- Steroid-sparing immunosuppressive agents:
  - Azathioprine
  - Cyclosporine
  - Mycophenolate mofetil
  - Cyclophosphamide
  - Methotrexate
- Plasmapheresis
- Intravenous immunoglobulins
- Newer biologic agents:
  - Rituximab (Rituxan)
  - Anticytokine agents

ADDITIONAL TREATMENT

General Measures

Care should be taken to prevent and manage side effects of immunosuppressive therapy such as gastric prophylaxis, blood sugar and blood pressure monitoring, and purified protein derivative (PPD) tuberculosis screening.

Issues for Referral

Systemic treatment of ocular manifestations should be comanaged with the patient's primary doctor and/or rheumatologist.

Additional Therapies

- Anticoagulation for vasoocclusive disease or APA syndrome
  - Aspirin
  - Warfarin

SURGERY/OTHER PROCEDURES

- Treat complications of proliferative retinopathy:
  - Panretinal photocoagulation
  - Vitrectomy

IN-PATIENT CONSIDERATIONS

Initial Stabilization

Consider inpatient admission for pulse IV methylprednisolone: 1g/day

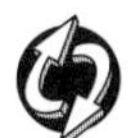

ONGOING CARE

FOLLOW-UP RECOMMENDATIONS

Patient Monitoring

- The antimalarial agents are associated with bull's eye maculopathy leading to impairment of visual acuity, color vision, and visual field.
- All patients initiating antimalarial therapy should receive counseling about risk of retinopathy and have baseline eye exam: visual acuity, dilated fundus examination, Amsler, Humphrey 10-2, optional tests (color, fundus photos, fluorescein angiography, multifocal electroretinogram [ERG])
- Risk factor for complications include dose >6.5 mg/kg hydroxychloroquine, >3 mg/kg chloroquine, duration >5 years, renal or liver disease, preexisting retinal disease, and age >60 years.
  - Low-risk patients do not require additional screening exams.
  - High-risk patients should have annual screening exams.
- Cessation of treatment may halt or even reverse sight-threatening complications.

PROGNOSIS

- Vision loss in 55% of patients with severe vasoocclusive retinopathy (4)[B]
- Optic neuritis outcomes highly variable, appear to improve with early initiation of steroid treatment (5)[B]

COMPLICATIONS

Visual loss, retinal detachment, optic neuropathy

REFERENCES

1. Helmick CG, Felson DT, Lawrence RC, et al. Estimates of the prevalence of arthritis and other rheumatic conditions in the United States. Part I. *Arthritis Rheum* 2008;58(1):15–25.
2. Montehermoso A, Cervera R, Font J, et al. Association of antiphospholipid antibodies with retinal vascular disease in systemic lupus erythematosus. *Semin Arthritis Rheum* 1999;28: 326–332.
3. Marmor MF, Carr RE, Easterbrook M, et al. Recommendations on screening for chloroquine and hydroxychloroquine retinopathy. A report by the American Academy of Ophthalmology. *Ophthalmology* 2002;109:1377–1382.
4. Jabs DA, Fine SL, Hochberg MC, et al. Severe retinal vaso-occlusive disease in systemic lupus erythematosus. *Arch Ophthalmol* 1986;104: 558–563.
5. Lin YC, Wang AG, Yen MY. Systemic lupus erythematosus-associated optic neuritis: clinical experience and literature review. *Acta Ophthalmol* 2009;87(2):204–210.

CODES

ICD9

- 370.33 Keratoconjunctivitis sicca, not specified as sjogren's
- 373.34 Discoid lupus erythematosus of eyelid
- 710.0 Systemic lupus erythematosus

CLINICAL PEARLS

- Episcleritis will blanch with topical phenylephrine whereas scleritis will not.
- Scleritis and vasoocclusive retinopathy require systemic treatment.
- Always consider infection when evaluating a lupus patient on immunosuppressive therapy presenting with a new manifestation or flare.

TALC RETINOPATHY

Paul S. Baker

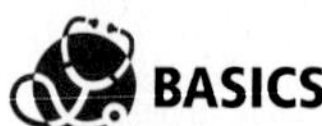

BASICS

DESCRIPTION

Characteristic retinopathy with small, intraretinal, whitish yellow, refractile deposits in patients who abuse intravenous drugs, especially those made from crushed tablets or powder (1)[B]

RISK FACTORS

Occurs in patients of any age

PATHOPHYSIOLOGY

- Drug addicts crush oral medications such as methylphenidate hydrochloride (Ritalin) or methadone hydrochloride and create an aqueous suspension for intravenous injection.
- Oral medications contain talc (hydrous magnesium silicate) as an inert filler.
- After intravenous administration, talc particles embolize to the pulmonary vasculature.
- With chronic intravenous drug abuse, collateral vasculature forms in the lung and allows talc particles to enter the systemic circulation.
- Talc particles embolize to other organs, including the eye.
- After many talc particles become lodged in the small arterioles of the retinal vasculature, an ischemic retinopathy develops.

ETIOLOGY

Intravenous drugs that contain talc particles

COMMONLY ASSOCIATED CONDITIONS

Intravenous drug abuse

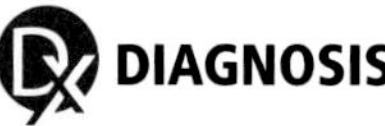

DIAGNOSIS

HISTORY

Chronic intravenous drug abuse, especially with crushed tablets or powder such as methylphenidate (Ritalin)

PHYSICAL EXAM

- Small, white, glistening crystals concentrated at end arterioles (intravascular space) throughout the retina, most prominent in the posterior pole.
- Ischemic retinopathy with capillary nonperfusion, including microaneurysms, cotton wool spots, and venous loops
- Severe cases can have optic disc and peripheral retinal neovascularization with vitreous hemorrhage (2)[B].
- Inspection of skin may reveal evidence of intravenous drug abuse.

DIAGNOSTIC TESTS & INTERPRETATION

Imaging

Fluorescein angiography is used to assess capillary nonperfusion and retinal neovascularization.

DIFFERENTIAL DIAGNOSIS

- Crystalline retinopathy
  - Cholesterol emboli (Hollenhorst plaque)
  - Canthaxanthin ingestion (oral tanning agent)
  - Tamoxifen (history of breast cancer)
  - Methoxyflurane anesthesia
  - Cystinosis
  - Parafoveal telangiectasia
  - Calcified drusen
  - Bietti's crystalline dystrophy
  - West African crystalline retinopathy
  - Intraretinal lipid exudates

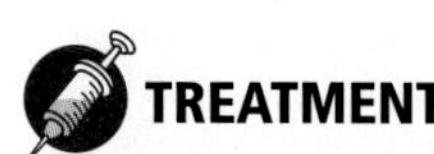

TREATMENT

ADDITIONAL TREATMENT

General Measures

- Patients should stop intravenous drug abuse.
- In the absence of retinal or optic nerve neovascularization, observation is appropriate.

SURGERY/OTHER PROCEDURES

- In the presence of peripheral nonperfusion and neovascularization, panretinal photocoagulation should be considered.
- Pars plana vitrectomy for non-clearing vitreous hemorrhage or visually significant tractional retinal detachment can be beneficial.

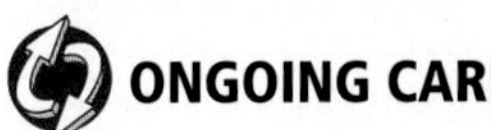

ONGOING CARE

FOLLOW-UP RECOMMENDATIONS

Yearly exam for asymptomatic talc retinopathy, more frequent if there is significant non-perfusion

PATIENT EDUCATION

Systemic and ocular risks of intravenous drug abuse

PROGNOSIS

- Visual prognosis is variable
- Visual acuity can be decreased because of macular ischemia, vitreous hemorrhage, macular fibrosis, and tractional retinal detachment (3)[B].
- In the absence of ongoing intravenous drug abuse, talc retinopathy has been shown to be static and nonprogressive (4)[B].

COMPLICATIONS

- Ischemic retinopathy
- Retinal and optic nerve neovascularization
- Vitreous hemorrhage
- Preretinal fibrosis/tractional retinal detachment

REFERENCES

1. Murphy SB, Jackson WB, Pare JA. Talc retinopathy. *Can J Ophthalmol* 1978;13:152–156.
2. Tse DT, Ober RR. Talc retinopathy. *Am J Ophthalmol* 1980;90:624–640.
3. Sharma MC, Ho AC. Macular fibrosis associated with talc retinopathy. *Am J Ophthalmol* 1999; 128:517–519.
4. Martidis A, Yung CW, Ciulla TA. Talc embolism: a static retinopathy. *Am J Ophthalmol* 1997;124: 841–843.

CODES

ICD9

362.10 Background retinopathy, unspecified

CLINICAL PEARLS

- White intraretinal particles within the retinal vasculature are characteristic of talc retinopathy.

TERSON'S SYNDROME

Mitchell S. Fineman

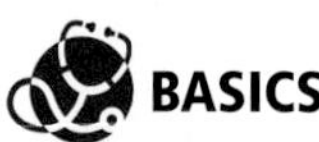

BASICS

DESCRIPTION

- Named after the French ophthalmologist Albert Terson who described the condition in 1900
- Originally defined as vitreous hemorrhage in the setting of subarachnoid hemorrhage
- Definition has evolved to include any intraocular hemorrhage associated with intracranial hemorrhage and increased intracranial pressure

EPIDEMIOLOGY

Incidence

Approximately 15% of patients with subarachnoid hemorrhage develop intraocular hemorrhage (1)[A].

RISK FACTORS

- Patients with higher grade intracranial hemorrhage are more likely to have Terson's syndrome.
- The presence of Terson's syndrome is associated with higher mortality and morbidity in patients with intracranial hemorrhage (2)[B].

GENERAL PREVENTION

- Modify risk factors associated with intracranial hemorrhage
  - Smoking cessation
  - Treatment of hypertension

PATHOPHYSIOLOGY

- Mechanism is controversial with several competing theories
  - Original theory suggested that intracerebral blood directly communicated with intraocular space via the optic nerve sheath.
  - Intracranial bleeding may result in elevated venous pressure that is transmitted to the intraocular vessels.
  - Elevated intracranial pressure is transmitted along optic nerve sheath resulting in rupture of the peripapillary vessels.

ETIOLOGY

Intracranial hemorrhage combined with intracranial hypertension leading to intraocular hemorrhage

DIAGNOSIS

HISTORY

- A history of intracranial hemorrhage and increased intracranial pressure is usually present.
- Visual changes are usually present
  - Decreased vision
  - Restricted peripheral vision
  - New-onset floaters
- Patients with impaired neurological status may not be able to provide a history.

PHYSICAL EXAM

- Visual acuity may range from 20/20 to light perception.
- Ocular findings are usually bilateral.
- Ophthalmic manifestations may include:
  - Vitreous hemorrhage
  - Subhyaloid hemorrhage
  - Sub-internal limiting membrane (ILM) hemorrhage
  - Retinal hemorrhage
  - Peripapillary hemorrhage

DIAGNOSTIC TESTS & INTERPRETATION

Imaging

- Neuroimaging studies in consultation with a Neurosurgical specialist
  - CT scan
  - MRI scan
  - Cerebral angiography
- B-scan ultrasonography is recommended if the ocular hemorrhage obscures visualization of the retina.

Diagnostic Procedures/Other

Cerebrospinal fluid examination may be helpful in equivocal cases.

Pathological Findings

- Histology of vitreous samples show red blood cells with few white blood cells.
- Epiretinal membranes with glial proliferation may be found.

DIFFERENTIAL DIAGNOSIS

- Vitreous hemorrhage due to other causes
- Proliferative diabetic retinopathy
- Sickle cell retinopathy
- Shaken baby syndrome Valsalva retinopathy

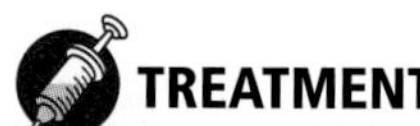

TREATMENT

ADDITIONAL TREATMENT

General Measures

- Treatment of the intracranial hemorrhage and control of intracranial pressure is managed by a neurosurgical specialist.
- Intraocular hemorrhage is managed with:
  - Observation with elevated head positioning to allow for spontaneous reabsorption
  - Avoidance of anticoagulant medications when medically possible

Pediatric Considerations

- The development of amblyopia in children with unilateral or asymmetric visual loss should be monitored closely.
- Early vitrectomy and/or patching of the fellow eye may be necessary to prevent amblyopia.

Issues for Referral

Any patient who presents with ocular findings consistent with Terson's syndrome should be referred immediately for urgent neurosurgical consultation

SURGERY/OTHER PROCEDURES

- YAG Laser vitreolysis to disrupt the posterior hyaloid face and promote absorption of the hemorrhage
  - This may increase the risk of epiretinal membrane formation.
- Pars plana vitrectomy surgery is indicated in the following situations:
  - Nonclearing vitreous hemorrhage
  - Retinal detachment associated with vitreous hemorrhage
  - Thick sub-ILM hemorrhage involving the fovea
  - Monocular patients with decreased vision
  - Children at risk for amblyopia

IN-PATIENT CONSIDERATIONS

Initial Stabilization

Managed by neurosurgical specialist

Admission Criteria

Determined by neurosurgical specialist

Discharge Criteria

Determined by neurosurgical specialist

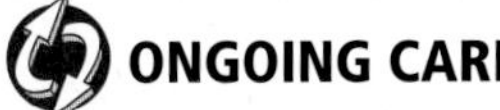

ONGOING CARE

FOLLOW-UP RECOMMENDATIONS

Resolution of the intraocular hemorrhage may take months without surgery

Patient Monitoring

Patients should be examined serially until the intraocular hemorrhage has cleared completely

PATIENT EDUCATION

Amsler grid monitoring may help to identify patients with epiretinal membrane development.

PROGNOSIS

- The visual prognosis in adults is excellent with >80% of patients recovering normal or near-normal vision (3)[B].
- Children have a more guarded visual prognosis because of the risk of amblyopia.
- Overall prognosis is related to the severity of the intracranial hemorrhage and the subsequent neurological sequelae.

COMPLICATIONS

- Risk of amblyopia in children under the age of 9 years
- Epiretinal membrane formation occurs as a late finding in a significant proportion of patients (4).
  - Subhyaloid or sub-ILM hemorrhage may stimulate glial cell proliferation.
  - May present years following resolution of the hemorrhage
  - Macular holes may also occur

REFERENCES

1. McCarron MO, Alberts MJ, McCarron P. A systematic review of Terson's syndrome: Frequency and prognosis after subarachnoid haemorrhage. *J Neurol Neurosurg Psychiatry* 2004;75:491–493.
2. Fountas KN, Kapsalaki EZ, Lee GP, et al. Terson hemorrhage in patients suffering aneurysmal subarachnoid hemorrhage: Predisposing factors and prognostic significance. *J Neurosurg* 2008;109:439–444.
3. Kuhn F, Morris R, Witherspoon CD, et al. Terson syndrome. Results of vitrectomy and the significance of vitreous hemorrhage in patients with subarachnoid hemorrhage. *Ophthalmology* 1998;105:472–477.
4. Schultz PN, Sobol WM, Weingeist TA. Long-term visual outcome in Terson syndrome. *Ophthalmology* 1991;98:1814–1819.

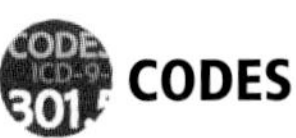

CODES

ICD9

- 360.43 Hemophthalmos, except current injury
- 379.23 Vitreous hemorrhage
- 432.9 Unspecified intracranial hemorrhage

CLINICAL PEARLS

- Terson's syndrome should be suspected in any patient presenting with neurological findings associated with intracranial hemorrhage.
- Patients with intracranial hemorrhage should have an ocular examination to screen for intraocular hemorrhage.
- Pediatric patients with Terson's syndrome should be closely monitored for the development of amblyopia.

THYGESON'S SUPERFICIAL PUNCTATE KERATOPATHY

Parveen K. Nagra

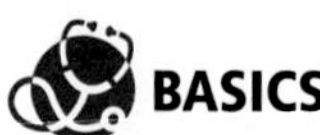

BASICS

DESCRIPTION

- Multiple, transient, whitish-grey, slightly elevated corneal epithelial opacities
- No stromal involvement, corneal edema, or conjunctival hyperemia
- Typically bilateral, may be asymmetric (1)[C]

EPIDEMIOLOGY

- Affects patients of all ages
- No sex predilection

Incidence/Prevalence

Rare

RISK FACTORS

None identified

Genetics

Associated with HLA DR3

PATHOPHYSIOLOGY

Unknown

DIAGNOSIS

HISTORY

- Patients often present with ocular irritation/foreign body sensation; may have photophobia.
- Vision may be slightly blurred or normal.
- Usually bilateral but may be asymmetric
- May be asymptomatic

PHYSICAL EXAM

- Slit-lamp examination
  - Conjunctival quiet or with minimal inflammation
  - Small, usually multiple, whitish, coarse corneal epithelial lesions with clear intervening epithelium and stroma
  - Lesions may have overlying punctate staining
  - Absence of anterior chamber inflammation

DIAGNOSTIC TESTS & INTERPRETATION

Lab

Clinical diagnosis, no additional testing required

Imaging

Imaging not required but could consider slit-lamp photographs and/or confocal microscopy (2)[C]

DIFFERENTIAL DIAGNOSIS

- Punctate epithelial keratitis
- Subepithelial infiltrates
- Infectious (bacterial) corneal infiltrate

TREATMENT

MEDICATION

First Line

- Mild topical steroid (e.g., fluorometholone 0.1%, loteprednol 0.2%) with very slow taper over months (1)[C]
- Topical cyclosporine
- Asymptomatic patients with few lesions may be observed.
- Topical lubrication (artificial tears/gel), usually in conjunction with steroids or alone in asymptomatic patients with few lesions

Second Line

- Soft contact lenses reported to provide symptomatic relief
- Treatment with idoxuridine contraindicated, (associated with subepithelial infiltrates)

ADDITIONAL TREATMENT

General Measures

- Topical steroids should be tapered very slowly, with some patients requiring long-term, infrequent use (i.e., weekly).
- Chronic condition marked by exacerbations and flare-ups over years

Issues for Referral

Consider referral to cornea specialist if diagnosis is unclear or patient is not responding to treatment

Additional Therapies

Antibiotics ineffective; trifluridine has been shown to be effective in some patients in early reports; idoxuridine is contraindicated

SURGERY/OTHER PROCEDURES

Has been noted to recur following LASIK, case reports suggest lower incidence of recurrence with PRK (3)[C]

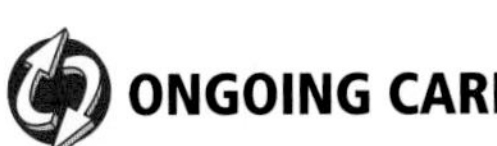

ONGOING CARE

FOLLOW-UP RECOMMENDATIONS

Regular follow-up with goal of slowly tapering steroids over months

PROGNOSIS

Excellent long-term prognosis

COMPLICATIONS

- Mild steroid use (and/or cyclosporine) is the mainstay of treatment but may be associated with side effects including elevated intraocular pressure and cataract formation.
- Anecdotal evidence suggests that steroid use may prolong the course of the disease.

REFERENCES

1. Nagra PK, Rapuano CJ, Cohen EJ, et al. Thygeson's superficial puncate keratitis: Ten years' experience. *Ophthalmology* 2004;111:34–37.
2. Cheng LL, Young AL, Wong AKK, et al. In vivo confocal microscopy of Thygeson's superficial punctate keratitis. *Clin Experiment Ophthalmol* 2004;32:325–340.
3. Netto MV, Chalita MR, Krueger RR. Thygeson's superficial punctate keratitis after laser in situ keratomileusis. *Am J Ophthalmol* 2004;138: 507–508.

ADDITIONAL READING

- Darrell RW. Thygeson's superficial punctate keratitis: Natural history and association with HLA DR3. *Trans Am Ophthalmol Soc* 1981;79:486–516.
- Tabbara KF, Ostler HB, Dawson C, et al. Thygeson's superficial punctate keratitis. *Ophthalmology* 1981;88:75–77.
- Thygeson P. Superficial punctate keratitis. *JAMA* 1950;144:1544–1549.

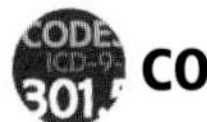

CODES

ICD9

370.21 Punctate keratitis

CLINICAL PEARLS

- Thygeson's superficial punctate keratopathy is a chronic condition marked by exacerbations and remissions over years.
- Mainstay of treatment is topical steroids and/or topical cyclosporine.
- Clinical diagnosis with excellent long-term visual prognosis

THYROID EYE DISEASE

Vladimir Yakopson
Jacqueline Carrasco

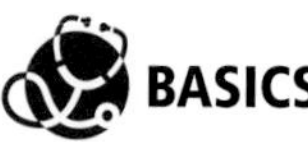

BASICS

DESCRIPTION

Thyroid eye disease (also referred to as Graves' ophthalmopathy, thyroid-related or associated orbitopathy or ophthalmopathy; TED) is an autoimmune process affecting extraocular muscles and orbital fat and connective tissues, resulting in a spectrum of findings including upper and lower lid retraction, proptosis (exophthalmos), restrictive strabismus, and, in the worst cases, optic neuropathy.

EPIDEMIOLOGY

Incidence

- Age-adjusted incidence of ophthalmopathy is 16/100,000 population per year for women and 2.9/100,000 population per year for men.
- Majority (up to 70%) of Graves' disease patients demonstrate extraocular muscle (EOM) enlargement on imaging although only ~50% show clinical signs and only 20–30% are clinically relevant manifestations (symptomatic).
- 3–5% of cases are severe/sight threatening
- Bilateral in 85–95%
- Bimodal age distribution
  - 5th and 7th decades of life
- More severe in men and older patients

RISK FACTORS

- Smoking
- Female gender
- Uncontrolled thyroid status (hyper- or hypothyroidism)
- Radioiodine therapy

Genetics

No known genetic predisposition identified at this time

GENERAL PREVENTION

- Smoking cessation is the most important modifiable risk factor.
- Smoking cessation or avoidance has been shown to reduce
  - Risk of developing TED
  - Severity of disease
  - Rate of recurrence of Graves' disease
  - Better response to immunosuppressive therapy
- 15% of patients treated with radioactive iodine showed progression of ophthalmopathy. This is reduced to 5% with concomitant oral prednisone treatment.

PATHOPHYSIOLOGY

Enlargement of EOMs and orbital fat leads to proptosis, lid retraction, corneal exposure, diplopia, and optic nerve compression at the orbital apex.

ETIOLOGY

An autoimmune disorder with stimulating autoantibodies binding to thyrotropin receptors in the orbit

COMMONLY ASSOCIATED CONDITIONS

- Hyperthyroidism
  - May occur concurrently, following diagnosis, or preceding diagnosis
  - TED is the most common extrathyroid sign of hyperthyroidism.
- Hypothyroidism
- Euthyroid state
- Myasthenia gravis

DIAGNOSIS

- Ophthalmic features in thyroid eye disease include various degrees of:
  - Lid retraction (scleral show)
  - Lid lag (lids do not move down with downgaze)
  - Lagophthalmos (incomplete lid closure)
  - Corneal exposure
  - Superior limbal keratitis (SLK)
  - Lid edema[1]
  - Redness of eyelids*
  - Conjunctival injection/redness*
  - Chemosis*
  - Inflammation of caruncle and/or plica*
  - Exophthalmos
  - Restrictive strabismus
  - Compressive optic neuropathy
- Systemic findings depend on thyroid state.[1]

HISTORY

- Inquire about
  - Acuity of onset
  - Periorbital ache*
  - Pain with eye movement*
  - Diplopia (primary gaze or extreme side gaze only?)
  - Tearing, irritation, and foreign body sensation
  - Change in vision

PHYSICAL EXAM

- Visual acuity
- Pupillary reaction (check for rAPD)
- Color plates
- Ocular motility (restriction of movement)
- Ocular alignment (measurable tropia)
- Presence of external signs (see Diagnosis)
- Hertel exophthalmometry (measures proptosis)
- Anterior segment exam, with careful attention to corneal surface and presence of SLK
- Funduscopy
  - Examine for evidence of optic nerve swelling or pallor
  - Presence of macular abnormalities (unrelated to TED but possibly contributing to visual loss, if present)

DIAGNOSTIC TESTS & INTERPRETATION

Lab

- TSH, T3, and Free T4
- Thyroid stimulating immunoglobulin (absence does not rule out disease. Positive test helps confirm diagnosis in mild disease; may be followed in treatment of Graves' disease)

Imaging

- CT of orbits (axial and coronal projections)
- Other conditions are ruled out (see Differential Diagnosis)
- EOM enlargement is assessed (inferior and medial recti are most commonly involved)
- Orbital apex is assessed for evidence of optic nerve compression.
- Radiologic proptosis can be measured and correlated with clinical findings.
- Quiescent disease often shows fatty infiltration of EOMs (EOMs appear tubular in cross section).

Diagnostic Procedures/Other

- Visual field testing (may have various defects in cases of optic neuropathy)
- Single binocular Visual Field Test
- Hess screen (measures strabismus)
- External photography
- Color plate deficiencies (decreased color perception may be an indicator of optic neuropathy)

Pathological Findings

- Extraocular muscles are separated by granular material consisting of collagen fibrils and glycosaminoglycans.
- Focal and diffuse mononuclear cell infiltrates within EOMs and orbital fat in active disease.
- Fibrotic changes in inactive disease

DIFFERENTIAL DIAGNOSIS

- Idiopathic orbital inflammation
- Orbital tumor
- Orbital vascular malformation (e.g., varix, lymphocele)
- Carotid–cavernous fistula
- Metastatic disease

Note: many of the above conditions are typically unilateral in presentation.

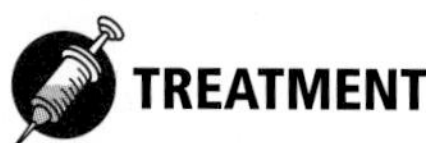

TREATMENT

ADDITIONAL TREATMENT

General Measures

- Treatment is determined by level of activity [Clinical Activity Score (CAS) is a validated tool] and severity of the disease.
- Presence of inflammatory signs and/or worsening of signs and symptoms suggests active disease (CAS >3).
- Severity is graded mild, moderate-to-severe, and sight-threatening (optic neuropathy or corneal ulceration/breakdown).
- May be observed if mild or asymptomatic, otherwise treated based on severity
- Lubrication with artificial tears for symptoms of corneal exposure (e.g., dry, gritty, foreign body sensation, tearing)
- Prisms for mild degrees of diplopia
  - Fresnel prisms—applied to back of spectacle lenses (con: decrease visual acuity, may cause glare)
  - Prisms may be also be ground into glasses (con: expensive, increase weight of lens)

[1] Items marked with * comprise the Clinical Activity Score. 1 point is assigned to each. CAS>3 indicates active disease

- **Moderately Severe Disease**
  - If active: immunosuppression with pulse i.v. or p.o. steroids (Level Ib evidence for IV pulse)
  - ~1 mg/kg per day starting dose for oral prednisone
  - Large cumulative doses (8–15 g) of i.v. methylprednisolone have led to death due to acute liver failure. (Level III) Total dose <4.25 g appears safe. Fewer side effects than p.o. steroids.
  - Orbital radiation (typical dose: 20 Gy) may also be used
  - Conflicting evidence regarding overall efficacy. Shown to be effective in improving motility and decreasing diplopia (Level Ib)
  - Also used to shorten overall course of disease and allow reconstructive surgery to be performed
- **Sight-Threatening Disease**
  - If due to corneal breakdown, it is imperative to restore adequate coverage of cornea with aggressive lubrication, tarsorrhaphy, etc.
  - If due to optic neuropathy
    - High-dose i.v. pulse steroids (Level III) followed by orbital decompression
    - Urgent decompression if unable to tolerate steroids or no response to i.v. steroids
- Once disease is **stable**, may proceed with reconstructive surgery

SURGERY/OTHER PROCEDURES

A stepwise approach: Orbital Decompression → Strabismus surgery → Eyelid surgery

- Orbital surgery may alter strabismus measurements; strabismus surgery may, in turn, affect eyelid position
- Not all patients will need all 3 types of surgery
- Some patients may skip one of the steps (e.g., a patient with severe proptosis and lid retraction)
- Orbital decompression
  - The orbit is a bony compartment with fixed volume (~35 cc)
  - Enlargement of EOMs may push the eye forward (proptosis), compress the optic nerve (optic neuropathy), and/or cause eyelid retraction.
  - Decompression surgery involves removing parts of bony orbital walls in order to allow the enlarged EOMs and orbital fat to prolapse into the surrounding sinuses (floor and medial wall decompression, most commonly performed) or fossae (temporal fossa with lateral wall decompression, anterior cranial fossa with roof decompression—rarely done, neurosurgical involvement mandatory)
  - Orbital fat may also be debulked at the same time
- Strabismus surgery
  - Goal is to realign the eyes in primary (straight ahead) and reading gaze
  - Diplopia in peripheral gazes may persist
  - Adjustable suture technique is used to verify alignment once patient is awake
  - May affect eyelid position [e.g., recession (weakening) of inferior rectus may worsen lower lid retraction]
- Eyelid surgery
  - Goal is to restore eyelid closure, coverage during blink, and reduce symptoms of exposure
  - Secondary goal is to improve cosmesis, restoring a more normal appearance (remove "thyroid stare")
  - Upper eyelids
    - Transcutaneous or transconjunctival approaches may be utilized
    - Upper eyelid retractors (Muller's muscle and/or levator palpebrae) are cut (recessed)
  - Lower eyelids
    - Lower lid retractors are recessed
    - Spacer graft (AlloDerm, buccal mucosa, banked sclera, etc.) may be used in severe cases to elevate lower lid position.

ONGOING CARE

FOLLOW-UP RECOMMENDATIONS

- Primary care provider and/or endocrinologist manage systemic thyroid disease
- Ophthalmologist with subspecialty involvement of an oculoplastic surgeon manages eye complications and surgery
- Others may include radiation oncologist, ENT, neuro-ophthalmology, and rarely neurosurgery

Patient Monitoring

Frequency depends on activity and severity of disease, ranging from once every 3–4 weeks to yearly if mild or stable.

PATIENT EDUCATION

- Patients are informed about the state of their disease (activity and severity) and advised as to the recommended treatment and prognosis.
- Smoking cessation is discussed and encouraged if applicable.

PROGNOSIS

- Most cases are mild and require supportive care and monitoring only.
- Smoking cessation is important in control of progression/severity of disease.

COMPLICATIONS

- Visual loss
- Persistent diplopia
- Disfigurement

ADDITIONAL READING

- Bahn RS. Graves' ophthalmopathy. *N Engl J Med* 2010;362(8):726–738.
- Bartalena L, Baldeschi L, Dickinson A, et al. European Consensus Statement of the European Group on Graves' Orbitopathy (EUGOGO) on Management of GO. *Eur J Endocrinol* 2008;158: 273–285.
- Bradley EA, Gower EW, Bradley DJ, et al. Orbital radiation for Graves' ophthalmopathy: A report by the American Academy of Ophthalmology. *Ophthalmology* 2008;115:398–409.
- Stiebel-Kalish H, Robenshtok E, Hasanreisoglu M, et al. Treatment modalities for Graves' ophthalmopathy: Systematic review and metaanalysis. *J Clin Endocrinol Metab* 2009;94:2708–2716.
- Wiersinga WM, Bartalena L. Epidemiology and prevention of Graves' ophthalmopathy. *Thyroid* 2002;12:855–860.
- Wiersinga WM. Management of Graves' ophthalmopathy. *Nat Clin Pract Endocrinol Metab* 2007;3:396–404.

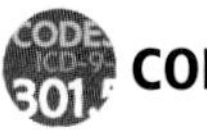

CODES

ICD9

- 242.00 Toxic diffuse goiter without mention of thyrotoxic crisis or storm
- 374.41 Lid retraction or lag
- 376.30 Exophthalmos, unspecified

CLINICAL PEARLS

- May occur in hyper-, hypo-, and euthyroid states
- Lid retraction is the most common sign.
- Number one cause of both unilateral and bilateral proptosis in adults
- Corneal exposure, optic neuropathy, and side effects of treatment (e.g., steroid-induced cataracts) can lead to visual loss.

T

THYROID OPTIC NEUROPATHY

Raed Behbehani

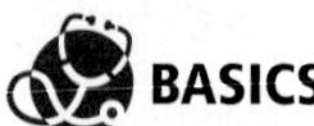

BASICS

DESCRIPTION

Thyroid eye disease (TED) is a chronic orbital inflammatory disease, commonly associated with hyperthyroidism (90%) but occasionally with hypo- or euthyroid status.

EPIDEMIOLOGY

Incidence

Female: Male ratio of 5:1 (16 women: 3 men per 100,000 population)

Prevalence

Occurs in 25–50% of patients with Graves' disease (hyperthyroidism)

RISK FACTORS

- Graves' disease
- Hashimoto's thyroiditis
- Smoking

Genetics

Genetic loci implicated include (HLA, 6p21-3), cytotoxic T-Lymphocyte antigen-4 (CTLA-4, 2q33), tumor necrosis factor (TNF), interferon-gamma, intracellular adhesion molecule (ICAM-10), and thyroid stimulating hormone receptor (TSH-R).

GENERAL PREVENTION

Avoid smoking (odds ratio for smokers vs. nonsmokers is 7.7)

PATHOPHYSIOLOGY

- Autoimmunity
  - Autoantibodies acting specifically on fibroblasts surface TSH-R and insulin-like growth factor-1 receptor (IGF-1R) (1)
  - Activated fibroblasts secrete chemokines and cytokines promoting lymphocyte migration and B-cell maturation.
  - Prostaglandin-E2 (PGE2), PGD-2, Interleukin-6 (IL-6), and IL-8 may stimulate orbital fibroblasts to produce glycosaminoglycans (GAG) and adipose tissue, increasing orbital mass.
- Smoking
  - Cigarette smoking has been found to be a risk factor for the development and severity of TED (2).

ETIOLOGY

Autoimmune (see pathophysiology)

COMMONLY ASSOCIATED CONDITIONS

- Hyperthyroidism (Graves' disease) in 90% of cases.
- Autoimmune conditions (diabetes, myasthenia gravis)

DIAGNOSIS

HISTORY

- Known thyroid disease with signs and symptoms (palpitations, weight loss, tremor, proximal muscle weakness)
- Proptosis
- Eyelid retraction
- Diplopia
- Ocular pain
- Red eye, foreign body sensation
- Vision loss
- Smoking
- Symptoms of associated myasthenia (double vision, ptosis, muscle weakness)

PHYSICAL EXAM

- Conjunctival redness over the insertion of the extraocular muscle insertion, exposure keratopathy superior limbic conjunctivitis, and dry eye.
- Chemosis
- Lid edema
- Exophthalmos
- Strabismus/ophthalmoplegia
- Optic neuropathy
- High intraocular pressure

DIAGNOSTIC TESTS & INTERPRETATION

Lab

Initial lab tests

- TSH, FT3, FT4, and thyroid stimulating immunoglobulin (TSI).
- Acetylcholine receptor antibody testing if ocular myasthenia is suspected

Follow-up & special considerations

Endocrinologic assessment for monitoring and correction of the thyroid status

Imaging

- CT scan of the orbit
  - Can be ordered (axial and coronal views) as a baseline or in atypical cases and can show enlarged extraocular muscle, orbital fat expansion, straightening of the optic nerve, and muscle crowding at the orbital apex
  - CT scan should be ordered in all cases of suspected thyroid compressive optic neuropathy to study the apical region of the orbit especially before orbital decompression.

Diagnostic Procedures/Other

- Complete ophthalmologic evaluation
  - Slit-lamp examination with fluorescein staining: Rule out exposure keratopathy
  - Goldman applanation tonometry in primary position and upgaze positions.
  - Pupillary evaluation: To detect RAPD in compressive optic neuropathy
  - Hertel exophthalmometry: To measure proptosis
  - Orthoptic evaluation: For diplopia due to strabismus
  - Dilated fundus examination: To assess the optic nerve
- Visual field assessment is important in case of compressive optic neuropathy.

Pathological Findings

The extraocular muscles reveal lymphocyte and plasma cell infiltration along with edema within the endomysium of the extraocular muscles.

DIFFERENTIAL DIAGNOSIS

- Orbital inflammatory diseases
  - Idiopathic orbital inflammatory disease (orbital pseudotumor)
  - Sarcoidosis
  - Wegener's granulomatosis
  - Orbital infiltration (lymphoma, metastatic disease)
- Ophthalmoplegia
  - Ocular myasthenia gravis

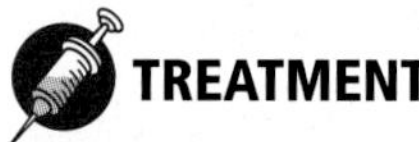

TREATMENT

MEDICATION

First Line

- Local symptomatic management (Mild disease)
  - Smoking cessation
  - Artificial tears, cold compressors
  - Patching or prisms for diplopia

Second Line

- Moderate–severe disease (severe congestive orbitopathy/exposure keratopathy/optic neuropathy)
  - Steroids: Oral dose of 60–100 mg can be administered over 2–3 months as a temporizing measure. Intravenous steroids on various pulse regimens for a cumulative dose of 8 g can also be given and appear to be more effective and better tolerated than oral steroids (3).

- Orbital radiotherapy: This can be given along with steroids for a cumulative dose 20 Gy, but the data on its efficacy is conflicting. It is not effective in treating proptosis but should be considered in patients with active disease with optic neuropathy refractory to maximal medical therapy and/or surgical decompression (4).
- Orbital decompression: Removal of parts of the orbital bony walls (medial, inferior, and lateral) and fat for compressive optic neuropathy or severe proptosis and corneal exposure
- Immunomodulatory drugs: Rituximab, rapamycin, and etanercept have been recently found beneficial in TED (5).

ADDITIONAL TREATMENT

General Measures

Uncontrolled thyroid function is associated with more severe TED.

Issues for Referral

- The complex nature of Graves' disease requires multidisciplinary team approach of endocrinologist/orbital surgeon/radiation oncologist.
- Corneal exposure and compressive optic neuropathy are sight-threatening signs and should be managed expeditiously by referral to an orbital/neuroophthalmology specialist.

Additional Therapies

Botulinum toxin can be give in the upper lids to relieve lid retraction or into the extraocular muscles as a temporizing measure for diplopia.

SURGERY/OTHER PROCEDURES

- Orbital decompression: A combination of medial/inferior/lateral bony walls can be decompressed in proptosis, exposure keratopathy, and optic neuropathy.
- Strabismus surgery is usually done following orbital decompression for diplopia.
- Lid surgery for lid retraction and dermatochalasis can be done with or following strabismus surgery.

ONGOING CARE

FOLLOW-UP RECOMMENDATIONS

- Patient with mild disease and no exposure keratopathy or optic neuropathy can be followed q 3–6 months.
- Patients with advanced exposure keratopathy and/or compressive optic neuropathy require immediate attention (steroids/radiation/orbital decompression).
- Patients receiving radioactive iodine ablation therapy for hyperthyroidism should be treated prophylactically with steroids to avoid activation of TED after treatment.
- Patients finishing radioactive ablation therapy should be treated quickly with thyroid hormone replacement as the sudden change to hypothyroidism can trigger TED activation.

Patient Monitoring

- Regular periodic ophthalmic evaluation including pupillary assessment, color vision, visual fields
- Patients with intermittent diplopia should be assessed for possible associated myasthenia gravis.
- IV steroids pulse regimen for active disease have been associated with hepatic toxicity especially in cumulative doses above 8 g. Liver function testing is recommended during IV steroid pulse therapy.
- Oral bisphosphonate should be given to patients requiring steroid treatment to prevent osteoporosis.

PATIENT EDUCATION

- Patients are told to watch for color desaturation or decreased vision (signs of optic neuropathy)
- Emphasize the importance of smoking cessation
- Graves' disease foundation (www.ngdf.org)

PROGNOSIS

- Rundle's curve
  - Active (inflammatory) phase (6 months to 5 years)
  - Inactive (Fibrotic) phase: Stable clinical signs for at least 6 months suggest that patient has entered the inactive phase.

COMPLICATIONS

- Corneal exposure/ corneal ulceration
- Compressive optic neuropathy
- Diplopia
- Glaucoma

REFERENCES

1. Lehmann GM, Garcia-Bates TM, Smith TJ, et al. Regulation of lymphocyte function by PPARgamma: Relevance to thyroid eye disease-related inflammation. *PPAR Res* 2008;2008:895901.
2. Cawood TJ, Moriarty P, O'Farelly C, et al. Smoking and thyroid-associated ophthalmopathy: A novel explanation of the biologic link. *J Clin Endocrinol Metab* 2007;92(1):59–64.
3. Zoumalan CI, Cockerham KP, Turbin RE, et al. Efficacy of corticosteroids and external beam radiation in the management of moderate to severe thyroid eye disease. *J Neuroophthalmol* 2007; 27:205–214.
4. Bradley EA, Gower EW, Bradley DJ, et al. Orbital radiation for Graves ophthalmopathy: A report by the American Academy of Ophthalmology. *Ophthalmology* 2008;115:398–409.
5. Khanna D, Chong KK, Afifiyan NF, et al. Rituximab treatment of patients with severe, corticosteroid-resistant thyroid-associated ophthalmopathy. *Ophthalmology* 2010;117: 133–139.

ADDITIONAL READING

- Perry JD, Feldon SE. Rationale for radiotherapy in thyroid eye disease. *Am J Ophthalmol* 2009;148: 818–819.
- Bahn RS. Graves' ophthalmopathy. *New Engl J Med* 2010;362:726–738.

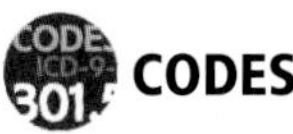

CODES

ICD9

- 242.00 Toxic diffuse goiter without mention of thyrotoxic crisis or storm
- 376.21 Thyrotoxic exophthalmos

CLINICAL PEARLS

- TED can be associated with vision-threatening complications such as exposure keratopathy and/or compressive optic neuropathy.
- Patients who do not display severe proptosis, especially older males, are at a higher risk for compressive optic neuropathy.
- Patients below the age of 40 years tend to have fat expansion, whereas patients over 60 years tend to have extraocular muscle swelling.
- TED course is divided into an active inflammatory phase and inactive fibrotic phase.
- Emergent treatment of vision threatening complications with steroids and/or orbital radiation and decompression is important to prevent permanent visual deficit.

TILTED DISC SYNDROME

Michael J. Bartiss

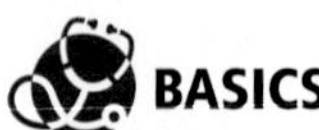

BASICS

DESCRIPTION

- Elevated superotemporal optic disc with posteriorly displaced inferonasal disc resulting in an oval appearance of the optic nerve head
- Long axis of disc obliquely oriented
- Situs inversus of retinal vessels, scleral crescent located inferiorly or inferonasally
- Thinning of the inferonasal retinal pigment epithelium and choroid is typically present.
- Often associated with incomplete bitemporal hemianopia (preferentially involving the superior quadrants) that, unlike chiasmal lesions, does not respect the vertical midline
- Kinetic perimetry testing demonstrates fairly normal fields with large and small isopters.
- Severely constricted medium isopters occur due to marked ectasia of the midperipheral fundus (which often normalizes with appropriate refractive correction).
- Typically accompanied by myopic astigmatism refractive error (secondary to fundus ectasia;)

RISK FACTORS

Genetics

Has been reported in patients with X-linked recessive congenital stationary night blindness (NYX in CSNB1 and CACNA1F in CSNB2)

PATHOPHYSIOLOGY

Staphylomatous defect surrounding the optic disc

ETIOLOGY

Cause unknown, but may have pathogenic relationship to retinochoroidal coloboma

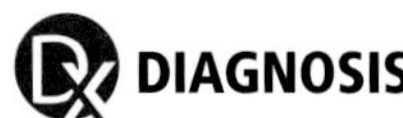

DIAGNOSIS

HISTORY

Congenital defect

PHYSICAL EXAM

- Full ocular examination including careful evaluation of the optic discs and evaluation for concomitant treatable amblyopia
- Careful evaluation of both eyes

DIAGNOSTIC TESTS & INTERPRETATION

Imaging

Initial approach

Neuro-imaging should be done in any patient with tilted disc syndrome whose visual field defect either respects the vertical midline or fails to preferentially involve the midperipheral kinetic perimetry isopter because suprasellar tumor must be ruled out

DIFFERENTIAL DIAGNOSIS

- Optic nerve dysplasia
- Optic nerve hypoplasia
- Optic nerve coloboma

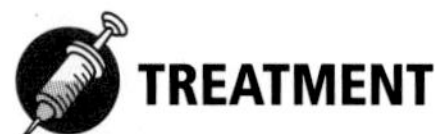

TREATMENT

MEDICATION

No medical treatment for the primary disorder

ADDITIONAL TREATMENT

General Measures

Appropriate refractive error correction as soon as indicated

Issues for Referral
Low vision evaluation and support as indicated in cases with significant bilateral involvement

COMPLEMENTARY & ALTERNATIVE THERAPIES
None proven or indicated

SURGERY/OTHER PROCEDURES
Amblyopia therapy and strabismus surgery as indicated

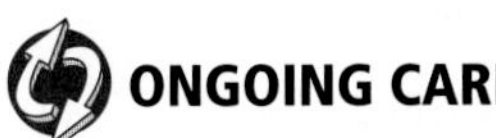

ONGOING CARE

FOLLOW-UP RECOMMENDATIONS
- Regular follow-ups to monitor for changes in refractive error
- As needed for amblyopia and strabismus monitoring and treatment
- Low vision care if indicated
- Kinetic visual field evaluation as soon as patient is capable of giving reliable responses

Patient Monitoring
Patient concerns about appearance if significant strabismus is present

PATIENT EDUCATION
Low vision intervention in patients with significant bilateral involvement

PROGNOSIS
Broad range of best corrected visual acuity

ADDITIONAL READING

- Nucci P, Mets MB, Gabianelli EB. Trisomy 4q with morning glory disc anomaly. *Ophthalmic Genetics*, 1990;11:143–145.
- Brodsky MC, Baker RS, Hamed LM. *Pediatric neuro-ophthalmology*. New York: Springer, 1996;59–61.
- Pollack S. The Morning Glory disc anomaly; contractile movement, classification, and embryogenesis. *Doc Ophthalmol* 1987;65: 439–460.
- Brown G, Tasman W. *Congenital anomalies of the optic disc*. New York: New York Grune & Stratton, 1983;171–178.

CODES

ICD9
- 368.47 Heteronymous bilateral field defects
- 743.57 Specified congenital anomalies of optic disc

CLINICAL PEARLS
- Work to maximize visual potential, especially in bilateral cases
- Protective eyewear if best corrected visual acuity is subnormal

T

TOXIC ANTERIOR SEGMENT SYNDROME (TASS)

Richard Tipperman

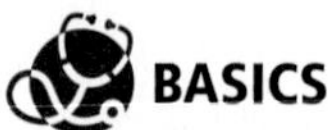

BASICS

DESCRIPTION

Toxic anterior segment syndrome (TASS) is a sterile postoperative inflammatory reaction which typically occurs 12–48 h following cataract or anterior segment surgery. It is caused by a noninfectious substance and is limited to the anterior segment of the eye. Gram stain and culture samples are negative and the condition is managed with intensive topical steroid treatment.

EPIDEMIOLOGY

Incidence of TASS is rare but typically occurs in "outbreaks" at a specific surgical center.

RISK FACTORS

- Any medication injected in or around the eye or placed topically at the time of surgery can be implicated in TASS.
- Preservatives and pH incompatibilities can lead to TASS as can contaminants from sterilization.
- Intraocular solutions with inappropriate chemical composition, concentration, pH, or osmolality
  - Preservatives
  - Denatured ophthalmic viscosurgical devices
  - Enzymatic detergents
  - Bacterial endotoxin
  - Oxidized metal deposits and residues
  - Intraocular lens residues

GENERAL PREVENTION

- Following appropriate protocols for instrument sterilization and cleaning
- Following appropriate protocols for administration and ordering of intra- and periocular medications

PATHOPHYSIOLOGY

The acute inflammatory response induces cellular necrosis and/or apoptosis as well as extracellular damage.

ETIOLOGY

See risk factors

COMMONLY ASSOCIATED CONDITIONS

Occurs at time of anterior segment surgery

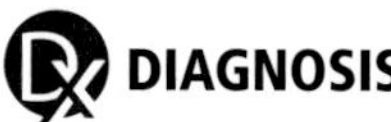

DIAGNOSIS

HISTORY

- Inflammatory process which starts within 12–24 h of cataract surgery
- Gram stain and cultures are negative.
- Improves with topical and/or oral steroids

PHYSICAL EXAM

- Severe anterior segment inflammation
- Hypopyon is often present.
- Limbus to limbus corneal edema is present.
- Vitreous cavity is rarely involved.
- Gonioscopy can be helpful to look for posterior synechiae.

DIAGNOSTIC TESTS & INTERPRETATION

Lab

Initial lab tests

Gram stain and culture

Follow-up & special considerations

Will be negative in TASS but can also be negative in infectious endophthalmitis

Pathological Findings

- Hypopyon
- Limbus to limbus corneal edema

DIFFERENTIAL DIAGNOSIS

Infectious endophthalmitis

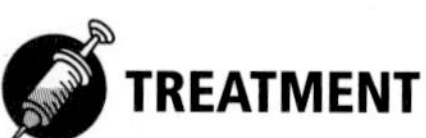

TREATMENT

MEDICATION

First Line

Topical steroids

Second Line

Oral steroids

ADDITIONAL TREATMENT

Issues for Referral

- Permanent corneal edema may require DSEK or PK.
- Scarring of trabecular meshwork may lead to glaucoma.

SURGERY/OTHER PROCEDURES

Permanent corneal edema may require surgery as described above

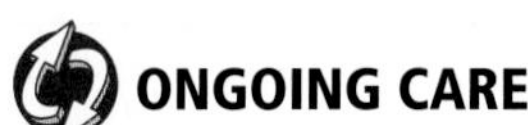

ONGOING CARE

PROGNOSIS
- Depends on severity of inflammation
- Patients can have permanent corneal edema
- Patients can have fixed and dilated pupil
- Patients can develop glaucoma

COMPLICATIONS
- Glaucoma
- Tonic pupil
- Persistent corneal edema

ADDITIONAL READING

- Mamalis N, Edelhauser HF, et al. Toxic anterior segment syndrome. *J Cataract Refract Surg* 2006;32:322–323.
- Kutty PK, Forster TS, Wood-Koob C, et al. Multistate outbreak of toxic anterior segment syndrome, 2005. *J Cataract Refract Surg* 2008;34:585–590.

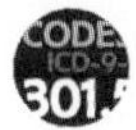

CODES

ICD9
- 360.19 Other endophthalmitis
- 364.05 Hypopyon
- 379.8 Other specified disorders of eye and adnexa

CLINICAL PEARLS
- As opposed to endophthalmitis, which typically occurs at 4–7 days postoperatively, TASS is usually seen in the 1st 24 h.
- Adnexal inflammation, which is commonly seen with infectious endophthalmitis, is not typical with TASS
- An inflammatory response in the vitreous cavity is uncommon in TASS and common in infectious endophthalmitis

TOXIC KERATOCONJUNCTIVITIS

Christine G. Saad

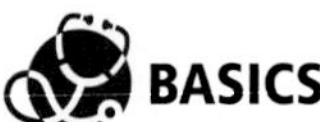

BASICS

DESCRIPTION

Toxic keratoconjunctivitis is an inflammation of the bulbar and palpebral conjunctiva with corneal involvement due to exposure to foreign substance(s).

RISK FACTORS

- Use of topical ophthalmic medications, eye cosmetics, and contact lenses. Further, periocular molluscum contagiosum
- Exposure to environmental irritants

GENERAL PREVENTION

Avoidance of known irritants

PATHOPHYSIOLOGY

Nonantigenic induction of lymphocytes resulting in mitotic and lymphoblastic transformation

ETIOLOGY

- Exposure to environmental irritants, topical ophthalmic medications, contact lenses and solutions, and eye cosmetics
- Prolonged use of ophthalmic medications including glaucoma medications (e.g., brimonidine, apraclonidine, pilocarpine), antivirals (e.g., trifluridine), antibiotics (e.g., neomycin, gentamicin), and cycloplegics (e.g., atropine, homatropine)
- Preservatives in ophthalmic medications and solutions(i.e., benzalkonium chloride)
- Preservative-containing soaking solutions and enzymatic cleansers in contact lens wearers
- Proteins that spill from molluscum contagiosum lesions

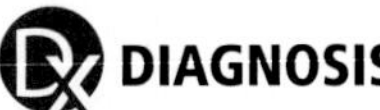

DIAGNOSIS

HISTORY

Ocular redness, burning, irritation, and tearing with gradual onset from initial exposure to irritant or use of ophthalmic agent

PHYSICAL EXAM

- Diffuse conjunctival injection associated with a follicular response
- Follicles are enlarged and inflamed and mostly noted in the inferior fornix and palpebral conjunctiva
- Punctate epithelial staining of the cornea
- Chemosis
- Mild periocular erythema or edema
- Periocular molluscum contagiosum lesions: Elevated, round, white lesions with an umbilicated center

DIAGNOSTIC TESTS & INTERPRETATION

Pathological Findings

True lymphoid follicles that contain germinal centers with lymphoblasts

DIFFERENTIAL DIAGNOSIS

Allergic, bacterial, or viral conjunctivitis, dry eye, blepharitis, and contact lens overwear

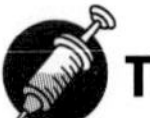

TREATMENT

MEDICATION

First Line

- Avoid exposure to, or discontinue use of, the offending agent, if possible
- Preservative-free artificial tears 4–8 times daily
- Artificial tear ointment at bedtime as needed

Second Line

- Mild topical steroid may be considered in severe cases that are not responsive to first-line therapy
  - Treatment with topical steroid should be initiated by an eye care provider.

ADDITIONAL TREATMENT

General Measures

- Identification and removal of offending agent
- Contact lens holiday. Use of another contact lens-care solution when contact lens use is resumed

Issues for Referral
- Failure to respond to treatment
- Referral to an eye care provider when there is visual impairment

SURGERY/OTHER PROCEDURES
Curettage or excision of molluscum contagiosum lesions

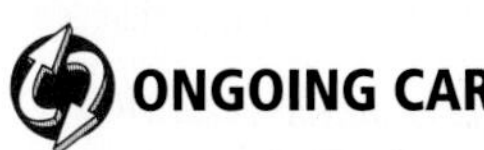

ONGOING CARE

FOLLOW-UP RECOMMENDATIONS
- Approximately 1 week following the initiation of treatment, although follow-up should be based on severity of disease and comorbidities
  - When glaucoma medications are stopped, closely monitor intraocular pressure

Patient Monitoring
Monitor vision. With topical steroid use, monitor intraocular pressure and intraocular lens

PATIENT EDUCATION
- Risks of topical steroid use include glaucoma, cataract formation, and predisposition to infection. Treatment with topical steroid should be a short-term treatment only.
- Patients should be advised to follow up sooner than advised if there is a progression in symptoms or if symptoms are accompanied by visual impairment.

PROGNOSIS
Generally good

COMPLICATIONS
Elevation of intraocular pressure when glaucoma medications are stopped

ADDITIONAL READING

- Dart J. Corneal toxicity: The epithelium and stroma in iatrogenic and factitious disease. *Eye (Lond.)* 2003;17:886–892.
- Lindquist T. Conjunctivitis: An overview and classification. In: Krachmer J, Mannis M, Holladay E, (eds). *Cornea*, 2nd ed. Elsevier Mosby, 2005.
- Rubenstein JB, Virasch V. Conjunctivitis: Infectious and noninfectious. In: Yanoff Duker, (ed). *Ophthalmology*, 3rd ed. Mosby, 2008.
- Wilkerson M, Lewis RA, Shields MB. Follicular conjunctivitis associated with apraclonidine. *Am J Ophthal* 1991;111:105.
- Wilson FM II. Adverse external ocular effects of topical ophthalmic therapy: An epidemiologic, laboratory, and clinical study. *Trans Am Ophthalmol Soc* 1983;81:854–965.
- Wilson FM II. Adverse external ocular effects of topical ophthalmic medications. *Surv Ophthalmol* 1979;24:57.

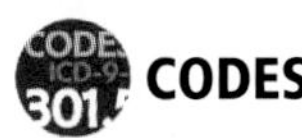

CODES

ICD9
370.49 Other keratoconjunctivitis, unspecified

T

TOXIC OPTIC NEUROPATHY (INCLUDING NUTRITIONAL)

Susan M. Ksiazek

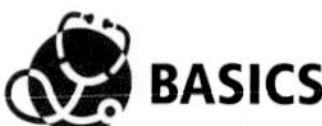

BASICS

DESCRIPTION

- Painless, bilateral vision loss including dyschromatopsia and central or centrocecal scotoma
- Exception is unilateral vision loss from phosphodiesterase inhibitors, which are possibly associated with ischemic optic neuropathy
- Typically slowly progressive; less often acute
  - Toxins [e.g., methanol, ethylene glycol, toluene, styrene, carbon monoxide, cyanide (from smoking and cassava)]
  - Drugs
    - Direct (e.g., ethambutol, disulfiram iodochlorohydroxyquinoline, alpha interferon, vincristine, amiodarone, cyclosporine, tacrolimus)
    - Indirect (phosphodiesterase inhibitors and infliximab)
  - Nutritional deficiencies (e.g., vitamin B12, thiamine, folate)
- System(s) affected: Nervous

EPIDEMIOLOGY

- Affects all ages, races, and economic strata
- Both sexes are equally affected
- Nutritional affects individuals from lower economic status and during times of war and famine
- More common in individuals on certain drugs, occupational exposure, smokers, and alcoholics

Incidence

- Varies on type, yet not known in most cases
  - Ethambutol optic neuropathy is 1.5% in 1 Korean study or 100,000 new cases annually (1)

Prevalence

Unknown but varies with type

RISK FACTORS

- Impaired renal disease with ethambutol
- Occupational exposure for toluene and styrene
- Smoking with toxic and nutritional causes
  - Pipe and cigar more than cigarettes
- Alcohol intake is often associated with nutritional causes

Genetics

Unknown

GENERAL PREVENTION

- Regular monitoring of patients on ethambutol
- B-complex vitamins and vitamin A reduces incidence in Cuba

PATHOPHYSIOLOGY

- Generally related to interference of mitochondrial function with oxidative stress
  - Demyelination of white matter—formic acid, a metabolite of methanol, is a mitochondrial toxin
  - Defective mitochondrial oxidative phosphorylation, with buildup of reactive oxygen species in the optic nerve in ethambutol and Cuban epidemic optic neuropathy
  - Chelates metal-containing enzymes used in the mitochondria with ethambutol, disulfiram, and penicillamine
  - Smoking may cause elevated cyanide
- Vascular changes at optic nerve head with phosphodiesterase inhibitors

ETIOLOGY

Multifactorial with both poor nutrition and toxicity playing roles

COMMONLY ASSOCIATED CONDITIONS

- Smoking and alcohol use are seen often but are not clearly demonstrated
  - Tobacco may be a toxin by itself
  - Alcohol is not a primary contributor; but is related to poor nutrition
- Pernicious anemia with vitamin B12 deficiency

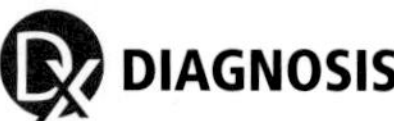

DIAGNOSIS

HISTORY

- Either acute (some nutritional and toxins) versus gradual progressive loss of color and central vision
  - Careful documentation of exposure to drug or toxin or dietary history (2)[B]

ALERT

Methanol and ethylene glycol poisoning presents initially with nausea and vomiting. Vision loss together with respiratory distress is delayed. Coma and death may follow if not recognized (1)[B]

PHYSICAL EXAM

- Decreased visual acuity and color perception
- Optic disc either normal or swollen acutely
  - Eventual pallor
  - Other neurologic signs depending on agent:
    - Keratopathy and hearing loss with nutritional deficiency
    - Myelopathy and dementia with vitamin B12 deficiency
    - Nausea, vomiting, respiratory distress, headache, confusion, abdominal pain, coma, death with methanol and ethylene glycol
    - Peripheral neuropathy with nutritional deficiency and disulfiram reaction
    - Ophthalmoplegia and nystagmus with cyclosporine

DIAGNOSTIC TESTS & INTERPRETATION

Lab

Initial lab tests

- Vitamin levels before treatment (thiamine and B12)
- Other labs when methanol or ethylene glycol is suspected agent
  - Elevated methanol ($>$20 mg/dL) or ethylene glycol ($>$20 mg/dL) levels
  - Oxalate crystals in urine with ethylene glycol
  - Serum bicarbonate $<$8 meq/L

Follow-up & special considerations

Frequent measure of blood methanol, CO_2, bicarbonate, pH, and potassium

Imaging

- MRI with and without gadolinium with attention to optic nerves and chiasm to exclude compressive causes (e.g., pituitary adenomas)
  - Bilateral putaminal hyperintense lesions on T2-weighted images with methanol poisoning

Diagnostic Procedures/Other

- Visual fields
- Color vision

Pathological Findings

- Affects the papillomacular bundle of the nerve fiber layer
- Initial swelling followed by atrophy

DIFFERENTIAL DIAGNOSIS

- Retinal diseases, specifically maculopathies
- Hereditary optic neuropathies
- Compressive optic nerve lesions

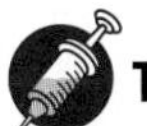

TREATMENT

MEDICATION

First Line

- Ethanol or fomepizole for methanol and ethylene glycol
- Dialysis for methanol and ethylene glycol
- Bicarbonate for pH <7.3
  - Thiamine injection with nutritional correction
  - Stop inciting drug
  - Supportive care (may include airway protection)

Second Line

- Well-balanced diet, high in protein (3)[C]
  - Supplement with B complex vitamins

ADDITIONAL TREATMENT

Issues for Referral

- Follow-up with ophthalmologist within 1 week of discharge
  - Social services depending on level of disability (vision and mobility)

COMPLEMENTARY & ALTERNATIVE THERAPIES

Steroids

IN-PATIENT CONSIDERATIONS

Initial Stabilization

- Metabolic acidosis with methanol and ethylene glycol poisoning
  - Coma and death from respiratory failure

Admission Criteria

- Central nervous system dysfunction
  - High suspicion of drug ingestion

IV Fluids

Crystalloids if blood pressure problems

Nursing

Awareness of a patient with poor vision and need to assist with basic activities (e.g., eating and walking)

Discharge Criteria

- Stabilized neurologically
- Stabilized from a renal standpoint

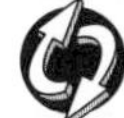

ONGOING CARE

FOLLOW-UP RECOMMENDATIONS

Vision rarely returns; when it does, it occurs slowly, over 3–9 months

Patient Monitoring

- ICU initially for severe toxicities
- Floor care with medically stable patients

DIET

High protein with B-complex vitamins

PATIENT EDUCATION

- With necessary treatment, that is, ethambutol for tuberculosis, call doctor if any spots or decrease in red color or ability to read appear
- Stop use of phosphodiesterase inhibitors if visual changes

PROGNOSIS

- Variable
- Some toxicities are fatal or result in neurologic deficits including blindness

COMPLICATIONS

- Neurologic effects depending on agent
  - Peripheral neuropathy with linezolid
  - Cognitive impairment with methanol, ethylene glycol, and vitamin B12

REFERENCES

1. Lee EJ, Kim SJ, Choung HK, et al. Incidence and clinical features of ethambutol-induced optic neuropathy in Korea. *J Neuroophthalmol* 2008;28:269–277.
2. Jammalamadaka D, Raissi S. Ethylene glycol, methanol and isopropyl alcohol intoxication. *Am J Med Sci* 2010;339:276–281.
3. Orssaud C, Roche O, Dufier JL. Nutritional optic neuropathies. *J Neurol Sci* 2007;262:158–164.

ADDITIONAL READING

- Carter JE. Anterior ischemic optic neuropathy and stroke with use of PDE-5 inhibitors for erectile dysfunction: cause or coincidence? *J Neurol Sci* 2007;262:89–97.
- Chang V, McCurdy D, Gordon LK. Enanercept associated optic neuropathy. *Graefes Arch Clin Exp Ophthalmol* 2007;35:680–682.
- Kerrison JB. Optic neuropathies caused by toxins and adverse drug reactions. *Ophthalmol Clin North Am* 2004;17:481–488.
- Kesler A, Pianka P. Toxic optic neuropathy. *Curr Neurol Neurosci Rep* 2003;3:410–414.
- Kessler L, Lucescu C, Pinget M, et al. Tacrolimus-associated optic neuropathy after pancreatic islet transplantation using a sirolimus/tacrolimus immunosuppressive regimen. *Transplantation* 2006;81:636–637.
- Lloyd MJ, Fraunfelder FW. Drug-induced optic neuropathies. *Drugs of Today* 2007;43:8217–8236.
- Purvin V, Kawasaki A, Borruat FX. Optic neuropathy in patients using amiodarone. *Arch Ophthalmol* 2006;124:696–701.
- Rucker JC, Hamilton SR, Bardenstein D, et al. Linezolid-associated toxic optic neuropathy. *Neurology* 2006;66:595–598.

CODES

ICD9

- 377.33 Nutritional optic neuropathy
- 377.34 Toxic optic neuropathy

CLINICAL PEARLS

- Early recognition and withdrawal of medication can reverse vision loss.
- Suspicion and early treatment of methanol or ethylene glycol can be life and vision saving.
- Ethambutol patients must be regularly monitored.

TOXOCARIASIS

Justis P. Ehlers

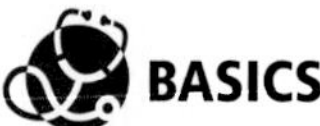

BASICS

DESCRIPTION
- Ocular toxocariasis is a helminthic disease that is a common cause of posterior uveitis, particularly in children.
- 3 major presentations:
  - Endophthalmitis
  - Peripheral granuloma
  - Posterior granuloma

EPIDEMIOLOGY
- Varies by region; actual incidence is unknown
- Constitutes 1–2% of pediatric uveitis
- Average age of onset is 7.5 years
- 80% of patients are <16 years of age

RISK FACTORS
- Exposure to soil contaminated with canine feces infected with *Toxocara canis* eggs
- Exposure to infected pets or animals

GENERAL PREVENTION
- Good hygiene
- Reducing exposure to contaminated environment
- Periodic treatment of pets

PATHOPHYSIOLOGY
Inflammatory response secondary to parasitic infection resulting in eosinophilic abscess and chronic granulomatous inflammation

ETIOLOGY
Toxocara canis, the dog roundworm, is the primary causative organism. Infectious eggs are ingested and the developing larvae move hematogenously to the eye or other organs.

COMMONLY ASSOCIATED CONDITIONS
- Visceral larval migrans
  - Systemic infection secondary to *Toxocara* resulting from migration of larvae throughout the body, particularly liver, brain, lung, and eye
  - Typically in children, 6 months to 3 years of age
  - History of contact with puppies and/or ingestion of soil
  - Often asymptomatic, but may have fever, weight loss, and coughing
  - Laboratory results may show leukocytosis with eosinophilia, elevated *Toxocara* IgG and IgM.
  - Prognosis usually excellent
  - Rarely associated with ocular toxocariasis

DIAGNOSIS

- Clinical features of ocular toxocariasis include:
  - Typically, young children but may occur in adults
  - Usually unilateral

HISTORY
- Exposure to puppies
- History of ingestion of soil or other contaminated substances (e.g., grass)
- Possible history of systemic infection
- Presence or absence of pain. *Toxocara*, even in the endophthalmitis form, is rarely painful and does not cause significant photophobia.

PHYSICAL EXAM
Ophthalmic Exam
- Variable, multiple presentations
  - Endophthalmitis
    - Vitreitis
    - Granulomatous keratic precipitates
    - Hypopyon may be present
    - Possible yellowish-white chorioretinal mass
    - Retinal detachment may be present
    - Leukocoria may be present
  - Peripheral granuloma
    - White elevated mass present in the peripheral retina and/or ciliary body region
    - Retinal dragging and formation of a falciform fold may occur
    - Macular heterotopia may be present
  - Posterior granuloma
    - Overlying vitreitis and inflammation may be present in the acute stage
    - White elevated mass typically 0.5–4 disc diameters in size
    - Often diagnosed at older age
  - Optic papillitis
    - Localized infection of the optic nerve
    - Disc edema with telangiectatic vessels
    - Possible subretinal exudate
    - Variable peripapillary nodule
- Other associated ophthalmic findings
  - Strabismus
  - Amblyopia
  - Leukocoria

DIAGNOSTIC TESTS & INTERPRETATION

Diagnostic Procedures/Other

- Thorough slit-lamp and indirect ophthalmoscopic exam are critical to diagnosis
- Ultrasonography is vital for evaluating leukocoria to help distinguish between other possible diagnoses (e.g., calcifications for retinoblastoma, hyaloid remnants for PHPV).
- CBC for eosinophilia is useful for visceral larval migrans, but is not useful for ocular disease.
- Serum and vitreous testing for *Toxocara* IgG
- Vitreous sample with cytopathologic examination for eosinophils

Pathological Findings

In ocular toxocariasis, granulomatous inflammation with eosinophilic abscess is often present. Significant quantities of eosinophils may be present in the vitreous and uveal tract.

DIFFERENTIAL DIAGNOSIS

- Retinoblastoma
- Coat's disease
- Persistent hyperplastic primary vitreous (PHPV)
- Retinopathy of prematurity
- Familial exudative vitreoretinopathy
- Toxoplasmosis

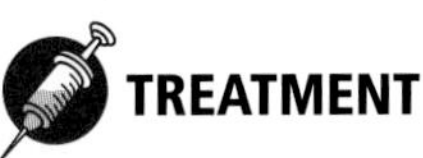

TREATMENT

MEDICATION

- Anti-helminthic medications are rarely used for ocular disease.
- Topical or periocular steroids may be used for control of ocular inflammation.
- Topical cycloplegics may be useful in cases with severe anterior segment inflammation.
- Oral steroids may also be employed in cases of severe inflammation.
- Amblyopia and strabismus should be addressed, as indicated.

SURGERY/OTHER PROCEDURES

- Diagnostic pars plana vitrectomy may be performed in cases with unclear etiology to obtain vitreous fluid for analysis.
- Pars plana vitrectomy may also be utilized to address various complications related to the infection (e.g., retinal detachment, severe vitreoretinal traction).
- Laser photocoagulation of the *Toxocara* larva has been reported.

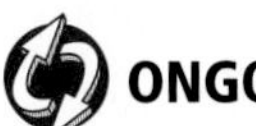

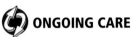

ONGOING CARE

FOLLOW-UP RECOMMENDATIONS

- Determined based on severity of inflammation and disease
- Consultation with vitreoretinal specialist and/or pediatric ophthalmologist may be appropriate depending on severity
- Monocular precautions (e.g., eye protection) for all patients with severe unilateral vision loss

PATIENT EDUCATION

- Centers for Disease Control Parasitic Disease Information: Toxocariasis (http://www.cdc.gov/NCIDOD/DPD/PARASITES/toxocara/factsht_toxocara.htm)
- The National Institute for Health and Clinical Excellence Clinical Knowledge Summaries: Toxocariasis (http://www.cks.nhs.uk/patient_information_leaflet/toxocariasis)

PROGNOSIS

- Depends on severity of inflammation and location of the infection in the eye
- Some patients will maintain excellent visual acuity with minimal sequelae and others may have severe complications requiring enucleation.

COMPLICATIONS

- Visual loss
- Retinal detachment
- Phthisis

ADDITIONAL READING

- Sabrosa NA, Zajdenweber M. Nematode infections of the eye: Toxocariasis, onchocerciasis, diffuse unilateral subacute neuroretinitis, and cysticercosis. *Ophthalmol Clin North Am* 2002;15:351–356.
- Shields JA. Ocular toxocariasis. A review. *Surv Ophthalmol* 1984;28:361–381.

CODES

ICD9

- 128.0 Toxocariasis
- 360.19 Other endophthalmitis
- 363.20 Chorioretinitis, unspecified

CLINICAL PEARLS

- Retinoblastoma can closely mimic some presentations of toxocariasis and must be ruled out.

TOXOPLASMOSIS

James H. Whelan

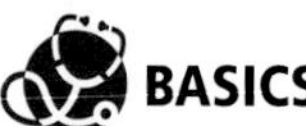

BASICS

DESCRIPTION

- Toxoplasmic chorioretinitis is usually a unifocal, full thickness chorioretinal lesion.
- Frequently arises from border of preexisting chorioretinal scar
- Associated with focal vitreous inflammation directly over the lesion
- Anterior segment findings may include mild iritis, large keratic precipitates, raised intraocular pressure.
- Signs and symptoms usually limited to the eye, cerebral form seen in HIV

EPIDEMIOLOGY

Incidence

- Majority of cases assumed to be congenital, although recent publications have challenged this
- There are documented reports of acquired disease in patients with a previously normal fundus and seronegative antibody titers.

Prevalence

- Most common cause of posterior uveitis
- Accounts for 90% of necrotizing retinitis

RISK FACTORS

- Ingestion of raw meat
- Exposure to cats
- HIV

GENERAL PREVENTION

- Avoid modifiable risk factors
- Consider using trimethoprim/sulfamethoxazole in patients with history of toxoplasmosis prior to cataract surgery

ETIOLOGY

- Infestation with an obligate intracellular protozoan, *Toxoplasma gondii*
- Parasite found in cats. Intermediate hosts include rodents and birds.
- Infestation is usually congenital (transplacental) and occasionally acquired.
- Predilection for the eye and brain.

COMMONLY ASSOCIATED CONDITIONS

- HIV
- Immunocompromised patients and the elderly

DIAGNOSIS

HISTORY

- Young healthy patients with recent onset of blurred vision.
  - Photophobia
  - Red eye
  - Floaters
- Ingestion of raw meat that contains tissue cysts.
- Exposure to cats
- HIV or Immunocompromise

PHYSICAL EXAM

Common ophthalmic features of toxoplasmosis chorioretinitis can include:

- Decreased vision
- Floaters
- Conjunctival erythema
- Moderate to severe vitreous inflammatory reaction
- Focal area of chorioretinal inflammation
- Unilateral pale retinal lesion, with adjacent chorioretinal scar
- Mild anterior uveitis
- Raised intraocular pressure
- Optic disc swelling

Less common ophthalmic features include:

- Pain with severe iridocyclitis
- Large keratic precipitates
- Neuroretinitis with macular star formation
- Retinal artery or vein occlusion
- Cystoid macular edema
- Retinal vasculitis
- Peri-arterial exudation, Kyrieleis arteritis

DIAGNOSTIC TESTS & INTERPRETATION

Lab

Initial lab tests

- Serum IgM and IgG antibodies can be evaluated for presumed acquired infections
- IgM found 2 weeks to 6 months after initial infection
- High percentages of general population are IgG seropositive
- Can compare antibody levels in serum to intraocular fluid (aqueous or vitreous) to confirm intraocular production.
- Polymerase chain reaction (PCR) of the aqueous humor may be useful in atypical cases
- Chest x-ray, luetic screening, Toxocara serology, and TB testing may be helpful when the diagnosis is uncertain.
- HIV testing in atypical cases or patients at risk

DIFFERENTIAL DIAGNOSIS

- Syphilis
- Tuberculosis
- Toxocariasis
- Sarcoidosis
- Acute retinal necrosis (ARN)
- Endophthalmitis
  - Endogenous
  - Exogenous

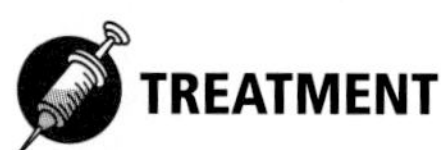

TREATMENT

MEDICATION

First Line

Treatment plan based on location and severity

- Small non-sight threatening lesions
  - Trimethoprim/sulfamethoxazole
  - Second-generation tetracycline
- Sight threatening lesions near disc (2–3 mm) or in macula
  - Pyrimethamine, PO 200 mg loading dose, then 25 mg PO daily
  - Sulfadiazine 2 g PO loading dose, then 1 g PO q.i.d
  - Folinic acid 10 mg PO every second day
    - Treatment duration is 5–6 weeks

- Steroids
  - Low dose (20–60 mg PO daily 2–3 weeks)
  - Required to reduce macular or optic nerve inflammation or swelling
  - Start minimum of 24 hours after initiation of antibiotics
    - Discontinue 7–10 days prior to stopping antibiotics
    - Avoid periocular steroids as they may cause scleritis
- Topical medications: If anterior segment inflammation ± raised IOP
  - Steroids, Prednisolone acetate 1% q.i.d
  - Cycloplegic agent, Homatropine 2% t.i.d
  - Antiglaucoma medications, Timolol maleate 0.5% b.i.d

Second Line

Sulfa allergy: Use Azithromycin, or Atovaquone, or Clindamycin.

ADDITIONAL TREATMENT

Additional Therapies

- Considerations for immunocompromised patients.
  - Frequently subclinical inflammation
  - May not have preexisting chorioretinal scars
  - Multifocal ± bilateral disease can be seen
  - Can be relentlessly progressive
  - Cerebral form more common, patients require CNS imaging studies
  - Delayed treatment can lead to diffuse spreading form mimicking ARN
  - Avoid systemic steroid use
  - May require long-term maintenance antibiotic therapy

Pregnancy Considerations

- Maternal fetal transmission can cause more severe ocular manifestations.
- Ophthalmic findings in the newborn
  - Microphthalmos
  - Bilateral macular scars
- CNS findings in the newborn
  - Convulsions
  - Paralysis
  - Hydrocephalus
  - Intracranial calcification
  - Stillbirth
  - Visceral involvement
- Pregnant women seronegative for Toxoplasmosis antibodies should avoid any contact with cats during pregnancy.
- Consult Obstetrician
- Treatment in Pregnancy:
  - Clindamycin 300–600 mg PO q.i.d
  - Spiramycin 3 g PO in 3–4 doses
  - Do not use Pyrimethamine

SURGERY/OTHER PROCEDURES

Vitrectomy may be required for dense vitreitis or other complications such as retinal detachment.

ONGOING CARE

FOLLOW-UP RECOMMENDATIONS

- Small non-sight threatening lesions require less stringent follow-up care, but should be assessed 1 week after initiating therapy and then every 2 weeks.
- Sight threatening infections near the optic nerve or macula should be assessed at 3 days and then weekly.
- Usual course of treatment is 6 weeks.
- Avoid delays in treating immunocompromised patients and remember these patients may require long-term antibiotics.

Patient Monitoring

- All patients should have a complete dilated ocular exam on each visit.
- Results of all blood tests and ancillary testing should be attained as soon as possible.
- Patients on Pyrimethamine require weekly CBC testing.
- Fasting blood glucose levels should be determined prior to starting systemic steroid treatment.

DIET

- All patients should be instructed to avoid eating raw or undercooked meat containing *Toxoplasma* cysts.
- Other dietary risks include raw milk or unfiltered chlorinated surface water.

PATIENT EDUCATION

- All patients should be aware that the major routes of transmission are:
  - Ingestion of contaminated foodstuffs; recommend adequate cooking of meat and care handling raw meat
  - Contamination of hands from disposing of cat feces or contaminated soil or sand boxes; recommend gloves or hand washing
  - Transplacental transmission from infected mother to fetus during gestation; pregnant women should avoid any contact with cats

PROGNOSIS

- 40% of patients may have permanent unilateral visual loss to 20/100 or less
- 90% of patients with macular lesions will experience severe vision loss
- 15% of patients may have mild visual loss (20/40–20/70)
- 5 year recurrence rate is ~80%
- Vision loss more associated with duration of active episode than number of recurrences

COMPLICATIONS

- Mild to severe vision loss
- Vitreous hemorrhage
- Secondary choroidal neovascularization
- Epiretinal membrane formation
- Chronic and relentless vitreitis
- Retinal tear and detachment
- Cystoid macular edema
- Cataract

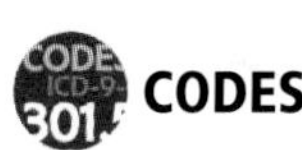

CODES

ICD9

- 130.2 Chorioretinitis due to toxoplasmosis
- 130.9 Toxoplasmosis, unspecified

TRACHOMA

Colleen P. Halfpenny

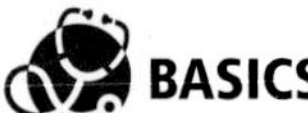

BASICS

DESCRIPTION

- A blinding infectious condition currently found in mostly undeveloped countries
- Consists of an active inflammatory stage in childhood followed by scarring sequelae in adulthood

EPIDEMIOLOGY

Incidence

Incidence varies widely by geographic area

Prevalence

- 1.2 billion people live in endemic areas in Africa, Middle East, southern Asia, India, Australia and the Pacific Islands
- 48.5% active trachoma concentrated in 5 countries: Ethiopia, India, Nigeria, Sudan, and Guinea.
- 50% of the global burden of trichiasis is concentrated in only 3 countries: China, Ethiopia, and Sudan.
- Active form affects 40.6 million people
- 8.1 million people have trichiasis
- Accounts for ~3% of world's blindness

RISK FACTORS

- Endemic areas
- Poverty
- Crowded living conditions
- Poor water supply
- Host immunity
- Active stage: Children Ages 2–5
- Late stage: Women
- Transmission:
  - Direct contact (eye-to-eye)
  - Indirect contact (shared clothes)
  - Eye seeking (synanthropic) muscoid fly
  - Coughing or sneezing

GENERAL PREVENTION

- Improved personal hygiene
- Improved environmental sanitation

PATHOPHYSIOLOGY

- Bacterial cytoplasmic inclusions infect conjunctival epithelial cells.
- Chronic conjunctival inflammation causes tarsal scarring, which causes lid deformities and trichiasis.
- Recurrent infectious keratitis secondary to exposure and trichiasis
- End stage occurs with corneal scarring

ETIOLOGY

Recurrent ocular infections with *Chlamydia trachomatis* (serotypes A, B, Ba, and C)

COMMONLY ASSOCIATED CONDITIONS

- Dry eyes
- Concurrent infection with *Hemophilus influenzae* conjunctivitis may cause more severe course.

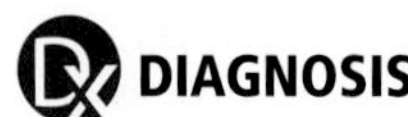

DIAGNOSIS

HISTORY

- Acute stage: asymptomatic, tearing, discharge, itching, foreign body sensation, and hyperemia
- Late stage: foreign body sensation, tearing, photophobia, and decreased vision

PHYSICAL EXAM

- Grading system (2):
- TF (trachomatous inflammation-follicular): follicles (≥5 of at least 0.5 mm diameter)
- TI (trachomatous inflammation-intense): inflammatory thickening of the tarsal conjunctiva obscuring half of normal conjunctival vessels
- TS (trachomatous scarring): white lines (Arlt's lines), bands or sheets of scarring of tarsal conjunctiva
- TT (trachomatous trichiasis): ≥1 eyelash(es) rubbing eyeball
- CO (corneal opacity): corneal opacity obscuring pupil margin
- Corneal vascularization/pannus
- Herbert's pits: Shallow limbal depressions, which are old ruptured follicles
- Entropion

DIAGNOSTIC TESTS & INTERPRETATION

Lab

Conjunctival scraping sent for:

- Polymerase chain reaction (PCR)
- Direct fluorescein-labeled monoclonal antibody (direct fluorescent antibody [DFA]) assay and enzyme immunoassay (EIA) of conjunctival smears
- Giemsa cytology

Pathological Findings

- Chlamydial inclusions in conjunctival epithelial cells
- Lymphoid follicles
- Loss of goblet cells
- Squamous cell metaplasia
- Subepithelial fibrous membrane formation

DIFFERENTIAL DIAGNOSIS

- Active phase:
  - Viral (e.g., adenoviral, HSV, VZV)
  - Bacterial (*Staph aureus*, *Moraxella*)
  - Medicamentosa/toxicity
  - Molluscum contagiosum
- Late stage:
  - Viral (e.g., adenoviral, HSV, VZV)
  - Bacterial (*Corynebacterium*)
  - Ocular cicatricial pemphigoid
  - Stevens–Johnson syndrome
  - Chemical injury

TREATMENT

MEDICATION

First Line

- SAFE strategy (3)[A]:
  - S = Surgery
  - A = antibiotics
  - F = facial cleanliness
  - E = environmental improvement
- Active, infectious disease (4)[A]:
  - Azithromycin: Children: 20 mg/kg oral single dose; Adults: 1 g oral single dose (1)[A]
  - Doxycycline: 100 mg b.i.d for 7 days
  - Tetracycline: 15 mg/kg/day for 14 days
- Late disease (5)[B]: Correction of eyelid deformities (bilamellar tarsal rotation procedure)
- Corneal opacity: Corneal transplantation (following lid procedure)

Second Line

Tetracycline ointment b.i.d for 3–6 days every month for 6-month course

ADDITIONAL TREATMENT

General Measures

- Education on the importance of facial cleanliness and hygiene
- Improved water supplies (e.g., water provision program, hand-dug wells, rainwater harvesting)
- Improved sanitation (e.g., household pit latrines)

Issues for Referral

Referral to health system capable of eyelid repair/reconstruction is critical

SURGERY/OTHER PROCEDURES

- Eyelid surgery
- Corneal transplantation: Poor prognosis if continued lid abnormalities or if corneal vascularization is present

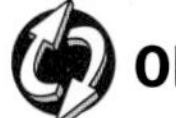

ONGOING CARE

FOLLOW-UP RECOMMENDATIONS

- Single, annual, high-coverage mass dose of oral azithromycin can interrupt the transmission of trachoma and also reduces childhood mortality in areas where trachoma is moderately prevalent (<35% in children; ref. 6, 7)
- Repeated biannual treatments in hyperendemic areas (>50% children) is probably needed for elimination (8).

PATIENT EDUCATION

- Hygiene education
- Medication compliance education

PROGNOSIS

- Approximately 20–45% of patients with recurrent active trachoma will develop late scarring
- Women and individuals with age >40 more likely to have scarring

COMPLICATIONS

Corneal blindness

REFERENCES

1. Mariotti SP, Pascolini D, Rose-Nussbaumer J. Trachoma: Global magnitude of a preventable cause of blindness. *Br J Ophthalmol* 2009;93: 563–568.
2. Thylefors B, Dawson CR, Jones BR, et al. A simple system for the assessment of trachoma and its complications. *Bull World Health Organ* 1987;65: 477–483.
3. Kuper H, Solomon AW, Buchan J, et al. A critical review of the SAFE strategy for the prevention of blinding trachoma. *Lancet Infect Dis* 2003;3: 372–381.
4. Bailey RJ, Arullendran P, Whittle HC, et al. Randomized controlled trial of single-dose oral azithromycin in treatment of trachoma. *Lancet* 1993;342:453–456.
5. Reacher M, Foster A, Huber J. *Trichiasis surgery for trachoma — the bilamellar tarsal rotation procedure. Geneva: World Health Organization,* 1993.
6. Solomon AW, Holland MJ, Alexander NDE, et al. Mass treatment with single-dose azithromycin for trachoma. *N Engl J Med* 2004;351:1962–1971.
7. Porco TC, Gebre T, Ayele B, et al. Effect of mass distribution of azithromycin for trachoma control on overall mortality in Ethiopian children: A randomized trial. *JAMA* 2009;302:962–968.
8. Lietman T, Porco T, Dawson C, et al. Global elimination of trachoma: How frequently should we administer mass chemotherapy? *Nat Med* 1999;5:572–576.

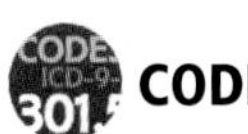

CODES

ICD9

- 076.9 Trachoma, unspecified
- 077.0 Inclusion conjunctivitis

CLINICAL PEARLS

- Early surgical intervention for treatment of trichiasis is imperative.
- Host immunity and concurrent bacterial infections play a role in active disease progressing to chronic sequelae.
- High-coverage mass distribution of oral azithromycin will greatly reduce the transmission of trachoma. The need for repeat treatments may depend on prevalence in this community.

TRANSIENT VISUAL LOSS

Mary Ellen P. Cullom

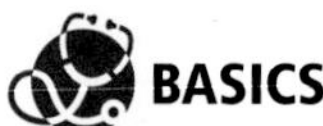

BASICS

DESCRIPTION
- Transient loss of vision in 1 or both eyes
  - Transient monocular visual loss(TMVL)
  - Transient binocular visual loss (TBVL)
  - System(s) affected: Central nervous system, ocular

RISK FACTORS
- Atherosclerosis
- Hypertension
- Diabetes mellitus
- Dyslipidemia
- Cardiac disease
- Obesity
- Hypercoagulable states
- Polymyalgia rheumatica
- Pregnancy
- Medications and drugs

Genetics
Hypercoagulability—Factor V Leiden (AD), antithrombin III deficiency (AD), protein S and C deficiency (AD), dysfibrogenemia (AD), hyperhomocystinemia (AD), and hemoglobin S (AR)

GENERAL PREVENTION
- Smoking cessation
- Control of hypertension
- Achieve and maintain glycemic control
- Treatment of dyslipidemia
- Anticoagulation of atrial fibrillation, high-risk cardioembolic disorders
- Exercise

PATHOPHYSIOLOGY
- TMVL
  - Ischemia of retina, optic nerve, choroid
  - Ocular—surface disease, angle-closure glaucoma, and hyphema
- TBVL
  - Transient ischemic attack–ischemia of occipital cortex
  - Migraine–cortical spreading depression
  - Seizure–neuronal hyperexcitability and hypersynchrony

ETIOLOGY
- TMVL
  - Ischemia
    - Atherosclerotic large-vessel disease–carotid or ophthalmic artery, aortic arch stenosis with decreased ocular perfusion or thromboembolism. Coincident hypotension may elicit symptoms
    - Cardioembolic–arrhythmia, valvular disease, thrombus, tumor with embolization to eye, etc.
    - Vasculitis–giant cell arteritis causing retinal artery occlusion or arteritic anterior ischemic optic neuropathy
    - Hypercoagulable states– retinal arteriolar or venous thrombosis. Cardiac thrombi
    - Carotid artery dissection–traumatic or spontaneous with occlusion or thromboembolism
    - Retinal artery vasospasm– retinal migraine. Especially in young adults. Associated headache or periorbital pain
    - Papilledema and optic disc drusen–edema causes decreased retinal perfusion
    - Central retinal vein occlusion–decreased venous outflow
  - Ocular disease
    - Angle-closure glaucoma, hyphema, surface disease
- TBVL
  - Ischemia: Vertebrobasilar insufficiency (VBI) secondary to atherosclerotic disease, cardioembolic source, or vertebrobasilar dissection. Hypotension often elicits symptoms.
  - Migraine
  - Seizure

COMMONLY ASSOCIATED CONDITIONS
- Atrial fibrillation
- Trauma–head and neck. Carotid and vertebrobasilar dissection
- Polymyalgia rheumatica–giant cell arteritis
- Hypotension

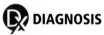

DIAGNOSIS

HISTORY
- TMVL versus TBVL- monocular or binocular visual loss. Patients with binocular hemianopic visual field loss will often incorrectly assign it to the eye with the temporal field loss and report monocular visual loss.
- Duration and frequency of visual loss–sudden or abrupt onset. Much overlap of duration
  - Seconds: Transient visual obscurations of papilledema or optic disc drusen. Ocular surface disease which improves with blinking or eye rubbing
  - Seconds to minutes: (30 sec to 30 min) Ischemic
  - Minutes: (10–60 min) migraine
  - Minutes–days: Seizures
  - Frequency of events–isolated or recurrent
- Description of visual loss
  - Positive visual phenomena
    - Photopsias (e.g., flashes, sparkles)–ischemia more likely to have negative visual phenomena
    - Scintillating fortification scotoma (migratory, bright, zigzag light)–migraine
    - Flickering, bright-colored shapes, geometric forms—seizures
  - Negative visual phenomena
    - Curtain, shade, altitudinal, or complete loss–ischemic TMVL
    - Blurry, foggy, hazy, patchy, dim–nonspecific, often ischemic TMVL
    - Dim, blurred, and complete–ischemic TBVL
- Precipitating factors
  - Orthostasis—hypotension produces symptoms in critical arterial stenosis.
  - Light-induced–severe carotid stenosis or giant cell arteritis
  - Head or neck trauma, chiropractic manipulation–carotid or vertebral dissection
- Associated symptoms
  - TMVL
    - Contralateral hemisensory or motor symptoms, lightheadedness, aphasia–carotid stenosis
    - Neck pain, headache, ipsilateral Horner's syndrome, contralateral sensory or motor symptoms–carotid dissection
    - Headache, scalp tenderness, jaw claudication, myalgias, diplopia–giant cell arteritis
    - Eye pain–retinal vasospasm in young adults with a prior history of migraine, angle-closure glaucoma
  - TBVL
    - Vertigo, diplopia, dysarthria, facial numbness–VBI
    - Severe headache or posterior neck pain with VBI symptoms–vertebrobasilar dissection
    - Headache following visual loss, nausea, vomiting, photophobia–migraine
    - Headache, altered consciousness, nausea, vomiting, blinking, nystagmus—seizure
- Drugs and medications
  - Prescription, over the counter, illicit, oral contraceptives, cocaine
- Family history
  - Cerebrovascular and cardiac disease
  - Migraine
  - Clotting disorders

PHYSICAL EXAM
- Vital signs
- Carotid auscultation–bruit in carotid stenosis
- Palpate superficial temporal artery–decreased pulse, cords, and tenderness in giant cell arteritis
- Visual acuity–may be reduced if permanent retinal or optic nerve ischemia
- Pupils—may have afferent papillary defect with permanent retinal or optic nerve ischemia
- Extraocular motility—may have cranial nerve palsy in giant cell arteritis
- Slit-lamp examination
  - Corneal dryness, keratitis
  - Narrow angles—angle-closure glaucoma
  - Hyphema
  - Neovascularization of iris or angle, flare in anterior chamber–ocular ischemic syndrome
- Tonometry–low intraocular pressure: ocular ischemic syndrome or high intraocular pressure: Angle-closure glaucoma
- Funduscopic exam
  - Optic nerve-disc edema, drusen
  - Retina
    - Cotton wool spots, retinal edema or hemorrhage, arteriolar narrowing, boxcarring or sheathing, venous dilation
    - Cholesterol emboli–yellowish orange, refractile, rectangular, often at vessel bifurcation. Source: Carotid or great vessels
    - Platelet—fibrin emboli–dull, grayish white, long. Source: Carotid, heart valves, coagulopathy
    - Calcific-chalk white, large, and round. Source: Heart valves, great vessels

DIAGNOSTIC TESTS & INTERPRETATION

Lab

- Automated visual field defect present if permanent retinal or optic nerve ischemia
- Elevated erythrocyte sedimentation rate and C-reactive protein. CBC: thrombocytosis in giant cell arteritis
- EKG–atrial fibrillation or sick sinus syndrome
- CBC, SPEP, PT, PTT, factor V Leiden, protein S and C, antithrombin III, homocystine, fibrinogen, antiphospholipid antibodies may identify hypercoagulable state, especially in young patients without risk factors for vascular disease.
- Lipid profile–elevated in atherosclerotic disease

Imaging

Initial approach

- TMVL
  - Carotid duplex ultrasonography–identifies degree of carotid stenosis and plaque morphology. May identify carotid dissection
  - Transthoracic echocardiography—detects mural thrombi, valvular and wall motion pathology, and tumors.
  - MRI brain–identifies parenchymal ischemic disease. May identify carotid dissection
  - CTA or MRA of brain and neck–mural thickening and luminal narrowing of carotid dissection. Can demonstrate carotid stenosis and plaque.
- TBVL
  - MRI brain–may demonstrate ischemic areas in posterior circulation distribution. Reserve for atypical presentation of migraine. See Migraine chapter.
  - CTA or MRA brain and neck: Stenosis or occlusion of vertebrobasilar system in patients with dissection
  - Transthoracic echocardiography–See TMVL above.

Follow-up & special considerations

- Transesophageal echocardiography–reserve for patients with high degree of suspicion of valvular disease, septal defects, and aortic arch disease
- Carotid angiography—differentiates 99% stenosis from complete occlusion
- Holter monitor–may identify intermittent arrhythmia

Diagnostic Procedures/Other

- Intravenous fluorescein angiogram–retinal, optic nerve, or choroidal ischemia
- Temporal artery biopsy—giant cell arteritis
- EEG–epileptiform activity in seizures

Pathological Findings

Temporal artery biopsy: inflammatory mononuclear cell infiltrate with destruction of internal elastic lamina; giant cells may be present

DIFFERENTIAL DIAGNOSIS

See Etiology

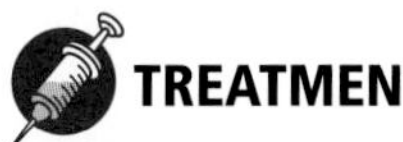

TREATMENT

MEDICATION

First Line

- Giant cell arteritis–See Giant cell arteritis chapter.
- Carotid stenosis >70%—ASA 325 mg/day, clopidogrel 75 mg/day, or ASA 25 mg plus dipyridamole 200 mg b.i.d.
- Carotid or vertebral dissection—anticoagulation with i.v. heparin followed by warfarin
- Cardiac disease—treatment of arrhythmia, valvular disease, CHF. Anticoagulation (target INR 2.5)
- Seizures–anticonvulsant therapy
- Vasospasm in young patients–calcium channel blockers

Second Line

Carotid or vertebral dissection–anti-platelet therapy if anticoagulation is contraindicated

SURGERY/OTHER PROCEDURES

Carotid stenosis 70–99% and good surgical candidate–carotid endarterectomy

IN-PATIENT CONSIDERATIONS

Admission Criteria

- Giant cell arteritis with visual loss
- Carotid or vertebral dissection
- Unstable cardiac arrhythmia

Nursing

Instruct patient to report any change in vision or neurologic status

Discharge Criteria

- TMVL (non-cardioembolic): Long-term antiplatelet therapy (1)[C]
- Atrial fibrillation, cardioembolic source, some hypercoagulable states: Long-term anticoagulation
- Giant cell arteritis: Oral prednisone taper over 1–2 years dictated by symptoms, sedimentation rate, and C-reactive protein.
- Discontinue cigarette smoking
- Blood pressure reduction
- Fasting blood glucose <126 mg/dL
- Treatment of hyperlipidemia

ONGOING CARE

FOLLOW-UP RECOMMENDATIONS

Patient Monitoring

- Follow-up with neuro-ophthalmology in 1 week
- Follow-up with neurology and/or cardiology as dictated by underlying disease

DIET

Avoid excessive alcohol use.

PROGNOSIS

- In most young patients (<45 years of age) with TMVL, no etiology will be found. Their risk of stroke is low (2)[C].
- In TMVL with 50–99% carotid stenosis who were treated medically the 3-year risk of ipsilateral stroke is 10% (3)[A].

COMPLICATIONS

- Cerebrovascular accident
- Myocardial infarction
- Death

REFERENCES

1. Albers GW, Hart RG, Lutsep HL, et al. AHA Scientific statement: Supplement to the guidelines for the management of transient ischemic attacks: A statement from the Ad Hoc Committee On Guidelines for the Management of Transient Ischemic Attacks, Stroke Council, American Heart Association. *Stroke* 1999;30:2502–2511.
2. Tippin J, Corbett JJ, Kerber RE, et al. Amaurosis fugax and ocular infarction in adolescents and young adults. *Ann Neurol* 1989;26:69–77.
3. Benavente O, Eliasziw M, Streifler JY, et al., for the North American Symptomatic Carotid Endarterectomy Trial Collaborators. Prognosis after transient monocular blindness associated with carotid artery stenosis. *N Engl J Med* 2001;345: 1084–1090.

CODES

ICD9

- 346.0 Migraine with aura
- 362.34 Amaurosis fugax
- 435.1 Vertebrobasilar insufficiency

CLINICAL PEARLS

- TMVL and TBVL are usually ischemic in origin.
- Atherosclerotic disease accounts for the majority of cases. Cardioembolic sources are less likely.
- TMVL in patients <45 is typically benign.

TRAUMATIC GLAUCOMA

Kathryn Burleigh Freidl
L Jay Katz
Anand V. Mantravadi

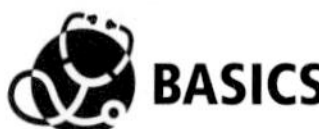

BASICS

DESCRIPTION

- Diverse mechanistic grouping of posttraumatic disorders that results in decreased aqueous outflow, elevated intraocular pressure (IOP), and subsequent optic neuropathy
- Early posttraumatic period mechanisms:
  - Hyphema
  - Angle recession
  - Inflammation
  - Lens subluxation
- Late posttraumatic period mechanisms:
  - Angle recession
  - Direct penetrating injury to angle structures

EPIDEMIOLOGY

Incidence

- Angle recession occurs in up to 75% of bluntly injured eyes.
  - Incidence is almost 100% in cases with traumatic hyphema
  - 10% of patients with angle recession >180° develop chronic glaucoma even many years after the trauma.

Prevalence

- 2.4 million eye injuries occur annually in the.
  - Males are 3 times more likely to sustain eye trauma than females

RISK FACTORS

- In children and young adults, the most common cause is playground accidents.
- In ages 30+, the leading causes are sporting accidents, assaults, and motor vehicle accidents (airbag deployment).

GENERAL PREVENTION

- Appropriate protective eyewear and headgear
- Public safety measures to prevent injuries

PATHOPHYSIOLOGY

Non-penetrating blunt trauma

- A blunt force initiates an anterior-to-posterior axial compression and subsequent equatorial expansion.
- Shearing forces exceed the elasticity of the anterior chamber structures
  - *Hyphema* results from rupture of iris and ciliary body vessels.
  - *Angle recession* occurs when the ciliary body tears between the circular and longitudinal muscles.
  - *Lens subluxation* can occur with disruption of zonular fibers. Forward rotation of the lens, protrusion of vitreous through ruptured zonules, or total dislocation of the lens into the anterior chamber may result in pupillary block and iris bombe.
  - The trabecular meshwork itself may be torn; subsequent scar tissue may obstruct outflow.
  - Inflammation levels vary based on injury severity.
    - Acutely, ciliary body swelling and inflammatory debris can contribute to pressure spikes.
    - Chronic inflammation may result in synechiae formation and chronic angle-closure glaucoma.

Penetrating Injuries

- Usually, in the acute setting, penetration of the globe is associated with hypotony, but it can cause direct damage to outflow channels. This may result in a chronic glaucoma after the initial injury is addressed.

ETIOLOGY

Traumatic glaucoma is most commonly caused by a blunt compression injury to the globe.

COMMONLY ASSOCIATED CONDITIONS

- Unilateral cataract
- Traumatic mydriasis
- Iridodialysis
- Cyclodialysis

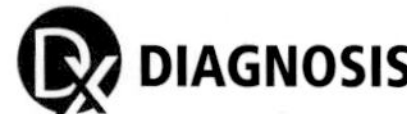

DIAGNOSIS

HISTORY

The inciting injury may not be recalled or may seem deceptively inconsequential.

PHYSICAL EXAM

- In the acute trauma setting, gonioscopy is difficult and sometimes impossible. The following may be seen:
  - Hyphema
  - Iridodialysis
  - Iris sphincter tears
  - Lens subluxation
  - Corneal edema
- Remote to the trauma, gonioscopy can demonstrate angle abnormalities such as recession and/or peripheral anterior synechiae. The following may also be noted:
  - Unilateral elevated IOP
  - Unilateral cataract ± phacodonesis

DIAGNOSTIC TESTS & INTERPRETATION

Lab

Initial lab tests

In cases of hyphema where sickle cell trait or disease is a possibility, hemoglobin electrophoresis should be performed.

Follow-up & special considerations

- Hyphema in sickle cell disease or trait requires special considerations:
  - Avoid carbonic anhydrase inhibitors
  - Avoid epinephrine
  - Poor prognosis if IOP uncontrolled >24 h
    - It is reasonable to hospitalize these patients for treatment and close observation.
    - If IOP is uncontrolled within the first 24 h, early surgical intervention is recommended.

Imaging

- Ultrasound biomicroscopy provides high-resolution imaging of the anterior chamber structures and can elucidate angle recession, iridodialysis, cyclodialysis, and zonular dehiscence.
- All patients with penetrating injury should receive a CT scan to rule out a retained foreign body.
- CT scanning may also be required to evaluate for comorbidities (orbital fractures).

Diagnostic Procedures/Other

- Traumatic glaucoma is a clinical diagnosis.
- Gonioscopy will elucidate damage to angle structures.
- Pachymetry is useful for determining the accuracy of IOP measurements.

Pathological Findings

- Angle recession has a characteristic tear between the longitudinal and circular muscles of the ciliary body.
- Abnormal corneal endothelial cell proliferation may occur in angle recession and, in some cases, has been noted to cover the meshwork with a hyaline membrane.

DIFFERENTIAL DIAGNOSIS

- Uveitis–glaucoma–hyphema syndrome
- ICE syndrome
- C-C fistula

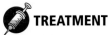

TREATMENT

MEDICATION

First Line

- For Elevated IOP:
  - Topical aqueous suppressants
    - β-Blockers, α_2-agonists, carbonic anhydrase inhibitors
  - Prostaglandins
    - Should be avoided in the acute setting when inflammation is present
    - Likely helpful in chronic angle recession glaucoma
  - Miotics should be avoided in traumatic glaucoma.
- For Hyphema:
  - Topical cycloplegia
  - Topical steroids
- For Pupillary Block from anterior lens dislocation:
  - Dilation of the pupil while the patient is supine may allow the lens to fall back.
  - Cataract extraction is the definitive treatment.

Second Line

- Systemic carbonic anhydrase inhydrase inhibitors
  - Acetazolamide
    - Diamox 125–250 mg p.o. q.i.d
    - Diamox Sequels 500 mg p.o. b.i.d
    - 500 mg i.v.
    - Do not exceed 1 g in a 24-h period.
    - Contraindicated in severe renal disease, hepatic disease, severe pulmonary obstruction, and adrenocortical insufficiency
  - Methazolamide 50–100 mg p.o. b.i.d
    - Contraindicated in renal insufficiency
- Systemic hyperosmotic
  - Mannitol 1.5—2 g/kg i.v. over a 30-min period
    - 20% solution (7.5–10 mL/kg)
    - 15% solution (10–13 mL/kg)
    - Do not exceed 500 mL in a 24-h period.
    - Contraindicated in anuria, progressive renal failure, CHF, severe dehydration, or intracranial bleeding

ADDITIONAL TREATMENT

Issues for Referral

- In cases of uncertain diagnosis, consultation with a glaucoma specialist is recommended.
- Referrals to the appropriate specialists may be necessary depending on the extent of the trauma and the structures involved.

SURGERY/OTHER PROCEDURES

- Surgical intervention is indicated when the maximally tolerated medical treatment has failed and the elevated IOP threatens the optic nerve.
- Surgery is also indicated when there is associated corneal blood staining.
- **Surgical Procedures in the acute setting:**
  - Anterior chamber wash-out
  - Filtration surgery with anterior chamber wash-out
  - In cases of papillary block from lens subluxation—cataract extraction
- **Surgical Procedures in the late posttraumatic period:**
  - Laser trabeculoplasty has shown disappointing long-term success rates (<25% at 36 months
  - Filtration surgery such as trabeculectomy or tube placement is more prone to fistula fibrosis in patients with history of trauma; use of an anti-metabolite is important to enhance the chances of long-term success.

ONGOING CARE

FOLLOW-UP RECOMMENDATIONS

- Normotensive eyes with angle recession >180° require routine reexamination at least once a year indefinitely.
- Eyes with elevated pressure following trauma should be seen every 4–6 weeks in the 1st year following the trauma.
- The decision to treat eyes with elevated pressure is based on the overall clinical picture, taking into account the following factors:
  - Severity of elevated IOP
  - Optic nerve appearance
  - Visual field findings

PATIENT EDUCATION

Patients should be advised of the importance of follow-up monitoring.

PROGNOSIS

Is variable and dependent on the success of maintaining a normotensive IOP and adequate patient monitoring

COMPLICATIONS

- Vision loss
- Traumatic cataract
- Loss of eye

ADDITIONAL READING

- Bazzaz S, Katz LJ, Myers JS. Post-traumatic glaucoma. In: Shaarawy TM, Sherwood MB, Hitchings RA, et al, eds: *Glaucoma: Medical diagnosis and therapy*, Vol. 1, Philadelphia: Saunders/Elsevier Limited, 2009:31–439.
- Canavan YM, Archer DF. Anterior segment consequences of blunt ocular injury. *Br J Ophthalmology* 1982;66:549–555.
- Kaufman JH, Tolpin DW. Glaucoma after traumatic angle recession: A ten-year prospective study. *Am J Ophthalmology* 1974;79:648–654.
- Macewan CJ. Eye injuries: A prospective survey of 5671 cases. *Br J Ophthalmol* 1989;73:888–894.
- Manners T, Salmon JF, Barron A, et al. Trabeculectomy with mitomycin C in the treatment of post-traumatic angle recession glaucoma. *Br J Ophthalmol* 2001;85:159–163.
- Melamed S, Ashkenazi I, Gutman I, et al. Nd:YAG laser trabeculopuncture in angle-recession glaucoma. *Ophthalmic Surg* 1992;23:31–35.
- Sihota R, Kumar S, Gupta V, et al. Early predictors of traumatic glaucoma after closed globe injury: Trabecular pigmentation, widened angle recess, and higher baseline intraocular pressure. *Arch Ophthalmol* 2008;126:921–926.
- Sullivan BR. Glaucoma, angle recession, *eMedicine*. Apr 29 2010. http://emedicine.medscape.com/article/1204999-overview
- Wolff SM, Zimmerman LE. Chronic secondary glaucoma. Association with retrodisplacement of iris root and deepening of the anterior chamber angle secondary to contusion. *Am J Ophthalmol* 1962;84:547–563.

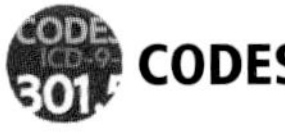

CODES

ICD9

- 364.41 Hyphema of iris and ciliary body
- 364.77 Recession of chamber angle of eye
- 365.65 Glaucoma associated with ocular trauma

T

TRAUMATIC OPTIC NEUROPATHY

Mary Ellen P. Cullom

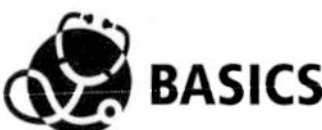

BASICS

DESCRIPTION

Traumatic optic neuropathy (TON) is an optic neuropathy which occurs after head or ocular trauma. 2 mechanistic etiologies are recognized.

- Direct TON

Trauma resulting from penetrating foreign body which damages optic nerve

- Indirect TON

Trauma transmits concussive force to optic nerve. No foreign body or penetration.

- Anterior indirect TON
  - Due to sudden anterior displacement or torsion of globe
  - Often has funduscopic signs (e.g., optic nerve avulsion, optic nerve edema, retinal edema, or central retinal artery and vein occlusion)
- Posterior indirect TON
  - Most common cause of TON
  - Due to frontal, orbital, or midfacial trauma
  - Almost always has normal optic nerve appearance

System(s) affected: Central nervous system

EPIDEMIOLOGY

- Predominant age: 20–40 years
- Predominant sex: Male
- Occurs in 1–5% of closed head injuries

PATHOPHYSIOLOGY

- Direct TON
  Penetrating foreign body damages nerve or causes hemorrhage. Hemorrhage compresses surrounding structures causing ischemia, axonal block, and axonal death.
  - Optic nerve transection
  - Optic nerve contusion or foreign body impingement
  - Compressive optic neuropathy secondary to orbital or intrasheath hemorrhage
- Indirect TON
  - Anterior indirect TON
    - Sudden anterior displacement of globe
    - Optic nerve avulsion, central retinal artery or vein occlusion
  - Posterior indirect TON
    - Trauma transmits concussive force to nerve.
    - Shearing, stretching, compression, or transection of optic nerve
    - Focal block of axonal conduction
    - Contusion necrosis
    - Ischemic necrosis
    - Late demyelination

ETIOLOGY

- Direct TON
  - Penetration foreign body (e.g., knife, bullet, BB)
  - Postoperative complication
    - Endoscopic sinus surgery
    - Maxillofacial surgery
    - Ocular surgery (e.g., retrobulbar anesthesia, orbital surgery, blepharoplasty)
- Indirect TON
  - Closed head injury
    - Motor vehicle accident
    - Bike accident
    - Falls
    - Assaults

COMMONLY ASSOCIATED CONDITIONS

- Loss of consciousness
- Intraorbital or intracranial foreign bodies
- Orbital hemorrhage
- Orbital, maxillofacial, or basilar skull fracture
- Optic canal fracture
- Intracranial hemorrhage

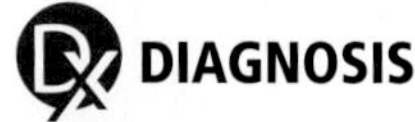

DIAGNOSIS

HISTORY

- Location of trauma
  - Frontal, orbital, or midfacial
- Mechanism of trauma
  - Direct TON
    - Foreign body
  - Indirect TON
    - Sudden deceleration injury
    - Trauma occasionally may seem insignificant
- Onset of visual loss
  - Immediately after injury or reported when patient regains consciousness
  - If delayed: Suspect expanding nerve sheath or orbital hemorrhage
- Associated symptoms:
  - Loss of consciousness
  - Anosmia, diabetes insipidus, other neurologic deficits imply skull base fracture

PHYSICAL EXAM

- Vital signs
- External Ocular Exam
  - Orbital findings:
    - Ecchymoses, edema, and emphysema
    - Proptosis
    - Penetrating wound or foreign body
- Ocular motility
  Ophthalmoplegia may be due to:
  - Muscle trauma
  - Orbital hemorrhage
  - Cranial nerve palsy (basilar skull fracture)
- Visual acuity
  - May range from 20/20 to no light perception
- Pupil exam
  - Critical for diagnosis, especially in an unconscious patient
  - Afferent papillary defect: present in unilateral TON. May be absent if there is bilateral TON
- Funduscopic exam
  - Optic nerve appears normal in posterior indirect TON
- Optic nerve avulsion, edema (unusual), central retinal artery and vein occlusion—anterior indirect TON

DIAGNOSTIC TESTS & INTERPRETATION

Lab

Initial lab tests

- Slit-lamp examination—exclude ruptured globe
- Tonometry—intraocular pressure may be elevated in orbital compartment syndrome or decreased in occult ruptured globe
- Visual fields
  - Automated or confrontation—a variety of defects (e.g., altitudinal, arcuate, paracentral, or central scotoma) may be present
- Color vision
  - Ishihara color plates—dyschromatopsia
  - Red desaturation—present
- Flash VEP—abnormal or absent in affected eye. Useful in unconscious patient.

Follow-Up & Special Considerations

- Low vision specialist for patients with poor visual outcome
- Occupational therapy for patients with poor visual outcome

Imaging

- CT scan
  - Imaging Recommendations
    - Axial and coronal planes
    - Thin sections and reconstructions
    - Attention to optic canal
    - Spiral CT—short scan time helpful in children
  - Orbital CT findings
    - Periorbital soft-tissue edema
    - Orbital hematoma
    - Optic nerve sheath hemorrhage
    - Optic nerve transection
    - Foreign body
    - Orbital, facial, or optic canal fracture
  - Head CT findings
    - Basilar skull fracture
    - Optic canal fracture
    - Epidural, subdural, subarachnoid, or cerebral hemorrhage

- MRI: Not always necessary. Better identifies soft-tissue findings
  - Imaging recommendations
    - First exclude metallic foreign body with CT or plain film
    - Gadolinium enhanced
    - Thin sections
  - Orbital MRI findings:
    - Optic nerve sheath hemorrhage
    - See orbital CT findings
  - Brain MRI findings:
    - Chiasmal edema and hemorrhage
    - See head CT findings

DIFFERENTIAL DIAGNOSIS
- Nonorganic visual loss
- Ruptured globe
- Retinal detachment

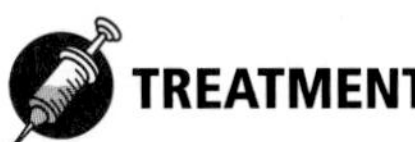

TREATMENT

MEDICATION
If patient seen within 8 h of injury
- Corticosteroids
  - High-dose steroids may be offered although there is no proven clinical benefit (1)[A]
  - Thorough discussion with patient and family
  - Methylprednisolone 30 mg/kg i.v. bolus followed by 5.4 mg/kg/h for 48 h (2)[A]
  - Histamine 2 blocker to protect gastric mucosa
  - Side effects: Peptic ulcer disease, gastrointestinal bleed, hyperglycemia, hypertension, weight gain, osteoporosis, and psychosis

ADDITIONAL TREATMENT
General Measures
- Cardiovascular and respiratory stabilization of patient
- Multidisciplinary approach: Consult otolaryngology, neurology, and/or neurosurgery if indicated

Issues for Referral
Neuro-ophthalmology in 2–3 days

COMPLEMENTARY & ALTERNATIVE THERAPIES
Observation alone of TON is a valid treatment option.

SURGERY/OTHER PROCEDURES
- Optic canal decompression
  - May be offered to patient although there is no proven clinical benefit (3)[A]
  - Consider if fracture fragment impinging on optic nerve.
  - Consider if no improvement in visual acuity after 48 h of i.v. steroids
  - Only at institutions with experienced surgeons
  - Avoid in the comatose patient
- Removal of foreign body or fracture fragment if optic nerve impingement
- Optic nerve sheath fenestration if optic nerve sheath hemorrhage is demonstrated on MRI
- Canthotomy/cantholysis if orbital compartment syndrome and optic nerve compression

IN-PATIENT CONSIDERATIONS
Initial Stabilization
Address cardiovascular or respiratory compromise

Admission Criteria
- Floor or ICU status determined by general neurologic status and severity of associated injuries
- Treatment with i.v. steroids
- Operative cases

Nursing
- Check visual acuity every 2 h for first 24 h, and thereafter daily.
- Instruct patient to report any decrease in vision.

Discharge Criteria
- Untreated TON
- Visually stable TON treated with i.v. steroids or operatively
- Neurologically stable

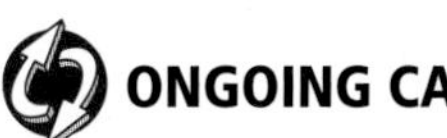

ONGOING CARE

FOLLOW-UP RECOMMENDATIONS
Neuro-ophthalmology in 2–3 days

PATIENT EDUCATION
- Report any decrease in vision or increase in swelling, proptosis, or pain to neuro-ophthalmologist
- If any change in mental status: Call 911

PROGNOSIS
- Variable: 32–57% of patients have improvement in vision.
- Better in patients with indirect TON than direct TON
- Poor if initial visual acuity is no light perception

COMPLICATIONS
- Decreased visual acuity, decreased color vision, and visual field defects
- Periorbital scarring
- Post-concussive syndrome

REFERENCES

1. Yu-Wai-Man P, Griffith PG. Steroids for traumatic optic neuropathy. *Cochrane Database Syst Rev* 2007:CD006032.
2. Bracken MB, Shepard MJ, Holford TR, et al. Administration of methyl prednisolone for 24 or 48 hours or trilizad mesylate for 48 hours in the treatment of acute spinal cord injury. Results of the Third National Acute Spinal Cord Injury Randomized Control Trial. National Acute Spinal Cord Injury Study. *JAMA* 1997;277:1597.
3. Yu-Wai-Man P, Griffiths PG. Surgery for traumatic optic neuropathy. *Cochrane Database Syst Rev* 2005:CD005024.

ADDITIONAL READING

- Levin LA, Beck RW, Joseph MP. The treatment of traumatic optic neuropathy: The International Optic Nerve Trauma Study. *Ophthalmology* 1999;106: 1268–1277.

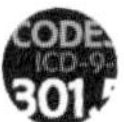

CODES

ICD9
- 377.39 Other optic neuropathy

CLINICAL PEARLS

- TON occurs after closed head trauma and penetrating orbital or intracranial injuries.
- The optic nerve typically appears normal but an afferent papillary defect is present (unless bilateral TON).
- No consensus exists regarding the management of TON; therefore, treatment must be individualized.

TRICHIASIS

Thaddeus S. Nowinski

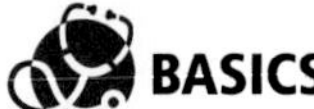

BASICS

DESCRIPTION

- Acquired misdirection or inturning of eyelashes in an otherwise normal eyelid margin position
- Distichiasis—abnormal hair growing from meibomian gland openings

EPIDEMIOLOGY

Incidence

- Cicatricial—ocular cicatricial pemphigoid (OCP)—females >males
- Average age 60–70 years

Prevalence

Cicatricial—OCP—1 in 15,000–20,000 (1)[C]

RISK FACTORS

Genetics

OCP—associated with HLA—DQB7*301

PATHOPHYSIOLOGY

- Distichiasis—hair grows from poorly differentiated pilosebaceous units
- Trachoma—Chlamydial infection
- Ocular pemphigoid—autoimmune

ETIOLOGY

- Usually unknown
- Scarring of eyelid margin
- Prostaglandin analog eyedrops
- OCP—a systemic autoimmune pemphigoid disorder that has ocular and nonocular manifestations
  - OCP thought to be a type 2 hypersensitivity reaction, genetically predisposed

COMMONLY ASSOCIATED CONDITIONS

- Uncommon:
  - Ocular pemphigoid
  - Trachoma

DIAGNOSIS

HISTORY

- Foreign body sensation
- Tearing
- Redness
- Previous chemical or physical trauma

PHYSICAL EXAM

- Inturned eyelashes abrading globe with normal position of eyelid margin
- Superficial punctuate keratopathy or corneal abrasions
- Chronic blepharitis
- Eyelid or conjunctival scarring
- Symblepharon—cicatricial—linear scar/fold of palpebral conjunctiva to bulbar conjunctiva, shortening of fornix
  - Scarring of upper eyelid tarsal conjunctiva on eyelid eversion (trachoma)

DIAGNOSTIC TESTS & INTERPRETATION

Imaging

Initial approach

- None
- OCP—ANA

Follow-up & special considerations

OCP—elevated soluble CD 8 glycoprotein, elevated tumor necrosis factor

Diagnostic Procedures/Other

Cicatricial—conjunctival biopsy

Pathological Findings

OCP—biopsy of conjunctiva for direct immunofluorescence studies or indirect immunofluorescence for presence of antibodies—positive in >80%

DIFFERENTIAL DIAGNOSIS

- Entropion
- Epiblepharon
- Epicanthus

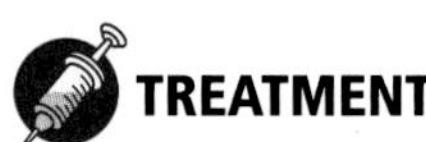

TREATMENT

MEDICATION

First Line

- Ocular lubrication
  - Frequent artificial tears, ophthalmic ointment
- Treat underlying blepharitis

Second Line

Single-dose oral azithromycin (1 g) for trachoma—household member treatment does not improve prognosis (2)[C]

ADDITIONAL TREATMENT

General Measures

Epilation of lashes—recurrence very common every 2–6 weeks

Issues for Referral

Ophthalmologist 1 week

Additional Therapies

- Bandage contact lens
- OCP—prednisone, dapsone, methotrexate, cyclophosphamide, CellCept, or doxycycline

SURGERY/OTHER PROCEDURES
- Procedures to destroy eyelash follicle
  - Electrolysis or cautery
  - Cryotherapy
  - Laser
  - Radiofrequency
- Surgical cutting procedures
  - Trephination, excision of follicles
  - Eyelid splitting and cryo
  - Eyelid resection
  - Eyelid margin rotation
  - Anterior lamellar resection

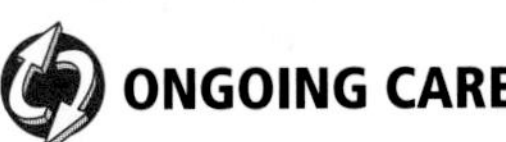

ONGOING CARE

FOLLOW-UP RECOMMENDATIONS
Eyelashes regrow in few weeks

Patient Monitoring
Ophthalmologist – outpatient

PATIENT EDUCATION
- Warning signs of ocular irritation
- Trachoma is one of the most important and prevalent eye diseases in the world

PROGNOSIS
- Lashes will almost always regrow; follicles are not damaged by epilation
- Trachoma—cycles of infection, inflammation, scarring, and increased trichiasis and entropion
- Ocular pemphigoid—stabilize if possible with

COMPLICATIONS

ALERT
Corneal abrasion, ulcer, scarring, opacity, perforation, vascularization, and blindness (3)[C]

REFERENCES

1. Landers J, Kleinschmidt A, Wu J, et al. Prevalence of cicatricial trachoma in an indigenous population of Central Australia: The Central Australian Trachomatous Study (CATTS). *Clin Experiment Ophthalmol* 2005;33:142–146.
2. West SK, West ES, Alemayehu W, et al. Single-dose azithromycin prevents trichiasis recurrence following surgery: Randomized trial in Ethiopia. *Arch Ophthalmol* 2006;124:309–314.
3. West ES, Munoz B, Imeru A, et al. The association between epilation and corneal opacity among eyes with trachomatous trichiasis. *Br J Ophthalmol* 2006;90:171–174.

ADDITIONAL READING

- Bieyen I, Dolman PJ. The Wies procedure for management of trichiasis or cicatricial entropion of either upper or lower eyelids. *Br J Ophthalmol* 2009;93:1612–1615.
- El Toukhy E, Lewallen S, Courtright P. Routine bilamellar tarsal rotation surgery for trachomatous trichiasis: Short-term outcome and factors associated with surgical failure. *Ophthal Plast Reconstr Surg* 2006;22:109–112.
- Moosavi AH, Mollan SP, Berry-Brincat A, et al. Simple surgery for trichiasis. *Ophthal Plast Reconstr Surg* 2007;23:296–297.
- Shiu M, McNab A. Cicatricial entropion and trichiasis in an urban Australian population. *Clin Experiment Ophthalmol* 2005;33:582–585.
- Wu AY, Thakker MM, Wladis EJ, et al. Eyelash resection procedure for severe, recurrent, or segmental cicatricial entropion. *Ophthal Plast Reconstr Surg* 2010;26:112–116.

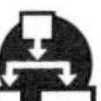

See Also (Topic, Algorithm, Electronic Media Element)
- www.asoprs.org
- Topics:
  - Entropion
  - Ocular Cicatricial Pemphigoid
  - Blepharitis
  - Trachoma

CODES

ICD9
- 374.05 Trichiasis of eyelid without entropion
- 694.61 Benign mucous membrane pemphigoid with ocular involvement
- 704.2 Abnormalities of the hair

CLINICAL PEARLS
- Trichiasis if untreated may lead to corneal scarring, infection, and permanent loss of vision.
- Eyelashes will regrow after epilation in a few weeks time.
- Suspect ocular pempigoid or trachoma in unusual cases

T

TUBERCULOSIS IN THE EYE

Jason Hsu

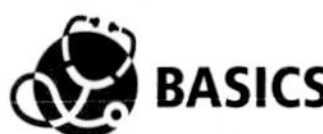

BASICS

DESCRIPTION

- Tuberculosis (TB) is a chronic infection caused by the acid-fast bacillus, *Mycobacterium tuberculosis.*
  - Systemic disease that mainly involves the lung
  - Extrapulmonary manifestations may occur with or without pulmonary TB
    - Sites include gastrointestinal tract, genito-urinary tract, cardiovascular system, skin, central nervous system, and eyes
  - Uveitis is the most common ophthalmic presentation, although any part of the eye may be affected.

EPIDEMIOLOGY

Incidence

- Annual incidence of tuberculosis is ~9.3 million patients worldwide
  - Heaviest case burden in developing countries
    - Annual incidence rate of 363 per 100,000 in Africa
    - Annual incidence rate of 32 per 100,000 in the US

Prevalence

- In 2007, an estimated 13.7 million people had active TB with 1.8 million deaths
  - Leading cause of death in patients with HIV and of infectious death in women of reproductive age

RISK FACTORS

- Silicosis
- Chronic renal failure
- Diabetes mellitus
- Low body weight
- Immunocompromised patients (e.g., acquired immune deficiency syndrome [AIDS], leukemia, Hodgkin's disease)

PATHOPHYSIOLOGY

Phlyctenulosis, interstitial keratitis, and retinal vasculitis may result from a hypersensitivity reaction to mycobacterial proteins

ETIOLOGY

- Inhalation of aerosolized droplets carrying *Mycobacterium tuberculosis*
  - 90% of infected persons never develop clinical disease.
    - 5% develop disease within first few years of exposure
    - 5% develop disease several years later due to altered host immunity (reactivation of latent infection)
  - Infectious organisms may disseminate from lungs hematogenously, resulting in extrapulmonary manifestations
    - Miliary TB (1.3% of reported cases) may result, described as millet-like seeding in the lungs and extrapulmonary tissues

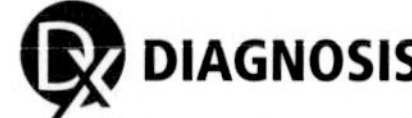

DIAGNOSIS

HISTORY

- Classic symptoms (pulmonary TB): chronic cough, blood-tinged sputum, fever, night sweats, and weight loss
- Vision loss, floaters, eye pain, red eye, and photophobia
- If orbital involvement is present, patient may also have diplopia and ophthalmoplegia

PHYSICAL EXAM

- Eyelid manifestations (usually in children):
  - Lupus vulgaris
    - Most common form of cutaneous TB
    - Reddish-brown nodules which blanch an "apple-jelly" color on palpation
  - May simulate a chalazion or look like a "cold abscess" (soft, fluctuant mass without inflammation)
- Tuberculous conjunctivitis:
  - Unusual and more often in children
  - May present with mucopurulent discharge, lid edema, and injection with marked lymphadenopathy (similar to Parinaud's oculoglandular syndrome)
  - Often chronic, which can lead to scarring

- Tuberculous episcleritis and scleritis:
  - Occurs rarely
  - Most common type: Focal necrotizing scleritis
    - Scleral perforation may occur
  - Posterior scleritis has been rarely reported
- Corneal manifestations:
  - Phlyctenulosis
    - Slightly raised, small, pinkish white to yellow nodules surrounded by dilated vessels, usually near limbus on conjunctiva or peripheral cornea
  - Sectoral interstitial keratitis
    - Typically unilateral
    - Peripheral stromal infiltrate with vascularization
  - Sclerosing keratitis
  - Tuberculous pannus (associated with ulcerative granulomas involving conjunctiva)
  - Corneal ulcer
- Anterior uveitis
  - Typically granulomatous with acute or chronic presentation
  - May have mutton fat keratic precipitates and posterior synechiae
  - Secondary glaucoma may occur
  - Iris or angle granulomas
    - Small translucent nodules at pupillary margin (Koeppe's nodules) may be seen with recurrent uveitis
  - Hypopyon or mass lesion in severe cases
- Intermediate uveitis
  - Chronic low-grade vitreitis, typically bilateral
  - May be associated with snowball opacities, snow banking, peripheral vascular sheathing, peripheral granulomas
- Posterior uveitis
  - Choroidal tubercles
    - Most common manifestation of intraocular TB
    - Results from hematogenous spread
    - Multiple grayish white to yellow lesions with indistinct borders (<5–50 in number)
    - Unilateral or bilateral
    - Usually localized to posterior pole
    - Size: 0.5–3 mm
    - Occasionally may grow into larger mass (choroidal tuberculoma)
    - Pigmented and atrophic scars upon resolution with distinct margins
    - Immunocompromised patients may have no concomitant inflammation
  - Choroidal tuberculoma
    - Solitary subretinal mass that may mimic choroidal tumor
    - Initially small, round, whitish lesion but may become yellowish
    - Size: 4–14 mm
    - Associated findings: hemorrhages, retinal folds, and exudative retinal detachment
  - Serpiginous-like choroiditis
    - Multifocal or diffuse plaque-like lesions
    - Typically have progressive course despite treatment
  - Retinal vasculitis
    - Associated findings: vitreitis, retinal hemorrhages, perivascular choroiditis, neovascularization, and neuroretinitis
    - May resemble Eales' disease but usually has more prominent intraocular inflammation
  - Eales's disease
    - Retinal vasculitis that mainly affects peripheral retina with recurrent vitreous hemorrhages and fibrovascular proliferation in the relative absence of intraocular inflammation
    - Seen in young, healthy adults
    - Perivascular exudates and hemorrhages may progress to venous thrombosis, neovascularization, and traction retinal detachment
- Endophthalmitis/panophthalmitis
  - Usually in children or severely ill adults in the setting of systemic TB and chronic illness, poor nutrition, or intravenous drug abuse
  - Severe inflammation may cause widespread destruction of ocular tissues
  - Anterior segment:
    - Corneal infiltrates
    - Hypopyon
  - Posterior segment:
    - Vitreitis
    - Choroidal detachment
    - Globe perforation may occur typically near equator in cases of panophthalmitis
- Tuberculous optic neuropathy and neuroretinitis
  - Optic nerve involvement may manifest as an optic nerve tubercle, papillitis, papilledema, optic neuritis, retrobulbar neuritis, neuroretinitis, or opticochiasmatic arachnoiditis

- Orbital manifestations:
  - Rare case reports
  - Clinical presentations:
    - Periostitis: Chronic ulceration or discharging sinus in periorbital region with discolored/thickened/edematous surrounding skin often adherent to underlying bone
    - Orbital soft-tissue tuberculoma or cold abscess without bony destruction: Proptosis and palpable orbital mass
    - Orbital TB with evidence of bony involvement: Proptosis, ophthalmoplegia, and palpable orbital mass
    - Orbital spread from paranasal sinuses: Proptosis, significant globe dystopia, palpable mass, ophthalmoplegia, and epistaxis
    - Dacryoadenitis: Limitation of eye movements, ptosis, proptosis, globe displacement, mass in region of lacrimal gland, and regional lymphadenopathy

DIAGNOSTIC TESTS & INTERPRETATION

Lab

Initial lab tests

- Tuberculin skin test (PPD)
  - High-risk groups (e.g., medical personnel, intravenous drug abusers): Induration >10 mm considered positive
  - Immunocompromised: Induration >5 mm considered positive
  - Low-risk groups: Induration >15 mm considered positive
  - False positives may occur in patients with prior BCG vaccination
    - Note that vaccination-induced reactions wane over time and are unlikely to persist for >10 years
  - May be falsely negative in up to 30% of patients with active TB, especially if immunocompromised
- Interferon-gamma release assays (e.g., QuantiFERON-TB test): Detects cellular response to TB antigens through measurement of interferon-gamma release
  - Reduced false positive rate in patients with prior BCG vaccination
- Sputum culture (if pulmonary symptoms)

Follow-up & special considerations

- In select cases, consider vitreous biopsy or diagnostic anterior chamber paracentesis:
  - May see acid-fast bacilli on smear or culture
    - May be falsely negative due to low yield of organisms from intraocular fluids
  - Polymerase chain reaction testing may improve detection and can be performed on even small samples.

Imaging

Initial approach

Chest X-ray (PA and lateral)

Follow-up & special considerations

Chest CT if chest X-ray is inconclusive

Diagnostic Procedures/Other

- Fluorescein angiography
  - Choroidal tubercles:
    - Hypofluorescent during transit phase with late hyperfluorescence
    - May also confirm a choroidal neovascular membrane or retinal angiomatous proliferation associated with a choroidal tubercle (acute phase or inactive lesion)
  - Choroidal tuberculoma:
    - Early hyperfluorescence with dilated capillary bed → leakage and pooling in late phase if there is surrounding exudative detachment
  - Serpiginous-like choroiditis:
    - Active edge with early hypofluorescence and late hyperfluorescence with diffuse staining
    - Healed lesions show transmission hyperfluorescence or blocked fluorescence from pigment epithelial proliferation
  - Retinal vasculitis:
    - Staining and leakage from vessel walls, primarily veins
    - Peripheral sweeps helpful for documenting capillary nonperfusion and neovascularization
- Indocyanine green angiography
  - Choroidal tubercles/tuberculoma
    - Active lesions hypofluorescent → iso- or hyperfluorescent border present in late phase
    - Resolving lesions become less hypofluorescent
    - Helpful in detecting subclinical lesions
  - Serpiginous-like choroiditis:
    - Active lesions are hypofluorescent throughout angiogram
- Optical coherence tomography
  - May be helpful if a choroidal neovascular membrane or cystoid macular edema is suspected
- B-scan ultrasonography
  - Choroidal tuberculoma:
    - Solid, elevated mass
    - Low to medium internal reflectivity
- Ultrasound biomicroscopy: May show ciliary body granulomas
- If orbital TB is suspected, CT head/orbit is the preferred imaging modality.
  - Biopsy confirmation is typically recommended (either open biopsy or fine needle aspiration biopsy)

Pathological Findings

- Granulomas with central caseous necrosis surrounded by epithelioid cells, Langerhans' giant cells, lymphocytes, and plasma cells
- Immunocompromised patients:
  - More of a purulent infection with necrotic and viable neutrophils, macrophages, and numerous bacteria

DIFFERENTIAL DIAGNOSIS

- Infectious
  - Toxoplasmosis
  - Syphilis
  - Lyme's disease
  - Cat scratch disease
  - Toxocariasis
  - Nocardiasis
  - Coccidiomycosis
  - Candidiasis
  - Brucellosis
  - Leptospirosis
  - Leprosy
- Noninfectious
  - Sarcoidosis
  - Behçet's disease
  - Autoimmune vasculitis
  - Tumors
  - Metastasis

TREATMENT

MEDICATION

First Line

- Multidrug anti-TB regimen is required to avoid resistance.
  - Typically: Isoniazid, rifampin, pyrazinamide, and ethambutol for 2–4 months
  - Subsequently: Isoniazid and rifampin for another 4–7 months
  - In cases of isolated ocular TB, some advocate the above therapy without ethambutol
- Systemic corticosteroids may limit damage from delayed-type hypersensitivity
  - Consider 4- to 6-week course
  - Must be used with anti-TB medications or could lead to panophthalmitis and systemic TB due to activation of latent infection
- Conjunctivitis: Anti-TB therapy
- Scleritis/episcleritis: Anti-TB therapy; systemic steroids may be used depending on severity
- Interstitial keratitis: Topical steroids, systemic with or without topical anti-TB therapy, and cycloplegics
- Phlyctenulosis: Topical steroids, anti-TB therapy, and cycloplegics
- Uveitis:
  - Use of anti-TB therapy decreases recurrence of uveitis
  - Anterior uveitis: Cycloplegics and topical steroids in addition to anti-TB therapy
  - Intermediate uveitis: Topical, periocular and/or oral steroids after anti-TB therapy is initiated
  - Posterior uveitis: Oral steroids after anti-TB is therapy initiated
    - May have paradoxical worsening of serpiginous-like choroiditis after initiation of anti-TB therapy
  - Eales' disease: Anti-TB therapy, when associated with clinical evidence of TB infection
    - If cystoid macular edema is present, intravitreal triamcinolone or bevacizumab may be used
    - Intravitreal bevacizumab helps induce regression of neovascularization
- Tuberculous optic neuropathy: Anti-TB therapy and oral steroids after anti-TB therapy is initiated
- Orbital TB: Anti-TB therapy

Second Line

- Streptomycin
- Rifabutin and rifapentine may be alternatives to rifampin
- Drugs that may be useful for drug-resistant TB:
  - Cycloserine, levofloxacin, moxifloxacin, gatifloxacin, amikacin, kanamycin, ethionamide, and capreomycin

SURGERY/OTHER PROCEDURES

- Retinal vasculitis/Eales' disease:
  - Laser photocoagulation of ischemic nonperfused retina
  - If non-clearing vitreous hemorrhage, may consider pars plana vitrectomy
- Orbital TB: Surgical intervention may be diagnostic, therapeutic (e.g., excision of bone and fistulous tract), or both (e.g., excisional biopsy)

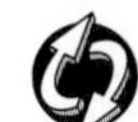

ONGOING CARE

FOLLOW-UP RECOMMENDATIONS

- Infectious disease specialist or internist experienced in managing TB
- Pulmonologist: In cases of suspected associated pulmonary TB
- Ophthalmologist: In cases with ocular or orbital involvement, or with ethambutol therapy to evaluate for toxicity

Patient Monitoring

- Local public health officials may need to be notified
  - In some locations, directly observed therapy (DOTS) is recommended to increase compliance with anti-TB therapy and to lower the risk of drug resistance
- Ocular side effects of anti-TB drugs
  - Isoniazid, pyrazinamide, and rifampin carry risk of hepatotoxicity
    - Liver function needs to be monitored during therapy
  - Ethambutol
    - Toxic effects: Optic neuritis, photophobia, and extraocular muscle paresis
    - Onset is usually 3–6 months after initiation of therapy
    - Dose dependent: Occurs in 1–2% of patients receiving 25 mg/kg/day but is rare with daily dose <15 mg/kg
    - Recommendation: Baseline ophthalmologic exam with visual field and color plate testing followed by monthly exams and testing if dose >15 mg/kg or every 3–6 months if lower dose
    - Self-monitoring with vision card: Instruct patient to stop ethambutol and undergo ophthalmic exam if visual acuity decreases
    - If no vision improvement 10–15 weeks after ethambutol is discontinued, consider parenteral hydroxocobalamin 40 mg/day for 10–28 weeks

PROGNOSIS

- With appropriate diagnosis and timely treatment, prognosis is often good
  - In advanced, neglected, or aggressive cases, the outcome may be poor despite appropriate therapy
- Orbital TB: Rarely, deaths have been reported due to extension of an orbital focus into the brain
  - Visual loss may occur in some cases due to optic atrophy

ADDITIONAL READING

- Thompson MJ, Albert DM. Ocular tuberculosis. *Arch Ophthalmol* 2005;123:844–849.
- Madge SN, Prabhakaran VC, Shome D, et al. Orbital tuberculosis: A review of the literature. *Orbit* 2008;27:267–277.
- Bansal R, Gupta A, Gupta V, et al. Role of anti-tubercular therapy in uveitis with latent/manifest tuberculosis. *Am J Ophthalmol* 2008;146:772–779.
- Gupta V, Gupta A, Arora S, et al. Presumed tubercular serpiginous-like choroiditis. *Ophthalmology* 2003;110:1744–1749.
- Gupta V, Gupta A, Rao NA. Intraocular tuberculosis—an update. *Surv Ophthalmol* 2007;52:561–587.

CODES

ICD9

- 017.30 Tuberculosis of eye, unspecified examination
- 363.13 Disseminated choroiditis and chorioretinitis, generalized
- 370.31 Phlyctenular keratoconjunctivitis

CLINICAL PEARLS

- Ocular TB can mimic various other eye diseases, necessitating a high level of clinical suspicion in order to make the correct diagnosis

T

TUBEROUS SCLEROSIS

Eugene Milder

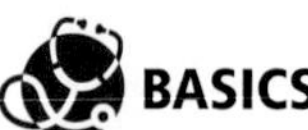

BASICS

DESCRIPTION
Tuberous sclerosis (TS) is a rare multisystem syndrome with a classic triad of findings including: Infantile seizures, adenoma sebaceum of facial skin, and mental retardation.

EPIDEMIOLOGY
Incidence
10–16 per 100,000 live births

Prevalence
7–12 per 100,000

RISK FACTORS
Family history

Genetics
Autosomal dominant

GENERAL PREVENTION
Genetic counseling

PATHOPHYSIOLOGY
Hamartin (gene: TSC1) and tuberin (gene: TSC2) on chromosome 9, act as a single unit in the mTOR signaling pathway controlling cell division and growth. Defects in these genes lead to unregulated hamartomatous growth in multiple body sites.

ETIOLOGY
Many different mutations have been identified in both the TSC1 and TSC2 genes.

COMMONLY ASSOCIATED CONDITIONS
None

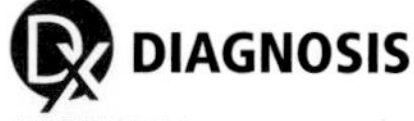

DIAGNOSIS

HISTORY
- Careful family history and physical exam of family members
- Infantile seizures/spasms
  - Usually last a few seconds and involve rapid nodding of the head and myoclonic spasms of the limbs
- Facial adenomatous rash
- Developmental delay

PHYSICAL EXAM
- Skin
  - Facial adenoma sebaceum
  - Ash-leaf spots (using a Wood's lamp)
  - Subungual fibromas
  - Café-au-lait spots (rare)
- Eye
  - Optic disc or peripheral retinal astrocytic hamartomas
  - Hypopigmented lesions
  - Coloboma (rare)
  - Papilledema (in cases of hydrocephalus)
  - Rarely: Vitreous hemorrhage, retinal neovascularization, retinal exudation or detachment, and vitreous seeding
- Oral cavity
  - Pitting of enamel
  - Gingival fibromas
- Pulmonary
  - Abnormal lung sounds
  - Evidence of pneumothorax

DIAGNOSTIC TESTS & INTERPRETATION
Lab
- Basic metabolic panel: Look specifically at renal function
- Urinalysis: Look for hematuria

Imaging
Initial approach
- MRI/CT (MRI is preferred)
  - Periventricular calcified subependymal nodules
- Echocardiogram
  - Cardiac rhabdomyoma
- Renal ultrasound
  - Renal angiomyolipoma
  - Polycystic kidney disease, renal cell carcinoma (rare)
- Chest X-ray/CT
  - Parenchymal and subpleural cystic changes, pneumothorax
- Skeletal X-ray
  - Sclerotic areas with focal calcification involving the skull and spine
  - Cysts in the phalanges of the hands and feet

Follow-up & special considerations
Routine surveillance for new tumors, or growth of existing tumors

Diagnostic Procedures/Other
- No reliable genetic testing available
- Patient is categorized as definite, probable, or suspect for TS on the basis of constellation of findings
  - Definite: 2 major features or 1 major feature plus 2 minor features
  - Probable: 1 major plus 1 minor feature
  - Suspect: 1 major feature or 2 or more minor features
- Major features
  - Facial angiofibromas
  - Ungual fibromas
  - Ash-leaf spots
  - Shagreen's patch
  - Multiple retinal astrocytic hamartomas
  - Cortical brain tuber
  - Subependymal brain nodule
  - Subependymal giant cell astrocytoma
  - Cardiac rhabdomyoma
  - Lymphangioleiomyomatosis of the lungs
  - Renal angiomyolipoma
- Minor features
  - Pitting of dental enamel
  - Gingival fibromas
  - Nonrenal hamartoma (liver, spleen, etc.)
  - Rectal hamartoma polyps
  - Bone cysts
  - Brain white matter "migration tracts"
  - Retinal hypopigmented patch
  - Multiple renal cysts
  - "Confetti" skin lesions

Pathological Findings
- CNS: Astrocytic hamartoma—large, well-differentiated, astrocytes with calcium
- Skin: Adenoma sebaceum—benign angiofibroma
- Skin: Ash-leaf spot: Amelanotic nevus
- Retina: Astrocytic hamartoma
  - Endophytic: in the nerve fiber layer
  - Exophytic: In the subretinal space
  - Can slowly enlarge, and rarely exude fluid causing retinal detachment or vitreous seeding (simulating retinoblastoma)
  - Composed of large pleomorphic astrocytes with focal calcification
- Renal: Angiomyolipoma—composed of HMB-45+ spindle cells; can occur in the renal medulla, cortex, or capsule
- Pulmonary: Lymphangioleiomyomatosis consists of a proliferation of HMB-45+ smooth muscle-like cells growing along the walls of airways and blood vessels.

DIFFERENTIAL DIAGNOSIS

- Differential diagnosis of a retinal astrocytic hamartoma
  - Retinoblastoma
  - Optic disc drusen
  - Retinal astrocytoma (solitary lesion, identical to retinal lesions of TS. Lesions in TS are often multiple)
  - Coats' disease
  - Toxocariasis
  - Myelinated nerve fiber layer

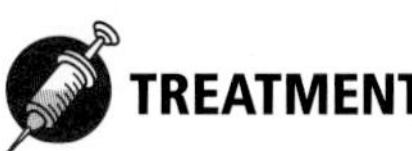

TREATMENT

MEDICATION

First Line

- Drugs to control symptoms
- Anti-epileptics for seizure control

Second Line

Rapamycin has been used (Experimental) in mice to reduce learning deficits in TS.

ADDITIONAL TREATMENT

General Measures

Routine surveillance for new tumors, or growth of existing tumors

Issues for Referral

- Pediatrics and Genetics for diagnosis and family counseling
- Neurology for seizures and CNS involvement
- Cardiology for rhabdomyoma
- Nephrology, if kidney involvement is severe
- Pulmonary, if lung involvement is severe
- Ophthalmology/retina examination to look for astrocytic hamartomas, often crucial for diagnosis

Additional Therapies

Genetic counseling for patient and family

SURGERY/OTHER PROCEDURES

- Neurosurgery for obstructive hydrocephalus
- Renal transplant for end-stage renal failure
- Lung transplant (rare) for severe lung involvement
- Pars plana vitrectomy (rare) for vitreous hemorrhage or retinal detachment

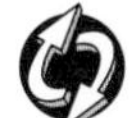

ONGOING CARE

FOLLOW-UP RECOMMENDATIONS

Routine surveillance for new tumors or growth of existing tumors

Patient Monitoring

- Monitor for changes in mental status or seizure control
- Monitor for changes in lung function

DIET

No special diet

PATIENT EDUCATION

- Tuberous Sclerosis Alliance
  - www.tsalliance.org/

PROGNOSIS

Life expectancy can be normal

COMPLICATIONS

- Cardiac rhabdomyomas can cause obstructive heart failure or arrhythmia, usually in infancy
- Renal failure can be progressive and require renal transplant
- Pulmonary involvement can be progressive
  - Can present with pneumothorax
  - Severe lymphangioleiomyomatosis of the lungs is more common in females
- Neurologic complications include hydrocephalus, severe mental retardation, and (rarely) status epilepticus
- Ocular complications are rare but can include visual field defects, vitreous hemorrhage, and retinal detachment

ADDITIONAL READING

- Roach ES, Smith M, Huttenlocher P, et al. Diagnostic criteria: Tuberous sclerosis complex, Report of the diagnostic criteria committee of the National Tuberous Sclerosis Association. *J Child Neurol* 1992;7:22–24.
- Rowley SA, O'Callaghan FJ, Osborne JP. Ophthalmic manifestations of tuberous sclerosis: A population-based study. *Br J Ophthalmol* 2001;85:420–423.
- Williams R, Taylor D. Tuberous sclerosis. *Surv Ophthalmol* 1985;30:143–153.

CODES

ICD9

- 362.89 Other retinal disorders
- 759.5 Tuberous sclerosis
- 759.6 Other congenital hamartoses, not elsewhere classified

CLINICAL PEARLS

- Hypopigmented macules ("Ash-leaf spots"), best seen with a Wood's lamp, are often the only finding of TS present at birth.
- Cardiac rhabdomyomas enlarge during late gestation and early infancy and tend to regress thereafter.
- Retinal astrocytic hamartoma, found in ~50% of TS patients, can occur as a solitary lesion in normal patients, but can be multiple and bilateral in TS.

UVEITIS-GLAUCOMA-HYPHEMA (UGH) SYNDROME

Andrea Knellinger Sawchyn
L. Jay Katz

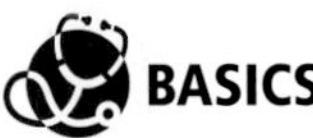

BASICS

DESCRIPTION

A secondary glaucoma resulting from elevated intraocular pressure (IOP) due to intraocular lens (IOL)–associated chronic inflammation and recurrent hyphemas

EPIDEMIOLOGY

Incidence

Uncommon

Prevalence

Unknown

RISK FACTORS

- Most common with iris-supported or closed-loop anterior chamber IOLs
- Malpositioned haptics of posterior chamber IOLs
- Subluxed IOLs

GENERAL PREVENTION

- Avoid using closed-loop anterior chamber IOLs
- Meticulous placement of posterior chamber lenses in the bag and appropriate lenses in the sulcus to avoid poorly positioned haptics.

PATHOPHYSIOLOGY

IOL-induced iris trauma leads to chronic intraocular inflammation and hemorrhage.

ETIOLOGY

A poorly positioned IOL causes iris chaffing and leads to inflammation and hemorrhage, resulting in elevated IOP.

COMMONLY ASSOCIATED CONDITIONS

Pseudoexfoliation

DIAGNOSIS

HISTORY

- History of cataract surgery with placement of an iris-sutured anterior chamber or a malpositioned posterior chamber IOL
- Transient blurring of vision
- Anticoagulation may exacerbate hemorrhage associated with IOL-induced iris chaffing (1)[C].

PHYSICAL EXAM

- Elevated IOP
- Anterior chamber IOL
- Poorly positioned or subluxed posterior chamber IOL
- Iritis
- Hyphema or microhyphema
- Iris transillumination defects
- Posterior synechiae
- Gonioscopy may be helpful in identifying malpositioned IOL haptics.
- Also perform gonioscopy to rule out neovascularization/peripheral anterior synechiae of the angle.

DIAGNOSTIC TESTS & INTERPRETATION

Lab

Consider checking the PT/INR in patients on anticoagulants to rule out supratherapeutic levels.

Imaging

Initial approach

- Ultrasound biomicroscopy (2)[C] may be used to identify IOL malpositioning and facilitate planning for surgical intervention.
- Optic disc photography or imaging (confocal scanning laser ophthalmoscopy, optical coherence tomography, scanning laser polarimetry)

Follow-up & special considerations

Repeat optic nerve photography or imaging periodically.

Diagnostic Procedures/Other

Visual fields

Pathological Findings

- Sterile anterior segment inflammation and hemorrhage
- Iris melanosomes on IOL haptics

DIFFERENTIAL DIAGNOSIS

- Trauma
- Neovascular glaucoma
- Uveitic glaucoma
- Swan syndrome (elevated IOP and recurrent hyphema associated with neovascularization of the corneoscleral surgical wound)
- Fuchs' heterochromic iridocyclitis
- Ghost cell glaucoma
- Intraocular tumors (such as malignant melanomas) resulting in recurrent hyphemas
- Juvenile xanthogranuloma

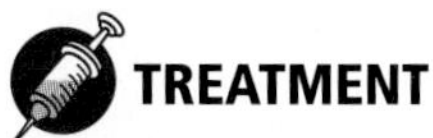

TREATMENT

MEDICATION

First Line

- Atropine 1%
- Topical steroids (e.g., prednisolone acetate)
- Topical beta-blockers (e.g., timolol, betaxolol), alpha-2 agonists (e.g., brimonidine), and/or carbonic anhydrase inhibitors (e.g., dorzolamide, brinzolamide)
- Prostaglandin analogues (e.g., travoprost, latanoprost, bimatoprost) may be used if other topical medications fail to provide adequate IOP control.

Second Line

- Oral or intravenous carbonic anhydrase inhibitors (e.g., acetazolamide)
- Intravenous hyperosmotics (e.g., mannitol)

ADDITIONAL TREATMENT

Issues for Referral

Consider referral to an experienced anterior segment surgeon if surgical intervention is warranted.

SURGERY/OTHER PROCEDURES

- Argon laser ablation of an isolated area of bleeding vessels may be attempted (3)[C].
- Lens exchange or repositioning and/or anterior chamber washout is often required (4)[C].
- Trabeculectomy or tube shunt if IOP remains uncontrolled

IN-PATIENT CONSIDERATIONS

Initial Stabilization

Control the IOP using the medications described previously.

Admission Criteria

Admission is rarely indicated. Consider admission if the IOP remains significantly elevated despite topical and oral medications.

Discharge Criteria

- Reasonable IOP
- Controlled eye pain

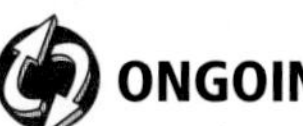

ONGOING CARE

FOLLOW-UP RECOMMENDATIONS

Timing of follow-up is dependent on IOP control.

Patient Monitoring

Periodically monitor IOP, optic nerve appearance, and visual fields.

PROGNOSIS

- Variable depending on:
  - Time to diagnosis and treatment
  - Preexisting optic nerve damage

COMPLICATIONS

- Glaucomatous visual field loss
- Decreased acuity related to IOL position, glaucomatous optic neuropathy, or both

REFERENCES

1. Schiff FS. Coumadin related spontaneous hyphemas in patients with iris-fixated pseudophakos. *Ophthalmic Surg* 1985;16:172–173.
2. Piette S, Canlas OA, Tran HV, et al. Ultrasound biomicroscopy in uveitis-glaucoma-hyphema syndrome. *Am J Ophthalmol* 2002;133:839–841.
3. Magaragal LE, Goldberg RE, Uram M, et al. Recurrent microhyphema in the pseudophakic eye. *Ophthalmology* 1983;90:1231–1234.
4. Carlson AN, Steward WC, Tso PC. Intraocular lens complications requiring removal or exchange. *Surv Ophthalmol* 1998;42:417–440.

ADDITIONAL READING

- Mamalis N, Crandall AS, Pulsipher MW, et al. Intraocular lens explantation and exchange: A review of lens styles, clinical indications, clinical results, and visual outcome. *J Cataract Refract Surg* 1991;17:811–818.
- Mamalis N. Explantation of intraocular lenses. *Curr Opin Ophthalmol* 2000;11:289–295.

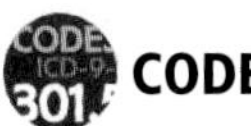

CODES

ICD9

- 364.41 Hyphema of iris and ciliary body
- 365.62 Glaucoma associated with ocular inflammations

CLINICAL PEARLS

- Recurrent hyphemas and/or iritis in a pseudophakic patient should prompt the clinician to rule out iris and angle neovascularization and carefully evaluate IOL position.
- Ultrasound biomicroscopy may be useful in assessing the position of posterior chamber IOLs.
- Topical steroids, cycloplegics, and IOP-lowering medications are the first line of treatment of uveitis–glaucoma–hyphema (UGH) syndrome but definitive management may require IOL repositioning or exchange.

VITAMIN A DEFICIENCY/XEROPHTHALMIA

Marlon Maus

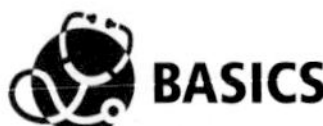

BASICS

DESCRIPTION

- Xerophthalmia (Greek for dry eyes) is a condition of severe dry eye generally referring to the disease caused by vitamin A deficiency (VAD).
- Other conditions can also be associated with dry eyes (keratoconjunctivitis sicca). (See Differential Diagnosis.)
- Ocular signs of xerophthalmia due to VAD include night blindness, conjunctival and corneal xerosis (dryness), Bitot's spots, keratomalacia, corneal ulceration, corneal scars, and retinal changes.
- VAD is a major public health nutrition problem in the developing world particularly Southern Asia and Africa. It especially affects young children also causing limited growth, weakened immune defenses, and increased risk of death.

EPIDEMIOLOGY

Incidence

Clinical xerophthalmia is extremely rare in the U.S. and other developed countries.

Prevalence

The WHO reported 2.8 million preschool children with clinical xerophthalmia worldwide accounting for 20,000–100,000 new cases of childhood blindness each year.

RISK FACTORS

- VAD particularly when associated with protein deficiency
  - Children aged 1–6 years and pregnant women are especially at risk.
  - Patients with AIDS may be at greater risk for VAD.
  - Vegan and other severe dietary restrictions may also pose a greater risk for deficiency.

GENERAL PREVENTION

- Adequate vitamin A intake, preferably through a balanced diet
- The Food and Nutrition Board at the Institute of Medicine recommends the following:
  - Infants 400–500 μg/day
  - Children 300–600 μg/day
  - Adolescents and adults 700–900 μg/day
  - Women who are pregnant or producing breast milk (lactating) need higher amounts.

PATHOPHYSIOLOGY

- Vitamin A is a fat-soluble vitamin ingested in the diet in two forms: as retinol itself from animal sources or as the provitamin carotene from plant sources.
- Adequate body stores of zinc and protein are necessary for the formation of retinol-binding protein (RBP), without which vitamin A cannot be transported to its target tissues.
  - In the retina, vitamin A serves as a precursor to the visual pigments of the photoreceptors.
  - It is necessary for conjunctival mucosa and corneal stromal integrity.
- VAD leads to atrophic changes in the normal mucosal surface, with loss of goblet cells, and replacement of the normal epithelium.

ETIOLOGY

VAD

COMMONLY ASSOCIATED CONDITIONS

- Protein deficiency
- Malnutrition
- Immune deficiency

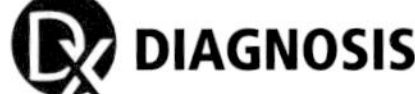

DIAGNOSIS

HISTORY

- A history of malnutrition or malabsorption leading to a VAD state
- Night blindness is an early symptom.
- Dry eyes can usually be diagnosed by the symptoms alone: dryness, foreign body sensation, burning, itching, ocular pain, mucus formation, red eye, visual disturbances, and easily fatigued eye.
- The diagnosis of xerophthalmia is mostly clinical, and a high degree of suspicion is required.

PHYSICAL EXAM

- A slit lamp examination should be performed to diagnose dry eyes and to document any damage to the eye.
- A Schirmer's test can measure the amount of tears bathing the eye. This test is also useful to determine the severity of the condition. A 5-minute Schirmer's test, using a standard 5 × 35-mm paper strip, with and without anesthesia showing wetting under 5 mm is considered diagnostic for dry eyes (1)[B].
- A tear breakup time (TBUT) test measures the time it takes for tears to break up in the eye. A breakup time of less than 10 seconds is considered abnormal.
- Abnormal staining of the cornea and conjunctiva with fluorescein or rose bengal 1% is also a useful diagnostic test.

DIAGNOSTIC TESTS & INTERPRETATION

Lab

- Serum vitamin A levels of 35 μmol/dL or less (2)
- Total and holo-RBP (complex of vitamin A and RBP) for serum RBP tend to correlate with measures of serum vitamin A (3)[C].
- Conjunctival impression cytology is a technique useful for detecting preclinical xerophthalmia. It is a noninvasive method of obtaining a specimen to assess the histological appearance of the superficial conjunctival layers.

Pathological Findings

Conjunctival biopsy shows epidermidalization with surface keratinization; a reduction of goblet cell density and squamous metaplasia can also be documented with impression cytology.

DIFFERENTIAL DIAGNOSIS

The differential diagnosis includes other conditions that can be associated with dry eyes (keratoconjunctivitis sicca) such as radiation, Sjögren's syndrome, systemic lupus erythematosus, rheumatoid arthritis, scleroderma, sarcoidosis, amyloidosis, hypothyroidism, and the use of some medications including antihistamines, nasal decongestants, tranquilizers, and antidepressant.

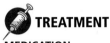

TREATMENT

MEDICATION

Oral treatment consists of 200,000 IU of vitamin A in oil followed the next day with an additional dose of 200,000 IU (4)[B]. In the presence of severe corneal disease or malabsorption, the preferable dose is 100,000 IU water-miscible vitamin A intramuscularly followed the next day and every 1 to 2 weeks with an oral dose (5)[B].

ADDITIONAL TREATMENT

General Measures

- Supportive treatment of symptoms usually includes use of artificial tears in the form of eye drops, increasing the humidity of the environment with humidifiers, use of goggles, and wearing wraparound glasses when outdoors to minimize the effects of wind.
- Lacrimal drainage punctal plugs can be used to increase the tear lake.
- Prevention and treatment of secondary bacterial infections from ulcers
- Topical retinoic acid (0.1%) can be used to promote healing; however, this can increase scaring so it should be used with caution (6)[B].

Issues for Referral

- Corneal and conjunctival ulcers, bacterial infections, and corneal melting all require immediate care by an ophthalmologist. Retinal changes also may need to be attended to.
- Associated conditions, such as immune deficiency, malnutrition, and malabsorption syndromes may require subspecialty referral.

SURGERY/OTHER PROCEDURES

- Surgery plays a limited role in xerophthalmia. Keratomalacia (corneal melting) is usually inoperable and mostly residual, visually significant scars are amenable to corneal transplants.
- Many patients in developing countries are generally too weak and malnourished to tolerate surgery.

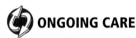

ONGOING CARE

FOLLOW-UP RECOMMENDATIONS

- Repeated external ophthalmic and funduscopic exams are warranted to document adequate, sustained healing and prevention of relapses.
- In children, sustained healing of severe xerophthalmia requires addressing the underlying protein deficiency.

DIET

- Vitamin A comes from animal sources, such as eggs, meat, milk, cheese, cream, liver, kidney, cod, and halibut fish oil.
- Vegetable sources of beta-carotene are carrots, pumpkin, sweet potatoes, winter squashes, cantaloupe, pink grapefruit, apricots, broccoli, spinach, and most dark green, leafy vegetables. The more intense the color of a fruit or vegetable, the higher the beta-carotene content. Bioavailability of vegetable sources may be less than that of animal sources.
- Strains of genetically modified rice rich in vitamin A have been developed to help decrease deficiencies in developing countries.

PROGNOSIS

- Response to adequate therapy is quick and often dramatic. Night blindness and corneal signs and symptoms resolve very rapidly particularly in less advanced disease.
- In the absence of severe corneal scarring, visual acuity can be expected to recover completely.

COMPLICATIONS

- Permanent corneal scarring with loss of vision and even loss of an eye from perforation and infection can result from advanced or untreated disease.
- If decreased visual acuity is not addressed in young children permanent amblyopia may develop.

REFERENCES

1. Horwath-Winter J, Berghold A, Schmut O, et al. Evaluation of the clinical course of dry eye syndrome. *Arch Ophthalmol* 2003;121(10): 1364–1368.
2. World Health Organization. Report of a joint WHO/UNICEF/USAAID/HKI/IVACG meeting. *"Control of Vitamin A deficiency"*. Geneva, Switzerland: World Health Organization, 1982.
3. Smith J, Steinemann TL. Vitamin A deficiency and the eye. *Int Ophthalmol Clin* 2000;40:83–91.
4. Sommer A, Muhilal H, Tarwotjo I. Protein deficiency and treatment of xerophthalmia. *Arch Ophthalmol* 1982;100:785–787.
5. Sommer A, Tarwotio I, Muhilal, et al. Oral versus intramuscular vitamin A in the treatment of xerophthalmia. *Lancet* 1980;315:557–559.
6. Sommer A. Treatment of corneal xerophthalmia with topical retinoic acid. *Am J Ophthalmol* 1983;95:349–352.

ADDITIONAL READING

- Calonge M. The treatment of dry eye. *Surv Ophthalmol* 2001;45(S2):S227–S239.
- Sommer A. Vitamin A deficiency and clinical disease: A historical overview. *J Nutr* 2008;138:1835–1839.

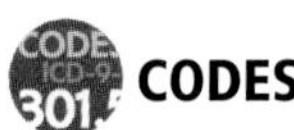

CODES

ICD9

- 264.8 Other manifestations of vitamin a deficiency
- 372.53 Conjunctival xerosis

VITREORETINAL LYMPHOMA

Carol L. Shields

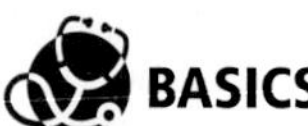

BASICS

DESCRIPTION

- Vitreoretinal lymphoma (VR lymphoma) is a high-grade type of non-Hodgkin's lymphoma that involves the retina and vitreous.
- The term "primary intraocular lymphoma" is commonly used in the literature to refer to this condition. This term is somewhat of a misnomer and should be avoided as uveal lymphoma (a distinct clinical entity) can be primary and is also intraocular.

EPIDEMIOLOGY

Incidence

- VR lymphoma is rare with an estimated incidence of 30–50 cases per 10 million population.
- There has been an increase in the incidence of VR lymphoma within the past several decades in both the immunocompetent and immunocompromised populations.

RISK FACTORS

- Immunodeficiency states: Organ transplantation, HIV infection, and congenital immunodeficiency.
- Age: VR lymphoma primarily affects the middle-aged and elderly, although cases in children have been reported.

Genetics

See "Molecular gene analysis" under "Diagnostic tests and interpretation".

ETIOLOGY

Infection by Epstein-Barr virus, herpesvirus, and *Toxoplasma gondii* has been implicated in the induction of primary central nervous system (PCNS) or VR lymphoma, but results are inclusive at this time.

COMMONLY ASSOCIATED CONDITIONS

- PCNS lymphoma: VR lymphoma is strongly associated with and is considered a subtype of PCNS lymphoma.
  - It is estimated that of patients with PCNS lymphoma, 15–25% have VR lymphoma at diagnosis and another 25% develop VR lymphoma during subsequent follow-up.
  - 60–80% of patients presenting with VR lymphoma will develop PCNS lymphoma.
- Systemic lymphoma: VR lymphoma secondary to systemic lymphoma is rare.
  - Intraocular lymphoma secondary to systemic lymphoma generally affects the uvea (see "Choroidal metastasis" under "Differential diagnosis").

DIAGNOSIS

HISTORY

- Patients present with symptoms of floaters or blurred vision.
- Eye pain, redness, and photophobia are uncommon.

PHYSICAL EXAM

- The most common features of VR lymphoma include chronic vitreous cellular infiltration and yellowish sub-retinal pigment epithelium (RPE) infiltrates in combination or as isolated findings.
  - Sub-RPE infiltrates are initially small and focal and might resemble soft drusen but can enlarge and coalesce into larger plaques over time.
  - Resolution of sub-RPE infiltrates is usually accompanied by residual RPE atrophy.
  - Spontaneous resolution of sub-RPE infiltrates has rarely been reported.
- Other less common findings include anterior chamber reaction, keratic precipitates, vitreous hemorrhage, retinal vascular infiltration, and optic disc edema.
- 80% of cases are bilateral but ocular involvement can be asymmetrical.
- PCNS lymphoma generally affects the frontal lobe.
  - Neurologic findings include behavioral and cognitive changes (most common), headache, seizure, hemiparesis, cerebellar dysfunction, and cranial nerve palsies.

DIAGNOSTIC TESTS & INTERPRETATION

Lab

- All patients with suspected VR lymphoma require cerebrospinal fluid (CSF) analysis to exclude PCNS lymphoma.
  - 25% of patients with brain lésions identified on magnetic résonance Imaging (MRI) have lymphoma cells in their CSF.

Imaging

- All patients with suspected VR lymphoma require CNS imaging to exclude PCNS lymphoma.
  - Brain lesions are low signal on T1-weighted and high signal in T2-weighted MRI images.

Diagnostic Procedures/Other

- Routine cytology: Allows evaluation of cell morphology (see under "Pathological findings") (1)[B].
- Immunophenotyping (immunohistochemistry): Uses monoclonal antibodies to analyze surface markers of lymphoma cells (CD19+, CD20+, CD22+, CD79a+, BCL-2+, MUM1/IRF4+, BCL-6+) to establish B-cell monoclonality.
  - Can be performed on slide-mounted sample or with flow cytometry.
  - Light-chain immunoglobulins (kappa or lambda) are other cell surface markers that can be studied by immunohistochemistry; ratio of kappa/lambda or lambda/kappa >3 is suggestive of B-cell lymphoma.
- Molecular gene analysis: Immunoglobulin heavy chain (IgH) gene rearrangement demonstrated by polymerase chain reaction can be used to establish monoclonality of B-cell lymphoma. t (14:18) translocation involving the bcl-2 gene has also been reported.
- Cytokine analysis: High levels of interleukin-10 (IL-10) are seen in the vitreous of eyes with RV lymphoma, whereas IL-6 (and IL-12) is increased in eyes with inflammatory conditions. IL-10:IL-6 ratio >1.0 is suggestive of B-cell lymphoma.

Pathological Findings

- Majority of VR lymphomas are B-cell non-Hodgkin lymphomas subtyped as diffuse large B-cell lymphoma, according to the World Health Organization lymphoma classification.
- The malignant cells are medium to large pleomorphic cells with high nuclear/cytoplasmic ratios and prominent nucleoli.
- Sample for analysis can be obtained from the vitreous (needle biopsy, vitrectomy) or from the sub-RPE infiltrates (needle biopsy, chorioretinal biopsy).
  - The obtained sample should be handled with care and transferred to the laboratory as quickly as possible to minimize degeneration of fragile lymphoma cells.
  - Use of cell culture media instead of saline can increase the diagnostic yield.
  - Prior steroid treatment can induce lysis of lymphoma cells. Discontinuing steroid use before biopsy may increase the diagnostic yield.
  - The malignant cells are accompanied by large numbers of non-neoplastic cells (small reactive lymphocytes, histiocytes) and necrotic debris making detection of lymphoma cells more challenging.
  - Multiple tissue biopsies may be required to establish the correct diagnosis.

DIFFERENTIAL DIAGNOSIS

- Inflammatory/infectious conditions (Multifocal choroiditis, bird-shot chorioretinitis, acute posterior multifocal placoid pigment epitheliopathy, multiple evanescent white dot syndrome, Vogt-Koyanagi-Harada syndrome, toxoplasmosis, sarcoidosis, tuberculosis, syphilis, viral retinitis, etc)
  - RV lymphoma is the most common cause of masquerade syndrome and should be considered in the differential diagnosis of chronic ocular inflammatory conditions in the elderly.
  - VR lymphoma can initially and temporarily respond to steroid treatment with decrease in vitreous cells and improvement of symptoms leading to misdiagnosis of inflammatory condition.
- Choroidal metastasis: Multifocal choroidal metastasis can simulate the sub-RPE infiltrates of lymphoma but lacks the vitreous cellular infiltration.

- Choroidal lymphoma: Is a distinct entity and although most cases present with diffuse homogenous choroidal thickening, some can manifest yellowish–orange multifocal choroidal infiltrates that can be confused with the sub-retinal infiltrates of VR lymphoma. Features of choroidal lymphoma that help differentiate it from VR lymphoma include:
  - Can be associated with anterior epibulbar (subconjunctival) extension of lymphoma manifesting as salmon patches
  - Does not manifest significant vitreous cellular infiltration
  - B-scan ultrasound generally shows acoustically hollow diffuse choroidal thickening with occasional posterior epibulbar (extraocular) extension of tumor. In contrast, eye wall thickening seen on B-scan ultrasonography of VR lymphoma is generally focal and less pronounced with no extraocular extension.
  - In contrast to VR lymphoma, which is high-grade and aggressive, choroidal lymphoma is low-grade and slowly progressive with good life prognosis.
  - Has no association with PCNS lymphoma but can be associated with systemic non-Hodgkin's lymphoma, especially in some bilateral cases

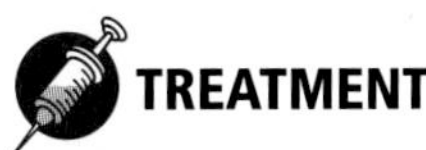

TREATMENT

MEDICATION

PCNS Lymphoma

First Line

- Patients with PCNS lymphoma are usually treated with high-dose intravenous methotrexate (MTX) with or without intrathecal chemotherapy or whole-brain radiation.
  - Combined chemotherapy and radiotherapy offers a better life prognosis compared with radiotherapy alone but is associated with high rates of delayed neurotoxicity especially in patients >60 years of age.

Second Line

- Newer agents used for systemic treatment of PCNS lymphoma, usually in combination with high-dose MTX, include:
  - Rituximab (anti-CD20 antibody)
  - Ifosfamide/trofosfamide (nitrogen mustard alkylating agents)

VR Lymphoma

- There is no general agreement on the optimal treatment for VR lymphoma.
- Patients with combined VR and PCNS lymphoma require systemic/CNS therapy as described above.
- Treatment options for patients with isolated VR lymphoma include systemic chemotherapy, local ocular therapy (radiation, intravitreal injection), or a combination of both (2)[B].

First Line

- Low-dose EBRT (35–40 Gy) has been shown to be very effective in treatment of VR lymphoma (3)[B].
  - Radiation complications are generally mild and tolerable and include dry eye, cataract, and radiation retinopathy.

Second Line

- Intravitreal MTX (400 mcg/0.1 mL) has been used successfully for treatment of VR lymphoma (4)[B].
  - Requires multiple injections of intravitreal MTX over many months.
  - Is associated with complications such as corneal keratopathy, cataract, neovascular glaucoma, and inflammatory reaction
  - Intravitreal rituximab (1 mg/0.1 mL) has been used in limited number of patients but long-term safety and efficacy is not yet known (5) [B].

SURGERY/OTHER PROCEDURES

Complete pars plana vitrectomy not only provides enough vitreous sample for diagnostic procedures (see under "Diagnostic tests & interpretation"), but also allows earlier visual rehabilitation in patients with severe vitreous haziness.

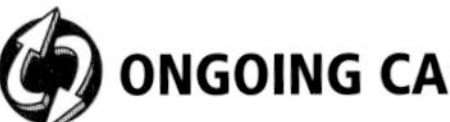

ONGOING CARE

FOLLOW-UP RECOMMENDATIONS

Patient Monitoring

- All patients with isolated VR lymphoma are at high risk for development of PCNS lymphoma and require long-term CNS monitoring.
- Regardless of the method of treatment, all patients with treated VR lymphoma require close ocular monitoring for early detection of lymphoma recurrence and for treatment complications.

PATIENT EDUCATION

Patients should report any onset of new or recurrent ocular symptoms (see in "Symptoms" under "Diagnosis") or neurologic symptoms (see in "Physical exam" under "Diagnosis") without delay.

- www.fighteyecancer.com
- www.eyecancerinfo.com

PROGNOSIS

- Presence of PCNS lymphoma imparts a poor prognosis for life (2–3 years).
- Extensive macular sub-RPE infiltrates lead to development of macular RPE alterations and are associated with poor a visual prognosis.

REFERENCES

1. Raparia K, Chang CC, Chévez-Barrios P. Intraocular lymphoma: Diagnostic approach and immunophenotypic findings in vitrectomy specimens. *Arch Pathol Lab Med* 2009;133: 1233–1237.
2. Jahnke K, Korfel A, Komm J, et al. Intraocular lymphoma 2000–2005: Results of a retrospective multicentre trial. *Graefes Arch Clin Exp Ophthalmol* 2006;244:663–669.
3. Berenbom A, Davila RM, Lin HS, et al. Treatment outcomes for primary intraocular lymphoma: Implications for external beam radiotherapy. *Eye* 2007;21:1198–1201.
4. Frenkel S, Hendler K, Siegal T, et al. Intravitreal methotrexate for treating vitreoretinal lymphoma: 10 years of experience. *Br J Ophthalmol* 2008;92:383–388.

ADDITIONAL READING

- Choi JY, Kafkala C, Foster CS. Primary intraocular lymphoma: A review. *Semin Ophthalmol* 2006;21:125–133.
- Coupland SE, Chan CC, Smith J. Pathophysiology of retinal lymphoma. *Ocul Immunol Inflamm* 2009;17:227–237.
- Coupland SE, Damato B. Understanding intraocular lymphomas. *Clin Experiment Ophthalmol* 2008;36:564–578.

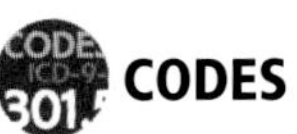

CODES

ICD9

200.50 Primary central nervous system lymphoma, unspecified site, extranodal and solid organ sites

CLINICAL PEARLS

- VR lymphoma is the most common cause of masquerade syndrome and should be considered in the differential diagnosis of all cases of chronic posterior uveitis, especially in the elderly.
- Because of high rate of development of PCNS lymphoma (up to 80%), patients presenting with isolated VR lymphoma require regular long-term monitoring for CNS involvement.

VOGT-KOYANAGI-HARADA'S SYNDROME (UVEOMENINGITIS)

Sunir J. Garg

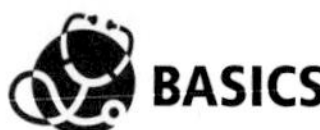

BASICS

DESCRIPTION

- Bilateral granulomatous panuveitis with skin, meningeal, and auditory-vestibular involvement
- Usually occurs in more darkly pigmented individuals

EPIDEMIOLOGY

Incidence

- Rare
- More common in young patients (teens to early 40s)
- Slight female preponderance
- Occurs more often in the Spring and Fall

Prevalence

Very uncommon

RISK FACTORS

- Occurs most commonly in patients from the Middle East, South and East Asia, Latin America, and in Native Americans
- Rarely seen in Caucasians or patients from Africa

Genetics

HLA-DRB1*0405, HLA-DR4, and HLA-Dw53 have been identified as risk factors.

PATHOPHYSIOLOGY

T-cell mediated autoimmune disorder against melanocytes, specifically against tyrosinase and tyrosinase-related proteins.

ETIOLOGY

Unknown. Epstein-Barr virus has been suggested as a possible trigger, and injury to the skin has also been suggested as an inciting injury.

COMMONLY ASSOCIATED CONDITIONS

See Diagnosis, signs and symptoms.

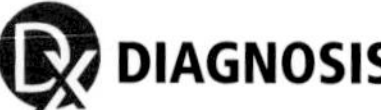

DIAGNOSIS

HISTORY

Usually CNS findings first.

- History of blurred vision in one or both eyes, ocular pain, photophobia, and floaters.
- CNS: Heartache, stiff neck, periocular discomfort, vertigo, tinnitus, and dysacusis
- Later findings: Hair loss; skin/hair depigmentation, sensitivity to touch of the hair/skin
- The American Uveitis Society criteria for VKH are:
  - No history of ocular trauma
  - No other evidence of another disease process
  - Early or late ocular disease as listed below
  - Neurologic/auditory findings (subjective or objective)
  - Skin findings: Poliosis, vitiligo, alopecia

PHYSICAL EXAM

- Bilateral granulomatous panuveitis, often with serous retinal detachments, dense vitreitis, optic disc edema, and Dalen-Fuchs nodules
  - In chronic disease, disturbance of the retinal pigment epithelium can cause a sunset glow fundus
  - Skin findings of poliosis, vitiligo, alopecia
  - Auditory dysfunction

DIAGNOSTIC TESTS & INTERPRETATION

Lab

Rule out other causes: Syphilis (FTA-ABS), Lyme titers, Tuberculosis (PPD), Sarcoid (ACE, Chest x-ray/CT)

Imaging

Initial approach

- Fluorescein angiography (FA) is very helpful – delayed choroidal filling with pinpoint areas of hyperfluorescence later (starry sky) and optic disc leakage
- B-scan ultrasonography: Nonspecific choroidal thickening (helps to distinguish from posterior scleritis, uveal effusion syndrome, choroidal metastasis)
- Optical coherence tomography may show exudative retinal detachment (nonspecific).

Follow-up & special considerations

Weekly until inflammation under control, then every 3 months until off immunosuppression and inflammation free.

Diagnostic Procedures/Other

- Lumbar puncture: Pleocytosis occurs in up to 84% of patients.
- Detailed auditory testing to rule out other causes of central hearing loss

Pathological Findings

Diffuse granulomatous inflammation of the choroid with sparing of the choriocapillaris (in contrast to sympathetic ophthalmia).

DIFFERENTIAL DIAGNOSIS

- Sympathetic ophthalmia (history of ocular trauma/surgery)
- Central serous chorioretinopathy
- Uveal metastasis
- Idiopathic uveal effusion
- Posterior scleritis
- Sarcoidosis
- Syphilis
- Lyme
- Tuberculosis
- Ocular lymphoma

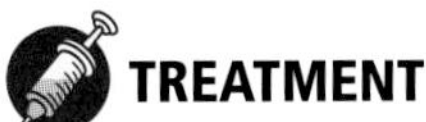

TREATMENT

MEDICATION

First Line

Prompt, aggressive corticosteroid treatment is critical (approximately 1–2 mg/kg/d initially). IV corticosteroids may hasten resolution and should be considered in severe cases. If inflammation present for more than 2–3 months on more than 10 mg daily, consider second line agent.

Second Line

- As patients may have inflammation for many months or years, given the risks of chronic prednisone use greater than 10 mg/d, early use of immunomodulatory therapy should be strongly considered.
- Agents such as azathioprine, mycophenolate mofetil (CellCept), cyclosporine, and anti-Tumor Necrosis Factor (TNF) agents (Remicade and Humira) are effective.
- A steroid implant (Retisert, fluocinolone acetonide, Bausch and Lomb) may be considered.

ADDITIONAL TREATMENT

Issues for Referral

Prompt referral to a uveitis specialist.

SURGERY/OTHER PROCEDURES

- Cataract surgery: The eye should be inflammation free for 3 months before surgery. Patients may still develop posterior synechiae.
- Uncommon. For complications of VKH: Draining chronic subretinal fluid, subfoveal choroidal neovascular membrane therapy with intravitreal injection of anti-VEGF agent, photodynamic therapy, or submacular surgery

IN-PATIENT CONSIDERATIONS

Initial Stabilization

High dose corticosteroids.

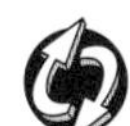

ONGOING CARE

FOLLOW-UP RECOMMENDATIONS

Every week until inflammation free, then every 3 months until inflammation free off immunosuppressive medications.

PROGNOSIS

Guarded. Prompt, aggressive therapy with use of steroid sparing agents can be vision saving.

COMPLICATIONS

- Permanent vision loss
- Cataract formation, glaucoma, chronic retinal detachment, subretinal fibrosis, subfoveal choroidal neovascular membrane formation can occur.

ADDITIONAL READING

- Read RW, Holland GN, Rao NA, et al. Revised diagnostic criteria for Vogt-Koyanagi-Harada disease: report of an international committee on nomenclature. *Am J Ophthalmol* 2001;131(5): 647–652.
- Lertsumitkul S, Whitcup SM, Nussenblatt RB, et al. Subretinal fibrosis and choroiral neovascularization in Vogt-Koyanagi-Harada syndome. *Graefes Arch Clin Exp Ophthalmol* 1999;237:1029–1045.

CODES

ICD9

- 360.12 Panuveitis
- 364.24 Vogt-koyanagi syndrome

CLINICAL PEARLS

- Bilateral granulomatous panuveitis with skin, meningeal, and auditory-vestibular involvement
- Patients must have no history of ocular trauma.
- Aggressive systemic treatment is very effective in preventing vision loss.

VON HIPPEL-LINDAU DISEASE

Jeremy D. Wolfe
Alok Bansal

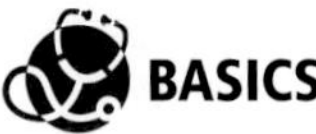

BASICS

DESCRIPTION

- Von Hippel-Lindau (VHL) disease is an inherited cancer predisposition syndrome characterized by various tumors affecting multiple organ systems (see 'Commonly Associated Conditions').
- The primary ophthalmic finding, retinal capillary hemangioblastoma, is common; it is frequently an early manifestation of VHL disease.

EPIDEMIOLOGY

Incidence

1 in 40,000–54,000 live births (1,2)

Prevalence

- VHL disease is rare, affecting approximately 7,000 patients in the US (3)
- Retinal capillary hemangioblastomas is found in approximately 37–59% of patients with VHL (3,4)

RISK FACTORS

Genetics

- Autosomal dominant
- High penetrance
- Chromosome 3 (3p25–26)

GENERAL PREVENTION

Genetic counseling

PATHOPHYSIOLOGY

- The VHL gene functions as a tumor suppressor gene.
- Tumor formation results from lack of function of the gene.
- Tumor formation thought to follow two-hit model (similar to retinoblastoma).
- Clinical phenotype of ocular manifestations in VHL may vary based on precise gene mutation (4).

COMMONLY ASSOCIATED CONDITIONS

- Hemangioblastoma
  - Retinal
  - Cerebellar
  - Spinal cord
- Visceral lesions
  - Renal cell carcinoma
  - Pheochromocytoma
  - Renal cysts
  - Pancreatic cysts
  - Islet cell tumors
  - Epididymal cystadenoma
  - Bilateral endolymphatic sac tumors
  - Adnexal papillary cystadenoma of probable mesonephric origin (APMO)

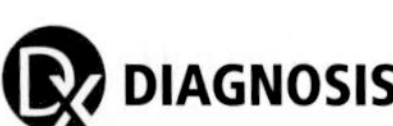

DIAGNOSIS

HISTORY

- Family history is paramount as VHL is inherited in an autosomal dominant manner, however, full penetrance does not occur until approximately age 65 years. If history is equivocal consider examination of family members.
- A detailed review of systems may reveal complaints related to any of the potential associated disorders (see 'Commonly Associated Conditions'). However, many of the associated conditions are asymptomatic in VHL disease and therefore screening protocols have been developed (see "Follow-up Recommendations').

PHYSICAL EXAM

- Classification of retinal capillary hemangioblastomas is based on location.
- Peripheral endophytic
  - Most common
  - Reddish–orange circumscribed tumor (one or more)
  - Progressive enlargement
  - Dilated, tortuous feeding, and draining vessels
  - Intraretinal and subretinal exudation (frequently in macula)
  - Possible tractional retinal detachment
- Juxtapapillary
  - Less common
  - May appear as discrete red/pink lesions at the disc margin (endophytic) or as diffuse gray/pink thickening that may blur the disc borders (exophytic)
- Systemic/visceral
  - CNS hemangioblastoma
    - Cerebellum (75%) and spinal cord (15%) are most common locations
  - Pheochromocytoma
    - Typically bilateral and multiple in VHL disease
    - Palpitations, anxiety, headaches, sweating, hypertension
  - Renal cysts
    - Potential malignant transformation
  - Renal cell carcinoma
    - Bilateral in large majority (90%) of cases in VHL disease
    - Typically lack pain or hematuria
  - Pancreatic cysts
    - Secretory versus non-secretory
  - Cystadenoma of epididymis or broad ligament
    - Asymptomatic and largely benign
    - Rarely a cause of infertility
  - Endolymphatic sac tumor
    - Locally aggressive, benign cystadenoma
    - May present with impaired hearing, tinnitus, and vertigo

DIAGNOSTIC TESTS & INTERPRETATION

Lab

- Urinary catecholamines
- Genetic evaluation

Imaging

Initial approach

- Fundus photos
- Fluorescein angiography (FA)
  - Rapid arterial phase
  - Diffuse leakage in mid and late frames
- Systemic evaluation
  - Brain/spine MRI
  - Abdominal CT/MRI/ultrasound

Follow-up & special considerations

May use retinal fundus photos to follow progression or assess response to treatment for retinal capillary hemangioblastoma.

Diagnostic Procedures/Other

- Ultrasonography (ocular)
  - Acoustically solid with variable reflectivity (medium or high reflectivity)
- CT
  - Thin section, contrast enhanced CT is sensitive for early renal lesions
- MRI
  - Most useful for detecting CNS hemangioblastoma
  - Hyperintense on T1
  - Hypointense on T2
  - Enhance with contrast
- Diagnostic Criteria
  - Based upon presence of retinal or CNS capillary hemangioblastoma, visceral lesions, and family history
  - With positive family history, only 1 hemangioblastoma (retinal or CNS) or visceral lesion required
  - Negative family history requires 2 hemangioblastomas or a hemangioblastoma and a visceral lesion
- National Cancer Institute classification
  - Type I – Pheochromocytoma absent
  - Type II – Pheochromocytoma present (further subdivisions of Type II exist)

Pathological Findings

- Spindle cells, small blood vessels, clear stromal cells
- Stromal cells appear to be cells of origin

DIFFERENTIAL DIAGNOSIS

Retinal Capillary Hemangioblastoma

- Coats' disease
- Racemose hemangioma
- Retinal arterial macroaneurysm
- Retinal cavernous hemangioma
- Vasoproliferative tumor

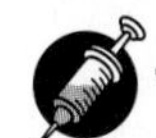

TREATMENT

SURGERY/OTHER PROCEDURES

- Most common procedures/therapy
  - Laser photocoagulation
  - Cryotherapy
- Less common procedures/therapy
  - Photodynamic therapy
  - External beam radiotherapy
  - Proton beam radiotherapy
  - Plaque radiotherapy
- New or experimental therapy (4)[C]
  - Systemic anti-VEGF
  - Local anti-VEGF
- Visceral/systemic
  - CNS angiomas are typically observed but may be surgically excised if symptomatic
  - Small renal cell carcinomas (<3 cm) may be observed, larger lesions are typically removed with nephron-sparing surgery
  - Functional pheochromocytomas are excised with adrenal sparing surgery
  - Early removal of endolymphatic sac tumors may prevent hearing loss

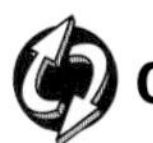

ONGOING CARE

FOLLOW-UP RECOMMENDATIONS

- Patients with or at risk for VHL (5)[B]
  - Ophthalmoscopy yearly
  - Urinary catecholamine yearly
  - MRI of brain and spine every 2 years
  - Abdominal ultrasound every year
  - Abdominal CT every 1–2 years
- Ophthalmologist (likely retina or oncology) to follow ocular lesions and implement treatment when appropriate
- Referral to geneticist and/or oncologist with an interest/expertise in VHL

PROGNOSIS

- Risk of severe bilateral vision loss (legal blindness) is low (approximately 5%).
- Risk of severe unilateral vision loss (20/200) is approximately 25%.
  - Risk increases with age, juxtapapillary tumors, and increased tumor number.
- Morbidity/mortality commonly associated with CNS lesions or renal cell carcinoma.
  - Average life expectancy of approximately 50 years
  - Appropriate screening may reduce morbidity and mortality.

REFERENCES

1. Maher ER, Iselius L, Yates JR, et al. Von Hippel-Lindau disease: A genetic study. *J Med Genet* 1991;28:443–447.
2. Neumann HP, Wiestler OD. Clustering of features of von Hippel–Lindau syndrome: Evidence for a complex genetic locus. *Lancet* 1991;337: 1052–1054.
3. Singh AD, Shields CL, Shields JA. Von Hippel-Lindau disease. *Surv Ophthalmol* 2001;46:117–142.
4. Wong WT, Chew EY. Ocular Von Hippel-Lindau disease: Clinical update and emerging treatments. *Curr Opin Ophthalmol* 2008;19:213–217.
5. Choyke PL, Glenn GM, Walther MM, et al. Von Hippel–Lindau disease: Genetic, clinical, and imaging features. *Radiology* 1995;194:629–642.

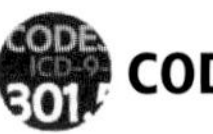

CODES

ICD9

759.6 Other congenital hamartoses, not elsewhere classified

CLINICAL PEARLS

- VHL is a cancer predisposition syndrome characterized by multiple tumors including retinal capillary hemangioblastoma, CNS hemangioblastoma, pheochromocytoma, and renal cell carcinoma.
- Following appropriate follow-up and screening protocols may reduce morbidity and mortality.
- Multiple treatments exist for retinal capillary hemangioblastomas, with a good overall visual prognosis.

WEGENER'S GRANULOMATOSIS

Bhairavi V. Kharod

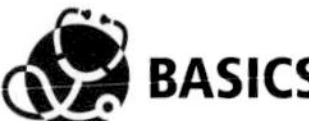

BASICS

DESCRIPTION

- Wegener's granulomatosis is a necrotizing vasculitic syndrome of small-sized blood vessels that affects multiple organs.
- Most commonly affected organs include kidney, lung, upper respiratory tract, eyes, ears, and skin.
- Dr. Friedrich Wegener first described the disease in 1936.

EPIDEMIOLOGY

Incidence

The reported annual incidence of Wegener's granulomatosis is 10 per million population.

Prevalence

The prevalence of Wegener's granulomatosis in the US is approximately 3 per 100,000 persons.

RISK FACTORS

- Wegener's granulomatosis is primarily a disease of Caucasian patients and rarely affects African Americans.
- A slight male preponderance is also reported.

Genetics

Some alleles have been identified as protective factors against Wegener's granulomatosis, although further research is being performed to identify any genetic association.

GENERAL PREVENTION

Early diagnosis is crucial to prevent end-organ damage and life-threatening complications.

PATHOPHYSIOLOGY

- The hallmark of this disease is necrotizing granulomas of small vessels.
- Evidence suggests that Wegener's granulomatosis is an autoimmune inflammatory process, in which the cytoplasmic variants of antineutrophilic cytoplasmic antibodies (cANCAs) are directed at neutrophil proteinase 3 (PR3). Neutrophils and endothelial cells are thought to be both targets and promoters of inflammation.

ETIOLOGY

The etiology of Wegener's granulomatosis remains unknown, although several chromosomes are being investigated for possible loci predisposing to this disease.

COMMONLY ASSOCIATED CONDITIONS

- Wegener's granulomatosis is a multisystem disease.
- Classic features are vasculitis, glomerulonephritis, and granulomas of the upper and lower respiratory tract.

DIAGNOSIS

HISTORY

- The onset of Wegener's granulomatosis is variable; it may be indolent or may have a rapid and severe onset.
- Approximately 80–90% of patients have symptoms of a cold, runny nose, or sinusitis that fail to respond to therapy or last longer than usual.
- Patients may report nasal membrane ulcerations and crusting, hearing problems, decline in vision, cough (with or without hemoptysis), rash and/or skin sores, fever, malaise, loss of appetite, weight loss, arthralgias, night sweats, and hematuria.

PHYSICAL EXAM

- Ophthalmic findings:
  - Ocular symptoms are the first manifestation in 20% of patients. Approximately half of the patients with Wegener's granulomatosis develop ocular involvement over the course of the disease.
  - Orbital involvement has been reported in 45–70% of patients. Orbital inflammation can cause pain, diplopia, proptosis, and loss of vision.
  - Common ocular findings include tearing due to nasolacrimal duct obstruction, peripheral ulcerative keratitis, scleritis, and episcleritis.
  - Uveitis, retinal vasculitis, retinal artery occlusion, optic nerve vasculitis, optic neuropathy, restricted movement of extraocular muscles, yellow eyelid lesions, and conjunctival scarring may also be found.
  - Proptosis in the setting of upper and lower respiratory disease is highly suggestive of Wegener's granulomatosis.
- Systemic findings:
  - Patients may be febrile and appear ill.
  - Neurologic: Patients may have mononeuritis multiplex, neuropathy, stroke, seizure, cerebritis, or meningitis.
  - Ears, nose, and throat: Sinusitis and nasal mucosal disease are the most common findings. Other findings include purulent or sanguinous nasal discharge, otitis media, hearing loss from auditory tube dysfunction, deformation or destruction of the nose (saddle nose), subglottic stenosis.
  - Oral involvement is rare; however, "strawberry gingival hyperplasia" is classic of this disease.
  - Skin: palpable purpura, papules, subcutaneous nodules, ulcerations resembling pyoderma gangrenosum, petechiae, vesicles, pustules, hemorrhagic bullae, digital necrosis, subungual splinter hemorrhages, and genital ulcers resembling squamous cell carcinoma have been reported.
  - The lower extremities are most commonly affected.
  - Renal: rapidly progressive glomerulonephritis owing to chronic renal failure
  - Pulmonary: pulmonary nodules or infiltrates, pulmonary hemorrhage leading to hemoptysis
  - Arthritis

DIAGNOSTIC TESTS & INTERPRETATION

Lab

- cANCA blood test in the presence of signs and symptoms of Wegener's granulomatosis is highly suggestive of this disease. ANCA is reported to be positive in only 67% of patients with Wegener's granulomatosis.
- Anemia, mild leukocytosis, and elevated ESR are nonspecific findings.
- Urinalysis may also show hematuria, erythrocyte casts, and proteinuria in patients with glomerulonephritis.

Imaging

Initial approach

Chest radiographs may show infiltrates, nodules, masses, or cavities. The presence of hilar adenopathy alone is not compatible with the diagnosis of Wegener's granulomatosis.

Follow-up & special considerations

- CT of the chest is more sensitive than chest radiography and can often show abnormalities in the presence of a normal radiograph.
- Sinonasal CT studies should include both soft tissue and bone algorithms. Findings include mucosal thickening, opacification, air–fluid level, bony destruction (mainly of the nasal septum), and sclerosing osteitis.
- Orbital MRI may demonstrate granulomatous infiltration of the orbit.
- MRI of the brain may show diffuse linear dural thickening, and local dural thickening contiguous with orbital, nasal, and paranasal disease. In few cases, granulomatous lesions in brain parenchyma are observed. Pituitary gland and infundibulum involvement are also reported.

Diagnostic Procedures/Other

The definitive diagnosis of Wegener's granulomatosis is established by performing a tissue biopsy.

Pathological Findings

A classic triad of vasculitis, granuloma, and large areas of necrosis (geographic necrosis) admixed with acute and chronic inflammatory cells is diagnostic of Wegener's granulomatosis.

DIFFERENTIAL DIAGNOSIS

- Wegener's granulomatosis may often be confused with chronic sinusitis, atypical bacterial pneumonia, thoracic aspergillosis, and primary or metastatic lung cancer.
- Other conditions to be considered include the following:
  - Microscopic polyangiitis
  - Churg–Strauss syndrome
  - Goodpasture's syndrome
  - Systemic lupus erythematosus
  - Sarcoidosis

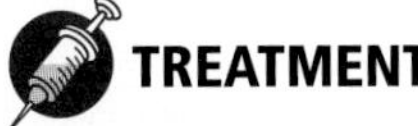

TREATMENT

MEDICATION

First Line

- Untreated Wegener's granulomatosis is fatal.
- Often, the initial therapy for patients is prednisone (initiated at 1 mg/kg daily). This dose is maintained for 1–2 months and then tapered.
- Cyclophosphamide is initiated at 2 mg/kg daily and continued for at least 6–12 months. Patients can then be switched to azathioprine (2 mg/kg/day). Approximately 90% of patients improve with this treatment and 75% remit.
- 50% of the patients who remit may relapse.
- Oral daily cyclophosphamide causes serious toxicity including cytopenia, infection, and hemorrhagic cystitis. Long-term use of cyclophosphamide in patients with Wegener's granulomatosis significantly increases the risk of cancers, especially bladder cancer and lymphoma.
- Monthly intravenous cyclophosphamide is less toxic but is also reported to be less effective.

Second Line

- Weekly methotrexate is an effective alternative for patients with non–life-threatening Wegener's granulomatosis. This regimen is reported to be beneficial in maintaining remission.
- Trimethoprim–sulfamethoxazole is considered by some to cause reduction in the relapse rate, especially when the disease is limited to the upper respiratory tract. Furthermore, it is considered beneficial in preventing pneumonia secondary to *Pneumocystis carinii*.
- Azathioprine has also been used as an alternative immunosuppressant.
- Plasmapheresis has been reported to be beneficial in cases of pulmonary hemorrhage.
- Calcium supplements should be given to any patient on steroids to prevent bone loss.
- Gastrointestinal prophylaxis should also be considered in patients on steroids.

ADDITIONAL TREATMENT

General Measures

Early diagnosis and treatment are crucial to decreasing morbidity and mortality in patients with Wegener's granulomatosis.

Issues for Referral

Patients with this disease should be referred to otolaryngologists, pulmonologists, nephrologists, and dermatologists.

IN-PATIENT CONSIDERATIONS

Initial Stabilization

- Patients with Wegener's granulomatosis may present with acute respiratory failure, pericarditis, myocardial infarction, or acute renal failure.
- A patient with subglottic stenosis should receive a tracheotomy.
- For a patient presenting with proptosis or declining vision, orbital and sinus imaging should be done immediately.

Admission Criteria

- Patient with any life-threatening complication should be admitted for further management.
  - For a patient presenting with proptosis and declining vision, an oculoplastics consult along with ENT consult should be obtained immediately for admission. Urgent surgical decompression may be necessary in case of progressive proptosis causing optic nerve damage.

ONGOING CARE

FOLLOW-UP RECOMMENDATIONS

- Patients have to be monitored very closely in the initial stages of Wegener's granulomatosis until the patient is in remission.
  - Close monitoring of blood work and urinalysis is necessary to detect complications of immunosuppressive therapy.

Patient Monitoring

- CBC count should be performed weekly for the first 1–2 months in patients on oral cyclophosphamide.
- Urinalysis, serum creatinine, urine protein and creatinine ratios, and erythrocyte sedimentation rates should be monitored monthly for the first several months.
- cANCA titers are screened every 3–6 months. In case of clinical relapse, cANCA is checked more frequently.

DIET

Patients should be advised of salt and water retention when on glucocorticoids.

PATIENT EDUCATION

- Patients on oral cyclophosphamide should drink ample fluids and attempt to void every 4 hours to maintain high urine output and reduce the risk of hemorrhagic cystitis.
- Patients should be advised to take oral cyclophosphamide in the morning to avoid high bladder concentrations in the middle of the night when fluid intake is minimal.
- Patients should be advised to report to their doctors for any signs of cold, sinusitis, fever, or hematuria.
- Women of child-bearing age should be advised to not start a pregnancy in the presence of active disease.

PROGNOSIS

With advanced treatments and earlier diagnosis, Wegener's granulomatosis patients have improved prognosis.

COMPLICATIONS

- Chronic renal insufficiency is reported in approximately 35% patients.
- Renal failure can lead to dialysis or kidney transplant.
- Permanent morbidity from disease or its treatment is reported in more than 80% of patients.
- Nasal deformity occurs in approximately half the patients with Wegener's granulomatosis.
- Subglottic stenosis occurs in 35% of patients.

REFERENCES

1. Mohammed AJ, Jacobsson LT, Westman KW, et al. Incidence and survival rates in Wegener's granulomatosis, microscopic polyangiitis, Churg-Strauss syndrome and polyarteritis nodosa. *Rheumatology (Oxford)* 2009;48(12):1560–1565.
2. Cotch MF, Hoffman GS, Yerg DE, et al. The epidemiology of Wegener's granulomatosis. Estimates of the five-year period prevalence, annual mortality, and geographic disease distribution from population-based data sources. *Arthritis Rheum* 1996;39(1):87–92.
3. Cocco G, Gasparyan AY. Myocardial ischemia in Wegener's granulomatosis: Coronary atherosclerosis versus vasculitis. *Open Cardiovasc Med J* 2010;4:57–62.

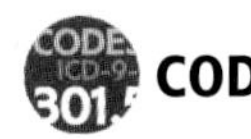

CODES

ICD9

- 370.00 Corneal ulcer, unspecified
- 376.00 Acute inflammation of orbit, unspecified
- 446.4 Wegener's granulomatosis

CLINICAL PEARLS

- Wegener's granulomatosis is marked by necrotizing granulomas of small vessels.
- Systemic findings include sinusitis, progressive glomerulonephritis, hearing loss, saddle nose deformity, pulmonary nodules, skin rash, neurologic signs, and constitutional symptoms such as fever and malaise.
- Ophthalmic features are characterized by inflammation and can involve any part of the adnexa or eye.
- Untreated Wegener's granulomatosis is fatal. Treatment is aimed at immunosuppression.

WEILL-MARCHESANI

Brandon B. Johnson

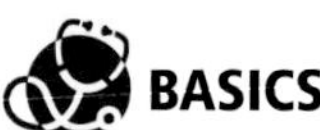

BASICS

DESCRIPTION

- A rare connective tissue disorder associated with short stature, brachydactyly (short digits), joint stiffness, and eye anomalies.
  - Intraocular abnormalities include microspherophakia, ectopia lentis, glaucoma, and lenticular myopia

EPIDEMIOLOGY

Prevalence

- Not well documented
  - Listed as a "rare" disease by the Office of Rare Diseases (ORD) of the National Institutes of Health (occurs in<200,000 people in the US)

RISK FACTORS

Family history

Genetics

- Autosomal dominant and recessive inheritance have been described.
  - Fibrillin-1 mutations on chromosome 15q21 have been reported with autosomal dominant transmission (1)[C].
  - *ADAMTS10* mutations on chromosome 19p are present in families with autosomal recessive inheritance (2)[C].

GENERAL PREVENTION

Genetic counseling to inform family planning

PATHOPHYSIOLOGY

- Mesodermal dysgenesis causes extremely long and loose zonules, which give rise to lens-related complications (3)[C] including the following:
  - Lenticular myopia from a globular lens
  - Pupillary block as the lens moves forward and contacts the iris
  - Secondary iris bombe and anterior chamber shallowing lead to angle-closure glaucoma.
  - Ectopia lentis from zonular dehiscence can lead to luxation into anterior chamber.

ETIOLOGY

Extracellular matrix proteins important in the development of the lens, skin, and heart are dysfunctional.

DIAGNOSIS

HISTORY

A family history of Weill–Marchesani syndrome or manifestations of the syndrome

PHYSICAL EXAM

- Microspherophakia and brachydactyly must be present (4)[C].
  - Other features suggesting Weill–Marchesani syndrome include joint restriction and short stature.
  - Cardiac anomalies can be associated with this condition such as patent ductus arteriosus, mitral and aortic valve stenosis, prolonged QTc, and mitral valve prolapse.

DIAGNOSTIC TESTS & INTERPRETATION

Lab

Initial lab tests

Molecular genetic testing is available for *ADAMTS10*.

Follow-Up & Special Considerations

Consider consultation with medical geneticist.

Imaging

Initial approach

- Cardiac echocardiogram and EKG
- Consider plain films of digits/joints

Follow-up & special considerations

Consider cardiology consult especially if echo/EKG is abnormal.

Pathological Findings

Zonules are long and loose due to mesodermal dysgenesis often leading to dehiscence.

DIFFERENTIAL DIAGNOSIS

OTHER

- Marfan syndrome
- Homocystinuria
- Sulfite oxidase deficiency
- Hyperlysinemia
- Simple dominant ectopia lentis
- Ectopia lentis et pupillae
- Glaucoma-lens ectopia–microspherophakia–stiffness–shortness (GEMSS) syndrome
- Klinefelter syndrome
- Mandibulofacial dysostosis
- Alport syndrome
- Trauma
- Buphthalmos
- Aniridia
- Familial ectopia lentis
- Persistent fetal vasculature
- Coloboma
- Syphilis
- Xanthine oxidase deficiency
- Molybdenum cofactor deficiency
- Hyperlysinemia
- Methylenetetrahydrofolate reductase deficiency

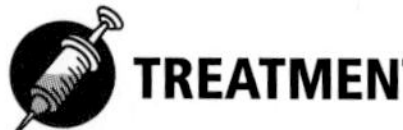

TREATMENT

MEDICATION

Medical treatment of pupillary block glaucoma is difficult due to the unpredictable effects of miotic and mydriatic agents.

ALERT

- Use of miotic agents can induce pupillary block glaucoma in patients with microspherophakia and intact lens (3)[C]
- There are reports of angle closure with the use of mydriatics such as cyclopentolate (5)[C]
- Intraocular pressure can be controlled using topical beta-blockers, alpha-2 agonists, carbonic anhydrase inhibitors, and prostaglandins.
  - Lowering of intraocular pressure in the pediatric population is first achieved through the use of topical beta-blockers such as timolol. If monotherapy is insufficient, these medications can be combined with carbonic anhydrase inhibitors such as dorzolamide. Alpha-2 agonists such as brimonidine are contraindicated in children younger than 2 years due to serious side effects (i.e., lethargy, sleepiness). Prostaglandins such as latanoprost are less effective in children.

SURGERY/OTHER PROCEDURES
- Early identification and surgical removal of dislocated lens are important; however, surgical complications including vitreous loss have been described (3)[C]. Pars plana lensectomy and vitrectomy may minimize complications.
- Prophylactic peripheral iridectomy at an early age may be required to protect against pupillary block glaucoma (3)[C]

IN-PATIENT CONSIDERATIONS
Initial Stabilization
- Acute angle-closure glaucoma should never be treated with miotics due to their loosening of zonular support.
  - Preoperative interventions should be aimed at relieving pupillary block and lowering intraocular pressure while definitive surgical management is planned.
  - Topical timolol is a first-line intraocular pressure–lowering medication in children. Consider adding carbonic anhydrase inhibitors as well as hyperosmotics if intraocular pressure control is insufficient.
  - Laying the patient supine and using ocular massage over a closed lid can facilitate posterior displacement of lens.

Admission Criteria
Patients with acute angle-closure glaucoma secondary to ectopia lentis should be admitted for surgical management of luxated lens.

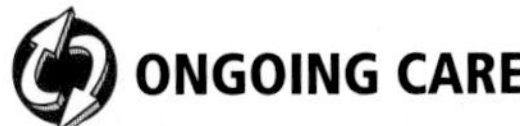

ONGOING CARE

FOLLOW-UP RECOMMENDATIONS
- Patients with an intact lens should be closely monitored by an ophthalmologist for lens dislocation and glaucoma.
- If patient undergoes surgery for luxated lens, follow postoperatively as needed.

PATIENT EDUCATION
- Patients with intact lens should be counseled regarding their risk of chronic and acute angle-closure glaucoma.
- Acute angle closure warning signs
  - Eye pain
  - Headache
  - Conjunctival injection
  - Blurred vision
  - Nausea

PROGNOSIS
- 90% of Weill–Marchesani lenses will eventually dislocate (1)[C]. Lensectomy is recommend for secondary glaucoma, subluxation, and severe lenticular myopia.
  - 80% will suffer pupillary block glaucoma (1)[C]. Prophylactic peripheral iridotomy is recommended to reduce this risk.

COMPLICATIONS
- Surgical complications include difficulty performing lensectomy, intraocular lens implantation, and vitreous loss (6)[C].
- Complications of angle closure include nerve damage, loss of visual field, CRAO, corneal decompensation.

REFERENCES

1. Faivre L, Gorlin RJ, Wirtz MK, et al. In frame fibrillin-1 gene deletion in autosomal dominant Weill-Marchesani syndrome. *J Med Genet* 2003;40:34–36.
2. Dagoneau N, Benoist-Lasselin C, Huber C, et al. ADAMTS10 mutations in autosomal recessive Weill-Marchesani syndrome. *Am J Hum Genet* 2004;75:801–806.
3. Ritch R, Wand M. Treatment of the Weill-Marchesani syndrome. *Ann Ophthalmol* 1981;13: 665–667.
4. Marchesani O. Brachydaktylie und angeborene Kugellinse als Systemerkrankung. *Klin Monatsbl Augenheilkd* 1939;103:392.
5. Wright K, Chrousos G. Weill-Marchesani syndrome with bilateral angle-closure glaucoma. *J Pediatr Ophthalmol Strabismus* 1985;22:129–132.
6. Taylor J. Weill-Marchesani syndrome complicated by secondary glaucoma-case management with surgical lens extraction. *Aust N Z J Ophthalmol* 1996;24(3):275–278.

ADDITIONAL READING

- Willi M, Kut L, Cotlier E. Pupillary-block glaucoma in the Marchesani syndrome. *Arch Ophthalmol* 1973;90:504–508.

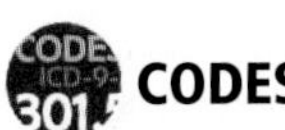

CODES

ICD9
- 743.36 Congenital anomalies of lens shape
- 743.37 Congenital ectopic lens
- 759.89 Other specified congenital anomalies

CLINICAL PEARLS
- Thorough family history and physical exam are important in the diagnosis of Weill–Marchesani syndrome.
- Both miotic and mydriatic agents can precipitate pupillary block angle-closure glaucoma in Weill-Marchesani syndrome.
- Angle-closure glaucoma secondary to pupillary block usually requires lensectomy.
- Prophylactic treatment includes peripheral iridotomy (prophylactic lensectomy has not been studied).

WILSON'S DISEASE

Suzanne K. Jadico

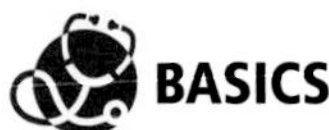

BASICS

DESCRIPTION

- Wilson's disease (WD) is an autosomal recessive defect in cellular copper transport characterized by dramatic build-up of intracellular hepatic copper with subsequent hepatic, neurologic, and other systemic abnormalities.
- Also called: Copper storage disease, hepatolenticular degeneration

EPIDEMIOLOGY

- Manifests as liver disease in children, peaking at ages 10–13 years
- Manifests as neuropsychiatric illness in young adults aged 19–20 years
- Males and females affected equally in all ethnic groups.

Incidence

The gene frequency is 0.56% with a carrier frequency of 1 in 90 (see Genetics section).

Prevalence

Approximately 1 case in 30,000 in most populations

RISK FACTORS

Genetics

- Inherited as an autosomal recessive trait
- Genetic defect localized to chromosome 13, which codes for the ATP7B protein (1).
  - Can be affected by mutations at many different sites
  - Mediates copper transport by sequestering copper into vesicles, which undergo exocytosis across the plasma membrane.
- Normal variations in the *PRNP* gene modify the course of WD.
  - *PRNP* gene codes for prion protein, which is involved in copper transport.
  - Normal variation in the *PRNP* gene may delay the age of onset of WD or affect clinical manifestations.

GENERAL PREVENTION

Genetic counseling

PATHOPHYSIOLOGY

- Impaired transport of copper from the liver into bile leads to excess copper accumulation in the liver.
- Excess copper may act as a prooxidant.
  - Promotes free radical formation
  - Progressive hepatic damage manifests as asymptomatic liver function test (LFT) abnormality, chronic hepatitis, portal hypertension, acute liver failure, and eventual cirrhosis.
- Once cirrhosis occurs, free copper leaks into the bloodstream.
  - Accumulates in and damages other tissues
  - Neuropsychiatric, hematologic, renal, and other organ system disease manifestations
- Incorporation of copper into apoceruloplasmin to form ceruloplasmin is also impaired, accounting for the decreased serum ceruloplasmin.

ETIOLOGY

See Genetics section.

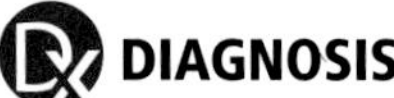

DIAGNOSIS

HISTORY

- Clumsiness
- Difficulty speaking
- Involuntary shaking
- Drooling
- Personality changes
- Depression
- Easy bruising
- Fatigue
- Nausea
- Joint pain
- Impotence
- Night blindness
- Family history of WD

PHYSICAL EXAM

- Signs of acute or chronic liver failure and portal hypertension
  - Yellowing of the skin and eyes (jaundice)
  - Hepatomegaly
  - Swelling of arms and legs
- Neurologic symptoms
  - Tremor
  - Ataxia
  - Parkinsonism
  - Dystonia
  - Cerebellar and pyramidal signs
  - Impairment of vertical eye movements, in particular vertical pursuits, more often than vertical optokinetic nystagmus and vertical saccades (2)
- Kayser–Fleischer ring
  - Brownish or gray–green rings that represent fine pigmented granular deposits of copper in Descemet's membrane in the cornea close to the limbus
  - Formation begins first at superior pole, then the inferior pole, and ultimately circumferentially
- Renal dysfunction
  - Kidney stones
  - Fanconi syndrome (proximal tubular dysfunction) causes abnormal number of amino acids excreted in the urine (aminoaciduria).

DIAGNOSTIC TESTS & INTERPRETATION

Lab

- Liver enzymes: mildly to moderately elevated, often with aspartate aminotransferase (AST) > alanine aminotransferase (ALT)
- Blood ceruloplasmin
  - An extremely low serum ceruloplasmin level (<5 mg/dL) is strong evidence for the diagnosis.
  - A serum ceruloplasmin concentration <20 mg/dL in a patient who also has Kayser–Fleischer rings is diagnostic (1)[B].
  - Serum ceruloplasmin alone has a low positive predictive value, only 6% in one study (3)
    - Low serum ceruloplasmin levels also found in asymptomatic WD heterozygotes, marked renal or enteric protein loss, end-stage liver disease of any cause, and other rare disease of copper deficiency
  - Normal ceruloplasmin does not rule out WD
    - Can be elevated in the presence of acute liver inflammation, pregnancy, and estrogen supplementation
- Basal 24-h urinary excretion of copper
  - 24-h urinary copper excretion of >100 μg is typical in symptomatic patients (normal <40 μg/day).
  - Penicillamine challenge useful in symptomatic children if urinary copper excretion is <100 μg/24 h
  - Values of >1,600 μg copper/24 h following the administration of 500 mg of D-penicillamine are found in WD (4)[B].
- Serum copper concentration
  - Nonceruloplasmin-bound copper levels are greater than 25 μg/dL in the majority of untreated patients with WD (normal <15 μg/dL).
  - Values may be influenced by a variety of conditions; therefore, the sensitivity, specificity, and positive predictive value have not been well-established.
- Slit lamp exam
  - Kayser–Fleischer rings, dependent upon type of presentation (1)
    - Present in 50–60% of patients who present with isolated hepatic involvement
    - Present in 98% of patients who present with neurologic involvement
    - Absence of Kayser–Fleischer rings does not exclude the diagnosis.
    - Not absolutely specific for WD; reported in other chronic cholestatic diseases.
  - Sunflower cataracts, representing copper deposits in the lens
  - Rarely, optic neuritis or pallor of the optic disc

Imaging
- Brain CT
  - Slit-like, low-attenuation foci involving the basal ganglia, particularly the putamen
  - Larger regions of low attenuation in the basal ganglia, thalamus, or dentate nucleus
  - Widening of the frontal horns of the lateral ventricles and diffuse cerebral and cerebellar atrophy
- Brain MRI
  - More sensitive than CT in detecting early lesions
  - Focal abnormalities in the white matter, pons, and deep cerebellar nuclei are typically bilateral with low signal intensity on T1-weighted images, representing cell loss and gliosis.
  - Decreased signal intensity in the putamen and other parts of the basal ganglia may represent either copper or iron ferritin deposition.

Diagnostic Procedures/Other
- Liver biopsy
  - Essential for diagnosis in absence of Kayser–Fleischer rings or neurologic abnormalities
  - Quantitative copper determination (1)
    - Levels of more than 250 μg/g of dry weight found even in asymptomatic patients.
    - Normal hepatic copper concentration (15–55 μg/g) excludes the diagnosis.
- Genetic testing currently limited to screening of family members for an identified mutation detected in the index patient.

Pathological Findings
- Liver biopsy
  - Ranges from fatty infiltration to cirrhosis
  - May appear similar to chronic active hepatitis
  - Histochemical staining of liver specimens for copper is of little diagnostic value.

DIFFERENTIAL DIAGNOSIS
- Hepatitis
  - Acute or chronic hepatitis of any etiology, commonly mimicking autoimmune hepatitis
- Neuropsychiatric disorders

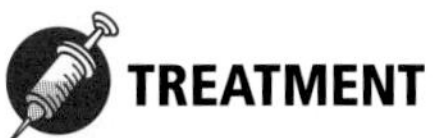

TREATMENT

MEDICATION
First Line
- Chelating agents: Remove excess copper from body.
  - Penicillamine (Cuprimine, Depen) (5)[B]
    - Adult: Initial 1.5–2 g PO qday; Maintenance: 750 mg to 1 g/day PO q.i.d.
    - Pediatric: 25 mg/kg PO qday
    - Extensive side effects including skin problems, bone marrow suppression, worsening of neurological symptoms, and birth defects.
    - Must be administered with pyridoxine 25 mg PO qday
  - Trientine (Syprine) 250–500 mg PO t.i.d. (6)[B]
    - If unable to tolerate penicillamine
    - Risk of bone marrow suppression and worsening neurologic symptoms
    - Should be administered with zinc

Second Line
- Zinc acetate (150–300 mg PO qday) prevents your body from absorbing copper from the food.
  - Approved for maintenance after initial chelation therapy
  - Drug of choice in presymptomatic, pregnant, and pediatric populations

ADDITIONAL TREATMENT
General Measures
See Diet section

Issues for Referral
Consultation with a hepatologist recommended

SURGERY/OTHER PROCEDURES
- Liver transplantation
  - Primarily reserved for treatment of patients with fulminant liver failure or end-stage liver cirrhosis despite chelation therapy

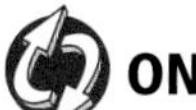

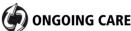

ONGOING CARE

FOLLOW-UP RECOMMENDATIONS
Patient Monitoring
- Weekly for the first 4–6 weeks following initiation of chelation therapy
  - Physical examination, 24-h urinary copper excretion assay, CBC, urinalysis, serum-free copper measurement, and renal and LFTs
- Bimonthly evaluations through the first year, followed by yearly examinations thereafter
- Yearly slit lamp examination to document fading of Kayser–Fleischer rings

DIET
- Limit dietary copper intake
  - Avoid liver, shellfish (especially lobster), mushrooms, nuts, legumes, and chocolate
  - Avoid copper pots, pans, or containers
  - Replace well water with purified water if the copper content is greater than 0.2 ppm.
- Avoid alcohol and hepatotoxic drug therapy

PATIENT EDUCATION
- Wilson's Disease Association
  - http://www.wilsonsdisease.org/home.html

PROGNOSIS
- Fatal if not treated in a timely manner
- If treated early, symptomatic recovery is often complete with a normal life expectancy.
- Residual dysarthria and mild dystonia are relatively common in neurological WD.
- Lifelong chelation therapy is necessary.

COMPLICATIONS
- Chronic liver failure and cirrhosis can lead to bleeding from varices, hepatic encephalopathy, hepatorenal syndrome, and coagulation abnormalities.
- Fulminant liver failure may occur, especially due to medication noncompliance.

REFERENCES

1. El-Youssef M. Wilson disease. *Mayo Clin Proc* 2003;78(9):1126–1136.
2. Ingster-Moati I, Bui Quoc E, Pless M, et al. Ocular motility and Wilson's disease: A study on 34 patients. *J Neurol Neurosurg Psychiatry* 2007;**78**:1199–1201.
3. Cauza E, Maier-Dobersberger T, Polii C, et al. Screening for Wilson's disease in patients with liver diseases by serum ceruloplasmin. *J Hepatol* 1997;27:358.
4. Roberts EA, Schilsky ML. Diagnosis and treatment of Wilson disease: An update. *Hepatology* 2008;47:2089.
5. Durand F, Bernuau J, Giostra E, et al. Wilson's disease with severe hepatic insufficiency: Beneficial effects of early administration of D-penicillamine. *Gut* 2001;48:849–852.
6. Dahlman T, Hartvig P, Lofholm M, et al. Long-term treatment of Wilson's disease with triethylene tetramine dihydrochloride (trientine). *QJM* 1995;88:609–616.

ADDITIONAL READING

- Gow PJ, Smallwood RA, Angus PW, et al. Diagnosis of Wilson's disease: An experience over three decades. *Gut* 2000;46:415–419.
- Medici V, Rossaro L, Sturniolo GC. Wilson disease—A practical approach to diagnosis, treatment and follow-up. *Dig Liver Dis* 2007;39(7): 601–609.

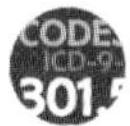

CODES

ICD9
- 275.1 Disorders of copper metabolism
- 371.14 Kayser-fleischer ring

CLINICAL PEARLS

- WD is an autosomal recessive defect in cellular copper transport characterized by hepatic and neurologic abnormalities.
- Diagnosis is made with LFTs, blood ceruloplasmin levels, 24-h urine copper levels, slit lamp exam identification of Kayser–Fleischer rings, and liver biopsy.
- Treatment necessitates lifelong copper chelating therapy.

W

WYBURN–MASON SYNDROME

Lawrence Y. Ho

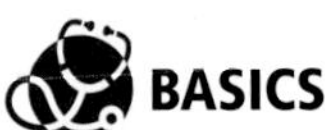

BASICS

DESCRIPTION

- Also known as Bonnet–Dechaume–Blanc syndrome, congenital retinocephalic vascular malformation syndrome, or racemose hemangiomatosis
- Congenital, neurocutaneous condition usually characterized by unilateral CNS, ocular, and skin arteriovenous malformations (AVMs)

EPIDEMIOLOGY

Incidence

Rare

Prevalence

Unknown

RISK FACTORS

None

Genetics

Sporadic, no known locus

PATHOPHYSIOLOGY

- AVMs are abnormal vessel communications between arteries and veins.
- It may involve capillaries, arterioles, venules, arteries, or veins and are a result of defective vascular development.

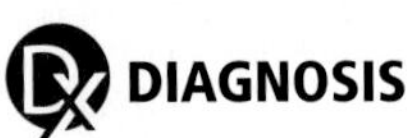

DIAGNOSIS

HISTORY

- Can be asymptomatic
- Ophthalmologic symptoms
  - Impaired vision
  - Eye discomfort
  - Double vision
  - Conjunctival injection
  - Decreased visual field
  - Involuntary eye movements
- CNS symptoms
  - Mental status changes
  - Headache
  - Emesis
  - Seizures
  - Weakness
- Dermatologic symptoms
  - Birthmark
- Other symptoms
  - Epistaxis
  - Oral bleeding, for example, during dental extraction

PHYSICAL EXAM

- Ophthalmologic findings
  - Decreased visual acuity
  - May have afferent papillary defect
  - Elevated intraocular pressure (IOP)
  - Dilated conjunctival vessels
  - Arteriovenous communications are divided into three groups:
    - Group 1: Interposition of an abnormal capillary plexus between major vessels
    - Group 2: Direct arteriovenous communication without interposition of capillaries
    - Group 3: More extensive arteriovenous shunts often associated with vision loss
  - Vessel sheathing
  - Absent spontaneous venous pulsations
  - Optic atrophy
  - Optic nerve edema
  - Strabismus
  - Nystagmus
  - Proptosis
- CNS findings
  - Bruit
  - Cranial nerve paresis
  - Hemiparesis
  - Hemianopsia
  - Intracranial hemorrhage
  - AVMs of the cerebrum and brainstem
- Dermatologic findings
  - Facial angiomas, nevi, or pigmented lesions
- Other findings
- AVMs of the maxilla, pterygoid fossa, or mandible

DIAGNOSTIC TESTS & INTERPRETATION

Lab

Initial lab tests

- Complete ophthalmologic examination with indirect ophthalmoscopy
- Fluorescein angiography shows rapid arteriovenous transit without leakage
- Optical coherence tomography (1)[C]

Follow-Up & Special Considerations

Follow for development of ocular complications

Imaging

Initial approach

- MRI
- Magnetic Resonance Angiography (MRA)

Follow-up & special considerations

Follow for development of neurologic complications

Diagnostic Procedures/Other

Clinical diagnosis

Pathological Findings

- Retinal histology
  - Retinal vessels were thickened with fibromuscular media and wide, fibrohyaline adventitial coats.
  - Retinal vessels may occupy entire thickness of retina touching retinal pigment epithelium.
  - Loss of nerve fibers and ganglion cells

DIFFERENTIAL DIAGNOSIS

- Hypertension
- Retinal neovascularization
- Intraretinal microvascular abnormalities
- Retinal vessel collaterals
- Retinal telangiectasias
- Sturge–Weber syndrome
- Von Hippel–Lindau disease
- Rendu–Osler–Weber disease
- Familial retinal arteriolar tortuosity
- Congenital unilateral retinal macrovessels

TREATMENT

MEDICATION

- Topical medications for increased IOP:
  - Beta-blockers
  - Carbonic anhydrase inhibitors
  - Prostaglandin analogues
  - Alpha-2 receptor agonists
  - Miotic agents
- Systemic medications for increased IOP
  - Carbonic anhydrase inhibitors
  - Hyperosmotic agents
- Treatment of amblyopia with patching +/− cycloplegia
- Anticonvulsant medications for seizures

ADDITIONAL TREATMENT

General Measures

- Spontaneous involution may occur.
- Monitor for ocular or neurologic complications.

Issues for Referral

- Neurology referral if retinal AVMs are noted
- Dermatology referral for skin lesions

SURGERY/OTHER PROCEDURES

- Ophthalmic surgery
  - Scatter panretinal photocoagulation for neovascular complications following vein occlusions (2)[C]
  - Glaucoma filtration or cyclodestructive procedures for cases failing medical management (2)[C]
  - Vitrectomy for nonclearing vitreous hemorrhage
  - Strabismus surgery when indicated
- Neurosurgical intervention (3)[C]
  - Endovascular embolization
  - Surgical resection
  - Radiosurgical procedures

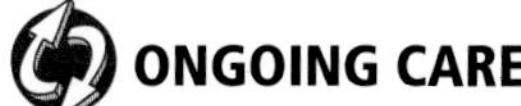

ONGOING CARE

FOLLOW-UP RECOMMENDATIONS

- Continued observation by:
  - Ophthalmologist
  - Neurologist/neurosurgeon
  - Dermatologist

DIET

Regular

PATIENT EDUCATION

- National Institutes of Health Office of Rare Diseases Research
  - http://rarediseases.info.nih.gov/
- National Organization for Rare Disorders (NORD)
  - http://www.rarediseases.org/

PROGNOSIS

Depends on location and severity of lesions

COMPLICATIONS

- Vision loss
- Vein occlusions
- Neovascular glaucoma secondary to vein occlusion
- Secondary glaucoma due to increased episcleral venous pressure
- Vitreous hemorrhage
- Intracranial hemorrhage/stroke
- Seizures
- Uncontrolled oral bleeding

REFERENCES

1. Saleh M, Gaucher D, Sauer A, et al. Spectral optical coherence tomography analysis of a retinal arteriovenous malformation (Wyburn-Mason syndrome). *J Fr Ophtalmol* 2009;32(10):779–780.
2. Mansour AM, Wells CG, Jampol LM, et al. Ocular complications of arteriovenous communications of the retina. *Arch Ophthalmol* 1989;107(2): 232–236.
3. Achrol AS, Guzman R, Varga M, et al. Pathogenesis and radiobiology of brain arteriovenous malformations: Implications for risk stratification in natural history and posttreatment course. *Neurosurg Focus* 2009;26(5):E9.

ADDITIONAL READING

- Bonnet P, Dechaume J, Blanc E. L'aneurysme cirsoide de la retine (aneurysme vasemeaux). *J Med Lyon* 1937;18:165–178.
- Schmidt D, Pache M, Schumacher M. The congenital unilateral retinocephalic vascular malformation syndrome (Bonnet-Dechaume-Blanc syndrome or Wyburn-Mason syndrome): Review of the literature. *Surv Ophthalmol* 2008;53(3):227–249.
- Wyburn-Mason R. Arteriovenous aneurysm of midbrain and retina, facial naevi and mental changes. *Brain* 1943;66:163–203.

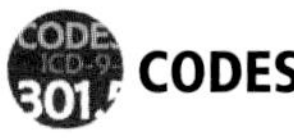

CODES

ICD9

- 369.9 Unspecified visual loss
- 743.58 Vascular anomalies, congenital
- 747.81 Congenital anomalies of cerebrovascular system

CLINICAL PEARLS

- Rare, sporadic neurocutaneous syndrome characterized by CNS, ocular, and dermatologic AVMs
- Usually occurs unilaterally
- Referral to neurologist for evaluation once retinal AVMs are seen
- Lifelong monitoring for ocular and neurologic complications
- Medical and surgical treatments are available for complications of Wyburn–Mason syndrome.

X-LINKED RETINOSCHISIS

Avni Vyas

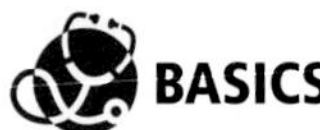

BASICS

DESCRIPTION

X-linked retinoschisis is a genetic disorder of the retina that primarily affects males in the 1st decade leading to decreased vision, foveal schisis, and peripheral retinoschisis in both eyes.

EPIDEMIOLOGY

Prevalence

It is an uncommon disease that has been described in multiple countries, with the highest carrier prevalence reported in Finland: 14 per 10,000 people (1)[A].

RISK FACTORS

Genetics

X-linked recessive disorder with full penetrance

PATHOPHYSIOLOGY

Gene mutations that encode retinoschisis (RS1) cause this disease (2).

ETIOLOGY

- A primary defect in the Müller cell has been proposed as the etiology of this disease process.
- An abnormality of retinal and choroidal vascular development has also been proposed to cause the retinoschisis cavities.

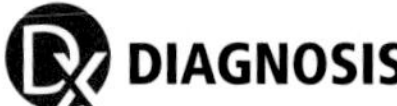

DIAGNOSIS

HISTORY

- X-linked retinoschisis occurs almost exclusively in males who typically present in the first decade of life with decreased vision, strabismus, and nystagmus.
- It may present as early as infancy with nystagmus.

PHYSICAL EXAM

- Foveal retinoschisis is the most characteristic ophthalmoscopic finding and is present in virtually all patients. Radiating striae in the internal limiting membrane (ILM) and foveal microcysts are typically seen. In older patients, pigmentary changes and retina pigment epithelial (RPE) atrophy often evolve over time.
- In approximately 50% of patients, peripheral retinoschisis is present, often inferotemporally. The splitting typically affects the superficial retinal layers.
- Vascular changes such as sheathing, microvascular abnormalities, and retinal neovascularization are sometimes seen.
- Up to 29% of patients have hyperopia and/or strabismus.
- Vitreous hemorrhage and retinal detachment are complications of X-linked retinoschisis. Vitreous hemorrhage can occur from rupture of poorly supported retinal blood vessels or less frequently from neovascularization.

DIAGNOSTIC TESTS & INTERPRETATION

Lab

- The electroretinogram (ERG) shows reduced b-wave amplitude in all patients. The a-wave is initially normal but may be reduced in older patients. In advanced cases, the ERG can be virtually unrecordable.
- Visual field testing generally demonstrates a relative central scotoma and absolute scotomas corresponding to the peripheral schisis cavities.

Imaging

Optical coherence tomography (OCT) can be performed to further assess the foveomacular schisis changes. Although X-linked retinoschisis has traditionally been associated with nerve fiber layer schisis, one study indicates that the schisis cavities can affect multiple layers (nerve fiber layer, inner nuclear layer, outer nuclear layer/outer plexiform layer) and the entire macula (3)[A].

DIFFERENTIAL DIAGNOSIS

- Acquired retinoschisis
- Retinitis pigmentosa
- Retinal vasculitis
- Goldmann–Favre syndrome: Foveal schisis is also seen. However, the inheritance pattern is autosomal recessive. Patients typically have severe nyctalopia and reduced a- and b-waves on ERG.

TREATMENT

MEDICATION

- There is no cure for this disorder.
- Refractive error, strabismus, and amblyopia should be treated appropriately.
- Prophylactic laser photocoagulation treatment of schisis cavities has been associated with an increased incidence of rhegmatogenous retinal detachment and, therefore, is not recommended.
- Repair of retinal detachments with vitrectomy and internal tamponade has shown the best results (4). Repair with scleral buckling has had variable outcomes.
- Panretinal photocoagulation is effective in managing neovascularization.
- Vitreous hemorrhage typically clears spontaneously. In cases of dense or nonclearing hemorrhages, vitrectomy may be considered, and should be performed earlier in the amblyogenic age groups.
- Some case reports have suggested a benefit of topical dorzolamide in the treatment of foveal cystic-appearing lesions with improvement in visual acuity (5)[A].

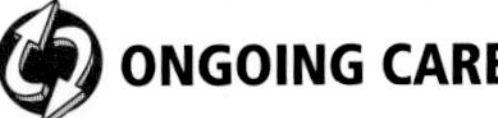

ONGOING CARE

FOLLOW-UP RECOMMENDATIONS

- This is a chronic, slowly progressive disorder.
- Patients should be followed regularly to monitor for complications.

PATIENT EDUCATION

All affected patients and their families should undergo genetic counseling.

PROGNOSIS

Vision loss progresses slowly with retention of reasonable vision until the 5th or 6th decade when visual acuity may worsen secondary to macular atrophy.

COMPLICATIONS

Up to 20% of patients will develop retinal detachment, and up to 40% will develop vitreous hemorrhage.

REFERENCES

1. George ND, Yates JR, Moore AT. X linked retinoschisis. *Br J Ophthalmol* 1995;79:697–702.
2. Sergeev YV, Caruso RC, Meltzer MR, et al. Molecular modeling of retinoschisin with functional analysis of pathogenic mutations from human x-linked retinoschisis. *Hum Mol Genet* 2010;19(7):1302–1313.
3. Yu J, Ni Y, Keane PA, et al. Foveomacular schisis in juvenile X-linked retinoschisis: An optical coherence tomography study. *Am J Ophthalmol* 2010;149(6): 973–978.
4. Garg SJ, Lee HC, Grand MG. Bilateral macular detachments in X-linked retinoschisis. *Arch Ophthalmol* 2006;124(7):1053–1055.
5. Apushikin MA, Fishman GA. Use of dorzolamide for patients with X-linked retinoschisis. *Retina* 2006;26:741–745.

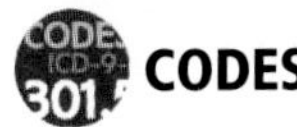

CODES

ICD9

- 361.10 Retinoschisis, unspecified
- 362.73 Vitreoretinal dystrophies

CLINICAL PEARLS

- X-linked retinoschisis is a cause of cystoid macular edema in otherwise healthy adult males. The OCT shows significant cystoid change, but the fluorescein angiogram is not impressive.

OPTIC NERVE GLIOMA (OPG)

Matthew D. Kay

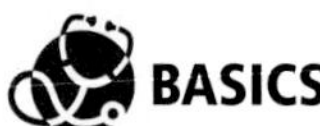

BASICS

DESCRIPTION
- Most common infiltrative lesion of the optic nerve (ON).

EPIDEMIOLOGY
Incidence
- 1% of all intracranial tumors
- 3% of orbital tumors
- 4% of all gliomas
- Occurs in 15% of patients with NF1
- Represents 65% of intrinsic optic nerve tumors
- 90% recognized by second decade of life
- Also known as optic pathway glioma (OPG)

RISK FACTORS
- Neurofibromatosis type 1 (NF1) in 25–30% of cases of OPG.

Genetics
- Localized to chromosome 17 if associated with NF1 (autosomal dominant)

GENERAL PREVENTION
- N/A

PATHOPHYSIOLOGY
- Progressive growth with infiltration and compression of the ON, producing visual loss
  - May affect ON anywhere along its course from globe through optic tract

ETIOLOGY
- Neoplastic infiltration of ON

COMMONLY ASSOCIATED CONDITIONS
- NF1 present in 25–30% of OPG

DIAGNOSIS

HISTORY
- Progressive painless visual loss +/− proptosis and/or diplopia
- History of NF1

PHYSICAL EXAM
- Demonstrates features of an optic neuropathy: Decreased visual acuity, decreased color vision, nerve fiber bundle-type visual field defects though may have temporal defects or homonymous defect if concurrent involvement of the optic chiasm or tract respectively, afferent pupillary defect if unilateral or asymmetric optic nerve involvement
- Optic nerve may be pale or edematous based upon location of tumor with anterior involvement producing ON edema while posterior orbital, canalicular, or intracranial lesions demonstrate ON pallor
- May have proptosis, strabismus, or nystagmus
- May have stigmata of NF1 (e.g., Lisch nodules, café au lait spots, dermal neurofibromas)

ALERT
Malignant transformation of an OPG essentially only occurs in patients who have previously undergone radiation therapy for their tumor.

DIAGNOSTIC TESTS & INTERPRETATION
Imaging
Initial approach
- MRI brain and orbits with and without contrast including T1 post-contrast images with fat suppression
  - MRI demonstrating characteristic features generally sufficient to establish diagnosis
  - Fusiform or occasionally diffuse enlargement of the intraorbital optic nerve
  - Intense enhancement common
  - "Kinking" of the optic nerve within the orbit
  - "Pseudo-CSF" signal on T2 images secondary to perineural arachnoidal gliomatosis in patients with NF1

Follow-up & special considerations
- Follow-up MRI q 6–12 months initially with decreased frequency once long-term stability is established

Diagnostic Procedures/Other
- Biopsy of the lesion may occasionally be indicated if radiographic diagnosis unclear especially in the absence of NF1

Pathological Findings
- Juvenile pilocytic astrocytoma composed of benign astrocytic infiltration occasionally with surrounding reactive leptomeningeal hyperplasia

DIFFERENTIAL DIAGNOSIS
- Optic nerve sheath meningioma
- Optic neuritis
- Sarcoidosis

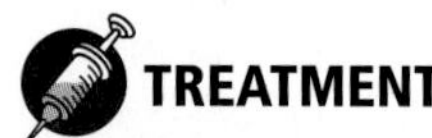

TREATMENT

MEDICATION
First Line
- Observation without treatment unless clear evidence of progression with extension into the chiasm, opposite ON, or hypothalamus
  - Chemotherapy reserved for patients <6 years old if they meet the above criteria

ADDITIONAL TREATMENT

General Measures

- Radiation therapy utilized for patients >6 years old if they demonstrate radiographic progression as listed under First Line Treatment above.

Issues for Referral

- Evaluation for NF1 if no prior diagnosis

Additional Therapies

- Treat amblyopia if present

SURGERY/OTHER PROCEDURES

- Resection generally reserved for tumors confined to ON with poor or no vision, for gross cosmetically unacceptable proptosis in a blind eye, or for tumors confined to the ON but demonstrate radiographic growth which is threatening chiasm
  - Exophytic components can be debulked
  - Ventriculoperitoneal shunt can be placed for hydrocephalus if present

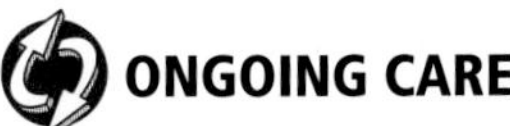

ONGOING CARE

FOLLOW-UP RECOMMENDATIONS

- Call for visual changes

Patient Monitoring

- Serial clinical examination of ON function including formal perimetry (if patient old enough to perform reliably) every 6–12 months or as dictated by clinical course
- OCT

PATIENT EDUCATION

- Discuss genetics with family and association with NF1

PROGNOSIS

- Generally good when lesion confined to ON (5% mortality)
- 50% mortality if OPG with hypothalamic involvement
- Sporadic OPG are more aggressive than NF1
  - Malignant ON gliomas are rare and tend to occur only in adults with most patients becoming completely blind and dying within 1 year regardless of treatment

COMPLICATIONS

- Blindness
- Amblyopia
- Late malignant transformation of tumor almost exclusively in patients who previously received radiation therapy for OPG
- Numerous adverse effects of radiation therapy or chemotherapy if administered

ADDITIONAL READING

- Lee AG. Neuroophthalmological management of optic pathway gliomas. *Neurosurg Focus* 2007; 23(5):E1.
- Volpe NJ. Compressive and infiltrative Optic Neuropathies, in Miller NR, Newman NJ (eds): *Walsh and Hoyt's Clinical Neuro-ophthalmloogy,* 6th ed, 2005:397–403.
- Weber AL, Klufas R, Pless M. Imaging evaluation of the optic nerve and visual pathway. *Neuroimaging Clinics of North America* February 1996;6(1): 143–177.

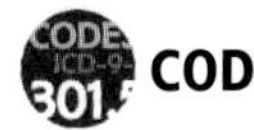

CODES

ICD9

- 192.0 (Benign neoplasm of cranial nerve)
- 225.1 Benign neoplasm of cranial nerves
- 237.9 Neoplasm of uncertain behavior of other and unspecified parts of nervous system

CLINICAL PEARLS

- Characteristic ON "kinking" on MRI is almost exclusively seen in NF1.
- Relatively high incidence of NF1 in patients with OPG.

INDEX